Brief Contents

TENTH EDITION

MOSBY'S TEXTBOOK FOR
NURSING ASSISTANTS

SHEILA A. SORRENTINO, PhD, RN   LEIGHANN N. REMMERT, MS, RN

ELSEVIER

ELSEVIER

3251 Riverport Lane
St. Louis, Missouri 63043

Notices

Practitioners and researchers must always rely on their own experience and knowledge in evaluating
and using any information, methods, compounds or experiments described herein. Because of rapid
advances in the medical sciences, in particular, independent verification of diagnoses and drug
dosages should be made. To the fullest extent of the law, no responsibility is assumed by Elsevier,
authors, editors or contributors for any injury and/or damage to persons or property as a matter of
products liability, negligence or otherwise, or from any use or operation of any methods, products,
instructions, or ideas contained in the material herein.

Previous editions copyrighted 2017, 2012, 2008, 2004, 2000, 1996, 1992, 1987, and 1984.

Library of Congress Cataloging-in-Publication Data
Sorrentino, Sheila A., author.
 Mosby's textbook for nursing assistants / Sheila A. Sorrentino,
Leighann N. Remmert.—Tenth edition.
     p. ; cm.
 Textbook for nursing assistants
 Includes bibliographical references and index.
 ISBN 978-0-323-65560-6 (pbk. : alk. paper)—ISBN 978-0-323-65561-3 (hardcover : alk. paper)
 I. Remmert, Leighann N., author.   II. Title.   III. Title: Textbook for nursing assistants.
 [DNLM: 1. Nurses' Aides.   2. Nursing Care.   WY 193]
 RT84
 610.7306'98—dc23
                    2015036852

Senior Content Strategist: Nancy O'Brien
Senior Content Development Manager: Luke Held
Senior Content Development Specialist: Kelly Skelton
Publishing Services Manager: Catherine Jackson
Book Production Specialist: Kristine Feeherty
Design Direction: Margaret Reid

Working together
to grow libraries in
developing countries

www.elsevier.com • www.bookaid.org

The cycle of life continues ...

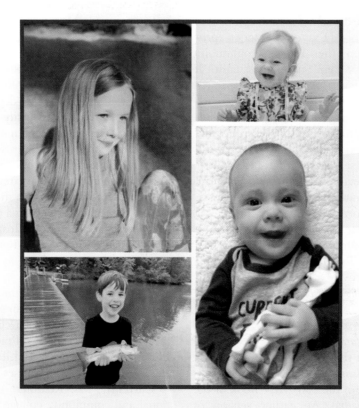

Loved ones are lost and children are born bringing joy and new memories ...

Kylie Brooke, Weston Anthony, Emma Rose, Mason Anthony, and all those yet to be ...

With much love,

Aunt Sheila

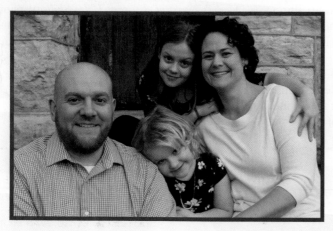

To the ones I cherish most ...

Shane, Olivia, and Ava

With all my love,

Leighann (Mom)

About the Authors

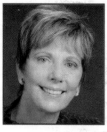

Sheila A. Sorrentino was instrumental in the development and approval of CNA-PN-ADN career-ladder programs in the Illinois community college system and has taught at various levels of nursing education—nursing assistant, practical nursing, associate degree nursing, and baccalaureate and higher degree programs. Her career includes experiences in nursing practice and higher education—nursing assistant, staff nurse, charge and head nurse, nursing faculty, program director, assistant dean, and dean.

A Mosby author and co-author of several nursing assistant titles since 1982, Dr. Sorrentino's titles include:
- *Mosby's Textbook for Nursing Assistants* (ed 1–10)
- *Mosby's Essentials for Nursing Assistants* (ed 1–6)
- *Mosby's Textbook for Long-Term Care Nursing Assistants* (ed 1–6)
- *Mosby's Textbook for Nursing Assistive Personnel* (ed 1–2)
- *Mosby's Basic Skills for Nursing Assistants*
- *Mosby's Textbook for Medication Assistants*

She was also involved in the development of an early version of *Mosby's Nursing Assistant Video Skills* and *Mosby's Nursing Video Skills*, winner of the 2003 AJN Book of the Year Award (electronic media). An earlier version of nursing assistant video skills won an International Films Award on caregiving.

Dr. Sorrentino has a Bachelor of Science degree in nursing, a Master of Arts degree in education, a Master of Science degree in nursing, and a PhD in higher education administration. She is a member of Sigma Theta Tau International, the Honor Society of Nursing. Her past community activities include the Rotary Club of Anthem (Anthem, Arizona), the Provena Senior Services Board of Directors (Mokena, Illinois), the Central Illinois Higher Education Health Care Task Force, the Iowa-Illinois Safety Council Board of Directors, and the Board of Directors of Our Lady of Victory Nursing Center (Bourbonnais, Illinois).

She received an alumni achievement award from Lewis University for outstanding leadership and dedication in nursing education. She is also a member of the Illinois State University College of Education Hall of Fame.

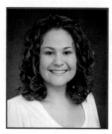

Leighann N. Remmert is a nursing assistant instructor in central Illinois. She has taught adult learners and high school nursing assistant students in the classroom and clinical settings.

Ms. Remmert has a Bachelor of Science degree in nursing from Bradley University (Peoria, Illinois) and a Master of Science degree in nursing education from Southern Illinois University Edwardsville (Edwardsville, Illinois).

Ms. Remmert's background includes the roles of nursing assistant/technician, nurse extern, staff nurse, charge nurse, nurse preceptor, and trauma nurse specialist. She acquired diverse clinical experience as a nursing assistant/technician and extern at St. John's Hospital (Springfield, Illinois). As a registered nurse, Ms. Remmert concentrated in the area of emergency nursing at Memorial Medical Center (Springfield, Illinois).

As an educator, Ms. Remmert supervised, instructed, and evaluated student learning in various long-term care and acute care settings as a clinical nursing instructor at the Capital Area School of Practical Nursing (Springfield, Illinois). A former Basic Life Support instructor, Ms. Remmert taught CPR courses for the community.

Currently, Ms. Remmert instructs students in vocational and community college nursing assistant programs in central Illinois. Through her teaching, she emphasizes the importance of professionalism and work ethics, safety, teamwork, communication, and accountability. Valuing the role of the nursing assistant and treating the person with dignity, care, and respect are integral to her instruction.

Ms. Remmert is co-author of *Mosby's Textbook for Nursing Assistants* (ed 8–10), *Mosby's Essentials for Nursing Assistants* (ed 4–6), and *Mosby's Textbook for Medication Assistants*. She was a consultant on *Mosby's Textbook for Long-Term Care Nursing Assistants* (ed 6) and served as a content adviser for *Mosby's Nursing Assistant Video Skills* (version 4.0).

Ms. Remmert is a member of Sigma Theta Tau International, the Honor Society of Nursing, and the Certified Nursing Assistant Educator's Association (Illinois, Central Region).

Acknowledgments

Many individuals help us develop an accurate, up-to-date, and timely publication. Therefore we extend a "thank you" and appreciation to:

- The Christian Village (Lincoln, Illinois) for hosting photo shoots.
- Steven Territo and Ryan Edgecombe for their efforts coordinating the photo shoots at The Christian Village.
- Karen Carter and Janet Ginger for coordinating student involvement in our photo shoot.
- Friends, colleagues, and former students who participated in our photo shoot: Lillian Beams, Kacey Bennett, Karen Carter, Kelsey Cowan, Anita Davis, Austin Garriott, Chastity Henderson, Ted Jordan, Ivy Pierce, and Madlen Tanner.
- Lorraine French, Ken French, Bill Gossett, and R. Jean Gossett for their involvement in our photo shoot.
- Mike DeFilippo (St. Louis, Missouri), our favorite photographer. The things we ask Mike to do require acrobatic movements and magic!
- Jeanne Robertson for her talented artistry, attention to detail, and prompt revisions.
- Memorial Medical Center (Springfield, Illinois) for providing the ICU photo.
- Lanny Nelson and the staff of PostNet Anthem (Anthem, Arizona), especially Florencey, for their timely and efficient printing services. Beyond helpful!
- The reviewers who made comments and offered suggestions to improve our textbook. See "Reviewers" list below.
- Susan Broadhurst (New Orleans, Louisiana) for her role as copy editor. She accommodates our style well.
- Graphic World for their proofreading efforts. The task requires attention to detail.
- And finally the Elsevier/Mosby staff involved:
  - Nancy O'Brien, Senior Content Strategist
  - Kelly Skelton, Senior Content Development Specialist
  - Kristine Feeherty, Book Production Specialist
  - Margaret Reid, Senior Book Designer

To all individuals who contributed to this effort in any way, we are sincerely grateful.

Sheila A. Sorrentino
Leighann N. Remmert

REVIEWERS

Karen J. Amoscato, MA, RN, RCP, RDMS
Registered Nurse - CNA Instructor
Valley Academy for Career & Technology Education (VACTE)
Cottonwood, Arizona

Mary L. Barr, RN
Lancaster County Career & Technology Center
Willow Street, Pennsylvania

Demy Blake, RN MSN Ed.
Nurse Educator
South Dade Technical College
Homestead, Florida

Fatima Demonteverde Reyes, RN, MS, CCRN
Program Coordinator
Avid CNA School, Streamwood, Illinois
Visiting Professor, Chamberlain College of Nursing, Addison, Illinois
Nursing Supervisor, Alexian Brothers Medical Center, Elk Grove Village, Illinois

Jessica Olachea, RN, BSN
Registered Nurse
Lynchburg, Virginia

Rachana J. Patel, RN, DSD
American Red Cross Instructor
CNA Program Instructor and Director
Mission Trails Regional Occupational Program/Soledad
Soledad, California

Suzanne Pinos, MSN, RN
Professor I, Nursing
Palm Beach State College
Lake Worth, Florida

Darlene Seay, RN, BSN, MSEd
Nurse Aide Evaluator for Credentia
Nurse Aide Instructor and Coordinator
Piedmont Va. Community College and Nelson County High School
Charlottesville and Lovingston, Virginia

Angela M. Spencer, BS, MPA
Administrator, Nursing
Chicago Community Learning Center
Chicago, Illinois

Instructor Preface

The tenth edition of *Mosby's Textbook for Nursing Assistants* serves several purposes.

- Prepares students to function as nursing assistants in nursing centers, hospitals, and home care settings.
- Assists faculty in meeting educational goals.
- Serves as a resource when preparing for the competency evaluation.
- Serves as a resource for nursing assistants wanting to review or learn new information for safe care.

The following foundational principles are presented in specific chapters while values, objectives, and organizational strategies are integrated in content and key features throughout the book. (See "Student Preface," p. xi for key features.)

- Patients and residents are *persons* with dignity having a past, a present, and a future. Such persons are physical, social, psychological, and spiritual beings with basic needs and protected rights.
- Nursing assistant roles, functions, and limitations are described in federal and state laws with dependence on effective delegation and good work ethics.
- Body structure and function, body mechanics, preventing infection, and safety and comfort measures form an essential knowledge base.
- Communication skills enhance relationships with the nursing and health teams, patients and residents, and families and visitors.
- The nursing assistant has a key role in the nursing process.

CONTENT ISSUES

Content decisions are based on changes in laws or in guidelines and standards issued by federal and state governments, accrediting agencies, and national organizations. So are changes to state curricula and competency evaluations.

Student learning needs and abilities, instructor desires, work-related issues, course/program and book length, and student cost also are among the many factors considered.

New Content
Chapter 1: Health Care Agencies
- Memory Care Units

Chapter 3: The Nursing Assistant
- PROMOTING SAFETY AND COMFORT: Certification

Chapter 4: Delegation
- PROMOTING SAFETY AND COMFORT: Delegation

Chapter 5: Ethics and Laws
- Table 5-1 Elder Abuse

Chapter 6: Student and Work Ethics
- Box 6-4 Bullying

Chapter 8: Health Team Communications
- Table 8-1 Parts of the Medical Record
- DELEGATION GUIDELINES: The Nursing Process

Chapter 9: Medical Terminology *(new)*
- Table 9-2 Defining Medical Terms
- Table 9-3 Common Abbreviations

Chapter 10: Body Structure and Function
- Table 10-1 Endocrine System

Chapter 11: Growth and Development
- Table 11-1 Milestones—Infancy (Birth to 1 Year)
- Table 11-2 Milestones—Toddlerhood (1 to 3 Years)
- Table 11-3 Milestones—Preschool (3 to 6 Years)

Chapter 13: Safety
- CARING ABOUT CULTURE: Lead Poisoning
- FOCUS ON CHILDREN AND OLDER PERSONS: Choking
- FOCUS ON LONG-TERM CARE AND HOME CARE: Fire Safety (Hoarding)

Chapter 14: Preventing Falls
- PROMOTING SAFETY AND COMFORT: Position Change Alarms

Chapter 15 Restraint Alternatives and Restraints
- PROMOTING SAFETY AND COMFORT: Safe Restraint Use
- PROMOTING SAFETY AND COMFORT: Risks From Restraint Use
- FOCUS ON COMMUNICATION: Laws, Rules, and Guidelines

Chapter 16: Preventing Infection
- PROMOTING SAFETY AND COMFORT: Bloodborne Pathogen Standard

Chapter 17: Isolation Precautions *(new)*

Chapter 23: Oral Hygiene
- Box 23-1 Oral Hygiene—Early Childhood

Chapter 27: Urinary Needs
- DELEGATION GUIDELINES: Normal Urination
- Female Urinals

Chapter 28: Urinary Catheters
- DELEGATION GUIDELINES: Catheters
- Catheter-Associated UTIs

Chapter 29: Bowel Needs
- Emptying Ostomy Pouches
- DELEGATION GUIDELINES: Emptying Ostomy Pouches
- PROMOTING SAFETY AND COMFORT: Emptying Ostomy Pouches
- PROCEDURE: Assisting the Person to Empty an Ostomy Pouch

Chapter 31: Fluid Needs
- Electrolytes

Key Terms

- Acid reflux (Chapter 50)
- Addiction (Chapter 52)
- Affected side (Chapter 26)
- Antiseptic (Chapter 39)
- Bed rest (Chapter 34)
- Biopsy (Chapter 47)
- Cardiopulmonary resuscitation (CPR) (Chapter 58)
- Comminuted fracture (Chapter 48)
- Delegated nursing responsibility (Chapter 4)
- Delegation (Chapter 4)
- Detoxification (Chapter 52)
- Discrimination (Chapter 60)
- Electrolytes (Chapter 31)
- Frostbite (Chapter 58)
- Garment (Chapter 26)
- Gay (Chapter 55)
- Gravity (Chapter 28)
- Groin (Chapter 27)
- Hygiene (Chapter 23)
- Hypothermia (Chapter 58)
- Informed consent (Chapter 5)
- Milestone (Chapter 11)
- Misappropriation (Chapter 3)
- Mouth care (Chapter 23)
- Musculo-skeletal disorder (MSD) (Chapter 18)
- Personal protective equipment (PPE) (Chapter 17)
- Position change alarm (Chapter 14)
- Reasonable accommodation (Chapter 60)
- Referred pain (Chapter 35)
- Reflex (Chapter 10)
- Resuscitate (Chapter 58)
- Routine nursing task (Chapter 4)
- Stage (Chapter 11)
- Stimulus (Chapter 10)
- Supra-pubic catheter (Chapter 28)
- Surgical site infection (SSI) (Chapter 39)
- Survey (Chapter 1)
- Unaffected side (Chapter 26)
- Under-garment (Chapter 26)

Key Abbreviations

- **AD** Autonomic dysreflexia
- **APRN** Advanced practice registered nurse
- **ASC** Ambulatory surgery center
- **BON** Board of nursing
- **CAUTI** Catheter-associated urinary tract infection
- ***C. diff*** *Clostridioides difficile; Clostridium difficile*
- **CPSC** Consumer Product Safety Commission
- **FAS** Fetal alcohol syndrome
- **FASDs** Fetal alcohol spectrum disorders
- **ICD** Implanted cardioverter defibrillator
- **ISTAP** International Skin Tear Advisory Panel
- **MRN** Medical record number
- **MSDS** Material safety data sheet
- **NFPA** National Fire Protection Association
- **OAB** Over-active bladder

Key Abbreviations—cont'd

- **PPS** Prospective Payment Systems
- **PROM** Passive range of motion
- **SSI** Surgical site infection
- **STI** Sexually transmitted infection
- **TDV** Teen dating violence
- **UI** Urinary incontinence

New Figures

- **Figure 1-2** Parts of a health care system.
- **Figure 6-3** A watch with a second (sweep) hand.
- **Figure 8-1** A nursing assistant uses an electronic medical record.
- **Figure 8-2** A sample progress note.
- **Figure 9-1** Prefixes, roots, and suffixes are combined to form medical terms.
- **Figure 13-6** Steps for drug disposal in the household trash.
- **Figure 13-7** Sources of and clues to possible carbon monoxide problems.
- **Figure 16-15 A,** FDA-cleared sharps containers.
- **Figure 17-1** PPE is outside the person's room.
- **Figure 19-14** Re-positioning in a reclining chair.
- **Figure 21-5** A medical (patient) recliner.
- **Figure 21-6** Controls for staff use are on the outer part of the rail.
- **Figure 21-15** Over-bed table.
- **Figure 21-16** A bedside stand.
- **Figure 22-19** Making a toe pleat.
- **Figure 23-3** Toothpaste amounts in early childhood.
- **Figure 23-12** Charting sample—oral hygiene.
- **Figure 24-3** Rash in a skin fold.
- **Figure 24-16** A shower bench.
- **Figure 24-24** Cleaning the penis. **B,** Clean the shaft with downward strokes.
- **Figure 24-25** A bruise. Report bruising to the nurse.
- **Figure 24-26** The left foot and leg are swollen. Report swelling to the nurse.
- **Figure 24-27** Charting sample—skin care.
- **Figure 25-7** Shampooing at the sink with a shampoo tray.
- **Figure 27-10** Urinal holder.
- **Figure 27-11** Using the male urinal. **A,** Standing. **B,** In bed.
- **Figure 27-12** Female urinal.
- **Figure 28-3** Supra-pubic catheter.
- **Figure 28-6** Catheter securing devices.
- **Figure 28-8** Drainage bag holder.
- **Figure 29-14** An ostomy pouch with a clamp.
- **Figure 29-15** Cleaning the outlet of an ostomy pouch.

- **Figure 30-4 A,** Nectar-thick liquid. **B,** Honey-thick liquid. **C,** Pudding-thick (spoon-thick) liquid.
- **Figure 31-1** Edema in the lower leg. The nurse applies pressure to the body part to check for edema.
- **Figure 33-21** Using a watch with a second (sweep) hand to count for 30 seconds.
- **Figure 34-27** Walker tennis balls on the rear legs of a walker.
- **Figure 36-2** A sample nursing assistant admission checklist.
- **Figure 38-3** A urine specimen kit.
- **Figure 38-5** Collecting a specimen from a urinary catheter.
- **Figure 39-4** An antiseptic is applied to the skin to prevent infection.
- **Figure 39-6** Surgical clippers.
- **Figure 40-7** Skin tears. **A,** No skin loss. **B,** Partial flap loss. **C,** Total flap loss.
- **Figure 40-24** Removing a dressing.
- **Figure 40-26** Applying a dressing.
- **Figure 41-5** Blanchable and non-blanchable skin.
- **Figure 41-9** Slough.
- **Figure 41-10** Eschar.
- **Figure 48-12** A comminuted fracture is broken into 3 or more pieces.
- **Figure 48-23** Osteoporosis in the spine.
- **Figure 49-9** COPD. Chronic bronchitis causes inflammation and mucus in the airways. Emphysema damages the inner walls of alveoli.
- **Figure 50-4** Inflammatory bowel disease.
- **Figure 51-2** *Shading* shows the flank area.
- **Figure 54-2** A child with cerebral palsy.
- **Figure 56-4** Car seat guidelines.
- **Figure 56-6** A safe sleep setting can reduce SIDS risk.
- **Figure 58-9** Sequence of adult CPR.
- **Figure 58-14** AED with a key to lower the shock dosage for a child.

FEATURES AND DESIGN

For features and design elements, see "Student Preface," p. xi.

May this book serve you and your students well. We aim to provide current information for teaching and learning safe and effective care during a time of dynamic change in health care.

Sheila A. Sorrentino, BSN, MA, MSN, PhD, RN
Leighann N. Remmert, BSN, MS, RN

Student Preface

This book with special features (pp. xii-xv) was designed to help you learn. This preface gives study guidelines to help you use the book. To study effectively, use a study system with these steps.

- Survey or preview
- Question
- Read and record
- Recite and review

SURVEY OR PREVIEW

Preview or survey the reading assignment for a few minutes. This gives an idea of what the assignment covers. It also helps you to recall what you know about the subject. Carefully look over the assignment. Preview the chapter title, objectives, key terms and abbreviations, headings, subheadings, and key ideas in italics. Also survey the boxes and chapter review questions.

QUESTION

Questioning sets a purpose for reading. Form questions to answer while reading. Questions should relate to how the information applies to care or possible test questions. Use the headings and subheadings to form questions. *What*, *why*, or *how* questions are helpful. Avoid questions with 1-word answers. If a question does not help you study, change the question.

READ AND RECORD

You read to:

- Gain new information.
- Connect new information to what you already know.
- Find answers to your questions.

Break the assignment into small parts. Then answer your questions as you read each part. Underline or highlight important information. This reminds you of what you need to learn. Review the marked parts later. Make notes by writing down important information in the margins or in a notebook. Use words and statements to prompt your memory about the material.

To remember what you read, organize information into a study guide. Create diagrams or charts to show relationships or steps in a process. Note taking in an outline also is very useful. For example:

1. Main heading
   A. Second level
   B. Second level
      (1) Third level
      (2) Third level

RECITE AND REVIEW

Finally, recite and review. Use your notes and study guides. Answer your questions and others from reading and answering chapter "Review Questions." Answer all questions out loud (recite).

Reviewing is more about *when* to study rather than *what* to study. You decided *what* to study during your preview, question, and reading steps. It is best to review right after the first study session, 1 week later, and before a quiz or test.

We hope you enjoy learning and your work. You and your work are important. You and the care you give make a difference in the person's life!

Sheila A. Sorrentino
Leighann N. Remmert

SPECIAL FEATURES

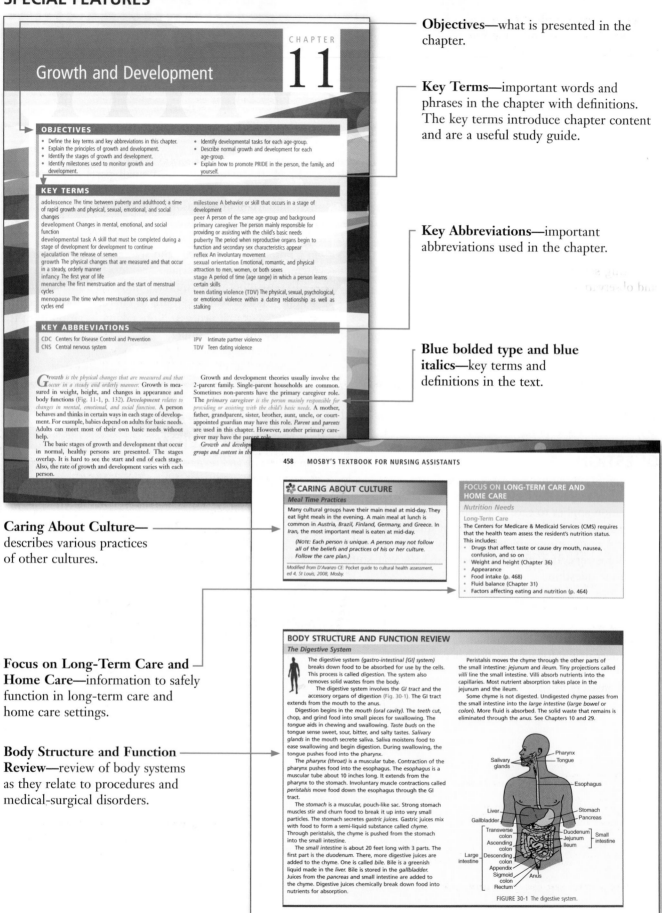

Objectives—what is presented in the chapter.

Key Terms—important words and phrases in the chapter with definitions. The key terms introduce chapter content and are a useful study guide.

Key Abbreviations—important abbreviations used in the chapter.

Blue bolded type and blue italics—key terms and definitions in the text.

Caring About Culture—describes various practices of other cultures.

Focus on Long-Term Care and Home Care—information to safely function in long-term care and home care settings.

Body Structure and Function Review—review of body systems as they relate to procedures and medical-surgical disorders.

Focus on Communication—suggests what to say and questions to ask when interacting with patients, residents, visitors, and the nursing team.

Color illustrations and photographs—visually present key ideas, concepts, and procedure steps.

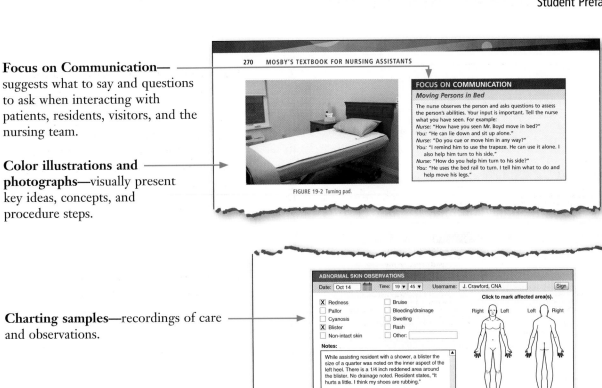

270 MOSBY'S TEXTBOOK FOR NURSING ASSISTANTS

FIGURE 19-2 Turning pad.

FOCUS ON COMMUNICATION

Moving Persons in Bed

The nurse observes the person and asks questions to assess the person's abilities. Your input is important. Tell the nurse what you have seen. For example:

Nurse: "How have you seen Mr. Boyd move in bed?"
You: "He can lie down and sit up alone."
Nurse: "Do you cue or move him in any way?"
You: "I remind him to use the trapeze. He can use it alone. I also help him turn to his side."
Nurse: "How do you help him turn to his side?"
You: "He uses the bed rail to turn. I tell him what to do and help move his legs."

Charting samples—recordings of care and observations.

ABNORMAL SKIN OBSERVATIONS

Date: Oct 14   Time: 19 ▼ 45 ▼   Username: J. Crawford, CNA   [Sign]

Click to mark affected area(s).

[X] Redness   [ ] Bruise
[ ] Pallor   [ ] Bleeding/drainage
[ ] Cyanosis   [ ] Swelling
[X] Blister   [ ] Rash
[ ] Non-intact skin   [ ] Other: _____

Notes:
While assisting resident with a shower, a blister the size of a quarter was noted on the inner aspect of the left heel. There is a 1/4 inch reddened area around the blister. No drainage noted. Resident states, "It hurts a little. I think my shoes are rubbing."

Nurse notified: M. Polk, RN

Right   Left   Left   Right

FIGURE 41-22 Charting sample.

Focus on Math—math involved in various care measures and procedures.

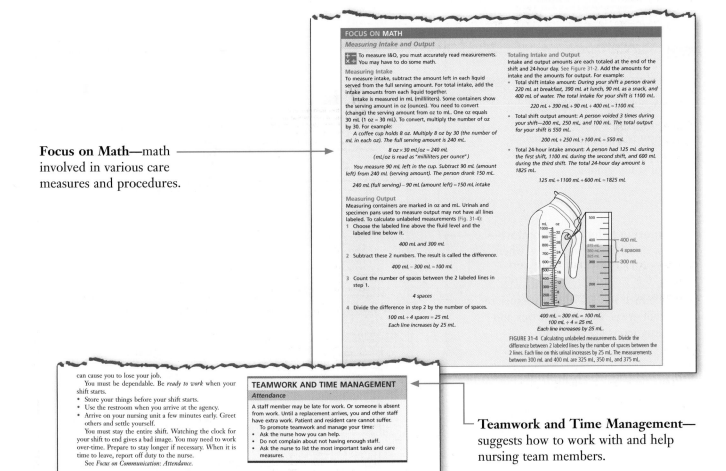

FOCUS ON MATH

Measuring Intake and Output

To measure I&O, you must accurately read measurements. You may have to do some math.

Measuring Intake
To measure intake, subtract the amount left in each liquid served from the full serving amount. For total intake, add the intake amounts from each liquid together.

Intake is measured in mL (milliliters). Some containers show the serving amount in oz (ounces). You need to convert (change) the serving amount from oz to mL. One oz equals 30 mL (1 oz = 30 mL). To convert, multiply the number of oz by 30. For example:

A coffee cup holds 8 oz. Multiply 8 oz by 30 (the number of mL in each oz). The full serving amount is 240 mL.

8 oz × 30 mL/oz = 240 mL
(mL/oz is read as "milliliters per ounce")

You measure 90 mL left in the cup. Subtract 90 mL (amount left) from 240 mL (serving amount). The person drank 150 mL.

240 mL (full serving) − 90 mL (amount left) = 150 mL intake

Measuring Output
Measuring containers are marked in oz and mL. Urinals and specimen pans used to measure output may not have all lines labeled. To calculate unlabeled measurements (Fig. 31-4):
1 Choose the labeled line above the fluid level and the labeled line below it.

400 mL and 300 mL

2 Subtract these 2 numbers. The result is called the *difference.*

400 mL − 300 mL = 100 mL

3 Count the number of spaces between the 2 labeled lines in step 1.

4 spaces

4 Divide the difference in step 2 by the number of spaces.

100 mL ÷ 4 spaces = 25 mL
Each line increases by 25 mL.

Totaling Intake and Output
Intake and output amounts are each totaled at the end of the shift and 24-hour day. See Figure 31-2. Add the amounts for intake and the amounts for output. For example:

• Total shift intake amount: *During your shift a person drank 220 mL at breakfast, 390 mL at lunch, 90 mL as a snack, and 400 mL of water. The total intake for your shift is 1100 mL.*

220 mL + 390 mL + 90 mL + 400 mL = 1100 mL

• Total shift output amount: *A person voided 3 times during your shift—200 mL, 250 mL, and 100 mL. The total output for your shift is 550 mL.*

200 mL + 250 mL + 100 mL = 550 mL

• Total 24-hour intake amount: *A person had 125 mL during the first shift, 1100 mL during the second shift, and 600 mL during the third shift. The total 24-hour day amount is 1825 mL.*

125 mL + 1100 mL + 600 mL = 1825 mL

400 mL − 300 mL = 100 mL
100 mL ÷ 4 = 25 mL
Each line increases by 25 mL.

FIGURE 31-4 Calculating unlabeled measurements. Divide the difference between 2 labeled lines by the number of spaces between the 2 lines. Each line on this urinal increases by 25 mL. The measurements between 300 mL and 400 mL are 325 mL, 350 mL, and 375 mL.

can cause you to lose your job.

You must be dependable. Be *ready to work* when your shift starts.
• Store your things before your shift starts.
• Use the restroom when you arrive at the agency.
• Arrive on your nursing unit a few minutes early. Greet others and settle yourself.

You must stay the entire shift. Watching the clock for your shift to end gives a bad image. You may need to work over-time. Prepare to stay longer if necessary. When it is time to leave, report off duty to the nurse.

See *Focus on Communication: Attendance.*

TEAMWORK AND TIME MANAGEMENT

Attendance

A staff member may be late for work. Or someone is absent from work. Until a replacement arrives, you and other staff have extra work. Patient and resident care cannot suffer.

To promote teamwork and manage your time:
• Ask the nurse how you can help.
• Do not complain about not having enough staff.
• Ask the nurse to list the most important tasks and care measures.

Teamwork and Time Management—suggests how to work with and help nursing team members.

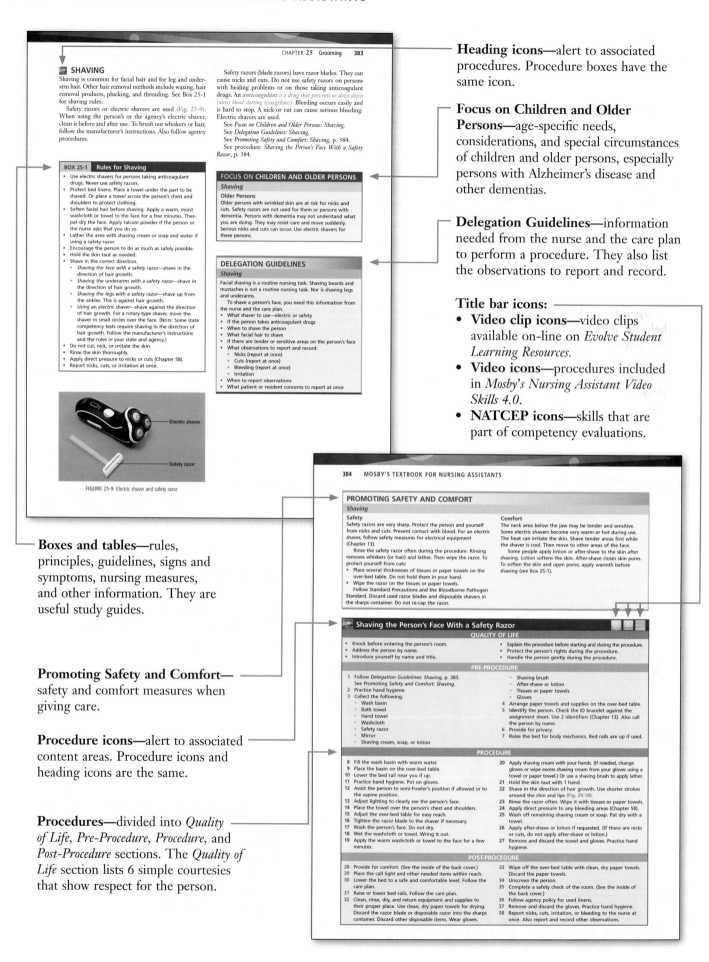

Heading icons—alert to associated procedures. Procedure boxes have the same icon.

Focus on Children and Older Persons—age-specific needs, considerations, and special circumstances of children and older persons, especially persons with Alzheimer's disease and other dementias.

Delegation Guidelines—information needed from the nurse and the care plan to perform a procedure. They also list the observations to report and record.

Title bar icons:
- **Video clip icons**—video clips available on-line on *Evolve Student Learning Resources.*
- **Video icons**—procedures included in *Mosby's Nursing Assistant Video Skills 4.0.*
- **NATCEP icons**—skills that are part of competency evaluations.

Boxes and tables—rules, principles, guidelines, signs and symptoms, nursing measures, and other information. They are useful study guides.

Promoting Safety and Comfort—safety and comfort measures when giving care.

Procedure icons—alert to associated content areas. Procedure icons and heading icons are the same.

Procedures—divided into *Quality of Life, Pre-Procedure, Procedure,* and *Post-Procedure* sections. The *Quality of Life* section lists 6 simple courtesies that show respect for the person.

The following text appears within the sample textbook pages shown in the figure:

SHAVING

Shaving is common for facial hair and for leg and underarm hair. Other hair removal methods include waxing, hair removal products, plucking, and threading. See Box 25-1 for shaving rules.

Safety razors or electric shavers are used (Fig. 25-9). When using the person's or the agency's electric shaver, clean it before and after use. To brush out whiskers or hair, follow the manufacturer's instructions. Also follow agency procedures.

Safety razors (blade razors) have razor blades. They can cause nicks and cuts. Do not use safety razors on persons with healing problems or on those taking anticoagulant drugs. An *anticoagulant is a drug that prevents or slows down* (anti) *blood clotting* (coagulate). Bleeding occurs easily and is hard to stop. A nick or cut can cause serious bleeding. Electric shavers are used.

See *Focus on Children and Older Persons: Shaving.*
See *Delegation Guidelines: Shaving.*
See *Promoting Safety and Comfort: Shaving,* p. 384.
See procedure: *Shaving the Person's Face With a Safety Razor,* p. 384.

BOX 25-1 Rules for Shaving

- Use electric shavers for persons taking anticoagulant drugs. Never use safety razors.
- Protect bed linens. Place a towel under the part to be shaved. Or place a towel across the person's chest and shoulders to protect clothing.
- Soften facial hair before shaving. Apply a warm, moist washcloth or towel to the face for a few minutes. Then pat dry the face. Apply talcum powder if the person or the nurse asks that you do so.
- Lather the area with shaving cream or soap and water if using a safety razor.
- Encourage the person to do as much as safely possible.
- Hold the skin taut as needed.
- Shave in the correct direction.
  - *Shaving the face with a safety razor*—shave in the direction of hair growth.
  - *Shaving the underarms with a safety razor*—shave in the direction of hair growth.
  - *Shaving the legs with a safety razor*—shave up from the ankles. This is against hair growth.
  - *Using an electric shaver*—shave against the direction of hair growth. For a rotary-type shaver, move the shaver in small circles over the face. (NOTE: Some state competency tests require shaving in the direction of hair growth. Follow the manufacturer's instructions and the rules in your state and agency.)
- Do not cut, nick, or irritate the skin.
- Rinse the skin thoroughly.
- Apply direct pressure to nicks or cuts (Chapter 58).
- Report nicks, cuts, or irritation at once.

FOCUS ON CHILDREN AND OLDER PERSONS

Shaving

Older Persons
Older persons with wrinkled skin are at risk for nicks and cuts. Safety razors are not used for them or persons with dementia. Persons with dementia may not understand what you are doing. They may resist care and move suddenly. Serious nicks and cuts can occur. Use electric shavers for these persons.

DELEGATION GUIDELINES

Shaving

Facial shaving is a routine nursing task. Shaving beards and mustaches is not a routine nursing task. Nor is shaving legs and underarms.

To shave a person's face, you need this information from the nurse and the care plan.
- What shaver to use—electric or safety
- If the person takes anticoagulant drugs
- When to shave the person
- What facial hair to shave
- If there are tender or sensitive areas on the person's face
- What observations to report and record:
  - Nicks (report at once)
  - Cuts (report at once)
  - Bleeding (report at once)
  - Irritation
- When to report observations
- What patient or resident concerns to report at once

FIGURE 25-9 Electric shaver and safety razor.

Electric shaver

Safety razor

PROMOTING SAFETY AND COMFORT

Shaving

Safety
Safety razors are very sharp. Protect the person and yourself from nicks and cuts. Prevent contact with blood. For an electric shaver, follow safety measures for electrical equipment (Chapter 13).

Rinse the safety razor often during the procedure. Rinsing removes whiskers (or hair) and lather. Then wipe the razor. To protect yourself from cuts:
- Place several thicknesses of tissues or paper towels on the over-bed table. Do not hold them in your hand.
- Wipe the razor on the tissues or paper towels.
  Follow Standard Precautions and the Bloodborne Pathogen Standard. Discard used razor blades and disposable shavers in the sharps container. Do not re-cap the razor.

Comfort
The neck area below the jaw may be tender and sensitive. Some electric shavers become very warm or hot during use. The heat can irritate the skin. Shave tender areas first while the shaver is cool. Then move to other areas of the face.

Some people apply lotion or after-shave to the skin after shaving. Lotion softens the skin. After-shave closes skin pores. To soften the skin and open pores, apply warmth before shaving (see Box 25-1).

Shaving the Person's Face With a Safety Razor

QUALITY OF LIFE

- Knock before entering the person's room.
- Address the person by name.
- Introduce yourself by name and title.

- Explain the procedure before starting and during the procedure.
- Protect the person's rights during the procedure.
- Handle the person gently during the procedure.

PRE-PROCEDURE

1. Follow *Delegation Guidelines: Shaving,* p. 383. See *Promoting Safety and Comfort: Shaving.*
2. Practice hand hygiene.
3. Collect the following.
   - Wash basin
   - Bath towel
   - Hand towel
   - Washcloth
   - Safety razor
   - Mirror
   - Shaving cream, soap, or lotion
   - Shaving brush
   - After-shave or lotion
   - Tissues or paper towels
   - Gloves
4. Arrange paper towels and supplies on the over-bed table.
5. Identify the person. Check the ID bracelet against the assignment sheet. Use 2 identifiers (Chapter 13). Also call the person by name.
6. Provide for privacy.
7. Raise the bed for body mechanics. Bed rails are up if used.

PROCEDURE

8. Fill the wash basin with warm water.
9. Place the basin on the over-bed table.
10. Lower the bed rail near you if up.
11. Practice hand hygiene. Put on gloves.
12. Assist the person to semi-Fowler's position if allowed or to the supine position.
13. Adjust lighting to clearly see the person's face.
14. Place the towel over the person's chest and shoulders.
15. Adjust the over-bed table for easy reach.
16. Tighten the razor blade to the shaver if necessary.
17. Wash the person's face. Do not dry.
18. Wet the washcloth or towel. Wring it out.
19. Apply the warm washcloth or towel to the face for a few minutes.
20. Apply shaving cream with your hands. (If needed, change gloves or wipe excess shaving cream from your gloves using a towel or paper towel.) Or use a shaving brush to apply lather.
21. Hold the skin taut with 1 hand.
22. Shave in the direction of hair growth. Use shorter strokes around the chin and lips (Fig. 25-10).
23. Rinse the razor often. Wipe it with tissues or paper towels.
24. Apply direct pressure to any bleeding areas (Chapter 58).
25. Wash off remaining shaving cream or soap. Pat dry with a towel.
26. Apply after-shave or lotion if requested. (If there are nicks or cuts, do not apply after-shave or lotion.)
27. Remove and discard the towel and gloves. Practice hand hygiene.

POST-PROCEDURE

28. Provide for comfort. (See the inside of the back cover.)
29. Place the call light and other needed items within reach.
30. Lower the bed to a safe and comfortable level. Follow the care plan.
31. Raise or lower bed rails. Follow the care plan.
32. Clean, rinse, dry, and return equipment and supplies to their proper place. Use clean, dry paper towels for drying. Discard the razor blade or disposable razor into the sharps container. Discard other disposable items. Wear gloves.
33. Wipe off the over-bed table with clean, dry paper towels. Discard the paper towels.
34. Unscreen the person.
35. Complete a safety check of the room. (See the inside of the back cover.)
36. Follow agency policy for used linens.
37. Remove and discard the gloves. Practice hand hygiene.
38. Report nicks, cuts, irritation, or bleeding to the nurse at once. Also report and record other observations.

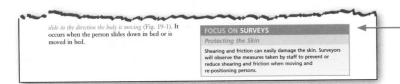

slide in the direction the body is moving (Fig. 19-1). It occurs when the person slides down in bed or is moved in bed.

FOCUS ON SURVEYS

Protecting the Skin

Shearing and friction can easily damage the skin. Surveyors will observe the measures taken by staff to prevent or reduce shearing and friction when moving and re-positioning persons.

Focus on Surveys—questions that surveyors may ask you or what they may observe you doing.

Focus on PRIDE: The Person, Family, and Yourself—builds on chapter content to help you promote *pride* in the person, the family, and yourself. The first letter of each section spells *PRIDE*.

- *Personal and Professional Responsibility*—how to have pride in yourself through personal and professional behaviors and development.
- *Rights and Respect*—how to promote the person's rights and respect him or her as a person with dignity and value.
- *Independence and Social Interaction*—ways to help the person remain or attain independence and interact socially with others.
- *Delegation and Teamwork*—how to work efficiently with and help nursing team members.
- *Ethics and Laws*—laws affecting nursing care and doing the right thing when dealing with patients, residents, and co-workers.

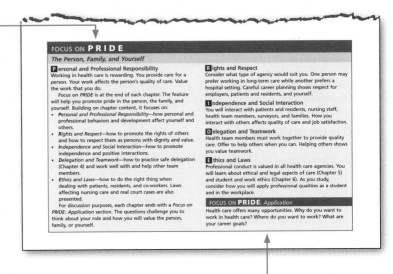

FOCUS ON P R I D E

The Person, Family, and Yourself

P ersonal and Professional Responsibility
Working in health care is rewarding. You provide care for a *person*. Your work affects the person's quality of care. Value the work that you do.

Focus on PRIDE is at the end of each chapter. The feature will help you promote pride in the person, the family, and yourself. Building on chapter content, it focuses on:
- *Personal and Professional Responsibility*—how personal and professional behaviors and development affect yourself and others.
- *Rights and Respect*—how to promote the rights of others and how to respect them as persons with dignity and value.
- *Independence and Social Interaction*—how to promote independence and positive interactions.
- *Delegation and Teamwork*—how to practice safe delegation (Chapter 4) and work well with and help other team members.
- *Ethics and Laws*—how to do the right thing when dealing with patients, residents, and co-workers. Laws affecting nursing care and real court cases are also presented.

For discussion purposes, each chapter ends with a *Focus on PRIDE: Application* section. The questions challenge you to think about your role and how you will value the person, family, or yourself.

R ights and Respect
Consider what type of agency would suit you. One person may prefer working in long-term care while another prefers a hospital setting. Careful career planning shows respect for employers, patients and residents, and yourself.

I ndependence and Social Interaction
You will interact with patients and residents, nursing staff, health team members, surveyors, and families. How you interact with others affects quality of care and job satisfaction.

D elegation and Teamwork
Health team members must work together to provide quality care. Offer to help others when you can. Helping others shows you value teamwork.

E thics and Laws
Professional conduct is valued in all health care agencies. You will learn about ethical and legal aspects of care (Chapter 5) and student and work ethics (Chapter 6). As you study, consider how you will apply professional qualities as a student and in the workplace.

FOCUS ON PRIDE: *Application*

Health care offers many opportunities. Why do you want to work in health care? Where do you want to work? What are your career goals?

Focus on PRIDE: Application—how to apply information in Focus on PRIDE. Questions are intended for personal thought or classroom discussion.

Review Questions—study guides to review what you have learned. Use them to study for a test or for the competency evaluation. Answers are at the back of the book. See p. 885.

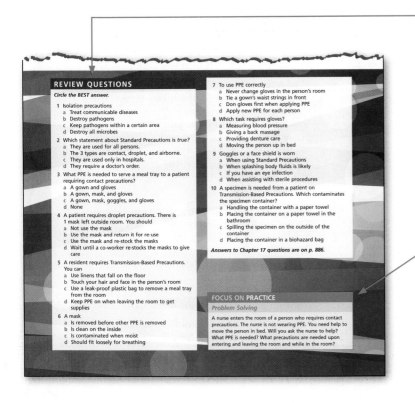

REVIEW QUESTIONS

Circle the BEST answer.

1 Isolation precautions
  a Treat communicable diseases
  b Destroy pathogens
  c Keep pathogens within a certain area
  d Destroy all microbes
2 Which statement about Standard Precautions is *true*?
  a They are used for all persons.
  b The 3 types are contact, droplet, and airborne.
  c They are used only in hospitals.
  d They require a doctor's order.
3 What PPE is needed to serve a meal tray to a patient requiring contact precautions?
  a A gown and gloves
  b A gown, mask, and gloves
  c A gown, mask, goggles, and gloves
  d None
4 A patient requires droplet precautions. There is 1 mask left outside room. You should
  a Not use the mask
  b Use the mask and return it for re-use
  c Use the mask and re-stock the masks
  d Wait until a co-worker re-stocks the masks to give care
5 A resident requires Transmission-Based Precautions. You can
  a Use linens that fall on the floor
  b Touch your hair and face in the person's room
  c Use a leak-proof plastic bag to remove a meal tray from the room
  d Keep PPE on when leaving the room to get supplies
6 A mask
  a Is removed before other PPE is removed
  b Is clean on the inside
  c Is contaminated when moist
  d Should fit loosely for breathing

7 To use PPE correctly
  a Never change gloves in the person's room
  b Tie a gown's waist strings in front
  c Don gloves first when applying PPE
  d Apply new PPE for each person
8 Which task requires gloves?
  a Measuring blood pressure
  b Giving a back massage
  c Providing denture care
  d Moving the person up in bed
9 Goggles or a face shield is worn
  a When using Standard Precautions
  b When splashing body fluids is likely
  c If you have an eye infection
  d When assisting with sterile procedures
10 A specimen is needed from a patient on Transmission-Based Precautions. Which contaminates the specimen container?
  a Handling the container with a paper towel
  b Placing the container on a paper towel in the bathroom
  c Spilling the specimen on the outside of the container
  d Placing the container in a biohazard bag

Answers to Chapter 17 questions are on p. 886.

FOCUS ON PRACTICE

Problem Solving

A nurse enters the room of a person who requires contact precautions. The nurse is not wearing PPE. You need help to move the person in bed. Will you ask the nurse to help? What PPE is needed? What precautions are needed upon entering and leaving the room and while in the room?

Focus on Practice: Problem Solving—follow the Review Questions. A situation is presented that you may encounter as a student or in the work setting. For classroom discussion or self-study, questions follow about what you should do, how you should act, or how you can improve the situation.

Contents

Health Care Agencies

- Define the key terms and key abbreviations in this chapter.
- Describe the types, purposes, and organization of health care agencies.
- Describe the health team and nursing team members.
- Describe the nursing service department.

- Describe 5 nursing care patterns.
- Describe the programs that pay for health care.
- Explain your role in meeting standards.
- Explain how to promote PRIDE in the person, the family, and yourself.

KEY TERMS

acute illness An illness of rapid onset and short duration; the person is expected to recover

assisted living residence (ALR) Provides housing, personal care, support services, health care, and social activities in a home-like setting to persons needing some help with daily activities

case management A nursing care pattern; services for the person's care needs are obtained and monitored from admission through discharge and into the home or long-term care setting

chronic illness A long-term health condition that may not have a cure; it can be controlled and complications prevented with proper treatment

functional nursing A nursing care pattern focusing on tasks and jobs; each nursing team member is assigned certain tasks and jobs

health team The many health care workers whose skills and knowledge focus on the person's total care; interdisciplinary health care team

hospice A health care agency or program that promotes comfort and quality of life for the dying person and his or her family

licensed practical nurse (LPN) A nurse who has completed a practical nursing program and has passed a licensing test; called *licensed vocational nurse (LVN)* in California and Texas

licensed vocational nurse (LVN) See "licensed practical nurse (LPN)"

nursing assistant A person who has passed a nursing assistant training and competency evaluation program (NATCEP); performs delegated nursing tasks under the supervision of a licensed nurse

nursing team Those who provide nursing care—RNs, LPNs/LVNs, and nursing assistants

patient-focused care A nursing care pattern; services are moved from departments to the bedside

primary nursing A nursing care pattern; an RN is responsible for the person's total care

registered nurse (RN) A nurse who has completed a 2-, 3-, or 4-year nursing program and has passed a licensing test

survey The formal review of an agency through the collection of facts and observations

surveyor A person who collects information by observing and asking questions

team nursing A nursing care pattern; an RN leads a team of nursing staff; the RN decides the amount and kind of care each person needs

terminal illness An illness or injury from which the person will not likely recover

KEY ABBREVIATIONS

ALR	Assisted living residence	LVN	Licensed vocational nurse
APRN	Advanced practice registered nurse	PPS	Prospective Payment Systems
DON	Director of nursing	RN	Registered nurse
LPN	Licensed practical nurse	SNF	Skilled nursing facility

Health care agencies (Box 1-1, p. 2) vary in size, services, and staff. The *person* is always the focus of care.

Health care agencies must follow local, state, and federal laws and rules. This is to ensure safe care.

AGENCY PURPOSES

Some agencies have a narrow focus. Surgery centers are an example. Surgeries and medical procedures are done in a non-hospital setting. The person returns home the same day or the next day. Other agencies have many purposes and services.

BOX 1-1	Types of Health Care Agencies

- Hospitals
- Long-term care centers (nursing homes, nursing facilities, nursing centers)
- Memory care facilities
- Home care agencies; home health care agencies
- Surgery centers
- Urgent care centers
- Adult day-care centers
- Assisted living residences
- Board and care homes
- Rehabilitation and sub-acute care facilities
- Hospices
- Doctors' offices
- Clinics
- Centers for persons with mental health disorders
- Centers for persons with intellectual and developmental disabilities
- Drug and alcohol treatment centers
- Crisis centers for rape, abuse, suicide, and other emergencies

The purposes of health care are:

- *Health promotion.* The goal is to reduce the risk of physical or mental illness. People learn about healthy living—diet, exercise, and the warning signs and symptoms of illness are included. They learn how to manage and cope with health problems.
- *Disease prevention.* Immunizations prevent some infectious diseases. Polio, measles, mumps, smallpox, and hepatitis B are examples. Life-style changes can promote health. For example, high blood pressure can cause heart attacks and strokes. Diet and exercise help to lower blood pressure.
- *Detection and treatment of disease.* Diagnostic tests, physical exams, surgery, emergency care, and drugs are used. Respiratory, physical, and occupational therapies are common. The nursing team observes signs and symptoms and gives care.
- *Rehabilitation and restorative care.* This involves returning persons to their highest possible level of physical and mental function and to independence. *Independence means not relying on or needing care from others.* The process starts when the person first seeks health care. The person learns or re-learns skills needed to live, work, and enjoy life. Maintaining function is important. Help is given to make needed home changes.

These purposes are related. For example: having chest pain, a person goes to an emergency room. After an exam and tests, the doctor diagnoses a heart attack. The person is admitted to the hospital for treatment. He or she learns about heart attack risk factors, diet, drugs, life-style, activity, and coping with fears and concerns. A rehabilitation program begins. Activity starts slowly and may progress from walking to jogging and swimming. Successful treatment and rehabilitation promote health and may prevent another heart attack.

Student Learning

Agencies are often learning sites for students. Students assist in the purposes of health care. They are involved with and provide care.

TYPES OF AGENCIES

Nursing assistants work in many settings. Some work in doctors' offices and clinics. Most work in the following agencies.

Hospitals

Hospitals provide emergency care, surgery, nursing care, x-ray procedures and treatments, and laboratory testing. Respiratory, physical, occupational, speech, and other therapies are provided. Hospital care is either in-patient or out-patient.

- *In-patient care*—health care a person receives when admitted to an agency. At least 1 over-night stay is involved. See Figure 1-1.
- *Out-patient (ambulatory) care*—medical or surgical care received when a person is not admitted to an agency. The person does not stay over-night.

People of all ages need hospital care. They have babies, surgery, physical and mental health disorders, and broken bones. Some are dying.

Hospital patients have acute, chronic, or terminal illnesses.

- *Acute illness is an illness of rapid onset and short duration. The person is expected to recover.* A heart attack is an example.
- *Chronic illness is a long-term health condition that may not have a cure. The illness can be controlled and complications prevented with proper treatment.* Arthritis is an example.
- *Terminal illness is an illness or injury from which the person will not likely recover.* The person will die (Chapter 59). Cancers not responding to treatment are examples.

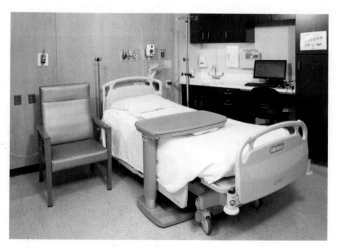

FIGURE 1-1 A hospital room.

Rehabilitation and Sub-Acute Care Agencies

Hospital stays are often short. Some people do not need hospital care but are too sick or disabled to go home. Care needs fall between hospital care and long-term care. Along with rehabilitation, complex equipment and care measures are often needed. See Chapter 45.

Some hospitals and long-term care centers have rehabilitation and sub-acute care units. Others are separate agencies. Many persons are able to return home. Others need long-term care.

Long-Term Care Centers

Some persons cannot care for themselves at home but do not need hospital care. Long-term care centers are designed to meet their needs. Care needs range from simple to complex. Medical, nursing, dietary, recreation, rehabilitation, and social services are provided.

Persons in long-term care centers are called *residents*. They are not *patients*. The center is their short- or long-term home.

Most residents are older. Many have chronic diseases, poor nutrition, memory problems, or poor health. Not all residents are old. Some are disabled from birth defects, accidents, or disease. Hospital patients are often discharged while recovering from illness or surgery. Some need home care. Others need long-term care until able to go home. Others need end-of-life care (Chapter 59).

Nursing Centers. A *nursing center (nursing facility, nursing home)* provides medical, nursing, dietary, recreation, rehabilitation, and social services. *Skilled nursing facilities (SNFs)* provide complex care for severe health problems. SNF residents need time to recover or rehabilitation. Others never go home.

Memory Care Units. A memory care unit is designed for persons with Alzheimer's disease and other dementias (Chapter 53). Such persons suffer increasing memory loss and confusion. Over time, they cannot tend to simple personal needs. Wandering is common. The unit is usually closed off from other parts of the center. The closed unit provides a safe setting where residents can wander freely.

Assisted Living Residences

An *assisted living residence (ALR) provides housing, personal care, support services, health care, and social activities in a home-like setting to persons needing some help with daily activities* (Chapter 57). Some ALRs are part of nursing centers or retirement communities (Chapter 12).

The person has a room, an apartment, or a cottage. Three meals a day and 24-hour supervision are provided. So are housekeeping, laundry, social, recreational, transportation, and some health care services. Help is given with personal care and drugs.

Mental Health Centers

Some persons have problems with life events. Others present dangers to themselves or others because of how they think and behave. Out-patient mental health care is common. Some need short-term or long-term in-patient care.

Home Care Agencies

Health care services are provided to people where they live. Services range from health teaching and supervision to bedside nursing care. Physical therapy, rehabilitation, and food services are common. Hospitals, health care systems, public health departments, and private businesses offer home care.

People of all ages need home health care. Some persons need end-of-life care at home.

Hospices

A *hospice is a health care agency or program that promotes comfort and quality of life for the dying person and his or her family.* Hospice patients no longer respond to treatments aimed at cures. Usually they have less than 6 months to live.

The physical, emotional, social, and spiritual needs of the person and family are met. The focus is on comfort, not cure. Children and pets can visit. Family and friends can assist with care.

Hospice care is provided by hospitals, nursing centers, and home care and hospice agencies.

Health Care Systems

Agencies join together as 1 provider of care. A system usually has hospitals, nursing centers, home care agencies, hospice settings, and doctors' offices (Fig. 1-2, p. 4). An ambulance service and medical supply store for home care are common. The system serves a community or larger region.

The goal is to meet all health care needs. A person uses system providers as needed. See Box 1-2 for an example.

BOX 1-2   **Using a Health Care System**

A health care system owns:

- 3 hospitals
- Doctors' offices
- A home care service
- An ambulance service
- A medical supply store
- A nursing center

A patient sees a hospital emergency room doctor because of sudden dizziness and right-sided weakness. Admitted to the hospital, the patient was having a stroke.

After 2 weeks of rehabilitation, the patient returns home by ambulance. The family obtains needed care items from the medical supply store—hospital bed, wheelchair, and other items.

The home care agency arranges for the patient's nursing needs. A nursing assistant will help with daily hygiene and grooming needs. A nurse will visit 3 times a week.

Because of another stroke, the patient is taken to the hospital by ambulance. After hospital care and rehabilitation, the patient and family agree to nursing center care.

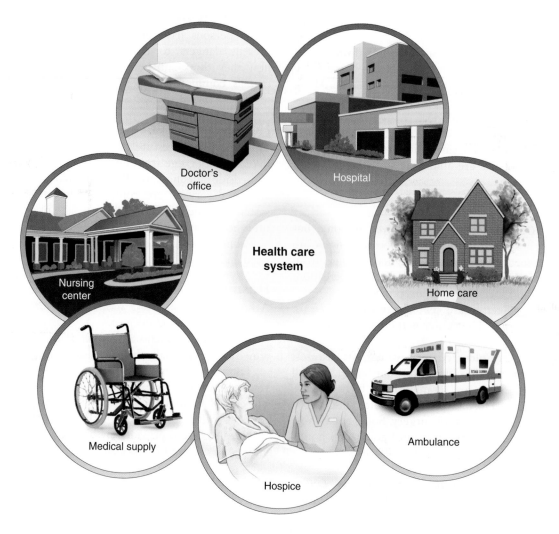

FIGURE 1-2 Parts of a health care system.

ORGANIZATION

An agency has a governing group called the *board of trustees* or *board of directors*. The board makes policies. The focus is safe care at the lowest possible cost. Local, state, and federal laws are followed.

An administrator manages the agency. He or she reports directly to the board. Directors or department heads manage certain areas (Fig. 1-3). For example, a director of nursing manages the nursing department. A human resources director handles personnel matters such as hiring staff. A social services director meets the social needs of the person and family.

See *Focus on Long-Term Care and Home Care: Organization.*

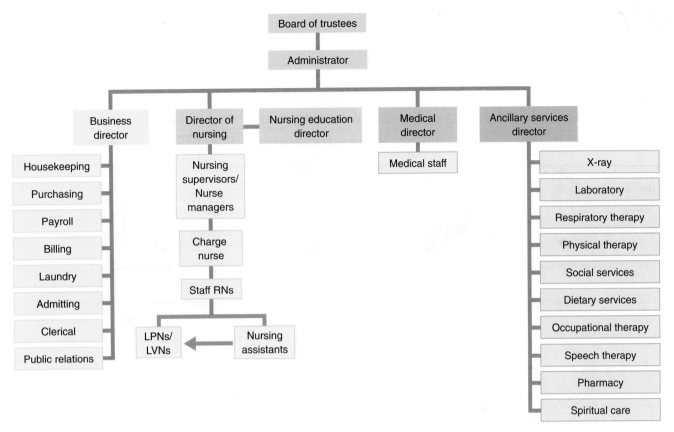

FIGURE 1-3 Sample organizational chart of a health care agency. Titles and departments may vary among states and agencies.

The Health Team

The *health team* (interdisciplinary health care team) involves the many health care workers whose skills and knowledge focus on the person's total care (Table 1-1, p. 6). The goal is to provide quality care. The person is the focus of care.

Many team members are involved in the care of each person. Coordinated care is needed. A registered nurse (RN) usually leads this team.

See *Focus on Communication: The Health Team.*

FOCUS ON COMMUNICATION

The Health Team

Team members have different roles. They communicate often. You may have questions or concerns about a person and his or her care. Tell the team leader. The leader will communicate with health team members.

TABLE 1-1	Health Team Members
Title	**Description**
Activities director/recreational therapist	Plans and directs recreation treatment programs to help maintain or improve a person's physical, social, and emotional well-being.
Audiologist	Treats hearing, balance, and ear problems.
Cleric (clergyman; clergywoman)	Assists with spiritual needs.
Clinical nurse specialist (CNS)	Advanced practice registered nurse (APRN) who consults in a specialty. Geriatrics, critical care, diabetes, rehabilitation, and wound care are examples. Can prescribe drugs in some states.
Dental hygienist	Cleans teeth and provides preventive care.
Dentist	Treats problems with the teeth, gums, and related parts of the mouth.
Dietitian and nutritionist	Assesses and plans for nutritional needs to promote health and manage disease. Teaches about diet and healthy eating.
Home health aide/personal care aide	Assists persons in home settings with daily activities—laundry, bedmaking, grocery shopping, meals, hygiene, dressing, and grooming.
Licensed practical/vocational nurse (LPN/LVN)	Provides nursing care and gives drugs under the direction of RNs and doctors.
Medical or clinical laboratory technologist/technician	Collects specimens. Performs tests on blood, urine, and other body fluids, secretions, and excretions.
Medical records and health information technician	Maintains the quality and security of medical records. Codes patient information for billing purposes.
Medication assistant-certified (MA-C)	Gives drugs as allowed by state law under the supervision of a licensed nurse.
Nurse practitioner (NP)	An APRN with specialized graduate education who diagnoses and treats common health problems. May prescribe some drugs and treatments.
Nursing assistant	Assists nurses and gives care. Supervised by a licensed nurse.
Occupational therapist (OT)	Assists persons to learn or retain skills needed for daily living and working.
Occupational therapy assistant	Performs tasks and services as directed by an OT.
Pharmacist	Fills drug orders and advises about safe prescription use. Consults with doctors and nurses about drug actions and interactions.
Physical therapist (PT)	Assists ill and injured persons with movement, pain management, and rehabilitation.
Physical therapy assistant (PTA)	Performs tasks and services as directed by a PT.
Physician (doctor)	Diagnoses and treats diseases and injuries.
Physician's assistant (PA)	Performs exams, diagnoses, and provides treatments under a doctor's direction.
Podiatrist	Prevents, diagnoses, and treats foot, ankle, and lower leg problems.
Radiographer/radiologic technologist	Takes images using x-rays and other equipment.
Registered nurse (RN)	Assesses, makes nursing diagnoses, plans, implements, and evaluates nursing care. Supervises LPNs/LVNs and nursing assistants.
Respiratory therapist	Assists in treating lung and heart disorders. Gives respiratory treatments and therapies.
Social worker	Deals with social, emotional, and environmental issues affecting illness and recovery. Coordinates community agencies to assist the person and family.
Speech-language pathologist/speech therapist	Diagnoses and treats communication and swallowing disorders.

Modified from Bureau of Labor Statistics, U.S. Department of Labor: Occupational outlook handbook, September 4, 2019.

Nursing Service

Nursing service is a large department (see Fig. 1-3). The director of nursing (DON) is an RN. (*Director of nursing services, chief nurse executive, vice president of nursing,* and *vice president of patient services* are some other titles.) Usually a bachelor's or higher degree is required. The DON is responsible for the entire nursing staff and the nursing care given.

Nursing supervisors and nurse managers (usually RNs) over-see a work shift, nursing unit, or certain nursing function. They are responsible for all nursing care and the actions of nursing staff in their areas.

- Work shift—8-, 10-, and 12-hour shifts are common.
- Nursing unit—surgical, medical, intensive care, pediatric, and mental health units are examples. Operating and recovery areas, emergency room, and maternity department are others.
- Nursing function—staff development, restorative nursing, infection control, and continuous quality care are examples.

Nursing units usually have RN *charge nurses* for each shift. LPNs/LVNs can be charge nurses in some states. The charge nurse is responsible for all nursing care and nursing staff actions during that shift. Staff RNs report to the charge nurse. LPNs/LVNs report to staff RNs or to the charge nurse. You report to the nurse supervising your work.

Nursing education staff:

- Plan and present educational programs (in-service programs). This includes those that meet federal and state educational requirements.
- Provide new and changing information.
- Show how to use new equipment and supplies.
- Review policies and procedures on a regular basis.
- Educate and train nursing assistants.
- Conduct new employee orientation programs.

THE NURSING TEAM

The *nursing team involves those who provide nursing care— RNs, LPNs/LVNs, and nursing assistants.* All focus on the physical, social, emotional, and spiritual needs of the person and family.

Registered Nurses

A *registered nurse (RN) has completed a 2-, 3-, or 4-year nursing program and has passed a licensing test.*

- Community college programs—2 years
- Hospital-based diploma programs—2 or 3 years
- College or university programs—4 years

Graduates take a licensing test offered by their state board of nursing. They receive a license and become *registered* after passing the test. RNs must have a license recognized by the state in which they work.

RNs assess, make nursing diagnoses, plan, implement, and evaluate nursing care (Chapter 8). They provide care and delegate (Chapter 4) nursing care and tasks to the nursing team. They evaluate how nursing care affects each person. RNs teach the person and family how to improve health and independence.

RNs follow the doctor's orders. They may delegate them to other nursing team members. RNs do not prescribe treatments or drugs. However, RNs can become *clinical nurse specialists* or *nurse practitioners*. Depending on state law, these RNs have limited diagnosing and prescribing functions.

RNs work as charge or staff nurses, nurse supervisors or managers, DONs, agency administrators, and instructors. Those and other career options depend on education, abilities, and experience.

Licensed Practical Nurses and Licensed Vocational Nurses

A *licensed practical nurse (LPN) has completed a practical nursing program and has passed a licensing test.* Hospitals, community colleges, vocational schools, and technical schools offer programs. Programs are 10, 12, or 18 months long. Some high schools offer 2-year programs.

Graduates take a licensing test for practical nursing. After passing the test, they have a license to practice and the title of *licensed practical nurse. Licensed vocational nurse (LVN) is used in California and Texas.* LPNs/LVNs must have a license recognized by the state where they work.

LPNs/LVNs are supervised by RNs and doctors. They have fewer responsibilities and functions than RNs do. They need less supervision when the person's condition is stable and care is simple. They assist RNs with acutely ill persons and complex procedures.

Nursing Assistants

A *nursing assistant has passed a nursing assistant training and competency evaluation program (NATCEP).* Nursing assistants *perform delegated nursing tasks under the supervision of a licensed nurse.* Nursing assistants are discussed in Chapter 3.

NURSING CARE PATTERNS

The *nursing care pattern* used depends on how many persons need care, the staff, and the cost. See Figure 1-4.

- *Functional nursing. Focuses on tasks and jobs. Each nursing team member is assigned certain tasks and jobs.* For example, 1 nurse gives all drugs. Another gives all treatments. Nursing assistants give baths, make beds, and serve meals.
- *Team nursing. An RN leads a team of nursing staff. The RN decides the amount and kind of care each person needs.* The team leader delegates the care of certain persons to other nurses and nursing assistants. Delegation (Chapter 4) decisions depend on the person's needs and team member abilities. Team members report observations and the care given to the team leader.
- *Primary nursing. The primary nurse (an RN) is responsible for the person's total care.* The nursing team assists as needed. The RN gives nursing care and makes discharge plans for home or long-term care. Needed patient teaching is provided.
- *Case management. Services for the person's care needs are obtained and monitored from admission through discharge and into the home or long-term care setting.* The case manager communicates with doctors, the health team, insurance companies, and community agencies. Case managers work with certain doctors, certain age-groups, or persons with certain health problems. Heart disease, diabetes, and cancer are examples.
- *Patient-focused care. Services are moved from departments to the bedside.* Besides nursing care, the nursing team performs basic skills usually done by other health team members. For example, an RN draws a blood sample. This reduces the number of staff involved and the care costs.

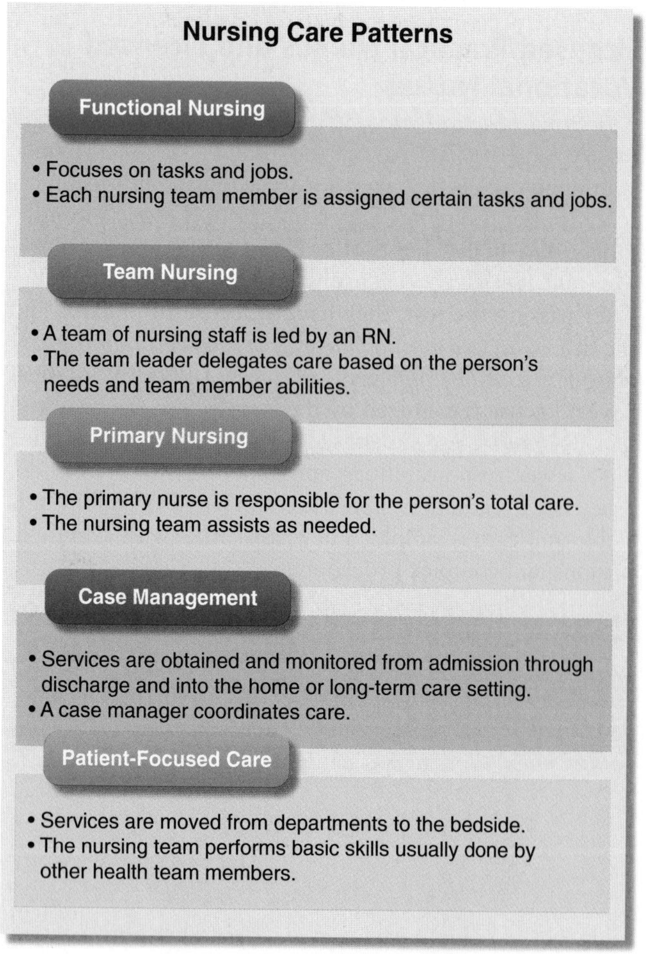

PAYING FOR HEALTH CARE

Health care is costly. Some people avoid health care because they cannot pay. Others pay doctor bills but go without food or drugs. Health insurance covers some costs. Rarely are all costs covered.

These programs help pay for health care.

- *Private insurance* is bought by individuals and families.
- *Group insurance* is bought by groups or organizations for individuals. This is often an employee benefit.
- *Medicare* is a federal program for persons 65 years of age or older. Some younger people with certain disabilities qualify. Part A is for hospital, nursing center, hospice, and home care costs. Part B is for doctor visits, ambulance services, medical equipment, mental health care, and some drugs. Part B is voluntary. The person pays a monthly premium for Part B.
- *Medicaid* is jointly funded by the federal government and the states. People and families with low incomes usually qualify. It covers children and older, blind, and disabled persons.
- *The Patient Protection and Affordable Care Act of 2010* is commonly called "Obamacare" after President Barack Obama and the *Affordable Care Act (ACA)*. Some people do not qualify for Medicare or Medicaid. They can buy insurance through health insurance exchanges. These are market-places for buying health insurance. Exchanges are run by the federal government, by states, or both.

See *Promoting Safety and Comfort: Paying for Health Care.*

Nursing Care Patterns

Functional Nursing
- Focuses on tasks and jobs.
- Each nursing team member is assigned certain tasks and jobs.

Team Nursing
- A team of nursing staff is led by an RN.
- The team leader delegates care based on the person's needs and team member abilities.

Primary Nursing
- The primary nurse is responsible for the person's total care.
- The nursing team assists as needed.

Case Management
- Services are obtained and monitored from admission through discharge and into the home or long-term care setting.
- A case manager coordinates care.

Patient-Focused Care
- Services are moved from departments to the bedside.
- The nursing team performs basic skills usually done by other health team members.

FIGURE 1-4 Nursing care patterns.

PROMOTING SAFETY AND COMFORT

Paying for Health Care

Safety

Some conditions can be prevented with proper care. Medicare pays a lower rate for such conditions if they are acquired during a hospital stay. Pressure injuries (Chapter 41) and certain types of falls, trauma, and infections are examples. You must help prevent such conditions.

Prospective Payment Systems

The Centers for Medicare & Medicaid Services (CMS) uses Prospective Payment Systems (PPS). *Prospective* means *before*. PPS limit care costs for Medicare and Medicaid services. The amount paid for a specific service is fixed. If costs are less than the amount paid, the agency keeps the extra money. If costs are greater, the agency takes the loss.

Different PPS are used for hospitals, home health care agencies, SNFs, rehabilitation centers, and other health care agencies. Each system determines the amount paid.

MEETING STANDARDS

Health care agencies must meet standards set by federal and state governments and accrediting agencies. Standards relate to policies, procedures, and quality of care. An agency must meet standards for:

- *Licensure.* A state license is required to operate and provide care.
- *Certification.* This is required to receive Medicare and Medicaid funds.
- *Accreditation.* This is voluntary. It signals quality and excellence.

The Survey Process

Surveys are done to see if standards are met. A *survey is the formal review of an agency through the collection of facts and observations.* Survey teams are made up of surveyors. A *surveyor is a person who collects information by observing and asking questions.*

A survey team will:

- Review policies, procedures, and medical records.
- Interview staff, patients and residents, and families.
- Observe how care is given.
- Observe if dignity and privacy are promoted.
- Check for cleanliness and safety.
- Make sure staff meet state requirements. (Are doctors and nurses licensed? Are nursing assistants on the state registry?)

If standards are met, the agency receives a license, certification, or accreditation. Sometimes problems (*deficiencies*) are found. The agency usually has 60 days or less to correct the problem. The agency can be fined for uncorrected or serious deficiencies. Or it can lose its license, certification, or accreditation.

Your Role

You have an important role in meeting standards and in the survey process. You must:

- Provide quality care.
- Protect the person's rights.
- Provide for the person's and your own safety.
- Help keep the agency clean and safe.
- Act in a professional manner.
- Have good work ethics.
- Follow agency policies and procedures.
- Answer questions honestly and completely.
  See *Focus on Surveys: Your Role.*

FOCUS ON **SURVEYS**

Your Role

A surveyor may ask you questions. If so, be polite. Answer questions honestly and completely. If you do not understand a question, ask that it be re-phrased. Do not guess. Tell the surveyor where you can find the answer. You can say: "I will ask the nurse."

For example, a surveyor approaches you.

Surveyor: "May I ask you some questions?"

You: "Yes. I am happy to answer your questions."

Surveyor: "Thank you. First, when do you practice hand hygiene?"

You: "I wash my hands before and after contact with a patient. I also wash my hands when they are dirty and after taking off gloves."

Surveyor: "Thank you. Next, what are 2 appropriate patient identifiers?"

You: "I don't understand. Can you re-phrase the question?"

Surveyor: "Yes. Name 2 things you can use to identify a patient."

You: "Okay. Thank you. I can use the patient's full name and date of birth. I cannot use the room number."

Surveyor: "I have 1 last question. In a disaster, where would you find the Emergency Preparedness Plan?"

You: "I'm not sure. I will ask the charge nurse where to find it."

FOCUS ON **PRIDE**

The Person, Family, and Yourself

P ersonal and Professional Responsibility

Working in health care is rewarding. You provide care for a *person*. Your work affects the person's quality of care. Value the work that you do.

Focus on PRIDE is at the end of each chapter. The feature will help you promote pride in the person, the family, and yourself. Building on chapter content, it focuses on:

- *Personal and Professional Responsibility*—how personal and professional behaviors and development affect yourself and others.
- *Rights and Respect*—how to promote the rights of others and how to respect them as persons with dignity and value.
- *Independence and Social Interaction*—how to promote independence and positive interactions.
- *Delegation and Teamwork*—how to practice safe delegation (Chapter 4) and work well with and help other team members.
- *Ethics and Laws*—how to do the right thing when dealing with patients, residents, and co-workers. Laws affecting nursing care and real court cases are also presented.

For discussion purposes, each chapter ends with a *Focus on PRIDE: Application* section. The questions challenge you to think about your role and how you will value the person, family, or yourself.

R ights and Respect

Consider what type of agency would suit you. One person may prefer working in long-term care while another prefers a hospital setting. Careful career planning shows respect for employers, patients and residents, and yourself.

I ndependence and Social Interaction

You will interact with patients and residents, nursing staff, health team members, surveyors, and families. How you interact with others affects quality of care and job satisfaction.

D elegation and Teamwork

Health team members must work together to provide quality care. Offer to help others when you can. Helping others shows you value teamwork.

E thics and Laws

Professional conduct is valued in all health care agencies. You will learn about ethical and legal aspects of care (Chapter 5) and student and work ethics (Chapter 6). As you study, consider how you will apply professional qualities as a student and in the workplace.

FOCUS ON **PRIDE**: *Application*

Health care offers many opportunities. Why do you want to work in health care? Where do you want to work? What are your career goals?

REVIEW QUESTIONS

Circle the BEST answer.

1 Helping persons return to their highest physical and mental function is called
   a Maintaining independence
   b Promoting health
   c Preventing disease
   d Rehabilitation

2 Rehabilitation starts when the
   a Person is ready to leave the agency
   b Person first seeks health care
   c Doctor writes the order
   d Health team thinks the person is ready

3 A health care program for dying persons is a
   a Hospice
   b Home care agency
   c Skilled nursing facility
   d Hospital

4 You work in an assisted living residence. You
   a Give care in the person's home
   b Care for patients recovering from surgery
   c Help persons with their daily activities
   d Care for persons with acute illnesses

5 Who controls policy in a health care agency?
   a The survey team
   b The board of directors
   c The health team
   d Medicare and Medicaid

6 Who is responsible for the entire nursing staff and safe nursing care?
   a The case manager
   b The director of nursing
   c The charge nurse
   d The RN

7 You are a member of
   a The health team and the nursing team
   b The health team and the medical team
   c The nursing team and the medical team
   d The board of trustees

8 The nursing team includes
   a Doctors
   b Pharmacists
   c Physical and occupational therapists
   d RNs, LPNs/LVNs, and nursing assistants

9 Nursing assistants are supervised by
   a Licensed nurses
   b Other nursing assistants
   c The health team
   d The medical director

10 The nursing assistant's role is to
   a Meet Medicare and Medicaid standards
   b Perform delegated tasks
   c Follow the doctor's orders
   d Manage care

11 Your agency uses a team nursing care pattern. Which is *true*?
   a An RN is the team leader.
   b An RN gives all care.
   c Each staff member is assigned certain tasks.
   d The nursing team performs health team functions.

12 Medicare is for persons who
   a Are 65 years of age or older
   b Need nursing center care
   c Have group insurance
   d Have low incomes

13 Which is required for an agency to operate and provide care?
   a Accreditation
   b Certification
   c A license
   d A survey

14 Which is voluntary for health care agencies?
   a Licensure
   b Certification
   c Accreditation
   d Surveys

15 Surveys are done to
   a Reduce health care costs
   b See if agencies meet set standards
   c Educate the nursing team
   d Determine the amount paid by insurers

16 A surveyor asks you some questions. You should
   a Refer all questions to the nurse
   b Answer as the DON tells you to
   c Give as little information as possible
   d Give honest and complete answers

Answers to Chapter 1 questions are on p. 885.

FOCUS ON **PRACTICE**

Problem Solving

The nurse supervising you has not returned from a meal break. You have a question about a patient's care. Your nursing department is organized as shown in Figure 1-3. What will you do?

The Person's Rights

People want to know about their health problems and treatment. They want to understand and take part in treatment decisions. As patients and residents, they have certain rights.

PATIENT RIGHTS

The Patient Care Partnership: Understanding Expectations, Rights, and Responsibilities is from the American Hospital Association. The document explains the person's rights and expectations during hospital stays. The relationship between the doctor, health team, and patient is stressed. See Box 2-1.

RESIDENT RIGHTS

The *Omnibus Budget Reconciliation Act of 1987 (OBRA)* is a federal law. It applies to all 50 states. The Centers for Medicare & Medicaid Services (CMS) enforces OBRA.

OBRA requires that nursing centers provide care in a manner and in a setting that maintains or improves each person's quality of life, health, and safety. Nursing assistant training and competency evaluation are part of OBRA (Chapter 3). Resident rights are a major part of OBRA.

Residents have rights as United States citizens. For example, they have the right to vote. They also have rights relating to their every-day lives and care in a nursing center. These rights are protected by federal and state laws.

Nursing centers must protect and promote the person's rights. The center cannot interfere with a resident's rights. Some residents cannot exercise their rights. Then a representative (spouse, partner, adult child, court-appointed guardian) does so. A *representative is a person with the legal right to act on the patient's or resident's behalf when he or she cannot do so for himself or herself.*

Nursing centers must inform residents of their rights—orally and in writing. Residents are also informed of the rules about their conduct and responsibilities in the center. The information is given before or during admission to the center, as needed during the person's stay, and when laws or center rules change.

Resident rights and other information are given in the language and format the person uses and understands.
- An interpreter is used if the person speaks and understands a foreign language or communicates by sign language.
- Written translations are provided in the foreign languages common in the center's geographic area.
- Medical terms are avoided to the extent possible.
- Sign language and communication aids are used as necessary.
- Large-print texts are available for persons with vision problems.

BOX 2-1	The Patient Care Partnership—Understanding Expectations, Rights, and Responsibilities (A Summary)

High-Quality Care
- The hospital provides needed care with skill, compassion, and respect.
- The patient has the right to know the identities of:
  - Doctors, nurses, and other staff
  - Students and other trainees

Clean and Safe Setting
- There are policies and procedures to:
  - Avoid mistakes.
  - Prevent abuse or neglect.
- The patient is told of unexpected or significant events.
  - What happened
  - Needed changes in care

Involvement in Care
- The patient has the right to make informed decisions about treatment choices.
  - What are the benefits and risks of each treatment?
  - Is the treatment experimental or part of a research study?
  - What can be expected from treatment?
  - How might long-term effects of treatment affect quality of life?
  - What will the patient and family need to do after discharge?
  - What are the costs for uncovered services or providers?
- The patient has the right to consent to or refuse treatment. The person is told of the effects of refusing treatment.
- The patient is expected to give information about:
  - Past illnesses, surgeries, or hospital stays
  - Allergic reactions
  - Drugs or dietary supplements that are taken
  - Health insurance plan admission requirements
- The patient's health care goals, values, and spiritual beliefs are respected. The patient is responsible for sharing his or her wishes with the doctor, family, and health team.

Involvement in Care—cont'd
- The patient is expected to communicate about who makes decisions when he or she is unable.
  - *Power of attorney, living will,* or *advance directive* documents are shared with the doctor, family, and health team (Chapter 59).
  - Help is provided with making difficult decisions. Counselors or chaplains are available.

Protection of Privacy
- The hospital protects the confidentiality of:
  - The patient's relationships with the doctor and health team
  - Information about the patient's health and care
- A "Notice of Privacy Practices" is provided describing:
  - How patient information is used, disclosed, and protected
  - How to obtain a copy of hospital records about patient care

Preparing to Leave the Hospital
- Sources for follow-up care are identified. The hospital's financial interest in any referrals is disclosed.
- Hospital activities are coordinated with community caregivers. The hospital requests permission to share care information.
- Information and training are given about self-care at home.

Help With Bills and Insurance Claims
- The hospital files insurance, Medicare, or Medicaid claims.
- Patients can contact the business office about insurance coverage.
- The hospital tries to find financial help or make other arrangements if the person is without health coverage. The patient provides needed information to obtain coverage or assistance.

Modified from American Hospital Association: The patient care partnership: understanding expectations, rights, and responsibilities.

Resident rights (Box 2-2, p. 14) are posted throughout the center. Those affecting your role are described in this chapter.

Sometimes an ombudsman is needed to protect the person's rights. An *ombudsman* is someone who supports or promotes the needs and interests of another person. See *Focus on PRIDE: The Person, Family, and Yourself* (p. 19).

See *Focus on Surveys: Resident Rights.*

FOCUS ON SURVEYS

Resident Rights

Resident rights are a major focus of surveys. Surveyors observe staff behaviors and actions. They listen to staff comments and remarks. Always assume they are doing so. What you say and do must promote quality of life, health, and safety. For example, a surveyor may observe:
- How you prevent exposure of the person's body
- How you help a person dress for the season and time of day
- How you label clothing
- If you knock on a person's door before entering the room
- If you change a person's music or TV without permission
- If you move personal items without permission
- How you address and speak to a person

You will learn how to protect the person's rights as you study this and other chapters. Always act and speak in a professional manner.

BOX 2-2	Resident Rights

- To be treated with dignity and respect. And to receive quality care.
- To exercise rights as a center resident and as a United States citizen.
- To be informed orally and in writing of rights and center rules. This is done in a language the person understands.
- To access all his or her records.
- To obtain copies of his or her records. This is at the resident's expense.
- To refuse treatment.
- To refuse to take part in experimental research. This is the development and testing of new treatments and drugs.
- To make advance directives (Chapter 59).
- To be informed of Medicare benefits and services. This includes costs covered and not covered.
- To file complaints with the appropriate state agency about abuse, neglect, and the mis-use of property.
- To be informed of center services and charges.
- To choose a doctor.
- To know the doctor's name, specialty, and contact information.
- To be informed of his or her health status and medical condition.
- To be informed of:
  - Any accident or injury that may need medical attention
  - A change in physical, mental, or psycho-social status
  - The need to stop, change, or add a treatment
  - A decision to transfer or discharge the person
  - A room or roommate change
  - A change in rights under federal or state law
- To manage personal and financial affairs.
- To be informed in advance about care and treatment. This includes changes in care and treatment.
- To have privacy and confidentiality:
  - Of personal and medical records
  - Of treatment and care
  - Of written and phone communications
  - During visits with family and friends
  - When meeting with resident groups

- To voice grievances and have them solved promptly.
- To see the results of federal and state surveys and plans to correct problems or areas of weakness.
- To perform or refuse to perform services for the center.
- To send and receive un-opened mail. To buy supplies to send mail.
- To receive information about protecting persons with intellectual and developmental disabilities and mental health disorders.
- To have and use personal items and clothing.
- To take drugs without help if able.
- To refuse to change to a different room.
- To be free from restraints (Chapter 15).
- To be free from abuse (verbal, sexual, physical), bodily punishment, involuntary seclusion, and other abuse or mistreatment (Chapter 5).
- To be cared for in a manner and setting that maintains or enhances quality of life.
- To choose activities, schedules, and health care that meet his or her interests and needs.
- To interact with community members inside and outside the center.
- To make choices about his or her life in the center.
- To organize and take part in resident groups.
- To take part in social, religious, and community activities.
- To have a setting and services that consider his or her needs and choices.
- To be informed of his or her health and medical condition in a language that he or she understands. That language is used when taking part in care planning.
- To have a clean, comfortable, and home-like setting. This includes temperature, lighting, and sound levels.
- To attain or maintain his or her highest level of function.
- To have closet space.
- To visit with a spouse or partner, family, and friends at any reasonable hour.

Information

The *right to information* means access to all records about the person. Medical records, contracts, incident reports, and financial records are included. The request can be oral or written.

The person has the right to be fully informed of his or her health condition. The person must also have information about his or her doctor. This includes the doctor's name, specialty, and contact information.

Report any information request to the nurse. *You do not give the information described above to the person or family* (Chapter 3).

See *Focus on Communication: Information.*

FOCUS ON COMMUNICATION

Information

You may be asked about a person's care. You must not give out information. This is the nurse's responsibility. You can say:

I am sorry. I am not allowed to give that information. I will report your request to the nurse.

Communicate the request promptly. You can tell the person:

I told the nurse about your question. The nurse will speak with you soon.

Refusing Treatment

The person has the *right to refuse treatment*. *Treatment means the care provided to maintain or restore health, improve function, or relieve symptoms.* A person cannot be treated without consent (Chapter 5).

The center must:

- Find out what the person is refusing and why.
- Explain the problems that can result from the refusal.
- Offer other treatment options.
- Continue to provide all other services.

Advance directives are part of the right to refuse treatment (Chapter 59). They include living wills and instructions about life support. *Advance directives* are written instructions about health care when the person is not able to make such decisions.

Report any treatment refusal to the nurse. The nurse may change the person's care plan (Chapter 8).

Privacy and Confidentiality

Residents have the *right to personal privacy*. Staff must maintain privacy of the person's body. Expose the person's body only as necessary. Only staff directly involved in care and treatment are present. Consent is needed for others to be present. For example, a person's consent is needed for a student to observe a treatment.

Privacy is maintained for all personal care measures. Bathing, dressing, and elimination are examples. To protect privacy:

- Close privacy curtains, doors, and window coverings.
- Remove residents from public view.
- Provide clothes or drape the person to prevent unnecessary exposure of body parts.
- Practice the measures listed in Chapter 5.

Leaving the person without a gown, clothing, or bed covers violates the right to privacy. So does an open door when the person uses the bathroom, commode, urinal, or bedpan.

Residents have the right to visit in private—where others cannot see or hear them. If requested, the center must provide private space. Offices, chapels, dining rooms, and meeting rooms are options.

Residents have the right to make phone calls in private (Fig. 2-1). The calls must not be over-heard. Privacy is provided for phone calls in offices or at the nurses' station. Phones are at the correct height for use by persons in wheelchairs. Phones for hard of hearing persons are also available. Some residents have their own phones.

The person has the right to send and receive mail without others interfering. No one can open mail the person sends or receives without the person's consent. Un-opened mail is given to the person within 24 hours of delivery to the center. Out-going mail is delivered to the postal service within 24 hours on days of regular delivery or pick-up services.

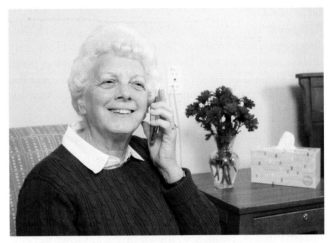

FIGURE 2-1 A resident is talking privately on her phone.

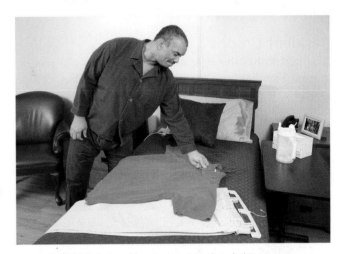

FIGURE 2-2 A resident is choosing what clothing to wear.

Information about the person's care, treatment, and condition is kept confidential. So are medical and financial records. Consent is needed for their release to other agencies or persons.

You must provide privacy and protect confidentiality. Doing so shows respect and protects the person's dignity. See Chapters 5 and 6.

Personal Choice

Residents have the *right to make their own choices*. This includes:

- Choosing doctors
- Choosing friends and visitors
- Helping to plan care and treatment
- Choosing activities, schedules, and care:
  - When to go to bed and when to get up
  - What to wear (Fig. 2-2)
  - How to spend time
  - What to eat

Personal choice promotes quality of life, dignity, and self-respect. Allow personal choice whenever safely possible.

Grievances

Residents have the *right to voice concerns, questions, and complaints about treatment and care*. The problem may involve another person. It may be about care that was given or not given. The center must promptly try to correct the matter. No one can punish the person in any way for voicing a grievance.

Work

The person does not work for care, care items or other things, or privileges. The person is not required to perform services for the center.

However, the person has the *right to work or perform services if he or she desires*. Some people like to garden, repair or build things, clean, sew, mend, or cook. Other persons need work for rehabilitation or activity reasons. The care plan reflects the person's desire or need to work. Residents volunteer or are paid for their services.

Resident Groups

The person has the *right to form and take part in resident groups*. Families can meet with other families. These groups can plan activities, discuss concerns, take part in educational events, and suggest center improvements. They can support and comfort group members.

Residents have the right to take part in social, cultural, religious, and community events. They have the right to help in getting to and from such events.

Personal Items

Residents have the *right to keep and use personal items*. This includes clothing and some furnishings. The items allowed depend on space needs and the health and safety of others.

Treat the person's property with care and respect. The items may lack value to you but have meaning to the person. They also relate to personal choice, dignity, a home-like setting, and quality of life.

The person's property is protected. Items are labeled with the person's name. The center must investigate reports of lost, stolen, or damaged items. Sometimes the police help. The person and family are advised to keep jewelry and costly items at home.

Protect yourself and the center from being accused of stealing. Do not go through a closet, drawers, purse, or other space without the person's knowledge and consent. A nurse may ask you to inspect closets and drawers. Center policy should require that a co-worker and the person or legal representative be present. They witness your actions. Follow center policy for reporting and recording the inspection.

Freedom From Abuse, Mistreatment, and Neglect

Residents have the *right to be free from verbal, sexual, physical, and mental abuse* (Chapter 5). *Abuse* means:
- The willful infliction of injury, unreasonable confinement, intimidation, or punishment that results in physical harm, pain, or mental anguish. *Intimidation* means to threaten to hurt or punish.
- Depriving the person of the goods or services needed for well-being.

They also have the right to be free from *involuntary seclusion*.
- *Separating a person from others against his or her will*
- *Keeping the person to a certain area*
- *Keeping the person away from his or her room without consent*

No one can abuse, neglect, or mistreat a resident. This includes center staff, volunteers, and staff from other agencies or groups. It also includes other residents, family members, visitors, and legal representatives. Centers must investigate suspected or reported cases of abuse. They cannot employ persons who:
- Were found guilty of abusing, neglecting, or mistreating others by a court of law.
- Have a finding entered into a state's nursing assistant registry (Chapter 3) about abuse, neglect, mistreatment, or wrongful acts involving the person's money or property (Chapter 5). A *finding* means that a state determined that the employee abused, neglected, mistreated, or wrongfully used the person's money or property.

Freedom From Restraint

Residents have the *right not to have body movements restricted*. Restraints and certain drugs can restrict body movements (Chapter 15). Some drugs are restraints because they affect mood, behavior, and mental function. Sometimes residents are restrained to protect them from harming themselves or others. A doctor's order is needed for restraint use. Restraints are not used for staff convenience or to discipline a person. They are used only if required to treat medical symptoms.

Quality of Life

Residents have the *right to quality of life*. They must be cared for in a manner and setting that promotes dignity and respect for self. Staff must provide care in a manner that maintains or enhances self-esteem and feelings of self-worth. Care must promote physical, mental, and social well-being. Protecting resident rights promotes quality of life. It shows respect for the person.

Be polite and courteous. Good, honest, and thoughtful care enhances quality of life. Box 2-3 lists OBRA-required actions that promote dignity and privacy.

See *Focus on Communication: Quality of Life*.

BOX 2-3	Promoting Dignity and Privacy—OBRA-Required Actions

Courteous and Dignified Interactions

- Use the right tone of voice.
- Use good eye contact.
- Stand or sit close enough as needed.
- Use the person's proper name and title. For example: "Mrs. Crane." Or use the name the person prefers.
- Gain the person's attention before interacting with him or her.
- Use touch if the person approves.
- Respect the person's social status.
- Listen with interest to what the person is saying.
- Do not yell at, scold, or embarrass the person.

Privacy and Self-Determination

- Drape properly during care and procedures to avoid exposure and embarrassment.
- Use privacy curtains or screens during care and procedures.
- Close the room door during care and procedures. Also close window coverings.
- Knock on the door before entering. Wait to be asked in.
- Close the bathroom door when the person uses the bathroom.
- Drape properly in a chair.

Personal Choice and Independence

- Person smokes in allowed areas.
- Person takes part in activities of his or her interest.
- Person takes part in scheduling activities and care.
- Person gives input into the care plan about preferences and independence.
- Person is involved in a room or roommate change.
- The person's items are moved or inspected only with the person's consent.

Courteous and Dignified Care

- Assist with dressing in the right clothing for time of day and personal choice.
- Promote independence and dignity in dining.
- Respect private space and property. For example, change TV stations or music only with the person's consent.
- Assist with walking and transfers. Do not interfere with independence.
- Assist with hygiene and grooming preferences. Do not interfere with independence.
  - Appearance is neat and clean.
  - Hair is styled as the person prefers.
  - The person is clean shaven or has a groomed beard and mustache.
  - Nails are trimmed and clean.
  - Dentures, hearing aids, eyeglasses, and other devices are used correctly.
  - Clothing is clean.
  - Clothing fits and is properly fastened.
  - Shoes, hose, and socks are on properly and fastened.
  - Extra clothing is worn for warmth as needed. Sweaters and lap blankets are examples.

FOCUS ON COMMUNICATION

Quality of Life

Every person deserves to be addressed in a manner that shows dignity and respect. Address the person by title and last name. For example: Mr. Baker, Mrs. Harty, or Dr. Collins. Do not use a person's first name or another name unless the person requests it. Avoid using terms like *sweetheart, honey, grandpa,* and *dear.*

Environment. Residents have the *right to a safe, clean, comfortable, and home-like setting.* The person can have and use personal items to the extent possible. Doing so promotes personal choice and a home-like setting.

The setting, services, and staff must meet the person's needs and preferences. They must promote independence, dignity, and well-being. The center must try to change schedules, call systems, and room arrangements to meet the person's desires and needs. For example, a person:

- Prefers a shower, not a tub bath.
- Wants a shower before breakfast.
- Is afraid of falling in the shower and elsewhere.
- Is uneasy about a staff member giving care.
- Cannot reach or use the call light.
- Cannot reach personal items.
- Does not like the food served.

Activities. Residents have the *right to activities that enhance each person's physical, mental, and psycho-social well-being.* The center provides religious services for spiritual health. Activities are meaningful when they:

- Reflect the person's needs, interests, culture, background, and life-style.
- Are enjoyed by the person.
- Help the person feel useful or produce something useful.
- Provide a sense of belonging.

Activities involve large groups (bingo), small groups (a card game), or 2 people. The person may do something alone. Letter writing and computer games are examples.

See *Focus on Communication: Activities.*
See *Teamwork and Time Management: Activities.*
See *Focus on Surveys: Activities.*

FOCUS ON COMMUNICATION

Activities

You assist residents to and from activity programs. You may need help doing so. Politely ask a co-worker to help you. Share the following with your co-worker.

- What time you need help.
- How much of the co-worker's time you need—5 minutes, 10 minutes, and so on.
- The residents you need help with.
- If the person walks or uses a wheelchair.
- What adaptive (assistive) devices are used. Eyeglasses, hearing aids, canes, and walkers are examples.

Always say "please" when asking for help. And thank the person for helping you. For example:

Jane, can you please help me assist 2 residents to the concert? It starts at 2:00, so I'll need your help at 1:45. Mr. Harris needs his glasses, hearing aid, and walker. Mrs. Janz uses a wheelchair. She needs her glasses. The blanket for her lap is in the wheelchair. The concert is over at 3:00. Can you help me then, too? Thanks so much for helping me.

FOCUS ON SURVEYS

Activities

Surveyors may ask you about:

- Your role in getting residents ready for a group activity.
  - How do you make sure the person is dressed and ready for an activity?
  - How do you provide needed transportation?
- Your role in helping with activities of daily living during an activity. For example, does the person need to use the bathroom? Does the person need help eating?
- Your role in helping a person with an individual activity. For example, you play cards with a person. Do you have needed supplies? Is the person properly positioned? Do you provide good lighting?
- How are activities provided when the activities staff members are not available?

TEAMWORK AND TIME MANAGEMENT

Activities

Know when an activity begins and ends. Before assisting residents to activities:

- Assist with elimination needs and hand hygiene.
- Assist with grooming such as brushing and combing hair. A person may want to apply perfume or make-up.
- Have the person wear the correct clothing and footwear for the activity.
- Provide needed adaptive (assistive) devices. Eyeglasses, hearing aids, canes, and walkers are examples.

Allow 15 to 20 minutes to assist residents to and from the activity. Help co-workers as needed.

Residents may need help with activities (Fig. 2-3). If not, use activity time wisely. Provide needed care and visit residents who cannot leave their rooms. You can clean and straighten rooms, bathrooms, shower rooms, and utility rooms.

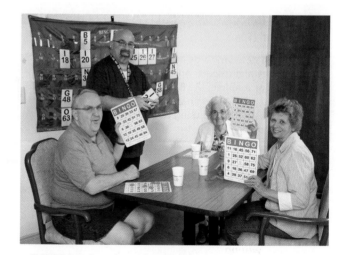

FIGURE 2-3 A nursing assistant is helping residents with an activity.

FOCUS ON **PRIDE**

The Person, Family, and Yourself

Personal and Professional Responsibility
You are responsible for the care you give. You can help improve each person's quality of life, health, and safety. Take pride in the quality of your work.

Rights and Respect
The *Older Americans Act* is a federal law. It requires a long-term care ombudsman program in every state. An *ombudsman supports or promotes the needs and interests of another person.*

Ombudsmen act on behalf of persons receiving health care. They protect a person's health, safety, welfare, and rights. They:
- Investigate and resolve complaints.
- Provide services to assist the person.
- Assist with hospital access or discharge concerns.
- Provide information about long-term care services.
- Monitor nursing care and conditions.
- Provide support to resident and family groups.
- Help the person and family resolve family conflicts.
- Help the center manage difficult problems.

Residents have the right to communicate privately with anyone of their choice. They can share concerns with anyone outside the center.

Nursing centers must post contact information for local and state ombudsmen. A resident or family may share a concern with you. Follow center policies and procedures for contacting an ombudsman. Ombudsman services are useful when:
- There is a concern about a person's care or treatment.
- Someone interferes with a person's rights, health, safety, or welfare.

Independence and Social Interaction
Encourage social interaction. Tell the person about activities and offer help to and from activities. Also respect the person's right to privacy during visits with others and phone calls. These actions promote independence, self-worth, and quality of life.

Delegation and Teamwork
Health care agencies must meet the person's needs and preferences. Schedules, care assignments, and room arrangements may need to change to meet the person's needs. Flexibility, good teamwork, and communication are required to provide quality care.

Ethics and Laws
Every person has the right to keep personal information private. This includes information about health care. The *Health Insurance Portability and Accountability Act of 1996 (HIPAA)* protects the privacy and security of a person's health information. HIPAA is discussed further in Chapter 5.

FOCUS ON **PRIDE**: *Application*

You have an important role in protecting the person's rights. Identify 3 ways you can promote the person's right to:
- Personal choice
- Privacy and confidentiality
- A safe, clean, and comfortable setting

REVIEW QUESTIONS

Circle **T** *if the statement is TRUE or* **F** *if it is FALSE.*

1 T F The *Patient Care Partnership: Understanding Expectations, Rights, and Responsibilities* is a federal law concerned with hospital care.

2 T F OBRA applies to all 50 states.

3 T F Nursing center residents have rights as U.S. citizens.

4 T F Residents are informed of their rights only in writing.

5 T F Residents have the right to choose their own doctors.

6 T F You should open the person's mail within 24 hours of delivery to the center.

7 T F A resident complains about the food. The center must try to provide desired foods.

8 T F Residents must provide some type of work for the center.

9 T F Resident groups can discuss ideas for activity programs.

10 T F An employee was found guilty of abusing a resident. The center can continue to employ the person.

11 T F You can restrain a resident to provide care.

12 T F A staff member tells a resident: "I don't have time to help you." The statement promotes quality of life.

Continued

REVIEW QUESTIONS—cont'd

Circle the BEST answer.

13 These statements are about hospital care. Which is *correct?*
 a Patients must file their own insurance claims.
 b The health team makes care decisions when the person is unable.
 c Patients must allow students to provide care.
 d Patients have the right to make informed treatment choices.

14 A son has the legal right to act on his mother's behalf. The son is his mother's legal
 a Ombudsman
 b Representative
 c Caregiver
 d Health care provider

15 A daughter wants to read her father's medical record. What should you do?
 a Give her the medical record.
 b Ask the resident if she can read the record.
 c Tell the nurse.
 d Tell her that she cannot do so.

16 A resident refuses to have a shower. What should you do?
 a Tell him or her that a shower cannot be refused.
 b Tell the family.
 c Comply, but say that the person must shower tomorrow.
 d Tell the nurse.

17 Which violates the person's right to privacy?
 a Closing the bathroom door when the person uses the bathroom
 b Opening window blinds when assisting with bathing
 c Covering the person for personal care
 d Asking the person's permission to observe a treatment

18 A resident has a phone and wants to make a call. What should you do?
 a Leave the room.
 b Tell the nurse.
 c Have the person use the phone at the nurses' station.
 d Close the privacy curtain so you can finish your tasks in the room.

19 Who decides how to style a person's hair?
 a The person
 b The nurse
 c You
 d The ombudsman

20 Residents have the right to
 a Bring weapons into the center
 b Mistreat other residents
 c Use other residents' personal items
 d Voice complaints about care

21 A resident brought some items from home. They are
 a Sent home with the family
 b Labeled with the person's name
 c Arranged as you prefer
 d Shared with the person's roommate

22 Residents have the right to be free from
 a Disease
 b Grievances
 c Involuntary seclusion
 d Rules

23 Who selects activities for a resident?
 a The nurse
 b You
 c The person's representative
 d The person

24 A nursing center must provide
 a A safe, clean, and comfortable setting
 b An indoor smoking area
 c A bed near a window
 d A noise-free setting

25 Which action promotes dignity?
 a Restraining the person
 b Making clothing choices for the person
 c Scolding the person
 d Listening to the person

26 Which is the correct way to address a person?
 a "Hello, sweetie."
 b "Hello."
 c "Hello, Mrs. Smith."
 d "Hello, grandpa."

27 Which promotes privacy?
 a Entering a person's room without knocking
 b Closing the privacy curtain for a procedure
 c Leaving the door open during personal care
 d Looking through the person's belongings

28 A long-term care ombudsman
 a Is employed by the nursing center
 b Investigates resident complaints
 c Grants a nursing center a license or certification
 d Can prevent a resident from leaving the center

Answers to Chapter 2 questions are on p. 885.

FOCUS ON PRACTICE
Problem Solving

A resident refuses to eat. What will you do? Does the resident have the right to refuse to eat? What is the nursing center's responsibility?

The Nursing Assistant

OBJECTIVES

- Define the key terms and key abbreviations in this chapter.
- Explain the history and trends affecting nursing assistants.
- Explain the laws that affect nursing assistants.
- Describe the training and competency evaluation requirements for nursing assistants.
- Identify the information in the nursing assistant registry.
- List the reasons for denying, suspending, or revoking a nursing assistant's certification, license, or registration.

- Explain how to obtain certification, a license, or registration in another state.
- Describe what nursing assistants can do and their role limits.
- Describe the standards for nursing assistants developed by the National Council of State Boards of Nursing.
- Explain why a job description is important.
- List the nursing assistant job titles used in some agencies.
- Explain how to promote PRIDE in the person, the family, and yourself.

KEY TERMS

certification Official recognition by a state that standards or requirements have been met

endorsement A state recognizes the certificate, license, or registration issued by another state; reciprocity or equivalency

equivalency See "endorsement"

job description A document that describes what the agency expects you to do

misappropriation The dishonest use of property

nursing task Nursing care or a nursing function, procedure, skill, or activity

reciprocity See "endorsement"

KEY ABBREVIATIONS

BON	Board of nursing	OBRA	Omnibus Budget Reconciliation Act of 1987
CNA	Certified nursing assistant; certified nurse aide	RN	Registered nurse
LNA	Licensed nursing assistant	RNA	Registered nurse aide
LPN	Licensed practical nurse	SRNA	State registered nurse aide
LVN	Licensed vocational nurse	STNA	State tested nurse aide
NATCEP	Nursing assistant training and competency evaluation program		

Federal and state laws and agency policies combine to define your roles and functions. To give safe care, you need to know:

- What you can and cannot do
- Rules and standards of conduct affecting your work
- Your role limits

Laws, job descriptions, and the person's condition shape your work. So does the amount of supervision you need.

HISTORY AND CURRENT TRENDS

For decades, nursing assistants have helped nurses with basic nursing care. Often called nurse's aides, they helped with bathing, grooming, elimination, bedmaking, and other needs. Until the 1980s, training was not required by law. Nurses gave on-the-job training. Some hospitals, nursing centers, and schools offered courses.

Team nursing was common. A team leader (registered nurse; RN) assigned care to nurses and nursing assistants. Assignments depended on each person's needs and condition. They also depended on the staff member's education and experience.

Primary nursing emerged in the 1980s. RNs planned and gave care. Many hospitals hired only RNs. Meanwhile, nursing centers relied on nursing assistants for resident care.

Home care increased during the 1980s. To reduce costs, hospital stays were shorter. Discharged hospital patients often needed care at home.

Managing health care costs is a growing concern. A staffing mix can help reduce costs. Nursing centers, home care agencies, and many hospitals hire RNs, licensed practical nurses/licensed vocational nurses (LPNs/LVNs), and nursing assistants.

FEDERAL AND STATE LAWS

The U.S. Congress makes federal laws for all 50 states to follow. State legislatures make state laws. For example, the Texas legislature makes state laws for Texas. The Alaska legislature does so for Alaska. You must know the federal and state laws affecting your work. The laws provide direction for what you can do.

See Chapter 5 for other laws affecting your work.

Nurse Practice Acts

Each state has a nurse practice act. A nurse practice act:
- Defines RN and LPN/LVN and their scope of practice.
- Describes RN and LPN/LVN education and licensing requirements.
- Protects the public from persons practicing nursing without a license. Persons who do not meet the state's requirements cannot perform nursing functions.

A nurse practice act is enforced by the state's board of nursing (BON). The BON can deny, revoke, or suspend a nurse's license. The intent is to protect the public from unsafe nurses. Reasons include:
- Being convicted of a crime in any state
- Selling or distributing drugs
- Using a person's drugs for oneself
- Placing a person in danger from the over-use of alcohol or drugs
- Demonstrating grossly negligent nursing practice
- Being convicted of abusing or neglecting children or older persons
- Violating a nurse practice act and its rules and regulations
- Demonstrating incompetent behaviors
- Aiding or assisting another person to violate a nurse practice act and its rules and regulations
- Making medical diagnoses
- Prescribing drugs and treatments
- See "Maintaining Competence," p. 24.

Nursing Assistants.

Some nurse practice acts regulate nursing assistant roles, functions, education, and certification requirements. Other states have separate laws for nursing assistants. The laws are enforced by BONs or similar boards.

If you do something beyond the legal limits of your role, you could be practicing nursing without a license. This means serious legal problems for you, your supervisor, and the agency.

You must function with skill and safety. Like nurses, you can have your certification (license, registration) denied, revoked, or suspended. (See "Certification.")

The Omnibus Budget Reconciliation Act of 1987

The *Omnibus Budget Reconciliation Act of 1987 (OBRA)* is a federal law. It applies to all 50 states.

OBRA sets minimum requirements for nursing assistant training and evaluation. Each state must have a nursing assistant training and competency evaluation program (NATCEP). A nursing assistant must successfully complete a NATCEP to work in a nursing center, hospital long-term care unit, or home care agency receiving Medicare funds.

The Training Program.

OBRA requires at least 75 hours of instruction. Some states require more hours. Classroom and at least 16 hours of supervised practical training are required (Fig. 3-1). Practical training (clinical practicum or clinical experience) occurs in a laboratory or clinical setting. Students perform nursing tasks on another person. A nurse supervises this training.

The training program includes the knowledge and skills needed to give basic nursing care. Areas of study include:
- Communication
- Infection control
- Safety and emergency procedures
- Residents' rights
- Basic nursing skills and personal care skills—skin care, dressing, elimination, feeding, and so on
- Transferring, positioning, and turning methods
- Helping the person walk
- Range-of-motion exercises
- Signs and symptoms of common diseases
- Caring for cognitively impaired persons (those with thinking and memory problems)
  See *Focus on Communication: The Training Program.*

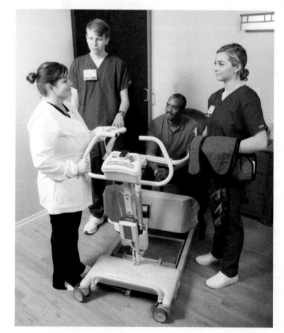

FIGURE 3-1 Nursing assistant training program. An instructor demonstrates a skill to her students.

Competency Evaluation.

The competency evaluation has a written test and a skills test (Appendix A, p. 889).

- The written test has multiple-choice questions. Each has 4 choices. Only 1 answer is correct. The number of questions varies from state to state.
- For the skills test, you perform certain skills learned in your training program.

You take the competency evaluation after your training program. Your instructor knows the testing service used in your state and how to schedule the evaluation and pay the required fee. If working in a nursing center, the employer pays the fee. Otherwise you pay the fee.

Your training prepares you for the competency evaluation. If you listen, study hard, and practice safe care, you should do well. If the first attempt was not successful, you can re-test. OBRA allows at least 3 attempts to successfully complete the evaluation.

Each testing service has a candidate handbook. Review the handbook carefully as you prepare for the competency evaluation.

Nursing Assistant Registry.

OBRA requires a nursing assistant registry in each state. It is the official record or listing of persons who have successfully completed that state's approved NATCEP. The registry must have at least the following information about each nursing assistant.

- Full name, including maiden name and any married names.
- Identifying information.
- Date the competency evaluation was passed.
- Information about findings of abuse, neglect, or misappropriation. (*Misappropriation is the dishonest use of property* [stealing, theft]. See Chapter 5.) The nature of the offense and supporting evidence are documented. If a hearing was held, the date and its outcome are included. The person has the right to include a statement disputing the finding. All information stays in the state's registry for at least 5 years or as required by the state. Findings reported to the federal government are permanent. They may appear in a background check report.

OBRA requires removing registry entries for persons who have not worked as nursing assistants for 24 consecutive months. Entries remain for findings of abuse, neglect, or dishonest use of property.

Any health care agency can access registry information. You also receive a copy of your registry information. The copy is sent when the first entry is made and when information is changed or added. You can correct wrong information.

Certification. *Certification is the official recognition by a state that standards or requirements have been met.* After successfully completing your state's NATCEP, you have the title used in your state. Titles include:

- Certified nursing assistant (CNA) or certified nurse aide (CNA). CNA is used in most states.
- Licensed nursing assistant (LNA).
- Registered nurse aide (RNA).
- State registered nurse aide (SRNA).
- State tested nurse aide (STNA).

Nursing assistants can have their certification (licenses, registration) disciplined for actions that are harmful or dangerous to the public or a person's health. A state may deny, revoke, or suspend a certification (license, registration.) See Box 3-1, p. 24.

See *Promoting Safety and Comfort: Certification.*

BOX 3-1	Discipline Reasons

- Violating professional boundaries with a patient, resident, or family member. See "Professional Boundaries" in Chapter 5.
- Engaging in sexual conduct with a patient, resident, or family member.
- Leaving an assignment or abandoning a person. The nursing assistant did not notify the nurse that he or she was leaving.
- Failing to accurately record the care given.
- Making a false or incorrect entry in a person's health record.
- Failing to follow agency policies and procedures for patient or resident safety.
- Failing to protect a person's safety or welfare.
  - The person is at risk from actual or potentially incompetent care.
  - The nursing assistant did not report the risk to the nurse or agency administrator.
- Failing to report observations to the nurse in a timely manner. See Chapter 8.
- Violating a person's rights or dignity.
- Violating a person's privacy by sharing his or her information.
- Neglecting or abusing a person. The abuse can be physical, verbal, emotional, or financial.
- Asking for or borrowing money or property from a patient, resident, or family member.
- Taking money, property, or personal items without permission from:
  - A patient or resident
  - A family member
  - A co-worker
  - The agency
  - A member of the public
- Requesting payment for services not performed from a person or the agency.
- Using or being under the influence of alcohol, a drug, or other substance while on duty when:
  - Judgment is impaired.
  - Safe function is affected.
- Accepting or performing a task or function that he or she was not trained to perform.
- Removing from the agency, without authorization:
  - Narcotics or other drugs
  - Supplies or equipment
  - Health records

- Obtaining, possessing, using, or selling any narcotic, controlled substance, or illegal drug. Doing so violates agency policy or any federal or state law.
- Allowing or helping a person use the nursing assistant's certificate (license, registration) or identity.
- Making false or misleading advertisements about his or her practice as a nursing assistant.
- Offering or providing paid nursing assistant services without a nurse supervisor.
- Threatening, harassing, or exploiting a person. To *exploit* means *to use or take advantage of another person.*
- Using violent or abusive behavior in the work setting.
- Failing to cooperate with the BON during an investigation by:
  - Not providing a complete, written explanation about the matter in question.
  - Not responding to a BON-issued subpoena. *Subpoena* comes from the Latin word for *under penalty.* It is a legal request to provide specific documents or to testify in court or at a hearing before a government agency.
  - Not completing and returning a BON-issued questionnaire by a certain date.
  - Not informing the BON of a change of address or phone number within a certain number of days.
- Engaging in fraud or deceit about:
  - The competency evaluation
  - An application or renewal of his or her certification (license, registration)
- Making a false or inaccurate statement to the BON or the BON's representative during an investigation.
- Making a false or misleading statement on an employment or credential application about his or her:
  - Previous employment
  - Work experience
  - Education
  - Credentials (qualifications)
- Failing to notify the BON of any criminal conviction, plea arrangement, or deferred judgment within a certain time frame. He or she includes:
  - Identifying information
  - Certification (license, registration) number
  - Date of the conviction, plea arrangement, or deferred judgment
  - Nature of the offense
- Practicing in any manner that gives the BON reasonable cause to believe a person or the public may be harmed.

Modified from National Council of State Boards of Nursing, Inc.: NCSBN model rules, Chicago, 2017, Author.

Maintaining Competence. OBRA requires that agencies provide 12 hours of education to nursing assistants every year. Performance reviews also are required. That is, your work is evaluated. These requirements help ensure that you have the current knowledge and skills to give safe, effective care.

OBRA has requirements to ensure the competence of nursing assistants who have not worked for 24 months. It does not matter how long you worked as a nursing assistant before. What matters is how long you did *not* work. States can require:

- A new competency evaluation
- Both re-training and a new competency evaluation
  See *Teamwork and Time Management: Maintaining Competence.*
  See *Focus on Surveys: Maintaining Competence.*

TEAMWORK AND TIME MANAGEMENT

Maintaining Competence

Educational programs are commonly called *in-service programs* or *in-service training*. Some are required; others are optional. In-service announcements and schedules are posted on nursing units, in staff locker rooms and lounges, by the time clock, and on websites. Know where the agency posts in-service information. Check those areas often.

In-services are scheduled before, during, or after your shift. If before work, plan to arrive early. If after work, plan to stay late. Arrange for transportation and childcare as needed (Chapter 6).

If an in-service is during your shift, plan with your co-workers. Some staff stay on the unit while others attend the in-service. Staff on the unit tend to all patients and residents. Share any information about special care with the staff providing the care. After returning to the unit, thank your co-workers for helping you. Help your co-workers when they attend in-services.

FOCUS ON SURVEYS

Maintaining Competence

Surveyors must make sure that nursing assistants are competent to give safe care. They will:
- Check if nursing assistants have completed a NATCEP.
- Ask nursing assistants:
  - Where they received their training
  - The length of their training
  - How long they have worked in the agency
- Observe if nursing assistants:
  - Maintain or improve the person's independent functioning.
  - Perform range-of-motion exercises (Chapter 34).
  - Transfer the person from bed to a wheelchair safely (Chapter 20).
  - Observe, describe, and report the person's behavior and condition to the nurse (Chapter 8).
  - Follow instructions.
  - Practice infection control (Chapters 16 and 17) and safety measures (Chapters 13 and 14).

Working in Another State

To work in another state, you must meet that state's NATCEP requirements. First, contact the state agency responsible for NATCEPs and the nursing assistant registry. To find that agency, do 1 of the following.
- Contact your current nursing assistant registry.
- Search on-line to locate the state agency.

Then apply to the desired state agency for endorsement (reciprocity, equivalency) as a CNA (LNA, RNA, SRNA, STNA). *Endorsement (reciprocity, equivalency) means that a state recognizes the certificate, license, or registration issued by another state.* This means that:
- Your application is reviewed to see if you meet the state's requirements.
  - Your certification (license, registration) is current and in good standing.
  - You meet that state's education, work, and legal requirements.
- Certification (a license, registration) is granted if the requirements are met.

Follow the application instructions. Expect to:
- Complete required forms.
- Provide proof of successfully completing a nursing assistant training program. A school transcript or grade report may be required. Or you may need to send a copy of the certificate of course completion from your training program. Do not send the original.
- Request written registry verification from the state in which you are currently certified (licensed, registered). Pay the required fee.
- Provide fingerprints.
- Pay the required application fee.

A criminal background check is done. Registry information is checked. Expect an investigation if a criminal history is revealed. Or if the registry check shows findings of abuse, neglect, misappropriation, or other action against you.

You must be truthful. False or misleading information may result in:
- Denial of certification (a license, registration)
- Disciplinary action
- A fine

The application review results in 1 or more of the following.
- Being granted or denied certification (a license, registration).
- Having to take a NATCEP competency evaluation. This may be the written test, the skills test, or both.
- Having to take the entire NATCEP in that state (training program and competency evaluation).

ROLES AND RESPONSIBILITIES

OBRA, nurse practice acts and other state laws, and legal and advisory opinions direct what you can do. To protect persons from harm, you must understand what you can do, what you cannot do, and the legal limits of your role. This is called *scope of practice* or *range of functions*.

Licensed nurses supervise your work. You perform nursing tasks related to the person's care. A *nursing task is nursing care or a nursing function, procedure, skill, or activity.* (See Chapter 4.) Often you function without a nurse in the room. At other times you help nurses give care. The rules in Box 3-2 will help you understand your role.

The range of functions for nursing assistants varies among states and agencies. Before performing a nursing task make sure that:

- Your state allows nursing assistants to do so.
- It is in your job description.
- You have the education and training to do so.
- A nurse is available to answer questions and to guide and assist you as needed.

Box 3-3 describes the limits of your role—tasks that you should never do. State laws differ. Know what you can do in the state in which you are working. For example, you move from Utah to Maryland. You must learn Maryland's laws. Or you might work in 2 states. For example, you work in Illinois and Iowa. You must know the laws of both states.

Your job description reflects your state's laws and rules. An agency can further limit what you can do. So can a nurse based on the person's needs. However, no agency or nurse can expand your range of functions beyond what your state's laws and rules allow.

See *Focus on Long-Term Care and Home Care: Roles and Responsibilities.*

BOX 3-3   Role Limits

- **Never give drugs.** This includes drugs given:
  - Orally, rectally, vaginally, and by injection
  - By application to the skin, eyes, ears, and nose
  - Directly into the bloodstream or through an intravenous (IV) line

  Nurses give drugs. Many states allow nursing assistants to give some drugs after completing a state-approved medication assistant training program. The function must be in your job description. And you must have the necessary supervision.
- **Never insert tubes or objects into body openings. Do not remove them from the body.** You must not insert tubes into the person's bladder, esophagus, trachea, nose, ears, bloodstream, or surgically created body openings. Exceptions to this rule are the procedures you will study during your training. Giving enemas is an example. To give enemas, the task must be in your job description. And you must have the necessary supervision.
- **Never take oral or phone orders from doctors.** Politely give your name and title, and ask the doctor to wait for a nurse. Promptly find a nurse to speak with the doctor.
- **Never tell the person or family the person's diagnosis or medical or surgical treatment plans.** This is the doctor's responsibility. Nurses may clarify what the doctor has said.
- **Never diagnose or prescribe treatments or drugs for anyone.** Doctors, physician's assistants, and some advanced practice nurses (Chapter 1) diagnose and prescribe.
- **Never supervise others including other nursing assistants.** This is a nurse's responsibility. You will not be trained to supervise others. Supervising others can have serious legal problems.
- **Never ignore an order or request to do something.** This includes nursing tasks that you can do, those you cannot do, and those beyond your legal limits. Promptly and politely explain to the nurse why you cannot carry out the order or request. The nurse assumes you are doing what you were told to do unless you explain otherwise. You cannot neglect the person's care.

BOX 3-2   Rules for Nursing Assistants

- You are an assistant to the nurse.
- A nurse assigns and supervises your work.
- You report observations about the person's physical and mental status to the nurse (Chapter 8). Report changes in the person's condition or behavior at once.
- The nurse decides what is done or not done for a person. You do not make these decisions.
- Review directions and the care plan (Chapter 8) with the nurse before going to the person.
- Perform only the nursing tasks that you are trained to do.
- Ask a nurse to guide and assist you if you are not comfortable performing a nursing task.
- Perform only the nursing tasks that your state and job description allow.

FOCUS ON LONG-TERM CARE AND HOME CARE

Roles and Responsibilities

Home Care

You provide personal care and home services. Home services may include:

- Laundry. You wash, iron or fold, and mend clothing and linens. This may include family laundry.
- Shopping for groceries and household items.
- Preparing and serving meals. You plan menus, follow diets, and feed the person if necessary.
- Light housekeeping. You do not do heavy housekeeping. This includes moving heavy furniture, waxing floors, shampooing carpets, washing windows, and cleaning rugs or drapes. You do not carry firewood, coal, or ash containers.

Nursing Assistant Standards

All NATCEPs include the range of functions required by OBRA. Some states allow other functions. NATCEPs also prepare nursing assistants to meet the standards listed in Box 3-4.

Job Description

The *job description is a document that describes what the agency expects you to do* (Fig. 3-2, p. 28). It also states educational requirements and your job title. (See "Nursing Assistant Job Titles.")

Always obtain a written job description when you apply for a job. Ask questions about it during your job interview (Chapter 60). Before accepting a job, tell the employer about:

* Functions you did not learn
* Functions you cannot do for moral or religious reasons

Clearly understand what is expected before taking a job. Do not take a job that requires you to:

* Act beyond the legal limits of your role.
* Function beyond your training limits.
* Perform acts that are against your morals or religion.

No one can force you to do something beyond the legal limits of your role. Sometimes jobs are threatened for refusing to follow a nurse's orders. Often staff obey out of fear. That is why you must understand:

* Your roles and responsibilities
* What you can safely do
* The things you should never do
* Your job description
* The ethical and legal aspects of your role (Chapter 5) See *Focus on Communication: Job Description.*

FOCUS ON COMMUNICATION

Job Description

Your training prepares you for certain nursing tasks. The agency may not let you do everything you learned. Other agencies may want you to do things not learned. Use your job description to discuss these issues with the nurse.

For example, a job description includes changing a dressing (Chapter 40). You did not learn this skill in your training program. You can say:

I see changing dressings in my job description. I did not learn to do that. Will I be trained to perform this skill?

Carefully review your job description. Know what you can and cannot do. Ask if you have questions.

BOX 3-4	Nursing Assistant Standards

The nursing assistant:

* Performs nursing tasks within the range of functions allowed by the state's nurse practice act and its rules.
* Is honest and shows integrity. (*Integrity* involves following a code of ethics. See Chapter 5.)
* Accepts or refuses nursing tasks based on his or her education and training and the nurse's directions. See Chapter 4.
* Is accountable for his or her behavior and actions while assisting the nurse and helping patients and residents.
* Assists the nurse in observing patients and residents. Also assists in identifying their needs.
* Communicates:
  * Progress toward completing nursing tasks
  * Problems in completing nursing tasks
  * Changes in the person's status
* Asks the nurse to clarify what is expected when unsure.
* Uses educational and training opportunities as available.
* Practices safety measures to protect the person, others, and self.
* Respects the person's rights, concerns, decisions, and dignity.
* Functions as a member of the health team. Helps implement the care plan (Chapter 8).
* Respects the person's property and the property of others.
* Protects confidential information unless required by law to share the information.

Modified from National Council of State Boards of Nursing, Inc.: NCSBN model rules, Chicago, 2017, Author.

Nursing Assistant Job Titles. After successfully completing a NATCEP, you have the title used by law and the nursing assistant registry in your state (see "Certification"). For job purposes, agencies often use other titles. Your job title depends on the setting and your roles and functions in the agency. Examples are listed in Box 3-5.

BOX 3-5	Nursing Assistant Job Titles

* Clinical technician
* Health care assistant
* Health care technician
* Nurse technician
* Nursing care partner
* Nursing support technician
* Patient care assistant
* Patient care attendant
* Patient care monitor
* Patient care technician
* Patient care worker
* Support partner

POSITION DESCRIPTION/PERFORMANCE EVALUATION

Job Title: Certified Nursing Assistant (CNA), Skilled Nursing Facility   Supervised by: Licensed Nurse

Prepared by: _____   Date: _____   Approved by: _____   Date: _____

Job Summary: Provides direct and indirect resident care activities under the direction of an RN or LPN. Assists residents with activities of daily living, provides for personal care and comfort, and assists in the maintenance of a safe and clean environment for an assigned group of residents.

DUTIES AND RESPONSIBILITIES:

E=Exceeds the Standard   M=Meets the Standard   NI=Needs Improvement

Demonstrates Competency in the Following Areas:	E	M	NI
Assists in the preparation for admission of residents.	2	1	0
Assists in and accompanies residents in the admission, transfer, and discharge procedures.	2	1	0
Provides morning care, which may include bed bath, shower or whirlpool, oral hygiene, combing hair, back massage, dressing resident, changing bed linen, cleaning over-bed table and bedside stand, straightening room, and other general care as necessary throughout the day.	2	1	0
Provides evening care, which includes hand/face washing as needed, oral hygiene, back massage, pericare, freshening linen, cleaning over-bed table, straightening room, and other general care as needed.	2	1	0
Notifies RN/LPN when resident complains of pain.	2	1	0
Assists with post-mortem care.	2	1	0
Assists nurses in treatment procedures.	2	1	0
Provides general nursing care such as positioning residents, turning residents, applying/utilizing special equipment, assisting in use of bedpan or commode, and ambulating the residents.	2	1	0
Performs all aspects of resident care in an environment that optimizes resident safety and reduces the likelihood of medical/health care errors.	2	1	0
Measures and records temperature, pulse, respiration, weight, blood pressure, and intake-output.	2	1	0
Makes rounds with outgoing shift. Knows whereabouts of assigned residents.	2	1	0
Makes rounds with oncoming shift to ensure the unit is left in good condition.	2	1	0
Adheres to policies and procedures of the center and the Department of Nursing.	2	1	0
Participates in socialization activities on the unit.	2	1	0
Turns and positions residents as ordered and/or as needed, making sure no rough surfaces are in direct contact with the body. Moves and turns with proper and safe body mechanics and with available resources.	2	1	0
Checks for reddened areas or skin breakdown and reports to RN or LPN.	2	1	0
Ensures residents are dressed properly and assists, as necessary. Ensures that clothing is properly stored in bedside stand or on hangers in closet. Ensures that all residents are clean and dry at all times.	2	1	0
Checks unit for adequate linen. Cleans linen cart. Provides clean linen and clothing. Makes beds.	2	1	0
Treats residents and their families with respect and dignity.	2	1	0
Follows center policies and procedures when caring for persons who are restrained.	2	1	0
Prepares residents for meals. Serves and removes food trays. Assists with meals or feeds residents, if necessary.	2	1	0
Distributes drinking water and other nourishments to residents.	2	1	0
Performs general care activities for residents on Isolation Precautions.	2	1	0
Answers residents' call lights promptly. Anticipates residents' needs and makes rounds to assigned residents.	2	1	0
Assists residents with handling and care of clothing and other personal property (including dentures, eyeglasses, contact lenses, hearing aids, and prosthetic devices).	2	1	0
Transports residents to and from various departments, as requested.	2	1	0
Reports and, when appropriate, records any changes observed in condition or behavior of residents and unusual incidents.	2	1	0
Participates in and contributes to Resident Care Conferences.	2	1	0
Follows directions, both oral and written, and works cooperatively with other staff members.	2	1	0

FIGURE 3-2 Sample job description. Note that the job description is also a performance evaluation tool. (Modified from Medical Consultants Network, Inc., Englewood, Colo.)

POSITION DESCRIPTION/PERFORMANCE EVALUATION—cont'd

	E	M	NI
Establishes and maintains interpersonal relationships with residents, family members, and other center personnel while assuring confidentiality of resident information.	2	1	0
Has the ability to acquire knowledge of and develop skills in basic nursing procedures and simple charting.	2	1	0
Attends in-service education programs, as assigned, to learn new treatments, procedures, skills, etc.	2	1	0
Maintains personal health in order to prevent absence from work due to health problems.	2	1	0

Professional Requirements:

	E	M	NI
Meets dress code standards. Appearance is neat and clean.	2	1	0
Completes annual education requirements.	2	1	0
Maintains regulatory requirements.	2	1	0
Meets center's standards for attendance.	2	1	0
Consistently completes and maintains assigned duties.	2	1	0
Wears identification while on duty.	2	1	0
Practices careful, efficient, and non-wasteful use of supplies and linen. Follows established charge procedure for resident charge items.	2	1	0
Attends annual review and department in-services, as scheduled.	2	1	0
Attends at least 75% of staff meetings. Reads and returns all monthly staff meeting minutes.	2	1	0
Represents the center in a positive and professional manner.	2	1	0
Actively participates in the Continuous Quality Improvement (CQI) activities.	2	1	0
Complies with all center policies regarding ethical business practices.	2	1	0
Communicates the mission, ethics, and goals of the center, as well as the focus statement of the department.	2	1	0
Possesses a genuine interest and concern for older and disabled persons.	2	1	0

TOTAL POINTS _____ _____ _____

Regulatory Requirements:

- High school graduate or equivalent
- Current Certified Nursing Assistant (CNA) certification
- Current Basic Life Support for Healthcare Providers certification within three (3) months of hire date

Language Skills:

- Ability to read and communicate effectively in English
- Additional languages preferred

Skills:

- Basic computer knowledge

Physical Demands:

- See "Physical Demands" policy.

I have received, read, and understand the Position Description/Performance Evaluation above.

_____   _____
Name/Signature   Date Signed

FIGURE 3-2, cont'd

FOCUS ON **PRIDE**

The Person, Family, and Yourself

Personal and Professional Responsibility

Personal and professional qualities allow you to do your job well. Communication skills, patience, compassion, and teamwork are examples. You will learn about other qualities when you study work ethics in Chapter 6.

Rights and Respect

Most NATCEPs involve practice in a clinical setting. Sometimes a patient or resident refuses to have a student. Or the person refuses to allow a student to watch a procedure. The person's right to refuse must be respected.

Independence and Social Interaction

You will practice many skills in the classroom or laboratory before going to the clinical setting. Practice as if you were with a real patient or resident. Practice what to say and how to act. Practice the skill many times. This will help you feel more comfortable and confident in the clinical setting.

Delegation and Teamwork

Delegation deals with what you are asked to do (Chapter 4). To safely assist the nurse, you must know what you can and cannot do. Do not be discouraged by what you *cannot* do. Value what you *can* do. Your attitude affects your work. Take pride in your role.

Ethics and Laws

Some nursing assistants work in more than 1 setting. Some are also emergency medical technicians (EMTs). EMTs give emergency care outside of health care settings. State laws and rules for EMTs and nursing assistants differ. For example, you work as an EMT and a nursing assistant. Your state laws allow EMTs to start intravenous (IV) lines. Nursing assistants do not start IVs.

The ability to do something does not give the right to do so in all settings. There are legal limits to your role. Be proud of the advanced skills and training you may have. But when working as a nursing assistant, follow your state's laws and rules for nursing assistants.

FOCUS ON **PRIDE**: *Application*

Your NATCEP involves a skills test. An evaluator will observe you performing certain skills. How will you prepare for the test?

REVIEW QUESTIONS

*Circle **T** if the statement is **TRUE** or **F** if it is **FALSE**.*

1 T F   OBRA requires a nursing assistant training and competency evaluation program in every state.

2 T F   You are allowed 1 attempt to pass your state's competency evaluation.

3 T F   Each state must have a nursing assistant registry.

4 T F   You have not worked for 3 years. Your certification (license, registration) is still current.

5 T F   All states have the same training and evaluation requirements.

6 T F   An agency can expand your range of functions beyond what is allowed in your state.

*Circle the **BEST** answer.*

7 A state's nurse practice act is regulated by
   a The state's board of nursing
   b OBRA
   c Medicare
   d Medicaid

8 What state law affects what nursing assistants can do?
   a Standards for nursing assistants
   b Medicaid
   c OBRA
   d Nurse practice act

9 Your nursing assistant certification (license, registration) can be revoked for
   a Refusing a nursing task for moral reasons
   b Asking the nurse questions
   c Performing acts beyond your role
   d Keeping the person's information confidential

10 As a nursing assistant, you
   a Must perform all tasks as directed by the nurse
   b Make decisions about a person's care
   c Need a written job description before employment
   d Give a drug when a nurse tells you to

11 As a nursing assistant, you
   a Can take verbal or phone orders from doctors
   b Report observations to the nurse
   c Can remove tubes from the person's body
   d Can ignore a nursing task if it is not in your job description

REVIEW QUESTIONS—cont'd

12 Who assigns and supervises your work?
   a A nurse
   b The health team
   c Another nursing assistant
   d You

13 You are responsible for
   a Supervising other nursing assistants
   b Telling the person his or her diagnosis
   c Knowing what you can safely do
   d Deciding what treatments are needed

14 You perform a task not allowed by your state. Which is *true*?
   a If a nurse asked you to do the task, there is no legal problem.
   b You could be practicing nursing without a license.
   c You can perform the task if it is in your job description.
   d If you complete the task safely, there is no legal problem.

15 Which describes what an agency expects you to do?
   a Nurse practice act
   b Range of functions
   c Scope of practice
   d Job description

Answers to Chapter 3 questions are on p. 885.

FOCUS ON PRACTICE

Problem Solving

You are training in the clinical setting. A resident refuses care from students. The person asks that students leave the room during a procedure. How might you and the other students react? What should you tell your instructor?

Delegation

OBJECTIVES

- Define the key terms and key abbreviations in this chapter.
- Identify which nurses can delegate nursing tasks.
- Describe the delegation process.
- Explain your role in the delegation process.

- Describe the *Five Rights of Delegation* for nursing assistants.
- Explain how to accept or refuse a delegated task.
- Explain how to promote PRIDE in the person, the family, and yourself.

KEY TERMS

accountable To answer to one's self and others about his or her choices, decisions, and actions

delegate To authorize or direct a nursing assistant to perform a nursing task

delegated nursing responsibility A nursing task that a nurse transfers to a nursing assistant when it does not require a nurse's professional knowledge or judgment

delegation The process a nurse uses to direct a nursing assistant to perform a nursing task; allowing a nursing assistant to perform a nursing responsibility that is beyond the nursing assistant's usual role and not routinely done by the nursing assistant

nursing task Nursing care or a nursing function, procedure, skill, or activity

routine nursing task A nursing task that is part of a nursing assistant's routine job description and commonly assigned to the nursing assistant; a nursing task that was learned in a nursing assistant training and competency evaluation program (NATCEP)

KEY ABBREVIATIONS

APRN	Advanced practice registered nurse	**NATCEP**	Nursing assistant training and competency evaluation program
LPN	Licensed practical nurse	**RN**	Registered nurse
LVN	Licensed vocational nurse		

Nursing assistants function under the supervision of licensed nurses—advanced practice registered nurses (APRNs), registered nurses (RNs), or licensed practical nurses/licensed vocational nurses (LPNs/LVNs). Nurse practice acts give nurses the right to *assign* or *delegate* nursing tasks to nursing assistants. Definitions vary among state nurse practice acts, agency job descriptions, and national organizations such as the National Council of State Boards of Nursing and the American Nurses Association. You need to know the definitions used in your state.

The following definitions are used in this textbook.

- *Nursing task—nursing care or a nursing function, procedure, skill, or activity*
- *Routine nursing task:*
  - *A nursing task that is part of a nursing assistant's routine job description and commonly assigned to the nursing assistant*
  - *A nursing task that was learned in a nursing assistant training and competency evaluation program (NATCEP)*

- *Delegate—to authorize or direct a nursing assistant to perform a nursing task*
- *Delegated nursing responsibility—a nursing task that a nurse transfers to a nursing assistant when it does not require a nurse's professional knowledge or judgment*
- *Delegation:*
  - *The process a nurse uses to direct a nursing assistant to perform a nursing task*
  - *Allowing a nursing assistant to perform a nursing responsibility that is beyond the nursing assistant's usual role and not routinely done by the nursing assistant*

You will learn how to perform routine nursing tasks. Moving and transfer procedures, hygiene and grooming measures, and how to measure weight and height are examples. Such tasks are part of the routine care you give. Some states allow nurses to delegate nursing tasks that are not routinely done by nursing assistants—*delegated nursing responsibilities.* Inserting urinary catheters (Chapter 28) and giving tube feedings (Chapter 32) are examples.

Delegation Guidelines boxes accompany the procedures in this book. The guidelines list the information you need from the nurse and care plan before performing a routine task or a delegated nursing responsibility. They also list the observations to record and report to the nurse. Review the guidelines carefully to safely complete a task.

See *Promoting Safety and Comfort: Delegation.*

PROMOTING SAFETY AND COMFORT
Delegation

Safety

Routine nursing tasks and delegated nursing responsibilities must be allowed by your state and in your job description. If not learned in your NATCEP or something you do not do often, the agency must:

* Provide needed education and training about the task.
* Evaluate your ability to perform the task safely.
  Some nursing responsibilities cannot be delegated to you.
They include:

* The nursing process (Chapter 8)
  * Performing assessments
  * Developing care plans
  * Evaluating responses to care
* Providing education (teaching) to the person and family
* Performing nursing tasks that require a nurse's professional knowledge and judgment
* Making delegation decisions
* Supervising others
* Taking oral or phone orders from doctors or APRNs
* Giving drugs
* Inserting intravenous (IV) catheters (Chapter 32)
  See "Your Role in Delegation," p. 36.

WHO CAN DELEGATE

Licensed nurses can delegate.
* An APRN can delegate to RNs, LPNs/LVNs, and nursing assistants.
* An RN can delegate to LPNs/LVNs and nursing assistants.
* An LPN/LVN can delegate to nursing assistants if allowed by the state's nurse practice act.

A nurse's delegation decisions must protect the person's (patient or resident) health and safety. The delegating nurse is legally accountable to the patient or resident. *Accountable means to answer to one's self and others about his or her choices, decisions, and actions.* The delegating nurse is accountable for delegation decisions. The delegating nurse must make sure the task was completed safely and correctly.

Nursing assistants cannot delegate. You cannot delegate any task to other nursing assistants or to any other worker. You can ask someone to help you. But you cannot ask or tell someone to do your work. Also, you cannot re-assign a task or re-delegate a nursing responsibility to another nursing assistant or other worker.

See *Promoting Safety and Comfort: Who Can Delegate.*

PROMOTING SAFETY AND COMFORT
Who Can Delegate

Safety

Delegation requires a nurse's knowledge and judgment. Routine nursing tasks and delegated nursing responsibilities must be:

* *Within the nurse's scope of practice.* For example, pulling out loose teeth is not within a nurse's scope of practice. The nurse cannot tell you to pull out a person's loose tooth.
* *Within the nursing assistant range of functions allowed by your state.* For example, your state does not allow nursing assistants to cut toenails. The nurse cannot delegate cutting toenails to you.
* *Listed in your job description.* For example, your state allows nursing assistants to give enemas. The task is in your job description. The nurse can delegate the task to you. The nurse must know the tasks allowed by your job description.
  You must know what you can and cannot do (Chapter 3). You must refuse a task that you were not trained to do. You also must refuse a task that is:
* Beyond the nurse's scope of practice
* Beyond the nursing assistant range of functions allowed by your state
* Not in your job description
  See "Refusing a Task," p. 36.

DELEGATION PROCESS

For safe delegation, the person's needs, the nursing task, and the staff member doing the task must fit (Fig. 4-1). The nurse decides if the task is safe for you to do. The person's needs and the task may require a nurse's knowledge, judgment, and skill. You may be asked to assist.

Delegation decisions must result in the best care for the person. Otherwise the person's health and safety are at risk. To make delegation decisions, the nurse follows a process (Fig. 4-2, p. 34).

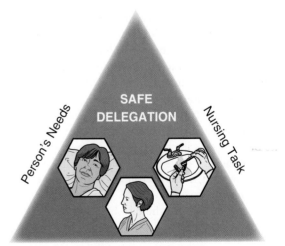

FIGURE 4-1 The nurse considers the person's needs, the task, and the staff member's abilities when making delegation decisions.

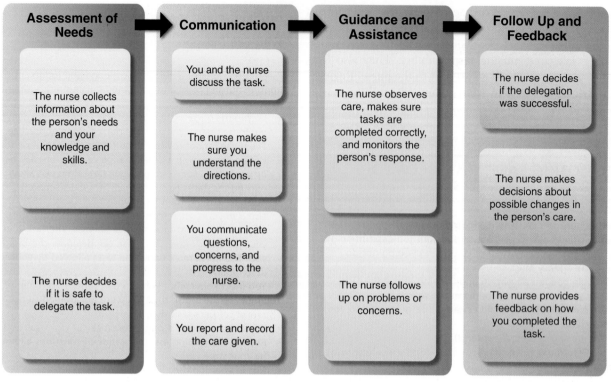

FIGURE 4-2 The delegation process.

Assessment of Needs

The nurse needs to understand the person's needs. And the nurse needs to know your knowledge, skills, and job description.

To assess the person's needs, the nurse answers these questions.

- What are the person's needs? How complex and urgent are they? How can they vary?
- What are the most important long-term and short-term needs?
- How much judgment is needed to meet the person's needs and give care?
- How predictable is the person's health status? How does the person respond to health care?
- What problems might arise from the task? How severe might they be?
- What actions are needed if a problem occurs? How complex are the needed actions?
- What emergencies might arise? How likely might they occur?
- How involved is the person and family in health care decisions?
- How will delegating the task help the person? What are the risks?

To assess your knowledge and skills, the nurse answers these questions.

- What knowledge and skills are needed to safely perform the task?
- What is in your job description?
- What are the conditions affecting the task?
- What is expected after the task?
- What problems might the person develop during the task?
- What problems can arise from the task?

The nurse decides if you can safely perform the task. It must be safe for the person and you. If unsafe, the nurse stops the delegation process. If safe for the person and you, the nurse continues the delegation process.

Communication

This step involves the nurse and you. The nurse must give you clear and complete directions about:

- How to perform and complete the task
- What observations to report and record
- When to report observations
- What patient or resident concerns to report at once
- Priorities for tasks
- What to do if the person's condition changes or needs change

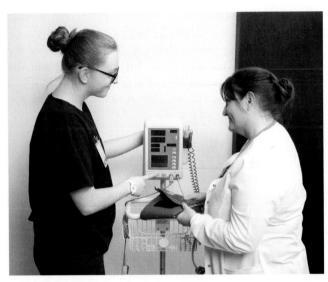

FIGURE 4-3 A nurse and nursing assistant discuss a nursing task.

The nurse asks questions to make sure you understand. The nurse may ask you to explain what you will do. Do not be insulted by such questions. The intent is to protect the person and you.

Before performing a delegated task, discuss the task with the nurse (Fig. 4-3). Make sure that you:

- Ask questions about the task and what you are expected to do.
- Tell the nurse if you have not done the task before or not often.
- Ask for needed training or supervision.
- Re-state what is expected of you.
- Re-state what patient or resident concerns to report to the nurse.
- Explain how and when you will report progress in completing the task.
- Know how to call the nurse for an emergency.
- Know what to do during an emergency.

After completing a task, report and record the care given. Also report and record your observations. See "Reporting and Recording" in Chapter 8.

See *Focus on Long-Term Care and Home Care: Communication.*

Guidance and Assistance

The nurse supervises your work. The nurse must be available to guide and assist you as needed. The nurse:

- Observes the care you give as needed.
- Makes sure that you complete the task correctly.
- Observes the person's condition and response to care. The frequency of the nurse's observations depends on:
  - The person's health status and needs
  - If the person's condition is stable (not likely to change) or unstable (likely to change)
  - If the nurse can predict the person's responses and risks to care
  - The setting where the task occurs
  - The resources and support available
  - If the task is simple or complex

The nurse follows up on problems or concerns. For example, the nurse takes action if:

- You did not complete the task in a timely manner.
- The task did not meet expectations.
- There is a change in the person's condition.

The nurse is alert for possible changes in the person's condition. With your help, the nurse can act before the person's condition changes.

Depending on the person's needs, the nurse might need to assist you with the task. Or the nurse can decide to perform the task.

After you complete the task, the nurse may review and discuss what happened with you. This helps you learn. If something similar happens again, you have ideas about how to adjust.

Follow Up and Feedback

To *follow up* means *to review and take needed action*. The nurse decides if the delegation was successful. The nurse answers these questions.

- Was the task done correctly?
- Did the person respond as expected?
- Was the result as desired? Was the result good or bad?
- Did you and the nurse have timely and effective communication?
- What went well? What were the problems?
- Does the care plan need to change (Chapter 8)?
- Did the nurse give feedback? *Feedback* means *to respond*. The nurse tells you what you did correctly and about any errors. Feedback helps you learn and improve the care you give.

YOUR ROLE IN DELEGATION

You must protect the person from harm. You have 2 choices when delegated a task. You either *accept* or *refuse* a task. Use the *Five Rights of Delegation* in Box 4-1.

BOX 4-1	The *Five Rights of Delegation* for Nursing Assistants

The Right Task
- Does your state allow you to perform the task?
- Is the task in your job description?
- Were you trained to do the task?

The Right Circumstance
- Do you have experience with the task given the person's condition and needs?
- Do you understand the purposes of the task for the person?
- Can you perform the task safely under the current circumstances?
- Do you have needed equipment and supplies?
- Do you know how to use the equipment and supplies?

The Right Person
- Are you comfortable performing the task?
- Do you have concerns about performing the task?

The Right Directions and Communication
- Did the nurse give clear directions and instructions?
- Did you review the task with the nurse?
- Do you understand what the nurse expects?

The Right Supervision and Evaluation
- Is a nurse available to answer questions?
- Is a nurse available if the person's condition changes or if problems occur?
- Did the nurse evaluate the result?

Modified from National Council of State Boards of Nursing, Inc.: The five rights of delegation, Chicago, as referenced in National guidelines for nursing delegation, April 29, 2019, National Council of State Boards of Nursing and American Nurses Association.

Accepting a Task

When you agree to perform a routine nursing task or a delegated nursing responsibility, you are responsible for your actions. What you do or fail to do can harm the person. *You must complete the task safely.* Ask for help if you are unsure or have questions. Report to the nurse what you did and your observations.

Refusing a Task

You have the right to refuse and not accept a delegated task. You should refuse when:

- The task is beyond the range of functions for nursing assistants allowed by your state.
- The task is not in your job description.
- You were not trained to do the task.
- The task could harm the person.
- The person's condition has changed.
- You do not know how to use the supplies or equipment.
- Directions are not ethical or legal.
- Directions are against agency policies.
- Directions are not clear or complete.
- A nurse is not available to guide and assist you as needed.

Use common sense. This protects you and the person. Ask yourself if what you are doing is safe for the person.

Never ignore an order or a request to do something. Share your concerns with the nurse. For tasks within the legal limits of your role and in your job description, the nurse can help increase your comfort. The nurse can:

- Answer your questions.
- Demonstrate the task.
- Show you how to use supplies and equipment.
- Help you as needed.
- Observe you doing the task.
- Check on you often.
- Arrange for needed training.

Do not refuse a task because you do not like it or do not want to do it. You must have sound reasons. Otherwise, you place the person at risk for harm. You could lose your job.

See *Focus on Communication: Refusing a Task.*

FOCUS ON COMMUNICATION

Refusing a Task

A nurse may delegate a task that was not part of your training. The task is in your job description. You can say:

I know this task is in my job description, but I did not learn it in school. Can you show me what to do and then observe me doing it? That would really help me.

A nurse may ask you to do something that is not in your job description. With respect, you must firmly refuse the nurse's request. For example: the nurse brings in a patient's morning drugs. The patient is in the bathroom. The nurse asks you to give the drugs when the patient comes out of the bathroom. If you give the drugs, you are performing a nursing responsibility outside the limits of your role. With respect, firmly refuse to follow the nurse's direction. You can say:

I'm sorry, but I cannot give a person drugs. I was not trained to give drugs, and the task is not in my job description. Can I help you with something else?

FOCUS ON **PRIDE**

The Person, Family, and Yourself

P ersonal and Professional Responsibility
You must communicate delegation concerns to the nurse. If uncertain about your ability to safely perform a delegated task, tell the nurse. Take pride in protecting the person from harm.

You are also responsible for keeping your skills up-to-date. See "Maintaining Competence" in Chapter 3.

R ights and Respect
Feedback helps you learn and improve in your role as a nursing assistant. Receive feedback in a respectful manner.
* Listen carefully.
* Have good eye contact.
* Consider ways you can improve.
* Avoid arguing or being defensive.
* Thank the nurse for the feedback.

I ndependence and Social Interaction
Delegation experiences promote positive interactions when staff:
* Communicate openly.
* Trust each other.
* Help and encourage each other.
* Work toward a common goal.

D elegation and Teamwork
State nurse practice acts vary about delegation and what nursing assistants can do. Your agency will define delegation and identify *routine nursing tasks* that are commonly part of nursing assistant assignments. Such tasks are learned in your NATCEP. Your agency will also identify nursing tasks that are beyond the routine role of the nursing assistant but can be safely delegated—*delegated nursing responsibilities.*

Examples of delegated nursing responsibilities may include procedures related to:
* Urinary catheters (Chapter 28)
* Enemas (Chapter 29)
* Nutritional support and IV therapy (Chapter 32)
* Measuring blood glucose (Chapter 38)
* Wound care (Chapter 40)
* Oxygen therapy (Chapter 43)

Before performing a delegated nursing responsibility, make sure that:
* Your state allows you to perform the task.
* The procedure is in your job description.
* You have the necessary education and training.
* The agency has determined that you are competent to perform the task safely.
* You review the task with the delegating nurse.
* The delegating nurse is available to answer questions and to guide and assist you as needed.

Carefully review the *Delegation Guidelines* boxes that accompany the procedures in this book. A procedure will be identified as either a *routine nursing task* or a *delegated nursing responsibility.*

E thics and Laws
Nurses are legally responsible for making safe and ethical delegation decisions. You are responsible for your decision to accept or refuse a task and for completing the task.

FOCUS ON **PRIDE**: Application

How do staff relationships affect the delegation process? How do positive interactions benefit the nursing team and person?

REVIEW QUESTIONS

Circle T if the statement is TRUE or F if it is FALSE.

1 T F   Nursing assistants can delegate.

2 T F   A delegated task must be safe for the person.

3 T F   Delegated nursing responsibilities are tasks not routinely done by nursing assistants.

4 T F   The nurse is accountable for delegation decisions.

5 T F   If a task is in your job description, the nurse must delegate it to you.

6 T F   You must have clear directions before performing a task.

Circle the BEST answer.

7 As a nursing assistant, you
   a Must accept all tasks delegated by the nurse
   b Make decisions about a person's care
   c Must know what tasks are in your job description
   d Give a drug when a nurse tells you to

8 You are responsible for
   a Completing tasks safely
   b Assessing the person's needs
   c Supervising other nursing assistants
   d Deciding what treatments are needed

9 In the delegation process, communication involves
   a Observing care
   b Determining who should perform a task
   c Deciding if the task was successful
   d Asking questions about a task

10 Which statement about the nurse's guidance and assistance is *true*?
    a The nurse must be with you when you provide care.
    b The nurse must make sure you complete tasks correctly.
    c Simple tasks require more assistance than complex ones.
    d More guidance is required when the person's condition is stable.

11 A patient begins having trouble swallowing. The nurse decides not to delegate feeding to you. Why?
    a The task is beyond the legal limits of your role.
    b You are not trained to do the task.
    c The nurse does not trust you to do the task safely.
    d The person's circumstances have changed.

12 A nurse delegates a task to you. You must
    a Complete the task
    b Re-assign the task if you are busy
    c Decide to accept or refuse the task
    d Ignore the request if you do not know what to do

13 You can refuse to perform a task if
    a The task is within the legal limits of your role
    b The task is in your job description
    c You do not like the task
    d A nurse is not available to guide or assist you as needed

14 You decide to refuse a task. What should you do?
    a Communicate your concerns to the nurse.
    b Delegate the task to a nursing assistant.
    c Ignore the request.
    d Talk to the director of nursing.

Answers to Chapter 4 questions are on p. 885.

FOCUS ON PRACTICE

Problem Solving

A nurse delegates a task that you have not done before. What must you do to safely accept the task? What must you do if you need to refuse the task?

Ethics and Laws

OBJECTIVES

- Define the key terms and key abbreviations in this chapter.
- Describe ethical conduct.
- Describe a code of conduct for nursing assistants.
- Explain how to maintain professional boundaries.
- Explain how to prevent negligent acts.
- Give examples of false imprisonment, defamation, assault, battery, and fraud.

- Describe how to protect the right to privacy.
- Explain the correct use of electronic communications.
- Explain the purpose of informed consent.
- Describe elder and child abuse and intimate partner violence.
- Explain your role in relation to wills.
- Explain how to promote PRIDE in the person, the family, and yourself.

KEY TERMS

abuse
- The willful infliction of injury, unreasonable confinement, intimidation, or punishment that results in physical harm, pain, or mental anguish
- Depriving the person (or the person's caregiver) of the goods or services needed to attain or maintain well-being

assault Intentionally attempting or threatening to touch a person's body without the person's consent

battery Touching a person's body without his or her consent

boundary crossing
- A brief act or behavior of being over-involved with the person
- The intent of the act or behavior is to meet the person's needs

boundary sign An act, behavior, or thought that warns of a boundary crossing or boundary violation

boundary violation An act or behavior that meets your needs, not the person's

child abuse and neglect The intentional harm or mistreatment of a child under 18 years old:
- Involves any recent act or failure to act on the part of a parent or caregiver
- Results in death, serious physical or emotional harm, sexual abuse, or exploitation
- Presents a likely or immediate risk for harm

civil law Laws concerned with relationships between people

code of ethics Rules, or standards of conduct, for group members to follow

crime An act that violates a criminal law

criminal law Laws concerned with offenses against the public and society in general

defamation Injuring a person's name and reputation by making false statements to a third person

elder abuse Any knowing, intentional, or negligent act by a caregiver or any other person to an older adult that causes harm or serious risk of harm

ethics Knowledge of what is right conduct and wrong conduct

false imprisonment Unlawful restraint or restriction of a person's freedom of movement

fraud Saying or doing something to trick, fool, or deceive a person

informed consent The process by which a person receives and understands information about a treatment or procedure and is able to decide if he or she will receive it

intimate partner violence (IPV) Physical violence, sexual violence, stalking, or psychological aggression by a current or former partner

invasion of privacy Violating a person's right not to have his or her name, photo, or private affairs exposed or made public without giving consent

law A rule of conduct made by a government body

libel Making false statements in print, in writing (including e-mail and text messages), through pictures or drawings, through broadcast (radio, TV, or video), posted on-line on websites, or through video sites and social media sites

malpractice Negligence by a professional person

neglect When a caregiver or responsible person fails to:
- Protect a vulnerable person from harm
- Provide food, water, clothing, shelter, health care, and other activities of daily living to a vulnerable person

negligence An unintentional wrong in which a person did not act in a reasonable and careful manner and a person or the person's property was harmed

professional boundary That which separates helpful actions and behaviors from those that are not helpful

professional sexual misconduct An act, behavior, or comment that is sexual in nature

protected health information Identifying information and information about the person's health care that is maintained or sent in any form (paper, electronic, oral)

self-neglect A person's behaviors and way of living that threaten his or her health, safety, and well-being

KEY TERMS—cont'd

slander Making false statements through the spoken word, sounds, sign language, or gestures

standard of care The skills, care, and judgments required by a health team member under similar conditions

tort A wrong committed against a person or the person's property

vulnerable adult A person 18 years old or older who has a disability or condition that makes him or her at risk to be wounded, attacked, or damaged

will A legal document of how a person wants property distributed after death

KEY ABBREVIATIONS

CDC Centers for Disease Control and Prevention

HIPAA Health Insurance Portability and Accountability Act of 1996

IPV Intimate partner violence

OBRA Omnibus Budget Reconciliation Act of 1987

Nurse practice acts, your training and job description, and safe delegation serve to protect patients and residents from harm (Chapters 3 and 4). Protecting them from harm also involves laws, rules, and standards of conduct. They form the ethical and legal aspects of care.

ETHICAL ASPECTS

Ethics is knowledge of what is right conduct and wrong conduct. Ethics involves choices or judgments about what should or should not be done. An ethical person behaves and acts in the right way. He or she does not cause another person harm.

Ethical behavior also involves not being prejudiced or biased. To be *prejudiced* or *biased* means *making judgments and having views before knowing the facts.* Judgments and views often are based on one's values and standards. They are based on culture, religion, education, and experiences. The person's situation and yours may be very different. For example:

- Children think their mother needs nursing home care. In your culture, children care for older parents at home.
- An older man does not want life-saving measures. You believe that everything must be done to save a life.

Do not judge the person by your values and standards. Do not avoid persons whose standards and values differ from your own.

Ethical problems involve choices. What is the right thing to do? For example:

- A co-worker is in an empty room drinking from a cup. You smell alcohol. The co-worker asks you not to tell anyone.
- A resident has bruises all over her body. She told the nurse that she fell. She tells you that her family is very mean to her. She asks you not to tell the nurse.

Codes of Ethics

Professional groups have codes of ethics. A *code of ethics has rules, or standards of conduct, for group members to follow.* Also called *codes of conduct*, professional nursing organizations have codes of ethics for nurses. The rules of conduct in Box 5-1 can guide your thinking, actions, and behavior. See Chapter 6 for student and work ethics.

BOX 5-1	Code of Conduct for Nursing Assistants

- Respect each person as an individual.
- Know the limits of your role and knowledge.
- Perform only the tasks within the legal limits of your role.
- Perform only the tasks that you have been trained to do.
- Perform no act that will harm the person.
- Take drugs only if prescribed and supervised by a health care provider—doctor, dentist, physician's assistant, advanced practice registered nurse.
- Follow the nurse's directions to your best possible ability.
- Follow agency policies and procedures.
- Complete each task safely.
- Be loyal to your employer and co-workers.
- Act as a responsible citizen at all times.
- Keep the person's information confidential.
- Protect the person's privacy.
- Protect the person's property.
- Consider the person's needs to be more important than your own.
- Report errors and incidents honestly and at once.
- Be responsible for your actions.

Professional Boundaries

A *boundary* limits or separates something. A fence forms a boundary. You stay inside or outside of the fenced area. As a nursing assistant, you enter into a helping relationship with patients, residents, and families. The helping relationship has professional boundaries.

Professional boundaries separate helpful actions and behaviors from those that are not helpful (Fig. 5-1). The boundaries create a helpful zone. If your actions and behaviors are outside of the helpful zone, you are over-involved or under-involved with the person.

If you are *under-involved*, the following can occur.
- Disinterest—you lack interest in the person.
- Avoidance—you avoid the person.
- Neglect—you do not properly care for the person (p. 46).

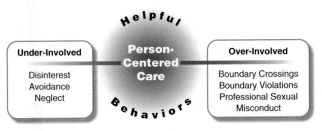

Professional Boundaries

FIGURE 5-1 Professional boundaries guide your actions and behavior. Your focus is on helping the person. Being under-involved or over-involved is not helpful. (Modified from National Council of State Boards of Nursing, Inc.: *A nurse's guide to professional boundaries*, Chicago, 2018, Author.)

If you are *over-involved*, the following can occur.
- *Boundary crossing—a brief act or behavior of being over-involved with the person. The intent of the act or behavior is to meet the person's needs.* The act or behavior may be thoughtless or something you did not mean to do. Or it could have purpose if it meets the person's needs. For example, you give a crying patient a hug. The hug meets the person's needs at the time. If the hug meets your needs, the act is wrong. Also, it is wrong to hug the person every time you see him or her.
- *Boundary violation—an act or behavior that meets your needs, not the person's.* The act or behavior is not ethical. It violates the code of conduct in Box 5-1. The person can be harmed. Boundary violations include:
  - Abuse (p. 45).
  - Giving a lot of information about yourself. You tell the person about your personal relationships or problems.
  - Keeping secrets with the person.
- *Professional sexual misconduct—an act, behavior, or comment that is sexual in nature.* It is sexual misconduct even if the person consents or makes the first move.

Some boundary violations and some types of professional sexual misconduct also are crimes (p. 42). To maintain professional boundaries, follow the rules in Box 5-2. You must be alert to boundary signs. *Boundary signs are acts, behaviors, or thoughts that warn of a boundary crossing or boundary violation* (see Box 5-2).

See *Focus on Communication: Professional Boundaries*, p. 42.

BOX 5-2	**Professional Boundaries**

Maintaining Professional Boundaries
- Follow the code of conduct in Box 5-1. Maintain a professional relationship at all times.
- Talk to the nurse if you sense a boundary sign, crossing, or violation.
- Avoid caring for family, friends, and people you know. This may be hard to do in a small community. Tell the nurse if you know the person. The nurse may change your assignment.
- Do not make sexual comments or jokes.
- Do not use offensive language.
- Use touch correctly (Chapter 7). Touch or handle sexual and genital areas only for needed care. The areas include the breasts, nipples, perineum, buttocks, thighs, and anus.
- Do not visit or spend extra time with someone who is not part of your assignment.
- The following apply to patients, residents, and families.
  - Do not date, flirt with, kiss, or have a sexual relationship with them.
  - Do not discuss your sexual relationships with them.
  - Do not say or write things that could suggest a romantic or sexual relationship with them.
  - Do not accept gifts, loans, money, credit cards, or other valuables from them.
  - Do not give gifts, loans, money, credit cards, or other valuables to them.

Maintaining Professional Boundaries—cont'd
  - Do not borrow from them. This includes money, personal items, and transportation.
  - Do not develop a personal relationship or friendship with them.
  - Do not share personal or financial information with them.
  - Do not help with their finances.
  - Do not take a person home with you. This includes for holidays or other events.
- Ask yourself these questions before you date or marry a person for whom you provided care. Be aware of the risk for professional sexual misconduct.
  - When were you involved with the person's care?
  - Was the person's care short-term or long-term?
  - What kind and how much information do you have about the person? How will that information affect your relationship with the person?
  - Will the person need more care in the future?
  - Does dating or marrying the person place the person at risk for harm?

Boundary Signs
- You think about the person when not at work.
- You organize your work and provide other care around the person's needs.
- You spend time and visit with the person during breaks, meal times, when off duty, and so on.

Continued

BOX 5-2	Professional Boundaries—cont'd

Boundary Signs—cont'd

- You trade assignments to provide the person's care.
- You give more attention to the person at the expense of others.
- You believe that no one else understands the person and his or her needs.
- The person gives you gifts or money.
- You give the person gifts or money.
- You share information about yourself or your work situation with the person.
- You flirt with the person.
- You make comments with a sexual message.
- You tell the person "off-color" jokes.
- You notice more touch between you and the person.
- You use foul, vulgar, or offensive language when talking to the person.

Boundary Signs—cont'd

- You and the person have secrets.
- You choose the person's side during family or staff disagreements.
- You select what to report and record. You do not give complete information.
- You do not like questions about your care or your relationship with the person.
- You change how you dress or your appearance when you will work with the person.
- You receive gifts from the person after he or she leaves the agency.
- You have contact with the person after he or she leaves the agency.

FOCUS ON COMMUNICATION

Professional Boundaries

Some patients, residents, and families send thank-you cards and letters. Some offer thank-you gifts—candy, cookies, money, gift certificates, flowers, and so on. Accepting gifts is a boundary violation. When offered a gift, you can say:

- "Thank you for thinking of me. It's very kind of you. However, it is against center policy to accept gifts. I do appreciate your offer."
- "Thank you for wanting me to have the flowers from your friend. They are lovely. However, it is against hospital policy to receive gifts. May I help you find a way to take them home?"

LEGAL ASPECTS

Ethics is about what you *should or should not do*. Laws tell you what you *can and cannot do*. A *law is a rule of conduct made by a government body.* The U.S. Congress and state legislatures make laws. Enforced by the government, laws protect the public welfare.

Criminal laws are concerned with offenses against the public and society in general. An act that violates a criminal law is called a crime. If found guilty of a crime, the person is fined or sent to prison. Murder, robbery, stealing, rape, kidnapping, and abuse (p. 45) are crimes.

Civil laws are concerned with relationships between people. Contracts and nurse practice acts are examples. A person found guilty of breaking a civil law usually has to pay a sum of money to the injured person.

Tort comes from the French word meaning *wrong*. Torts are part of civil law. A *tort is a wrong committed against a person or the person's property.* Some torts are *unintentional.* Harm was not intended. *Intentional* torts are done on purpose. Harm was intended. Some torts are also crimes.

What you do or do not do can lead to legal action if you harm a person or a person's property. You are legally responsible (liable) for your own actions. Sometimes refusing to follow the nurse's directions is your right and duty (Chapter 4).

Unintentional Torts

Negligence is an unintentional wrong. The negligent person did not act in a reasonable and careful manner. A person or the person's property was harmed. The person causing the harm did not intend or mean to cause harm. The person failed to do what a reasonable and careful person *would have done.* Or he or she did what a reasonable and careful person *would not have done.*

Malpractice is negligence by a professional person. A person has professional status because of his or her education and the services provided. Nurses, doctors, dentists, and pharmacists are examples.

Standards of Care. Health team members are expected to give care at a certain level. For example, nurses are expected to give a level of care higher than nursing assistants. A *standard of care refers to the skills, care, and judgments required by a health team member under similar conditions.* Standards of care come from:

- Laws, including nurse practice acts and those relating to nursing assistants.
- Textbooks.
- Agency policies and procedures. *Policies* are guides for staff conduct. *Procedures* explain how to perform certain tasks or skills.
- Manufacturer's instructions for equipment and supplies.
- Job descriptions.
- Approval and accrediting agency standards. The Centers for Medicare & Medicaid Services is an example of an approving agency.
- Standards and guidelines from government agencies. See Chapter 16 for guidelines from the Centers for Disease Control and Prevention (CDC).

The following harmful actions could lead to charges of negligence.

- You fail to test the water temperature for a shower. The water is too hot. The person is burned.
- A resident needs help to the bathroom. You do not answer the call light promptly. Getting up without help, the resident falls and breaks an arm.

- You do not follow the manufacturer's instructions for using a mechanical lift. The patient slips out of the lift, falls to the floor, and fractures a hip.
- A patient complains of chest pain. You do not tell the nurse. The person has a heart attack and dies.
- Two residents have the same last name. You do not identify the person before a procedure. You perform the procedure on the wrong person. Both residents are harmed. One had a procedure that was not ordered. The other did not have a needed procedure.

Intentional Torts

Intentional torts are meant to be harmful and may be crimes.

- *Defamation is injuring a person's name and reputation by making false statements to a third person.*
  - *Libel is making false statements in print, in writing (including e-mail and text messages), through pictures or drawings, through broadcast (radio, TV, or video), posted on-line on websites, or through video sites and social media sites.* See "Wrongful Use of Electronic Communications," p. 44.
  - *Slander is making false statements through the spoken word, sounds, sign language, or gestures.*
- *False imprisonment is the unlawful restraint or restriction of a person's freedom of movement.* It involves:
  - Threatening to restrain a person
  - Restraining a person
  - Preventing a person from leaving the agency
- *Assault is intentionally attempting or threatening to touch a person's body without the person's consent.* The person fears bodily harm. Threatening to "tie down" a person is an example of assault.
- *Battery is touching a person's body without his or her consent.* The person must consent to any procedure, treatment, or other act that involves touching the body. The person has the right to withdraw consent at any time. See "Informed Consent," p. 45.
- *Fraud is saying or doing something to trick, fool, or deceive a person.* The act is fraud if it does or could harm a person or the person's property. Telling someone that you are a nurse is fraud. So is giving wrong or incomplete information on a job application.
- *Invasion of privacy is violating a person's right not to have his or her name, photo, or private affairs exposed or made public without giving consent.* You must treat the person with respect and ensure privacy. Only staff involved in the person's care should see, handle, or examine his or her body. See Box 5-3 for measures to protect privacy.

  See *Focus on Communication: Intentional Torts (Invasion of Privacy).*

  See *Promoting Safety and Comfort: Intentional Torts,* p. 44.

BOX 5-3	Protecting the Right to Privacy

- Keep all information about the person confidential.
- Cover the person when in hallways and elevators.
- Ask visitors to leave the room when care is given.
- Screen the person. Close the privacy curtain as in Figure 5-2. Close the room door and window coverings to give care.
- Close the bathroom door for elimination or hygiene.
- Expose only the body part involved in a task.
- Do not discuss the person or the person's treatment with anyone except the nurse supervising your work.
- Do not open the person's mail.
- Allow the person to visit with others in private.
- Allow the person to use the phone in private.
- Follow agency policies and procedures to protect privacy.

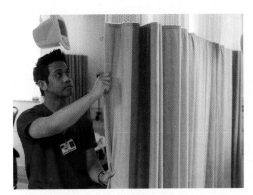

FIGURE 5-2 Pulling the privacy curtain around the bed helps protect the person's privacy.

FOCUS ON **COMMUNICATION**

Intentional Torts (Invasion of Privacy)

The *Health Insurance Portability and Accountability Act of 1996 (HIPAA)* protects the privacy and security of a person's health information. *Protected health information refers to identifying information and information about the person's health care that is maintained or sent in any form (paper, electronic, oral).* Failure to follow HIPAA rules can result in fines, penalties, and criminal actions including jail time.

To avoid HIPAA violations:

- Always follow agency policies and procedures.
- *Never take photos or videos of patients or residents or any person in the health care or home care setting.* Sharing photos or videos or posting them on video sites or social media sites is a very serious violation of HIPAA.
- *Never send an e-mail or text message or post anything on a website, video site, or social media site about a patient, resident, family member, or visitor.* Sharing information is a very serious violation of HIPAA.
- *Never write anything for a newspaper, magazine, or print source about a patient, resident, family member, or visitor.*
- *Never broadcast (through TV, radio, or video) anything about a patient, resident, family member, or visitor.*
- *Only discuss the person's health information with staff directly involved in the person's care.*
- See "Wrongful Use of Electronic Communications," p. 44.

  You may be asked questions about the person or the person's care. Direct any questions about the person or the person's care to the nurse. Also follow the rules for using computers and other electronic devices (Chapter 8).

PROMOTING SAFETY AND COMFORT

Intentional Torts

Safety

To protect yourself from defamation, never make false statements about a patient, resident, family member, visitor, co-worker, or any other person. This includes:

- Through e-mails or text messages
- On websites, video sites, or social media sites
- In newspapers, magazines, or other print sources
- Through broadcasts (TV, radio, or film)
- With words, sounds, signs, gestures, or any form of communication

Examples of defamation include:

- Implying or suggesting that a person uses drugs
- Saying that a person is insane or mentally ill
- Posting on-line that a co-worker was fired for hitting a resident
- Implying or suggesting that a person steals money from the staff

Also protect yourself from being accused of assault and battery. Explain to the person what you are going to do and get the person's consent. Consent may be verbal—"yes" or "okay." Or it can be a gesture—a nod, turning over for a back massage, or holding out an arm for you to take a pulse.

Wrongful Use of Electronic Communications

Electronic communications include e-mail, text messages, faxes, websites, video sites, and social media sites. Video and social media sites include Facebook, Twitter, LinkedIn, YouTube, Instagram, blogs and comments to blog postings, chat rooms, bulletin boards, and so on. Other forms of electronic communications are expected in the future.

Correct use of electronic communications is essential in your personal life and as a nursing assistant. Follow the rules in Box 5-4. Do so whether using a computer, wireless phone, camera, or other electronic device at home, at school, at work, or in any other setting. Wrongful use of electronic communications can result in job loss and loss of your certification (license, registration) for:

- Defamation
- Invasion of privacy
- HIPAA violations
- Violating the right to confidentiality (Chapter 6)
- Patient or resident abuse
- Unprofessional or unethical conduct

Wrongful use of electronic communications may be violations of federal and state laws that protect privacy and confidentiality. HIPAA is an example. Besides losing your certification (license, registration), wrongful use can result in:

- Civil action resulting in a fine
- Criminal action resulting in a fine or jail time

See *Focus on Communication: Wrongful Use of Electronic Communications.*

BOX 5-4	Electronic Communications

- Follow agency policies for using electronic communications.
- Remember that:
  - Anything you send or post electronically can be sent to or shared with someone other than the intended person.
  - Electronic communications last forever. They can be retrieved for legal purposes.
  - Private information shared with the intended person still violates the rights to privacy and confidentiality.
  - Referring to a person by nickname, room number, diagnosis, or other means but not by name still violates the rights to privacy and confidentiality.
- Protect privacy and maintain confidentiality at all times.
- Never take photos or videos of the person or any part of the person's body.
- Never send in any way information about the person or images (photos, videos, art) of the person.
- Never identify patients or residents by name.
- Never share information that can lead to the person being identified.
- Maintain professional boundaries. Avoid electronic contact with patients and residents, former patients and residents, and family members.
- Do not use electronic communications to share or discuss workplace issues or co-workers.
- Tell the nurse at once if you may have violated the person's right to privacy or confidentiality. If you suspect that a co-worker has done so, also tell the nurse.
- See "Gossip" in Chapter 6.
- See "Unethical Student Behavior" in Chapter 6.
- See "Electronic Devices" in Chapter 8.

Modified from National Council of State Boards of Nursing: A nurse's guide to the use of social media, *Chicago, 2018, Author.*

FOCUS ON COMMUNICATION

Wrongful Use of Electronic Communications

The following are examples of wrongful use of electronic communications.

- Laura is a nursing assistant student. On the last day of clinical, she asks 2 residents if she can take a photo with them. Laura posts the photo on a social media site with this comment: "Done with clinical! I'll miss my residents."
- Justin works on a cancer unit. A patient posts on a blog about a tiring day of treatments. Justin posts: "Chemo can wear you down. Maybe the new medicine will help you rest. Hope you feel better tomorrow. See you then."
- Sara works in home care. She sends a text message to a friend that says: "I'll be done at 22 Third Street at noon. Want to get lunch?"

What did Laura, Justin, and Sara do wrong?

Often wrongful use of electronic communications is not intentional. You must be very careful. Your communication must protect privacy and confidentiality at all times.

Informed Consent

Informed consent is the process by which a person receives and understands information about a treatment or procedure and is able to decide if he or she will receive it. A person has the right to decide what will be done to his or her body and who can touch his or her body. The doctor is responsible for informing the person about all aspects of treatment. Consent is informed when the person clearly understands:
* The reason for a treatment, procedure, or care measure
* What will be done and how
* Who will do it
* The expected outcomes
* Other treatment, procedure, or care options
* The effects of not having the treatment, procedure, or care measure

Persons under legal age (usually 18 years) cannot give consent. Nor can persons who are mentally incompetent—unconscious, sedated, or confused. Or they have certain mental health disorders. Informed consent is given by a responsible party—a spouse, parent, daughter, son, guardian, or legal representative.

A general consent to treatment is signed when the person enters the agency. Special consents are required for admission to secured memory care units (Chapter 53). Surgeries and some procedures performed by the doctor require special consents. The doctor informs the person about all aspects of the procedure. The nurse may have this responsibility.

You are never responsible for obtaining written consent. In some agencies, you can witness the signing of a consent. When a witness, you are present when the person signs the consent.

See *Focus on Communication: Informed Consent.*

FOCUS ON COMMUNICATION

Informed Consent

There are different ways to give consent.
* *Written consent.* The person signs a form agreeing to a treatment or procedure. You are not responsible for obtaining written consent.
* *Verbal consent.* The person states aloud that he or she consents. "Yes" and "okay" are examples.
* *Implied consent.* For example, you ask a person if you can check his or her blood pressure. The person extends an arm. The movement implies consent.

Before any procedure or task, explain the steps to the person. This is how you obtain verbal or implied consent. Also explain each step during a procedure. This allows the person to refuse at any time.

REPORTING ABUSE

Some persons are mistreated or harmed on purpose. This is abuse. Abuse is a crime. *Abuse is:*
* *The willful infliction of injury, unreasonable confinement, intimidation, or punishment that results in physical harm, pain, or mental anguish.* **Intimidation** means *to make afraid with threats of force or violence.* Abuse includes involuntary seclusion (Chapter 2).
* *Depriving the person (or the person's caregiver) of the goods or services needed to attain or maintain well-being.*

Abuse can occur at home or in a health care agency. All persons must be protected from abuse. This includes persons in a coma.

The abuser is often a family member or caregiver—spouse, partner, brother or sister, adult child, and others. The abuser can be a friend, neighbor, landlord, or other person. Both men and women are abusers. Both men and women are abused.

State laws, accrediting agencies, and the *Omnibus Budget Reconciliation Act of 1987 (OBRA)* do not allow agencies to employ persons who were convicted of abuse, neglect, or mistreatment. Before hiring, the agency must thoroughly check the applicant's work history, references, and any criminal records.

The agency also checks the nursing assistant registry for findings of abuse, neglect, or mistreatment. It also is checked for financial abuse (p. 48).

See *Focus on Communication: Reporting Abuse.*
See *Focus on Surveys: Reporting Abuse*, p. 46.

FOCUS ON COMMUNICATION

Reporting Abuse

Abused persons may confide in you. They may ask you to keep it a secret. For example, a person says: "If I tell you something, will you promise not to tell anyone?" Never promise to keep abuse a secret from the nurse. Be honest. Do not say you will keep a secret and then report it to the nurse. You can say: "For your safety, some things I must tell the nurse. What did you want to tell me?" If the person refuses to tell you, notify the nurse.

If you suspect abuse, tell the nurse. Give as much detail as you can. For example: "I am concerned about Ms. Sloan. She is very quiet today. When I asked about her visit with her family, she didn't answer. She refused her bath. And when I helped her to the bathroom, I saw bruises on her back."

FOCUS ON SURVEYS

Reporting Abuse

Abuse is a major part of surveys. Surveyors look for signs of abuse through interviews, observations, and medical records.

Agencies must have procedures to:

- Screen staff applicants for a history of abuse, neglect, or mistreatment of residents. This includes information from:
  - Previous or current employers
  - Nursing assistant registries or licensing boards
- Train staff on how to prevent abuse.
- Identify and correct situations in which abuse is more likely to occur.
- Identify events, patterns, and trends that may signal abuse. Bruises, falls, and staff yelling are examples.
- Investigate abuse.
- Protect patients and residents from harm during an investigation.
- Report and respond to claims of abuse or actual abuse.

Vulnerable Adults

Vulnerable comes from the Latin word *vulnerare*, which means *to wound*. *Vulnerable adults are persons 18 years old or older who have disabilities or conditions that make them at risk to be wounded, attacked, or damaged.* They have problems caring for or protecting themselves due to:

- A mental, emotional, physical, intellectual, or developmental disability. See Chapter 54.
- Brain damage.
- Changes from aging.

All patients and residents, regardless of age or care setting, are vulnerable. Older persons and children (p. 50) are at risk for abuse.

See *Focus on Long-Term Care and Home Care: Vulnerable Adults.*

FOCUS ON LONG-TERM CARE AND HOME CARE

Vulnerable Adults

Home Care

A caregiver or responsible party may neglect a vulnerable adult. *Neglect is when a caregiver or responsible person fails to:*

- *Protect a vulnerable person from harm*
- *Provide food, water, clothing, shelter, health care, and other activities of daily living to a vulnerable person*

Some persons neglect themselves. *Self-neglect is when the person's behaviors and way of living threaten his or her health, safety, and well-being.*

Causes of self-neglect include declining health and chronic disease. Other causes are disorders that impair judgment or memory—Alzheimer's disease, dementia, depression, drug or alcohol abuse, and other mental health disorders (Chapters 52 and 53). Some persons refuse care.

Persons at risk for self-neglect include those who:

- Live alone.
- Are women. More women live alone than men.
- Are depressed.
- Are confused.
- Are older.
- Have alcohol or drug problems.
- Have a history of poor hygiene or living conditions.

The person has the right to personal choice, to make decisions for himself or herself, and to be independent. However, report warning signs of self-neglect to the nurse.

- Not enough food, water for drinking, heat, or other necessities. Other necessities include indoor plumbing, running water, working toilet, electricity, and so on.
- Safety hazards in the home. See Chapter 13.
- Unclean living conditions—filth, odors (urine, feces, trash, food), soiled bedding or clothing, human or animal urine or feces, pests (mice, rats, ants, fleas, and other insects), and so on.
- Needed home repairs.
- Hoarding—saving, hiding, or storing things. For example, the person saves newspapers, magazines, food containers, shopping bags, and so on. The hoarding can present fire, pest (mice, rats, ants, fleas, and other insects), and other safety hazards.
- Failing to take needed drugs.
- Refusing to seek medical treatment for serious illnesses.
- Dehydration—poor urinary output, dry skin, dry mouth, confusion.
- Weight loss.
- Poor hygiene. The person has dirty hair, nails, or skin. He or she smells of urine or feces.
- Skin rashes or pressure injuries (Chapter 41).
- Not wearing the correct clothing for the weather. Wearing dirty or torn clothing.
- Not having dentures, eyeglasses, hearing aids, walkers, wheelchairs, commodes, or other needed devices.
- Signs of confusion, disorientation, hallucinations, or delusions (Chapters 52 and 53).
- Mis-using drugs or alcohol.
- The person's health or living conditions seem worse.
- Untreated health problems.

Elder Abuse

An *elder*, as defined by the CDC, is an *older adult 60 years of age or older. Elder abuse is any knowing, intentional, or negligent act by a caregiver or any other person to an older adult. The act causes harm or serious risk of harm.* There are many forms and signs of elder abuse. See Table 5-1 and Box 5-5 (p. 48). Often more than 1 form of abuse is present.

See *Focus on Long-Term Care and Home Care: Elder Abuse.*

FOCUS ON LONG-TERM CARE AND HOME CARE

Elder Abuse

Home Care

Abandonment is always serious. However, it is most serious in home care. Unlike in hospitals and nursing centers, often you are the only caregiver in the home. If you leave before completing your assignment, there is no one to give care. The person is left alone without needed care. Serious harm could result. You could have your certification (license, registration) revoked or suspended for abandonment in any setting.

TABLE 5-1	Elder Abuse	
Type	Description	Examples
Physical abuse	The intentional use of physical force that results in: • Acute or chronic illness • Injury • Pain • Impaired function • Distress • Death	• Biting • Burning • Choking • Corporal punishment—punishment inflicted directly on the body (beatings, lashings, whippings, and so on) • Force-feeding • Grabbing • Hair-pulling • Hitting • Kicking or stomping • Pinching • Punching • Pushing or shoving • Restraint—physical or chemical • Scratching • Shaking • Slapping • Striking—with or without an object • Suffocation
Sexual abuse or abusive sexual contact	Forced or unwanted sexual interaction of any kind with an older adult or an incapacitated person. *(Incapacitated means being unconscious or lacking awareness.)* The interaction may: • Be completed or attempted. • Involve touching or non-touching.	• Contact: • Between the penis and the vulva (female external genitalia) or anus • Between the mouth and the penis, vulva, or anus • Penetration of the vagina or anus by another person using a hand, finger, or other object • Touching directly or through clothing of the genitalia, anus, groin, breast, inner thigh, or buttocks • Forced nudity • Forced watching of sexual acts • Harassing a person about sex or his or her sexuality • Taking sexually oriented photos or videos
Emotional or psychological abuse	Any verbal (oral or written) or nonverbal behavior that causes mental pain, anguish, fear, or distress.	• Yelling, screaming, or shouting at the person • Insults and name-calling • Scolding or criticizing • Threats of punishment or harm • Humiliation, harassment, or ridicule • Treating or talking to the person like an infant or child • Not speaking to the person • Unkind gestures • Saying things to frighten the person • Confining the person to a certain area • Threatening to with-hold care

Continued

TABLE 5-1	Elder Abuse—cont'd	
Type	Description	Examples
Neglect	Failure of a caregiver or responsible person to: • Protect a vulnerable person from harm. • Provide food, water, clothing, shelter, health care, and other activities of daily living to a vulnerable person.	• Dirty clothing • Poor hygiene • Leaving the person lying or sitting in urine or feces • Lacking appropriate clothing for the weather • Cluttered or dirty home • Hoarding • Home in need of repairs • Fire or safety hazards in the home • Lacking needed utilities—water, electricity, plumbing, heating/cooling
Financial abuse	Exploitation—to mis-use a person's money, property, or assets. Misappropriation—the illegal, dishonest, unfair, or wrongful use of a person's money, property, or assets for one's own use.	• Forging a person's signature • Mis-use or theft of money or possessions • Using a person's credit card, debit card, or bank account • Changing names on a will, bank account, insurance policy, deed, or other financial or legal document • Taking money from a person's wallet
Abandonment	Deserting or leaving a vulnerable adult alone without someone being responsible for the person or his or her care. Involves 4 points: • Accepting an assignment to care for a person or group of persons • Accepting the assignment for a certain time • Removing yourself from the care setting—home, hospital, or nursing center • Failing to report off to a staff member who will assume responsibility for care	• Leaving the agency before your shift ends without telling the nurse • Failing to report to a home care assignment • Leaving without completing a home care assignment • Sleeping on the job

BOX 5-5	Signs of Elder Abuse

- The person reports mistreatment or shows signs of abuse (Fig. 5-3). See Table 5-1.
- Living conditions are not safe, clean, or adequate. See *Focus on Long-Term Care and Home Care: Vulnerable Adults.*
- Personal and oral hygiene are lacking (Chapters 23 and 24). The person is not clean. Clothes are dirty.
- Weight loss—signs of poor nutrition and poor fluid intake.
- Adaptive (assistive) devices are missing or broken—eyeglasses, hearing aids, dentures, cane, walker, and so on.
- Medical needs are not met.
- Frequent injuries—injuries are strange or seem impossible.
- Old and new injuries—bruises, pressure marks, welts, scars, fractures, punctures, and so on.
- Problems walking or sitting.
- Bleeding, bruising, irritation, itching, or pain around the breasts, inner thighs, or genital or anal area.
- Torn, stained, or bloody under-garments.
- Burns on the feet, hands, buttocks, or other parts of the body. Cigarettes and cigars cause small circle-like burns.
- Pressure injuries (Chapter 41) or contractures (Chapter 34).
- Emotional problems (Chapter 52):
  - Panic attacks
  - Post-traumatic stress disorder
  - Quiet; withdrawn from others and normal activities
  - Does not want to talk or answer questions
  - Depression
  - Suicide thoughts or attempts
  - Fear, anxiety, or agitation (Chapter 53)
  - Inappropriate, unusual, or aggressive sexual behavior (Chapter 55)
- Sudden changes in alertness.
- Sudden changes in finances.
- The person is restrained. Or the person is locked in a certain area for long periods.
- The person cannot reach toilet facilities, food, water, and other needed items.
- Private conversations are not allowed. The caregiver is present during all conversations.
- Strained or tense relationships with a caregiver.
- Frequent arguments with a caregiver.
- The person seems anxious to please the caregiver.
- Drugs are not taken properly. Drugs are not bought. Or too much or too little of the drug is taken.
- Emergency room visits may be frequent.
- The person may change doctors often. Some people do not have a doctor.

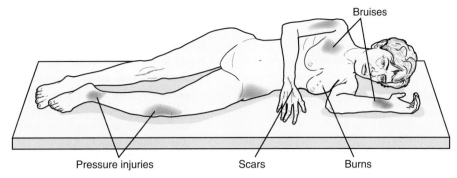

FIGURE 5-3 Some signs of physical elder abuse.

Reporting Elder Abuse. Federal and state laws require the reporting of elder abuse. If abuse is suspected, it must be reported. Where and how to report abuse varies among states. If you suspect abuse, share your concerns and observations with the nurse. Be as detailed as possible. The nurse contacts health team members as needed.

The nurse also contacts community agencies that investigate elder abuse. They act at once if the problem is life-threatening. Sometimes the police or courts are involved.

Helping abused older persons is not always easy or possible. Some abuse is not reported or recognized. Or investigators cannot gain access to the person. A victim may want to protect the abuser, especially if the abuser is a spouse, partner, or adult child. Some victims are embarrassed or believe abuse is deserved. A victim may fear what will happen. He or she may think that the present situation is better than no care at all. Some people fear not being believed if they report the abuse themselves.

Box 5-6 lists some prosecuted cases of elder abuse. If you are involved, an investigation can lead to 1 or more of the following.
- Job loss
- Loss of certification (license, registration)
- Being convicted of a crime
  See *Focus on Long-Term Care and Home Care: Reporting Elder Abuse.*

FOCUS ON LONG-TERM CARE AND HOME CARE

Reporting Elder Abuse

Long-Term Care
OBRA requires these actions if abuse is suspected within the center.
- The matter is reported at once to:
  - The administrator
  - Other investigative agencies as required by federal and state laws
- All claims of abuse are thoroughly investigated.
- The center must prevent further potential for abuse while the investigation is in progress.
- Investigation results are reported to the center administrator and required agencies within 5 days of the incident.
- Corrective actions are taken if the claim is found to be true.

BOX 5-6   Prosecuted Cases of Elder Abuse

- A resident was complaining of pain while being cleaned. To stop him from complaining, a nursing assistant stuck a rag down his throat.
- A patient was screaming. To stop the patient from screaming, a nurse poured water down her throat.
- A nursing assistant beat and kicked a 92-year-old man who was lying on the floor.
- A nursing assistant stepped on a resident's face.
- A person was visiting his grandmother. While there, he sexually abused a patient with head injuries.
- A nursing assistant dragged a female patient in a wheelchair into a room. The nursing assistant forced the patient to have sex with him.
- A nursing assistant teased and taunted a resident with dementia.
- A health care worker repeatedly insulted an older woman because her son was gay.
- A nursing assistant forced a person to urinate in bed. Then the nursing assistant made fun of the person.
- Two older women lived in a board and care home. Both had Alzheimer's disease. They were left in a room with blood splattered on the walls. The carpet was caked with feces, vomitus, and urine. The women were partially dressed. One was tied to the bed with a sheet.
- A nursing assistant failed to feed a resident who could not feed herself. A video camera caught the nursing assistant dumping the person's food into trash cans.
- A resident could not talk. She totally depended on the staff for care. She did not have a bowel movement for 26 days. She was given a laxative every 3 days. No other treatment was given for her constipation.
- Caregivers willfully neglected to give drugs to residents.

Modified from Elder abuse and neglect: prosecution and prevention, *San Francisco, American Society on Aging.*

Child Abuse and Neglect

Child abuse and neglect is the intentional harm or mistreatment of a child under 18 years old.
- *Involves any recent act or failure to act on the part of a parent or caregiver.*
- *Results in death, serious physical or emotional harm, sexual abuse, or exploitation.*
- *Presents a likely or immediate risk for harm.*

Child abuse and neglect occur in low-, middle-, and high-income families. The abuser's education level may be low or high. Often the abuser is a household member or caregiver—parent, parent's partner, brother or sister, foster parent, nanny, babysitter. Usually an abuser is someone the family knows. Risk factors for abusing children include:
- Stress
- Family crisis (divorce, unemployment, low income, moving, crowded living conditions, intimate partner violence, p. 52)
- Single-parenting
- Teenage parenting
- Several young children under 5 years of age
- Physical or mental illness, including depression
- Drug or alcohol abuse
- Abuser history of abuse or neglect as a child
- Discipline beliefs that include physical punishment
- Lack of emotional attachment to the child
- Poor parent-child relationships
- A child with birth defects, chronic illness, or a physical, intellectual, or developmental disability
- A child with a personality or behaviors that the abuser considers "different" or not acceptable
- Unrealistic expectations for the child's behavior or performance
- Lack of understanding about children's needs, child development, and parenting skills
- Families that move often and do not have family or friends nearby

Types of Child Abuse and Neglect.
Child abuse and neglect have many forms. Often more than 1 type is present.
- *Physical abuse* is injuring the child on purpose. It can cause bruising, fractures, or death. See Table 5-1.
- *Neglect* is failing to provide for a child's basic needs.
  - *Physical neglect*—failure to provide food, shelter, or supervision.
  - *Medical neglect*—failure to provide needed medical or mental health treatment. (Some religious beliefs do not allow medical care. State laws vary on what is considered medical neglect.)
  - *Educational neglect*—failure to educate a child or provide special education needs.
  - *Emotional neglect*—failure to meet the child's needs for affection and attention. Includes letting a child use alcohol or other drugs.

- *Sexual abuse* is using, persuading, forcing, or exposing a child to engage in sexual contact, activity, or behavior. There may be oral, genital, vaginal, anal, buttock, thigh, or breast involvement.
  - *Rape or sexual assault*—forced sexual acts with a person against his or her will.
  - *Molestation*—sexual advances toward a child. It includes kissing, touching, or fondling sexual areas. The abuser may kiss, touch, or fondle the child. Or the child is forced to kiss, touch, or fondle the abuser.
  - *Incest*—sexual activity between family members. The abuser may be a parent, brother or sister, aunt or uncle, cousin, or grandparent.
  - *Child pornography*—taking photos or videos of a child involved in sexual acts or poses.
  - *Child prostitution*—forcing a child to engage in sexual acts for money. Usually the child is forced to have many sexual partners.
- *Emotional abuse* is injuring the child mentally or his or her sense of self-worth. The abuser constantly criticizes, threatens, or rejects the child. The abuser may with-hold love, support, or guidance. The child has changes in behavior, emotional responses, thinking, reasoning, learning, and so on. The child may show anxiety, depression, withdrawal, or aggressive behaviors. Emotional abuse is almost always present with other forms of abuse.
- *Substance abuse* is part of child abuse and neglect in some states. Pre-natal exposure (during pregnancy) is 1 form of substance abuse. Others involve alcohol abuse, drug abuse, and illegal drug activity. A *controlled substance* is a drug or chemical substance whose possession and use are controlled by law. Substance abuse involves:
  - Making a controlled substance in the presence of a child or on the premises occupied by a child.
  - Allowing a child to be where there are chemicals or equipment used to make or store a controlled substance.
  - Selling, distributing, or giving drugs or alcohol to a child.
  - Using a controlled substance (a caregiver) that impairs the caregiver's ability to care for the child.
  - Exposing the child to equipment and supplies for using, selling, or distributing drugs.
  - Exposing the child to other drug-related activities.
- *Abandonment* is when the parent's identity or whereabouts are unknown. The child is left in circumstances that cause serious harm. Or the parent fails to maintain contact with the child or provide support for the child.

| BOX 5-7 | Child Abuse and Neglect—Signs and Symptoms |

General Behaviors

- **The Child**
  - Reports bad treatment or abuse by a parent or caregiver.
  - Has sudden changes in behavior.
  - Has sudden changes in school performance.
  - Has learning problems or problems concentrating. The problem is not caused by a physical or mental health disorder.
  - Has untreated health problems.
  - Seems watchful; seems to wait for something bad to happen.
  - Lacks adult supervision.
  - Is overly agreeable or obedient.
  - Is quiet, withdrawn, or uninvolved.
  - Arrives early at school or stays late.
  - Does not want to go home from school, activities, or someone's house.
  - Fears a parent or certain person; does not want to be around a parent or certain person.
- **The Parent**
  - Denies that the child has problems at school or home.
  - Blames the child for problems at school or home.
  - Asks teachers or caregivers to use harsh discipline.
  - Describes the child as bad, worthless, or a burden.
  - Demands physical or academic performance above the child's abilities.
  - Shows little concern for the child.
  - Relies on the child for care, attention, or emotional satisfaction.
- **Parent and Child**
  - Rarely touch or look at each other.
  - View their relationship as poor or bad.
  - State that they do not like each other.

Physical Abuse

- **The Child**
  - Has injuries that are not explained—burns, bites, bruises, broken bones, black eyes.
  - Has fading bruises or other marks after being gone from school.
  - Is scared, anxious, depressed, withdrawn, or aggressive.
  - Fears parents and does not want to go home.
  - Shrinks (cowers) when an adult approaches.
  - Has changes in eating and sleeping habits.
  - Reports injury by a parent or caregiver.
  - Abuses animals or pets.
- **The Parent**
  - Gives different or confusing stories about an injury. Or does not give an explanation.
  - Uses harsh discipline.
  - Has a history of abusing animals or pets.

Neglect

- **The Child**
  - Begs or steals food or money.
  - Is dirty or has a severe body odor.
  - Lacks the correct clothing for the weather.
  - Abuses alcohol or drugs.
  - States that no one is at home to provide care.
  - Is often absent from school.
  - Lacks medical or dental care. Does not have needed eyeglasses.
- **The Parent**
  - Seems to have little interest in the child.
  - Shows little or no emotion or is depressed.
  - Has behaviors that are bizarre or not logical.
  - Abuses alcohol or drugs.

Sexual Abuse

- **The Child**
  - Has trouble walking or sitting.
  - Has bleeding, bruising, or swelling in sexual areas.
  - Refuses to go to school.
  - Has nightmares or wets the bed.
  - Has a sudden change in appetite.
  - Has sexual knowledge or behavior that is unusual or does not fit with his or her age.
  - Is pregnant or has a sexually transmitted disease (Chapter 51) especially under the age of 14.
  - Runs away.
  - Reports sexual abuse.
  - Attaches to strangers or new adults quickly.
- **The Parent**
  - Tries to be the child's friend instead of a parent.
  - Makes up excuses to be alone with the child.
  - Tells the child about his or her personal problems or relationships.

Emotional Abuse

- **The Child**
  - Has extremes in behavior—overly agreeable or demanding, quiet and withdrawn, or aggressive.
  - Acts much younger or older than his or her age. For example, the child shows infant-like behaviors (rocking, head-banging). Or the child acts like a parent to other children.
  - Has physical or emotional developmental delays (Chapter 11).
  - Is depressed.
  - Has suicidal thoughts.
  - Has trouble bonding with others.
- **The Parent**
  - Blames, criticizes, or scolds the child often.
  - Describes the child negatively.
  - Rejects the child.

Modified from Child Welfare Information Gateway: What is child abuse and neglect: recognizing the signs and symptoms, *Washington, DC, April 2019, Children's Bureau.*

Reporting Child Abuse and Neglect. Box 5-7 lists the signs of child abuse and neglect. Report any changes in the child's body or behavior. Child and parent behaviors may alert to something wrong.

Child abuse is complex. Many more behaviors, signs, and symptoms are present than discussed here. You must be alert for signs and symptoms of child abuse. All states require the reporting of suspected child abuse. However, someone should not be falsely accused.

If you suspect child abuse, share your concerns with the nurse. Give as much detail as you can. The nurse contacts the health team and child protection agencies as needed.

Intimate Partner Violence

The CDC describes *intimate partner violence (IPV)* *as physical violence, sexual violence, stalking, or psychological aggression by a current or former partner.* Also called domestic abuse, domestic violence, intimate partner abuse, partner abuse, and spousal abuse—IPV occurs in relationships. IPV includes dating violence and teen dating violence (Chapter 11).

In IPV, 1 partner has power and control over the other through abuse. The partner may be a current or former spouse, boyfriend or girlfriend, dating partner, or sexual partner. Partners can be heterosexual or same-sex couples. IPV does not require a sexual relationship.

The abuse may range from 1 event to chronic, severe violence over several years. Rarely is IPV a 1-time event.

IPV causes fear and harm. Usually more than 1 type of IPV is present. The CDC describes 4 main types of IPV.

- *Physical violence*—the intentional use of physical force that may cause death, disability, injury, or harm. Physical violence includes the following actions or forcing a person to commit such acts.
  - Pushing, shoving, throwing, grabbing, or shaking
  - Biting
  - Choking
  - Hair-pulling
  - Hitting, slapping, scratching, or punching
  - Burning
  - Using a weapon
  - Using restraints
  - Using one's body, size, or strength against a person
- *Sexual violence*—any of the following acts that occur *without the victim's consent*, whether attempted or completed. This includes when the person cannot give consent because of being incapacitated by alcohol or drugs. The alcohol or drug use may be voluntary or involuntary.
  - Rape or penetration of the victim—unwanted vaginal, oral, or anal penetration. Physical force is used against the victim or there are threats of physical harm.
  - The victim was forced to sexually penetrate someone else—the perpetrator or another person. A *perpetrator* is someone who commits an illegal, criminal, or evil act.
  - Non-physical pressured unwanted penetration—the victim was pressured verbally to consent to penetration. The victim was intimidated (filled with fear) or authority (power) was mis-used against the victim.
  - Unwanted sexual contact—touching the victim or making the victim touch the perpetrator. The touch is direct or through clothing on the genitals, anus, groin, breast, inner thigh, or buttocks.
  - Non-contact unwanted sexual experiences—non-physical sexual events such as exposure to pornography, sexual harassment, and threats of sexual violence. It also includes the unwanted filming, taking, or sharing of sexual photographs.

- *Stalking*—a pattern of repeated, unwanted attention and contact that causes fear or concern for one's safety or the safety of another (family, friend). Examples include:
  - Phone calls, e-mails, or text messages
  - Leaving unwanted cards, letters, flowers, or other items
  - Watching or following from a distance
  - Spying
  - Showing up in places when the victim does not want to see the person
  - Sneaking into the victim's home or car
  - Damaging the victim's property
  - Harming or threatening the victim's pet
  - Threatening to physically harm the victim
- *Psychological aggression*—intending to mentally or emotionally harm the victim through verbal and nonverbal communication. Or the intent may be to control the person.
  - Name-calling, humiliation, and so on
  - Control—limiting access to transportation, money, friends, and family; monitoring whereabouts
  - Threats of physical or sexual violence
  - Control of reproductive or sexual health—refusing to allow birth control, forced pregnancy termination, and so on
  - Exploiting a victim's weakness—immigration status, disability, and so on
  - Presenting false information (mind games) so the victim questions his or her memory or thinking

Both men and women can be victims. However, most victims are women. There is no set age, race, culture, religion, educational level, income level, or marital status for IPV. Patients and residents can suffer from IPV. For example, a husband slaps his wife during a hospital visit. Or a wife uses her husband's money for herself rather than buying his needed medicine. You, yourself, may be a victim of IPV. Box 5-8 lists the risk factors and warning signs of IPV.

Intimate partner violence is a complex safety issue. The victim often hides the abuse. He or she may protect the abuser. State laws vary about reporting IPV. However, the health team has an ethical duty to give information about safety and community resources. If you suspect IPV, tell the nurse. The nurse gathers information to help the person.

See *Focus on Children and Older Persons: Intimate Partner Violence.*

See *Focus on Long-Term Care and Home Care: Intimate Partner Violence.*

See *Promoting Safety and Comfort: Intimate Partner Violence.*

BOX 5-8	Intimate Partner Violence

Risk Factors—The Victim or Abuser

- Low self-esteem
- Low income
- Low educational level
- Young age
- Problem behavior as a youth
- Heavy alcohol or drug use
- Depression
- Anger and hostility
- Antisocial or borderline personality traits (Chapter 52)
- History of physical abuse
- Few friends; being kept away from friends
- Unemployment
- Emotional dependence and insecurity
- Belief in strict gender roles—men are dominant and aggressive in relationships; men make family decisions; women stay at home and do not work; women are submissive (obey, follow orders) to men
- Desire for power and control in relationships

Risk Factors—The Victim or Abuser—cont'd

- Emotional dependence, insecurity
- Being a victim of abuse
- Having poor parenting as a child
- Having been physically disciplined as a child
- Marital conflicts—fights, tension, other struggles
- Divorce or marital separation
- Control by 1 partner over another
- Financial stress or hardship
- Unhealthy family relationships or interactions

Warning Signs

- Unwanted physical or sexual contact
- Threats to you, your children, family members, or pets
- Threats of suicide to get you to do something
- Using or threatening to use a weapon against you
- Keeping or taking your paycheck
- Saying things to put you down or make you feel bad
- Keeping you from seeing family or friends
- Keeping you from going to work

Modified from Centers for Disease Control and Prevention: Intimate partner violence: risk and protective factors for perpetration, Atlanta, last reviewed October 23, 2018.

FOCUS ON **CHILDREN AND OLDER PERSONS**

Intimate Partner Violence

Children

Teenagers can be victims of dating violence (Chapter 11). The CDC describes *teen dating violence as physical, sexual, or psychological or emotional violence within a dating relationship. It includes stalking.* Teen dating violence can occur:

- In person or electronically
- With a current or former dating partner

Victims of teen dating violence are at risk for depression and anxiety, unhealthy behaviors (tobacco, drug, and alcohol use), and antisocial behaviors (Chapter 52). Suicide thoughts and attempts are other risks.

PROMOTING SAFETY AND COMFORT

Intimate Partner Violence

Safety

Intimate partner violence occurs in relationships. Partners may be:

- Married
- Not married but living together
- Dating
- Divorced or separated
- Female and male; male and male; female and female

If you are a victim of abuse, call 911 or the police. Tell the police everything that happened—the abuser, what happened, marks on your body, and so on. Answer their questions honestly and completely. The police can help you and your children to a safe place. They can give you information about IPV, IPV programs and shelters, and how to develop a personal safety plan.

FOCUS ON **LONG-TERM CARE AND HOME CARE**

Intimate Partner Violence

Long-Term Care

Under OBRA, the resident has the right to be free from abuse, mistreatment, and neglect. If a resident is abused by anyone, the abuse must be reported. This includes abuse by a partner.

WILLS

A *will is a legal document of how a person wants property distributed after death.* You can ethically and legally witness a will signing. Or you can refuse without fear of legal action.

You cannot prepare wills. Politely refuse if asked to do so. Explain that you do not have the legal knowledge or ability to prepare a will. Report the request to the nurse. The nurse will discuss contacting a lawyer with the person or family.

Do not witness a will signing if you are named in the will. Doing so prevents you from getting what was left to you. As a witness, be prepared to testify that:

- The person was of sound mind when the will was signed.
- The person stated that the document was his or her last will.

Many agencies do not let staff witness wills. Know your agency's policy before you agree to witness a will. If you have questions, ask the nurse. If you witness a will, tell the nurse.

FOCUS ON **PRIDE**

The Person, Family, and Yourself

P ersonal and Professional Responsibility

States have laws about *mandatory reporters. Mandatory* means *required.* For example, health care providers may be required to report suspected abuse or neglect of children, vulnerable adults, and elders. Tell the nurse if you suspect abuse or neglect.

Some states require that all persons report suspected mistreatment. Other states allow voluntary reporting. You or someone you know may be in danger. Or you suspect abuse or neglect.

- For dangerous or life-threatening situations—call 911.
- For child abuse or neglect—contact your local child protective services office or the police. Call the Childhelp National Child Abuse Hotline at 1-800-4-A-CHILD (1-800-422-4453).
- For intimate partner violence—the National Domestic Violence Hotline has resources and information. You can call 1-800-799-SAFE (1-800-799-7233) or visit www.thehotline.org.
- For sexual violence—call the National Sexual Assault Hotline at 1-800-656-HOPE (1-800-656-4673).
- For elder abuse, neglect, or exploitation—visit the National Center on Elder Abuse's website.

R ights and Respect

The person has the right to be free from abuse, mistreatment, and neglect. Abuse can take many forms. For example:

- A person constantly crying out for help is left alone with the door closed.
- A person is told to be nice or care will not be given.
- A person is turned in a rough and hurried manner.
- A person lies in a wet and soiled bed all night.
- A person uses the call light a lot. It is removed from the room.
- A person is told that family does not visit because the person is mean.

I ndependence and Social Interaction

You will interact closely with patients, residents, and families. You may begin to know them well. Social and professional relationships differ. Maintain professional boundaries (p. 41).

D elegation and Teamwork

Working within the limits of your role protects persons from harm. You must understand your roles and responsibilities to know when a task is outside these limits. Accepting a task beyond the legal limits of your role can lead to negligence.

E thics and Laws

The following is a real account of an intentional tort committed by a nursing assistant.

A licensed nursing assistant (LNA) worked at a nursing center. Her license was suspended for using a resident's credit card without the resident's knowledge or consent. The LNA signed the resident's name to charges for about $1490. The LNA also took and used a nurse's credit card. Criminal charges of false impersonation were filed against the LNA.

The LNA was charged with:

- *Failing to comply with federal or state laws and rules*
- *Abusing or neglecting a patient*
- *Misappropriating patient property (p. 48)*
- *Being unfit or incompetent to function as a nursing assistant by reason of any cause*
- *Engaging in conduct of a character likely to deceive, defraud, or harm the public*

The LNA's license was suspended indefinitely. This means that the LNA:

- *Had to give her license to the Board.*
- *Could ask the Board to re-instate her license, but she had to prove that:*
  - *She posed no danger to the public or the practice of nursing.*
  - *She would safely and competently perform an LNA's duties.*
  - *She meets the requirements for license renewal and re-instatement.*

(State of Vermont Board of Nursing, 2000.)

FOCUS ON **PRIDE**: *Application*

A code of conduct guides your thinking and behavior. Write a personal code of conduct stating what you expect of yourself as a nursing assistant.

REVIEW QUESTIONS

Circle the BEST answer.

1 Ethics is
a Making judgments before you have the facts
b Knowledge of right and wrong conduct
c A behavior that meets your needs, not the person's
d A health team member's skill, care, and judgment

2 Which is ethical behavior?
a Sharing information about a person with a friend
b Accepting gifts from a resident's family
c Reporting errors
d Calling your family before answering a call light

3 On your days off, you call the agency to check on a patient. This is a
a Professional boundary
b Tort
c Boundary violation
d Boundary sign

4 To maintain professional boundaries, focus on
a Helping the person
b Meeting your needs
c Being biased
d Showing that you care

5 You help with a friend's hospital care. This is a
a Professional boundary
b Boundary crossing
c Tort
d Crime

6 Abuse is a crime.
a True
b False

7 These statements are about negligence. Which is *true?*
a It is an intentional tort.
b The negligent person acted in a reasonable manner.
c The person or the person's property was harmed.
d A prison term is likely.

8 Threatening to touch the person's body without the person's consent is
a Assault
b Battery
c Defamation
d False imprisonment

9 Restraining a person's freedom of movement is
a Neglect
b Invasion of privacy
c Defamation
d False imprisonment

10 Sharing a resident's photo on a social media site is
a Fraud
b Allowed with the family's consent
c A violation of HIPAA
d Allowed if you obtain informed consent

11 You tell others that you are nurse. This is
a Negligence
b Fraud
c Libel
d Slander

12 Informed consent is when the person
a Fully understands all aspects of treatment
b Signs a consent form
c Is admitted to the agency
d Agrees to a procedure

13 Self-neglect is when
a A caregiver harms a person
b The person's behaviors put him or her at risk for harm
c A person is deprived of food, clothing, hygiene, and shelter
d The person does not receive attention or affection

14 You scold an older person for not eating lunch. This is
a Physical abuse
b Neglect
c Battery
d Emotional or psychological abuse

15 A home care nursing assistant keeps the person's money after shopping for groceries. This is
a Allowed as a tip for services
b A boundary crossing
c Unprofessional but legal
d Financial abuse

16 Which is a sign of elder abuse?
a Stiff joints and joint pain
b Weight gain
c Poor personal hygiene
d Forgetfulness

17 Depriving a child of food, clothing, and shelter is
a Physical abuse
b Neglect
c Abandonment
d Emotional abuse

18 An older adult has a black eye and bruises on the face. These are signs of
a Physical abuse
b Sexual abuse
c Neglect
d Substance abuse

Continued

REVIEW QUESTIONS—cont'd

19 A child is dirty and has a body odor. These are signs of
   a Physical abuse
   b Sexual abuse
   c Neglect
   d Substance abuse

20 Bruising around a child's genitalia is a sign of
   a Physical abuse
   b Sexual abuse
   c Neglect
   d Substance abuse

21 These statements are about intimate partner violence. Which is *true*?
   a It always involves physical harm.
   b It is usually a 1-time event.
   c One partner has control over the other partner.
   d Only 1 type of abuse is usually present.

22 You suspect a resident was abused. You should
   a Tell the nurse
   b Call the police
   c Tell the family
   d Ask the person about the abuse

Answers to Chapter 5 questions are on p. 885.

FOCUS ON PRACTICE
Problem Solving

A resident in your nursing center asks you to bring your children to visit. How will you respond? How do professional boundaries protect the person?

Student and Work Ethics

CHAPTER

6

OBJECTIVES

- Define the key terms and key abbreviation in this chapter.
- Describe the qualities and traits of a successful nursing assistant.
- Describe good health and hygiene practices.
- Explain how to look professional.
- Explain how to plan for childcare and transportation.
- Describe ethical behavior on the job.
- Explain how to manage stress.

- Explain how to problem solve and deal with conflict.
- Explain the aspects of harassment.
- Explain how to resign from a job.
- Identify the common reasons for losing a job.
- Explain the reasons for drug testing.
- Describe unethical student behavior and possible consequences.
- Explain how to promote PRIDE in the person, the family, and yourself.

KEY TERMS

bullying Repeated attacks or threats of fear, distress, or harm by a bully toward a target

burnout A job stress resulting in being physically or mentally exhausted, having doubts about your abilities, and having doubts about the value of your work

confidentiality Trusting others with personal and private information

conflict A clash between opposing interests or ideas

courtesy A polite, considerate, or helpful comment or act

gossip To spread rumors or talk about the private matters of others

harassment To trouble, torment, offend, or worry a person by one's behavior or comments

priority The most important thing at the time

professionalism Following laws, being ethical, having good work ethics, and having the skills to do your work

stress The response or change in the body caused by any emotional, psychological, physical, social, or economic factor

stressor The event or factor that causes stress

teamwork Staff members work together as a group; each person does his or her part to give safe and effective care

work ethics Behavior in the workplace

KEY ABBREVIATION

NATCEP   Nursing assistant training and competency evaluation program

As a student and a nursing assistant, you must act and function in a professional manner. *Professionalism involves following laws, being ethical, having good work ethics, and having the skills to do your work.* Laws and ethics are discussed in Chapter 5. *Laws* are rules of conduct made by government bodies. *Ethics* deals with right and wrong conduct. It involves choices and judgments about what to do or what not to do. An ethical person does the right thing.

Work ethics deals with behavior in the workplace. Certain behaviors (conduct), choices, and judgments are expected. Work ethics involves:
- How you look
- What you say
- How you behave
- How you treat and work with others
- The qualities and traits shown and described in Figure 6-1, p. 58

In this chapter, *work ethics* applies to you as a student. For student success, practice good work ethics in the classroom and clinical setting and with instructors and fellow students.

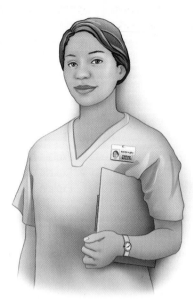

Caring—having concern for the person; making the person's life happier, easier, or less painful

Cheerful—greeting and talking to others in a pleasant manner

Conscientious—being careful, alert, and exact in following instructions; giving thorough care; protecting the person's property

Considerate—respecting the person's physical and emotional feelings; being kind to patients, residents, families, and the health team

Cooperative—helping and working with others willingly; taking an "extra step" during busy and stressful times

Courteous—being polite to patients, residents, families, and the health team

Dependable—reporting to work on time and as scheduled; completing assigments; keeping obligations and promises

Empathy—seeing things from the person's point of view; putting yourself in the person's place

Enthusiastic—being eager, interested, and excited about your work

Honest—reporting the care given, your observations, and any errors accurately

Patient—coping with problems and delays; staying calm rather than getting upset, annoyed, or angry; not rushing the person or a co-worker

Respectful—treating the person with respect and dignity at all times; respecting the person's rights, values, beliefs, and feelings; showing respect for the health team

Self-aware—knowing your feelings, strengths, and weaknesses; understanding yourself so you can understand patients and residents

Trustworthy—keeping information confidential; not gossiping about patients, residents, families, or the health team

FIGURE 6-1 Good work ethics involves these qualities and traits.

HEALTH, HYGIENE, AND APPEARANCE

Patients, residents, families, and visitors expect you to look, act, and be healthy. For example, a person must stop smoking. Yet because you smoke, you and your clothes smell of smoke. If you do not look or smell clean, people wonder if you give good care. Your health, hygiene, and appearance need careful attention.

Your Health

To learn and give safe and effective care, you must be physically and mentally healthy. The following affect your health.

- *Diet.* You need a balanced diet (Chapter 30). Eat a good breakfast. To maintain your weight, balance calorie intake with your energy needs. To lose weight, have fewer calories than your energy needs. Avoid foods high in fat, oil, and sugar. Also avoid salty foods and "crash" diets.
- *Sleep and rest.* Most adults need 7 to 8 hours of sleep daily. Fatigue, lack of energy, and being irritable mean you need more rest and sleep.
- *Body mechanics.* You will bend, carry heavy objects, and move and turn persons. Use your muscles correctly and avoid stress and strain on your body (Chapter 18).

- *Exercise.* Exercise promotes muscle tone, circulation, and weight control. Walking, running, swimming, and hiking are good forms of exercise. Regular exercise promotes physical and mental health. Consult your doctor before starting a vigorous exercise program.
- *Your eyes.* You must read instructions and measurements correctly. Wrong readings and measurements can harm the person. Have your eyes examined. Wear needed eyeglasses or contact lenses. Have good lighting for reading and fine work.
- *Smoking.* Smoke odors stay on your breath, hands, clothing, and hair. Hand-washing and good hygiene are needed.
- *Drugs.* Some drugs affect thinking, feeling, behavior, and function. Working under the influence of drugs affects the person's safety and yours. Take only prescribed drugs in the prescribed way.
- *Alcohol.* Alcohol is a drug that affects thinking, balance, coordination, and alertness. Never go to work under the influence of alcohol. Do not drink alcohol while working. Alcohol affects the person's safety and yours.

Your Hygiene

Your hygiene needs careful attention. Bathe daily. Use a deodorant or antiperspirant to prevent body odors. Brush your teeth often—upon awakening, before and after meals, and at bedtime. Use mouthwash to prevent breath odors. Shampoo often. Keep fingernails clean, short, and smoothly and neatly shaped.

Menstrual hygiene is important. Change tampons or sanitary pads often, especially for heavy flow. Wash your genital area with soap and water at least once a day. Also practice good hand-washing.

Foot care prevents odors and infection. Wash your feet daily. Dry thoroughly between the toes. Cut toenails straight across after bathing or soaking them.

Your Appearance

How you look affects what people think about you and the agency. If staff or students are clean and neat, people think the agency is clean and neat. They think the agency is unclean when staff or students are messy and unkempt. People also question the quality of care given.

You need to look clean, neat, and professional. See Box 6-1 and Figure 6-2, p. 60.

BOX 6-1	**Professional Appearance**

- Practice good hygiene.
- Follow the dress code of your agency or training program for:
  - Uniforms
  - Jewelry
  - Shoes
  - Hair
  - Nails, make-up, and fragrances

Uniforms

- Wear required uniforms. Do not wear home or social attire at work or as a student in the clinical setting. This includes tight, revealing, or sexual clothing. Halter tops, tank tops, low-cut tops, tops with arm slits, jeans, shorts, short skirts, low-rise pants, leggings, yoga pants, or high-cut pants are not worn.
- Uniforms fit well and are modest in length and style. Do not wear tight, revealing, or sexual-looking uniforms.
  - Women—do not show cleavage, tops of breasts, or upper thighs.
  - Men—do not wear tight pants. Do not expose your chest. Open just the top button of your shirt.
- Keep uniforms clean, pressed, and mended. Sew on buttons. Repair zippers, tears, and hems.
- Wear a clean uniform and clean under-garments daily.
- Wear appropriate under-garments for your body shape and uniform.
  - Under-garments are clean and fit properly.
  - Under-garments are the correct color for your skin tone.
  - Colored (red, pink, blue, and so on) and patterned under-garments are not worn. They can be seen through white and light-colored uniforms.
- Wear clean socks or stockings that fit well. Change them daily.
- Wear your name badge or photo ID (identification) according to the dress code. The badge or ID is usually worn above the waist where it can be seen by others (see Fig. 6-2). Agencies may use first and last names or only first names. Your student ID will have your school's name.
- Cover tattoos (body art) with your uniform. Tattoos (body art) may offend others.

Jewelry

- Wear only allowed jewelry.
  - Wedding and engagement rings may be allowed. Do not wear rings that can scratch a person.
  - Bracelets are not allowed. They can scratch a person.
  - Necklaces and dangling earrings are not allowed. Confused or combative persons and young children might pull on them.
  - One set of small, simple earrings is usually allowed.
- Do not wear jewelry in visible piercings—eyebrows, nose, lips, cheek, tongue, or other sites.
- Wear a wristwatch with a second (sweep) hand (Fig. 6-3, p. 60).

Shoes

- Wear shoes that fit, are comfortable, give needed support, and have slip-resistant soles.
  - Do not wear sandals or open-toed shoes.
- Wear clean shoes. Wash or replace shoes and laces as needed.

Hair

- Have a simple, attractive hair-style.
  - Hair is off your collar and away from your face. This includes men with long hair.
- Use simple pins, barrettes, hair ties, clips, bands, or other devices to keep long hair up and in place. This includes men with long hair.
- Keep beards and mustaches clean and trimmed.

Nails, Make-Up, and Fragrances

- Keep fingernails clean, short, and smoothly and neatly shaped. Long or jagged nails can scratch a person.
- Do not wear nail polish. Chipped nail polish may provide a place for microbes to grow.
  - If nail polish is allowed, wear only a light-colored polish.
- Do not wear non-natural nails. Fake and artificial nails and nail extenders are examples. Nails must be natural.
- Use make-up that is modest in amount and moderate in color. Avoid a painted and severe look.
- Do not wear perfume, cologne, or after-shave lotion. The scents (fragrances) may offend, nauseate, or cause breathing problems in patients and residents.

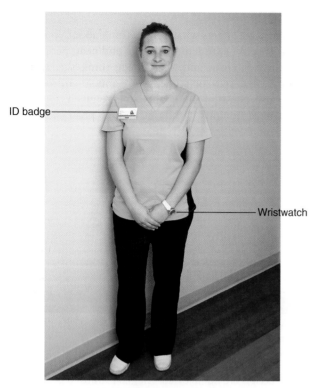

ID badge

Wristwatch

FIGURE 6-2 The nursing assistant is well groomed. Her uniform and shoes are clean. Her hair has a simple style—away from her face and off of her collar. She wears an ID badge and wristwatch. She does not wear jewelry.

PREPARING FOR SCHOOL OR WORK

Being dependable is important as a student and an employee. As a student, you are preparing yourself for work. The classroom and clinical settings help you develop dependable behaviors. To be dependable as a student:

* Arrive on time for class and clinical experiences. Arrive early to store your things, use the restroom, and gather needed items for class or clinical. Be ready for class or clinical to start.
* Complete and turn in assignments on time.
* Pay attention and follow directions.
* Stay for the entire class or clinical experience. To be dependable in the work setting, you must:
* Work when scheduled.
* Get to work on time.
* Stay the entire shift.

Absences and tardiness (being late) can affect your success in school. Your state's nursing assistant training and competency evaluation program (NATCEP) requires a certain number of hours. You must complete the required number of hours.

Absences and tardiness are also common reasons for losing a job. Childcare and transportation issues often interfere with getting to school and work. You need to plan carefully. See "Attendance."

Childcare

Someone needs to care for your children when you leave for school or work, while you are at school or work, and before you get home. Also plan for emergencies.

* Your childcare provider is ill or cannot care for your children that day.
* A child becomes ill or injured while you are at school or work.
* You will be late getting home from school or work.

Transportation

Plan for getting to and from school or work. If you drive, keep your car in good working order. Keep enough gas in the car. Or leave early to get gas.

Carpooling is an option. Carpoolers depend on each other. If the driver is late, everyone is late for school or work. If 1 person is not ready, everyone is late for school or work. Carpool with people you trust to be ready on time. Be on time as a driver and as a passenger.

Know bus or train schedules. Know what bus or train to take if delays occur. Always carry enough money for fares to and from school or work.

Have a back-up transportation plan. Your car may not start, the carpool driver may not be going that day, or public transportation may not run.

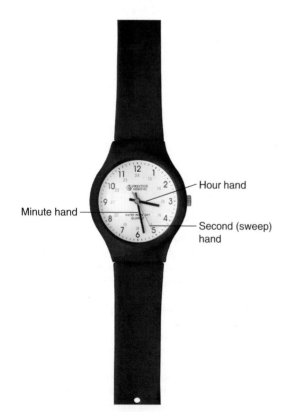

Minute hand

Hour hand

Second (sweep) hand

FIGURE 6-3 A watch with a second (sweep) hand. (Courtesy Prestige Medical, Northridge, California.)

TEAMWORK

Teamwork means that staff members work together as a group. Each person does his or her part to give safe and effective care. Teamwork involves:

- Working when scheduled.
- Being cheerful and friendly.
- Completing assignments.
- Helping others willingly.
- Being kind to others.

You are an important member of the health and nursing teams. Quality of care is affected by how you work with others and how you feel about your job. Some days it might seem that you are doing more than others. Other days, your co-workers may feel that you are not doing enough. Avoid comparing your assignments to what others are doing. Each staff member has a role individually and as a team member.

Attendance

Report to work when scheduled and on time. The entire unit is affected when just 1 person is late. Call the agency if you will be late or cannot go to work. Follow the attendance policy in your employee handbook. Poor attendance can cause you to lose your job.

You must be dependable. Be *ready to work* when your shift starts.

- Store your things before your shift starts.
- Use the restroom when you arrive at the agency.
- Arrive on your nursing unit a few minutes early. Greet others and settle yourself.

You must stay the entire shift. Watching the clock for your shift to end gives a bad image. You may need to work over-time. Prepare to stay longer if necessary. When it is time to leave, report off duty to the nurse.

See *Focus on Communication: Attendance.*
See *Teamwork and Time Management: Attendance.*
See *Focus on Long-Term Care and Home Care: Attendance.*

FOCUS ON COMMUNICATION

Attendance

Illness, a family death, and other emergencies may require an absence. You must tell your instructor or the agency about your absence. Otherwise you could have an unexcused absence from your NATCEP. If working, you could lose your job. To report an absence:

- *Call well before class, clinical, or your shift begins.* See the attendance policy in your student or employee handbook for when to call. At least 2 hours ahead is common.
- *Know who to call.* Students call their instructors. Charge nurses, nurse managers, or supervisors handle absences in the work setting. You may need your call transferred. For example: "Hello. This is Terry Jones. Please transfer me to the charge nurse." You must give information to the right person.
- *Give the reason for your absence.* Be honest. You can say: "I am sorry. I will be absent from work (class, clinical) today. I have a fever and a cough."
- *Give the length of your absence.* People often miss 1 or 2 days for illness or a family emergency. Longer absences require more communication.

TEAMWORK AND TIME MANAGEMENT

Attendance

A staff member may be late for work. Or someone is absent from work. Until a replacement arrives, you and other staff have extra work. Patient and resident care cannot suffer.

To promote teamwork and manage your time:
- Ask the nurse how you can help.
- Do not complain about not having enough staff.
- Ask the nurse to list the most important tasks and care measures.

FOCUS ON LONG-TERM CARE AND HOME CARE

Attendance

Home Care

You must complete home care assignments. Never leave in the middle of an assignment or before someone from the next shift arrives. Leaving before completing an assignment is *abandonment* (Chapter 5).

Sometimes problems occur in the home setting. Try to finish the assignment. Explain the problem to the nurse who will try to make needed changes. Do not walk out on (abandon) the person. Walking out (abandonment) is abuse, unsafe for the person, and very unethical behavior (Chapter 5).

See "Workplace Violence" in Chapter 13.

Your Attitude

You need a good attitude. Show that you enjoy your work. Listen to others. Be willing to learn. Stay busy and use your time well.

You and your work are important and have value. Nurses, patients, residents, and families rely on you for good care. They want you to be pleasant and respectful.

Always think before you speak. These statements signal a bad attitude.

- "That's not my resident (patient)."
- "I can't. I'm too busy."
- "I didn't do it."
- "I don't feel like it."
- "It's not my fault."
- "Don't blame me."
- "It's not my turn. I did it yesterday."
- "Nobody told me."
- "That's not my job."
- "You didn't say that you needed it right away."
- "I did more than she (he) did."
- "I work harder than anyone else."
- "No one appreciates what I do."
- "I'm tired of this place."
- "Is it time to leave yet?"
- "Good luck. I had a horrible day."

Gossip

To *gossip means to spread rumors or talk about the private matters of others.* Gossiping is unprofessional and hurtful. To avoid gossip:

- Remove yourself from where people are gossiping.
- Do not make or repeat any comment that can hurt any person—patient or resident, family member, visitor, co-worker, fellow student, instructor, the school or agency, and so on.
- Do not make or write false statements about another person. See Chapter 5.
- Do not talk about patients, residents, family members, visitors, co-workers, fellow students, instructors, the school or agency, or others at home or in social settings.
- Do not send or post comments about others or the school or agency by e-mail, instant messaging, text messaging, video sites, social media, or other electronic means. This is especially true of hurtful, false, or private comments. See "Wrongful Use of Electronic Communications" in Chapter 5.

Confidentiality

The person's information is private and personal. *Confidentiality means trusting others with personal and private information.* The person's information is shared only among staff involved in his or her care. The person has the right to privacy and confidentiality. Agency, family, co-worker, and student information also is confidential.

Share information only with the nurse or your instructor. Do not talk about patients, residents, families, the agency, or co-workers when others are present. Do not talk about them in hallways, elevators, dining areas, or outside the agency. Others may over-hear you and eavesdrop. To *eavesdrop* means *to listen in or over-hear what others are saying.* It invades a person's privacy.

Patients, residents, and visitors are very alert to comments. They think you are talking about them or their loved ones. This leads to wrong information and wrong impressions about the person's condition. You can easily upset or hurt the person or family. Be very careful about what, how, when, and where you say things.

Many agencies have intercom systems. They allow for communication between the bedside and the nurses' station (Chapter 21). The person uses the intercom to call for help. The intercom is answered at the nurses' station. The nursing team also uses the intercom to communicate with each other. Be careful what you say. The intercom is like a loud speaker. Others nearby can hear what you are saying.

See *Focus on Communication: Confidentiality.*

FOCUS ON COMMUNICATION

Confidentiality

Your family and friends may ask about patients, residents, families, or staff. For example, your mother says: "I heard my neighbor is in your nursing home. Do you know what's wrong?"

Do not share any information with your family and friends. Doing so violates the person's right to privacy and confidentiality (Chapters 2 and 5). You can say:

I'm sorry, but I can't tell you about anyone in the center. It is unprofessional and against center policies. And it violates the person's right to privacy and confidentiality. Please don't ask me about anyone in the center.

Speech and Language

Your speech and language must be professional. Some words used in home and social settings are not proper in class, the clinical setting, and at work. Such words may offend patients, residents, families, visitors, and co-workers. Remember:

- Do not swear or use foul, vulgar, slang, sexual, or abusive language.
- Speak softly and gently.
- Speak clearly. Hearing problems are common.
- Do not shout or yell.
- Do not fight or argue with a patient or resident, family member, visitor, co-worker, your instructor, or a fellow student.

Courtesies

A *courtesy is a polite, considerate, or helpful comment or act.* Courtesies take little time or energy. Even the smallest kind act can brighten someone's day.

- Address others by Miss, Mrs., Ms., Mr., or Doctor. Or use the name the person prefers. Do not call your instructor by his or her first name.
- Say "please." Begin or end each request with "please."
- Say "thank you" when someone does something for you or helps you.
- Apologize. Say "I'm sorry" when you make a mistake or hurt someone. Even little things—like bumping someone in the hallway—need an apology.
- Be thoughtful. Compliment others. Wish others a happy birthday, day or weekend off, or holiday.
- Wish the person and family well when they leave the agency. "Stay well" and "stay healthy" are examples.
- Hold doors and elevator doors open for others. If at the door first, open the door and let others pass through.
- Let patients, residents, families, and visitors enter elevators first.
- Stand to greet families and visitors.
- Help others willingly when asked.
- Give praise. When a co-worker or student does something that impresses you, tell that person. Also tell your co-workers or other students.
- Do not take credit for another person's deeds. Give the person credit for the action.

Personal Matters

Personal matters must not interfere with your job. Otherwise care is neglected. You could lose your job. To keep personal matters out of the workplace:

- Make phone calls during meals and breaks.
- Do not let family and friends visit you on the unit. If they must see you, meet them during a meal or break.
- Make appointments (doctor, dentist, lawyer, and others) for your days off.
- Do not use agency computers, printers, fax machines, copiers, or other equipment for your personal use.
- Do not take the agency's supplies (pens, paper, and others) for your personal use.
- Do not discuss personal problems.
- Control your emotions. If you need to cry or express anger, do so in private. Get yourself together quickly and return to your work.
- Do not borrow money from or lend it to co-workers or fellow students. This includes meal money and bus or train fares. Borrowing and lending can lead to problems with co-workers and students.
- Do not sell things or engage in fund-raising. For example, do not sell your child's candy or raffle tickets to co-workers or other students.
- Turn off personal phones and other electronic devices.
- Do not send or check e-mails, text messages, or other electronic messages.

Meals and Breaks

Meal breaks are usually 30 minutes. Other breaks are usually 15 minutes. Meals and breaks are scheduled with some staff always on the unit. Staff on the unit cover for the staff away on break.

Staff members depend on each other. Leave for and return from breaks on time. Other staff need their turn. Do not take longer than allowed. Tell the nurse when you leave and return to the unit.

Staff or student break rooms usually have tables and chairs, a microwave, refrigerator, and sink. Some have coffee makers, cups, and utensils. Do not leave a mess. Clean up after yourself before leaving the break room. Follow school or agency policies for keeping food and drinks in the refrigerator. Discard or take home food and food containers daily.

Job Safety

You must protect patients, residents, families, visitors, co-workers, and yourself from harm. Negligent acts affect the safety of others (Chapter 5). Safety practices are presented throughout this book. The following guidelines apply to everything you do.

- Understand the roles, functions, and responsibilities in your job description.
- Follow agency rules, policies, and procedures.
- Know what is right and wrong conduct.
- Know what you can and cannot do.
- Develop the desired qualities and traits in Figure 6-1.
- Follow the nurse's directions and instructions.
- Question unclear directions and things you do not understand.
- Help others willingly when asked.
- Ask for any training you might need.
- Report accurately—measurements, observations, the care given, the person's complaints, and any errors (Chapters 8 and 13).
- Be responsible for your actions. Admit when you are wrong or make mistakes. Do not blame others. Do not make excuses. Learn what you did wrong and why. Try to learn from your mistakes.
- Handle the person's property carefully and prevent damage.
- Follow the safety measures in Chapter 13 and throughout this book. Also see the *Promoting Safety and Comfort* boxes throughout this book.

Planning Your Work

Some care measures and nursing unit tasks are done at certain times. Others are done at the end of the shift. Deciding what to do and when is called *priority setting*. A *priority is the most important thing at the time.* To set your priorities, decide:

- Who has the greatest or most life-threatening needs.
- What task the nurse or person needs done first.
- What tasks need to be done at a certain time.
- What tasks need to be done when your shift starts and at the end of your shift.
- How long it takes to complete a task.
- How much help you need to complete a task.
- Who can help you and when.

Priorities change as the person's needs change. A person's condition can improve or worsen. New patients and residents are admitted. Others are transferred to other nursing units or discharged. These and many other factors can change priorities.

Setting priorities becomes easier with experience. Ask your instructor or the nurse to help you set priorities. Plan your work to give safe, thorough care and to use your time well (Box 6-2).

BOX 6-2	Planning Your Work

- Discuss priorities with the nurse.
- Know the routine of your shift and nursing unit.
- Follow unit policies for shift reports. In an *end-of-shift report,* the nurse gives a report to the on-coming shift (Chapter 8).
- List tasks that are on a schedule. For example, some persons are turned or offered the bedpan every 2 hours.
- Judge how much time you need for each person and task.
- Identify tasks to do while patients and residents are eating, visiting, or involved with activities or therapies.
- Plan care around meal times, visiting hours, and therapies. Consider recreation and social activities.
- Identify when you will need help from a co-worker. Ask a co-worker to help you. Give the time when you will need help and for how long.
- Schedule equipment or rooms for the person's use. The shower room is an example.
- Review your assignment sheet (Chapter 8). Gather needed supplies ahead of time.
- Do not waste time. Stay focused on your work.
- Leave a clean work area. Make sure rooms and utility areas are neat and orderly.
- Be a self-starter. Have initiative. Ask others if they need help. Follow unit routines, stock supply areas, and clean utility rooms. Stay busy.

STRESS

Stress is the response or change in the body caused by any emotional, psychological, physical, social, or economic factor. Stress is normal. It occurs every minute of every day and in everything you do.

A *stressor is the event or factor that causes stress.* Many stressors are pleasant—a child playing, a party, laughing with family and friends, a nice day. Some are not pleasant—illness, injury, family problems, death of loved ones, divorce, money concerns. School and some parts of your job are stressful.

No matter the cause—pleasant or unpleasant—stress affects the whole person (Chapter 7).

- Physically—sweating, rapid heart rate, faster and deeper breathing, increased blood pressure, dry mouth, and so on
- Mentally—anxiety, fear, anger, dread, apprehension, and defense mechanisms (Chapter 52)
- Socially—changes in relationships, avoiding others, needing others, blaming others, and so on
- Spiritually—changes in beliefs and values and strengthening or questioning one's beliefs in God or a higher power

Prolonged or frequent stress threatens physical and mental health. Some problems are often minor—headaches, stomach upset, sleep problems, muscle tension, and so on. Others are life-threatening—high blood pressure, heart attack, stroke, ulcers, and so on.

School, job, and personal stresses affect your family, friends, studies, or work. Stress affects you, the care you give, the person's quality of life, and how you relate to co-workers.

Burnout

Burnout is a job stress resulting in:
- *Being physically or mentally exhausted*
- *Having doubts about your abilities*
- *Having doubts about the value of your work*

Burnout occurs over time. Causes, signs, and symptoms are listed in Box 6-3. Burnout can cause physical and mental health problems. They include fatigue, sleep problems, depression, anxiety, alcohol or substance abuse, heart disease, diabetes, stroke, and weight gain. Problems can develop at home and with personal relationships.

BOX 6-3	**Burnout—Causes, Signs, and Symptoms**

Causes of Burnout
- Schedules, assignments, or workloads that you find difficult
- Not being comfortable with your supervisor or co-workers
- Being harassed, bullied, or heavily criticized by your supervisor or a co-worker
- Conflicts with how problems and grievances are handled
- Not liking your job or the agency
- Having skills that are greater than or lesser than what the job requires
- Lacking emotional support at work, at home, or socially
- Lacking balance between work and home, family, and social life

Signs and Symptoms of Burnout
- Lack of energy
- Sense of dread about going to work; not wanting to go to work
- Sleep problems
- Forgetfulness
- Problems concentrating
- Frequent illness—infection, cold, influenza
- Physical symptoms:
  - Chest pain
  - Rapid or irregular heartbeat
  - Shortness of breath
  - Gastro-intestinal pain
  - Dizziness
  - Fainting
  - Headaches
  - Loss of appetite
- Anxiety
- Anger
- Depression
- Irritability
- Wanting to be alone
- Calling in sick; going to work late

Managing Stress

To reduce or cope with stress:
- Exercise regularly. Physical and mental benefits include cardiovascular health, weight control, tension release, emotional well-being, and relaxation.
- Get enough rest and sleep.
- Eat healthy.
- Plan personal and quiet time for you. Read, take a hot bath, go for a walk, meditate, or listen to music. Do what makes you feel good.
- Use common sense about what you can and cannot do. Do not try to do everything that others ask you to do. Consider the amount of time and energy that you have.
- Do 1 thing at a time. You may feel overwhelmed with demands. List each thing to do. Set priorities.
- Do not judge yourself harshly. Do not try to be perfect or expect too much from yourself.
- Give yourself praise. You do good and wonderful things every day.
- Have a sense of humor. Laugh at yourself. Laugh with others. Spend time with those who make you laugh.
- Have a social life that does not include co-workers.
- Talk to the nurse if your work or a person is causing too much stress. The nurse can help you deal with the matter.

Dealing With Conflict

People bring their values, attitudes, opinions, experiences, and expectations to school and work settings. Differences often lead to conflict. *Conflict is a clash between opposing interests or ideas.* People disagree and argue. There are misunderstandings and unrest.

Conflicts arise over issues or events. Work schedules, absences, and the amount and quality of work are examples. The problems must be resolved (settled, worked out, solved). Otherwise, unkind words or actions may occur. The learning or work setting becomes unpleasant. Care is affected.

Resolving Conflict. *Problem solving* steps are used to resolve conflict.

- Step 1: Define the problem. *A nurse ignores me.*
- Step 2: Collect information about the problem. Do not include unrelated information. *The nurse does not look at me. The nurse does not talk to me. The nurse does not respond when I ask for help. The nurse does not ask me to help with tasks that require 2 people. The nurse talks to other staff members.*
- Step 3: Identify possible solutions. *Ignore the nurse. Talk to my supervisor. Talk to co-workers about the problem. Change jobs.*
- Step 4: Select the best solution. *Talk to my supervisor.*
- Step 5: Carry out the solution. *See below.*
- Step 6: Evaluate the results. *See below.*

Communication and good work ethics help prevent and resolve conflicts. Identify and solve problems before they become major issues. To deal with conflict:

- Ask your instructor or supervisor for time to talk privately. Explain the problem. Give facts and specific examples. Ask for advice to solve the problem.
- Approach the person with whom you have the conflict. Ask to talk privately. Be polite and professional.
- Agree on a time and place to talk.
- Talk in a private setting. No one should hear you or the other person.
- Explain the problem and what is bothering you. Give facts and specific behaviors. Focus on the problem. Do not focus on the person.
- Listen to the person. Do not interrupt.
- Identify ways to solve the problem. Offer your thoughts. Ask for the other person's ideas.
- Set a date and time to review the matter.
- Thank the person for meeting with you.
- Carry out the solution.
- Review the matter as scheduled.

See *Focus on Communication: Resolving Conflict.*

FOCUS ON COMMUNICATION

Resolving Conflict

Dealing with conflict is hard for many people. However, letting the problem continue will make the matter worse. The following may help you start talking to the person. Always ask the person involved if you can talk privately.

- "You say 'no' when I ask you to help me. I help you when asked. This bothers me. Can we talk privately for a few minutes?"
- "I heard you tell Sam that I was sitting in a resident's room. You seemed angry when you said it. Can we talk privately? I want to explain why I was sitting and find out why that bothers you."
- "The new schedule shows me working every weekend this month. Please tell me why. The employee handbook says that we work every other weekend."
- "We were late for class 2 times this week when you drove. How can I help so that we are not late?"

HARASSMENT

Harassment means to trouble, torment, offend, or worry a person by one's behavior or comments. Harassment can be sexual or involve age, race, ethnic background, religion, or disability. Respect others. Do not offend others with gestures, remarks, use of touch, or through electronic communications. Do not offend others with jokes, photos, or other images (pictures, drawings, cartoons, and so on). Harassment is not legal.

You have the right not to be harassed. No co-worker or student (in your NATCEP or otherwise) should be allowed to harass or bully you. The same applies to a co-worker, instructor, other school instructors or staff, and clinical staff. If you believe that you are being harassed or bullied, talk to your supervisor, instructor, or school counselor. Follow the steps in "Resolving Conflict."

See *Focus on Communication: Harassment.*

FOCUS ON COMMUNICATION

Harassment

You have the right to feel safe and not threatened. If comments make you uncomfortable, you can say: "Please don't say things like that. It's unprofessional." If someone's actions make you uneasy, you can say: "Please don't do that. It's unprofessional." Leave the area. Report the person's statements or actions to the nurse or your instructor.

Sexual Harassment

Sexual harassment involves unwanted sexual behaviors by another. The behavior may be a sexual advance or a request for a sexual favor. Some remarks, comments, and touch are sexual. The behavior affects work and comfort. In extreme cases, a job (or grade) is threatened if sexual favors are not granted.

Sexual harassment can take the form of sexting. *Sexting* combines the words *sex* and *texting*. Sexting involves creating, sending, and posting sexual text messages, photos, or videos of oneself or others. Phones and other electronic devices are used.

Victims of sexual harassment may be men or women. Men harass women or men. Women harass men or women. If you feel sexually harassed, report the matter to the nurse and the human resources officer. As a student, tell your instructor and school counselor.

Be careful about what you say or do. Even innocent remarks and behaviors can be viewed as sexual harassment. You might not be sure about your own or another person's remarks or behaviors. If so, talk to your instructor or the nurse. You cannot be too careful.

Bullying

Bullying is repeated attacks or threats of fear, distress, or harm by a bully toward a target. A bully tries to gain power and control over a target. Bullying can occur in work, classroom, clinical, or social settings. See Box 6-4 for the types of bullying.

Bullying can result in injury, emotional distress, and even death. Victims of bullying are at risk for depression, anxiety, sleep problems, and poor school or work performance. Those who bully are at risk for substance abuse, school or work problems, and violence.

Talk to your instructor or supervisor if you are being bullied. He or she will try to help you with the situation.

RESIGNING FROM A JOB

A job closer to home, better pay, or new opportunities may prompt you to leave your job. School, children, and illness are other reasons. Whatever your reason for resigning, tell your employer. Agency policy may require:

- A written notice
- A resignation letter
- Completing a form in the human resources office

A 2-week notice is a good practice. Do not leave without notice. Include the following in your notice.

- Reason for leaving
- The last date you will work
- Comments thanking the employer for the opportunity to work in the agency

An exit interview (on or before your last day) or an exit survey is common practice. You are asked about the agency, your job, and how the agency can improve.

BOX 6-4	Bullying

- *Physical bullying.* Physical attacks are used. Hitting, kicking, punching, shoving, slapping, and tripping are examples. Physical bullies are usually stronger and bigger than their targets.

- *Verbal bullying.* Words are used. Name-calling, insults, and teasing are used to hurt and humiliate the target. (*Humiliate* means *to cause shame or a loss of pride, self-respect, or dignity.*) Targets are chosen by the way they look, act, or behave.

- *Emotional bullying.* A bully tries to hurtfully exclude a target from a group. The target is shunned or is the victim of hurtful rumors.

- *Cyber-bullying.* Electronic means are used—e-mail, chat rooms, instant messaging, text messaging, videos, photos, and social media sites. The bully sends, posts, or shares things that are negative, harmful, hurtful, false, or mean about the target. Often cruel, cyber-bullying can occur 24 hours a day.

- *Sexual bullying.* A person, often a female, is targeted with repeated and harmful actions of a sexual nature. Examples include name-calling, making crude and vulgar comments or gestures, touching without consent, and suggesting sexual acts. Such actions may be directed at appearance, body shape, or sexual activity. Also see "Sexual Harassment."

- *Prejudicial bullying.* To be *prejudiced* means *to have an opinion or an attitude about a matter without factual knowledge.* The focus may be a target's race, ethnicity, religion, or sexual orientation (Chapter 55). The bully may engage in physical, verbal, emotional, cyber, or sexual bullying.

Modified from Gordon S: 6 types of bullying every parent should know about, *updated March 30, 2019, verywellfamily.com and referenced in Miller M:* 5 ways to prevent bullying on college campuses, *June 2, 2016, campusanswers.com.*

LOSING A JOB

You must perform your job well and protect patients and residents from harm. No pay raise or losing your job results from poor performance. Failing to follow agency policy is often grounds for termination. So is failing to get along with others. Box 6-5 lists the many reasons why you can lose your job. To protect your job, function at your best. Always practice good work ethics.

DRUG TESTING

Drug and alcohol use affect patient, resident, and staff safety. Quality of care suffers. Drug or alcohol users are late to work or absent more often than staff who do not use such substances. Therefore drug testing policies are common. Review your agency's policy for when and how you might be tested.

UNETHICAL STUDENT BEHAVIOR

Your NATCEP and school will likely have a code of conduct (Chapter 5). Violating the code of conduct is unethical behavior. Many of the reasons listed in Box 6-5 are violations of your school's and NATCEP's code of conduct. As a result, your school and NATCEP may take 1 or more of the following actions.

- Dismiss you from the school or NATCEP
- Issue a failing grade
- Not recommend that you take the competency evaluation (written and skills tests)

Act in an ethical manner at all times. Always try to do the right thing. If you do, you will be a successful nursing assistant.

BOX 6-5	Common Reasons for Losing a Job

- Poor attendance—not going to work or excessive tardiness (being late).
- Abandonment—leaving the job during your shift.
- Falsifying a record—job application or a person's record.
- Violent behavior in the workplace.
- Weapons in the workplace—guns, knives, explosives, or other dangerous items.
- Having, using, or distributing alcohol or drugs in the work setting. This excludes having or using drugs ordered by your doctor.
- Taking a person's drugs for your own use or giving them to others.
- Harassment (p. 66).
- Offensive speech and language.
- Stealing or destroying the agency's or a person's property.
- Disrespect to patients, residents, families, visitors, co-workers, or supervisors.
- Abusing or neglecting a person.
- Invading a person's privacy.
- Failing to maintain patient, resident, family, agency, or co-worker confidentiality. This includes access to computer and other electronic information.
- Wrongful use of electronic communications (Chapter 5).
- Using the agency's supplies and equipment for your own use.
- Defamation—see Chapter 5 and "Gossip" (p. 62).
- Abusing meal breaks and break time.
- Sleeping on the job.
- Violating the agency's dress code.
- Violating any agency policy or care procedure.
- Tending to personal matters while on duty.

FOCUS ON **PRIDE**

The Person, Family, and Yourself

Personal and Professional Responsibility

You are responsible for your behavior in the workplace. How you act makes a difference. An *Employee Handbook* of OSF Saint Francis Medical Center (Peoria, Ill.) said it well.

> *You are what people see when they arrive here; yours are the eyes they look into when they're frightened and lonely. Yours are the voices people hear when they ride the elevators, when they try to sleep, and when they try to forget their problems. You are what they hear on their way to appointments which could affect their destinies, and what they hear after they leave those appointments. Yours are the comments people hear when you think they can't.*
>
> *Yours is the intelligence and caring that people hope they'll find here. If you're noisy, so is the medical center. If you're rude, so is the medical center. And if you're wonderful, so is the medical center.*

You can help the person feel cared for, safe, and secure. By practicing good work ethics, you can make others' lives happier, easier, and less painful.

Rights and Respect

Conflict with other students and co-workers will arise. Do not gossip, put others down, or talk about people behind their backs. These behaviors are disrespectful and not professional.

Independence and Social Interaction

Smile and greet patients and residents by name. Politely introduce yourself. Display a caring and friendly manner all the time. Remain calm and helpful in stressful situations. These actions promote good relationships and reflect well on you and the agency.

Delegation and Teamwork

Your work ethics affect the team. Greet co-workers pleasantly. Help others willingly. After completing tasks, ask if you can help with anything else. Be someone others enjoy working with.

Ethics and Laws

As a student and nursing assistant, you are responsible for following the ethical guidelines in this chapter. Patients, residents, families, visitors, and co-workers depend on you for safe and effective care.

FOCUS ON **PRIDE**: *Application*

Think of a person you enjoy working with. What qualities do you value in a co-worker? How will you apply these qualities in your work?

REVIEW QUESTIONS

Circle T *if the statement is TRUE and* F *if it is FALSE.*

1 T F You wear needed eyeglasses. This helps protect the person's safety.

2 T F Childcare requires planning before going to school.

3 T F Being on time for work means arriving at the agency when your shift starts.

4 T F You share confidential information with a friend. You could lose your job.

5 T F You must be careful what you say over the intercom system.

6 T F You do not follow the agency's dress code. You could lose your job.

7 T F You can use your phone to send text messages during your clinical experiences.

8 T F You must follow the agency's attendance policy.

9 T F Harassment is legal in the workplace.

10 T F Excluding a student and spreading rumors are forms of bullying.

11 T F The agency cannot test you for drug use.

Circle the BEST answer.

12 Which will help you do your job well?
a Sleeping 3 to 4 hours daily
b Avoiding exercise
c Using drugs and alcohol
d Having good nutrition

13 Which is a good hygiene practice?
a Bathing weekly
b Wearing strongly scented perfume or cologne
c Brushing teeth after meals
d Having long and polished fingernails

14 You are getting ready for clinical. Which is a good practice?
a Styling hair up and off your collar
b Wearing jewelry
c Wearing your name badge at waist level
d Having tattoos exposed

15 Which statement reflects a good attitude?
a "It's not my fault."
b "I can help you."
c "That's not my job."
d "I did it yesterday. It's your turn."

16 A co-worker tells you that a doctor and nurse are dating. This is
a Gossip
b Eavesdropping
c Confidential information
d Sexual harassment

17 Which is professional speech and language?
a Using vulgar words
b Shouting
c Arguing
d Speaking clearly

18 Which is a courteous act?
a Telling co-workers they did a good job
b Calling a resident "Honey"
c Taking credit for a co-worker's work
d Closing an elevator door as a person approaches

19 You are on a meal break. Which is *true?*
a You cannot make personal phone calls.
b Family members cannot meet you.
c The nurse needs to know that you are off the unit.
d You can take a few extra minutes if needed.

20 When planning your work
a Discuss priorities with the nurse
b Delegate tasks you will not have time to do
c Do not ask co-workers for help
d Plan care so that you can watch the person's TV

21 These statements are about stress. Which is *true?*
a Personal stress does not affect work.
b Stress affects the whole person.
c All stress is unpleasant.
d Stress is abnormal.

22 Thinking about work makes you irritable and anxious. Which action is *best?*
a Ignore the feelings.
b Resign from your job.
c Call in absent.
d Try healthy coping strategies.

23 You have extra work because a co-worker is often late. To resolve the conflict
a Explain the problem to your supervisor
b Refuse to work with the person
c Ignore the problem
d Complain about the person to co-workers

24 Which statement about harassment is *true?*
a Giving a resident a compliment is harassment.
b Joking about a person's religion is not harassment.
c Harassment can occur through text messages.
d Only women are victims of harassment.

25 You are often late for work. Which is *true?*
a Tardiness is excused if you give the reason.
b You may be fined.
c You can make up the time by skipping your break.
d You can lose your job.

26 To show good ethics as a student
a Resolve other students' conflicts
b Follow your NATCEP's dress code
c Report an absence when you return to school
d Tell your family about residents at your clinical site

Answers to Chapter 6 questions are on p. 885.

FOCUS ON **PRACTICE**

Problem Solving

A co-worker did not show up for work. You and the other staff members have extra work. How do you respond? How will you plan, prioritize, and manage the extra work?

Communicating With the Person

OBJECTIVES

- Define the key terms in this chapter.
- Identify the parts that make up the whole person.
- Explain how to properly address the person.
- Explain Abraham Maslow's theory of basic needs.
- Explain how culture and religion influence health and illness.
- Identify the emotional and social effects of illness.
- Describe the persons cared for in health care agencies.
- Identify the elements needed for good communication.
- Describe how to use verbal and nonverbal communication.

- Explain the methods and barriers to good communication.
- Explain how to communicate with persons who have special needs.
- Explain why family and visitors are important to the person.
- Identify courtesies given to the person, family, and friends.
- Explain how to communicate with persons who have behavior problems.
- Explain how to promote PRIDE in the person, the family, and yourself.

KEY TERMS

bariatrics The field of medicine focused on the treatment and control of obesity

body language Messages sent through facial expressions, gestures, posture, hand and body movements, gait, eye contact, and appearance

comatose Being unable to respond to stimuli

communication The exchange of information—a message sent is received and correctly interpreted by the intended person

culture The characteristics of a group of people—language, values, beliefs, habits, likes, dislikes, customs—passed from 1 generation to the next

disability Any lost, absent, or impaired physical or mental function

esteem The worth, value, or opinion one has of a person

geriatrics The field of medicine concerned with the problems and diseases of old age and older persons

holism A concept that considers the whole person; the whole person has physical, social, psychological, and spiritual parts that are woven together and cannot be separated

morbid obesity Weighing 100 pounds or more over one's normal weight

need Something necessary or desired for maintaining life and mental well-being

nonverbal communication Communication that does not use words

obesity Having an excess amount of total body fat; body weight is 20% or more above what is normal for the person's height and age

obstetrics The field of medicine concerned with the care of women during pregnancy, labor, and childbirth and for 6 to 8 weeks after birth

optimal level of function A person's highest potential for mental and physical performance

paraphrasing Re-stating the person's message in your own words

pediatrics The field of medicine concerned with the growth, development, and care of children—newborns to teenagers

psychiatry The field of medicine concerned with mental health disorders

religion Spiritual beliefs, needs, and practices

self-actualization Experiencing one's potential

self-esteem Thinking well of oneself and seeing oneself as useful and having value

verbal communication Communication that uses written or spoken words

The patient or resident is the most important person in the agency. Each person is unique and has value. You must treat the person with respect—as someone who thinks, acts, feels, and makes decisions. Each has needs, fears, and rights. Each has suffered losses—loss of home, family, friends, and body functions.

Good communication is needed to give effective care. *Communication is the exchange of information—a message sent is received and correctly interpreted by the intended person.*

You communicate with the person every time you give care. You give information to the person. The person gives information to you.

An understanding of the whole person is important. Many other factors affect communication—basic needs, culture and religion, illness and disability, and family are examples.

THE WHOLE PERSON

Holism means *whole.* **Holism** *is a concept that considers the whole person. The whole person has physical, social, psychological, and spiritual parts. These parts are woven together and cannot be separated* (Fig. 7-1).

Each part relates to and depends on the others. As a social being, a person speaks and communicates with others. Physically, the brain, mouth, tongue, lips, and throat structures must function for speech. Communication is also psychological. It involves thinking and reasoning.

Health care involves the whole person. To consider only the physical part is to ignore the person's ability to think, make decisions, and interact with others. It also ignores experiences, life-style, culture, religion, joys, sorrows, and needs.

Disability and illness affect the whole person. For example, a person needs help with physical needs in a nursing center. No longer at home, family relationships are changed. The person is angry. Life changes cause the person to doubt spiritual beliefs. The health team plans care to address the person's physical, emotional, social, and spiritual problems.

Addressing the Person

You must know and respect the whole person for effective, quality care. Too often a person is referred to as a room number. For example: "12A needs the bedpan" rather than "Mrs. Olson in 12A needs the bedpan." This strips the person of his or her identity.

To address patients and residents with dignity and respect:

- Greet the person by title—Mrs. Jones, Mr. Wills, Miss Parker, Ms. Norris, or Dr. Gonzalez. Then ask what name the person prefers.
- Do not use their first names or any other name unless they ask you to.
- Do not call them Grandma, Papa, Sweetheart, Honey, or other names.

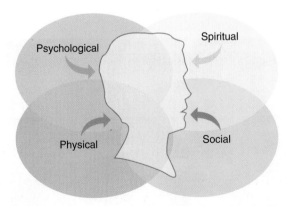

FIGURE 7-1 A person is a physical, psychological, social, and spiritual being. The parts over-lap and cannot be separated.

BASIC NEEDS

A **need** *is something necessary or desired for maintaining life and mental well-being.* According to psychologist Abraham Maslow, basic needs must be met for a person to survive and function. The needs are arranged from the lowest level to the highest level (Fig. 7-2, p. 72). Lower-level needs must be met before higher-level needs.

Disease, injury, or advanced age may prevent people from meeting their own needs. Ill or injured persons usually seek health care.

- *Physical needs.* Oxygen, food, water, elimination, rest, and shelter are needed to live and survive. A person dies within minutes without oxygen. Without food or water, weakness and illness occur within a few hours. The kidneys and intestines must function. If not, poisonous wastes build up in the blood and can cause death. Without enough rest and sleep, a person becomes very tired. Without shelter, the person is exposed to extremes of heat and cold.
- *Safety and security needs.* The person needs to feel safe from harm, danger, and fear. Health care often involves strange equipment, pain, and discomfort. People feel more secure if they know what will happen. For each task, even a simple bath, the person should know:
  - Why it is needed
  - Who will do it
  - How it will be done
  - What sensations or feelings to expect
- *Love and belonging needs.* These needs relate to love, closeness, affection, and meaningful relationships with others. Family, friends, and the health team can meet love and belonging needs.
- *Self-esteem needs.* **Esteem** *is the worth, value, or opinion one has of a person.* **Self-esteem** *means to think well of oneself and to see oneself as useful and having value.* People often lack self-esteem when ill, injured, older, or disabled. For example:
  - An older man worked a farm and raised a family. Now he cannot dress or feed himself.
  - A woman lost her hair from cancer treatments. She does not feel pretty or whole.
- *The need for self-actualization.* **Self-actualization** *means experiencing one's potential.* It involves learning, understanding, and creating to the limit of a person's ability. This is the highest need. Rarely, if ever, is it totally met. Most people constantly try to learn and understand more. This need can be postponed and life will continue.

See *Focus on Communication: Basic Needs (Self-Esteem Needs),* p. 72.

See *Focus on Long-Term Care and Home Care: Basic Needs (Safety and Security Needs),* p. 72.

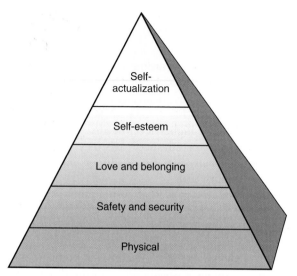

FIGURE 7-2 Basic needs for life as described by Maslow. (Redrawn from Maslow AH, Frager RD (Editor), Fadiman J (Editor): *Motivation and personality*, ed 3. © 1987. Reprinted with permission of Ann Kaplan.)

FOCUS ON COMMUNICATION

Basic Needs (Self-Esteem Needs)

You must treat all persons with respect. While it takes more time, encourage them to do as much for themselves as possible. This helps increase self-esteem.

FOCUS ON LONG-TERM CARE AND HOME CARE

Basic Needs (Safety and Security Needs)

Long-Term Care

Some people feel safe and secure in a nursing center. They have help when needed and staff to protect them. Others feel scared or confused. They are in a strange place with strange routines. Strangers care for them.

Show new residents their setting. Listen to their concerns. Explain all routines and tasks. You may have to repeat information often—sometimes for days or weeks until the person feels safe and secure. Be patient, kind, and understanding.

CULTURE AND RELIGION

Culture is the characteristics of a group of people—language, values, beliefs, habits, likes, dislikes, and customs. They are passed from 1 generation to the next. A person's culture influences communication and health beliefs and practices. Culture also affects thinking and behavior when health care is needed.

People come from many cultures, races, and nationalities. Their family practices and food choices may differ from yours. So might their hygiene habits and clothing styles. Some speak a foreign language. Some cultures have beliefs about what causes and cures illness. They may perform rituals to rid the body of disease. Many cultures have health beliefs and rituals about dying and death (Chapter 59).

Religion relates to spiritual beliefs, needs, and practices. Religions may have beliefs about daily living, behaviors, relationships with others, diet, healing, days of worship, birth and birth control, drugs, and death.

Many people find comfort and strength from religion during illness. They may want to pray and observe religious practices. Hospitals and nursing centers offer religious services and have areas for prayer (Fig. 7-3). Assist the person to attend services as needed.

A person may want to see a cleric (Chapter 1). If so, tell the nurse. Make sure the room is neat and orderly. Have a chair ready for the cleric. Provide privacy during the visit.

The person's care plan (Chapter 8) includes the person's cultural and religious practices. You must respect the person's culture and religion. Learn about their beliefs and practices. This helps you understand the person and give better care.

A person may not follow all the beliefs and practices of his or her culture or religion. Some people do not practice a religion. Each person is unique. Do not judge the person by your standards. And do not force your ideas on the person.

See *Caring About Culture: Culture and Religion.*

See *Focus on Communication: Culture and Religion.*

See *Focus on Long-Term Care and Home Care: Culture and Religion.*

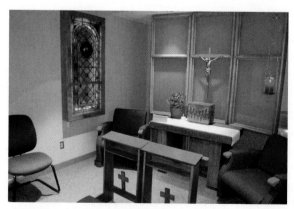

FIGURE 7-3 A hospital chapel provides a quiet area for prayer. (Courtesy Gene Vogelgesang, Illinois Valley Community Hospital, Peru, Illinois.)

🌸 CARING ABOUT CULTURE

Culture and Religion

Health Care Beliefs

Some *Mexican Americans* believe that illness is caused by prolonged exposure to hot or cold. If hot causes illness, cold is used for cure. Likewise, hot is used for illnesses caused by cold. Hot conditions include fever, infection, rashes, sore throat, diarrhea, and constipation. Cold conditions include cancer, joint pain, earache, and stomach cramps.

The hot-cold balance is also a belief of some *Vietnamese Americans*. Illnesses, food, drugs, and herbs are hot or cold. Hot is given to balance cold illnesses. Cold is given for hot illnesses.

Sick Care Practices

Folk practices are common among some *Vietnamese Americans*. They include *cao gio* ("rub wind")—rubbing the skin with a coin to treat the common cold. Skin pinching (*bat gio*—"catch wind") may be done for headaches and sore throats. Herbs, oils, and soups are used for many signs and symptoms.

Some *Russian Americans* practice folk medicine. For headaches, an ointment may be placed behind the ears and temples and at the back of the neck. Treatment for back pain may involve placing a dough of dark rye flour and honey on the spine.

Some *Mexican Americans* use folk healers. A *yerbero* may use herbs and spices to prevent or cure disease. A *curandero* (*curandera* if female) may deal with serious physical and mental illnesses.

(NOTE: Each person is unique. A person may not follow all of the beliefs and practices of his or her culture. Follow the care plan.)

Modified from Giger JN: Transcultural nursing: assessment and intervention, ed 6, St Louis, 2013, Mosby.

FOCUS ON **COMMUNICATION**

Culture and Religion

The person's care plan communicates practices to include in his or her care. Check the care plan for the person's preferences.

Show interest in the person's culture and religion. You can ask the person to explain a belief or practice to you. For example:

- "Your cross is pretty. Does it have a special meaning for you?"
- "I see that you like your food prepared a certain way. Why is that important to you?"
- "I understand that you are from France. Can you teach me some French words?"

FOCUS ON **LONG-TERM CARE AND HOME CARE**

Culture and Religion

Home Care

Culture is reflected in the home. Homes vary in size, neatness, furnishings, and price. Whether rich or poor, treat each person and family with respect, kindness, and dignity. Do not judge the person's life-style, habits, religion, or culture.

PERSONS YOU WILL CARE FOR

People of all ages need health care. They are often grouped by their problems, needs, and age (Table 7-1). Through quality care and good communication, you assist the person in regaining or maintaining his or her *optimal level of function. This is the person's highest potential for mental and physical performance.*

Encourage the person to be as independent as possible. Focus on what the person can do, not what he or she cannot do. See "Persons With Special Needs," p. 81.

TABLE 7-1	Persons You Will Care For
Group	**Description**
Mothers and newborns	• *Obstetrics—the field of medicine concerned with the care of women during pregnancy, labor, and childbirth and for 6 to 8 weeks after birth.* • Pre-natal (before birth) care is given in clinics and doctors' offices. • Mothers are admitted to hospital obstetric (maternity) units for labor and delivery. • Problems can occur during and after pregnancy and childbirth. • See Chapter 56.
Children	• *Pediatrics—the field of medicine concerned with the growth, development, and care of children—newborns to teenagers.* • Pediatric units are designed and equipped for the needs of children (usually up to age 16) and parents (Fig. 7-4, p. 74).
Adults with medical problems	• The focus is on illnesses, diseases, and injuries not needing surgery. • Health problems are acute, chronic, or terminal (Chapter 1).

Continued

TABLE 7-1	Persons You Will Care For—cont'd
Group	**Description**
Persons having surgery	• Care is given before, during, and after surgery. • Surgeries are simple (removal of an appendix) to complex (heart surgery). • See Chapter 39.
Persons with mental health disorders	• *Psychiatry*—the field of medicine concerned with mental health disorders. • Problems range from mild to severe. • Some persons need help coping with life stresses. Others present dangers to self and others.
Persons needing bariatric care	• *Bariatrics*—the field of medicine focused on the treatment and control of obesity. • *Obesity*—having an excess amount of total body fat. Body weight is 20% or more above what is normal for the person's height and age. • *Morbid obesity*—weighing 100 pounds or more over one's normal weight. • The person is at high risk for many serious health problems.
Persons in special care units	• Special care units are designed to treat and prevent life-threatening problems. • Emergency rooms and intensive care, coronary care, burn, and kidney dialysis units are examples (Fig. 7-5).
Persons needing rehabilitation or sub-acute care	• The person needs rehabilitation or more recovery time than hospital care allows. • See Chapter 45.
Older persons	• *Geriatrics*—the field of medicine concerned with the problems and diseases of old age and older persons. • See Chapter 12.
Persons needing long-term care	• *Alert, oriented persons*—know who and where they are. Care needs depend on their physical problems. • *Confused and disoriented persons*—are mildly to severely confused and disoriented. This may be a short-term or long-term problem. See Chapter 53. • *Persons needing complete care*—cannot meet their own needs. Require total help with all activities of daily living (ADL). Some cannot understand or say what they need or want. • *Short-term residents*—are recovering from fractures or other injuries, acute illness, or surgery. May need tube feedings, wound care, or other treatments or therapies (physical, occupational, speech, language, respiratory). The goal is optimal level of function and to return home. • *Persons needing respite care*—*respite* means *rest or relief*. The person living at home goes to a nursing center for a short stay. His or her caregiver gets relief for a vacation, business, or rest. Respite care can be a few days to several weeks. • *Life-long residents*—may have disabilities from birth defects or childhood or adult diseases or injuries. There may be physical impairments, intellectual impairments, or both. Life-long assistance, support, and special devices are needed. • *Persons with mental health disorders*—have problems with behaviors and function. Self-care and independent living may be impaired. Some persons have both physical and mental health disorders. • *Persons who are terminally ill*—the goal is quality end-of-life care for persons who are dying. See Chapter 59.

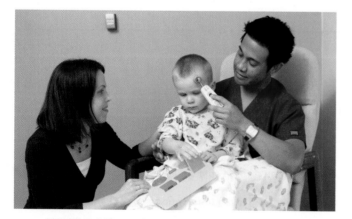

FIGURE 7-4 The nursing assistant gives care to a sick child.

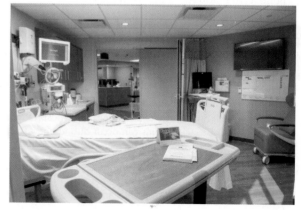

FIGURE 7-5 A room in an intensive care unit. (Courtesy Memorial Medical Center, Springfield, Illinois.)

EFFECTIVE COMMUNICATION

You communicate with the person every time you give care. You give information to the person. The person gives information to you. Your body sends messages all the time—at the bedside, in hallways, at the nurses' station, in the dining room, and elsewhere. The person and family are aware of what you say and do. Good work ethics and understanding the person are needed for good communication. What you say and what you do are also important. Follow the rules in Box 7-1.

See *Focus on Children and Older Persons: Effective Communication.*

BOX 7-1	Communicating With the Person

- Use words that have the same meaning for you and the person.
- Avoid medical terms and words not familiar to the person.
- Communicate in a logical and orderly manner. Do not wander in thought.
- Give facts and be specific.
- Be brief and concise.
- Understand and respect the patient or resident as a person.
- View the person as a physical, psychological, social, and spiritual human being.
- Appreciate the person's problems and frustrations.
- Respect the person's rights, religion, and culture.
- Give the person time to understand the information that you give.
- Repeat information as often as needed. Repeat what you said. Use the exact same words. Do not give the person a new message to process. If the person does not seem to understand after repeating, re-phrase the message. This is very important for persons with hearing problems.
- Ask questions to see if the person understood you.
- Be patient. People with memory problems may ask the same question many times. Do not say that you are repeating information.
- Include the person in conversations when others are present. This includes when a co-worker is assisting with care.

FOCUS ON CHILDREN AND OLDER PERSONS

Effective Communication

Communicating with persons who have dementia is often hard. The Alzheimer's Disease Education and Referral Center (ADEAR) recommends the following. Also see Chapter 53.

- Gain the person's attention before speaking. Say the person's name. Make eye contact.
- Choose simple words and short sentences.
- Use a gentle, calm voice.
- Do not talk to the person as you would a baby.
- Do not talk about the person as if he or she is not there.
- Keep distractions and noise to a minimum.
- Help the person focus on what you are saying.
- Give the person time to respond. Do not interrupt.
- Try to provide the word the person is struggling to find.
- State questions and instructions in a positive way.

Verbal Communication

Verbal communication uses written or spoken words. You talk to the person. You share information and find out how the person feels. Most verbal communication involves the spoken word. Follow these rules.

- Face the person. Look directly at the person.
- Position yourself at the person's eye level. Sit or squat by the person as needed.
- Control the loudness and tone of your voice.
- Speak clearly, slowly, and distinctly.
- Do not use slang or vulgar words.
- Repeat information as needed.
- Ask 1 question at a time. Wait for an answer.
- Do not shout, whisper, or mumble.
- Be kind, courteous, and friendly.

The written word is useful for persons who cannot speak or hear but can read. The nurse and care plan tell you how to communicate with the person. The devices shown in Figure 7-6 (p. 76) are often used. The person may have poor vision. When writing messages:

- Keep them simple and brief.
- Use a black felt pen on white paper.
- Print in large letters.
- Use black and a large font (print size) if using a computer or other electronic device.

Some persons cannot speak or read. Ask questions that have "yes" or "no" answers. The person can nod, blink, or use other gestures for "yes" and "no." Follow the care plan. A picture board may be helpful (Fig. 7-7, p. 77). Persons who are deaf may use sign language. See Chapter 46.

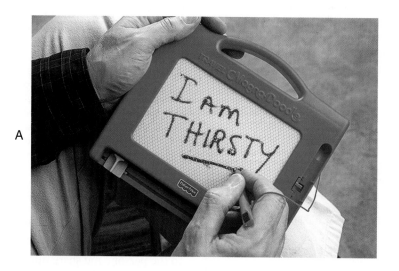

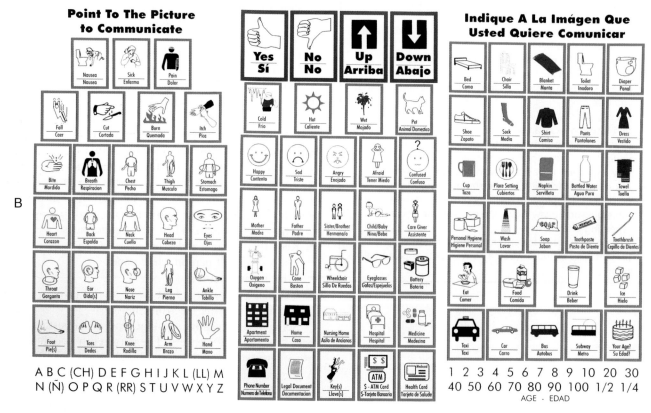

FIGURE 7-6 Communication aids. **A,** Magic Slate. **B,** Picture board in English and Spanish.

● ESTOY/TENGO
I AM

○ Dificultad para respirar *Short Of Breath*	○ Inseguro/a (con lo que está sucediendo) *Unsure (Of What Is Happening)*
○ Frustrado/a *Frustrated*	○ Arcadas *Gagging*
○ Náuseas *Nauseous*	○ Dolor *In Pain*
○ Ansiedad *Anxious*	○ Mareado/a *Light-Headed*
○ Decepcionado/a *Disappointed*	○ Miedo *Afraid*
○ Cansado/a *Tired*	○ Solo/a *Lonely*
○ Somnoliento/a *Drowsy*	○ Enfadado/a *Angry*
○ Mejor *Better*	○ Mojado/a *Wet*
○ Sed *Thirsty*	○ Peor *Worse*
○ Calor *Hot*	○ Hambre *Hungry*
○ Frío *Cold*	

● QUIERO
I WANT

EZ BOARD DE VIDATAK
SISTEMA INNOVADOR DE COMUNICACIÓN PARA PACIENTES

EZ BOARD BY VIDATAK
AN INNOVATION IN PATIENT COMMUNICATION

○ Que me hagan una succión *Suctioned*	○ Más control *More Control*	○ Sentirme reconfortado/a *To Be Comforted*
○ Sentarme *To Sit Up*	○ Recostarme *To Lie Down*	○ Orar *Prayer*
○ Agua *Water*	○ Hielo *Ice*	○ Ejercicio físico *Exercise*
○ Bañarme *Bath*	○ Champú *Shampoo*	○ Crema para el cuerpo *Lotion*
○ Anteojos *Eyeglasses*	○ Un cepillo para el pelo *Hairbrush*	○ Masaje *Massage*
○ Calcetines *Socks*	○ Un orinal *Urinal*	○ Chata para orinar *Bedpan*
○ Hacer una llamada *Make A Call*	○ Llamar a la enfermera, Ver TV *Call Light, TV*	○ Almohada *Pillow*
○ Darme vuelta a la derecha *To Turn Right*	○ Darme vuelta a la izquierda *To Turn Left*	○ Enciendan la luz *Lights On*
○ Que apaguen la luz *Lights Off*	○ Que bajen las luces *Lights Dim*	○ Cobija *Blanket*
○ En silencio *It Quiet*	○ Dormir *To Sleep*	○ Descansar *To Rest*

● QUIERO VER A UN/A
I WANT TO SEE

○ Médico *Doctor*	○ Terapeuta respiratorio *Respiratory Therapist*	
○ Enfermera *Nurse*	○ Terapeuta físico *Physical Therapist*	○ Capellán *Chaplain*
○ Asistente *Assistant*	○ Trabajador social *Social Worker*	○ Mi familia *My Family*

● QUIERO LIMPIARME
I WANT TO CLEAN

○ La boca *Mouth*	○ Los dientes *Teeth*	○ La cara *Face*
○ La nariz *Nose*	○ Las manos *Hands*	○ El cabello *Hair*

!	1	2	3	4	5	6	7	8	9	0	-	+	=	¡Gracias! *Thank You*
Q	W	E	R	T	Y	U	I	O	P	[	]			¡Te quiero mucho! *I Love You*
A	S	D	F	G	H	J	K	L	:	'				
Z	X	C	V	B	N	M	,	.	?					VIDATAK EZ BOARD

SPACE

Para prevenir infecciones, se ruega no usar esta pizarra con diferentes pacientes. For infection control purposes, please do not reuse this board between patients.

C

FIGURE 7-6, cont'd C, Communication board in Spanish.

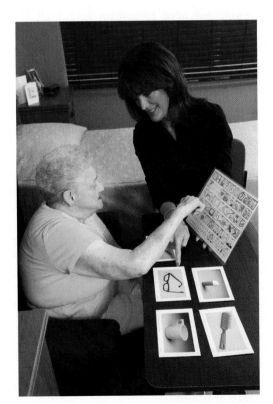

FIGURE 7-7 A therapist helps a resident use a picture board and picture cards to communicate.

Nonverbal Communication

Nonverbal communication does not use words. Gestures, facial expressions, posture, body movements, touch, and smell are used. Nonverbal messages more accurately reflect a person's feelings than words do. They are usually involuntary and hard to control. A person may say one thing but act another way. Watch the person's eyes, hand movements, gestures, posture, and other actions. They may tell you more than words.

See *Caring About Culture: Nonverbal Communication,* p. 78.

Touch. Touch is an important form of nonverbal communication. It conveys comfort, caring, love, affection, interest, trust, concern, and reassurance. Touch means different things to different people. The meaning depends on age, gender (male or female), experiences, and culture.

Cultural groups have rules or practices about touch. They relate to who can touch, when it can occur, and where to touch the body. See *Caring About Culture: Nonverbal Communication (Touch Practices),* p. 78.

Some people do not like being touched. However, stroking or holding a hand can comfort a person. Touch should be gentle—not hurried, rough, or sexual. To use touch, follow the person's care plan. Remember to maintain professional boundaries.

See *Focus on Children and Older Persons: Touch,* p. 78.

CARING ABOUT CULTURE

Nonverbal Communication

Touch Practices

Touch practices vary among cultural groups. Touch may be viewed as a friendly gesture in the *Philippine* culture. Touch is often used in *Mexico*. Some people believe that using touch while complimenting a person is important. It is thought to neutralize the power of the evil eye *(mal de ojo)*.

Persons from the *United Kingdom* may reserve touch for persons they know well. Within limits, touch may be acceptable in *Poland*. Its use depends on age, gender, and relationship.

In *India,* men shake hands with other men but not with women. For a greeting, women place their palms together and bow slightly.

In *Vietnam,* a person's head may be touched by others. It is considered the center of the soul. Men do not touch women they do not know. Men commonly shake hands with men.

In *China,* a nod or slight bow is given during introductions. Health care workers of the same gender are preferred.

In *Ireland,* a firm handshake is preferred. Usually only family and close friends are embraced.

Facial Expressions

Through facial expressions, *Americans* may communicate:

* *Coldness*—there is a constant stare. Face muscles do not move.
* *Fear*—eyes are wide open. Eyebrows are raised. The mouth is tense with the lips drawn back.
* *Anger*—eyes are fixed in a hard stare. Upper lids are lowered. Eyebrows are drawn down. Lips are slightly compressed.
* *Tiredness*—eyes are rolled upward.
* *Disapproval*—eyes are rolled upward.
* *Disgust*—eyes are narrowed. The upper lip is curled. There are nose movements.
* *Embarrassment*—eyes are turned away or down. The face is flushed. The person pretends to smile. He or she rubs the eyes, nose, or face. He or she twitches the hair, beard, or mustache.
* *Surprise*—the person has a direct gaze with raised eyebrows.

Italian, Jewish, African American, and *Hispanic* persons are known to smile readily. They may use many facial expressions and gestures for happiness, pain, or displeasure. *Irish, English,* and *Northern European* persons tend to have less facial expression.

In some cultures, facial expressions mean the opposite of what the person feels. For example, *Asians* may conceal negative emotions with a smile.

(NOTE: Each person is unique. A person may not follow all of the beliefs and practices of his or her culture. Follow the care plan.)

Modified from Giger JN: Transcultural nursing: assessment and intervention, ed 6, St Louis, 2013, Mosby. Modified from D'Avanzo CE: Pocket guide to cultural health assessment, ed 4, St Louis, 2008, Mosby.

FOCUS ON CHILDREN AND OLDER PERSONS

Touch

Children

Touch soothes and comforts infants and young children. They like to be held, stroked, rocked, patted, and cuddled. Older children and teenagers like to give and receive hugs.

Contact must be professional, casual, and with consent. It must not be sexual or involve sexual areas.

Body Language. People send messages through their *body language.*

* *Facial expressions* (see *Caring About Culture: Nonverbal Communication [Facial Expressions]*)
* *Gestures*
* *Posture*
* *Hand and body movements*
* *Gait*
* *Eye contact*
* *Appearance* (dress, hygiene, jewelry, perfume, cosmetics, body art and piercings, and so on)

Many messages are sent through body language. Slumped posture may mean the person is not happy or not feeling well. Denying pain, a person may protect the affected body part by standing, lying, or sitting in a certain way.

Your actions, movements, and facial expressions send messages. Your body language should show interest, caring, respect, and enthusiasm.

Often you will need to control your body language. Control reactions to odors from body fluids, secretions, excretions, or the person's body. The person cannot control some odors. Embarrassment increases if you react to odors.

Communication Methods

Certain methods help you communicate with others. They result in better relationships. More information is gained about the person.

Listening. Listening means to focus on verbal and non-verbal communication. You use sight, hearing, touch, and smell. You focus on what the person is saying. You observe nonverbal clues. They can support or not support what the person says. For example, a person says: "I want to stay here so my family won't have to care for me." You see tears and the person looks away from you. The person's verbal says *happy*; nonverbal shows *sadness*.

Listening requires that you care and have interest. Follow these guidelines.

* Face the person.
* Have good eye contact with the person. See *Caring About Culture: Communication Methods (Eye Contact Practices)*.
* Lean toward the person (Fig. 7-8). Do not sit back with your arms crossed.
* Respond to the person. Nod your head. Say: "uh huh," "mmm," and "I see." Repeat what the person says. Ask questions.
* Avoid the communication barriers (p. 80).

CARING ABOUT CULTURE

Communication Methods

Eye Contact Practices

In the *American* culture, eye contact usually signals a good self-concept. It also shows openness, interest in others, attention, honesty, and warmth. Lack of eye contact can mean:

- Shyness
- Embarrassment
- Lack of interest
- Low self-esteem
- Humility
- Rudeness
- Guilt
- Dishonesty

For some *Asian* and *American Indian* cultures, eye contact is impolite. It is an invasion of privacy. In certain *Indian* cultures, eye contact is avoided with persons of higher or lower socio-economic class.

Long, direct eye contact may be considered rude in *Mexico*. In some parts of *Vietnam*, it is not respectful to look at another person while talking. Blinking means that a message is received. In the *United Kingdom*, looking directly at a speaker usually means the listener is paying attention.

Silence

In some *English* and *Arabic* cultures, silence is used for privacy. Among *Russian*, *French*, and *Spanish* cultures, silence may mean agreement between parties. In some *Asian* cultures, silence is a sign of respect, particularly to an older person.

(NOTE: Each person is unique. A person may not follow all of the beliefs and practices of his or her culture. Follow the care plan.)

Modified from Giger JN: Transcultural nursing: assessment and intervention, ed 6, St Louis, 2013, Mosby. Modified from D'Avanzo CE: Pocket guide to cultural health assessment, ed 4, St Louis, 2008, Mosby.

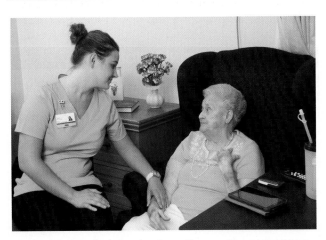

FIGURE 7-8 Listen by facing the person. Have good eye contact. Lean toward the person.

Paraphrasing. *Paraphrasing is re-stating the person's message in your own words.* You use fewer words than the person did. Paraphrasing:

- Shows you are listening.
- Lets the person see if you understand the message.
- Promotes more communication.

The person usually responds to your statement. For example:

Mrs. Hayes: My son was crying after talking to the doctor. I don't know what they said.
You: Your son was crying?
Mrs. Hayes: They must have talked about my tumor.

Direct Questions. Direct questions focus on certain information. You ask what you need to know. Some direct questions have "yes" or "no" answers. Others require more information. For example:

You: Mr. Walker, do you want to shower this morning?
Mr. Walker: Yes.
You: Mr. Walker, when would you like to do that?
Mr. Walker: Could we start in 15 minutes? I want to call my son first.
You: Yes, we can start in 15 minutes. Did you have a bowel movement today?
Mr. Walker: No.
You: You said you didn't eat much breakfast. What did you eat?
Mr. Walker: I had toast and coffee. I didn't feel like eating.

Open-Ended Questions. Open-ended questions lead or invite the person to share thoughts, feelings, or ideas. The person controls the topic and the information given. Answers require more than a "yes" or "no." For example:

- "What do you like about living with your son?"
- "What was your husband like?"
- "What do you like about being retired?"

Clarifying. Clarifying helps you understand the message. You can ask the person to repeat the message, say you do not understand, or re-state the message. For example:

- "Could you say that again?"
- "I'm sorry. I don't understand what you mean."
- "Are you saying that you want to go home?"

Focusing. Focusing deals with a certain topic. It is useful when a person rambles or wanders in thought. For example, a person talks at length about places to eat. You need to know why the person did not eat much breakfast. To focus on breakfast you say: "Let's talk about breakfast. You said you didn't feel like eating."

Silence. Silence is a powerful way to communicate. Sometimes you do not need to say anything. This is true during sad times. Just being there shows you care. At other times, silence gives time to think, organize thoughts, or choose words. It also helps when the person is upset and needs to gain control. Silence on your part shows caring and respect for the person's situation and feelings.

Pauses or long silences may seem uncomfortable. You do not need to talk when the person is silent. The person may need silence.

See *Caring About Culture: Communication Methods (Silence).*

Communication Barriers

Communication barriers prevent the sending and receiving of messages. Communication fails.

- *Unfamiliar language.* You and the person must use and understand the same language. If not, messages are not accurately interpreted. See *Evolve Student Learning Resources* for useful "Spanish Vocabulary and Phrases."
- *Cultural differences.* The person may attach different meanings to verbal and nonverbal communication. See *Caring About Culture: Communication Barriers.*
- *Changing the subject.* Someone changes the subject when the topic is uncomfortable.
- *Giving your opinion.* Opinions involve judging values, behaviors, or feelings. Let others express feelings and concerns without adding your opinion. Do not make judgments or jump to conclusions.
- *Talking a lot when others are silent.* Talking too much is usually because of nervousness and discomfort with silence. Silences have meaning. They show acceptance, rejection, and fear. They also show the need for quiet and time to think.
- *Failure to listen.* Do not pretend to listen. It shows lack of interest and caring. This causes poor responses. You miss important complaints or symptoms to report to the nurse.
- *Pat answers.* "Don't worry." "Everything will be okay." "Your doctor knows best." These show a lack of caring about the person's concerns, feelings, and fears.
- *Illness and disability.* Speech, hearing, vision, cognitive function, and body movements are often affected. Verbal and nonverbal communication is affected.
- *Age.* Values and communication styles vary among age-groups. See *Focus on Communication: Communication Barriers.*

✿ CARING ABOUT CULTURE

Communication Barriers

To communicate with persons from other cultures:

- Learn about the beliefs and values of the person's culture. You can ask the nurse, the person, and family. The person's care plan includes cultural beliefs and customs.
- Do not judge the person by your attitudes, values, beliefs, and ideas.
- Do the following when communicating with foreign-speaking persons.
  - Convey comfort by your tone of voice and body language.
  - Do not speak loudly or shout. It will not help the person understand English.
  - Speak slowly and distinctly.
  - Keep messages short and simple.
  - Be alert for words the person seems to understand.
  - Use gestures and pictures.
  - Repeat the message in other ways.
  - Avoid using medical terms and abbreviations.
  - Be alert for signs the person is pretending to understand. Nodding and "yes" to all questions are signs that the person does not understand what you are saying.

(NOTE: Each person is unique. A person may not follow all of the beliefs and practices of his or her culture. Follow the care plan.)

Modified from Giger JN: Transcultural nursing: assessment and intervention, ed 6, St Louis, 2013, Mosby.

FOCUS ON COMMUNICATION

Communication Barriers

Persons from different cultures may speak a language you do not understand. In the health care setting, the nurse may prefer to use a translator from the agency.

Trained translators know medical terms. Family or friends may state something other than what was meant. Receiving wrong information is a risk. Also, having family or friends translate violates the right to privacy. The *Health Insurance Portability and Accountability Act of 1996 (HIPAA)* protects the right to privacy and security of a person's health information (Chapter 5). Privacy is protected when using the agency's translator.

PERSONS WITH SPECIAL NEEDS

Each person is unique. Special knowledge and skills may be required to meet the person's needs.

Persons With Disabilities

A *disability is any lost, absent, or impaired physical or mental function.* Temporary or permanent, a disability can develop at any age. Children can develop hearing problems from ear infections. Head injuries can impair cognitive function. Spinal cord injuries can affect movements. And loud noise (music, machines) is linked to hearing loss.

To communicate with persons who have disabilities, see persons:

* Who have speech disorders—Chapter 46
* Who are hard of hearing—Chapter 46
* Who are blind—Chapter 46
* Who are confused—Chapter 53
* With Alzheimer's disease and other dementias—Chapter 53

Common courtesies and manners (*etiquette*) apply to any person with a disability. See Box 7-2 for disability etiquette.

BOX 7-2	Disability Etiquette

* Show the same courtesies to the person as you would to anyone else.
* Provide for privacy.
* Touch or handle the person's wheelchair only with his or her consent.
* Do not hang on or lean on a person's wheelchair.
* Treat adults as adults. Use the person's first name only if he or she asks you to do so. Do the same for others present.
* Do not pat a person who is in a wheelchair on the head.
* Speak directly to the person. Do not direct questions for the person to his or her companion.
* Do not be embarrassed for using words related to the disability. For example, you say: "Did you see that?" to a person with a vision problem.
* Sit or squat to talk to a person in a wheelchair or in a chair. You and the person are at eye level.
* Ask if help is needed before acting. If the answer is "no," respect the person's wishes. If the person wants help, ask what to do and how to do it.
* Think before giving directions to a person in a wheelchair. Think about distances, weather conditions, stairs, curbs, steep hills, and other obstacles.
* Let the person set the pace in walking, talking, or other activities.

Modified from Easter Seals, Disability etiquette, *2019.*

The Person Who Is Comatose

Comatose means being unable to respond to stimuli. (A *stimulus* is something that causes the person to change, react, or respond.) The person who is comatose is unconscious. The person cannot respond to others. Often the person can hear and can feel touch and pain. Pain may be shown by grimacing or groaning. Assume that the person hears and understands you. Use touch and give care gently. Practice these measures.

* Knock before entering the person's room.
* Tell the person your name, the time, and the place every time you enter the room.
* Follow the same schedule every day.
* Explain what you are going to do. Explain care measures step-by-step as you do them.
* Tell the person when you are completing care.
* Use touch to communicate care, concern, and comfort.
* Tell the person what time you will be back to check on him or her.
* Tell the person when you are leaving the room.

FAMILY AND FRIENDS

Family and friends help meet basic needs. They offer support and comfort. They lessen loneliness and help meet emotional needs. Some also help with the person's care. The presence or absence of family or friends affects the person's quality of life.

The person has the right to visit with others in private and without unneeded interruptions. You may need to give care when visitors are there. Protect the right to privacy. Do not expose the person's body in front of others. Politely ask them to leave the room. Show them where to wait. Promptly tell them when they can return. A partner or family member may want to help you. If the patient or resident consents, you can let the person stay.

Treat family and friends with courtesy and respect. They have concerns about the person's condition and care. They need support and understanding. However, do not discuss the person's condition with them. Refer their questions to the nurse.

Visiting rules depend on agency policy and the person's condition. Parents can usually visit with children whenever they want. Dying persons usually can have family present all the time. Know your agency's visiting policies and what is allowed for the person.

Visitors may have questions about the chapel, gift shop, lounge, dining room, or business office. Know the location, special rules, and hours of these areas.

A visitor may upset or tire a person. Report your observations to the nurse. The nurse will speak with the visitor about the person's needs.

See *Caring About Culture: Family and Friends,* p. 82.

See *Focus on Children and Older Persons: Family and Friends,* p. 82.

See *Focus on Long-Term Care and Home Care: Family and Friends,* p. 82.

CARING ABOUT CULTURE

Family and Friends

In *Vietnam*, family members may be involved in the person's hospital care. They stay at the bedside and sleep in the person's bed or on straw mats. In *Vietnam* and *China*, family members may provide food, hygiene, and comfort.

(NOTE: Each person is unique. A person may not follow all of the beliefs and practices of his or her culture. Follow the care plan.)

Modified from D'Avanzo CE: *Pocket guide to cultural health assessment,* ed 4, St Louis, 2008, Mosby.

FOCUS ON CHILDREN AND OLDER PERSONS

Family and Friends

Older Persons

Sometimes older brothers, sisters, and cousins live together. They provide companionship and share living expenses. They help each other during illness or disability.

Some older parents live with their children—in the child's home or the parent's home. The older parent may be healthy, need some supervision, or be ill or disabled. Living with a child can help the older person feel safe and secure. The adult child may need to assist or give care to the parent.

See "Living With Family" in Chapter 12.

FOCUS ON LONG-TERM CARE AND HOME CARE

Family and Friends

Home Care

Family personalities and attitudes affect the mood in the home. Families may have good or poor relationships. Mental or physical illness, drug or alcohol abuse, unemployment, and delinquency may affect the family. Some families have problems coping with or accepting the person's illness or disability.

Your supervisor explains family problems to you. Do not get involved. Be professional and have empathy. Do not give advice, take sides, or make judgments about family conflicts. Maintain professional boundaries at all times.

BEHAVIOR ISSUES

Many patients, residents, and families accept illness, injury, and disability. Others do not adjust well. They have some of the following behaviors (Fig. 7-9). These behaviors are new for some people. For others, they are part of one's personality.

- *Anger.* Anger is a common emotion. Causes include fear, pain, and dying and death. Loss of function and loss of control over health and life are causes. Anger is a symptom of some diseases that affect thinking and behavior. Some people are generally angry. Verbal outbursts, shouting, raised voices, and rapid speech are common. Some people are silent. Others are not cooperative. Nonverbal signs include rapid movements, pacing, clenched fists, and a red face. Glaring and getting close to you when speaking are other signs. Violent behaviors can occur.
- *Demanding behavior.* Nothing seems to please the person. The person is critical of others. He or she wants care at a certain time and in a certain way. Loss of independence, loss of health, and loss of control of life are causes. So are unmet needs.
- *Self-centered behavior.* Only the person's needs are important. The needs of others are ignored. The person expects time and attention from others. The person becomes impatient if needs are not met.
- *Aggressive behavior.* The person may swear, bite, hit, pinch, scratch, or kick. Fear, anger, pain, and dementia are causes. Protect the person, others, and yourself from harm (Chapter 13).
- *Withdrawal.* The person has little or no contact with others. He or she spends time alone and does not take part in social or group events. This may signal physical illness or depression. Some people are not social. They prefer to be alone.
- *Inappropriate sexual behavior.* Some people make inappropriate sexual remarks. Or they touch others in the wrong way. Some disrobe or masturbate in public. These behaviors may be on purpose. Or they are caused by disease, confusion, dementia, or drug side effects.

You cannot avoid the person or lose control. Good communication is needed. Behaviors are addressed in the care plan. The care plan may include some of the guidelines in Box 7-3.

See *Focus on Communication: Behavior Issues.*

See *Teamwork and Time Management: Behavior Issues.*

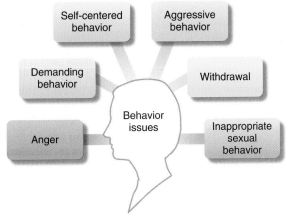

FIGURE 7-9 Behavior issues are a response to illness, injury, or disability, or they are life-long.

| BOX 7-3 | Dealing With Behavior Issues |

- Recognize frustrating and frightening situations. Put yourself in the person's situation. How would you feel? How would you want to be treated?
- Treat the person with dignity and respect.
- Answer questions clearly and thoroughly. Ask the nurse to answer questions you cannot answer.
- Keep the person informed. Tell the person what you are going to do and when.
- Do not keep the person waiting. Answer call lights promptly. If you tell the person that you will do something, do it promptly.
- Explain the reason for long waits. Ask if you can get or do something to increase the person's comfort.
- Stay calm and professional, especially if the person is angry or hostile. Often the person is not angry at you. He or she is angry at another person or situation.
- Do not argue with the person.
- Listen and use silence. The person may feel better if able to express his or her feelings.
- Protect yourself from violent behaviors (Chapter 13).
- Report the person's behavior to the nurse. Discuss how to deal with the person.

FOCUS ON COMMUNICATION

Behavior Issues

Anger is a common response to illness and disability. The person may be angry with the situation. You might have problems dealing with anger directed at you. Act professionally. Stay calm. Listen to his or her concerns. Give needed care. Try not to take angry statements personally. If a person says hurtful things, you can kindly say: "Please don't say those things. I'm trying to help you." Tell the nurse about the person's behavior.

Caring for demanding or angry persons can be hard. Ask the nurse or co-workers to help if needed.

TEAMWORK AND TIME MANAGEMENT

Behavior Issues

Persons who are demanding can take a lot of time. A simple task, such as filling a water mug, can take several minutes. The mug may be too full or not full enough. The water may be too warm or too cold. Or the person may have a list of other care needs.

Learn to recognize these situations. Offer to help co-workers with the person or other tasks. Hopefully they also will help you.

FOCUS ON **PRIDE**

The Person, Family, and Yourself

Personal and Professional Responsibility

Improving communication is on-going. You may be uncomfortable with patient or resident interactions at first. To develop communication skills:

- Use methods such as listening and clarifying.
- Pay attention to the nonverbal messages you send.
- Avoid the communication barriers.
- Know where to find communication aids. See Figure 7-6 or use translation lists with useful words or phrases (see *Evolve Student Learning Resources*).
- Learn from your mistakes.

  With practice, you will communicate more effectively. This is a valuable skill.

Rights and Respect

Each patient or resident has needs and concerns. Each person is unique and has value. Try to understand the person. Listen and use good communication. Treat the person with dignity and respect.

Independence and Social Interaction

Illness and disability affect the whole person. Normal, daily activities that bring pleasure, worth, and contact with others may be hard or impossible. Work, driving, meals, yard work, hobbies, and social events are examples. The person may feel angry, upset, and useless when help is needed with routine functions.

Fears of death, chronic illness, and loss of function are common. A broken leg may bring fears of a limp. Surgery may bring fears of cancer. A stroke may affect the ability to talk. Some people talk about being afraid. Others do not share their feelings. Body language may communicate that the person is stressed or troubled.

You can help the person feel safe, secure, and loved.

- Greet the person by name.
- Talk to the person while giving care. Explain care measures step-by-step.
- Take an extra minute to talk or just listen.
- Encourage as much independence as possible. Focus on the person's abilities, not his or her disabilities.
- Use touch appropriately. Hold a hand or give a hug while maintaining professional boundaries.
- Show that you are willing to help. Respond to the person's needs promptly.
- Allow private time with visitors.

Delegation and Teamwork

Caring for persons with behavior issues requires teamwork. Staff may become frustrated. The health team works together to manage such persons. A supportive and encouraging team makes caring for persons with behavior issues easier.

Ethics and Laws

You will care for persons with different ideas, values, and life-styles. These shape the person's character and identity. Do not force your views and beliefs on the person or insult the person. Respect the person as a whole. This includes his or her cultural and religious practices.

FOCUS ON **PRIDE**: *Application*

Imagine yourself as a patient or resident. What would you want the staff to know about you? Ask 1 or 2 others what would be important to them. How does understanding the person allow you to give better care?

REVIEW QUESTIONS

Circle the BEST answer.

1 Holism focuses on
   a The person's care plan
   b The person's physical, safety and security, and self-esteem needs
   c The person as a physical, psychological, social, and spiritual being
   d The person's cultural and spiritual needs

2 Which basic need is the *most* essential?
   a The need to feel safe
   b The need to feel valued
   c The need for affection
   d The need for food

3 A person says: "I'm falling!" Which needs are *most* important at the time?
   a Self-actualization needs
   b Safety and security needs
   c Love and belonging needs
   d Self-esteem needs

4 A person has a garden behind the nursing center. This relates to
   a Self-actualization
   b Self-esteem
   c Love and belonging
   d Safety and security

Continued

REVIEW QUESTIONS—cont'd

5 Which statement about culture and religion is *true*?
  a Cultural and religious practices are not allowed in health care.
  b A person must follow all beliefs and practices of his or her culture or religion.
  c Culture and religion influence health and illness practices.
  d Culture and religion do not influence food choices.

6 Which is *true*?
  a Mental health disorders are the focus of pediatrics.
  b Sick children are the focus of obstetrics.
  c The diseases of aging are the focus of geriatrics.
  d Childbirth is the focus of pediatrics.

7 Alert and oriented residents need nursing center care because they
  a Are very disabled and confused
  b Have trouble remembering things
  c Have physical problems
  d Need surgery

8 Which is *true*?
  a Nonverbal communication uses the written or spoken word.
  b Verbal communication is the truest reflection of a person's feelings.
  c Body language cannot be controlled.
  d Touch means different things to different people.

9 To communicate with the person you should
  a Use medical words and phrases
  b Change the subject often
  c Give your opinions
  d Be quiet when the person is silent

10 Which shows that you are listening?
  a You sit with your arms crossed.
  b You have eye contact with the person.
  c You do not ask questions.
  d You use communication barriers.

11 Which is an open-ended question?
  a "What hobbies do you enjoy?"
  b "Do you want to wear your red sweater?"
  c "Would you like eggs and toast for breakfast?"
  d "Do you want to sit in your chair?"

12 You ask: "What name do you prefer?" This is
  a A communication barrier
  b A direct question
  c Paraphrasing
  d An open-ended question

13 Focusing is useful when
  a A person is rambling
  b You want to make sure you understand the message
  c You want the person to share thoughts and feelings
  d A person is silent

14 Which promotes communication?
  a "Don't worry."
  b "Everything will be fine."
  c "This is a good nursing center."
  d "Why are you crying?"

15 Which is a barrier to communication?
  a Focusing
  b Asking questions
  c Pretending to listen
  d Using familiar language

16 A person uses a wheelchair. For effective communication, you should
  a Lean on the wheelchair
  b Pat the person on the head
  c Direct questions to the companion
  d Sit or squat next to the person

17 A person is comatose. Which action is *correct*?
  a You assume that the person cannot hear.
  b You explain what you are going to do.
  c You use listening and silence to communicate.
  d You enter the room without knocking.

18 A person has many visitors. Which is *true*?
  a They can help meet basic needs.
  b You can discuss the person's condition with them.
  c You can answer their questions about the person's care.
  d You decide who stays in the room when care is given.

19 A visitor seems to tire a person. What should you do?
  a Ask the person to leave.
  b Tell the nurse.
  c Stay in the room to observe the person and visitor.
  d Find out the visitor's relationship to the person.

20 A person wants care given at a certain time and in a certain way. Nothing seems to please the person. The person is most likely demonstrating
  a Angry behavior
  b Withdrawn behavior
  c Demanding behavior
  d Aggressive behavior

21 A person is demonstrating problem behavior. You should
  a Put yourself in the person's situation
  b Ignore the behavior
  c Ask the person to be nicer
  d Avoid the person

22 When interacting with the person
  a Focus on the person's illness or disability
  b Be silent while giving care
  c Use names like "Dear" and "Honey"
  d Take time to listen

Answers to Chapter 7 questions are on p. 885.

FOCUS ON PRACTICE

Problem Solving

A resident was admitted to the center last month. The resident is withdrawn, impatient, and angry toward the staff. Explain possible reasons for the behaviors. How will you manage the behaviors and provide quality care?

OBJECTIVES

- Define the key terms and key abbreviations in this chapter.
- Explain why health team members need to communicate.
- Describe the rules for good communication.
- Explain the purpose, parts, and information found in the medical record.
- Describe the legal and ethical aspects of medical records.
- Describe the 5 steps in the nursing process.
- Explain your role in the nursing process.
- Explain the difference between objective and subjective data.

- Identify the observations and information you need to report to the nurse.
- List the rules for recording.
- Explain how electronic devices are used in health care.
- Explain how to protect the right to privacy when using electronic devices.
- Describe how to answer phones.
- Use the 24-hour clock.
- Explain how to promote PRIDE in the person, the family, and yourself.

KEY TERMS

assessment Collecting information about the person; see "nursing process"

chart See "medical record"

clinical record See "medical record"

electronic health record (EHR) An electronic version of a person's medical record; electronic medical record

electronic medical record (EMR) See "electronic health record"

end-of-shift report A report that the nurse gives at the end of the shift to the on-coming shift; change-of-shift report

evaluation To measure if goals in the planning step were met; see "nursing process"

implementation To perform or carry out nursing interventions (nursing measures, nursing actions, nursing tasks) in the care plan; see "nursing process"

medical record The legal account of a person's condition and response to treatment and care; chart or clinical record

nursing care plan A written guide about the person's nursing care; care plan

nursing diagnosis A health problem that can be treated by nursing measures; see "nursing process"

nursing intervention An action or measure taken by the nursing team to help the person reach a goal; nursing action, nursing measure, nursing task

nursing process The method nurses use to plan and deliver nursing care; its 5 steps are assessment, nursing diagnosis, planning, implementation, and evaluation

objective data Information that is seen, heard, felt, or smelled by an observer; signs

observation Using the senses of sight, hearing, touch, and smell to collect information

planning Setting priorities and goals; see "nursing process"

progress note Describes the care given and the person's response and progress

recording The written account of care and observations; charting, documentation

reporting The oral account of care and observations

signs See "objective data"

subjective data Things a person tells you about that you cannot observe through your senses; symptoms

symptoms See "subjective data"

KEY ABBREVIATIONS

ADL	Activities of daily living	EPHI; ePHI	Electronic protected health information
BMs	Bowel movements		
CAA	Care Area Assessment	IDCP	Interdisciplinary care planning
CMS	Centers for Medicare & Medicaid Services	MDS	Minimum Data Set
EHR	Electronic health record	OASIS	Outcome and Assessment Information Set
EMR	Electronic medical record	PHI	Protected health information

Communication is needed for coordinated and effective care. Health team members share information about:

- What was done for the person
- What needs to be done for the person
- The person's response to treatment

For example, a patient needs comfort measures. The nurse plans to give a pain-relief drug and asks you to position the person. The nurse explains the plan to you and the patient. The nurse tells you when the drug is given and assesses the person's response. You position the person. The nurse records about pain. You report and record the care you gave. The nurse reports observations and care to the next nurse on duty.

Communication and care were coordinated. The person knew what to expect. Care was reported and recorded so team members know what was done.

You need to practice the aspects and rules of communication. Then you can communicate effectively with the nursing and health teams. For good communication, see Box 8-1.

BOX 8-1	**Communication Rules**

- Use words that have the same meaning for you and the message receiver. Avoid words with more than 1 meaning. Does "far" mean 50 feet or 100 feet?
- Ask about messages you do not understand. You will learn medical terms (Chapter 9). If you do not know a term, ask what it means. Or use a dictionary. You must understand the message for communication to occur.
- Be brief and concise. Do not add unrelated or unnecessary information. Stay on the subject. Do not wander in thought or get wordy.
- Give information in a logical and orderly way. Organize your thoughts. Present them step-by-step.
- Give facts and be specific. Reporting a pulse rate of 110 is more specific than the "pulse is fast."

THE MEDICAL RECORD

The *medical record (chart, clinical record) is the legal account of a person's condition and response to treatment and care.* Medical records are written on paper forms or electronically with computers or other electronic devices (Fig. 8-1). An *electronic health record (EHR) or electronic medical record (EMR) is an electronic version of a person's medical record.* Most agencies use EHRs (EMRs).

The health team uses the medical record to share information about the person. The record is a permanent legal document. Often it is used months or years later if the person's health history is needed. It can be used in court as legal evidence of the person's problems, treatment, and care.

Government and accrediting agencies review medical records to see if license, certification, or accrediting standards have been met. The record is also used to determine the amount paid for services (Chapter 1).

The record has different parts (Table 8-1, p. 88). Each part has the person's name, identification (ID) number, room and bed number, and other identifying information. The record tells about care provided and the person's response.

See *Focus on Long-Term Care and Home Care: The Medical Record*, p. 89.

Text continued on p. 90.

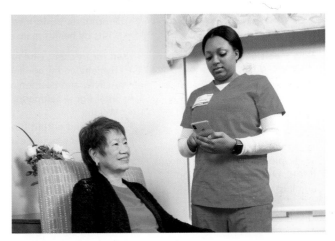

FIGURE 8-1 A nursing assistant uses an electronic medical record.

TABLE 8-1	Parts of the Medical Record
Part	**Description**
Admission record	Completed on admission (entry) into the agency. Contains personal and identifying information—legal name, birth date, age, biological sex (male or female), address, insurance information, marital status, nearest relative and legal representative, religion, place of worship, employer, diagnoses, date and time of admission, doctor's name. A signed general consent for treatment is included.
Advance directives	A document stating a person's wishes about end-of-life care (Chapter 59).
Health history	A record of the person's medical history. • Chief complaint—reason for seeking health care • History of current illness—onset (time, sudden or gradual) and signs and symptoms • Past health problems, surgeries, and injuries • Childhood illnesses • Allergies and type of reaction • Current drugs • Vaccinations • Family health history • Life-style—habits, diet, sleep, hobbies • Adaptive (assistive) devices used—dentures, eyeglasses, contact lenses, hearing aids, cane, walker, wheelchair, and so on • Ability to perform activities of daily living (ADL)—the activities usually done during a normal day in a person's life • Education and occupation
Nursing assessment	Data collected during the nurse's physical assessment (p. 91).
Nursing care plan; care plan	A guide about the person's nursing care (p. 93).
Nursing progress notes	*Progress notes describe the care given and the person's response and progress* (Fig. 8-2). For example, the nurse records: • Signs and symptoms • Information about treatments and drugs • Information about teaching and counseling • Procedures performed • Visits by health team members
Flow sheets and graphic sheets	Used for frequent care measures, measurements, and observations (Fig. 8-3). • Hygiene and grooming measures • Activity and positioning • Vital signs—temperature, pulse, respirations, and blood pressure • Weight • Intake and output (Chapter 31) • Urinary and bowel elimination
Medication administration record (MAR); electronic medication administration record (eMAR)	A record of drugs ordered, given, and not taken.
Physical examination	Information collected during the physical examination. The examination is done by a doctor, advanced practice registered nurse (APRN), or physician's assistant (PA).
Orders	Directions from the doctor, APRN, or PA about tests and care measures to be performed.
Progress notes (health team)	Reports from the health team—medical (doctor, APRN, PA); physical, occupational, speech-language, and recreational therapies; dietary; social services; and others.
Laboratory results	Results of tests done on blood, urine, and other body fluids and tissues.
X-ray reports	Results of x-ray tests.
Therapy records	Records for intravenous (IV), respiratory, wound care, and other therapies.
Consultation reports	Reports from other health care providers consulted by the person's doctor.
Special consents	Signed permissions for surgeries and procedures needing informed consent (Chapter 5).
Discharge summary	Information and instructions for the person when leaving the agency—wound care; drug prescriptions and changes; rest, activity, and exercise; diet; signs and symptoms to report; follow-up appointments.

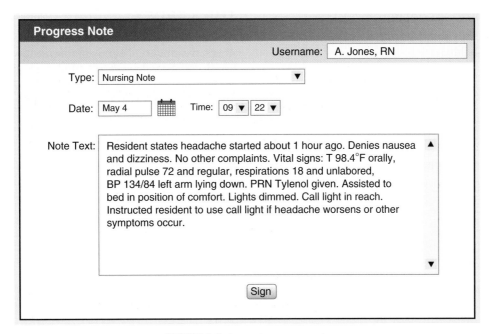

FIGURE 8-2 A sample progress note.

	06/16 12:00	06/16 13:00	06/16 13:10	06/16 13:20	06/16 15:00	06/16 15:10	06/16 15:15			
Vital Signs										
Temperature	98.4									
Pulse	72									
Respiration	18									
Blood Pressure	118/76									
O2SAT	99									
O2 L/M										
Intake/Output										
P.O. ORAL	240									
New Intake										
VOIDED URINE			250			200				
New Output										
NUTRITION:	SELF									
ELIMINATION:			TOILET			TOILET				
Activity										
ACTIVITY:	CHAIR	CHAIR	BATH	BED	AMBUL	BATH	BED			
POSITIONING:	SELF			BACK			RIGHT			
HYGIENE:		ORAL	PERI			PERI				
Safety SAFETY:	CALL	CALL	BELT	CALL	BELT	BELT	CALL			

Ready   Interface   CHART MENU   Reflex   Completed   Room: 274-1   Exit

FIGURE 8-3 A sample flow sheet. (Courtesy Abraham Lincoln Memorial Hospital, Lincoln, Ill.)

FOCUS ON LONG-TERM CARE AND HOME CARE

The Medical Record

Long-Term Care

The nurse writes progress notes for an unusual event, a problem, or a change in the person's condition. The Centers for Medicare & Medicaid Services (CMS) requires summaries of care at least every 3 months. They reflect the person's response to care and progress toward meeting care plan goals (p. 93). Some centers require summaries more often.

Home Care

A weekly record has sections for each day and for care activities. There are sections for personal care, activity, measurements, nutrition, household services, and procedures. You record on the day care was given.

Legal and Ethical Aspects

Agencies have policies about medical records and who can see them. Policies address:

- Who records
- When to record
- Ink color (paper charting)
- Abbreviations
- How to make and sign entries
- How to correct errors

Some agencies allow nursing assistants to record observations and care. Others do not. Follow your agency's policies.

Professional staff involved in a person's care can review charts. Cooks and laundry, housekeeping, and office staff do not need to read charts. Some agencies let nursing assistants read charts. If not, the nurse shares needed information.

You have an ethical and legal duty to keep information confidential. If not involved in the person's care, you have no right to read the person's chart. Doing so is an invasion of privacy.

Patients and residents have the right to the information in their medical records. The person or the person's legal representative may ask to see the chart. Tell the nurse. The nurse handles the request.

THE KARDEX

A *Kardex* summarizes information in the medical record—drugs, treatments, diagnoses, routine care measures, equipment, and special needs. The Kardex is a quick, easy source of information about the person (Fig. 8-4). It may be electronic or on paper as a card file. The Kardex is not part of the permanent medical record.

THE NURSING PROCESS

Nursing team members share information about the person's strengths, problems, nursing needs, and care. This information is shared through the nursing process. The *nursing process is the method nurses use to plan and deliver nursing care.* It has 5 steps.

- *Assessment*
- *Nursing diagnosis*
- *Planning*
- *Implementation*
- *Evaluation*

The person and nursing team need good communication. With good communication, nursing care is organized and has purpose. All nursing team members do the same things for the person. They focus on the same goals for the person.

The nursing process is on-going. New information is gathered and the person's needs may change. However, the

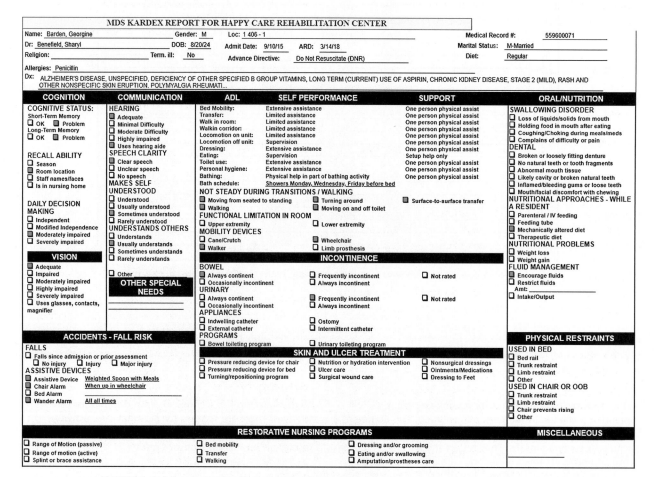

FIGURE 8-4 A sample Kardex. (Courtesy PointClickCare Technologies Inc., Mississauga, Ontario, Canada.)

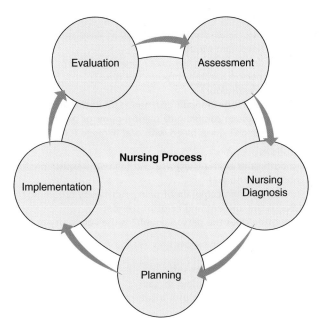

FIGURE 8-5 The nursing process is continuous.

steps are the same. You will see how the nursing process is continuous as each step is explained (Fig. 8-5).

You have a key role in the nursing process. Your observations are used for nursing diagnoses and planning. You may help develop care plans. In the implementation step, you perform tasks in the care plan. Your assignment sheet tells you what to do. Your observations are used for the evaluation step.

See *Delegation Guidelines: The Nursing Process.*

DELEGATION GUIDELINES

The Nursing Process

The nursing process is a nursing responsibility that cannot be delegated to you. You assist the nurse through the observations you make and the care you give.

Assessment

Assessment involves collecting information about the person. The nurse takes a health history about current and past health problems. The family's health history is important. Information from the doctor is reviewed. So are test results and past medical records.

The nurse assesses the person's body systems and mental status. You assist with assessment. You make observations as you give care and talk to the person.

Observation is using the senses of sight, hearing, touch, and smell to collect information.

- You *see* how the person lies, sits, or walks. You see flushed or pale skin. You see red and swollen body areas.
- You *listen* to the person breathe, talk, and cough. You use a stethoscope to measure blood pressure.
- Through *touch*, you feel if the skin is hot or cold, or moist or dry. You use touch to take a pulse.
- *Smell* is used to detect body, wound, and breath odors. You also smell odors from urine and bowel movements (BMs).

Objective data (signs) are seen, heard, felt, or smelled by an observer. You can feel a pulse. You can see urine color. *Subjective data (symptoms) are things a person tells you about that you cannot observe through your senses.* You cannot feel or see the person's pain, fear, or nausea.

Box 8-2 lists the observations to report at once. Box 8-3 (p. 92) lists the basic observations to make and report to the nurse. Note your observations as you make them. Use your notes when reporting to the nurse (p. 97).

You do not assess. The nurse uses your observations during the assessment step of the nursing process.

See *Focus on Long-Term Care and Home Care: Assessment.*

BOX 8-2	Observations To Report at Once

- A change in the person's ability to respond
  - A responsive person no longer responds.
  - A non-responsive person now responds.
- A change in the person's mobility
  - The person cannot move a body part.
  - The person can now move a body part.
- Complaints of sudden, severe pain
- A sore or reddened area on the skin
- Complaints of a sudden change in vision
- Complaints of pain or difficulty breathing
- Abnormal respirations
- Complaints of or signs of difficulty swallowing
- Vomiting
- Bleeding
- Dizziness
- Vital signs above or below normal ranges—temperature, pulse, respirations, and blood pressure (Chapter 33)

FOCUS ON LONG-TERM CARE AND HOME CARE

Assessment

Long-Term Care

The CMS requires the *Minimum Data Set (MDS)* for nursing center residents (Appendix B, p. 890). The MDS is an assessment tool. It provides information about the person. Examples include memory, communication, hearing and vision, physical function, and activities.

The nurse uses your observations for the MDS. The MDS is started when the person is admitted to the center. The MDS is updated before each care conference (p. 93). A new MDS is done once a year and for a significant change (decline or improvement) in the person's health status.

Home Care

Medicare-certified home health agencies use the *Outcome and Assessment Information Set (OASIS)*. It is used for adult home care patients. Besides assessment, OASIS is used for planning care.

BOX 8-3   Basic Observations

Ability to Respond
- Is the person easy or hard to wake up?
- Can the person give his or her name, the time, and location when asked?
- Does the person identify others correctly?
- Does the person answer questions correctly?
- Does the person speak clearly?
- Are instructions followed correctly?
- Is the person calm, restless, or excited?
- Is the person conversing, quiet, or talking a lot?

Movement
- Can the person squeeze your fingers with each hand?
- Can the person move arms and legs?
- Are movements shaky or jerky?
- Does the person complain of stiff or painful joints?

Pain or Discomfort
- Where is the pain located? (Have the person point to the pain.)
- Does the pain go anywhere else?
- How does the person rate the severity of the pain—mild, moderate, severe?
- How does the person rate the pain on a scale of 0 to 10 (Chapter 35)?
- When did the pain begin?
- What was the person doing when the pain began?
- How long does the pain last?
- How does the person describe the pain?
  - Sharp
  - Severe
  - Stabbing
  - Dull
  - Burning
  - Aching
  - Comes and goes
  - Depends on position
- Was a pain-relief drug given?
- Did the pain-relief drug relieve pain? Is pain still present?
- Can the person sleep and rest?
- What is the position of comfort?

Skin
- Is the skin pale or flushed?
- Is the skin cool, warm, or hot?
- Is the skin moist or dry?
- Does the skin appear mottled (blotchy, spotted with color)?
- What color are the lips and nail beds?
- Is the skin intact? Are there broken areas? If so, where?
- Are sores or reddened areas present? If yes, where?
- Are bruises present? If yes, where?
- Does the person complain of itching? If yes, where?

Eyes, Ears, Nose, and Mouth
- Is there drainage from the eyes? Drainage color?
- Are the eyelids closed? Do they stay open?
- Are the eyes reddened?
- Does the person complain of spots, flashes, or blurring?
- Is the person sensitive to bright lights?
- Is there drainage from the ears? Drainage color?
- Can the person hear? Is repeating necessary? Are questions answered correctly?

Eyes, Ears, Nose, and Mouth—cont'd
- Is there drainage from the nose? Drainage color?
- Can the person breathe through the nose?
- Is there breath odor?
- Does the person complain of a bad taste in the mouth?
- Does the person complain of painful gums or teeth?
- Do the person's gums bleed with oral hygiene (Chapter 23)?

Respirations
- Do both sides of the chest rise and fall with respirations?
- Is breathing noisy?
- Does the person complain of pain or difficulty breathing?
- What is the amount and color of sputum?
- How often does the person cough? Is the cough dry or productive?

Bowels and Bladder
- Is the abdomen firm or soft?
- Does the person complain of gas?
- Which does the person use: toilet, commode, bedpan, or urinal?
- What are the amount, color, and consistency of bowel movements (BMs)?
- What is the frequency of BMs?
- Can the person control BMs?
- Does the person have pain or difficulty urinating?
- What is the amount of urine?
- What is the color of urine?
- Is the urine clear? Are there particles in the urine?
- Does urine have a foul smell?
- Can the person control the passage of urine?
- What is the frequency of urination?

Appetite
- Does the person like the food served?
- How much of the meal is eaten?
- What foods does the person like?
- Can the person chew food?
- What is the amount of fluid taken?
- What fluids does the person like?
- How often does the person drink fluids?
- Can the person swallow food and fluids?
- Does the person complain of nausea?
- What is the amount and color of vomitus?
- Does the person have hiccups?
- Is the person belching?
- Does the person cough when swallowing?

Activities of Daily Living
- Can the person perform personal care without help?
  - Bathing?
  - Brushing teeth?
  - Combing and brushing hair?
  - Shaving?
- Does the person feed himself or herself?
- Can the person walk?
- What amount and kind of help is needed?

Bleeding
- Is the person bleeding? If yes, from where and how much?

Nursing Diagnosis

The nurse uses assessment information to make a nursing diagnosis. A *nursing diagnosis describes a health problem that can be treated by nursing measures.* See Box 8-4 for examples.

Nursing diagnoses and medical diagnoses are not the same. A *medical diagnosis* is the identification of a disease or condition by a doctor. Cancer, stroke, heart attack, and diabetes are examples. Doctors use drugs, therapies, and surgery to cure or heal.

BOX 8-4	Sample Nursing Diagnoses

Nursing diagnosis:
Bathing self-care deficit—inability to independently complete cleansing activities.

Defining characteristics:
- Impaired ability to access bathroom
- Impaired ability to access water
- Impaired ability to dry body
- Impaired ability to gather bathing supplies
- Impaired ability to regulate bath water
- Impaired ability to wash body

Nursing diagnosis:
Impaired bed mobility—limitation of independent movement from one bed position to another.

Defining characteristics:
- Impaired ability to move between long sitting and supine positions
- Impaired ability to move between prone and supine positions
- Impaired ability to move between sitting and supine positions
- Impaired ability to reposition self in bed
- Impaired ability to turn from side to side

Nursing diagnosis:
Impaired walking—limitation of independent movement within the environment on foot.

Defining characteristics:
- Impaired ability to climb stairs
- Impaired ability to navigate curbs
- Impaired ability to walk on decline
- Impaired ability to walk on incline
- Impaired ability to walk on uneven surface
- Impaired ability to walk required distance

Nursing diagnosis:
Urinary retention—inability to empty the bladder completely.

Defining characteristics:
- Absence of urinary output
- Bladder distention
- Dribbling of urine
- Dysuria
- Frequent voiding
- Overflow incontinence
- Residual urine
- Sensation of bladder fullness
- Small voiding

T. Heather Herdman/Shigemi Kamitsuru (Eds.), NANDA International, Inc. Nursing Diagnoses: Definitions and Classification 2018-2020, Eleventh Edition © 2017 NANDA International, ISBN 978-1-62623-929-6. Used by arrangement with the Thieme Group, Stuttgart/New York.

A person can have many nursing diagnoses. They deal with the person's physical, emotional, social, and spiritual needs. Nursing diagnoses may change as assessment information changes. Or new ones are added.

Planning

Planning involves setting priorities and goals.
- *Priorities*—what is most important for the person.
- *Goals*—what is desired for or by a person as a result of nursing care. Also called *objectives*, goals are aimed at the person's highest level of well-being and function.

Nursing interventions are chosen after goals are set. An *intervention* is an *action or measure*. A *nursing intervention (nursing action, nursing measure, nursing task) is an action or measure taken by the nursing team to help the person reach a goal.* A nursing intervention does not need a doctor's order. Nursing measures to prevent falls, provide hygiene, and promote comfort are examples.

The *nursing care plan (care plan) is a written guide about the person's nursing care.* It has the person's nursing diagnoses and goals. It also has the nursing measures or actions for each goal. A communication tool, the care plan:
- Communicates what care to give
- Helps ensure that nursing team members give the same care

The care plan is found in the written or electronic medical record (Fig. 8-6, p. 94). The plan is carried out. It may change as nursing diagnoses change.

See *Focus on Surveys: Planning.*

FOCUS ON SURVEYS

Planning

During a survey, you may be asked about the person's care plan. Give honest and complete answers. You may be asked about:
- The person's goals
- Nursing interventions
- How the nursing interventions are carried out
- How you give input about the person's care needs and your observations

---

Care Conferences. Care conferences are held to share information and ideas about the person's care. The purpose is to develop or revise the nursing care plan. Effective care is the goal. Nursing assistants may take part in the conference.

See *Focus on Communication: Care Conferences,* p. 94.

See *Focus on Long-Term Care and Home Care: Care Conferences,* p. 95.

Nursing Care Plan

Username: R. Thompson, RN   Date: June 6   Time: 10 ▼ 40 ▼   Sign

Nursing Diagnosis

Bathing self-care deficit—inability to independently complete cleansing activities

Defining characteristics:	Nursing interventions:
[X] Impaired ability to access bathroom	◉ Assist to the shower with a walker and gait belt.
[ ] Impaired ability to access water	◉ Use a shower chair.
[ ] Impaired ability to dry body	◉ Provide bathing supplies within reach.
[X] Impaired ability to gather bathing supplies	◉ Provide a long-handled sponge.
[ ] Impaired ability to regulate bath water	◉ Encourage the resident to wash self independently.
[ ] Impaired ability to wash body	◉ Remain in shower room. Provide for privacy with shower curtain.

Goal: Resident will safely perform bathing activities independently by 6/20.

Nursing Diagnosis

Impaired walking—limitation of independent movement within the environment on foot

Defining characteristics:	Nursing interventions:
[ ] Impaired ability to climb stairs	◉ Use a walker and gait belt for walking.
[ ] Impaired ability to navigate curbs	◉ Provide rest periods as needed.
[ ] Impaired ability to walk on decline	◉ Assist to and from the dining room 3 times daily.
[ ] Impaired ability to walk on incline	◉ Remind resident to call for help to the bathroom.
[ ] Impaired ability to walk on uneven surface	◉ Assist to and from the bathroom for elimination and grooming needs.
[X] Impaired ability to walk required distance	◉ Assist to and from the shower room for bathing.

Goal: Resident will safely walk to and from the dining room, bathroom, and shower room with assistance by 6/18.

FIGURE 8-6 A sample nursing care plan. Each nursing diagnosis has a goal. There are nursing interventions for each goal. (Nursing diagnoses, definitions, and defining characteristics from T. Heather Herdman/Shigemi Kamitsuru [Eds.], NANDA International, Inc. Nursing Diagnoses: Definitions and Classification 2018-2020, Eleventh Edition © 2017 NANDA International, ISBN 978-1-62623-929-6. Used by arrangement with the Thieme Group, Stuttgart/New York.)

FOCUS ON **COMMUNICATION**

Care Conferences

You see what patients and residents like and do not like and what they can and cannot do. They talk to you. They tell you about their families and interests. You make observations when you are with them. Share this information during care conferences.

Also share ideas about care. For example, you can say:

- "Mr. Antonio misses the fresh green beans and broccoli from his garden. Can we ask the family to bring those more often?"
- "Mrs. Clark can propel her wheelchair with her feet. Why do we push her wheelchair?"
- "Miss Walsh never talks when her family visits. She talks to her roommate often."

FOCUS ON LONG-TERM CARE AND HOME CARE

Care Conferences

Long-Term Care

The CMS requires 2 types of resident care conferences.

- *Interdisciplinary care planning (IDCP) conferences.* These are held to form care plans for new residents. They are also held regularly to review and update care plans. The RN, doctor, and other health team members attend.
- *Problem-focused conferences.* These are used when 1 problem affects a person's care. Only staff involved with the problem attend.

The person and family have the right to take part in planning conferences. The person may refuse actions suggested by the health team.

Problems identified on the MDS give *triggers* for the Care Area Assessment (CAA) (Appendix C, p. 892). Triggered care areas must be assessed more thoroughly.

The CMS requires a *comprehensive care plan.* It is a guide about the person's care. The plan has the person's problems, nursing diagnoses, goals, and actions to take.

For example, the MDS shows that a resident cannot do activities of daily living (ADL). A care plan is developed to solve the problem. The goal is for the resident to perform ADL. Actions to reach the goal are:

- Occupational therapy for ADL daily
- Physical therapy for exercises daily
- Nursing staff to walk the resident 20 yards twice daily

The care plan also has the person's strengths. For example, the resident can eat without help. This strength increases independence. The health team helps the resident to continue to eat without help.

Implementation

To *implement* means *to perform or carry out. In the implementation* step, *nursing interventions (nursing measures, nursing actions, nursing tasks) in the care plan are carried out.* Care is given.

Nursing care ranges from simple to complex. The nurse delegates tasks within your legal limits and job description. The nurse may delegate or ask you to assist with complex measures.

Assignment Sheets. The nurse communicates delegated tasks to you. An assignment sheet is used for this purpose (Fig. 8-7). The assignment sheet tells you about:

- Each person's care.
- What nursing interventions and tasks to do.
- Which nursing unit tasks to do. Cleaning utility rooms and stocking shower rooms are examples.

Talk to the nurse about an unclear assignment. Also check the care plan and Kardex for more information.

See *Focus on Communication: Assignment Sheets*, p. 96.

See *Teamwork and Time Management: Assignment Sheets*, p. 96.

Assignment Sheet

Date: 9–10
Shift: Day
Nursing assistant: J. Reed
Supervisor: M. Garcia, RN

Breaks: 1000   1400
Lunch: 1230
Unit Tasks: *Pass drinking water at 0900*
Clean utility room at 1430

***Check the care plan for other care measures and information**

Room # 501A Name: Mrs. Ann Lopez ID Number: S1514491530 Date of birth: 11/04/1934 VS: Daily at 0700 T _____ P _____ R _____ BP _____ Wt: Weekly (Monday at 0700) _____ Intake _____ Output _____ BM _____ Bath: Portable tub Shampoo Bed rails	**Functional status/care measures and procedures** Total assist with ADL Stand-pivot transfers Uses w/c Incontinent of bowel and bladder – uses briefs Passive ROM exercises to extremities twice daily Turn and re-position q2h when in bed Wears eyeglasses and dentures Diet: High fiber (total assist)
Room # 510B Name: Mr. Mark Lee ID Number: D4468947762 Date of birth: 12/29/1940 VS: 2 times daily, at 0700 and 1500 0700: T _____ P _____ R _____ BP _____ 1500: T _____ P _____ R _____ BP _____ Wt: Daily at 0700 _____ Intake _____ Output _____ BM _____ Bath: Shower	**Functional status/care measures and procedures** Independent with ADL Independent with ambulation Attends exercise group every morning Continent of bowel and bladder – q4h bathroom schedule to maintain continence Wears eyeglasses Coughing and deep-breathing exercises q4h Diet: Sodium-controlled (independent)

FIGURE 8-7 A sample assignment sheet. NOTE: This assignment sheet is a computer printout.

Evaluation

Evaluate means *to measure.* The *evaluation* step involves *measuring if the goals in the planning step were met.* Progress is evaluated. Goals may be met totally, in part, or not at all. Assessment information is used for this step. Changes in nursing diagnoses, goals, and the care plan may result.

REPORTING AND RECORDING

The health team communicates by reporting and recording. *Reporting* is the oral account of care and observations. *Recording* (charting, documentation) is the written account of care and observations.

Reporting and Recording Time

The 24-hour clock (military time or international time) has 4 digits (Fig. 8-8). The first 2 digits are for the hours. The last 2 digits are for minutes: 0110 = 1:10 AM. Colons and AM and PM are not used. Box 8-5 shows how *conventional time* is written in *24-hour time.*

See *Focus on Math: Reporting and Recording Time.*

See *Focus on Communication: Reporting and Recording Time.*

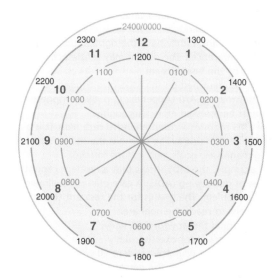

FIGURE 8-8 The 24-hour clock. The AM times are in orange. The PM times are in purple. NOTE: 12 noon is 1200; 12 midnight is 2400 or 0000.

BOX 8-5	24-Hour Clock		
AM		**PM**	
Conventional Time	24-Hour Time	Conventional Time	24-Hour Time
12:00 MIDNIGHT	0000 or 2400	12:00 NOON	1200
1:00 AM	0100	1:00 PM	1300
2:00 AM	0200	2:00 PM	1400
3:00 AM	0300	3:00 PM	1500
4:00 AM	0400	4:00 PM	1600
5:00 AM	0500	5:00 PM	1700
6:00 AM	0600	6:00 PM	1800
7:00 AM	0700	7:00 PM	1900
8:00 AM	0800	8:00 PM	2000
9:00 AM	0900	9:00 PM	2100
10:00 AM	1000	10:00 PM	2200
11:00 AM	1100	11:00 PM	2300

Reporting

Report care and observations to the nurse.
- When there is a change from normal or a change in the person's condition. Report these changes at once.
- When the nurse asks you to do so.
- Before leaving the unit for meals, breaks, or other reasons.
- Before the end-of-shift report (p. 98).
- After the end-of-shift report and before reporting off duty.

When reporting, follow the rules in Box 8-6.

See *Teamwork and Time Management: Reporting.*

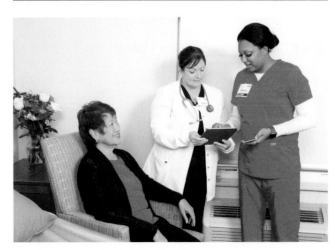

FIGURE 8-9 The nursing assistant uses notes to report to the nurse.

End-of-Shift Report. *The nurse gives a report at the end of the shift to the on-coming shift. This is called the **end-of-shift report** or change-of-shift report.* The nurse reports about:
- The care given
- The care to give during other shifts
- The person's current condition
- Likely changes in the person's condition
- New or changed orders

Some agencies have the entire nursing team hear the end-of-shift report as they come on duty. In other agencies, only nurses hear the report. After the report, nursing assistants receive needed information.

See *Teamwork and Time Management: End-of-Shift Report.*

See *Promoting Safety and Comfort: End-of-Shift Report.*

TEAMWORK AND TIME MANAGEMENT

End-of-Shift Report

The staff going off duty and the staff coming on duty are present during shift changes—the end of one and the start of another. All on-coming staff may attend the end-of-shift report. If so, staff going off duty answer call lights, provide care, and tend to routine tasks. If only nurses attend the report, nursing assistants of the on-coming shift help with those tasks.

The end-of-shift requires good teamwork. Continue to do your job. Your attitude is important. If going off duty, avoid saying or thinking:
- "I'm ready to go home. Let them do it."
- "It's their turn. I've been here all day (evening or night)."
- "No one helped us when we came on duty."

Some agencies have clear duties for the 2 shifts. For example, those going off duty know about the patients or residents. They continue to answer call lights. Waiting to receive report, the on-coming shift performs routine tasks and collects needed supplies and equipment.

PROMOTING SAFETY AND COMFORT

End-of-Shift Report

Safety

You may not hear the end-of-shift report as you come on duty. You answer call lights and give care before the nurse shares information with you. For safe care:
- Check the care plan and Kardex before granting a request. The person's condition or care plan may have changed. There may be new orders.
- Ask a nurse about the care needs of new patients or residents. If a need is urgent, politely interrupt the end-of-shift report to ask your questions.
- Do not take directions or orders from another nursing assistant. Remember, nursing assistants cannot supervise or delegate to other nursing assistants.

You may answer call lights during the end-of-shift report as you go off duty. Be sure to report observations, care measures, requests, and so on before you leave. For example, you assist a resident onto the bedpan before going home. The nursing team of the on-coming shift needs to know so they can check on the person. Otherwise the person could be left on the bedpan for a long time, causing the person harm.

Recording

When recording (documenting, charting), you must communicate clearly and thoroughly. Follow the rules in Box 8-7. Anyone reading your charting should know:
- What you observed
- What you did
- The person's response

See *Focus on Communication: Recording.*

FOCUS ON COMMUNICATION

Recording

"Small," "moderate," "large," "long," and "short" mean different things to different people. Is small the size of a dime or a quarter? In health care, different meanings can cause serious problems. Give accurate descriptions and measurements. If not sure, ask the nurse to look at what you are trying to describe.

BOX 8-7	Rules for Recording

General Rules

- Follow agency policies and procedures for recording. Ask for needed training.
- Check the name and identifying information on the chart. You must record on the correct chart.
- Include the date and time for each recording. Use 24-hour time or conventional time (AM or PM) according to agency policy.
- Use only agency-approved abbreviations (see "Abbreviations" in Chapter 9).
- Use correct spelling, grammar, and punctuation.
- Do not use ditto (") marks.
- Record only what you observed and did yourself. Do not record for another person.
- Never chart a procedure, treatment, or care measure until after it is completed.
- Be accurate, concise, and factual. Do not record judgments or interpretations. For example, "The person felt sad" is a judgment. "The person was crying" is factual.
- Record in a logical manner and in sequence.
- Be descriptive. Avoid terms with more than 1 meaning.
- Use the person's exact words when possible. Use quotation marks ("...") for a direct quote.
- Chart changes from normal or changes in the person's condition. Also chart that you told the nurse (include the nurse's name), what you said, and the time you made the report.
- Do not omit (leave out) information.
- Record safety measures. Examples include placing the call light within reach, assisting the person when up, or reminding a person not to get out of bed.
- Sign or save all entries as required by agency policy. For paper entries, include your name and title.

On Computer

- Log in using your username and password. Do not use another person's username.
- Check the time your entry is made. Make sure it is the right time.
- Check for accuracy. Review your entry before saving.
- Save your entries. Un-saved data will be lost.
- Follow the manufacturer's instructions to change or un-chart a mistaken entry. Most electronic systems keep a record of original entries and changes.
- Log off after charting. This prevents others from charting under your username.
- See "Electronic Devices," p. 100.

On Paper

- Make sure each form and page has the person's name and other identifying information.
- Always use ink. Use the ink color required by the agency.
- Make sure writing is readable and neat.
- Never erase or use correction fluid (white out). Draw a line through the incorrect part. Date and initial the line. Write "mistaken entry" over it if this is agency policy. Then re-write the part. Follow agency policy for correcting errors. See Figure 8-10.
- Do not skip lines. Draw a line through the blank space of a partially completed line or to the end of the page (see Fig. 8-10). This prevents others from recording in a space with your signature.

Date	Time	Nursing Margin / Other Depts Margin
7/26	1045	Requested assistance to lie down. States, "I don't feel well. I have a little upset stomach."
		Denies pain. VS taken. T-99(0). P-76 regular rate and rhythm. R-18 unlabored.
		BP 134/84 L arm lying down. Call light within reach. Paula Jones, RN notified at 1040
		of resident's complaint and VS. Mary Jensen, CNA
7-26	1100	Asleep in bed. Appears to be resting comfortably. Color good. No signs of
		discomfort or distress noted at this time. Paula Jones, RN
7-26	1145	Refused to go to the dining room for lunch. Complains of nausea.
		Denies abdominal pain. Has not had an emesis. Abdomen soft to
		palpation. Good bowel sounds. VS taken. T-98.2 99.2. P-76 regular [Mistaken entry 7-26, PJ]
		rate and rhythm. R-18 unlabored. BP-134/84. States she will try to
		eat something. Full liquid room tray ordered. Paula Jones, RN

FIGURE 8-10 Progress note on paper. A mistaken entry is corrected by drawing a single line through the incorrect part.

Electronic Recording. Electronic health or medical records improve access to medical records. Recording may be done in patients' or residents' rooms, in hallways, at the nurses' station, or on portable or hand-held devices (p. 100).

Users log in (sign in) to access the record. You will be trained to use your agency's system.

ELECTRONIC DEVICES

Electronic devices are used to store and send information to the health team. Such devices include:

- Desktop, mobile, and work-station computers (Fig. 8-11). A keyboard and mouse are used to input or access data. Or an electronic pen or pencil is used.
- Lap-tops. These are portable devices. The user works directly on the screen or uses a keyboard and mouse.
- Tablets and hand-held devices. Held in the palm of 1 hand, the other hand is used to work on the screen. See Figure 8-9.
- Fax machines. These devices are used to send and receive paper documents.

Follow agency policies when using electronic devices. Use only your username and password. You must keep protected health information (PHI) and electronic protected health information (EPHI; ePHI) confidential.

Follow the rules in Box 8-8 and the ethical and legal rules about privacy, confidentiality, and defamation (Chapters 5 and 6) when using electronic devices.

See *Teamwork and Time Management: Electronic Devices.*

TEAMWORK AND TIME MANAGEMENT
Electronic Devices

Electronic devices are often used for measurements such as blood pressures, temperatures, and heart rates. Some electronic devices for measuring vital signs (Chapter 33) send measurements directly to the EHR (EMR). The system alerts the nursing staff to abnormal vital signs.

Such systems save time and reduce recording errors. Quality care and safety are increased. Records are more accurate and complete. Staff are more efficient.

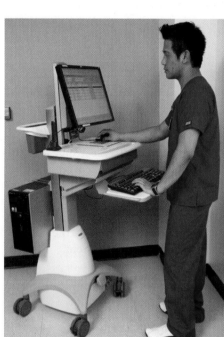
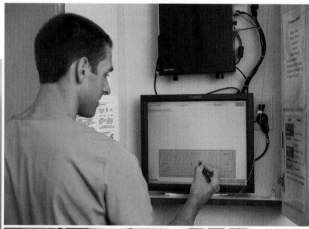
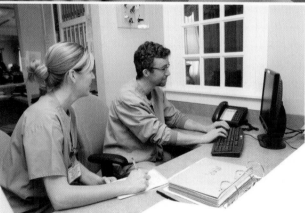

FIGURE 8-11 Examples of electronic devices used by the health team.

BOX 8-8	Electronic Devices

Computers, Lap-Tops, Tablets, and Hand-Held Devices

- See "Wrongful Use of Electronic Communications" in Chapter 5.
- Do not tell anyone your username or password. With your information, others can access, record, send, receive, or store PHI (EPHI; ePHI) under your name. It will be hard to prove you did not do so.
- Do not write down, post, or expose your username or password. This is for your security. For example, do not write them on a note pad or post them at your work station.
- Change your password often. Follow agency policy.
- Do not use another person's username or password.
- Follow the rules for recording (see Box 8-7).
- Enter data carefully. Double-check your entries.
- Prevent others from seeing the screen.
  - Place the screen so it cannot be seen by others.
  - Be aware of anyone standing behind you.
  - Stand or sit with your back to the wall if using a mobile computer.
  - Do not leave a device unattended.
- Log off after making an entry.
- Do not leave printouts where others can read or pick them up.
- Shred or destroy printouts, assignment sheets, or worksheets. Place such documents in a wastebasket marked CONFIDENTIAL INFORMATION for shredding. Follow agency policy.
- Send e-mail and messages only to those needing the information.
- Do not e-mail information or messages that require immediate reporting. Give the report in person. The person may not read the e-mail in a timely manner.
- Do not use e-mail or messages to report confidential information. This includes addresses, phone numbers, and Social Security numbers. The computer system may not be secure.
- Remember that any communication can be read or heard by someone other than the intended person.

Computers, Lap-Tops, Tablets, and Hand-Held Devices—cont'd

- Remember that deleted communications can be retrieved by authorized staff.
- Do not use agency devices for personal use. Do not:
  - Send personal e-mail messages.
  - Send or receive e-mail or messages that are offensive, not legal, or sexual.
  - Send or receive e-mail for illegal activities, jokes, politics, gambling (including football and other pools), chain letters, or other non-work activities.
  - Post information, opinions, or comments on websites or video or social media sites.
  - Upload, download, or send materials containing a copyright, trademark, or patent.
- Remember that the agency has the right to monitor your use of electronic devices. This includes Internet use.
- Do not open another person's e-mail or messages.
- Follow agency policy for mis-directed e-mails.

Faxes

- See "Wrongful Use of Electronic Communications" in Chapter 5.
- Use the agency's "cover sheet." The sheet has instructions about:
  - The confidentiality of PHI (EPHI; ePHI)
  - The receiver's responsibilities about PHI (EPHI; ePHI)
  - The receiver's responsibilities for a fax received in error (mis-directed fax)
- Complete the "cover sheet" according to agency policy. The following are common.
  - Name of the person to receive the fax
  - Receiver's fax number
  - Date
  - Number of pages being faxed
  - Department name
  - Name and phone number of the person sending the fax
- Follow agency policy for a mis-directed fax.
- Do not leave sent or received faxes unattended in the fax machine or lying around.

PHONE COMMUNICATIONS

You will answer phones at the nurses' station or in the person's room. Use good communication skills. Your tone of voice, speech clarity, and attitude are important. Be professional and courteous. Also practice good work ethics. Follow the agency's policy and the guidelines in Box 8-9, p. 102.

See *Focus on Long-Term Care and Home Care: Phone Communications.*

FOCUS ON LONG-TERM CARE AND HOME CARE

Phone Communications

Home Care

Answer phones in patients' homes with "hello." This is to protect the person, family, and you. Too much information is shared when you give the person's name ("Price residence") or your name and title.

People call homes for many reasons. Some make sales calls or ask for donations. Others have criminal intent. Some criminals target vulnerable people. Saying that you are a home health assistant means that an ill, older, or disabled person is in the home.

Do not give your name or the person's name until you know who is calling and why. Make sure it is someone you or the person wants to talk to—the person's family or friend, your supervisor, or a caller expected by the person.

BOX 8-9	Answering Phones

- Answer the call after the first ring if possible. Be sure to answer by the fourth ring.
- Do not answer in a rushed or hasty manner.
- Give a courteous greeting. Identify the agency or nursing unit and give your name and title. For example: "Good morning, 3 center. Pat Wills, nursing assistant."
- Follow agency policy for answering phones in patient or resident rooms.
- Note this information to take a message.
  - The caller's name and phone number (include the area code and extension number)
  - The date and time
  - Who the message is for
- Repeat the message and phone number back to the caller.
- Ask the caller to "Please hold" if necessary. First find out who is calling and the caller's number. Then ask if the caller can hold. Do not put callers with an emergency on hold.

- Do not lay the phone down or cover the receiver with your hand when not speaking to the caller. The caller may over-hear confidential conversations.
- Return to a caller on hold within 30 seconds. Ask if the caller can wait longer or if the call can be returned.
- Do not give confidential information to any caller. Patient, resident, and employee information is confidential. Refer such calls to the nurse.
- Transfer the call if appropriate.
  - Tell the caller that you are going to transfer the call.
  - Give the name of the department or the name of the person who should answer the phone if appropriate.
  - Get the caller's name and number in case the call gets disconnected.
  - Give the caller the phone number to call in case the call gets disconnected or the line is busy.
- End the conversation politely. Thank the person for calling and say good-bye.
- Give the message to the appropriate person.

FOCUS ON **PRIDE**

The Person, Family, and Yourself

P ersonal and Professional Responsibility
You are responsible for what you report and record. It must be accurate. If allowed to chart, follow the rules in Box 8-7.

R ights and Respect
The person has the right to take part in care planning. The person also has the right to refuse actions suggested by the nursing and health teams. The goal is a plan of care that meets the person's needs and preferences.

I ndependence and Social Interaction
Health team communications are not limited to reporting and recording. You interact in the nurses' station, patient and resident rooms, hallways, break room, cafeteria, parking lot, and so on. Treat co-workers with kindness and respect. Have a good attitude. Be someone others enjoy working with!

D elegation and Teamwork
Assignment sheets communicate the nursing tasks and unit tasks delegated to you. If you have a problem with an assignment or task, share your reason with the nurse. Not liking an assignment or task is not a good reason. The nurse will decide if a change is needed.

E thics and Laws
Legal action can be taken against persons who record false information. For example:

A licensed nursing assistant (LNA) worked at a home health and hospice agency. On November 9, she recorded on a time sheet that she was in a patient's home for about 30 minutes. However, the patient was in the hospital from November 8 through November 14.

The LNA admitted to unprofessional conduct. Her conduct violated Administrative Rules of the Board of Nursing for:
- *Making inaccurate or misleading entries*
- *Failing to comply with federal or state laws or rules*
  The LNA was given a reprimand by the Board.
  (State of Vermont Board of Nursing, 2003.)

A reprimand means that the Board considered her conduct to be improper. However, the Board did not limit her right to work as an LNA.

FOCUS ON **PRIDE**: *Application*
Explain why accurate and timely reporting and recording are important. What problems may occur from incorrect or delayed reporting or recording?

REVIEW QUESTIONS

Circle T if the statement is TRUE or F if it is FALSE.

1 T F You help with a person's care. Recording on the person's medical record violates the right to privacy.

2 T F Medical records can be used to prove the care given.

3 T F You can access all medical records in the agency.

4 T F The nursing process is the method nurses use to plan and deliver nursing care.

5 T F Measures in the care plan are carried out in the assessment step of the nursing process.

6 T F When using a computer, the person's privacy must be protected.

7 T F You can give information about the person over the phone.

8 T F You can post your username and password in your work area.

9 T F The agency can monitor your computer use.

10 T F You should leave faxes in the fax machine for the nurse to read.

REVIEW QUESTIONS—cont'd

Circle the BEST answer.

11 To communicate well, you should
   a Use terms with many meanings
   b Give long descriptions
   c Use unfamiliar terms
   d Give facts and be specific

12 A person is discharged from the agency. The medical record is
   a Destroyed
   b Sent home with the family
   c Permanent
   d No longer private

13 Where does the nurse describe the nursing care given?
   a Admission record
   b Health history
   c Progress notes
   d Kardex

14 You need to know if a resident uses a hearing aid. You should
   a Check the Kardex
   b Read the progress notes
   c Look through the person's belongings
   d Interrupt the end-of-shift report to ask the nurse

15 You need to record a patient's vital signs every hour. Where should you record the measurements?
   a Nursing assessment
   b Medication administration record
   c Discharge summary
   d Flow sheet

16 Your role in the nursing process involves
   a Reporting observations
   b Making nursing diagnoses
   c Writing the care plan
   d Evaluating if goals are met

17 Which is a symptom?
   a Redness
   b Vomiting
   c Pain
   d Pulse rate of 78

18 Which should you report at once?
   a The person can no longer move a body part.
   b The person answers questions correctly.
   c The person has a breath odor.
   d The person walked to the dining room.

19 The care plan is
   a Written by the doctor
   b The measures to help the person
   c The same for all persons
   d Not changed after it is developed

20 To communicate delegated tasks to you, the nurse uses
   a The care plan
   b The Minimum Data Set
   c An assignment sheet
   d Care conferences

21 Which statement about recording is *correct?*
   a Avoid using the person's exact words.
   b Record only what you did and observed.
   c Use correction fluid for a mistaken entry.
   d Chart a procedure before completing it.

22 In the evening, the clock shows 9:26. In 24-hour clock time this is
   a 9:26 PM
   b 1926
   c 0926
   d 2126

23 In the morning, the clock shows 7:45. In 24-hour clock time this is
   a 0745
   b 1945
   c 745
   d 7:45 AM

24 You have access to the agency's computer. Which is *true?*
   a You should log off after making an entry.
   b E-mail is used for reports the nurse needs at once.
   c You can use another person's username.
   d You can use the computer for your personal needs.

25 A phone rings at the nurses' station. Which greeting is *best?*
   a "Good morning. This is Joey."
   b "North hall."
   c "Good morning, North hall. Joey Wilson, nursing assistant, speaking."
   d "Hello."

Answers to Chapter 8 questions are on p. 885.

FOCUS ON PRACTICE

Problem Solving

A resident has become weak since you last provided care. The resident now needs more help to transfer from bed to chair. You were not told about the change at the start of your shift. Why is this a problem? How could it have been prevented?

Medical Terminology

OBJECTIVES

- Define the key terms in this chapter.
- Identify the word parts that make up medical terms.
- Explain how to define medical terms.
- Locate the 4 abdominal regions.
- Explain the terms used to describe body position.
- Define common abbreviations and health care terms.
- Explain how to promote PRIDE in the person, the family, and yourself.

KEY TERMS

abbreviation A shortened form of a word or phrase
anterior At or toward the front of the body or body part; ventral
distal The part farthest from the center or from the point of attachment
dorsal See "posterior"
lateral Away from the mid-line; at the side of the body or body part
medial At or near the middle or mid-line of the body or body part
posterior At or toward the back of the body or body part; dorsal

prefix A word element at the beginning of a word; it changes the meaning of the word
proximal The part nearest to the center or to the point of attachment
root A word element containing the basic meaning of the word
suffix A word element at the end of a word; it changes the meaning of the word
ventral See "anterior"
word element A part of a word

Medical terms and abbreviations are used in health care. Understanding the basics of medical terminology is important for your training and work.

If you do not understand a word, phrase, or abbreviation, ask a nurse for its meaning. Otherwise, communication does not occur. A medical dictionary is useful to learn new words.

MEDICAL TERMS

Like all words, medical terms are made up of *parts of words or word elements*—prefixes, roots, and suffixes. Most are from Greek or Latin. Word elements are combined to form medical terms (Fig. 9-1).

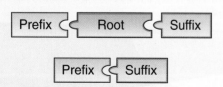

FIGURE 9-1 Prefixes, roots, and suffixes are combined to form medical terms. (Modified from Leonard PC: *Building a medical vocabulary with Spanish translations,* ed 10, St Louis, 2018, Elsevier.)

Prefixes, Roots, and Suffixes

A *prefix is a word element at the beginning of a word. It changes the meaning of the word.* For example, the prefix *hemi* (half) is placed before *plegia* (paralysis) to make *hemiplegia*. It means paralysis on half of the body. Prefixes are used with other word elements. Prefixes are not used alone.

The *root is the word element that contains the basic meaning of the word.* It is combined with another root, a prefix, or a suffix. A vowel (an *o* or an *i*) may be added when 2 roots are combined or when a suffix is added to a root. *Cardi(o)* is a root that means heart. *Neur(o)* is a root that means nerve. The vowel makes the word easier to pronounce.

A *suffix is a word element at the end of a word. It changes the meaning of the word.* Suffixes are not used alone. For example, *colonoscopy* means examination of the large intestine using a scope. It was formed by combining the root *colon(o)* (colon, large intestine) and the suffix *scopy* (examination using a scope).

See Table 9-1 for a list of common prefixes, roots, and suffixes. Studying word elements will help you understand the meanings of medical terms.

TABLE 9-1	Word Elements			
Prefix	**Meaning**		**Prefix**	**Meaning**
a-, an-	without, not, lack of		peri-	around
ab-	away from		poly-	many, much
ad-	to, toward, near		post-	after, behind
ante-	before, forward, in front of		pre-	before, in front of, prior to
anti-	against		pro-	before, in front of
auto-	self		re-	again, backward
bi-	double, two (2), twice		retro-	backward, behind
brady-	slow		semi-	half
circum-	around		sub-	under, beneath
contra-	against, opposite		super-	above, over, excess
cyan-	blue		supra-	above, over
de-	down, from, off, opposite		tachy-	fast, rapid
dia-	across, through, apart		trans-	across
dis-	apart, free from		uni-	one (1)
dys-	bad, difficult, abnormal, painful		**Root (combining vowel)**	**Meaning**
ecto-	outer, outside		abdomin (o)	abdomen
en-	in, into, within		aden (o)	gland
endo-	inner, inside		adren (o)	adrenal gland
epi-	over, on, upon		angi (o)	vessel
erythro-	red		arteri (o)	artery
eu-	normal, good, well, healthy		arthr (o)	joint
ex-	out, out of, from, away from		bronch (o)	bronchus, bronchi
hemi-	half		card, cardi (o)	heart
hyper-	excessive, too much, high		cephal (o)	head
hypo-	under, decreased, less than normal		chole, chol (o)	bile
in-	in, into, within, not		chondr (o)	cartilage
inter-	between		col, colon (o)	colon, large intestine
intra-	within		cost (o)	rib
intro-	into, within		crani (o)	skull
leuko-	white		cyst (o)	bladder, cyst
macro-	large		cyt (o)	cell
mal-	bad, illness, disease		dent (i)	tooth
meg-	large		derm, dermat (o)	skin
micro-	small		duoden (o)	duodenum (part of the small intestine)
mono-	one (1), single		electr (o)	electricity
neo-	new		encephal (o)	brain
non-	not		enter (o)	intestines
olig-	small, scant		fibr (o)	fiber, fibrous
para-	beside, beyond, after		gastr (o)	stomach
per-	by, through			

Continued

TABLE 9-1	Word Elements—cont'd

Root (combining vowel)	Meaning
gloss (o)	tongue
gluc (o)	sweetness, glucose
glyc (o)	sugar
gyn, gyne, gyneco	woman
hem, hema, hemo, hemat (o)	blood
hepat (o)	liver
hydr (o)	water
hyster (o)	uterus
ile (o)	ileum (part of the small intestine)
ili (o)	ilium (part of the hip bone)
jejun (o)	jejunum (part of the small intestine)
lapar (o)	abdomen, loin, flank
laryng (o)	larynx (voice box)
lith (o)	stone
mamm, mast (o)	breast, mammary gland
meno	menstruation
my (o)	muscle
myel (o)	spinal cord, bone marrow
necr (o)	death
nephr (o)	kidney
neur (o)	nerve
ocul (o)	eye
onc (o)	tumor
oophor (o)	ovary
ophthalm (o)	eye
orth (o)	straight, normal, correct
oste (o)	bone
ot (o)	ear
ped (o)	child, foot
pharyng (o)	pharynx (throat)
phleb (o)	vein
pneum (o)	lung, air, gas
proct (o)	rectum
psych (o)	mind
pulmon (o)	lung
py (o)	pus
rect (o)	rectum
rhin (o)	nose

Root (combining vowel)	Meaning
salping (o)	eustachian tube, fallopian tube
splen (o)	spleen
stern (o)	sternum
stomat (o)	mouth
therm (o)	heat
thorac (o)	chest
thromb (o)	clot, thrombus
thyr (o)	thyroid
toxic (o)	poison, poisonous
toxo	poison
trache (o)	trachea (windpipe)
urethr (o)	urethra
urin (o)	urine
ur (o)	urine, urinary tract, urination
uter (o)	uterus
vas (o)	blood vessel, vas deferens
vascul (o)	blood vessel
ven (o)	vein
vertebr (o)	spine, vertebrae

Suffix	Meaning
-algia	pain
-asis	condition, usually abnormal
-cele	hernia, herniation, pouching
-centesis	surgical puncture to remove fluid
-cyte	cell
-ectasis	dilation, stretching
-ectomy	excision, removal of
-emesis	vomiting
-emia	blood condition
-genesis	development, production, creation
-genic	producing, causing
-gram	record
-graph	a diagram, a recording instrument
-graphy	making a recording
-iasis	condition of
-ism	a condition
-itis	inflammation
-logy	the study of
-lysis	destruction of, decomposition

TABLE 9-1	Word Elements—cont'd		Suffix	Meaning
Suffix	Meaning		-ptosis	falling, sagging, dropping down
-megaly	enlargement		-rrhage, rrhagia	excessive flow
-mentia	condition of the mind		-rrhaphy	stitching, suturing
-meter	measuring instrument		-rrhea	flow, discharge
-oma	tumor		-scope	examination instrument
-osis	condition		-scopy	examination using a scope
-pathy	disease		-stasis	maintenance, maintaining a constant level
-penia	lack, deficiency			
-phagia	to eat or consume, swallowing		-stenosis	narrowing
-phasia	speaking, speech		-stomy, -ostomy	creation of an opening
-phobia	an exaggerated fear		-tomy, -otomy	incision, cutting into
-plasty	surgical repair or re-shaping		-trophy	decline of a body part
-plegia	paralysis		-uria	urine
-pnea	breathing, respiration			

Defining Medical Terms

Medical terms are formed by combining word elements. Remember, prefixes are at the beginning. Suffixes are at the end. A root can be combined with prefixes, roots, and suffixes. Some words have only a prefix and suffix.

To define a term, separate the word into its elements (Table 9-2). To read the meaning:

1 Begin with the suffix. Read the meaning of the suffix.
2 Then go to the beginning of the word. Read the meaning of each word part up to the suffix.

For terms with only a prefix and suffix, read the meaning of the prefix. Then read the meaning of the suffix.

TABLE 9-2	Defining Medical Terms	
Medical Term	**Word Elements**	**Definition**
Aphasia	*a-* (without, lack of) + *-phasia* (speaking) [prefix] [suffix]	Lack of speaking ability
Cyanosis	*cyan-* (blue) + *-osis* (condition) [prefix] [suffix]	Condition of having a bluish color
Dysphagia	*dys-* (difficult) + *-phagia* (swallowing) [prefix] [suffix]	Difficulty swallowing
Dyspnea	*dys-* (difficult, painful) + *-pnea* (breathing) [prefix] [suffix]	Difficult or painful breathing
Electrocardiogram	*electr (o)* (electricity) + *cardi (o)* (heart) + *-gram* (record) [root] [root] [suffix]	Record of the electricity in the heart
Endocarditis	*endo-* (inner) + *card* (heart) + *-itis* (inflammation) [prefix] [root] [suffix]	Inflammation of the inner part of the heart
Gastrostomy	*gastr* (stomach) + *-ostomy* (creation of an opening) [root] [suffix]	A surgically created opening in the stomach
Mastectomy	*mast* (breast) + *-ectomy* (excision or removal) [root] [suffix]	Removal of a breast
Nephritis	*nephr* (kidney) + *-itis* (inflammation) [root] [suffix]	Inflammation of the kidney
Oliguria	*olig-* (scant, small amount) + *-uria* (urine) [prefix] [suffix]	A small amount of urine

ABDOMINAL REGIONS

The abdomen is divided into regions (Fig. 9-2). They are used to describe the location of body structures, pain, or discomfort. The regions are:

- Right upper quadrant (RUQ)
- Left upper quadrant (LUQ)
- Right lower quadrant (RLQ)
- Left lower quadrant (LLQ)

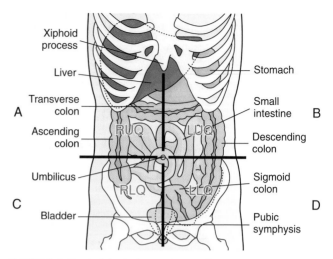

FIGURE 9-2 The 4 abdominal regions. **A,** Right upper quadrant (RUQ). **B,** Left upper quadrant (LUQ). **C,** Right lower quadrant (RLQ). **D,** Left lower quadrant (LLQ).

DIRECTIONAL TERMS

Certain terms describe the position of 1 body part in relation to another. These terms give the direction of the body part when a person is standing and facing forward. The arms are stretched out with the thumbs pointing outward. See Figure 9-3.

- *Anterior (ventral)*—at or toward the front of the body or body part
- *Posterior (dorsal)*—at or toward the back of the body or body part
- *Proximal*—the part nearest to the center or to the point of attachment
- *Distal*—the part farthest from the center or from the point of attachment
- *Lateral*—away from the mid-line; at the side of the body or body part
- *Medial*—at or near the middle or mid-line of the body or body part

ABBREVIATIONS

Abbreviations are shortened forms of words or phrases. They save time and space when recording. Each agency has a list of allowed abbreviations. Obtain the list when you are hired. Use only those on the list. If not sure about an abbreviation, write the term out in full. This promotes clear communication.

See Table 9-3 for a list of common abbreviations that you may use.

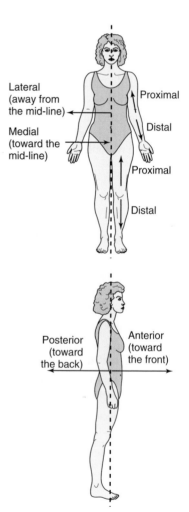

FIGURE 9-3 Directional terms describe the position of 1 body part in relation to another.

TABLE 9-3	Common Abbreviations		
Abbreviation	**Meaning**	**Abbreviation**	**Meaning**
abd	abdomen	lt; L	left
AC; a.c.	before meals	meds	medications
ADL	activities of daily living	mid noc	midnight
ad lib	as desired	min	minute
AIDS	acquired immunodeficiency syndrome	mL	milliliter
AM	morning	neg	negative
AMB; amb	ambulate (to walk); ambulatory (able to walk)	noc	night
amt	amount	NPO; npo	nothing by mouth (*nil per os*)
ap; AP	apical	O_2	oxygen
BM; bm	bowel movement	OOB	out of bed
BP	blood pressure	OR	operating room
BRP	bathroom privileges	os	mouth
c̄	with	OT	occupational therapy
C	centigrade; Celsius	oz; OZ	ounce
cal	calories	PC; p.c.	after meals
cath	catheter	per	by, through
CBR	complete bed rest	PM	afternoon
C/O; c/o	complains of	PO; po	by mouth; orally
CPR	cardiopulmonary resuscitation	prep	preparation
CS	central service; central supply	prn	when necessary
drsg	dressing	Pt; pt	patient
Dx	diagnosis	PT	physical therapy
ECG; EKG	electrocardiogram	q	every
ER; ED	emergency room; emergency department	qh	every hour
F	Fahrenheit	q2h, q3h, etc.	every 2 hours, every 3 hours, and so on
fl; fld	fluid	R	rectal temperature, respiration
Fx	fracture	R/O	rule out
GI	gastro-intestinal	ROM	range of motion; range-of-motion
h; hr	hour	rt; R	right
H_2O	water	s̄	without
HIV	human immunodeficiency virus	Spec; spec	specimen
ht	height	stat	at once, immediately
hx	history	tbsp	tablespoon
ICU	intensive care unit	TPR	temperature, pulse, and respirations
I&O	intake and output	tsp	teaspoon
IV	intravenous	U/a; U/A; u/a	urinalysis
L	liter	UTI	urinary tract infection
Lab	laboratory	VS; vs	vital signs
lb	pound	w/c	wheelchair
LOC	level of consciousness	Wt; wt	weight

COMMON TERMS AND PHRASES

Some terms and phrases apply to basic care, safety, or the person's condition. Because they are used throughout this book, they are defined in Table 9-4. Some are presented as key terms in other chapters.

TABLE 9-4	Common Health Care Terms and Phrases
Term	**Definition**
abnormal	Different from what is normal or usual
activities of daily living (ADL)	The activities usually done during a normal day in a person's life
aphasia	The total or partial loss (a) of the ability to use or understand language (phasia)
adpative (assistive) device	Any item used by the person or staff to promote the person's function or safety (hand rails, grab bars, mechanical lifts, canes, walkers, wheelchairs, devices for eating or dressing, and so on)
atrophy	The decrease (a) in size or the wasting away of tissue (trophy)
biological sex	Male or female
call light	Part of the call system allowing the person to signal the nurses' station for help
care plan	A written guide about the person's care
chronic	An on-going illness that is slow or gradual in onset; it has no known cure; it can be controlled and complications prevented with proper treatment
cognitive function	Involves memory, thinking, reasoning, ability to understand, judgment, and behavior
contracture	The lack of joint mobility caused by abnormal shortening of a muscle
dementia	The loss (de) of cognitive and social function (mentia) caused by changes in the brain
drug	A substance taken by mouth, injected, or applied to treat or prevent a disease or condition; medication, medicine
dysphagia	Difficulty (dys) swallowing (phagia)
dyspnea	Difficult, labored, or painful (dys) breathing (pnea)
feces	The semi-solid mass of waste products in the colon that is expelled through the anus; stool or stools
fever	Elevated body temperature
Fowler's position	A semi-sitting position; the head of the bed is raised between 45 and 60 degrees
incontinence	Not being able to control urination (urinary incontinence) or bowel movements (fecal incontinence)
orientation; oriented	Awareness of one's self and others, one's location, and the time; or awareness of one's surroundings
perineal	The genital and anal areas
pressure injury	Localized damage to the skin and underlying soft tissue; the injury is usually over a bony prominence or related to a medical or other device and results from pressure or pressure in combination with shear
semi-Fowler's position	The head of the bed is raised 30 degrees; or the head of the bed is raised 30 degrees and the knee portion is raised 15 degrees
stool	Excreted feces
supine	The back-lying or dorsal recumbent position
vital signs	Temperature, pulse, respirations, and blood pressure (and pulse oximetry [Chapter 43] and pain in some agencies)
voiding	Emptying urine from the bladder; urinating, urination

FOCUS ON **PRIDE**

The Person, Family, and Yourself

P ersonal and Professional Responsibility
To communicate in health care you must learn medical terms. You may feel overwhelmed at first. Start with the word elements in Table 9-1. Study a little at a time. Use a medical dictionary for words you do not understand and to learn new words. You will understand more as you study body structure, care measures, and disorders.

R ights and Respect
The person must be given information in a language he or she understands. The person may not know medical terms. Use familiar words when talking to the patient or resident.

I ndependence and Social Interaction
Only use abbreviations allowed by your agency. Social and texting abbreviations are not used.

D elegation and Teamwork
Assignment sheets often include medical terms and abbreviations. Review the assignment sheet example in Chapter 8. Do you understand the sheet better? Take pride in learning.

E thics and Laws
Never be afraid to ask for a term or abbreviation to be explained. You must know the meaning to provide safe care. A careful person asks for needed help. Negligence results when reasonable care is not taken and the person is harmed.

FOCUS ON **PRIDE**: *Application*

Identify ways to study word elements and medical terms. How do you plan to study? Do you study better alone or with someone? Ask another student how he or she plans to learn.

REVIEW QUESTIONS

Circle the BEST answer.

1 To define a medical term, what do you do *first?*
   a Read the meaning of the root.
   b Read the meaning of the suffix.
   c Separate the word into its parts.
   d Read the meaning of the prefix.

2 A suffix is
   a Placed at the beginning of a word
   b Placed after a root
   c A shortened form of a word or phrase
   d The main meaning of the word

3 Which word means a blood condition involving too much sugar?
   a Hepatitis (hepat-itis)
   b Tachycardia (tachy-cardia)
   c Hyperglycemia (hyper-glyc-emia)
   d Aphasia (a-phasia)

4 Which word means an excessive flow of blood?
   a Hemiplegia (hemi-plegia)
   b Cyanosis (cyan-osis)
   c Laparoscopy (laparo-scopy)
   d Hemorrhage (hemo-rrhage)

5 Which word means examination of the bladder using a scope?
   a Ileostomy (ileo-stomy)
   b Colonoscopy (colono-scopy)
   c Tracheostomy (tracheo-stomy)
   d Cystoscopy (cysto-scopy)

6 The stomach is located in the
   a RUQ
   b LUQ
   c RLQ
   d LLQ

7 Which term relates to the side of the body?
   a Anterior
   b Lateral
   c Posterior
   d Proximal

8 Which is *true?*
   a The shoulder is proximal to the elbow.
   b The toes are posterior.
   c The hip is distal to the knee.
   d The thumb is on the medial side of the hand.

9 You must complete a task *stat.* "Stat" means
   a At once, immediately
   b As desired
   c Without moving the person
   d When necessary, as needed

10 What are ADL?
   a The activities a person does daily
   b Devices used to assist with care
   c Foods allowed on the person's diet
   d Drugs a person takes daily

11 A person with dementia has
   a Difficulty swallowing
   b Painful or difficult breathing
   c Damage to the skin and tissues
   d Loss of cognitive and social function

12 Which definition is *correct?*
   a *Contracture* is the decrease in size or wasting away of tissue.
   b *Perineal* is the genital and anal areas.
   c *Supine* is a sitting position with the head of the bed raised 45 degrees.
   d *Voiding* is being unable to control urination.

Answers to Chapter 9 questions are on p. 885.

FOCUS ON **PRACTICE**

Problem Solving

You are training in the clinical setting. A person has an "NPO" sign above the bed. You do not remember what "NPO" means. What will you do? Why is it important for you to know?

Body Structure and Function

OBJECTIVES

- Define the key terms and key abbreviations in this chapter.
- Identify the basic structures of the cell.
- Explain how cells divide.
- Describe 4 types of tissues.

- Identify the structures and functions of each body system.
- Explain how to promote PRIDE in the person, the family, and yourself.

KEY TERMS

artery A blood vessel that carries blood away from the heart
capillary A very tiny blood vessel; nutrients, oxygen, and other substances pass from capillaries into the cells
cell The basic unit of body structure
digestion The process that breaks down food physically and chemically so it can be absorbed for use by the cells
hemoglobin The substance in red blood cells that carries oxygen and gives blood its red color
hormone A chemical substance secreted by the endocrine glands into the bloodstream
immunity Protection against a disease or condition; the person will not get or be affected by the disease
joint The point at which 2 or more bones meet to allow movement
menstruation The process in which the lining of the uterus *(endometrium)* breaks up and is discharged from the body through the vagina

metabolism How the body uses nutrients to provide energy and maintain body functions
organ Groups of tissue with the same function
peristalsis Involuntary muscle contractions in the digestive system that move food down the esophagus through the alimentary canal
reflex The body's response (function or movement) to a stimulus
respiration The process of supplying cells with oxygen and removing carbon dioxide from them
stimulus Anything that excites or causes a body part to function, become active, or respond
system Organs that work together to perform special functions
tissue A group of cells with similar functions
vein A blood vessel that returns blood to the heart

KEY ABBREVIATIONS

CNS	Central nervous system	**O₂**	Oxygen
CO₂	Carbon dioxide	**RBC**	Red blood cell
GI	Gastro-intestinal	**WBC**	White blood cell
mL	Milliliter		

Ideally, the human body is in *homeostasis*—a steady state. *(Homeo* means *sameness. Stasis* means *standing still.)* Various body functions and processes work to promote health and survival. Homeostasis is affected by illness, disease, and injury.

Knowing the body's normal structure *(anatomy)* and function *(physiology)* will help you understand signs, symptoms, and the reasons for care and procedures. You will give safe and more effective care.

See Chapter 12 for the changes in body structure and function that occur with aging.

CELLS, TISSUES, AND ORGANS

The basic unit of body structure is the cell. Cells have the same basic structure. Function, size, and shape may differ. Cells are very small. You need a microscope to see them. Cells need water, oxygen (O_2), and nutrients to live and function. Nutrients include proteins, fats, carbohydrates, vitamins, and minerals (Chapter 30).

Figure 10-1 shows the cell and its structures. The *cell membrane* is the outer covering. It encloses the cell and helps hold the cell's shape. The *nucleus* is the control center of the cell. It directs the cell's activities. The nucleus is in the center of the cell. The *cytoplasm* surrounds the nucleus. Cytoplasm contains smaller structures that perform cell functions. *Protoplasm* means "living substance." It refers to all structures, substances, and water within the cell. Protoplasm is a semi-liquid substance much like an egg white.

Chromosomes are thread-like structures in the nucleus. Each cell has 46 chromosomes. Chromosomes contain *genes*. Genes control the traits children inherit from their parents. Height, eye color, and skin color are examples.

The nucleus controls cell reproduction. Cells reproduce by dividing in half. The process of cell division is called *mitosis*. It is needed for tissue growth and repair. During mitosis, the 46 chromosomes arrange themselves in 23 pairs. As the cell divides, the 23 pairs are pulled in half. The 2 new cells are identical. Each has 46 chromosomes (Fig. 10-2).

Cells are the body's building blocks. *Groups of cells with similar functions combine to form tissues.*

- *Epithelial tissue* covers internal and external body surfaces. Tissue lining the nose, mouth, respiratory tract, stomach, and intestines is epithelial tissue. So are the skin, hair, nails, and glands.
- *Connective tissue* anchors, connects, and supports other tissues. It is in every part of the body. Bones, tendons, ligaments, and cartilage are connective tissue. Blood is a form of connective tissue.
- *Muscle tissue* stretches and contracts to let the body move.
- *Nerve tissue* receives and carries impulses to the brain and back to body parts.

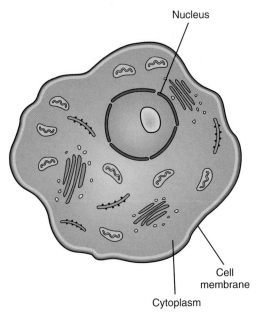

Nucleus

Cell membrane

Cytoplasm

FIGURE 10-1 Parts of a cell.

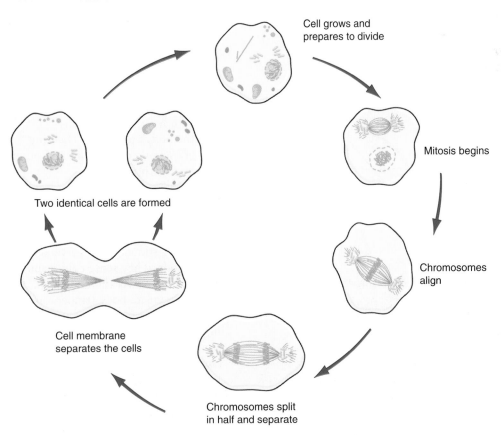

Cell grows and prepares to divide

Mitosis begins

Chromosomes align

Chromosomes split in half and separate

Cell membrane separates the cells

Two identical cells are formed

FIGURE 10-2 The process of cell division.

Groups of tissue with the same function form organs. An organ has 1 or more functions. Examples of organs are the heart, brain, liver, lungs, and kidneys. *Systems are formed by organs that work together to perform special functions* (Fig. 10-3).

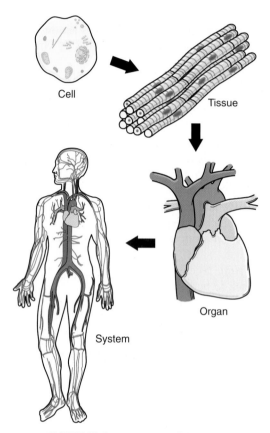

FIGURE 10-3 Organization of the body.

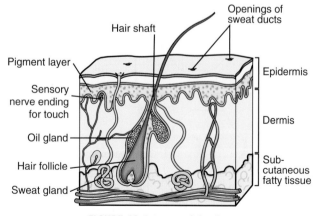

FIGURE 10-4 Layers of the skin.

THE INTEGUMENTARY SYSTEM

The *integumentary system*, or *skin*, is the largest system. *Integument* means *covering*. The skin covers the body. It has epithelial, connective, and nerve tissue. It also has oil glands and sweat glands. There are 2 skin layers (Fig. 10-4).

- The *epidermis* is the outer layer. It has living cells and dead cells. The dead cells were once deeper in the epidermis. They were pushed upward as the cells divided. Dead cells constantly flake off. They are replaced by living cells. Living cells die and flake off. Living cells of the epidermis contain *pigment*. Pigment gives skin its color. The epidermis has no blood vessels and few nerve endings.
- The *dermis* is the inner layer. It is made up of connective tissue. Blood vessels, nerves, sweat glands, and oil glands are found in the dermis. So are hair roots.

The epidermis and dermis are supported by *subcutaneous tissue*. The subcutaneous tissue is a thick layer of fat and connective tissue.

Oil glands and *sweat glands*, *hair*, and *nails* are skin appendages.

- Hair—covers the entire body, except the palms of the hands and the soles of the feet. Hair in the nose and ears and around the eyes protects these organs from dust, insects, and other foreign objects.
- Nails—protect the tips of the fingers and toes. Nails help fingers pick up and handle small objects.
- Sweat glands (*sudoriferous glands*)—help the body regulate temperature. Sweat consists of water, salt, and a small amount of wastes. Sweat is secreted through pores in the skin. The body is cooled as sweat evaporates.
- Oil glands (*sebaceous glands*)—lie near the hair shafts. They secrete an oily substance into the space near the hair shaft. Oil travels to the skin surface. This helps keep the hair and skin soft and shiny.

The skin has many functions.

- It is the body's protective covering.
- It prevents microorganisms and other substances from entering the body.
- It prevents excess amounts of water from leaving the body.
- It protects organs from injury.
- Nerve endings in the skin sense both pleasant and unpleasant stimulation. Nerve endings are over the entire body. They sense cold, pain, touch, and pressure to protect the body from injury.
- It helps regulate body temperature. Blood vessels *dilate* (widen) when temperature outside the body is high. More blood is brought to the body surface for cooling during evaporation. When blood vessels *constrict* (narrow), the body retains heat. This is because less blood reaches the skin.
- It stores fat and water.

THE MUSCULO-SKELETAL SYSTEM

The *musculo-skeletal system* provides the framework for the body. It lets the body move. This system also protects internal organs and gives the body shape.

Bones

The human body has 206 *bones* (Fig. 10-5). There are 4 types of bones.

- *Long bones* bear the body's weight. Leg bones are long bones.
- *Short bones* allow skill and ease in movement. Bones in the wrists, fingers, ankles, and toes are short bones.
- *Flat bones* protect the organs. They include the ribs, skull, pelvic bones, and shoulder blades.
- *Irregular bones* are the vertebrae in the spinal column. They allow various degrees of movement and flexibility.

Bones are hard, rigid structures. They are made up of living cells. Calcium and phosphorus are needed for bone formation and strength. Bones store these minerals for use by the body.

Bones are covered by a membrane called *periosteum*. Periosteum contains blood vessels that supply bone cells with O_2 and nutrients. Inside the hollow centers of the bones is a substance called *bone marrow*. Blood cells are formed in the bone marrow.

Joints

A *joint* *is the point at which 2 or more bones meet. Joints allow movement* (Chapter 34). *Cartilage* is connective tissue at the end of the long bones. It cushions the joint so that the bone ends do not rub together. The *synovial membrane* lines the joints. It secretes *synovial fluid*. Synovial fluid acts as a lubricant so the joint can move smoothly. Bones are held together at the joint by strong bands of connective tissue called *ligaments*.

There are 3 major types of joints (Fig. 10-6).

- A *ball-and-socket joint* allows movement in all directions. It is made of the rounded end of 1 bone and the hollow end of another bone. The rounded end of 1 fits into the hollow end of the other. The joints of the hips and shoulders are ball-and-socket joints.
- A *hinge joint* allows movement in 1 direction. The elbow is a hinge joint.
- A *pivot joint* allows turning from side to side. A pivot joint connects the skull to the spine.

Some joints cannot move. They connect the bones of the skull.

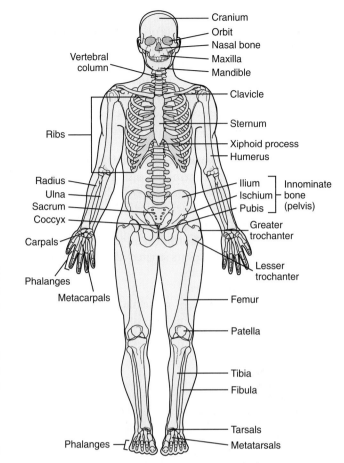

FIGURE 10-5 Bones of the body.

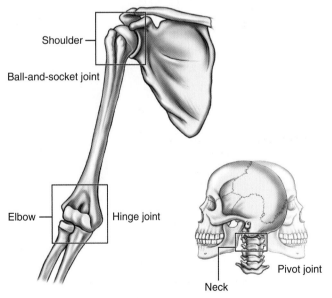

FIGURE 10-6 Types of joints. (Modified from Herlihy B: *The human body in health and illness,* ed 6, St Louis, 2018, Elsevier.)

Muscles

The body has over 500 *muscles* (Figs. 10-7 and 10-8). Some are voluntary. Others are involuntary.

- *Voluntary muscles* can be consciously controlled. Muscles attached to bones *(skeletal muscles)* are voluntary. Arm muscles do not work unless you move your arm; likewise for leg muscles. Skeletal muscles are *striated*. That is, they look striped or streaked.
- *Involuntary muscles* work automatically. You cannot control them. They control the action of the stomach, intestines, blood vessels, and other body organs. Involuntary muscles also are called *smooth muscles*. They look smooth, not streaked or striped.
- *Cardiac muscle* is in the heart. It is an involuntary muscle. However, it appears striated like skeletal muscle. Muscles have 3 functions.
- Movement of body parts
- Maintenance of posture or muscle tone
- Production of body heat

Strong, tough connective tissues called *tendons* connect muscles to bones. When muscles *contract* (shorten), tendons at each end of the muscle cause the bone to move. The body has many tendons. See the Achilles tendon in Figure 10-8. Some muscles constantly contract to maintain posture. When muscles contract, they use energy. Heat is produced. The more muscle activity, the greater the amount of heat produced. Shivering is how the body produces heat when exposed to cold. Shivering is from rapid, general muscle contractions.

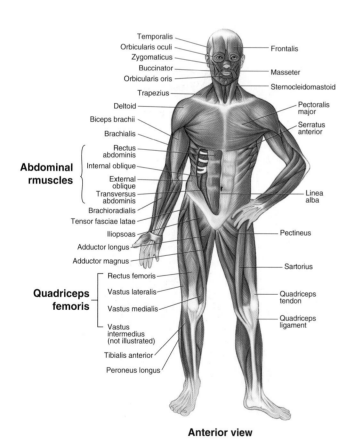

Anterior view

FIGURE 10-7 Anterior view of the muscles of the body. (From Herlihy B: *The human body in health and illness,* ed 6, St Louis, 2018, Elsevier.)

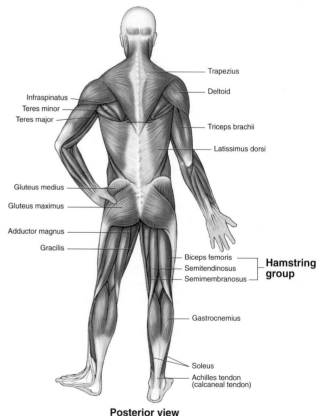

Posterior view

FIGURE 10-8 Posterior view of the muscles of the body. (From Herlihy B: *The human body in health and illness,* ed 6, St Louis, 2018, Elsevier.)

Sphincters are circular bands of muscle fibers. They *constrict* (narrow) a passage. Or they close a natural body opening. For example:

- The *lower esophageal sphincter* (Fig. 10-9) is between the esophagus and the stomach. It prevents food from moving back up into the esophagus.
- The *pyloric sphincter* (see Fig. 10-9) is an opening from the stomach into the small intestine. Closed, it holds food in the stomach for partial digestion. It opens to allow partially digested food to enter the small intestine.
- The *anal sphincter* keeps the anus closed. It opens for a bowel movement.
- *Urethral sphincters* seal off the bladder. This allows urine to collect in the bladder. The sphincters open for urination.

THE NERVOUS SYSTEM

The *nervous system* controls, directs, and coordinates body functions. Its 2 main divisions are:

- The *central nervous system (CNS)*. It consists of the brain and spinal cord (Fig. 10-10).
- The *peripheral nervous system*. It involves the nerves throughout the body (Fig. 10-11, p. 118).

Nerves connect to the spinal cord. Nerves carry messages or impulses to and from the brain. A *stimulus is anything that excites or causes a body part to function, become active, or respond. A **reflex** is the body's response (function or movement) to a stimulus.* A stimulus causes a nerve impulse. A reflex results. For example, eye irritation (stimulus) causes the eyelid to blink (reflex). Reflexes are involuntary, unconscious, and immediate. The person cannot control reflexes.

Nerves are easily damaged and take a long time to heal. Some nerve fibers have a protective covering called a *myelin sheath*. The myelin sheath also insulates the nerve fiber. Nerve fibers covered with myelin conduct impulses faster than those fibers without it.

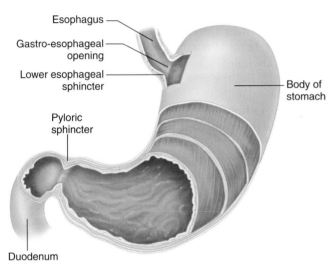

Esophagus
Gastro-esophageal opening
Lower esophageal sphincter
Body of stomach
Pyloric sphincter
Duodenum

FIGURE 10-9 Pyloric sphincter. (Redrawn from Patton KT, Thibodeau GA: *The human body in health and disease,* ed 7, St Louis, 2018, Elsevier.)

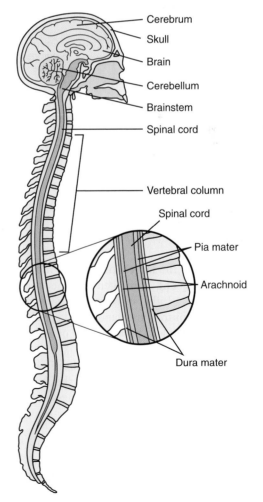

Cerebrum
Skull
Brain
Cerebellum
Brainstem
Spinal cord
Vertebral column
Spinal cord
Pia mater
Arachnoid
Dura mater

FIGURE 10-10 Central nervous system.

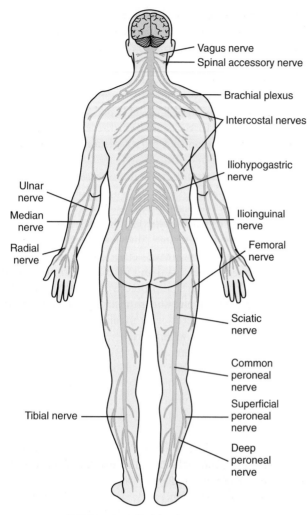

FIGURE 10-11 Peripheral nervous system.

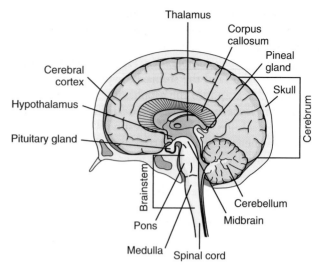

FIGURE 10-12 The brain.

The Central Nervous System

The *brain* and *spinal cord* make up the central nervous system. The brain is covered by the skull. The 3 main parts of the brain are the *cerebrum*, the *cerebellum*, and the *brainstem* (Fig. 10-12).

The cerebrum is the largest part of the brain. It is the center of thought and intelligence. The cerebrum is divided into 2 halves called *right* and *left hemispheres*. The right hemisphere controls movement and activities on the body's left side. The left hemisphere controls the right side.

The outside of the cerebrum is called the *cerebral cortex*. It controls the highest functions of the brain. These include reasoning, memory, consciousness, speech, voluntary muscle movement, vision, hearing, sensation, and other activities.

The cerebellum regulates and coordinates body movements. It controls balance and the smooth movements of voluntary muscles. Injury to the cerebellum results in jerky movements, loss of coordination, and muscle weakness.

The brainstem connects the cerebrum to the spinal cord. The brainstem contains the *midbrain, pons,* and *medulla*. The midbrain and pons relay messages between the medulla and the cerebrum. The medulla is below the pons. The medulla controls heart rate, breathing, blood vessel size, swallowing, coughing, and vomiting. The brain connects to the spinal cord at the lower end of the medulla.

The spinal cord lies within the spinal column. The cord is 17 to 18 inches long. It contains pathways that conduct messages to and from the brain.

The brain and spinal cord are covered and protected by 3 layers of connective tissue called meninges.
- The outer layer lies next to the skull. It is a tough covering called the *dura mater*.
- The middle layer is the *arachnoid*.
- The inner layer is the *pia mater*.

The space between the middle layer (arachnoid) and inner layer (pia mater) is the *arachnoid space*. The space is filled with *cerebrospinal fluid*. It circulates around the brain and spinal cord. Cerebrospinal fluid protects the central nervous system. It cushions shocks that could easily injure brain and spinal cord structures.

The Peripheral Nervous System

The peripheral nervous system has 12 pairs of *cranial nerves* and 31 pairs of *spinal nerves*. Cranial nerves conduct impulses between the brain and the head, neck, chest, and abdomen. They conduct impulses for smell, vision, hearing, pain, touch, temperature, and pressure. They also conduct impulses for voluntary and involuntary muscles. Spinal nerves carry impulses from the skin, extremities, and internal structures not supplied by the cranial nerves.

Some peripheral nerves form the *autonomic nervous system*. This system controls involuntary muscles and certain body functions. The functions include the heartbeat, blood pressure, intestinal contractions, and glandular secretions. These functions occur automatically.

The autonomic nervous system is divided into the *sympathetic nervous system* and the *parasympathetic nervous system*. They balance each other. The sympathetic nervous system speeds up functions. The parasympathetic nervous system slows functions. When you are angry, scared, excited, or exercising, the sympathetic nervous system is stimulated. The parasympathetic system is activated when you relax or when the sympathetic system is stimulated for too long.

The Sense Organs

The 5 senses are *sight, hearing, taste, smell,* and *touch*. Receptors for taste are in the tongue. They are called *taste buds*. Receptors for smell are in the nose. Touch receptors are in the dermis, especially in the toes and fingertips.

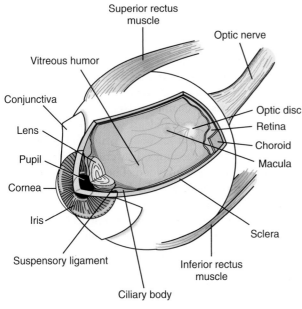

FIGURE 10-13 The eye.

The Eye. Receptors for vision are in the eyes (Fig. 10-13). The eye is easily injured. Bones of the skull, eyelids and eyelashes, and tears protect the eyes from injury.

The eye has 3 layers.
* The *sclera*, the white of the eye, is the outer layer. It is made of tough connective tissue.
* The *choroid* is the second layer. Blood vessels, the *ciliary muscle*, and the *iris* make up the choroid. The iris gives the eye its color. The opening in the middle of the iris is the *pupil*. Pupil size varies with the amount of light entering the eye. The pupil constricts (narrows) in bright light. It dilates (widens) in dim or dark places.
* The *retina* is the inner layer. It has receptors for vision and the nerve fibers of the *optic nerve*.

Light enters the eye through the *cornea*. It is the transparent part of the outer layer that lies over the eye. Light rays pass to the *lens*, which lies behind the pupil. The light is then reflected to the retina. Light is carried to the brain by the optic nerve.

The *aqueous chamber* separates the cornea from the lens. The chamber is filled with a fluid called *aqueous humor*. The fluid helps the cornea keep its shape and position. The *vitreous humor* is behind the lens. It is a gelatin-like substance that supports the retina and maintains the eye's shape.

The Ear. The *ear* is a sense organ (Fig. 10-14). It functions in hearing and balance. The ear has 3 parts—the *external ear, middle ear,* and *inner ear*.

The external ear (outer part) is called the *pinna* or *auricle*. Sound waves are guided through the external ear into the *auditory canal*. Glands in the auditory canal secrete a waxy substance called *cerumen*. The auditory canal extends about 1 inch into the *eardrum*. The eardrum (*tympanic membrane*) separates the external and middle ear.

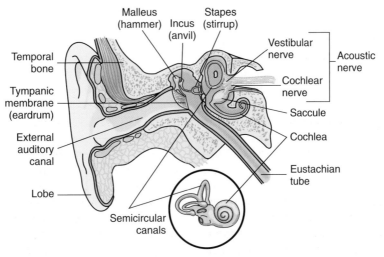

FIGURE 10-14 The ear.

The middle ear contains the *eustachian tube* and 3 small bones called *ossicles*. The eustachian tube connects the middle ear and the throat. Air enters the eustachian tube so there is equal pressure on both sides of the eardrum. The ossicles amplify sound received from the eardrum and transmit the sound to the inner ear. The 3 ossicles are:

- The *malleus*—looks like a hammer.
- The *incus*—looks like an anvil.
- The *stapes*—shaped like a stirrup.

The inner ear consists of *semicircular canals* and the *cochlea*. The cochlea contains fluid. The fluid carries sound waves from the middle ear to the *acoustic nerve*. The acoustic nerve then carries messages to the brain.

The 3 semicircular canals are involved with balance. They sense the head's position and changes in position. They send messages to the brain.

THE CIRCULATORY SYSTEM

The *circulatory system (cardiovascular system)* is made up of the *blood, heart,* and *blood vessels.* The heart pumps blood through the blood vessels. The circulatory system has many functions.

- Blood carries nutrients, hormones, and other substances to the cells.
- Blood transports (carries) the gases of respiration (p. 122). It brings O_2 to the cells.
- Blood removes waste products from cells.
- Blood plays a role in maintaining the body's fluid balance.
- Blood and blood vessels help regulate body temperature. The blood carries heat from muscle activity to other body parts. Blood vessels in the skin dilate to cool the body. They constrict to retain heat.
- The system produces and carries cells that defend the body from microbes that cause disease.

The Blood

The *blood* consists of blood cells and *plasma.* Plasma is mostly water. It carries blood to other body cells. Plasma also carries substances that cells need to function. This includes nutrients, hormones (p. 128), and chemicals.

Red blood cells (RBCs) are called *erythrocytes. Hemoglobin is a substance in RBCs that carries oxygen and gives blood its red color.* As RBCs circulate through the lungs, hemoglobin picks up O_2. Hemoglobin carries O_2 to the cells. When blood is bright red, hemoglobin in the RBCs is filled with O_2. As blood circulates through the body, O_2 is given to the cells. Cells release carbon dioxide (CO_2, a waste product). It is picked up by the hemoglobin. RBCs filled with CO_2 make the blood look dark red.

The body has about 25 trillion (25,000,000,000,000) RBCs. About 4½ to 5 million cells are in a cubic millimeter of blood (the size of a tiny drop). RBCs live for 3 to 4 months. They are destroyed by the liver and spleen as they wear out. New RBCs are formed in the bone marrow. About 1 million RBCs are produced every second.

White blood cells (WBCs) are called *leukocytes.* They have no color. They protect the body against infection. There are about 5000 to 10,000 WBCs in a cubic millimeter of blood. At the first sign of infection, WBCs rush to the infection site and multiply rapidly. The number of WBCs increases when there is an infection. Formed by the bone marrow, WBCs live about 9 days.

Platelets (thrombocytes) are needed for blood clotting. They are formed by the bone marrow. There are about 200,000 to 400,000 platelets in a cubic millimeter of blood. A platelet lives about 4 days.

The Heart

The *heart* is a muscle. It pumps blood through the blood vessels to the tissues and cells. The heart lies in the middle to lower part of the chest cavity toward the left side (Fig. 10-15) and is hollow with 3 layers (Fig. 10-16).

- The *pericardium* is the outer layer. It is a thin sac covering the heart.
- The *myocardium* is the second layer. It is the thick, muscular part of the heart.
- The *endocardium* is the inner layer. A membrane, it lines the inner surface of the heart.

The heart has 4 chambers (see Fig. 10-16). Upper chambers receive blood and are called *atria.* The *right atrium* receives blood from body tissues. The *left atrium* receives blood from the lungs. Lower chambers are called *ventricles.* Ventricles pump blood. The *right ventricle* pumps blood to the lungs for O_2. The *left ventricle* pumps blood to all parts of the body.

Valves are between the atria and ventricles. The valves allow blood flow in 1 direction. They prevent blood from flowing back into the atria from the ventricles. The *tricuspid valve* is between the right atrium and the right ventricle. The *mitral valve (bicuspid valve)* is between the left atrium and left ventricle.

Heart action has 2 phases.

- *Diastole.* It is the resting phase. Heart chambers fill with blood.
- *Systole.* It is the working phase. The heart contracts. Blood is pumped through the blood vessels when the heart contracts.

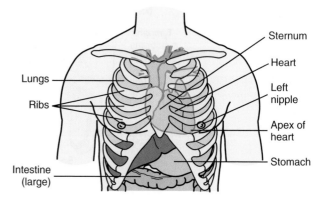

FIGURE 10-15 Location of the heart in the chest cavity.

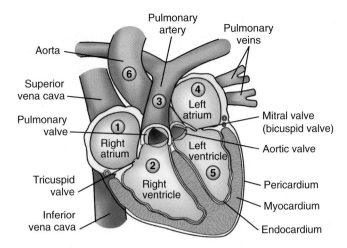

1. Venous blood, poor in O_2, enters the right atrium.
2. Blood flows through the tricuspid valve into the right ventricle.
3. The right ventricle pumps blood through the pulmonary artery to the lungs to pick up O_2.
4. Oxygen-rich blood from the lungs enters the left atrium.
5. Blood flows through the mitral valve into the left ventricle.
6. The left ventricle pumps blood through the aorta to other arteries.

FIGURE 10-16 Structures of the heart and blood flow through the heart.

The Blood Vessels

Blood flows to body tissues and cells through the blood vessels. There are 3 groups of blood vessels: *arteries*, *capillaries*, and *veins*.

Arteries are blood vessels that carry blood away from the heart. Arterial blood is rich in O_2. The *aorta* is the largest artery. It receives blood directly from the left ventricle. The aorta branches into other arteries that carry blood to all parts of the body (Fig. 10-17). These arteries branch into smaller parts within the tissues. The smallest branch of an artery is an *arteriole*.

Arterioles connect to capillaries. *Capillaries are very tiny blood vessels. Nutrients, oxygen, and other substances pass from capillaries into the cells.* The capillaries pick up waste products (including CO_2) from the cells. Veins carry waste products back to the heart.

Veins are blood vessels that return blood to the heart. They connect to the capillaries by *venules*. Venules are small veins. Venules branch together to form veins. The many veins also branch together as they near the heart to form 2 main veins—the *inferior vena cava* and the *superior vena cava* (see Fig. 10-17). Both empty into the right atrium. The inferior vena cava carries blood from the legs and trunk. The superior vena cava carries blood from the head and arms. Venous blood is dark red. It has little O_2 and a lot of CO_2.

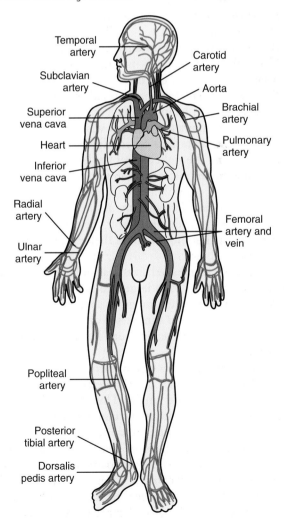

FIGURE 10-17 Arterial (red) and venous (blue) systems.

Blood flow through the heart is shown in Figure 10-16. From there:

1 Arterial blood is carried to the tissues by arterioles and to the cells by capillaries.
2 Cells and capillaries exchange O_2 and nutrients for CO_2 and waste products.
3 Capillaries connect with venules. Venules carry blood that has CO_2 and waste products.
4 Venules form veins.
5 Veins return blood to the heart.

THE LYMPHATIC SYSTEM

The lymphatic (lymph) system is a complex network that transports lymph throughout the body (Fig. 10-18). *Lymph* is a clear, thin, watery fluid. Lymph contains proteins and fats from the intestines. Lymph also contains white blood cells (WBCs). The lymphatic system:

- Collects extra lymph from the tissues and returns it to the blood. This helps maintain fluid balance. Water, proteins, and other substances normally leak out of the capillaries. The lymphatic system drains the extra fluid from the tissues. Otherwise, the tissues swell.
- Defends the body against infection by producing lymphocytes. *Lymphocytes* are a type of WBC that defends the body against microorganisms that cause infection (Chapter 16).
- Absorbs fats from the intestines and transports them to the blood.

Lymph is formed in the tissues. Lymph is transported by *lymphatic vessels*—lymphatic capillaries to lymphatic venules to the right lymphatic duct and the thoracic duct. Lymph then enters the blood in veins near the neck.

- The *right lymphatic duct* collects lymph from the right arm and from the right side of the head, neck, and chest. It empties into a vein on the right side of the neck.
- The *thoracic duct (left lymphatic duct)* collects lymph from the pelvis, abdomen, lower chest, and rest of the body. It empties into a vein on the left side of the neck.

Lymph nodes are shaped like beans. They range from the size of a pinhead to as large as a lima bean. They are found in the neck, underarm, groin area, chest, abdomen, and pelvis. Usually, you cannot see or feel lymph nodes. They swell when producing more lymphocytes to fight infection.

Lymph enters lymph nodes through the lymphatic vessels. The lymph nodes filter bacteria, cancer cells, and damaged cells from the lymph. This prevents such substances from entering and circulating throughout the body.

See Figure 10-18 for the location of the *thymus (thymus gland)*. Certain lymphocytes—T lymphocytes (T cells)—develop in the thymus. Such lymphocytes are important for immune system function (p. 127). The thymus reaches full growth at puberty. Then thymus tissue is slowly replaced by fat and connective tissue. By age 80, it is usually gone.

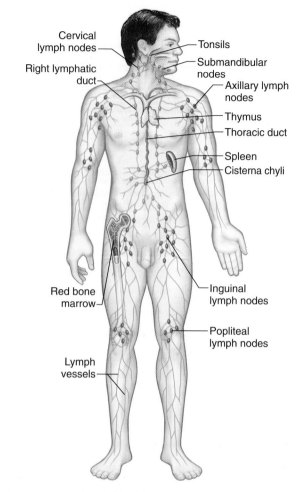

FIGURE 10-18 Lymphatic system. (From Patton KT, Thibodeau GA: *The human body in health and disease*, ed 7, St Louis, 2018, Elsevier.)

The *tonsils* are in the back of the throat. *Adenoids* are behind the nose. These structures trap microorganisms in the mouth and nose to help prevent infection.

The *spleen* is the largest structure in the lymphatic system. It is about the size of a fist. The spleen has a rich blood supply—about 500 milliliters (mL) (1 pint) of blood. The spleen:

- Filters and removes bacteria and other substances.
- Destroys old RBCs.
- Saves the iron found in hemoglobin when RBCs are destroyed.
- Stores blood. When needed, the blood is returned to the circulatory system.

THE RESPIRATORY SYSTEM

Oxygen (O_2) is needed to live. Every cell needs O_2. Air contains about 21% O_2. This meets the body's needs under normal conditions. The respiratory system (Fig. 10-19) brings O_2 into the lungs and removes carbon dioxide (CO_2). *Respiration is the process of supplying cells with oxygen and removing carbon dioxide from them.* Respiration involves *inhalation* (breathing in) and *exhalation* (breathing out). The terms *inspiration* (breathing in) and *expiration* (breathing out) also are used.

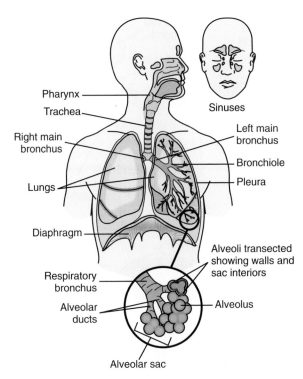

FIGURE 10-19 Respiratory system.

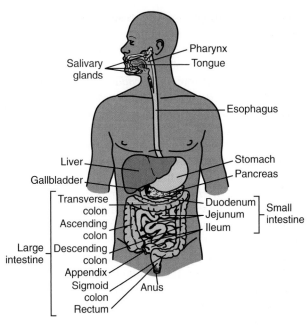

FIGURE 10-20 Digestive system.

Air enters the body through the *nose*. The air then passes into the *pharynx* (throat). It is a tube-shaped passageway for air and food. Air passes from the pharynx into the *larynx* (voice box). A piece of cartilage, the *epiglottis*, acts like a lid over the larynx. The epiglottis prevents food from entering the airway during swallowing. During inhalation the epiglottis lifts up to let air pass over the larynx. Air passes from the larynx into the *trachea* (windpipe).

The trachea divides into the *right bronchus* and the *left bronchus*. Each bronchus enters a lung. Upon entering the lungs, the bronchi divide many times into smaller branches called *bronchioles*. The bronchioles subdivide. They end up in tiny 1-celled air sacs called *alveoli*.

Alveoli look like small clusters of grapes. They are supplied by capillaries. The alveoli and capillaries exchange O_2 and CO_2. Blood in the capillaries picks up O_2 from the alveoli. Then the blood is returned to the left side of the heart and pumped to the rest of the body. Alveoli pick up CO_2 from the capillaries for exhalation.

The lungs are filled with alveoli, blood vessels, and nerves. Each lung is divided into lobes. The right lung has 3 lobes; the left lung has 2. The lungs are separated from the abdominal cavity by a muscle called the *diaphragm*.

Each lung is covered by a 2-layered sac called the *pleura*. One layer is attached to the lung and the other to the chest wall. The pleura secretes a very thin fluid that fills the space between the layers. The fluid prevents the layers from rubbing together during inhalation and exhalation. A bony framework made up of the ribs, sternum, and vertebrae protects the lungs.

THE DIGESTIVE SYSTEM

Digestion is the process that breaks down food physically and chemically so it can be absorbed for use by the cells. The digestive system is also called the gastro-intestinal (GI) system. The system also removes solid wastes from the body.

The digestive system involves the *alimentary canal (GI tract)* and the accessory organs of digestion (Fig. 10-20). The alimentary canal is a long tube. It extends from the mouth to the anus. Its major parts are the mouth, pharynx, esophagus, stomach, small intestine, and large intestine. Accessory organs are the teeth, tongue, salivary glands, liver, gallbladder, and pancreas.

Digestion begins in the *mouth (oral cavity)*. It receives food and prepares it for digestion. Using chewing motions, the *teeth* cut, chop, and grind food into small particles for digestion and swallowing. The *tongue* aids in chewing and swallowing. *Taste buds* on the tongue's surface contain nerve endings. Taste buds allow sweet, sour, bitter, and salty tastes to be sensed. *Salivary glands* in the mouth secrete *saliva*. Saliva moistens food particles to ease swallowing and begin digestion. During swallowing, the tongue pushes food into the *pharynx*.

The pharynx (throat) is a muscular tube. Swallowing continues as the pharynx contracts. Contraction of the pharynx pushes food into the *esophagus*. The esophagus is a muscular tube about 10 inches long. It extends from the pharynx to the *stomach*. *Involuntary muscle contractions in the digestive system move food down the esophagus through the alimentary canal* (**peristalsis**).

The stomach is a muscular, pouch-like sac. It is in the upper left part of the abdominal cavity. Strong stomach muscles stir and churn food to break it up into even smaller particles. A mucous membrane lines the stomach. It contains glands that secrete *gastric juices*. Food is mixed and churned with the gastric juices to form a semi-liquid substance called *chyme*. Through peristalsis, the chyme is pushed from the stomach into the small intestine.

The *small intestine* is about 20 feet long. It has 3 parts. The first part is the *duodenum*. There, more digestive juices are added to the chyme. One is called *bile*. Bile is a greenish liquid made in the *liver*. Bile is stored in the *gallbladder*. Juices from the *pancreas* and small intestine are added to the chyme. Digestive juices chemically break down food into nutrients to be absorbed.

Peristalsis moves the chyme through the 2 other parts of the small intestine: the *jejunum* and the *ileum*. Tiny projections called *villi* line the small intestine. Villi absorb nutrients into the capillaries. Most nutrient absorption takes place in the jejunum and the ileum.

Undigested chyme passes from the small intestine into the *large intestine (large bowel or colon)*. The colon absorbs most of the water from the chyme. The remaining semi-solid material is called *feces*. Feces contain a small amount of water, solid wastes, and some mucus and germs. These are the waste products of digestion. Feces pass through the colon into the *rectum* by peristalsis. Feces pass out of the body through the *anus*.

THE URINARY SYSTEM

The digestive system rids the body of solid wastes. The lungs rid the body of CO_2. Water and other substances leave the body through sweat. There are other waste products in the blood.

The urinary system (Fig. 10-21):
- Removes waste products from the blood.
- Maintains water balance within the body.
- Maintains electrolyte balance. *Electrolytes* are substances that dissolve in water—sodium, potassium, calcium, and magnesium.
  - Sodium is needed for fluid balance. The body retains water if sodium levels are high. Loss of sodium (through vomiting, diarrhea, some drugs, and so on) can result in dehydration.
  - Potassium is needed for the proper function of skeletal and cardiac muscles.
  - Calcium and magnesium are needed for normal nerve and muscle function and for bone and teeth formation.
- Maintains acid-base balance. A pH scale measures if a substance is acidic, neutral, or basic. A pH of 7 is neutral. Anything below 7 is acidic. Anything above 7 is basic. The blood must remain within a certain pH range (7.35–7.45) for normal body function.

The *kidneys* are 2 bean-shaped organs in the upper abdomen. Protected by the lower edge of the ribs, the kidneys lie against the back muscles on each side of the spine.

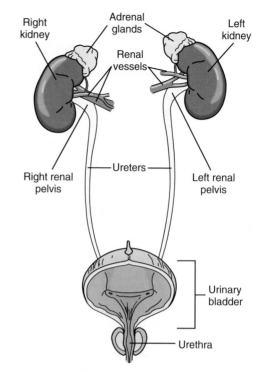

FIGURE 10-21 Urinary system.

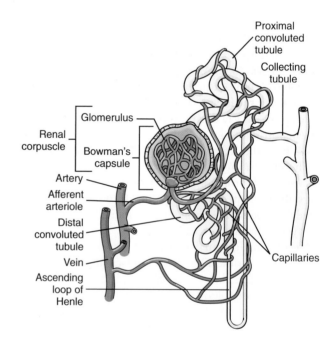

FIGURE 10-22 A nephron.

Each kidney has over a million tiny *nephrons* (Fig. 10-22). Each nephron is the basic working unit of the kidney. Each nephron has a *convoluted tubule*, which is a tiny coiled tube. Each convoluted tubule has a *Bowman's capsule* at 1 end. The capsule partly surrounds a cluster of capillaries called a *glomerulus*. Blood passes through the glomerulus and is filtered by the capillaries.

The fluid part of the blood is squeezed into the Bowman's capsule. The fluid then passes into the tubule. Most of the water and other needed substances are re-absorbed by the blood. The rest of the fluid and the waste products form *urine* in the tubule. Urine flows through the tubule to a *collecting tubule.* All collecting tubules drain into the *renal pelvis* in the kidney.

A tube called the *ureter* is attached to the renal pelvis of the kidney. Each ureter is about 10 to 12 inches long. The ureters carry urine from the kidneys to the *bladder.* The bladder is a hollow, muscular sac. It lies toward the front in the lower part of the abdominal cavity.

Urine is stored in the bladder until the need to urinate is felt. This usually occurs when there is about a half pint (250 mL) of urine in the bladder. Urine passes from the bladder through the *urethra.* The opening at the end of the urethra is called the *meatus.* Urine passes from the body through the meatus. Urine is a clear, yellowish fluid.

THE REPRODUCTIVE SYSTEM

Human reproduction results from the union of a male sex cell and a female sex cell. The male and female reproductive systems are different. This allows for the process of reproduction.

The Male Reproductive System

The male reproductive system is shown in Figure 10-23. The *testes (testicles)* are the male sex glands. Sex glands also are called *gonads.* The 2 testes are oval or almond-shaped glands. Male sex cells *(sperm)* are produced in the testes.

Testosterone, the male hormone, is produced in the testes. This hormone is needed for reproductive organ function. It also is needed for the development of the male secondary sex characteristics. There is facial hair; pubic and axillary (underarm) hair; and hair on the arms, chest, and legs. Neck and shoulder sizes increase.

The testes are suspended between the thighs in a sac called the *scrotum.* The scrotum is made of skin and muscle.

The *epididymis* is a coiled tube on top and to the side of each testis. Sperm travel from the testis to the epididymis. From the epididymis, sperm travel through a tube called the *vas deferens.* Each vas deferens joins a *seminal vesicle.* The 2 seminal vesicles store sperm and produce *semen.* Semen is a fluid that carries sperm from the male reproductive tract. The ducts of the seminal vesicles unite to form the *ejaculatory duct.* It passes through the *prostate gland.*

The prostate gland lies just below the bladder. It is shaped like a donut. The gland secretes fluid into the semen. As the ejaculatory ducts leave the prostate, they join the *urethra.* The urethra runs through the prostate gland. The urethra is the outlet for urine and semen. The urethra is contained within the *penis.*

The penis is outside of the body. The *glans* is at the end of the penis. The urethra opens at the end of the glans. A fold of skin *(prepuce* or *foreskin)* is at the end of the penis (Chapter 24).

The penis has *erectile* tissue. When a man is sexually excited, blood fills the erectile tissue. The penis enlarges and becomes hard and erect. The erect penis can enter a female's vagina. *Cowper's glands* are 2 pea-sized glands under the prostate. They produce a clear, colorless fluid before ejaculation (release of semen). The fluid cleanses the urethra, protects sperm from damage, and provides some lubrication for intercourse. With ejaculation, semen—containing sperm—is released into the vagina.

The Female Reproductive System

Figure 10-24 shows the female reproductive system. The female gonads are 2 almond-shaped glands called *ovaries.* An ovary is on each side of the uterus in the abdominal cavity.

The ovaries contain eggs called *ova.* Ova are the female sex cells. One ovum (egg) is released monthly during the woman's reproductive years. Release of an ovum is called *ovulation.*

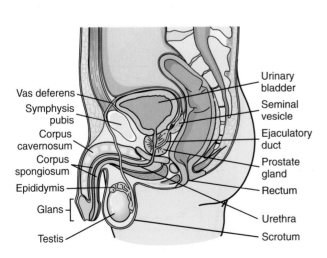

FIGURE 10-23 Male reproductive system.

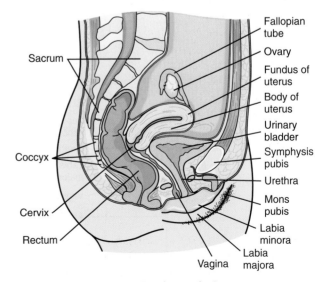

FIGURE 10-24 Female reproductive system.

The ovaries secrete the female hormones *estrogen* and *progesterone*. These hormones are needed for reproductive system function. They also are needed for the development of female secondary sex characteristics. These include increased breast size, pubic and axillary (underarm) hair, slight deepening of the voice, and widening and rounding of the hips.

When an ovum is released from an ovary, it travels through a *fallopian tube*. There are 2 fallopian tubes, 1 on each side. The tubes are attached at 1 end to the *uterus*. The ovum travels through the fallopian tube to the uterus.

The uterus is a hollow, muscular organ shaped like a pear. It is in the center of the pelvic cavity behind the bladder and in front of the rectum. The main part of the uterus is the *fundus*. The neck or narrow section of the uterus is the *cervix*. Tissue lining the uterus is the *endometrium*. The endometrium has many blood vessels. If sex cells from the male and female unite into 1 cell, that cell implants into the endometrium. There, the cell grows into a *fetus* (unborn baby) and receives nourishment.

The cervix of the uterus projects into a muscular canal called the *vagina*. The vagina opens to the outside of the body. It is just behind the urethra. The vagina receives the penis during intercourse. It also is part of the birth canal. Glands in the vaginal wall keep it moistened with secretions. The external vaginal opening is partially closed by a membrane called the *hymen*. The hymen can stretch or tear (rupture) from intercourse, injury, or surgery.

The external female genitalia are called the *vulva* (Fig. 10-25).

- The *mons pubis* is a rounded, fatty pad over a bone called the *symphysis pubis*. The mons pubis is covered with hair in the adult female.
- The *labia majora* and *labia minora* are 2 folds of tissue on each side of the vaginal opening.
- The *clitoris* is a small organ composed of erectile tissue. It becomes hard when sexually stimulated.

The *mammary glands (breasts)* secrete milk after childbirth. The glands are on the outside of the chest. They are made up of glandular tissue and fat (Fig. 10-26). The milk drains into ducts that open onto the *nipple*.

Menstruation. The endometrium is rich in blood to nourish the cell that grows into a fetus. If pregnancy does not occur, menstruation begins. *Menstruation is the process in which the lining of the uterus* (endometrium) *breaks up and is discharged from the body through the vagina.* It occurs about every 28 days. Therefore it is called the *menstrual cycle.*

The first day of the menstrual cycle begins with menstruation. Blood flows from the uterus through the vaginal opening. Menstrual flow usually lasts 3 to 7 days. Ovulation occurs during the next phase. An ovum matures in an ovary and is released. Ovulation usually occurs on or about day 14 of the cycle.

Meanwhile, estrogen and progesterone (the female hormones) are secreted by the ovaries. These hormones cause the endometrium to thicken for pregnancy. If pregnancy does not occur, the hormones decrease in amount. This causes the blood supply to the endometrium to decrease. The endometrium breaks up. It is discharged through the vagina. Another menstrual cycle begins.

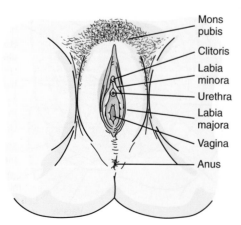

FIGURE 10-25 External female genitalia.

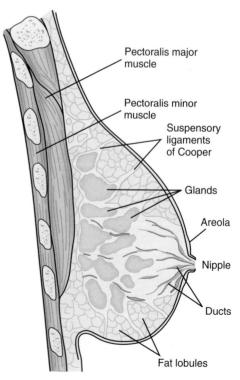

FIGURE 10-26 The female breast.

Fertilization

To reproduce, a male sex cell (sperm) must unite with a female sex cell (ovum). The uniting of the sperm and ovum into 1 cell is called *fertilization*. A sperm has 23 chromosomes. An ovum has 23 chromosomes. When the 2 cells unite, the fertilized cell has 46 chromosomes.

During intercourse, millions of sperm are deposited into the vagina. Sperm travel up the cervix, through the uterus, and into the fallopian tubes. If a sperm and an ovum unite in a fallopian tube, fertilization results. Pregnancy occurs. The fertilized cell travels down the fallopian tube to the uterus. After a short time, the fertilized cell implants into the thick endometrium and grows during pregnancy.

THE IMMUNE SYSTEM

The immune system protects the body from disease and infection. Abnormal body cells can grow into tumors. Sometimes the body produces substances that cause the body to attack itself. Microorganisms (bacteria, viruses, and other germs) can cause an infection. The immune system defends against threats inside and outside the body.

The immune system gives the body immunity. *Immunity means that a person has protection against a disease or condition. The person will not get or be affected by the disease.*

- *Specific immunity* is the body's reaction to a certain threat.
- *Non-specific immunity* is the body's reaction to anything it does not recognize as a normal body substance.

Special cells and substances function to produce immunity.

- *Antibodies*—normal body substances that recognize other substances. They are involved in destroying abnormal or unwanted substances.
- *Antigens*—substances that cause an immune response. Antibodies recognize and bind with unwanted antigens. This leads to the destruction of unwanted substances and the production of more antibodies.
- *Phagocytes*—white blood cells (WBCs) that digest and destroy microorganisms and other unwanted substances (Fig. 10-27).
- *Lymphocytes*—WBCs that produce antibodies. Lymphocyte production increases as the body responds to an infection.
  - *B lymphocytes (B cells)*—cause the production of antibodies that circulate in the plasma. The antibodies react to specific antigens.
  - *T lymphocytes (T cells)*—destroy invading cells. *Killer T cells* produce poisons near the invading cells. Some T cells attract other cells. The other cells destroy the invaders.

When the body senses an antigen from an unwanted substance, the immune system acts. Phagocyte and lymphocyte production increases. Phagocytes destroy the invaders through digestion. The lymphocytes produce antibodies that identify and destroy the unwanted substances.

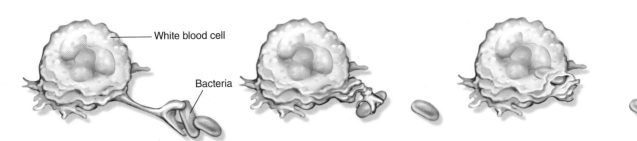

FIGURE 10-27 A phagocyte digests and destroys a microorganism. (Barbara Cousins; from Patton KT, Thibodeau GA: *Structure and function of the body*, ed 15, St Louis, 2016, Mosby.)

THE ENDOCRINE SYSTEM

The endocrine system is made up of glands called the *endocrine glands* (Fig. 10-28). *The endocrine glands secrete chemical substances called* **hormones** *into the bloodstream.* Hormones regulate the activities of other organs and glands in the body. See Table 10-1.

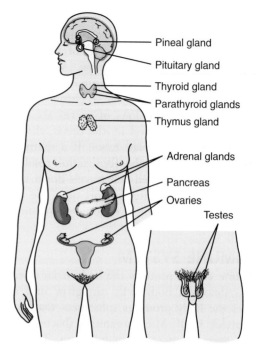

FIGURE 10-28 Endocrine system.

TABLE 10-1	Endocrine System
Gland	**Hormones and Actions**
Pituitary gland (master gland): • Small, cherry-sized gland at the base of the brain behind the eyes • 2 parts—*anterior pituitary lobe* and *posterior pituitary lobe*	Anterior pituitary lobe secretes: • *Growth hormone (GH)*—stimulates the growth of muscles, bones, and organs. • *Thyroid stimulating hormone (TSH)*—stimulates thyroid gland function. • *Adrenocorticotropic hormone (ACTH)*—stimulates adrenal gland function. • Hormones regulating growth, development, and function of the male and female reproductive systems. Posterior pituitary lobe secretes: • *Antidiuretic hormone (ADH)*—prevents the kidneys from excreting too much water. • *Oxytocin*—causes uterine contractions during childbirth.
Thyroid gland: • Butterfly-shaped gland in the neck below the larynx (voice box)	*Thyroid hormone (TH, thyroxine)* regulates *metabolism—how the body uses nutrients to provide energy and maintain body functions.* • Too little TH causes slow body processes, slow movements, and weight gain. • Too much TH causes increased metabolism, excess energy, and weight loss.
Parathyroid glands: • 4 total—2 lie on each side of the thyroid gland	*Parathormone* regulates calcium use. Calcium is needed: • For nerve and muscle function • To prevent *tetany*—a state of severe muscle contraction and spasm that can lead to death
Thymus: • Gland in the upper chest behind the sternum	*Thymosin*—needed for development and function of the immune system.
Pancreas: • Gland in the abdomen behind the stomach	*Insulin*—regulates the amount of sugar in the blood available for use by the cells. Without insulin, sugar cannot enter the cells. Excess sugar builds up in the blood causing *diabetes*.
Adrenal glands: • 2 glands—1 on top of each kidney • Each gland has 2 parts—*adrenal medulla* (inner part) and *adrenal cortex* (outer part)	Adrenal medulla secretes: • *Epinephrine and norepinephrine*—stimulate the body to quickly produce energy during emergencies. Heart rate, blood pressure, muscle power, and energy increase. Adrenal cortex secretes: • *Glucocorticoids*—regulate metabolism of carbohydrates and control the body's response to stress and inflammation. • *Mineralocorticoids*—regulate the amount of salt and water absorbed and lost by the kidneys. • Small amounts of male and female sex hormones.
Gonads: • *Testes*—male sex glands • *Ovaries*—female sex glands	• Male glands (testes) secrete *testosterone*. • Female glands (ovaries) secrete *estrogen* and *progesterone*.

FOCUS ON **PRIDE**

The Person, Family, and Yourself

Personal and Professional Responsibility

Taking care of yourself is a personal and professional responsibility. A healthy diet, exercise, and rest are needed. To care for others you need a strong and healthy body.

Rights and Respect

Patients and residents have the right to make decisions about their bodies. You may not agree with those decisions. But you must respect the person's choices. If the decision will cause no harm, comply with the request. For example, a person does not want to wear a sweater today.

If the person's decision may cause harm, tell the nurse at once. For example, a person refuses to eat. You tell the nurse. The person cannot be forced to eat. But the nurse can talk with the person about the decision, the consequences, and possible solutions.

Independence and Social Interaction

The body does not always work right. People become ill or injured. Sometimes the health team cannot prevent loss of function. Take pride in helping each person regain or maintain the highest level of function possible.

Delegation and Teamwork

The body works like a team. Each system has independent functions. But all systems interact and depend on each other. When a person has a problem with 1 body system, other systems are affected. Understanding each system and how the systems interact helps you provide better care.

Ethics and Laws

Sometimes a person is not able to make decisions about his or her own body. Spouses, parents, family members, or legal representatives may make decisions. Some persons have an advance directive (Chapter 59). Sometimes the court appoints a guardian for a short time. Finally, the agency's ethics committee may address complex issues. The person's safety and best interests must guide care decisions.

FOCUS ON **PRIDE**: *Application*

Body systems interact for normal function. Explain how the circulatory and respiratory systems interact. How might a problem in 1 system affect the other?

REVIEW QUESTIONS

Circle the BEST answer.

1 The basic unit of body structure is the
   a Cell
   b Neuron
   c Nephron
   d Ovum

2 The outer layer of the skin is called the
   a Dermis
   b Epidermis
   c Integument
   d Myelin

3 Which is a function of the skin?
   a Provides the protective covering for the body
   b Transports lymph
   c Forms blood cells
   d Provides the shape and framework for the body

4 Which allows movement?
   a Bone marrow
   b Synovial membrane
   c Joints
   d Ligaments

5 Skeletal muscles
   a Are under involuntary control
   b Appear smooth
   c Are under voluntary control
   d Appear striped and smooth

6 The highest functions in the brain take place in the
   a Cerebral cortex
   b Medulla
   c Brainstem
   d Spinal nerves

7 The ear is involved with
   a Regulating body movements
   b Balance
   c Smoothness of body movements
   d Controlling involuntary muscles

8 The liquid part of blood is the
   a Hemoglobin
   b Red blood cell
   c Plasma
   d White blood cell

9 Which part of the heart pumps blood to the body?
   a Right atrium
   b Left atrium
   c Right ventricle
   d Left ventricle

10 Which carry blood away from the heart?
   a Capillaries
   b Veins
   c Venules
   d Arteries

Continued

REVIEW QUESTIONS—cont'd

11 Which statement about the lymphatic system is *true*?
   a The tonsils are the largest structures in the lymphatic system.
   b Lymph transports oxygen and nutrients to cells.
   c The spleen filters and removes bacteria.
   d Extra lymph from the blood is moved to the tissues.

12 Oxygen and carbon dioxide are exchanged
   a In the bronchi
   b Between the alveoli and capillaries
   c Between the lungs and pleura
   d In the trachea

13 Digestion begins in the
   a Mouth
   b Stomach
   c Small intestine
   d Colon

14 Most nutrient absorption takes place in the
   a Stomach
   b Small intestine
   c Colon
   d Large intestine

15 Urine is formed by the
   a Jejunum
   b Kidneys
   c Bladder
   d Liver

16 Urine passes from the body through the
   a Ureters
   b Urethra
   c Anus
   d Nephrons

17 The male sex gland is called the
   a Penis
   b Semen
   c Testis
   d Scrotum

18 The male sex cell is the
   a Semen
   b Ovum
   c Gonad
   d Sperm

19 The female sex gland is the
   a Ovary
   b Cervix
   c Uterus
   d Vagina

20 The discharge of the lining of the uterus is called
   a The endometrium
   b Ovulation
   c Fertilization
   d Menstruation

21 The immune system protects the body from
   a Low blood sugar
   b Disease and infection
   c Loss of fluid
   d Stunted growth

22 The endocrine glands secrete
   a Hormones
   b Mucus
   c Semen
   d Antibodies

Answers to Chapter 10 questions are on p. 885.

FOCUS ON PRACTICE

Problem Solving

A patient has a disorder that affects the immune system. How does this affect body function? How will you provide care in a way that protects the person?

Growth and Development

OBJECTIVES

- Define the key terms and key abbreviations in this chapter.
- Explain the principles of growth and development.
- Identify the stages of growth and development.
- Identify milestones used to monitor growth and development.

- Identify developmental tasks for each age-group.
- Describe normal growth and development for each age-group.
- Explain how to promote PRIDE in the person, the family, and yourself.

KEY TERMS

adolescence The time between puberty and adulthood; a time of rapid growth and physical, sexual, emotional, and social changes

development Changes in mental, emotional, and social function

developmental task A skill that must be completed during a stage of development for development to continue

ejaculation The release of semen

growth The physical changes that are measured and that occur in a steady, orderly manner

infancy The first year of life

menarche The first menstruation and the start of menstrual cycles

menopause The time when menstruation stops and menstrual cycles end

milestone A behavior or skill that occurs in a stage of development

peer A person of the same age-group and background

primary caregiver The person mainly responsible for providing or assisting with the child's basic needs

puberty The period when reproductive organs begin to function and secondary sex characteristics appear

reflex An involuntary movement

sexual orientation Emotional, romantic, and physical attraction to men, women, or both sexes

stage A period of time (age range) in which a person learns certain skills

teen dating violence (TDV) The physical, sexual, psychological, or emotional violence within a dating relationship as well as stalking

KEY ABBREVIATIONS

CDC	Centers for Disease Control and Prevention	IPV	Intimate partner violence
CNS	Central nervous system	TDV	Teen dating violence

Growth is the physical changes that are measured and that occur in a steady and orderly manner. Growth is measured in weight, height, and changes in appearance and body functions (Fig. 11-1, p. 132). *Development relates to changes in mental, emotional, and social function.* A person behaves and thinks in certain ways in each stage of development. For example, babies depend on adults for basic needs. Adults can meet most of their own basic needs without help.

The basic stages of growth and development that occur in normal, healthy persons are presented. The stages overlap. It is hard to see the start and end of each stage. Also, the rate of growth and development varies with each person.

Growth and development theories usually involve the 2-parent family. Single-parent households are common. Sometimes non-parents have the primary caregiver role. The *primary caregiver is the person mainly responsible for providing or assisting with the child's basic needs.* A mother, father, grandparent, sister, brother, aunt, uncle, or court-appointed guardian may have this role. *Parent* and *parents* are used in this chapter. However, another primary caregiver may have the parent role.

Growth and development stages vary among experts. The groups and content in this chapter are broad and general.

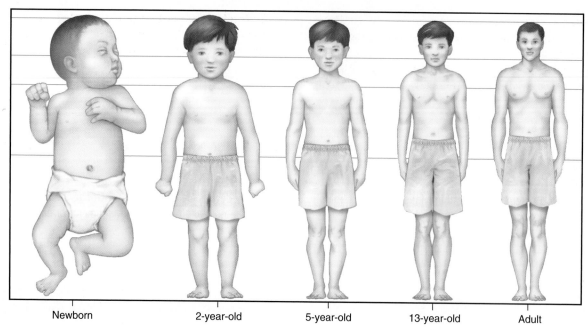

Newborn   2-year-old   5-year-old   13-year-old   Adult

FIGURE 11-1 Changes in appearance from birth to maturity. (From Patton KT, Thibodeau GA: *The human body in health and disease*, ed 7, St Louis, 2018, Elsevier.)

PRINCIPLES

Growth and development is a process affecting the whole person. Although they differ, growth and development:

- Overlap.
- Depend on each other.
- Occur at the same time.

For example, an infant coos or babbles (development) when the physical structures for speech are strong enough (growth). Basic principles of growth and development are:

- The process starts at fertilization and continues until death.
- The process proceeds from the simple to the complex. A baby sits before standing, stands before walking, and walks before running.
- The process occurs in certain directions.
  - From head to foot. Babies hold their heads up before sitting. They sit before standing.
  - From the center of the body outward. Babies control shoulder movements before controlling hand movements.
- The process occurs in a sequence, order, and pattern. A *stage* *is a period of time (age range) in which a person learns certain skills.* A stage cannot be skipped. Each stage is the basis for the next stage.
- *Milestones* track progress. A *milestone* *is a behavior or skill that occurs in a stage of development.* Milestones involve:
  - Physical growth and movement
  - Language and communication
  - Social and emotional changes
  - Cognitive changes (learning, thinking, and problem solving)

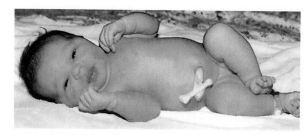

FIGURE 11-2 A newborn. (Courtesy Marjori M. Pyle for LifeCircle, Costa Mesa, Calif.)

- The rate of the process is uneven. It is not at a set pace. Growth is rapid during infancy. Some children develop fast. Others develop slowly.
- Each stage has its own characteristics and developmental tasks. A *developmental task* *is a skill that must be completed during a stage of development for development to continue.* For example, an infant must learn to walk in order to become less dependent as a toddler.

INFANCY (BIRTH TO 1 YEAR)

Infancy is the first year of life. Growth and development are rapid during this time. During this stage infants:

- Learn to walk.
- Learn to eat solid foods.
- Begin to talk and communicate with others.
- Learn to trust.
- Begin to have emotional relationships with parents, brothers, and sisters.
- Develop stable sleep and feeding patterns.

A baby is called a *neonate* or *newborn* from birth to 1 month (Fig. 11-2). (*Neo* means *new*; *nate* means *born*.) The average newborn weighs 6 to 9 pounds and is about 20 inches long. At 1 year the infant is about 29 inches.

Newborns have certain *reflexes (involuntary movements).* These reflexes decline and then disappear as the central nervous system (CNS) develops.

- *Moro reflex (startle reflex)*—occurs when the baby is startled by a loud noise, a sudden movement, or the head falling back. The arms are thrown apart. The legs extend and then flex. A brief cry is common. See Figure 11-3.
- *Rooting reflex*—occurs when the cheek is touched near the mouth (Fig. 11-4). The mouth opens and the head turns toward the touch. This reflex is needed for feeding. It guides the baby's mouth to the nipple.
- *Sucking reflex*—occurs when the lips are touched.
- *Palmar grasp reflex*—occurs when the palm is stroked. The fingers close firmly around the object (Fig. 11-5).
- *Step (dance) reflex*—occurs when the baby is held upright and the feet touch a surface. The feet move up and down and in stepping motions (Fig. 11-6).

See Table 11-1 (p. 134) for the milestones that normally occur by 2 months, 4 months, 6 months, 9 months, and 1 year.

Text continued on p. 136.

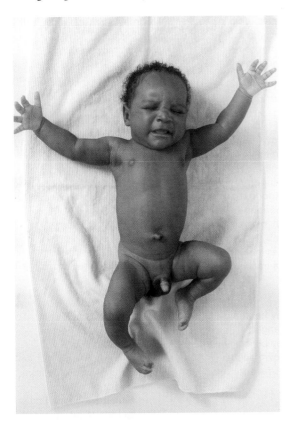

FIGURE 11-3 Moro reflex. (Courtesy Paul Vincent Kuntz, Texas Children's Hospital, as found in Hockenberry MJ, Wilson D: *Wong's nursing care of infants and children,* ed 10, St Louis, 2015, Mosby.)

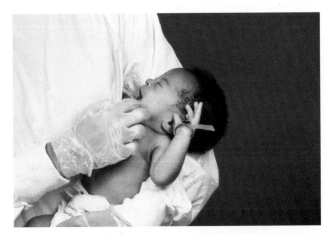

FIGURE 11-4 Rooting reflex. (From Seidel HM and others: *Mosby's guide to physical examination,* ed 3, St Louis, 1995, Mosby.)

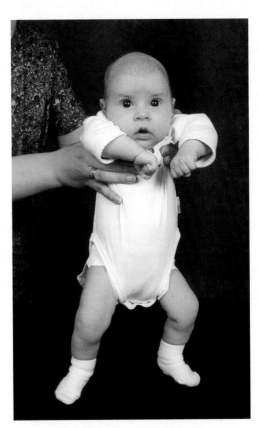

FIGURE 11-6 Step (dance) reflex.

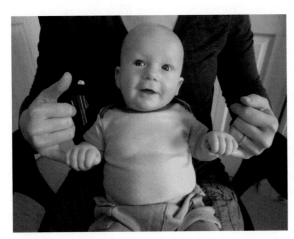

FIGURE 11-5 The palmar grasp reflex. (Courtesy Anne Skowronski, Mount Juliet, Tennessee.)

TABLE 11-1	Milestones—Infancy (Birth to 1 Year)		
Movement/Physical	Language and Communication	Social and Emotional	Learning, Thinking, Problem Solving
By 2 months • Can hold head up (Fig. 11-7) • Begins to push up when on stomach • Makes smoother arm and leg movements	• Coos • Makes gurgling sounds • Turns head toward sounds	• Begins to smile at others (Fig. 11-8) • Tries to look at parent • Sucks on hand to calm self	• Pays attention to faces • Begins to follow things with eyes • Recognizes others at a distance • Cries or fusses when activity does not change
By 4 months • Holds head steady when not supported • Pushes legs when feet are on a hard surface • May roll from front to back • Can hold and shake a toy • Swings at dangling toys • Brings hand to mouth • Pushes up to elbows when on stomach (Fig. 11-9)	• Begins to babble • Babbles with expression (smiles, frowns) • Copies sounds • Has different cries for hunger, pain, and being tired	• Smiles at others • Plays with others • Cries when playing stops • Copies some movements • Copies some facial expressions (smiles, frowns)	• Shows when happy or sad • Responds to affection • Reaches for a toy with 1 hand • Begins to develop hand-eye coordination (sees a toy and reaches for it) • Follows moving things • Watches faces • Recognizes familiar people and things at a distance
By 6 months • Rolls front to back and back to front • Begins to sit without support (Fig. 11-10) • Supports weight on legs and might bounce • Rocks back and forth • May crawl backward before going forward	• Makes sounds in response to sounds • Strings vowels together when babbling (ah, eh, oh) • Takes turns with parent while making sounds • Responds to his or her name • Makes sounds for joy and displeasure • Begins consonant sounds (m, b)	• Knows familiar faces • Begins to know if someone is a stranger • Responds to others' emotions • May often seem happy • Likes looking at self in a mirror	• Looks around at nearby things • Brings things to mouth • Is curious about things • Tries to get things out of reach • Begins to pass things from hand to hand
By 9 months • Stands while holding on • Can get into a sitting position • Sits without support • Pulls to stand • Crawls	• Understands "no" • Makes different sounds (mamamama; babababa) • Copies sounds and gestures of others • Points at things	• May be afraid of strangers • May be clingy with known adults • Has favorite toys	• Watches things fall • Looks for hidden items • Plays "peek-a-boo" • Puts things in mouth • Moves things smoothly from hand to hand • Uses thumb and index finger to pick up little things (pincer grasp) (Fig. 11-11)
By 1 year • Gets to sitting position with help • Pulls up to stand • Walks holding on to furniture (cruises) (Fig. 11-12) • May take a few steps without holding on • May stand alone	• Responds to simple requests • Uses simple gestures (shakes head for "no," waves "bye-bye") • Changes tone when making sounds • Says "mama," "dada," "uh-oh" • Tries to say words others say	• Is shy and nervous with strangers • Cries when parent leaves • Has favorite things and people • Shows fear in some situations • Hands a book when a story is wanted • Repeats sounds or actions for attention • Puts out arm or leg to help with dressing • Plays "peek-a-boo" and "pat-a-cake" type games	• Explores items by shaking, banging, throwing • Finds hidden things • Looks at correct picture when named • Copies gestures • Drinks from a cup • Brushes hair • Bangs 2 things together • Can put in and remove things from a container • Lets things go without help • Points with index finger • Follows simple directions ("pick up the toy")

Modified from Centers for Disease Control and Prevention: Milestones checklists.

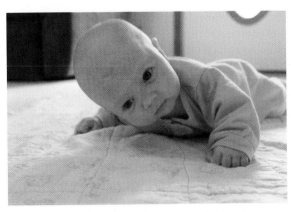

FIGURE 11-7 By 2 months, the infant can hold the head up.

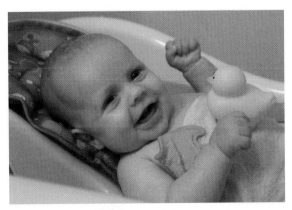

FIGURE 11-8 A 2-month-old smiles in response to others.

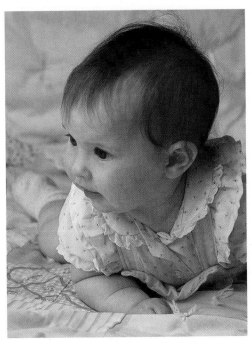

FIGURE 11-9 By 4 months, the infant can push up to the elbows when lying on the stomach.

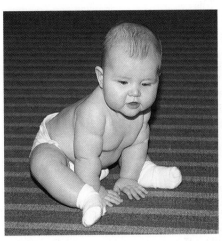

FIGURE 11-10 A 6-month-old begins to sit without support. (From James SR, Ashwill JW, Droske SC: *Nursing care of children: principles and practices,* ed 3, Philadelphia, 2007, Saunders.)

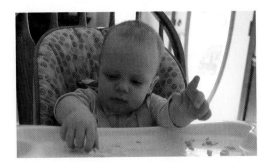

FIGURE 11-11 By 9 months, the infant uses a pincer grasp to pick up small objects.

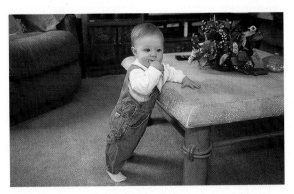

FIGURE 11-12 By 1 year, an infant can walk while holding on to furniture.

Infants are bottle-fed (formula-fed) or breast-fed. Solid foods are given at 4 to 6 months. Rice cereal mixed with breast-milk or formula is given first. Fruits, vegetables, and meats are introduced slowly. Foods are pureed and thin at first. Thicker and chunkier foods are given as more teeth erupt and chewing and swallowing skills increase. Teething often begins with the bottom front teeth. Weaning (stopping bottle or breast-feeding) may begin at the end of infancy.

The infant must develop a sense of trust. If successful, the infant trusts himself or herself and others. Trust develops with consistent care. The infant's physical and safety needs are met—feeding, comfort, warmth, touch, stimulation, and caring.

See *Promoting Safety and Comfort: Infancy (Birth to 1 Year)*.

PROMOTING SAFETY AND COMFORT
Infancy (Birth to 1 Year)

Safety

Infants cannot protect themselves. Safety measures for infants are presented in Chapters 13 and 56 and Appendix D. Also see *Focus on Children and Older Persons* boxes throughout this book.

TABLE 11-2   Milestones—Toddlerhood (1 to 3 Years)

Movement/Physical	Language and Communication	Social and Emotional	Learning, Thinking, Problem Solving
By 18 months • Walks alone • May walk up steps • May run • Pulls toys while walking • Can help undress self • Drinks from a cup • Eats with a spoon (Fig. 11-13)	• Says several words • Says "no" • Shakes head "no" • Points to show what he or she wants	• Likes to hand things to others in play • May have temper tantrums • May be fearful of strangers • Shows affection to known people • May cling to caregivers in new situations • Points at thing of interest • Explores with a parent nearby	• Knows what usual things are (phone, brush, spoon) • Points to others for attention • Pretends to feed a doll or stuffed animal • Points to a body part • Scribbles • Can follow simple commands ("sit down")
By 2 years • Stands on tip-toe • Kicks a ball • Begins to run • Climbs on and off furniture by self • Walks up and down stairs while holding on • Throws ball over-hand • Makes or copies straight lines and circles	• Points to named pictures or things • Knows names of familiar people • Knows names of body parts • Says 2- to 4-word sentences • Follows simple instructions • Repeats words said by others • Points to things in a book	• Copies adults and older children • Gets excited when with children • Shows increased independence • Shows defiant behavior (does what told not to do) • Plays beside other children • Begins to play with other children in chase games	• Finds hidden things • Begins to sort shapes and colors • Completes sentences and rhymes in known books • Plays simple make-believe games • Builds 4 or more block towers • Starts to prefer right or left hand • Follows 2-step instructions ("Pick up your shoes and put them in the closet.") • Names things in picture books
By 3 years • Climbs well • Runs easily • Rides a tricycle • Walks up and down stairs with 1 foot on each step	• Follows 2- to 3-step instructions • Can name most familiar things • Understands "in," "on," "under" • Says first name, age, and gender • Names a friend • Says "I," "me," "we," "you," and some plurals (cars, dogs, cats) • Talks well enough for others to understand • Converses with 2 to 3 sentences	• Copies adults and friends • Shows affection readily • Takes turns in games • Shows concern for crying person • Understands "mine," "his," "hers" • Shows range of emotions • Separates easily from a parent • May get upset with change in routine • Dresses and undresses self	• Can work toys with buttons, levers, moving parts • Plays make-believe with dolls, animals, people • Does puzzles with 3 or 4 pieces • Understands "2" • Copies a circle • Turns book pages 1 at a time • Builds 6 or more block towers • Opens and closes jar lids • Turns door handle

Modified from Centers for Disease Control and Prevention: Milestones checklists.

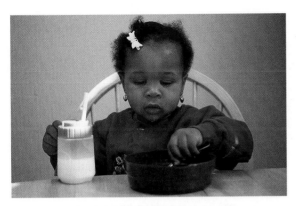

FIGURE 11-13 A toddler feeds herself.

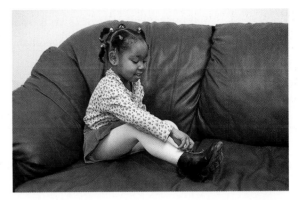

FIGURE 11-14 This 3-year-old can put on her shoes.

TODDLERHOOD (1 TO 3 YEARS)

Growth rate in toddlerhood is slower than during infancy. Toddlers learn to:

- Tolerate separation from the primary caregiver.
- Gain control of bowel and bladder function.
- Use words to communicate.
- Become less dependent on the primary caregiver.

See Table 11-2 for the milestones that normally occur during the toddler years.

Toddlers learn to walk well. They are curious and get into everything and anything. They touch, taste, smell, and climb to explore their settings. They go farther away from primary caregivers. They learn to do some things without a primary caregiver.

Computer play often begins in toddlerhood. Toddlers like to push keys, move a mouse, and play with levers and buttons on computer toys. Such actions help develop fine motor skills and hand-eye coordination.

Toilet training begins in toddlerhood. Bowel and bladder control is related to CNS development. Children must be mentally and physically ready for toilet training. Some are ready at 2 years. Others are ready at 2½ to 3 years of age.

Play skills increase. The child plays alongside other children but not with them. Toddlers are possessive and do not understand sharing.

Temper tantrums and saying "no" are common. Toddlers kick and scream to express anger and frustration. That is how they object when independence is challenged. Using "no" can frustrate primary caregivers. Almost every request may be answered "no," even if the child follows the request.

Toddlers learn separation from the primary caregiver. With discomfort, frustration, fear, or injury, they return to primary caregivers or cry for attention. If primary caregivers are consistently present when needed, children learn security. They learn to tolerate brief periods of separation.

PRESCHOOL (3 TO 6 YEARS)

Preschool children grow 2 to 3 inches per year. They gain about 5 pounds a year. Preschoolers are thinner, more coordinated, and more graceful than toddlers. Preschoolers:

- Increase their ability to communicate and understand others.
- Perform self-care.
- Learn gender differences and develop sexual modesty.
- Learn right from wrong and good from bad.
- Learn to play with others.
- Develop family relationships.

See Table 11-3 (p. 138) for the milestones that normally occur in the preschool years.

Personal care skills increase. Preschool children put on clothes and shoes and manage buttons (Fig. 11-14). They wash their hands, brush their teeth, feed themselves, and help with chores (setting the table).

Play is important. Preschool children enjoy crayons, cutting paper, pasting, and painting (Fig. 11-15, p. 138). They play with other children and learn to share (Fig. 11-16, p. 138). Imaginary friends and imitating adults are common. They like computer and board games, TV, riding toys (wagons, tricycles, bicycles), and playing "house" and "dress-up."

Gender differences are learned. Three-year-olds know that there are "boys" and "girls." Little girls may wonder how the penis works and why they do not have one. Little boys may wonder how girls can urinate without a penis.

TABLE 11-3	Milestones—Preschool (3 to 6 Years)		
Movement/Physical	**Language and Communication**	**Social and Emotional**	**Learning, Thinking, Problem Solving**
By 4 years • Hops and stands on 1 foot for up to 2 seconds • Catches a bounced ball most of the time • Can pour and cut with supervision • Mashes own food	• Follows some basic grammar rules • Uses "he" and "she" correctly • Sings a song or says a poem from memory ("Itsy Bitsy Spider," "Wheels on the Bus") • Tells stories • Says first and last name	• Enjoys new things • Plays "Mom" and "Dad" • Increasingly creative with make-believe play • Prefers playing with children rather than self (see Fig. 11-16) • Cooperates with children • May not know real from make-believe • Talks about likes and interests	• Names some colors and numbers • Understands the idea of counting • Starts to understand time • Understands "same" and "different" • Draws a person with 2 to 4 body parts • Uses scissors • Copies some capital letters • Plays board or card games • Remembers parts of a story and says what will happen next in a book
By 5 years • Stands on 1 foot for 10 or more seconds • Hops; may skip • Can do a somersault • Uses a fork and spoon; may use a table knife • Can use the toilet by self • Swings and climbs	• Speaks clearly • Tells a simple story • Uses full sentences • Uses future tense ("Grandma will be here.") • Says name and address	• Wants to please friends and be like friends • More likely to agree with rules • Sings, dances, and acts • Knows real from make-believe • Shows more independence • Is demanding at times; cooperative at other times	• Counts 10 or more things • Can draw a person with 6 or more body parts • Prints some letters or numbers • Copies a triangle or other shapes • Knows about every-day items like money and food

Modified from Centers for Disease Control and Prevention: Milestones checklists.

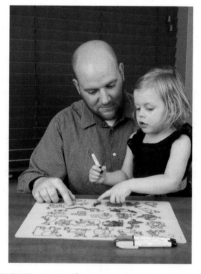

FIGURE 11-15 This 3-year-old enjoys coloring.

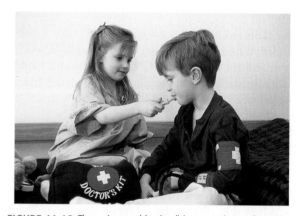

FIGURE 11-16 These 4-year-olds play "doctor and nurse" together.

Preschool children tend to tease, tattle, and tell fibs. When bad, they may blame others or an imaginary friend. Bragging, telling tales about family, and showing off are common. They are proud of achievements but have mood swings.

Rivalries with brothers and sisters are seen, especially when another child takes the child's things. Rivalries also occur when older children have more and different privileges. The family is often the focus of the child's frustrations. They enjoy doing things with primary caregivers (Fig. 11-17). Cooking, housekeeping, shopping, yard work, and sports are examples.

Five-year-olds learn to follow rules and be responsible. They are eager to do things right. They learn about manners, independence, and honesty. Fears lessen but nightmares and dreams are common.

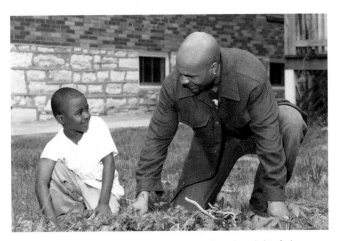

FIGURE 11-17 This 5-year-old does yard work with his father.

SCHOOL AGE (6 TO 9 OR 10 YEARS)

School-age children grow 2 to 3 inches a year. They gain 4½ to 6½ pounds a year. They need to:

- Develop the social and physical skills needed for playing games.
- Learn to get along with persons of the same age-group and background.
- Learn behaviors and attitudes common for one's gender.
- Learn basic reading, writing, and math skills.
- Develop a conscience and morals.
- Develop a good feeling and attitude about oneself.

Baby teeth are lost and permanent teeth erupt. This starts around age 6.

School-age children can run, jump, skip, hop, and ride a 2-wheeled bike. They can swim, skate, dance, and jump rope. Learning to play in groups, they can take part in team sports. Soccer, T-ball, baseball, football, and volleyball are examples (Fig. 11-18). They learn teamwork and sportsmanship and follow rules. Quiet play involves collections, board games, computer and video games, and crafts.

Reading, writing, grammar, and math skills develop. Sentences are longer and more complex. As reading skills increase, so do language skills. Children like to read and be read to.

Play activities have purpose and involve "work." School-age children like household tasks—cleaning, cooking, yard work. They also like crafts, building things, and scout groups. Rewards are important—good grades, trophies, payment for chores, scouting badges.

At about age 7, usually boys prefer playing with boys. Girls usually prefer playing with girls. From 8 to 9 years, play may involve boys and girls. Some show an interest in boy-girl relationships at about 8 to 9 years. However, children may deny such interest.

Peer groups develop. *Peers are persons of the same age-group and background.* Peer groups are important for love, belonging, and self-esteem needs. These children get along well with and need adults. However, they prefer peer group fads, opinions, and activities (Fig. 11-19).

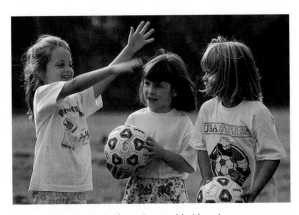

FIGURE 11-18 These 6-year-old girls enjoy soccer.

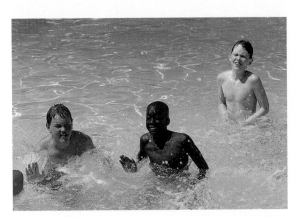

FIGURE 11-19 Belonging to a peer group is important to school-age children.

LATE CHILDHOOD (9 OR 10 TO 12 YEARS)

Late childhood (*pre-adolescence*) is the time between childhood and adolescence. Developmental tasks are like those for school-age children. In addition, pre-adolescents are expected to:

- Become independent of adults and learn to depend on oneself.
- Develop and keep friendships with peers.
- Understand physical, psychological, and social changes.
- Develop moral and ethical behavior.
- Develop greater muscular strength, coordination, and balance.
- Learn how to study.

Many permanent teeth erupt. Girls have a growth spurt. By age 12 years, they are taller and heavier than boys. Both boys and girls are more graceful and coordinated (Fig. 11-20). Muscle strength and physical skills increase. Skill in team sports is important.

Math and language skills increase. These children read for information and pleasure. They enjoy books and stories about romance, mystery, adventure, and science fiction.

The onset of puberty nears. *Puberty is the period when reproductive organs begin to function and secondary sex characteristics appear.* In girls, the hips widen and breast buds appear. Some 9-, 10-, and 11-year-old girls begin puberty. Boys show fewer signs of maturing sexually. Genital organs begin to grow. There is concern about body image.

Factual sex information is important. Information shared by friends is often not complete and not accurate. Parents and children may avoid the subject. When children ask questions, answers must be honest, complete, and in terms that children understand.

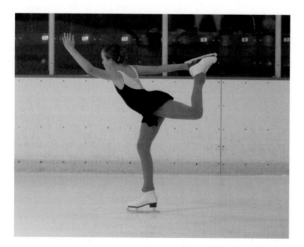

FIGURE 11-20 Movements are smooth and graceful in late childhood. (Courtesy Kevin Devine Photography, Kansas City, Missouri.)

Peer groups are the center of activities. The group affects attitudes and behavior. Friends of the same gender are preferred. Friends are loyal and share problems. A "best friend" is common. Interest in and feeling attraction to others begins.

These children are aware of the mistakes and faults of adults. Adult rules and standards are questioned. It is common to rebel against adults and test limits. Parents and children disagree. However, parents are needed for the child's development.

Bullying

Bullying is a form of youth violence. According to the Centers for Disease Control and Prevention (CDC), bullying involves:

- Unwanted aggressive behaviors by a person or group (not siblings or dating partners). Aggression may be verbal (name-calling, teasing, threatening), social (spreading rumors, leaving out of a group), or physical (hitting, tripping, spitting, breaking things).
- A real or a sense of a power imbalance. The bully has more power than or power over the victim.
- Repeated events or events that are likely to be repeated.

Most reported bullying occurs in school. It also happens on the playground, on the school bus, on the way to or from school, and in the community. Bullying also occurs electronically (cyber-bullying). See Chapter 6.

Physical, social, emotional, and educational harm and death can result. Victims are at risk for depression, anxiety, sleep problems, and problems adjusting in school. Bullies are at risk for substance use, school problems, and violence as a teenager and adult.

ADOLESCENCE (12 TO 18 YEARS)

Adolescence is the time between puberty and adulthood. There is rapid growth and physical, sexual, emotional, and social changes. The stage begins with puberty. Girls reach puberty between 9 and 16 years. Boys reach puberty between 13 and 15 years. Adolescents need to:

- Accept changes in the body and appearance.
- Develop appropriate relationships with others and begin to attract partners.
- Become independent from parents and adults.
- Prepare for marriage and family life.
- Prepare for a career.
- Develop the morals, attitudes, and values needed to function in society.

Boys and girls have a growth spurt. Both gain height and weight. They need about $9\frac{1}{2}$ hours of sleep because of such rapid growth. Girls usually complete physical development by age 17. Boys usually stop growing between 18 and 21 years.

Active oil glands lead to acne. Sweat glands are more active. Good hygiene is needed. Deodorants or antiperspirants prevent body odors.

Menarche marks the onset of puberty in girls. *Menarche is the first menstruation and the start of menstrual cycles* (Chapter 10). *Pregnancy can now occur.* Secondary sex characteristics appear. They include:

- Increase in breast size
- Pubic, axillary (underarm), and leg hair
- Slight deepening of the voice
- Widening and rounding of the hips

Ejaculation (the release of semen) signals the onset of puberty in boys. *Nocturnal emissions* ("wet dreams") occur. During sleep (*nocturnal*) the penis becomes erect. Semen is released (*emission*). *The male can father children.* Other secondary sex characteristics include:

- Facial, pubic, and axillary (underarm) hair
- Hair on the chest, arms, and legs
- Deepening of the voice
- Increases in neck and shoulder sizes

Accepting body changes and appearance occurs over time. Girls worry about weight gain. Breast development can embarrass girls, especially if breasts are large or small. Some do not like wearing a bra. Others wear clothes that show off the breasts. Boys may worry about genital size. Height is a concern for both genders. Being small limits play in some sports. Boys do not like being shorter than their peers. Tall girls may be embarrassed about being taller than other girls and boys.

Mood swings occur. Emotional reactions vary from high to low. They can be happy one moment and sad the next. Reactions to comments or events are hard to predict. They control emotions better later in this stage. Sometimes 14- to 18-year-olds are sad and depressed. However, they have more control over the time and place of emotional reactions.

Adolescents need to become independent of parents and other adults. They must learn to function, make decisions, and act responsibly without adult supervision. Many teenagers have part-time jobs or babysit (Fig. 11-21). They go to dances and parties, shop without an adult, and stay home alone. Many take part in school clubs and organizations.

Judgment and reasoning are not always sound. They still need guidance, discipline, and emotional and financial support from parents. The child and parents often disagree about behavior and activity restrictions and limits. Teens prefer doing things with their peers rather than with family. They tend to confide in and seek advice from adults other than their parents.

Interests and activities also reflect the need to develop intimate relationships. Adolescents may begin to feel or show a sexual orientation (Chapter 55). *Sexual orientation is emotional, romantic, and physical attraction to men, women, or both sexes.*

Teens like parties, dances, and other social events. Appearance is important (clothing, hair-styles). Teens experiment with make-up and hair-styles. They spend time talking to friends on the phone, texting, on social media sites, listening to music, and reading teen magazines.

Thoughts about careers and what to do after high school become a focus. Interests, skills, talents, and money are some factors that influence college or job choices.

Teens need to develop morals, values, and attitudes for living in society. They need to develop a sense about good and bad, right and wrong, and the important and unimportant. Parents, peers, culture, religion, the media, and school are influencing factors. Substance abuse, unwanted pregnancy, criminal acts, and suicide are risks for troubled teens.

Teen Dating

The age for dating varies. At first, dating involves school events, such as dances or football games. "Group dating" is common. The same group of girls is with the same group of boys. "Pairing off" as a couple replaces group dating. Couples may be sexual partners.

Parents and teens often disagree about dating. Parents worry about sexual activities, pregnancy, and sexually transmitted diseases. Teens usually do not understand or appreciate these concerns. Dating helps meet security, love and belonging, and self-esteem needs. Teens may have problems controlling sexual urges and considering the results of sexual activity.

See *Promoting Safety and Comfort: Teen Dating*, p. 142.

YOUNG ADULTHOOD (18 TO 40 YEARS)

Mental and social development continue during young adulthood. There is little physical growth. Adult height has been reached. Body systems are fully developed. Young adulthood involves:

- Choosing education and a career
- Selecting a partner
- Learning to live with a partner
- Becoming a parent and raising children
- Developing a satisfactory sex life

Most jobs require certain knowledge and skills. The education needed depends on career choice. Education usually increases job choices. Employment is needed for economic independence and to support a family.

Most adults marry at least once (Fig. 11-22, p. 142). Others choose to remain single. They may live alone or with friends of the same or other gender.

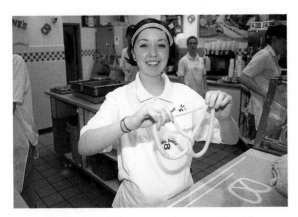

FIGURE 11-21 This teenager has a part-time job.

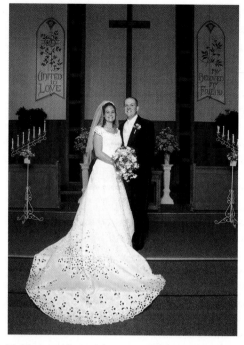

FIGURE 11-22 A wedding celebrates a couple's marriage. (Courtesy Dean Williams Photography, Springfield, Illinois.)

Birth control methods allow couples to plan when to have children and how many to have. Some pregnancies are not planned. Some couples choose not to have children. Physical problems in the man or woman can interfere with or prevent pregnancy.

Parents must agree on child-rearing practices and discipline methods. They need to adjust to the child and to the child's needs for parental time, energy, and attention.

MIDDLE ADULTHOOD (40 TO 65 YEARS)

This stage is more stable and comfortable. Children are usually grown and have moved away. Partners have time together. Worries about children and money are fewer.

Middle-age adults:

- Adjust to physical changes.
- Adjust to having grown children.
- Develop leisure-time activities.
- Adjust to aging parents.

Physical changes occur. Many are gradual and are not noticed. Others are seen early. Energy and endurance begin to slow down. So do metabolism and physical activities. Therefore weight control becomes a problem. Facial wrinkles and gray hair appear. Needing eyeglasses is common. Hair loss may begin. *Menstruation stops and menstrual cycles end (menopause).* It occurs between the ages of 45 and 55 years. Ovaries stop secreting hormones. The woman cannot have children.

Many diseases and illnesses can develop. The disorders become chronic and threaten life.

People marry for many reasons. They include love, emotional security, wanting a family, and sex. Some leave an unhappy home life. Some marry for social status, money, and companionship. Some marry to feel wanted, needed, and desirable.

Many factors affect partner selection. They include age, religion, interests, education, race, personality, and love. Some marriages or partnerships are happy and successful. Others are not. Partners must work together to build a relationship based on trust, respect, caring, and friendship.

Partners must learn to live together. Habits, routines, meals, and pastimes are changed or adjusted to "fit" the other person's needs. They learn to solve problems and make decisions together. They need to work toward the same goals. Open and honest communication is needed.

Sexual frequency, desires, practices, and preferences vary. For a satisfying and intimate relationship, partners must understand and accept the other's needs.

Children leave home for college, marry, move to their own homes, and start families. Adults have to let children go and adjust to being in-laws and grandparents (Fig. 11-23). Parents must let children lead their own lives. However, they provide emotional support when needed.

Spare time increases as parenting demands decrease. Hobbies and pastimes bring pleasure. They include gardening, fishing, painting, golfing, volunteer work, and being part of clubs and organizations (Fig. 11-24). These activities are even more important after retirement and during late adulthood.

Some middle-age adults have aging parents in poor health. Responsibility for aging parents may begin during this stage. Many middle-age adults deal with the death of parents.

LATE ADULTHOOD (65 YEARS AND OLDER)

Chapter 12 describes the many changes that occur in older persons. Older persons:

- Adjust to decreased strength and loss of health.
- Adjust to retirement and reduced income.
- Cope with a partner's death.
- Develop new friends and relationships.
- Prepare for one's own death.

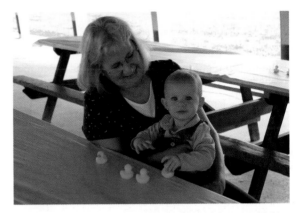

FIGURE 11-23 This woman enjoys time with her grandchild.

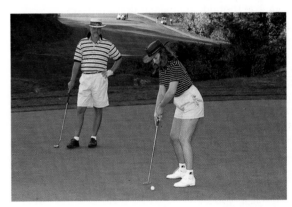

FIGURE 11-24 Middle-age adults usually have more time for leisure activities.

REVIEW QUESTIONS

Circle the BEST answer.

1 Changes in mental, emotional, and social function are called
   a Growth
   b Development
   c A reflex
   d A stage

2 These statements are about growth and development. Which is *true?*
   a They occur from complex to simple.
   b They occur at a set pace.
   c There is no order or pattern.
   d Each stage has its own characteristics.

3 Which reflexes does the infant need for feeding?
   a The Moro and startle reflexes
   b The rooting and sucking reflexes
   c The grasping and Moro reflexes
   d The rooting and palmar grasp reflexes

4 Which occurs first in infants?
   a Holding the head up
   b Rolling from front to back
   c Rolling from back to front
   d The pincer grasp

5 A 6-month-old can
   a Say 3 to 5 words
   b Understand simple instructions
   c Babble and make sounds
   d Respond to "no"

6 By 18 months a child can usually
   a Name body parts
   b Walk alone
   c Sort shapes and colors
   d Put on clothes and shoes

7 Toilet training begins
   a During infancy
   b During the toddler years
   c When the primary caregiver is ready
   d At the age of 4 years

8 The toddler can
   a Use a spoon and cup
   b Count items
   c Use scissors
   d Hop and skip

9 Playing with other children begins during
   a Infancy
   b The toddler years
   c The preschool years
   d The school-age years

10 Losing baby teeth usually begins at the age of
   a 4 years
   b 5 years
   c 6 years
   d 7 years

11 Peer groups become important to
   a Toddlers
   b Preschool children
   c School-age children
   d Young adults

12 Reproductive organs begin to function. Secondary sex characteristics appear. This is called
   a Late childhood
   b Puberty
   c Adolescence
   d Adulthood

13 Which is *true?*
   a Boys begin puberty earlier than girls.
   b Boys begin puberty between the ages of 9 and 11.
   c Little growth occurs during adolescence.
   d Menarche marks the onset of puberty in girls.

14 Dating usually begins
   a During late childhood
   b Before puberty
   c With "pairing off"
   d During adolescence

15 Teen dating violence
   a Can occur electronically or in person
   b Does not include stalking
   c Rarely occurs with teenagers
   d Often begins with physical violence

16 Adolescence is a time when parents and children
   a Talk openly about sex
   b Express love and affection
   c Disagree
   d Do things as a family

17 Young adulthood involves
   a Caring for aging parents
   b Making career choices
   c Physical growth and changes in body appearance
   d Adjusting to grown children

18 Middle adulthood ranges from
   a 20 to 35 years
   b 30 to 40 years
   c 35 to 45 years
   d 40 to 65 years

19 Middle adulthood is a time when
   a Families are started
   b Physical energy and free time increase
   c Children are grown and leave home
   d People need to prepare for death

20 Late adulthood involves
   a Retirement
   b Menopause
   c Stable health
   d Few changes

Answers to Chapter 11 questions are on p. 885.

FOCUS ON **PRACTICE**

Problem Solving

You are caring for an 18-month-old child. You take the child away from the mother for a weight measurement. You ask the child to stand on the scale. The child resists and says, "No." You try to place the child on the scale. The child cries and runs from you. Is this response normal? What could have been done to avoid this?

The Older Person

OBJECTIVES

- Define the key terms and key abbreviations in this chapter.
- Identify the psychological and social changes common in late adulthood.
- Describe the physical changes from aging and the care required.

- Describe housing options for older persons.
- Describe the gains and losses related to long-term care.
- Explain how to promote PRIDE in the person, the family, and yourself.

KEY TERMS

geriatrics The care of aging people
gerontology The study of the aging process

menopause The time when menstruation stops and menstrual cycles end; there has been at least 1 year without a menstrual period

KEY ABBREVIATIONS

ADU Accessory dwelling unit
CCRC Continuing care retirement community

CMS Centers for Medicare & Medicaid Services
ECHO Elder Cottage Housing Opportunity

Late adulthood ranges from 65 years of age and older. The oldest-old are 85 years of age and older. Aging is normal. Normal changes occur in body structure and function. Psychological and social changes also occur. *Gerontology is the study of the aging process. Geriatrics is the care of aging people.*

The risk for illness and injury increases with aging. Disability may result. Many older persons have 1 or more chronic diseases and disabilities. Disabilities can become more severe with aging and as the disease progresses. Quality of life is affected when disabilities interfere with every-day activities. They include:

- Managing money
- Shopping
- Preparing meals
- Taking prescribed drugs
- Tending to personal hygiene
- Dressing and undressing
- Feeding oneself
- Toileting (elimination)
- Moving about (mobility) in or outside the home
- Enjoying family and friends
- Enjoying leisure and recreational activities

Despite common myths, most older people adjust well and lead happy, meaningful lives. A *myth* is a widely believed story that is not true. See Box 12-1 (p. 146) for some common myths and facts about aging and older persons. Knowing the facts is important to give good care.

PSYCHOLOGICAL AND SOCIAL CHANGES

Graying hair, wrinkles, and slow movements are physical reminders of aging. They threaten self-esteem, self-image, self-worth, and independence.

Social roles change. A parent may rely on an adult child for care. Retirees may need activities to replace the work role. Adjusting to the deaths of parents, family members, and friends is common. The person faces his or her own death.

People adjust to aging in their own way. How they adjust depends on:

- Health status
- Life experiences
- Finances
- Education
- Social support systems

BOX 12-1	Aging—Myths and Facts

Myth: Older people lose their memory and have dementia.
Fact: Forgetting a name or misplacing an item happens at all ages and to everyone.

Myth: Older people are lonely.
Fact: Contact with family and friends is common. Many organizations and communities have social activities for older persons.

Myth: Older people are not sexual and cannot have relationships.
Fact: Healthy people with a desirable partner may continue to enjoy a fulfilling sex life. Sexuality, intimacy, love, and companionship are important.

Myth: Older people are crabby and rude.
Fact: Being happy and polite are factors of attitude and personality. Persons who were unhappy when younger are probably unhappy when older.

Myth: Most older people live in nursing centers.
Fact: Only a small number of older people live in nursing centers. Most live in a family setting with a spouse or partner, children, or other family members. Many live alone.

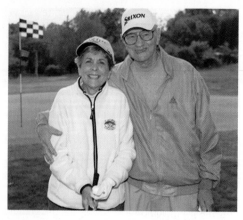

FIGURE 12-1 A retired couple enjoys golf as a leisure-time activity.

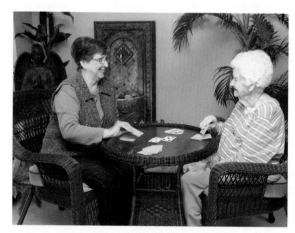

FIGURE 12-2 This retired woman is a nursing center volunteer.

Retirement

People usually retire between ages 62 and 66. Some retire earlier. Others work longer. Retirement allows time to relax and enjoy life (Fig. 12-1). Travel, leisure, and doing what one wants are retirement "benefits." Many people enjoy retirement. For others, poor health, disability, and medical bills can make retirement very hard.

Some retired people work part-time or do volunteer work (Fig. 12-2). Doing so meets love, belonging, and self-esteem needs. Friendships form. Daily events, leisure time, recreation, and companionship are shared with others.

Reduced Income. Retirement often means reduced income. Social Security benefits may provide the only income.

House or rent payments continue. Food, clothing, utility bills, entertainment, and taxes are other expenses. Car expenses, home repairs, drugs, and health care are other costs.

Reduced income may force life-style changes. Examples include:
- Limiting social and leisure events
- Buying cheaper food, clothes, and household items
- Moving to cheaper housing
- Living with children or other family
- Avoiding health care or needed drugs
- Relying on children or other family for money or needed items

Severe money problems can result. Some people have income from savings, investments, retirement plans, and insurance.

🌸 CARING ABOUT CULTURE

Foreign-Born Persons

Some older persons speak and understand a foreign language. Communication is with family and friends who speak the same language. They also share cultural values and practices. Family and friends may move away or die. The person may not have anyone to talk to. He or she may not be understood by others. The person may feel lonely and isolated.

Social Relationships

Social relationships change throughout life. (See *Caring About Culture: Foreign-Born Persons.*) Children grow up, leave home, and have families. Some live far away. Older family members and friends die, move away, or are disabled. Yet many older people have regular contact with children, grandchildren, family, and friends. Companionship with people their own age is important (Fig. 12-3).

Many older people adjust to social changes. Hobbies, religious and community events, and new friends provide enjoyment. Some community groups sponsor bus trips to ball games, shopping, plays, and concerts.

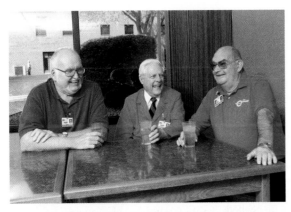

FIGURE 12-3 Older people enjoy being with others of their own age.

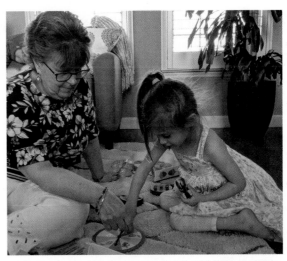

FIGURE 12-4 An older woman plays a game with her grandchild.

FOCUS ON **COMMUNICATION**

Social Relationships

The social changes of aging can cause loneliness. With nursing center care, the loneliness can seem greater. Staff and other residents do not replace family and friends. To provide social contact, you can:

- Suggest that the person contact a family member or friend. Offer to help with phone numbers and dialing. Many residents have their own phones.
- Keep the phone within reach. Calls or text messages can be placed or answered with greater ease.
- Suggest reading cards and letters. Offer to assist.
- Visit with the person a few times during your shift.
- Introduce new residents to other residents and staff.
- Encourage e-mail or video calls with family and friends. Some residents have computers with center-provided Internet access.

Grandchildren and family times can bring great love and joy (Fig. 12-4). They help the older person feel useful and wanted.

See *Focus on Communication: Social Relationships.*

Children as Caregivers

Sometimes parents and children change roles. The child cares for the parent. The older person may feel more secure or unwanted, in the way, and useless. Some lose dignity and self-respect. Tensions may occur among the child, parent, and other household members. Lack of privacy is a cause. So are disagreements and criticisms about housekeeping, raising children, meals, and friends.

Death and Grieving

A person may try to prepare for the death of a spouse or partner. When death occurs, the loss is crushing. No amount of preparation is ever enough for the emptiness and changes that result. The person loses a lover, friend, companion, and confidant. Grief may be very great. The person's life will likely change. Serious physical and mental health problems result. Some lose the will to live. Some attempt suicide.

The surviving spouse or partner may live alone. Others need to decide on housing options. (See "Housing Options.") Some people re-marry or have live-in arrangements with new partners.

Death of a Child. Sadly, newborns, infants, toddlers, school-age, and older children die. Death of a child at any age seems to be against the natural order of things. That is, parents should die before their children.

Parents of any age experience great grief when a child dies. As people live longer, some out-live their adult children. Their emotional needs are great. Often few family and friends are left to provide support and comfort.

PHYSICAL CHANGES

Physical changes of aging happen to everyone. See Table 12-1, p. 148. Body processes slow. Energy level and body efficiency decline. The rate and degree of changes vary with each person. They depend on diet, health, exercise, stress, environment, heredity, and other factors. Changes are slow over many years. Often they are not seen for a long time.

HOUSING OPTIONS

A person's home is more than a place to live. A home has family memories. It is a link to neighbors and the community. It brings pride and self-esteem.

Most older people live in their own homes. Many function without help. Others need help from family, home care, or community-based services for daily living and safety (Box 12-2, p. 150). Bathing, dressing, meals, housekeeping, shopping, and transportation are examples. Many services also provide social contact.

Some older persons choose smaller homes when children have left home. Others retire to warmer climates or move closer to children and family. Some choose other housing. Reduced income, taxes, home repairs, and yard work are factors. Some people cannot care for themselves.

Many housing options meet the needs of older people. A new home setting could maintain or improve quality of life.

See *Focus on Long-Term Care and Home Care: Housing Options*, p. 151.

Text continued on p. 151.

TABLE 12-1   The Aging Process: Physical Changes and Care Measures

Physical Changes	Care Measures
Nervous System	

Physical Changes — Nervous System

- Brain and spinal cord lose nerve cells
- Nerve cells send messages at a slower rate
- Reflexes slow
- Reduced blood flow to the brain
- Abnormal structures can form in the brain
- Brain tissue may shrink (atrophy)
- Changes in brain cells affect personality and mental function
- Shorter memory; forgetfulness; confusion may occur
- Trouble recalling recent events; long-ago events are easier to recall
- Slower ability to respond
- Dizziness
- Sleep patterns change
  - Difficulty falling asleep
  - Waking during the night
  - Less sleep is needed
  - Going to sleep early and waking early are common
- Reduced sensitivity to pain, pressure, and touch
- Smell and taste decrease
- Eyes and vision change
  - Eyelids thin and wrinkle
  - Less tear secretion
  - Pupils less responsive to light
  - Decreased vision at night or in dark rooms
  - Problems seeing green and blue colors
  - Poor vision; problems focusing on close objects
- Hearing loss
  - Changes in acoustic nerve
  - Eardrums atrophy
  - Earwax hardens and thickens; impacted earwax (wedged in the ear) can cause hearing loss
  - High-pitched sounds are hard to hear

Care Measures — Nervous System

- Practice safety measures to prevent injuries and falls.
- Remind the person to get up slowly from bed or chair.
- Follow the care plan to assist with memory, personality, or mental changes.
- Follow safety measures for heat and cold.
- Check for signs of skin breakdown and pressure injuries.
- Give good skin care.
- Prevent skin tears and pressure injuries.
- Follow the care plan to promote sleep. Day-time naps and rest may be needed.
- Have the person wear eyeglasses, contact lenses, and hearing aids as needed.
- Provide good room lighting and night-lights.
- See the following chapters for care measures.
  - Chapters 13 and 14—safety and preventing falls
  - Chapter 19—turning and moving
  - Chapter 20—getting in and out of bed or chair
  - Chapter 35—sleep
  - Chapter 40—skin tears
  - Chapter 41—pressure injuries
  - Chapter 42—heat and cold
  - Chapter 46—eyeglasses, contact lenses, and hearing aids
  - Chapters 52 and 53—mental changes and confusion

Integumentary System

Physical Changes — Integumentary System

- Skin becomes less elastic
- Skin loses strength
- Brown spots (age spots or liver spots) on the wrists and hands
- Fewer nerve endings affect temperature, pressure, and pain sensation
- Fewer blood vessels
- Fatty tissue layer is lost
- Skin thins and sags
- Skin is fragile and easily injured or burned
- Folds, lines, and wrinkles appear
- Blood vessels become more fragile
- Decreased secretion of oil and sweat glands
- Dry, itchy skin
- More sensitive to cold
- Nails become thick and tough
- Whitening or graying hair
- Facial hair in some women
- Loss or thinning of hair
- Drier hair

Care Measures — Integumentary System

- Protect from drafts and cold.
- Provide sweaters, lap blankets, socks, and extra blankets.
- Check thermostat settings. Higher settings are helpful.
- Provide for hygiene—shower or bath 2 times a week; partial baths on other days.
- Use mild soaps or soap substitutes to clean the underarms, genitals, and under the breasts. Soap is often avoided on the face, arms, legs, back, chest, and abdomen.
- Apply lotions and creams to prevent drying and itching.
- Provide nail and foot care.
- Prevent burns. Do not use hot water bottles or heating pads on the feet.
- Brush and shampoo hair as needed for hygiene and comfort. Shampoo frequency often decreases with age.
- Protect from prolonged sun exposure.
- See the following chapters for care measures.
  - Chapter 13—preventing burns
  - Chapters 24 and 25—hygiene, skin care, and grooming
  - Chapter 40—skin tears
  - Chapter 41—pressure injuries

TABLE 12-1	The Aging Process: Physical Changes and Care Measures—cont'd
Physical Changes	**Care Measures**

Musculo-Skeletal System

<ul><li>Muscles shrink *(atrophy)*</li><li>Muscle strength, tone, and contractility decrease</li><li>Bone mass decreases</li><li>Bones become weaker</li><li>Bones become brittle; can break easily</li><li>Vertebrae shorten</li><li>Joints become stiff and painful</li><li>Hip and knee joints become flexed (bent)</li><li>Gradual loss of height; trunk becomes shorter</li><li>Decreased mobility</li></ul>	<ul><li>Promote exercise and activity as ordered to prevent atrophy and loss of strength.</li><li>Assist with range-of-motion exercises as ordered (Chapter 34).</li><li>Encourage a diet high in protein, calcium, and vitamins as ordered.</li><li>Practice safety measures to prevent injuries and falls (Chapters 13 and 14).</li><li>Turn and move the person gently and carefully.</li><li>Assist the person in getting out of bed or chair as needed.</li><li>Provide support when walking as needed (Chapter 34).</li></ul>

Circulatory System

<ul><li>Heart pumps with less force</li><li>Heart valves thicken and become stiff</li><li>Heart rate may slow</li><li>Abnormal heart rhythms may occur</li><li>Heart may enlarge slightly</li><li>Heart walls thicken</li><li>Arteries narrow and become stiffer</li><li>Less blood flows through narrowed arteries</li><li>Weakened heart works harder to pump blood through narrowed vessels</li><li>Number of red blood cells decreases</li><li>Fatigue</li></ul>	<ul><li>Follow the person's activity limits.<ul><li>Promote exercise as ordered. Encourage the person to be as active as possible. Moderate daily exercise helps maintain health and well-being.</li><li>Assist with range-of-motion exercises as ordered.</li><li>Avoid over-exertion. The person should not walk far, climb many stairs, or carry heavy things. Encourage rest periods.</li><li>Encourage bed rest if ordered. *Bed rest* means *being confined to bed.*</li></ul></li><li>Keep personal care items, TV controls, phone, and other needed items within reach.</li></ul>

Respiratory System

<ul><li>Respiratory muscles weaken</li><li>Some lung tissue is lost</li><li>Lung tissue becomes less elastic</li><li>Chest is less able to stretch to breathe</li><li>Difficulty breathing *(dyspnea)*</li><li>Decreased strength for coughing and clearing the airway</li></ul>	<ul><li>Promote normal breathing.</li><li>Position the person for easier breathing. Semi-Fowler's or Fowler's position (Chapter 18) may be preferred.</li><li>Assist with coughing and deep-breathing exercises as ordered (Chapter 43).</li><li>Avoid heavy bed linens over the chest.</li><li>Turn and position the person according to the care plan. Persons on bed rest are re-positioned often.</li><li>Encourage activity as ordered.</li></ul>

Digestive System

<ul><li>Decreased saliva production</li><li>Difficulty swallowing *(dysphagia)*</li><li>Decreased appetite</li><li>Decreased secretion of digestive juices</li><li>Difficulty digesting fried and fatty foods</li><li>Indigestion</li><li>Loss of teeth</li><li>Decreased peristalsis causing *flatulence* (gas) and constipation</li></ul>	<ul><li>Provide oral hygiene and denture care to improve taste (Chapter 23).</li><li>Encourage diet as ordered (Chapter 30). Dry, fried, fatty, and hard-to-chew foods are avoided. The person may need food ground, chopped, or pureed.</li><li>Promote fluid intake as ordered (Chapter 31). Thickened liquids may be needed for persons with swallowing problems.</li><li>Follow the care plan to prevent *flatulence* (gas) and constipation (Chapter 29). High-fiber foods help prevent constipation. Some are hard to chew and irritate the intestines. Apricots, celery, and fruits and vegetables with skins and seeds are avoided.</li></ul>

Urinary System

<ul><li>Kidney function decreases</li><li>Reduced blood supply to kidneys</li><li>Kidneys atrophy</li><li>Bladder tissues less able to stretch</li><li>Bladder muscles weaken</li><li>Bladder may not empty completely</li><li>Urinary tract infections may occur</li><li>Urinary frequency, urgency, incontinence (loss of bladder control), or night-time urination may occur</li><li>Prostate gland enlarges (men)</li></ul>	<ul><li>Answer call lights promptly (Chapter 21).</li><li>Promote normal urination (Chapter 27).</li><li>Provide the bedpan, urinal, or commode as needed.</li><li>Follow the care plan to manage incontinence (Chapter 27).</li><li>Provide catheter care according to the care plan (Chapter 28).</li><li>Encourage fluids as ordered to prevent urinary tract infections. Most fluids should be taken before 5:00 PM (1700) to reduce the need to urinate at night.</li><li>Follow the person's bladder training program (Chapter 27).</li></ul>

Continued

TABLE 12-1	The Aging Process: Physical Changes and Care Measures—cont'd
Physical Changes	**Care Measures**
Reproductive System	

• Men
  • Testosterone decreases slightly
  • Erections take longer
  • Longer phase between erection and orgasm
  • Less forceful orgasms
  • Erections lost quickly
  • Longer time between erections
• Women
  • *Menopause—the time when menstruation stops and menstrual cycles end; there has been at least 1 year without a menstrual period*
  • Estrogen and progesterone decrease
  • Uterus, vagina, and genitalia atrophy
  • Thinning of vaginal walls
  • Vaginal dryness
  • Arousal takes longer
  • Less intense orgasms
  • Quicker return to pre-excitement state
	• Follow the care plan for the person with reproductive changes (Chapter 51).

BOX 12-2	In-Home and Community-Based Services

- *Adult day care*—a safe setting for those who cannot be alone during the day. Services may include personal care, social and recreational activities, meals, drug reminders, counseling, and home health aide services.
- *Adult protective services*—a state agency, it provides help to vulnerable adults and elders to stop or prevent abuse (Chapter 5).
- *Caregiver programs*—for older adults and for grandparents raising grandchildren. Programs offer information about available services, help obtaining support services, counseling, support groups, and other services.
- *Case management*—a case manager assesses the needs of the older person and family. Arrangements are made for needed services.
- *Companionship services*—volunteers provide supervision and support services as needed.
- *Emergency response systems*—in-home 24-hour alarm systems to call for emergency help. The person wears a necklace or bracelet with a button to push if help is needed. He or she is connected to an operator who will send help.
- *Financial counseling*—help with checking accounts, paying bills, taxes, and insurance claims and forms. Counseling is available about Social Security benefits, prescription drug programs, food stamps, and other programs.
- *Home health care*—nursing and physical, occupational, and speech therapies. The person may need help with such things as taking drugs, changing dressings, or catheter care.
- *Housekeeping services*—help with household tasks. Cleaning, changing linens, laundry, shopping, and preparing meals are examples.
- *Home repair and modification*—programs to keep the house in good repair. Roofing and plumbing are examples. See *Focus on Long-Term Care and Home Care: Housing Options* for home changes.

- *Hospice care*—Chapters 1 and 59. Nursing, comfort, and homemaker services are provided.
- *Legal assistance*—advice for some legal matters. Wills, advance directives (Chapter 59), renters' rights, and consumer problems are examples. A lawyer may represent the person in court.
- *Meal programs*—meals in-home or at a senior center, nutrition site, or other group setting.
- *Personal care*—help with eating, bathing, oral care, grooming, and dressing.
- *Rehabilitation*—therapies to assist the person to regain or maintain his or her highest level of functioning.
- *Respite care*—relieves caregivers of daily care for a short time.
- *Senior centers*—offer many social and recreational activities. Classes, day trips, travel groups, performing arts, and nature activities are examples. Services also include meals, counseling, legal help, health screenings, and transportation.
- *Phone reassurance*—regular phone contact with the person. The person is called at various times. If the person does not answer, someone is sent to the person's home. Also, the older person can call the service when help is needed.
- *Transportation*—rides to and from doctor visits, appointments, shopping, religious services, and other places.
- *Wellness programs*—blood pressure, blood sugar, and other tests are done to promote health. Sessions are held about fitness, nutrition, and other health topics.

FOCUS ON **LONG-TERM CARE AND HOME CARE**

Housing Options

Home Care

Simple changes can make a home safe, easy to use, and promote independence. The nurse discusses needed changes with the patient and family.

The Bathroom

- Non-slick flooring
- Grab bars by showers, tubs, and toilets
- Slip-resistant surfaces in showers and tubs (bath mats, slip-resistant bath strips)
- Rugs have non-slip backing and are secured to the floor outside the tub and shower and in front of the toilet; no throw rugs
- Hand-held shower nozzle or adjustable shower head
- Shower chair for shower or bathtub
- Transfer bench
- Lever-handle faucets
- Water controls close to the shower or tub entrance
- Anti-scald devices on faucets and shower heads
- Storage area for liquid soap and hair products is attached to the wall for easy access
- Towel bars or hooks raised or lowered for the person's reach
- Comfort-height toilet, raised toilet seat, or a toilet seat riser
- Chair placed in front of the sink for sitting
- Knee space under the sink for the person who sits
- Bright, non-glare lighting

The Bedroom

- Clear walking path in the room and to the bathroom; un-wanted and un-used furniture and items are removed
- Loose flooring is repaired
- Area rugs and cords are removed
- Phone on a nightstand
- Flashlight and extra batteries on a nightstand
- Remotes for the TV, fans, and lamps on a nightstand
- Bed rails if needed
- Night-lights
- Lit path to the bathroom
- Closet rods that adjust for height
- Lowered shelves or pull-down shelves
- Pull-out drawers, bins, and baskets in closets
- A commode chair near the bed for night-time use (Chapter 27)

The Kitchen

- Appliances within reach—side-by-side refrigerator/freezer, cook-top range, wall-mounted oven, dishwasher raised off the floor
- Stove controls on the front of the stove
- Stove controls clearly marked and easy to see
- Lowered shelves or pull-down or pull-out shelves
- Height of sink and countertops adjusted for the person's needs (lowered for wheelchair use; raised for the person who cannot bend easily)
- Anti-scald devices on faucets
- Lever-handle faucets
- Spray attachment to the sink—pots can be filled after placing them on the stove

Other

- Lever door handles on all doors
- Easy-to-grasp cabinet and drawer handles
- Hand rails on both sides of stairways and outside steps
- Keyless locking system
- Security system
- Shelves near outside doors—items can be set down to open the door
- Bright lights inside and outside entry-ways
- Motion-activated entrance lights
- Slip-free walk-ways and entry-ways
- House numbers that are easy to see from the street
- Automatic garage door opener
- Rocker light switches that turn on and off with a push
- Electrical outlets 18 inches above the floor
- Peepholes or view panels in doors at the correct height for the person
- Washer and dryer on the main floor
- Wall-mounted, fold-down ironing board
- Stair or platform lifts
- No scatter or throw rugs
- Thick carpeting replaced with low pile carpeting
- Furniture arranged for wheelchair use
- Phones in all rooms, including the bathroom
- Chairs throughout the home so the person can sit when tired, weak, dizzy, and so on
- Smoke alarms as required by local fire code
- Carbon monoxide alarms
- For poor eyesight—see Chapter 46
- For hearing loss—see Chapter 46
- For other safety measures—Chapter 13
- For fall prevention—Chapter 14

Living With Family

Sometimes older brothers, sisters, and cousins live together. They provide companionship and help during illness or disability. Living expenses are shared.

Some older persons live with their adult children. The older parent (parents) moves in with the child. Or the child moves to the parent's home. The parent may be healthy, may need some help, or may be ill or disabled. Some children give needed care or arrange for home care.

Living with family is a social change. Everyone in the home must adjust. If no spare bedroom, sleeping plans may change. A hospital bed may be needed. It can go in a living area, dining room, den, or bedroom.

The adult child's family needs time alone. Other family members may help give care. Respite care in a nursing center is an option (see Box 12-2). The person goes to a nursing center for a short time. This gives the family relief from the person's care. Home care agencies can provide nurses or home health aides. Many community and religious groups have volunteers who help give care.

Adult Day Care. Many children work even though the parent cannot stay alone. Adult day-care centers provide meals, supervision, and activities. Transportation, rehabilitation (Chapter 45), and dementia care (Chapter 53) are common.

Requirements vary. Some require the ability to walk. A cane or walker is allowed. Others allow wheelchairs. Most require some self-care abilities.

Card games, board games, movies, crafts, dancing, walks, exercise groups, and lectures are common activities (Fig. 12-5). Some provide bowling and swimming. All activities are supervised. Needed help is given.

Some day-care centers are inter-generational. Children and older persons are in the same center. They eat, play, and work together on activities. Young children bring much joy to older persons. They give older persons purpose, love, and affection. In turn, children learn about aging and receive love and affection.

Elder Cottage Housing Opportunity and Accessory Dwelling Units

Elder Cottage Housing Opportunity (ECHO) homes are small homes designed for older and disabled persons. The portable home is placed in the yard of a single-family home. Some ECHO homes attach to a house as a home addition. Government funding may be available.

An *accessory dwelling unit (ADU)* is a separate living area in a home or yard. It can be over a garage, in the basement, an addition to the house, or in a side or back yard. It has a kitchen, bedroom, and bathroom. Some have a small living room.

ADUs are also called "in-law apartments," "granny flats," "accessory apartments," "second units," and other names. ECHO homes and ADUs allow older persons to live independently but near family and friends.

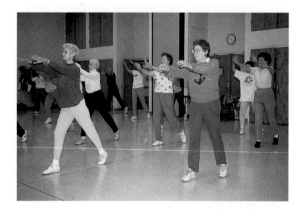

FIGURE 12-5 An adult day-care center activity.

Rental Options

Rental options include a single-family home, an apartment, a condo, a mobile home, or a room in a house. The renter pays rent and utility bills. The benefits of renting include:
- The renter does not have the responsibilities of home ownership.
- The owner (landlord) provides maintenance, yard work, snow removal, and repairs.
- The older person remains independent.
- The older person can keep personal items.

Downsides to renting include:
- Restrictions about having pets
- Relying on the landlord for repairs and maintenance
- Rent increases
- Ending rental agreements before the person wants to move
- Lack of gardening or yard work opportunities

Senior Citizen Housing. In many areas, state and federal funds support apartment complexes for older and disabled persons. Such persons have low to moderate incomes. Monthly rents depend on the person's monthly income.

Residential Hotels. The person rents a room or small apartment. Food services may include a dining room, cafeteria, or room service. Some hotels have recreational activities and emergency medical services. Most hotels are close to shopping, places of worship, and civic services.

Home-Sharing

Two or more people share a house or apartment. They share living spaces—kitchen, bathroom, living room. They share household chores and expenses. Or cooking, cleaning, and yard work are exchanged for rent.

Shared housing is a way to avoid living alone. It provides companionship. Some people feel safer when living with another person.

Group Settings

Group settings provide housing, in-home support services, and social activities. Services provided relate to personal care and independent living.
- Personal hygiene and grooming
- Meals
- Getting in and out of bed or chairs
- Using the bathroom
- Using the phone
- Housework
- Shopping
- Managing money

Assisted Living Residences. Assisted living residences are for persons needing help with daily living (Chapters 1 and 57). Residents have social contact with others in a home-like setting. Staff are available to assist 24 hours a day.

Board and Care Homes. Board and care homes (group homes; residential care facilities) are often private, single-family homes. The homes have been adapted for group living. Rooms are private or shared.

Homes are for older persons or for people with certain problems. Dementia, mental health disorders, and intellectual and developmental disabilities are examples.

Homes house 4 to 10 people or more. Personal care and meals are provided. Nursing and medical care are usually not provided on-site.

Adult Foster Care. An older person lives with a family. Or a single family home serves 4 to 5 persons with special needs. They may be older, disabled, or have mental health disorders. The person receives needed health care and help with personal care and independent living.

Adult Care Facilities. In this group setting, private apartments are designed for older people. Buildings have wheelchair access, hand rails, elevators, and other safety features.

Services are many. A doctor or nurse is on call. Someone checks on the person daily. A dining room is common. Rides are provided to places of worship, the doctor, or shopping areas. Tenants pay monthly rent.

Continuing Care Retirement Communities. Continuing care retirement communities (CCRCs; life care communities) offer many services in 1 location. They range from independent living units (houses or apartments) to 24-hour nursing care. CCRCs meet the changing needs of older persons living alone or with a partner.

When in an independent living unit, residents perform self-care and take their own drugs. Food service is provided. Help is nearby if needed. Many people travel or drive their own cars. Rides are provided for those who need them.

Services are added as the person's needs change. Over time, some persons need home care or nursing center care. The nursing center is within the CCRC. Many older couples find comfort in this plan. One partner needs nursing care. The other is close by and can visit often.

Nursing Centers

Nursing centers are options for persons who cannot care for themselves (Chapter 1). Some people stay in nursing centers until death. Others return home. The setting is as home-like as possible (Fig. 12-6).

The person needing nursing center care may suffer some or all of these losses.

- Loss of identity as a productive member of a family and community
- Loss of possessions—home, household items, car, and so on
- Loss of independence
- Loss of real-world experiences—shopping, traveling, cooking, driving, hobbies, and so on
- Loss of health and mobility

Feeling useless, powerless, and hopeless are common emotions. The health team helps the person cope with loss and improve quality of life. Treat the person with dignity and respect. Also practice good communication skills. Follow the care plan.

To receive Medicare or Medicaid funds, nursing centers must meet requirements of the *Omnibus Budget Reconciliation Act of 1987 (OBRA)*. OBRA protects the person's rights and promotes quality of life. The Centers for Medicare & Medicaid Services (CMS) has rules and regulations for OBRA. See Box 12-3.

Nursing centers serve to meet the needs of older and disabled persons. Aging changes and safety needs are considered in the design. Programs and services meet basic needs. Box 12-4 (p. 154) lists the features of a quality nursing center.

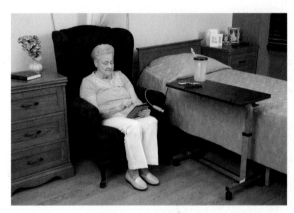

FIGURE 12-6 A nursing center is as home-like as possible. Some centers allow residents to bring their own bed and furniture from home.

BOX 12-3	**Environment Observations**

- The resident's needs and preferences are met.
- The call light system is functioning (Chapter 21).
- Sound levels are comfortable.
- Temperature levels are comfortable and safe.
- Lighting levels are proper and maintained.
- Resident rooms and the building are clean and in good condition—walls, floors, ceilings, drapes, furniture.
- Care equipment is in good repair and functions safely.
- Resident rooms are as home-like as possible. Personal belongings are allowed.
- Water temperatures are comfortable and at a safe level in resident rooms and in bathrooms and bathing areas.
- Bed and bath linens are clean and in good condition.
- The center is free of pests and rodents.
- Ventilation is adequate to control odors.
- Hand rails are securely affixed to the walls. Residents can access the hand rails.
- The center provides a safe, clean, and comfortable setting for residents, staff, and visitors.

Modified from Centers for Medicare & Medicaid Services: Environmental observations—FORM CMS-20061, *Baltimore, May 2017, U.S. Department of Health and Human Services.*

BOX 12-4   Features of a Quality Nursing Center

Basic Information
- The center is Medicare-certified.
- The center is Medicaid-certified.
- The administrator is licensed by the state.
- The center provides the level of care needed. Rehabilitation, dementia, ventilator, and hospice services are examples.
- The center is located close enough for family and friends to visit.
- The center gives information in writing about policies, services, extra charges, and fees. For example, is there an extra charge for beauty shop services?

Living Spaces
- The center is free from strong, unpleasant odors.
- The center appears clean and well-kept.
- The temperature is comfortable for the residents.
- The center has good lighting.
- Noise levels in the dining room and in common areas are comfortable.
- Smoking is not allowed. If allowed, it is restricted to certain areas.
- Furnishings in rooms and lounges are sturdy, comfortable, and attractive.
- Exits are clearly marked.
- The center has quiet areas where residents can visit with family and friends.
- All common areas, resident rooms, and doorways are designed for wheelchair use.
- The center has hand rails in the hallways.
- The center has grab bars in bathrooms.
- The center has smoke alarms and sprinklers.

Menus and Food
- Residents have food choices at meal times.
- The person's favorite foods are served.
- The center provides for special dietary needs.
- Nutritious snacks are available upon request.
- Staff help residents eat and drink if help is needed.

Staff
- The relationship between the staff and residents appears to be warm, polite, and respectful.
- All staff wear name tags.
- Staff knock on the person's door before entering the room.
- Staff refer to residents by name.
- The center offers a training and continuing education program for all staff.
- The center does background checks to make sure staff are not hired who:
  - Have been found guilty of abuse, neglect, or mistreatment of residents.
  - Have a finding of abuse, neglect, or mistreatment of residents in the state nurse aide registry.
- The center has licensed nurses 24 hours a day. An RN (registered nurse) is present at least 8 hours a day, 7 days a week.
- The center posts information about the number of nursing staff working. This includes the number of nursing assistants.

Staff—cont'd
- Nurses and nursing assistants work as a team to meet resident needs.
- Nursing assistants help plan the person's care.
- The center has a staff member to meet the social needs of residents.
- The nursing center has a social worker available to residents.
- The center will call the person's doctor for medical needs.
- The center's management team has worked together for at least 1 year. This includes the administrator and director of nursing.
- The resident's primary language is spoken by the staff. If not, an interpreter is available for the resident to communicate his or her needs.

Residents' Rooms
- Residents may have personal belongings and furniture in their rooms.
- Each resident has a storage space (closet and drawers) in his or her room.
- Each resident has a window in his or her room.
- Residents have access to a personal phone, TV, the Internet, and a computer.
- Residents have a choice of roommates.
- The center has policies and procedures to protect resident possessions. Cabinets and closets that lock are examples.

Activities
- Residents may choose a variety of activities. This includes residents who cannot leave their rooms.
- The center has outdoor areas for resident use. Staff help residents to go outside.
- The center has an active volunteer program.
- Residents help plan or choose activities.
- The resident chooses when to get up, go to sleep, or bathe.
- Residents can have visitors at any time. This includes during early or late hours.
- The center has procedures for when a resident wants to leave the center for a few hours or days.
- The center provides or arranges for a resident's religious and cultural needs.

Safety and Care
- Residents are clean and well-groomed.
- Residents are dressed correctly for the season or time of day.
- Residents may see their personal doctors.
- The center has an arrangement with a nearby hospital.
- Care plan meetings are held with residents and family members.
- The center has inspection reports—quality care, health, fire—available for residents to see.
- The center has corrected all problems on its last state inspection report.
- The center has policies and procedures related to the care of persons with dementia. This includes non-drug-based approaches.
- The center takes part in efforts to reduce the use of anti-psychotic drugs.

Modified from Centers for Medicare & Medicaid Services: Your guide to choosing a nursing home or other long-term care services & supports, CMS product no. 02174, revised April 2019.

FOCUS ON **PRIDE**

The Person, Family, and Yourself

Personal and Professional Responsibility

All older persons are not the same. Each person is unique. Treat each person as an individual. Also, communicate in a way that promotes dignity. Treat the person as an adult, not a child.

Rights and Respect

Simple actions can promote the older person's right to quality of life.

- Knock before entering the room.
- Make sure the person, clothes, and linens are clean and dry.
- Keep the room clean and orderly.
- Place soiled linens in the correct containers. Empty the containers often. Do not let them over-flow.
- Clean your work area and the bathroom after giving care.
- Help the person display belongings if asked. Do not touch the person's items without permission.
- Treat the person as if you were in his or her home.
- Respect the person and his or her setting.

Independence and Social Interaction

Older persons may feel alone and isolated. Loss of friends and loved ones, a new home setting, reduced income, and physical changes are causes. To promote social interaction:

- Encourage the person to talk about friends and family.
- Ask about hobbies and interests.
- Use touch to show caring. For example, gently place your hand on the person's shoulder or arm. Remember to maintain professional boundaries (Chapter 5).
- Take time to listen. Avoid seeming rushed.
  Some persons prefer quiet and privacy. They may avoid social contacts. Respect their wishes for privacy. Take pride in considering social needs.

Delegation and Teamwork

Co-workers often work together to assist older persons. A co-worker may be closer to your age, share your interests, relate to your work, share your native language, and so on. You must not ignore the person or speak in a foreign language. Focus on the person, not on others. This promotes a sense of belonging and self-worth.

Ethics and Laws

The Centers for Medicare & Medicaid Services (CMS) issues standards, rules, and regulations for nursing centers. Surveys are conducted for agency compliance. You may be observed or asked questions during a survey. Answer survey questions completely and honestly. Be professional and use good work ethics (Chapter 6).

FOCUS ON **PRIDE**: *Application*

List 5 changes that occur with aging. Describe how each affects the person. How would you modify care to meet the person's needs?

REVIEW QUESTIONS

Circle the BEST answer.

1 The study of the aging process is called
   a Geriatrics
   b Dysphagia
   c Gerontology
   d Dyspnea

2 Retirement usually means
   a Lowered income
   b Changes from aging
   c Less free time
   d Financial security

3 Which causes loneliness in older persons?
   a Having hobbies
   b Children moving away
   c Attending community events
   d Contact with other older persons

4 An adult child is an older parent's caregiver. This social change promotes
   a Independence
   b Privacy
   c Security
   d Usefulness

5 Which statement about a partner's death is *true*?
   a The surviving partner's life will not likely change.
   b Preparing for the event lessens grief.
   c Grief cannot cause physical problems.
   d Feelings of loss and emptiness occur.

6 Skin changes occur with aging. Care should include
   a Keeping the room cool
   b A daily bath with soap
   c Applying lotion
   d Bathing in hot water

Continued

REVIEW QUESTIONS—cont'd

7 An older person complains of cold feet. You should
 a Provide socks
 b Apply a hot water bottle
 c Soak the feet in hot water
 d Apply a heating pad

8 Musculo-skeletal changes occur with aging. Which is *true*?
 a Bones become firm.
 b Exercise promotes muscle atrophy.
 c Joints become stiff and painful.
 d Bed rest prevents loss of strength.

9 Aging causes changes in the nervous system. Which is *true*?
 a Less sleep is needed than when younger.
 b The person forgets events from long ago.
 c Sensitivity to pressure increases.
 d Confusion occurs in all older persons.

10 Changes occur in the eye with aging. Which is *true*?
 a Tear secretion increases.
 b There is no change in seeing colors.
 c There is more trouble focusing on far objects.
 d Vision is poor at night and in dark rooms.

11 Which is *true* of hearing loss in older persons?
 a Low-pitched sounds are hard to hear.
 b Acoustic nerve changes affect hearing.
 c Earwax cannot affect hearing.
 d Ear infections often cause hearing loss.

12 An older person has circulatory changes. Which care measure would you question?
 a Keep needed items nearby
 b Get a moderate amount of daily exercise
 c Avoid over-exertion
 d Take long walks

13 Respiratory changes occur with aging. Which is *true*?
 a Heavy bed linens are used.
 b The person is turned often if on bed rest.
 c The side-lying position is best for breathing.
 d Deep breathing is avoided.

14 Older persons should avoid dry foods because of
 a Decreases in saliva
 b Decreased appetite
 c Increased amounts of digestive juices
 d Increased peristalsis

15 Changes occur in the digestive system. Older persons should eat
 a Fruits and vegetables with skins and seeds
 b Dry and fatty foods
 c Raw apricots and celery
 d High-fiber foods

16 Changes occur in the urinary system. Which is *true*?
 a Kidneys increase in size.
 b Bladder muscles weaken.
 c The prostate gland in men shrinks.
 d Blood flow to the kidneys increases.

17 An older person is at risk for a urinary tract infection. The doctor ordered increased fluid intake. You should
 a Give most of the fluid before 1700 (5:00 PM)
 b Question the order
 c Start a bladder training program
 d Insert a catheter

18 Adult day-care centers
 a Provide meals, supervision, and activities
 b Provide housing and nursing care
 c Offer help for persons who cannot perform self-care
 d Provide personal care

19 A husband needs 24-hour nursing care. His wife needs an independent living unit. Which would meet their needs?
 a Adult foster care
 b Home health care
 c A continuing care retirement community
 d An assisted living residence

20 A quality nursing center
 a Is Medicare and Medicaid certified
 b Is owned by doctors and nurses
 c Has independent living units
 d Provides adult and child day care

Answers to Chapter 12 questions are on p. 885.

FOCUS ON **PRACTICE**

Problem Solving

A person has urinary incontinence and swallowing problems due to changes from aging. A co-worker uses the term "diaper" to describe incontinence products and "bib" for clothing protectors. The co-worker threatens to with-hold privileges if the person does not finish meals.

 Why should you treat the person as an adult and not a child? Describe ways to provide age-appropriate care. How will you respond to your co-worker's statements and actions?

Safety

OBJECTIVES

- Define the key terms and key abbreviations in this chapter.
- Describe accident risk factors.
- Explain why you identify a person before giving care.
- Explain how to correctly identify a person.
- Describe the safety measures to prevent burns, poisoning, and suffocation.
- Identify the signs and causes of choking.
- Explain how to prevent equipment accidents.
- Explain how to handle hazardous chemicals.

- Identify natural and human-made disasters.
- Describe fire prevention measures and oxygen safety.
- Explain what to do during a fire.
- Explain how to protect yourself from workplace violence.
- Describe your role in risk management.
- Perform the procedures described in this chapter.
- Explain how to promote PRIDE in the person, the family, and yourself.

KEY TERMS

coma A state of being unaware of one's setting and being unable to react or respond to people, places, or things

dementia The loss of cognitive and social function caused by changes in the brain

disaster A sudden, catastrophic event in which people are injured and killed and property is destroyed

electrical shock When electrical current passes through the body

elopement When a patient or resident leaves the agency without staff knowledge

ground That which carries leaking electricity to the earth and away from an electrical item

hazard Any thing in the person's setting that could cause injury or illness

hazardous chemical Any chemical that is a physical hazard or a health hazard

hemiplegia Paralysis (*plegia*) on 1 side (*hemi*) of the body

incident Any event that has harmed or could harm a patient, resident, visitor, or staff member

paralysis Loss of muscle function, sensation, or both

paraplegia Paralysis in the legs and lower trunk (*para* means *beyond; plegia* means *paralysis*)

poison Any substance harmful to the body when ingested, inhaled, injected, or absorbed through the skin

quadriplegia Paralysis in the arms, legs, and trunk (*quad* means *4; plegia* means *paralysis*); tetraplegia

suffocation When breathing stops from the lack of oxygen

tetraplegia See "quadriplegia" (*tetra* means *4; plegia* means *paralysis*)

workplace violence Violent acts (including assault or threat of assault) directed toward persons at work or while on duty

KEY ABBREVIATIONS

AED	Automated external defibrillator	**MRN**	Medical record number
CDC	Centers for Disease Control and Prevention	**MSDS**	Material safety data sheet
CMS	Centers for Medicare & Medicaid Services	**NFPA**	National Fire Protection Association
CO	Carbon monoxide	**OSHA**	Occupational Safety and Health Administration
CPR	Cardiopulmonary resuscitation	**PASS**	*Pull* the safety pin, *aim* low, *squeeze* the lever, *sweep* back and forth
DOB	Date of birth		
EMS	Emergency Medical Services	**PPE**	Personal protective equipment
F	Fahrenheit	**RACE**	Rescue, alarm, confine, extinguish
FBAO	Foreign-body airway obstruction	**RRS**	Rapid Response System
HCS	Hazard Communication Standard	**SDS**	Safety data sheet
ID	Identification		

Safety is a basic need. Patients and residents are at great risk for accidents and falls. (See Chapter 14 for falls.) Some accidents and injuries cause death.

The health team must provide for safety. Common sense and safety measures can prevent most accidents. You must protect patients, residents, visitors, co-workers, and yourself. The safety measures in this chapter apply to all health care settings and daily life.

The goal is to prevent accidents and injuries without limiting the person's mobility and independence. The care plan lists other safety measures. Safety measures must not interfere with the person's rights (Chapter 2).

See *Focus on Surveys: Safety.*

A SAFE SETTING

In a safe setting, there is little risk of illness or injury. The setting is free of hazards to the extent possible. The person feels safe and secure physically and mentally. The person has enough room and light to move about safely. The person and property are safe from fire and intruders. The person is not afraid and has few worries and concerns.

The person must receive the right care and treatment. Follow the person's care plan. Also practice the safety measures in this chapter.

See *Teamwork and Time Management: A Safe Setting.*

FOCUS ON SURVEYS

Safety

A survey team will observe the agency setting and patient or resident rooms.

- For potential or actual hazards. A *hazard is any thing in the person's setting that could cause injury or illness.* Examples include spills, loose hand rails, unanswered call lights, burnt-out bulbs, unsafe equipment, and other safety issues described in this and other chapters.
- For how staff respond to potential or actual hazards.
- If the care plan was followed on each shift for persons at risk.
- How staff supervise persons at risk.
- If a hazard was changed or removed.
  During staff interviews, a surveyor may ask you:
- About measures in the person's care plan to reduce the risk for an accident.
- When and how you report risks and hazards.
- When and how you correct an immediate hazard. A spill is an example.
- Agency procedures for removing or reducing a hazard.
  Always provide for safety. Know what to do if you find a hazard. Remember to give surveyors complete and honest answers. Surveys protect patients and residents.

TEAMWORK AND TIME MANAGEMENT

A Safe Setting

You can correct some safety hazards. Do so as soon as possible. For example:

- Wipe up spills right away. Do so even if you did not cause the spill.
- A person is sliding out of a wheelchair. Position the person correctly. Do so even if a co-worker is responsible for the person's care.
- A person has problems holding a coffee cup. Offer to help the person.
- Food is unattended in an oven. Turn off the oven. Then tell your co-worker the reason for your action.
  You cannot correct some safety issues. Follow agency policy to report such problems. They include:
- Electrical outlets or switches that do not work or are coming out of the wall
- Water leaks from windows, doors, ceilings, pipes, faucets, tubs, showers, toilets, water heaters, and other sources
- Toilets that do not work properly
- Water from faucets that does not warm up or is very hot
- Broken or damaged windows or furniture
- Windows and doors that do not work properly
- Knobs and handles that are broken or do not work properly
- Hand rails and grab bars that are loose or need repair
- Odd smells, odors, and sounds
- Signs of rodents, flies, ants, or other pests
- Lights and lamps that do not work or have burnt-out bulbs
- Flooring (carpeting, tiles, hardwood flooring) needing repair

ACCIDENT RISK FACTORS

Some people cannot protect themselves. They present dangers to themselves and others. Certain factors increase the risk of accidents and injuries.

- *Age.* Children and older persons are at risk for injuries. See *Focus on Children and Older Persons: Accident Risk Factors (Age).*
- *Awareness of surroundings.* Confused and disoriented persons may not understand what is happening to and around them. A coma can occur from illness or injury. *Coma is a state of being unaware of one's setting and being unable to react or respond to people, places, or things.*
- *Agitated and aggressive behaviors.* Pain can cause these behaviors. So can confusion, decreased awareness of surroundings, and fear of what may happen.
- *Vision loss.* Persons with poor vision can fall or trip over toys, rugs, equipment, furniture, and cords. Some cannot read container labels. Poisoning can result. Taking the wrong drug or the wrong dose can be harmful.
- *Hearing loss.* Persons with hearing loss may not hear warning signals or fire alarms. Some cannot hear approaching meal carts, drug carts, stretchers, or wheelchairs. They do not know to move to a safe place.

- *Impaired smell and touch.* Illness and aging affect smell and touch. The person may not detect smoke or gas odors. Burns are a risk from impaired touch. The person has problems sensing heat and cold. Some people have a decreased sense of pain. They may be unaware of injury. For example, a person does not feel a blister from shoes. Leg and foot circulation is poor. The blister can become a serious wound.
- *Impaired mobility.* Some diseases and injuries affect mobility. Aware of a danger, the person may not be able to move to safety. Some persons cannot walk or propel wheelchairs. Some persons are paralyzed.
  - *Paralysis means loss of muscle function, sensation, or both.*
  - *Paraplegia is paralysis in the legs and lower trunk. (Para means beyond. Plegia means paralysis.)*
  - *Quadriplegia (tetraplegia) is paralysis in the arms, legs, and trunk. (Quad and tetra mean 4. Plegia means paralysis.)*
  - *Hemiplegia is paralysis (plegia) on 1 side (hemi) of the body.*
- *Drugs.* Drug side effects may include loss of balance, drowsiness, and poor coordination. Reduced awareness, confusion, and disorientation may occur. The person may be fearful and uncooperative. Report behavior changes and the person's complaints to the nurse.

IDENTIFYING THE PERSON

Each person has different treatments, therapies, and activity limits. The wrong care can threaten life and health.

The person may receive an identification (ID) bracelet when admitted to the agency (Fig. 13-1). The bracelet has the person's name, ID number, room and bed number, date of birth (DOB), age, and doctor. Other identifying information and numbers are included. A medical record number (MRN)—used to identify the person's medical record—is an example.

FOCUS ON CHILDREN AND OLDER PERSONS

Accident Risk Factors (Age)

Children
Infants are helpless. Young children do not know safety from danger. They explore their settings, put objects in their mouths, and touch and feel new things. Falls, poisoning, choking, burns, and other accidents are risks. Practice the safety measures in Chapter 56 and Appendix D, p. 893.

Older Persons
Changes from aging increase the risk for falls and other injuries. See Chapter 12.

Some persons have dementia. *Dementia is the loss of cognitive and social function caused by changes in the brain* (Chapter 53). *(Cognitive relates to knowledge.)* Memory and the ability to think and reason are affected.

Persons with dementia are confused and disoriented. Awareness of surroundings is reduced. They may not understand what is happening to and around them. Judgment is poor. They no longer know safety from danger. They may access closets, cupboards, or other unsafe and unlocked areas. They may eat or drink cleaning products, drugs, or poisons. Accidents and injuries are great risks.

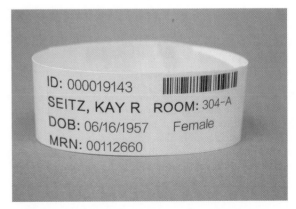

FIGURE 13-1 ID bracelet (ID–identification; DOB–date of birth; MRN–medical record number).

You use the ID bracelet to identify the person before giving care. Your assignment sheet states what care to give. To identify the person:

- Compare identifying information on the assignment sheet with that on the ID bracelet (Fig. 13-2). Carefully check the information. Some people have the same first and last names. For example, John Smith is a very common name.
- Use at least 2 identifiers. Some agencies require the person to state and spell his or her name and give his or her birth date. Others require using the person's ID number. You cannot use the person's room or bed number. Always follow agency policy.
- Call the person by name when checking the ID bracelet. This is a courtesy as you touch the person and before giving care. Just calling the person by name is not enough for identification. Confused, disoriented, drowsy, hard of hearing, or distracted persons may answer to any name.

See *Focus on Communication: Identifying the Person.*

See *Focus on Long-Term Care and Home Care: Identifying the Person.*

See *Promoting Safety and Comfort: Identifying the Person.*

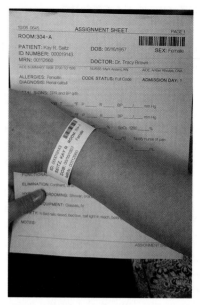

FIGURE 13-2 The ID bracelet is checked against the assignment sheet to accurately identify the person.

FOCUS ON **COMMUNICATION**

Identifying the Person

To identify the person, call the person by name. Ask to see the ID bracelet. For example: "Hello, Mr. Hall. May I see your ID bracelet?" Then ask for 2 identifiers. You can say: "Please tell me your full name and birth date." Compare the identifiers with the information on the ID bracelet and your assignment sheet.

Identifying oneself over and over again can be annoying. The person may say: "Do I have to say it again? You know who I am." Be polite. Explain why you check identity. You can say: "It is important to check so I give care to the right person. It is for your safety." Thank the person. Use his or her title and name. For example: "Thank you, Mr. Hall."

PROMOTING SAFETY AND COMFORT

Identifying the Person

Safety

Always identify the person before giving care. Do not identify the person and then leave the room for supplies and equipment. You could go to the wrong room and give care to the wrong person. The person needing care would not receive it. Harm could result.

Water, spilled food and fluids, and every-day wear and tear can damage ID bracelets. If you cannot read the information on the ID bracelet, tell the nurse. The nurse can have a new bracelet made.

Comfort

ID bracelets must not be too loose or too tight. You should be able to slide 1 or 2 fingers under a bracelet. If too loose or too tight, tell the nurse.

FOCUS ON **LONG-TERM CARE AND HOME CARE**

Identifying the Person

Long-Term Care

Alert and oriented residents may not wear ID bracelets. This is noted on the person's care plan. Follow center policy and the care plan to identify the person.

Some nursing centers have photo ID systems (Fig. 13-3). Taken on admission, the photo becomes part of the person's medical record. If your center uses such a system, learn to use it safely.

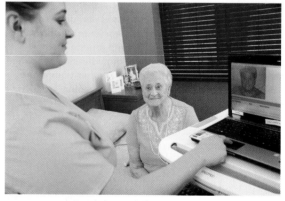

FIGURE 13-3 The nursing assistant uses the photo to identify the person.

PREVENTING BURNS

Burns are a leading cause of death among children and older persons. Smoking, spilled hot liquids, children playing with matches, grills, fireplaces, stoves, electrical items, and very hot water (sinks, tubs, showers) are common causes of burns. Burns from hot water can occur in seconds. The safety measures in Box 13-1 can prevent burns. See Chapter 58 for the emergency care of burns.

See *Focus on Children and Older Persons: Preventing Burns*, p. 162.

BOX 13-1   **Preventing Burns**

Smoke Alarms
- Have working smoke alarms on every level of the home, in each bedroom, and outside each bedroom or sleeping area.
- Test alarms every month.
- Replace batteries when Daylight Savings Time changes in the spring and fall. Use long-life batteries when possible. Replace batteries even if alarms are hard-wired.
- Use alarms with flashing strobe lights for hard of hearing persons.

Children
- Do not leave children home alone.
- Supervise young children at all times.
- Do not leave children alone in the kitchen, bathroom, or a room with a fireplace.
- Secure fireplaces with door guards or heat-resistant gates.
- Install barriers around fireplaces, ovens, and furnaces. Avoid glass screens that can become very hot and take a long time to cool down.
- Store matches, lighters, lamp oils, or other flammable materials in locked cabinets.
- Do not let children near stoves, space heaters, fireplaces, grills, radiators, registers, oil lamps, candles, curling irons, and other heat sources.
- Do not carry or hold a child while cooking.
- Keep space heaters and materials that can catch fire away from children.
- Teach children fire safety and fire prevention measures. Also teach the dangers of fire.
- Check metal playground equipment. Metal surfaces exposed to sunlight can heat to high temperatures. They can burn a child's face, hands, arms, legs, and buttocks.
- Check car seats, seat belts, and seat-belt buckles. If hot, they can burn children.
- Cover car seats with towels if you park in the sun. Also use a sun visor for the windshield.
- Protect children from sun exposure.
  - Use a sunscreen.
  - Cover exposed areas.
  - Limit time in the sun.

Kitchen and Cooking
- Do not let children help you cook.
- Use the back stove burners when cooking.
- Point pot and pan handles inward, toward the back. They point away from where people stand and walk.
- Stay in the kitchen when cooking. Turn off the stove if you have to leave the kitchen.
- Use a timer when baking, roasting, or simmering food. Check the food regularly.
- Do not leave cooking utensils in pots and pans.
- Do not wear long-sleeved or loose-fitting clothes.

Kitchen and Cooking—cont'd
- Keep things that can catch fire away from stoves. Examples include towels and paper towels, oven mitts, pot-holders, food packages, and curtains.
- Do not put wet food into frying pans or deep-fryers. Water causes the oil to splatter.
- Use dry oven mitts and pot-holders. Water conducts heat.
- Stay by the stove, oven, microwave oven, or grill when cooking. Do not leave cooking unattended.
- Open or uncover microwaved foods slowly. Steam can burn your fingers, hands, or face.
- Turn the oven and stove burners off when not in use.

Eating and Drinking
- Assist with eating and drinking as needed. Spilled hot food or liquids can cause burns.
- Be careful when carrying hot foods and liquids.
- Keep hot food and liquids away from counter and table edges. Use the center of the counter or table.
- Do not pour hot liquids near a person.

Water
- Set the water heater temperature no higher than 120°F (Fahrenheit).
- Have anti-scald devices on faucets and shower-heads.
- Turn on cold water first, then hot water. Turn off hot water first, then cold water.
- Measure bath or shower water temperature (Chapter 24). Check it before bathing a baby or before a person gets into the tub or shower.
- Check for "hot spots" in bath water. Move your hand back and forth in the water.

Appliances and Other Electrical Equipment
- See "Preventing Equipment Accidents" (p. 174).
- Do not allow the use of space heaters. If used, they must be at least 3 feet away from items that can burn. Turn off the heater before leaving the room.
- Do not let the person sleep with a heating pad or an electric blanket.
- Turn off and unplug irons, curling irons, electric rollers, and hair dryers when not in use.

Smoking
- Be sure patients and residents smoke only in smoking areas.
- Do not leave smoking materials at the bedside.
- Supervise the smoking of persons who cannot protect themselves.
- Do not allow smoking in bed.
- Do not allow smoking where oxygen is used or stored (Chapter 43).
- Be alert to ashes that may fall onto a person.

Other
- See "Fire Safety" (p. 178).
- Follow safety guidelines when applying heat and cold (Chapter 42).

PREVENTING POISONING

A *poison is any substance harmful to the body when ingested, inhaled, injected, or absorbed through the skin.* If too much is taken, any substance can be poisonous. Poisonings are intentional or unintentional.

- *Unintentional*—the person takes or gives a substance without intending to cause harm. This includes drugs or chemicals in excess amounts—an "over-dose."
- *Intentional*—the person takes (suicide) or gives (assault or homicide) a substance to cause harm.

Poisoning can cause illness, brain damage, coma, and death. Children and older persons are at risk. Drugs and household products are common poisons. Poisoning in adults may be from carelessness, confusion, or poor vision when reading labels. As a result, a person may take too much of a drug or ingest a harmful substance.

Common poisons include:
- Drugs (legal and illegal) and vitamins
- Household products—detergents, soaps, sprays, furniture polish, window cleaners, bleach, paint, paint thinner, toilet bowl and other cleaners, gasoline, kerosene, glue, and so on
- Personal care products—soaps, shampoos, hair conditioners, bath oils, powders, lotions, nail polish removers, sprays, make-up, perfumes, after-shave, deodorants, mouthwashes, and so on
- Fertilizers, insecticides, bug sprays, and so on
- Lead (p. 165)
- House plants
- Wild mushrooms
- Alcohol
- Carbon monoxide (p. 167)

The measures in Box 13-2 can prevent poisoning.

See *Focus on Long-Term Care and Home Care: Preventing Poisoning.*

See *Promoting Safety and Comfort: Preventing Poisoning,* p. 164.

BOX 13-2   Preventing Poisoning

All Ages

- Keep drugs and harmful products in high, locked areas (Fig. 13-4). Children and confused persons cannot see or reach them.
- Use prescription drugs correctly.
  - Only take drugs prescribed by a licensed health care professional.
  - Take drugs as prescribed. Do not take larger or more frequent doses. This is especially important for pain-relief drugs.
  - Do not share or sell drugs.
  - Read and follow all directions and warning labels. Have good lighting.
  - Keep drugs in their original bottles or containers.
- Buy products with child-resistant packaging.
- Keep child-resistant caps on all harmful products.
- Keep harmful products in their original containers. Do not use food containers.
- Leave the original label on harmful products (p. 176).
- Store personal care items according to agency policy. Soap, mouthwash, lotion, deodorant, and shampoo are examples. These items could cause harm when swallowed.
- Use and store harmful products according to the manufacturer's instructions (p. 176).
- Do not sniff chemical containers.
- Read all labels carefully before using the product.
- Do not leave harmful products unattended when in use.
- Do not mix cleaners or other household products together.
- Turn on fans and open windows when using cleaners and other household products.
- Point spray nozzles away from your face and other people.
- Do not store harmful products near food.
- Dispose of out-dated, unwanted, and un-used drugs and products. See *Focus on Long-Term Care and Home Care: Preventing Poisoning.*

All Ages—cont'd

- Use safety latches on kitchen, bathroom, utility, garage, basement, and workshop cabinets and drawers.
- Discard poisonous household plants. Or place them where persons at risk cannot reach them.
- Keep emergency numbers by the phone: Poison Control Center (1-800-222-1222), police, ambulance, hospital, and doctor.
- Prevent carbon monoxide poisoning (p. 167).

Children

- Keep children in your sight when using a harmful product.
- Teach children not to eat plants and unknown foods. Teach them not to eat leaves, stems, seeds, berries, nuts, or bark.
- Do not leave lamp oil or lamps or candles with lamp oil where children can reach them. Lamp oil is harmful if ingested.
- Practice safe drug use.
  - Do not call drugs or vitamins "candy."
  - Do not take drugs in front of children.
  - Do not put a dose on a counter or table where a child can reach it.
  - Do not leave drugs unattended if you need to do something else when taking drugs. Take children with you.
  - Secure child-safety caps on every drug.
  - Put drugs away after taking them. Put them out of the sight and reach of children.
  - Be aware that guests (including family and friends) may bring legal or illegal drugs into your home. Do not let children have access to purses, handbags, briefcases, backpacks, coat pockets, or similar items.
- Place warning stickers ("Mr. Yuk") on harmful substances (Fig. 13-5).
- Supervise children when visiting family and friends. Look for harmful products in and on counters, tables, bathrooms, and other areas and surfaces.
- Prevent lead poisoning (p. 165).

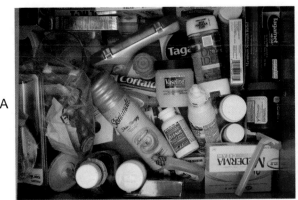 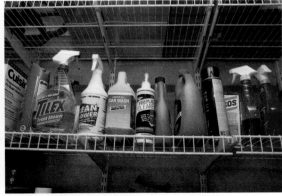

FIGURE 13-4 Harmful products must be kept in locked areas and out of the reach of children and persons who are confused. **A,** Bathroom drawers and cabinets hold many harmful products. **B,** Household cleaners can be harmful.

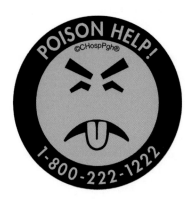

FIGURE 13-5 The "Mr. Yuk" warning sticker is placed on harmful products. (Courtesy Children's Hospital, Pittsburgh Poison Center, Pittsburgh, Pa.).

FOCUS ON **LONG-TERM CARE AND HOME CARE**

Preventing Poisoning

Home Care

Provide good lighting when patients take their drugs. Make sure they read prescription labels correctly and are taking the correct drug and dosage (Chapter 57).

Some products and drugs are out-dated, unwanted, or un-used. The nurse may have you check bathroom medicine cabinets, drawers, and counters for such items. Kitchen and bedrooms are checked too.

For safe disposal, obtain permission from the person and the nurse. Follow agency policy for disposal. For drugs, agency policy may involve 1 of these disposal methods.

- The disposal instructions on the label.
- Take-back programs.
  - National Prescription Drug Take-Back events are hosted by the U.S. Drug Enforcement Administration (DEA). Collection sites are set up in areas across the country.
  - Local law enforcement agencies sponsor take-back programs.

- Local waste management agency disposal options and guidelines.
- Household trash (Fig. 13-6, p. 164).
  1. *Mix* the drugs with an unpalatable substance. *(Palatable* means *taste. Unpalatable* means *to have an unpleasant or disagreeable taste.)* Dirt, cat litter, and coffee grounds are examples. Do not crush tablets or capsules.
  2. *Place* the mixture in a container. A sealed plastic bag is suggested.
  3. *Throw* the container in the household trash.
  4. *Scratch* out all personal information on the prescription label. Make it unreadable. Discard the empty bottle or package into the trash.
- Flushing. The nurse tells you what drugs can be flushed.

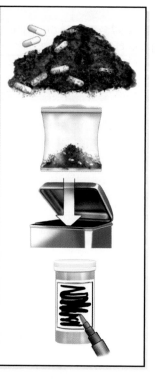

Follow these simple steps to dispose of drugs in the household trash

MIX
Mix drugs (do not crush tablets or capsules) with a bad tasting, unpleasant substance such as dirt, cat litter, or used coffee grounds.

PLACE
Place the mixture in a container such as a sealed plastic bag.

THROW
Throw the container in your household trash.

SCRATCH OUT
Scratch out all personal information on the prescription label of your empty bottle or empty drug packaging to make it unreadable. Then dispose of the container.

FIGURE 13-6 Steps for drug disposal in the household trash. (Redrawn from Food and Drug Administration: *Disposal of unused medicines: what you should know*, Silver Spring, Md.)

PROMOTING SAFETY AND COMFORT

Preventing Poisoning

Safety
Poisoning is an emergency. Some common signs and symptoms of poisoning are:

- Burns or redness around the mouth and lips
- A chemical odor to the breath
- Burns, stains, or odors on the person, on clothing, or around the person
- Empty drug bottles or spilled drugs
- Vomiting
- *Dyspnea*—difficulty *(dys)* breathing *(pnea)*
- Drowsiness
- Confusion
- Seizures (Chapter 58)

If you think a person has had contact with a poison, call the Poison Control Center—1-800-222-1222 or 911. Give the following information.

- Your location, name, phone number, and distance to the nearest hospital
- The person's signs and symptoms, condition (breathing; not breathing), and health problems
- The person's age and weight
- The substance, containers, or bottles involved
- How you think the substance entered the body
  - Swallowed
  - Inhaled or smelled
  - Injected
  - Skin contact
  - Splashed into the eyes

- When you think the substance entered the body
- Emergency care given
- If the person has vomited

During a poisoning emergency, follow the rules in Chapter 58 for basic emergency care. Also follow the directions given by the Poison Control Center. Such directions may include:

- *Poison in the eyes*—rinsing the eyes with running water.
- *Poison on the skin*—removing any clothing in contact with the poison. Rinsing the skin with running water.
- *Inhaled poison*—leaving the area. Get the person to fresh air at once.
- *Swallowed poison*—not having the person try to vomit or not giving the person anything to cause vomiting. Do not give the person anything to eat or drink unless told to do so by the Poison Control Center.

Call 911 to activate the Emergency Medical Services (EMS) system if the person stops responding, stops breathing, or has a seizure. Follow the guidelines for cardiopulmonary resuscitation (CPR) and rescue breathing (Chapter 58). See Chapter 58 for emergency care for seizures.

Lead Poisoning

Lead is a metal. It can be found in all parts of the environment. When in the body, it affects normal body functions. A very strong poison, it can injure the brain, nervous system, red blood cells, kidneys, liver, teeth, and bones. It can lower intelligence and cause learning and behavior problems.

See Box 13-3 (p. 166) for the sources of lead. Lead enters the body through:

- *Inhaling dust.* Windows may have lead-based paint. When windows are opened and closed, dust is created. Dust from soil may contain lead.
- *Ingestion.* Young children can eat, chew, and suck on non-food items containing lead. Toys and lead-painted surfaces—window sills and railings—are examples. They may eat paint chips. Water is a source of lead if plumbing materials contain lead.

Children under 6 years are at risk for lead poisoning. Lead can affect almost every body system. Signs and symptoms are usually gradual in onset. They are not always obvious. See Box 13-3 for signs, symptoms, and safety measures.

See *Caring About Culture: Lead Poisoning.*

See *Focus on Long-Term Care and Home Care: Lead Poisoning.*

✿ CARING ABOUT CULTURE

Lead Poisoning

Lead has been found in some folk medicines (traditional medicines) used by *East Indian, Indian, Middle Eastern, West Asian, Chinese,* and *Hispanic cultures.* Folk medicines may contain herbs, minerals, metals, and animal products. Lead and other metals are thought to help with arthritis, upset stomach, colic, vomiting, diarrhea, constipation, fertility problems, menstrual cramps, and other illnesses. Some are used for teething babies or to calm young children.

Lead can accidentally get into a folk medicine from grinding or coloring or from the package. Lead has been found in powders and tablets used in folk medicine.

Modified from Centers for Disease Control and Prevention: *Childhood lead poisoning prevention,* Atlanta, Ga., page reviewed July 30, 2019.

FOCUS ON **LONG-TERM CARE AND HOME CARE**

Lead Poisoning

Home Care
Dust and Paint

Household dust is a major source of lead. Window sills and window wells may contain high levels of leaded dust. The Centers for Disease Control and Prevention (CDC) recommends cleaning floors, window sills, window wells, and other surfaces every 2 to 3 weeks. The CDC recommends using a wet mop for floors and wet-wiping other surfaces.

The CDC also recommends keeping windows shut to avoid chipping painted surfaces. To open windows, the CDC suggests opening them from the top.

Water

Homes built before 1986 may have lead pipes and fixtures that are corroded—water taps, pipes in the house, pipes from the street to the house. *Corrosion* is when the metal dissolves or wears away from a chemical reaction between the water and plumbing. Lead can enter the water, especially hot water.

High levels of lead in tap water can cause health problems if lead enters the bloodstream. Because of their size, unborn babies, infants, and young children are at greater risk than adults. Infants who drink formula may be at high risk when formula is made with tap water.

Public water utilities can provide information about the amount of lead in water. The CDC also recommends that water be tested for lead. The CDC has steps to follow for using tap water for drinking or cooking when the water is contaminated with lead. The steps are especially important when water has been sitting in pipes for more than 6 hours.

- *When water is contaminated from inside the home:*
  1 Flush the water system. Run water from the tap to be used on *cold* for 1 to 2 minutes.
  2 Fill clean containers with water from the *cold* tap. The water can be used for drinking, cooking, or preparing baby formula.
- *When water is contaminated by pipes from the street:*
  1 Run shower taps on *cold* for 5 minutes or more.
  2 Run the kitchen tap on *cold* for another 1 or 2 minutes.
  3 Fill clean containers with water from the *cold* tap. The water can be used for drinking, cooking, or preparing baby formula.

You can use bottled water for drinking and cooking. Do not use water from the hot tap or boil the water. Hot water contains higher levels of lead than cold water. Boiling water will not reduce lead in the water.

BOX 13-3	Lead Poisoning

Sources of Lead Poisoning

- House paint before 1978. Children can swallow peeling paint and paint chips. When paint is stripped or sanded, lead dust is released into the air.
- Painted and plastic toys and decorations, especially those made outside of the United States.
- Toy jewelry made of lead.
- Candy imported from Mexico (includes candy wrappers).
- Imported candles.
- Lead bullets.
- Fishing sinkers.
- Curtain weights.
- Plumbing, pipes, and faucets. Lead can be found in drinking water if these devices contain lead.
- The soil near highways and houses. The soil may be contaminated with car exhaust and paint scrapings from houses.
- Hobbies that involve soldering, stained glass, making jewelry, pottery, and lead figures.
- Children's paint sets and art supplies.
- Pewter pitchers and dinnerware.
- Storage batteries.

Lead Poisoning in Children: Signs and Symptoms

- Abdominal pain; cramping
- Activity: decreased
- Anemia
- Appetite: poor or loss of
- Attention and learning problems
- Behavior problems; aggressive behavior
- Bowel problems: constipation and diarrhea
- Coma
- Coordination: poor
- Fatigue
- Growth: slowed
- Headaches
- Hearing loss
- Hyperactivity
- Irritability
- Kidney damage
- Language and speech problems
- Memory problems
- Muscle weakness
- *Pallor* (paleness)
- Reflexes: slow
- Seizures
- Sensations: reduced
- Sleep problems
- Sluggishness
- Vomiting
- Walking problems; staggering
- Weight loss

Safety Measures

- Prevent or discourage children from eating, chewing, or sucking on non-food items. They include the lead sources listed in this box.
- Do not let children play in dirt. Have them play in grassy or sandy areas.
- Assist the child with hand-washing before eating, after playing outside, and before going to bed.
- Wash toys often.
- Rinse pacifiers, baby bottles, and other items that fall to the floor.
- Prevent exposure to lead-based plumbing. See *Focus on Long-Term Care and Home Care: Lead Poisoning.*
- Prevent exposure to lead-based paint.
  - Keep children away from paint chips.
  - Keep children away from dust contaminated with lead paint.
  - Do not sweep or vacuum lead-based paint dust or paint chips.
  - Use a wet mop and wet cloths to clean up dust and paint chips.
  - Use a wet mop and wet cloths to clean furniture, window sills, and dusty surfaces.
  - Use duct tape to cover peeling or chipping paint. This is only a temporary measure. Peeling and chipping paint must be removed.
  - Do not bump into walls or furniture that may contain lead-based paint. This prevents dust and paint chips.
  - Do not open and close windows that have lead-based paint. This prevents dust and paint chips.
  - Keep the home as dust-free as possible.
- Prevent exposure to food contaminated with lead.
  - Do not use glazed pottery to cook food.
  - Do not eat foods that are stored or served in glazed pottery.
  - Do not eat foods that are canned outside the United States.
- Do not store wine, alcohol, or vinegar-based salad dressings in lead crystal decanters for long periods. Lead can get into the liquid.
- Prevent children from having contact with work or hobby materials that may contain lead. Welding, pottery, home building and repair, and automotive repair products and supplies are examples. So are children's paint sets and art supplies.
  - Store lead-based products where children cannot see or reach them.
  - Take shoes off before entering the home.
  - Shower and change clothes before contact with children.
  - Wash and store clothes contaminated with lead separately from others.
- Do not let children handle or play with old newspapers, magazines, or comic books. The ink may contain lead.

Carbon Monoxide Poisoning

Carbon monoxide (CO) is a deadly colorless, odorless, and tasteless gas. It is produced by the burning of fuel—gas, oil, kerosene, wood, charcoal (Fig. 13-7). Fuel-burning devices must work properly and be used correctly. Otherwise, dangerous levels of CO can build up in closed or semi-closed areas. Instead of breathing in oxygen, the person breathes in air filled with CO. Red blood cells pick up CO faster than oxygen. Oxygen does not get into the body. CO can quickly or slowly kill. If not fatal, brain and nervous system damage can result.

People and animals are at risk for CO poisoning. Sleeping or intoxicated persons can die before having symptoms. CO poisoning may be unintentional or intentional as a suicide attempt. See Box 13-4 (p. 168) for the signs and symptoms of CO poisoning and safety measures.

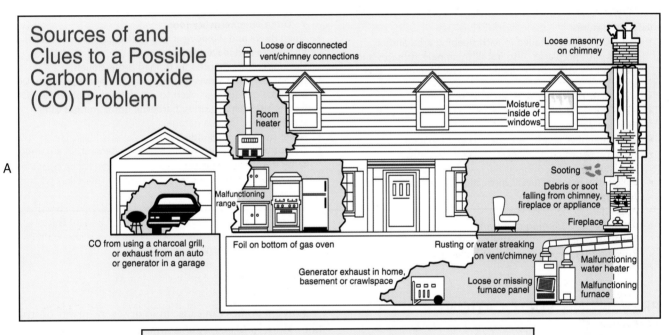

Examples of Carbon Monoxide Sources
- Fireplaces (wood and gas)
- Furnaces
- Gas clothes dryers
- Gas stoves and ovens
- Wood-burning stoves
- Gas water heaters
- Generators (portable)
- Grills and camp stoves used indoors (gas, charcoal)
- Lanterns
- Lawn mowers; weed trimmers
- Snow blowers
- Motor vehicles
- Space heaters (gas, kerosene)

FIGURE 13-7 A, Sources of and clues to possible carbon monoxide problems. **B,** Examples of carbon monoxide sources. (A from U.S. Consumer Product Safety Commission: *The invisible killer*, CPSC-464, Washington, DC.)

BOX 13-4	Carbon Monoxide Poisoning

Signs and Symptoms
- Breathing problems
- Cherry-pink skin
- Chest pain
- Confusion
- Dizziness
- Fainting
- Headache
- Nausea
- Sleepiness
- Slurred speech
- Vomiting
- Weakness

Safety Measures
- Have CO alarms installed in each sleeping area and in rooms with fireplaces. Also install them near furnaces and gas appliances (kitchens, laundry rooms, basements, and so on).
- Have vehicle exhaust systems checked regularly.
- Have the furnace inspected and repaired before every heating season.
- Have chimneys and flues inspected and repaired.
- Have fuel-burning appliances checked regularly.
  See Figure 13-7.
- Follow the manufacturer's instructions when using fuel-burning devices.

Safety Measures—cont'd
- Use the correct fuel for fuel-burning devices.
- Do not idle a vehicle, lawn mower, snow blower, weed trimmer, or other device in an open or closed area or garage. Fumes can leak into the house.
- Have fuel-burning devices, chimneys, and flues checked when people in the same building show signs and symptoms.
- Ventilate the room when using a space heater.
- If you or others have signs and symptoms:
  - Open doors and windows.
  - Turn off appliances.
  - Leave the home.
  - Go to an emergency room.
- Open doors and windows if you notice gas odors. Turn off appliances and leave the home.
- Have gas odors checked by trained professionals.
- Do not use a gas stove or oven to heat a home or room. Do not use a gas stove or oven to dry clothing or other items.
- Do not use charcoal grills, barbecue grills, and gas camp stoves indoors or in a garage.
- Never burn charcoal indoors.
- Do not use a generator indoors, in a basement, in a garage, or by a window, door, or vent.

PREVENTING SUFFOCATION

Suffocation is when breathing stops from the lack of oxygen. The person will die if he or she does not start breathing. Common causes include choking, drowning, inhaling gas or smoke, strangulation, and electrical shock (p. 174).

Measures to prevent suffocation are listed in Box 13-5. Clear the airway if the person is choking.

Choking

A foreign body (food or object) can obstruct (block) the airway. This is called *choking* or *foreign-body airway obstruction (FBAO)*. Air cannot pass through the airways into the lungs. The body does not get enough oxygen. Death can result.

Choking often occurs during eating. A large, poorly chewed piece of meat is a common cause. Laughing and talking while eating also are common causes. So is excessive alcohol intake.

Unconscious persons can choke. Common causes are aspiration of vomitus and the tongue falling back into the airway.

Foreign bodies can cause mild or severe airway obstruction. With *mild airway obstruction*, some air moves in and out of the lungs. The person is conscious and usually can speak. Often forceful coughing can remove the object. Breathing may sound like wheezing between coughs. For mild airway obstruction:
- Stay with the person.
- Encourage the person to keep coughing to expel the object.
- Do not interrupt the person's efforts to clear the airway. If the person is breathing and coughing, abdominal thrusts (p. 170) are not needed.
- If the obstruction persists, call for help.

A person with *severe airway obstruction* has difficulty breathing. Air does not move in and out of the lungs. The person may not be able to breathe, speak, or cough. If able to cough, the cough is of poor quality. When the person tries to inhale (breathe in), there is no noise or a high-pitched noise. The person may appear pale and *cyanotic* (bluish color). Severe airway obstruction is an emergency (p. 170).

See *Focus on Children and Older Persons: Choking*, p. 170.

BOX 13-5	Preventing Suffocation

All Age-Groups

- Cut foods into small, bite-sized pieces for persons who cannot do so themselves.
- Make sure dentures fit properly and are in place.
- Make sure the person can chew and swallow the food served.
- Report loose teeth or dentures.
- Check the care plan for swallowing problems before serving food (including snacks) or fluids. The person may ask for something that he or she cannot swallow.
- Tell the nurse at once if the person has swallowing problems.
- Do not give oral foods or fluids to persons with feeding tubes (Chapter 32).
- Follow aspiration precautions (Chapter 30).
- Do not leave a person unattended in a bathtub or shower.
- Remove the key from a gas fireplace. Store it out of reach.
- Move all persons from the area if you smell smoke.
- Position the person in bed properly (Chapter 18).
- Use bed rails correctly (Chapter 21).
- Use restraints correctly (Chapter 15).
- Prevent entrapment in the bed system (Chapter 21).
- Do not use power strips for care equipment.
- See "Preventing Equipment Accidents," p. 174.

Children

- Practice crib safety measures (Chapter 56 and Appendix D).
- Keep plastic bags away from children. This includes grocery bags, covers, garment bags, and dry-cleaning bags. Tie the bags in knots. Then discard them.
- Electrical safety:
  - Use safety plugs in outlets with caution. Children can remove and choke on them. And they can be misplaced when removed to use the outlet.
  - Keep electrical cords and electrical items out of the reach of children.
  - See "Preventing Equipment Accidents," p. 174.
- Sleep and position safety:
  - Position infants on their backs for sleep. This reduces the risk for sudden infant death syndrome (SIDS) (Chapter 56).
  - Do not use pillows to position infants or to prevent them from falling off of beds and furniture.
  - Remove pillows, loose sheets or blankets, comforters, quilts, sheepskin, stuffed toys, crib bumpers, sleep positioners, and other soft items from the crib when the baby is sleeping.
- Practice safe swaddling. To *swaddle* means *to snugly wrap the baby in a thin blanket or garment for safety and warmth*.
  - Use a sleep sack for warmth. A sleep sack is a wearable blanket.
  - Check that zippers or other fasteners are securely attached.
  - Avoid over-heating. Sweating, damp hair, flushed cheeks, rash, and rapid breathing are signs that the baby is too hot.
  - Stop swaddling if the baby can roll.
- Do not let babies sleep on soft surfaces (beds, sofas, chairs), recliners, bouncy chairs, or swings.
- Do not let children under the age of 6 sleep on a top bunk bed.
- Do not let babies or young children sleep with an adult or older child. Children can be rolled over or be caught between the mattress and wall.

Children—cont'd

- Food safety:
  - Do not feed an infant while he or she is lying down.
  - Do not leave a baby alone when drinking from a bottle. The baby could aspirate milk and choke.
  - Have children sit when they eat. They should not eat or suck on anything while lying down or playing.
  - Do not give infants and young children small, round, or hard foods. This includes hot dogs, nuts or peanuts, peanut butter, popcorn, grapes, raisins, hard candy, jellybeans, cough drops, gum, raw vegetables, raw and unpeeled fruit slices, dried fruits, and chunks of meat.
  - Remove pits, seeds, and small bones from fruits, vegetables, fish, chicken, and so on.
  - Give infants soft foods that do not require chewing.
  - Offer plenty of fluids to children while they are eating.
  - Do not let children play with dried beans or dried peas.
- Balloon safety:
  - Use Mylar balloons instead of latex ones.
  - Store latex balloons where children cannot see or reach them.
  - Do not let children inflate or deflate latex balloons.
  - Deflate and discard latex balloons after use.
  - Pick up and discard broken balloon pieces at once. Do not let children near them.
- Small object and toy safety:
  - Make sure toys are intact. They should not be broken, have cracks or chips, sharp or rough edges, need repair, and so on.
  - Give the child age-appropriate toys.
  - Check floors for small objects—buttons, coins, beads, marbles, pins, tacks, nails, screws, jewelry, and so on. Keep them out of a child's reach. Pick up and store or discard such objects. Children can choke on them. When checking floors, it is best to get on the floor on your hands and knees—the child's eye level.
  - Remove rubber knobs or tips from door stops.
  - Check toys for removable parts.
  - Do not let babies play with small toys or toys with small parts.
- Cord, string, and ribbon safety:
  - Do not string or hang any object on or near a crib. This includes a mobile, toy, or diaper bag. The child can get caught in it and strangle.
  - Never tie pacifiers or teethers around a child's neck.
  - Do not use bibs; clothes with ribbons, ties, or cords; or necklaces whenever the child is put in a crib or playpen.
  - Make sure dangling cords are not within a baby's reach. This includes cords from drapes, shades, and blinds.
- Other:
  - Keep appliance doors closed—ovens, refrigerators, clothes dryers, washing machines, freezers, dishwashers, coolers, and so on.
- See Chapter 56 for other child safety measures.

Older Persons

- Report signs and symptoms of weakness.
- Report signs or symptoms of difficulty swallowing (*dysphagia*).
- Be aware of chronic illnesses.

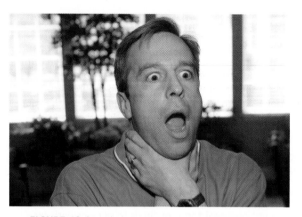

FIGURE 13-8 A choking person clutches at the throat.

Relieving Choking. When choking, the conscious person usually clutches at the throat (Fig. 13-8). Clutching at the throat is often called the *universal sign of choking*. The conscious person is very frightened. If the obstruction is not removed, the person will die.

Abdominal thrusts are used to relieve severe airway obstruction. Abdominal thrusts are quick, upward thrusts to the abdomen. Also known as the *Heimlich maneuver*, the thrusts force air out of the lungs and create an artificial cough. They are done to try to expel the foreign body from the airway.

You may observe a person choking. And you may perform emergency measures to relieve choking. Relief of choking occurs when the foreign body is removed. Or it occurs when you feel air move and see the chest rise and fall when giving rescue breaths (Chapter 58).

If you assist a choking person, report and record what happened. Include what you did and the person's response.

Chest thrusts are used for obese or pregnant persons (Fig. 13-9). If you are alone and choking, perform self-administered abdominal thrusts. See Box 13-6.

See *Focus on Children and Older Persons: Relieving Choking.*

See procedure: *Relieving Choking—Adult or Child (Over 1 Year of Age).*

See procedure: *Relieving Choking—In the Infant (Less Than 1 Year of Age),* p. 173.

Text continued on p. 174.

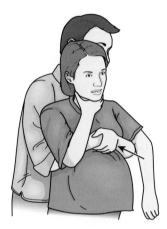

FIGURE 13-9 Chest thrusts to relieve choking in a pregnant woman.

BOX 13-6 Relieving Choking

Chest Thrusts for Obese or Pregnant Persons
1. Stand behind the person.
2. Place your arms under the person's underarms. Wrap your arms around the person's chest.
3. Make a fist. Place the thumb side of the fist on the middle of the sternum (breastbone).
4. Grasp the fist with your other hand.
5. Give chest thrusts until the object is expelled or the person becomes unresponsive.
6. If the person becomes unresponsive, have someone activate the Emergency Medical Services (EMS) system or the agency's Rapid Response System (RRS) if not already done. An RRS is a team that quickly responds to give care in life-threatening situations. Start cardiopulmonary resuscitation (CPR). See Chapter 58.

Self-Administered Abdominal Thrusts
1. Make a fist with 1 hand.
2. Place the thumb side of the fist above your navel and below the lower end of the sternum.
3. Grasp your fist with your other hand.
4. Press inward and upward quickly.
5. Press the upper abdomen against a hard surface if the thrust did not relieve the obstruction. Use the back of a chair, a table, or a railing.
6. Use as many thrusts as needed.

FOCUS ON CHILDREN AND OLDER PERSONS

Relieving Choking

Children

Respiratory infections can cause airway obstruction in infants and children. Airway structures become swollen. The airway narrows or becomes completely blocked. Air cannot enter the airway. The child needs emergency care at once.

The procedures that follow will not relieve airway obstruction caused by an infection. Do not try them if the child has a fever, rash, congestion, hoarseness, or other signs and symptoms of respiratory infection. You will waste precious time. Activate the EMS system or the agency's RRS. Give rescue breaths if the child is not breathing but has a pulse. Start CPR if the child is not responding, not breathing or not breathing normally (gasping), and has no pulse. See Chapter 58.

Abdominal thrusts are not given to infants. They can damage the liver and other organs. Back slaps (back blows) and chest thrusts are used for infants.

Guidelines for emergency care are updated as new information becomes available. You are responsible for following current guidelines. Updates can be found on-line at the American Heart Association's website.

Relieving Choking—Adult or Child (Over 1 Year of Age)

PROCEDURE

1 Ask the person if he or she is choking.
   a *If the person can cough or talk,* see p. 168 for mild airway obstruction.
   b *If the person is unresponsive,* you may not know the cause. Call for help and begin CPR. See Chapter 58.
   c *If the person nods "yes" and cannot talk,* continue to step 2.
2 Have someone call for help.
   a *In a public area,* have someone call 911 to activate the EMS system. Send someone to get an automated external defibrillator (AED) (Chapter 58).
   b *In an agency,* have someone call the agency's RRS and get a defibrillator (AED).
3 Give abdominal thrusts (Figs. 13-10 and 13-11, p. 172).
   a Stand or kneel behind the person.
   b Wrap your arms around the person's waist.
   c Make a fist with 1 hand.
   d Place the thumb side of the fist against the abdomen. The fist is slightly above the navel in the middle of the abdomen and well below the end of the sternum (breastbone). See Figure 13-10, *A.*
   e Grasp your fist with your other hand (see Fig. 13-10, *B*).
   f Press your fist into the abdomen with a quick, upward thrust (see Fig. 13-11).
   g Repeat thrusts until the object is expelled or the person becomes unresponsive.
4 *If the object is dislodged,* encourage hospital care. Injuries can occur from abdominal thrusts.

5 *If the person becomes unresponsive:*
   a Lower the person to the floor. Position the person supine (lying flat on the back).
   b Make sure the EMS or RRS was called.
      1) *If alone with a phone,* call while giving care.
      2) *If alone without a phone,* give about 2 minutes of CPR first. Then call the EMS or RRS and get an AED.
   c Start CPR. See Chapter 58. Do not check for a pulse.
      1) Give 30 chest compressions.
      2) Open the airway with the head tilt–chin lift method (Fig. 13-12, p. 172). Open wide the person's mouth. Look for an object. Remove the object if you can see it and can remove it easily.
      3) Give 2 breaths.
      4) Continue cycles of 30 compressions followed by 2 breaths. Look for an object every time you open the airway.
   d *If choking is relieved,* check for a response, breathing, and a pulse. (NOTE: Choking is relieved when you feel air move and see the chest rise and fall when giving breaths.)
      1) *If no response, no normal breathing, and no pulse*—continue CPR. Use the AED as soon as possible (Chapter 58).
      2) *If no response and no normal breathing but there is a pulse*—give rescue breaths. For an adult, give 1 breath every 5 to 6 seconds. For a child, give 1 breath every 3 to 5 seconds. Check for a pulse about every 2 minutes. If no pulse, begin CPR.
      3) *If the person has normal breathing and a pulse*—place the person in the recovery position if there is no response (Chapter 58). Continue to check the person until help arrives. Encourage hospital care.

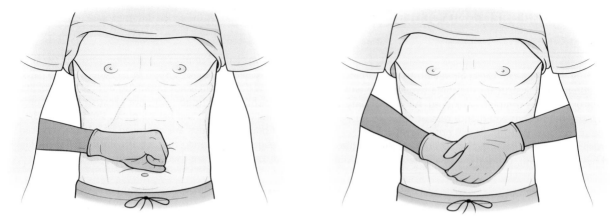

FIGURE 13-10 Hand positioning for abdominal thrusts. **A,** The fist is slightly above the navel in the mid-line of the abdomen. **B,** The other hand clasps the fist.

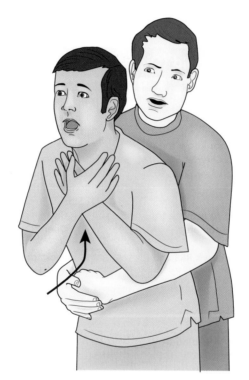

FIGURE 13-11 Abdominal thrusts with the person standing.

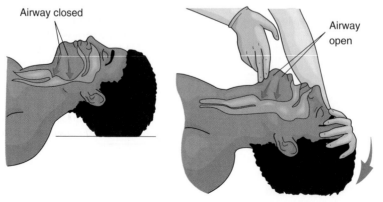

FIGURE 13-12 The head tilt–chin lift method opens the airway. One hand is on the person's forehead. Pressure is applied to tilt the head back. The chin is lifted with the fingers of the other hand.

Guidelines for emergency care are updated as new information becomes available. You are responsible for following current guidelines. Updates can be found on-line at the American Heart Association's website.

Relieving Choking—In the Infant (Less Than 1 Year of Age)
PROCEDURE

1 Have someone call for help.
   a *In a public area,* have someone call 911 to activate the EMS system. Send someone to get an AED. See Chapter 58.
   b *In an agency,* have someone call the agency's RRS and get a defibrillator (AED).
2 Kneel next to the infant. Or sit with the infant in your lap.
3 Expose the infant's chest and back. Perform this step only if it can be done easily.
4 Hold the infant face down over your forearm. (Support your arm on your thigh or lap.) The infant's head is lower than the chest. Support the head and jaw with your hand.
5 Give up to 5 forceful back slaps (back blows) (Fig. 13-13). Use the heel of your hand. Give the back slaps between the shoulder blades. (Stop the back slaps if the object is expelled.)
6 Turn the infant as a unit.
   a Continue to support the infant's face, jaw, head, neck, and chest with 1 hand.
   b Support the back and the back of the infant's head with your other hand. Your palm supports the back of the head.
   c Turn the infant as a unit. The infant is in a back-lying position on your forearm. Your forearm rests on your thigh. The infant's head is lower than the chest.
7 Give up to 5 chest thrusts (Fig. 13-14). The chest thrusts are quick and downward.
   a Place 2 fingers in the center of the chest just below the nipple line.
   b Give chest thrusts at a rate of about 1 every second.
   c Stop chest thrusts if the object is expelled.

8 Continue giving 5 back slaps followed by 5 chest thrusts until the object is expelled or the infant becomes unresponsive.
9 *If the infant becomes unresponsive:*
   a Send someone to activate the EMS system or RRS if not already done (step 1). If alone, do the following.
      1) *If alone with a phone,* call while giving care.
      2) *If alone without a phone,* give about 2 minutes of CPR first. Then call the EMS or RRS and get an AED.
   b Place the infant on a firm, flat surface.
   c Start CPR (Chapter 58). Do not check for a pulse. Give 30 chest compressions. (See Chapter 58 for infant CPR.)
   d Open the airway. Use the head tilt–chin lift method. Open the infant's mouth. Look for an object. Remove the object if you see it and can remove it easily. Use your fingers.
   e Give 2 breaths.
   f Continue cycles of 30 compressions followed by 2 breaths. Look for an object. Use your fingers to remove it if you see it and can remove it easily.
   g Continue CPR until help takes over or until choking is relieved.

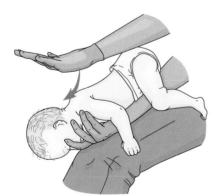

FIGURE 13-13 Back slaps (back blows). The infant is held face down and supported with 1 hand. The rescuer's forearm is supported on his or her thigh. Back slaps are given between the shoulder blades with the heel of 1 hand.

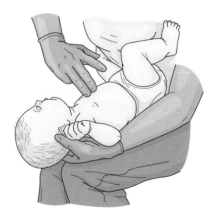

FIGURE 13-14 Chest thrusts. The infant is in the back-lying position. The rescuer uses 2 fingers to compress the center of the chest just below the nipple line.

PREVENTING EQUIPMENT ACCIDENTS

All equipment is unsafe if broken, not used correctly, not working properly, or in need of repair. This includes hospital beds. Inspect all equipment before use. Check all items for cracks, chips, and sharp or rough edges. They can cause cuts, stabs, or scratches. Follow the Bloodborne Pathogen Standard (Chapter 16).

Electrical Equipment

Frayed cords (Fig. 13-15, *A*) and over-loaded electrical outlets (Fig. 13-15, *B*) can cause fires, burns, and electrical shocks. *Electrical shock is when electrical current passes through the body.* It can burn the skin, muscles, nerves, and other tissues. It can affect the heart and cause death.

Three-pronged plugs (Fig. 13-16) are used on all electrical items. Two prongs carry electrical current. The third prong is the ground. A *ground carries leaking electricity to the earth and away from an electrical item.* Without a ground, leaking electricity can be conducted to the person. It can cause electrical shocks and possible death. If you receive a shock, report it at once. Do not use the item.

Warning signs of a faulty electrical item include:

* Shocks
* Loss of power or a power surge
* Dimming or flickering lights
* Sparks
* Sizzling or buzzing sounds
* Burning odor
* Loose plugs

Practice the safety measures in Box 13-7. Complete an incident report (p. 187) for an equipment-related accident. The *Safe Medical Devices Act* requires that agencies report equipment-related illnesses, injuries, and deaths.

Bariatric-Safe Equipment

Beds, chairs, wheelchairs, stretchers, toilets, commodes, and other equipment usually have a weight capacity of 250 to 350 pounds. Bariatric patients and residents can weigh from 250 pounds to over 1000 pounds. Bariatric equipment is labeled:

* BARIATRIC
* "EC" for "expanded capacity"
* With the weight limit suggested by the manufacturer

Do not use the item if the person's weight is greater than the weight capacity. Follow the nurse's directions and the care plan.

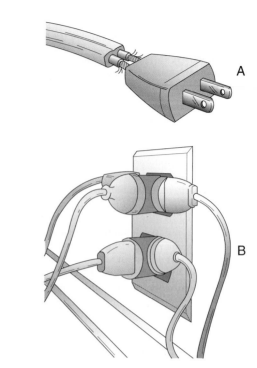

FIGURE 13-15 A, A frayed electrical cord. **B,** An over-loaded electrical outlet.

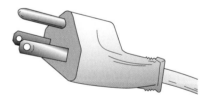

FIGURE 13-16 A 3-pronged plug.

BOX 13-7	Preventing Equipment Accidents

General Safety

- Follow agency policies and procedures.
- Follow the manufacturer's instructions. Use equipment correctly.
- Read all caution and warning labels.
- Do not use an unfamiliar item. Ask for training. Also ask a nurse to supervise you the first time you use the item.
- Use an item only for its intended purpose.
- Make sure the item works before you begin.
- Have all needed equipment before you begin. For example, you need an outlet to plug in an item.
- Do not use or give damaged items to patients or residents.
- Show a broken or damaged item to the nurse. Follow the nurse's instructions and agency policies for discarding items or sending them for repair.
- Do not try to repair broken or damaged items.
- Do not use broken or damaged items.

Electrical Safety

- Check cords and equipment for damage. Make sure they are in good repair.
- Use 3-pronged plugs on all electrical devices (see Fig. 13-16). Make sure all prongs are intact.
- Avoid using extension cords. If you need one, use it for only 1 device. This prevents over-loading a circuit.
- Do not use power strips for care equipment.
- Do not cover or run any cord under rugs, carpets, linens, or other materials.
- Connect a bed power cord directly to a wall outlet. Do not connect a bed power cord to an extension cord or power strip.
- Do not use the person's electrical items until they are safety checked. The maintenance staff does this.

Electrical Safety—cont'd

- Keep electrical items away from water.
- Keep work areas clean and dry. Wipe up spills right away.
- Do not touch electrical items if you are wet, if your hands are wet, if you are in water (tub, pool), or if you are standing in water. This includes using a phone when it is plugged into a charger.
- Do not put a finger or any item into an outlet.
- Use tamper-resistant outlets. If necessary, use outlet safety covers or plates over standard electrical outlets (Fig. 13-17, *A*). Use safety plugs with caution (Fig. 13-17, *B*). Children can remove and choke on outlet plugs or stick their fingers or small objects into outlet openings. Use power strip covers for power strips and attached cords.
- Turn off equipment before unplugging it. Sparks occur when electrical items are unplugged while turned on.
- Hold on to the plug (not the cord) when removing it from an outlet (Fig. 13-18).
- Do not give showers or tub baths during storms. Lightning can travel through pipes.
- Do not use electrical items or phones during storms.
- Do not use water to put out an electrical fire. If possible, turn off or unplug the item. Call 911 at once.
- Do not touch a person who is having an electrical shock. If possible, turn off or unplug the item. Call 911 or the RRS.
- Keep electrical cords away from heating vents and other heat sources.
- Turn off the device when done using the item.
- Unplug all devices when not in use.

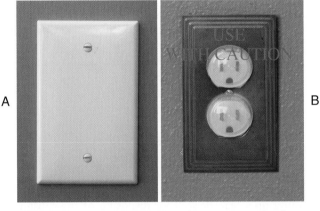

FIGURE 13-17 Outlet safety. **A,** Outlet safety cover. **B,** Outlet plugs. Use plugs with caution.

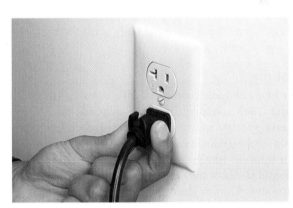

FIGURE 13-18 Hold on to the plug to remove it from the outlet.

Wheelchair and Stretcher Safety

Wheelchairs are useful for people who cannot walk or who have severe problems walking. Stretchers are used to transport persons who cannot sit up or must lie down. Stretchers are used in hospitals and by emergency medical personnel.

The person can fall from the wheelchair or stretcher. Or the person can fall during transfers to and from the wheelchair or stretcher. See Chapter 20 for wheelchair and stretcher safety.

HAZARDOUS CHEMICALS

A *hazardous chemical is any chemical that is a physical hazard or a health hazard. Physical hazards* can cause fires or explosions. *Health hazards* can cause health problems. Health hazards can:

- Cause cancer.
- Affect blood cell formation and function.
- Damage the kidneys, nervous system, lungs, skin, eyes, or mucous membranes.
- Cause birth defects, miscarriages, and fertility problems.

Exposure to hazardous chemicals can occur from equipment failures, container ruptures, or the release of a hazard into the workplace. Workplace hazards include:

- Latex gloves (Chapter 17)
- Thermometers and blood pressure equipment containing mercury (Chapter 33)
- Cleaners and disinfectants (Chapter 16)

The *Hazard Communication Standard (HCS)* is a policy of the Occupational Safety and Health Administration (OSHA). It requires container labeling (Fig. 13-19), safety data sheets (SDSs), and employee training. The standard also requires eyewash and total body wash stations where hazardous chemicals are used.

Labeling

Hazardous chemical containers have warning labels. The warning labels contain *pictograms*—symbols used to communicate specific information about a chemical hazard. See Figure 13-19 for examples.

If a warning label is removed or damaged, do not use the chemical. Show the container to the nurse and explain the problem. Do not leave the container unattended.

Health Hazard	Flame
• Carcinogen • Mutagenicity • Reproductive Toxicity • Respiratory Sensitizer • Target Organ Toxicity • Aspiration Toxicity	• Flammables • Pyrophorics • Self-Heating • Emits Flammable Gas • Self-Reactives • Organic Peroxides
Exclamation Mark	**Gas Cylinder**
• Irritant (skin and eye) • Skin Sensitizer • Acute Toxicity • Narcotic Effects • Respiratory Tract Irritant • Hazardous to Ozone Layer (Non-Mandatory)	• Gases Under Pressure
Flame Over Circle	**Skull and Crossbones**
• Oxidizers	• Acute Toxicity (fatal or toxic)

FIGURE 13-19 Some pictograms from the Occupational Safety and Health Administration. Depending on the chemical, the warning label contains the necessary pictograms and associated hazards. (Redrawn from OSHA Quick Card™, OSHA® Occupational Safety and Health Administration, U.S. Department of Labor, Washington, D.C.)

Safety Data Sheets

Every hazardous chemical has an SDS (material safety data sheet [MSDS] in some agencies). Information provided includes:

- Name and common names
- Hazards about the chemical
- Chemical ingredients
- Emergency measures
- Fire-fighting measures
- Accidental release measures
- Safe handling and storage measures
- Personal protection measures

Check the SDS before using a hazardous chemical, cleaning up a leak or spill, or disposing of the substance. Call for the nurse about a leak or spill right away. Do not leave a leak or spill unattended.

Employee Training

Your employer provides hazardous chemical training. You learn about hazards, exposure risks, and protection measures. You learn to read and use warning labels and the SDS.

Each hazardous chemical requires certain protection measures. See the safety measures in Box 13-8.

BOX 13-8	Hazardous Chemical Safety Measures

- Read and follow the safety measures on the warning label and SDS.
- Make sure each container has an undamaged warning label.
- Use a leak-proof container to carry or transport a hazardous chemical.
- Wear personal protective equipment (PPE) to clean up spills and leaks. Follow the warning label or SDS for what to wear (mask, gown, gloves, eye protection, safety boots).
- Clean up spills at once. Work from clean areas to dirty areas with circular motions.
- Dispose of hazardous chemicals in sealed bags or containers.
- Stand behind a lead shield during x-ray or radiation therapy procedures. Follow agency procedures to prevent radiation exposure.
- Do not enter a room while a person is having x-rays or radiation therapy.
- Wash your hands after handling hazardous chemicals.
- Work in well-ventilated areas to avoid inhaling gases.
- Use cleaning products safely.
  - Read and follow warnings and label directions.
  - Keep products in their original containers.
  - Make sure the area is well-ventilated.
  - Do not mix products. Mixing products can cause dangerous gases. For example, do not mix ammonia and bleach.
  - Close containers properly.
  - Put cleaning products away after use.
  - Do not store cleaning products near food.
  - Empty buckets, pails, basins, and other containers with cleaning solutions.
  - Do not use an empty container for other purposes or things.
- Dispose of or store a hazardous chemical according to the SDS.

FOCUS ON LONG-TERM CARE AND HOME CARE

Disasters

Home Care

A severe storm may occur when you are in a patient's home. For safety:

- Stay informed through local TV and radio stations. Satellite services may not have a signal with heavy storm clouds.
- Keep a flashlight with you for power outages.
- Move the patient, family, and yourself to a "safe room."
  - Basement
  - Room on the ground floor
  - Interior room away from outside walls, windows, and doors
  - Center hallway
  - Bathroom
  - Closet

FOCUS ON **SURVEYS**

Disasters

There may be unannounced disaster drills during a survey. They are done to test staff efficiency, knowledge, and response for a disaster.

A surveyor may ask you:

- About fire safety. See "Fire Safety" on p. 178. This includes:
  - What to do if a fire alarm goes off.
  - What to do if you find a fire in a person's room.
  - Where to find fire alarms and fire extinguishers.
  - How to use a fire extinguisher.
- What to do if a patient or resident is missing. See "Elopement" on p. 182.

DISASTERS

A *disaster* is a sudden, catastrophic event. People are injured and killed. Property is destroyed. Natural disasters include tornadoes, hurricanes, blizzards, earthquakes, volcano eruptions, floods, and some fires. Human-made disasters include auto, bus, train, and airplane accidents. They also include fires, bombings, power plant accidents, gas or chemical leaks, explosions, and wars.

Communities, fire and police departments, and health care agencies have disaster plans (emergency preparedness plans). They include caring for people needing treatment. The plan generally provides for:

- Discharging persons who can go home
- Assigning staff and equipment to an emergency area
- Assigning staff to transport persons from treatment areas
- Calling off-duty staff to work
- Evacuation procedures if the agency is damaged
  See *Focus on Long-Term Care and Home Care: Disasters.*
  See *Focus on Surveys: Disasters.*

Bomb Threats

Follow agency procedures for a bomb threat or if you find an item that looks or sounds strange. Bomb threats can be sent by phone, mail, e-mail, text message, messenger, or other means. Or the person can leave a bomb in the agency. If you see a stranger or strange item or package in the agency, tell the nurse at once. You cannot be too safe.

Fire Safety

Faulty electrical equipment and wiring, over-loaded electrical circuits, and smoking are major causes of fires. The health team must prevent fires and act quickly during a fire. See Box 13-9. Also see "Preventing Burns" (p. 161), "Preventing Equipment Accidents" (p. 174), and "Fire and Oxygen" (p. 180).

See *Focus on Long-Term Care and Home Care: Fire Safety.*

BOX 13-9	**Fire Prevention Measures**

- Follow the safety measures:
  - For oxygen use (p. 180)
  - To prevent equipment accidents (p. 174)
  - To prevent burns (p. 161)
- Practice smoking and ashtray safety.
  - Supervise persons who smoke. This is very important for persons who are confused, disoriented, or sedated.
  - Provide ashtrays for persons who are allowed to smoke. Deep, wide, and sturdy ashtrays on a sturdy table are best.
  - Keep ashtrays away from anything that can burn.
  - Empty ashtrays only when sure that all ashes, cigars, cigarettes, electronic cigarettes, and other smoking materials are out.
  - Empty ashtrays into a metal container partially filled with sand or water. Do not empty ashtrays into plastic containers or wastebaskets lined with paper or plastic bags.
  - Smoke only where allowed to do so. Do not smoke in patients' homes.
- Keep smoking materials, matches, lighters, candles, incense, flammable liquids and materials, and other fire sources away from children and confused or disoriented persons.
- Light matches carefully.
  - Be alert for sparks when lighting a match. Sparks can start a fire.
  - Keep your hair, clothing, and anything that will burn away from the match and flame.
- Do not leave cooking unattended on stoves, in ovens, in microwave ovens, or on grills.

- Practice safety measures for candles.
  - Do not use candles in bedrooms or other sleeping areas.
  - Use sturdy candle holders that will not tip over.
  - Place candle holders on sturdy, clutter-free surfaces.
  - Light candles carefully. Keep your hair and loose clothing away from the flame.
  - Do not burn a candle all the way down. Blow it out before it gets close to the holder.
  - Do not use candles where oxygen is used.
  - Keep candles at least 12 inches away from anything that can burn. This includes window coverings.
  - Blow out candles when you leave the room or go to bed.
  - Do not use candles during power outages. Use flashlights and battery-operated lighting.
  - Keep candles and incense away from flammable liquids and materials.
- Store flammable liquids outside in their original containers. Keep containers where children and confused or disoriented persons cannot reach them.
- Keep materials that will burn away from heat sources. Stacked newspapers, magazines, books, and paint rags are examples. Heat sources include space heaters, fireplaces, radiators, registers, candles, incense, and oil lamps.
- Do not smoke or light matches or lighters around flammable liquids or materials.
- Use clothes dryers safely.
  - Clean the lint filter before and after each use.
  - Use the correct plug and outlet.
  - Turn the dryer off when you leave the home.
  - Do not run dryers when people are sleeping.
- Follow the safety measures in this box when using incense.

FOCUS ON LONG-TERM CARE AND HOME CARE

Fire Safety

Home Care

According to the National Fire Protection Association (NFPA):

- Unattended cooking is the leading cause of kitchen fires.
- Most kitchen fires involve the stove.
- The risk of dying in a home fire caused by smoking materials increases with age.
- Smoking materials are the major cause of fires, injuries, and death when oxygen is used.
- The victim who dies in a fire may not be the one whose cigarette started the fire.
- Furniture fabrics, clothing, bedding, and hair can easily ignite from a spark or flame.
- Home candle fires occur most often in December.
- Many candle fires start in bedrooms.
- Most candle fires start when things are too close to a candle.
- A closed door may slow the spread of smoke, heat, or a fire.
- Many fire deaths happen in homes with no smoke alarms or alarms that do not work.
- Electric space heaters are leading causes of space heater fires.
- Many fires result because children can reach matches and lighters. All children are at risk for the unsafe use of fire.
- More than 2,500 people die each year in home fires.

Fire and the Use of Oxygen

Home care patients may need oxygen therapy. Remind the patient, family, and visitors about safety measures. See Chapter 43.

Smoke Alarms

Smoke alarms save lives, prevent injuries, and lessen property damage. Always locate them in a patient's home. They should be outside every sleeping area, in every bedroom, and on every floor. Make sure they are working. Tell the nurse, patient, and family if a smoke alarm does not work.

Special smoke alarms are available for persons who are deaf or hard of hearing. The following examples activate when a special smoke alarm sounds.

- Strobe lights that flash
- A pillow or bed shaker
- An alert device that has a loud, mixed, low-pitched sound

Preventing Fires

Cooking equipment is the leading cause of home fires. Practice safety measures to prevent burns (p. 161).

Space heaters present fire hazards. Electric and fuel-burning heaters are common. Practice these safety measures.

- Follow the manufacturer's instructions. Use the correct fuel.
- Light a gas space heater correctly.
  - Strike the match first.
  - Then turn on the gas.
- Do not use extension cords with space heaters.
- Keep heaters at least 3 feet away from any person and from window coverings, furniture, and anything that will burn.
- Place heaters on a solid, flat surface. Do not place heaters on stairs, in doorways, or where people walk.

Preventing Fires—cont'd

- Make sure the heater can automatically shut off if it tips over.
- Protect yourself and others from burns. Heaters are hot. Do not touch them. Keep them away from children and persons who cannot protect themselves.
- Prevent electrocution (being injured or killed by electrical shock). Keep electric heaters away from water. (Water conducts electricity.) Make sure the cord is in good repair.
- Do not leave heaters unattended. Turn off and unplug heaters before leaving the room or going to bed.
- Store fuel in the original container. Keep the fuel container outside.
- Refill the fuel container outside.
- Do not add fuel while the heater is running or hot. Do not over-fill the heater.

Hoarding

Hoarding is a disorder in which a person has difficulty discarding or getting rid of things. The person has a great need to save the items that might have little or no value. The home or living space becomes filled with stacks or piles of clutter. Often there are only narrow pathways from 1 room to another. Doors may be blocked.

The NFPA explains why hoarding increases danger for the person, others in the home, and firefighters.

- Items that can burn are close to the stove or oven.
- A heat source may be too close to things that can burn.
- Heat sources may be on unstable surfaces.
- Electrical wiring may be old or worn from heavy piles. Pests and rodents can chew on wires.
- Flames from smoking materials or candles may be close to clutter.
- Narrow and blocked pathways and doors may prevent escaping from a fire.
- Firefighters have difficulty moving through a home with clutter.
- Blocked windows and doors may trap firefighters.
- Falling objects can injure firefighters.
- The building can collapse on firefighters. Water to fight the fire increases the weight of the clutter.
- Clutter can block the way for firefighters to search for people and pets.

Fire Exits

Know 2 exits from each room and 2 exits from the building. Keep exits clear. Keep furniture and heavy items away from doors and windows. Doors and windows should open easily.

If a fire occurs, get the patient, family, and yourself out as fast as possible. Do not use elevators. In an apartment building, alert others to the fire. Use the fire alarm system and yell "FIRE" in the hallways. Manual fire alarms are usually near exits. Pull the bar or handle. Call 911 or the fire department when out of the building. Do not go back into the building.

Using a Fire Extinguisher

Locate fire extinguishers in the patient's home. Read the manufacturer's instructions. Make sure the device works. Tell the nurse, patient, and family if a fire extinguisher does not work.

Fire and Oxygen. Three things are needed for a fire.
- A spark or flame
- A material that will burn
- Oxygen

Air has some oxygen. However, some people need extra oxygen (Chapter 43). Safety measures are needed where oxygen is used and stored.
- NO SMOKING signs are on the door and near the bed.
- No one can smoke in the room.
- Smoking materials (cigarettes, electronic cigarettes, cigars, and pipes), matches, and lighters are removed from the room.
- Safety measures to prevent equipment accidents are followed (see Box 13-7).
- Wool blankets and synthetic fabrics that cause static electricity are removed from the room.
- The person wears a cotton gown or pajamas.
- Lit candles, incense, and other open flames are not allowed.
- Materials that ignite easily are removed from the room. They include oil, grease, nail polish remover, and so on.

Agencies have no-smoking policies and smoke-free areas. No smoking is allowed inside the buildings. Signs are posted on all entry doors. Some people ignore such rules. Remind them about the no-smoking rules.

See *Focus on Communication: Fire and Oxygen.*

FOCUS ON COMMUNICATION

Fire and Oxygen

You may have to remind a patient, resident, or visitor not to smoke inside the agency. You can simply say:
- "This is a smoke-free area. Here is an ashtray to put out your cigarette. I can show you the smoking area outside."
- "Please don't smoke inside the center. We have a smoking area outside the back entrance on hallway 2. I can show you the way."

Tell the nurse what happened and what you said and did. The nurse may need to speak with the person about not smoking.

What To Do During a Fire. Know your agency's fire emergency and evacuation procedures. Know where to find fire alarms, fire extinguishers, and emergency exits. Fire drills are held to practice emergency fire procedures. Remember the word *RACE* (Fig. 13-20).
- *R*—for *rescue.* Rescue persons in immediate danger. Move them to a safe place.
- *A*—for *alarm.* Sound the nearest fire alarm. Call 911 or the operator.
- *C*—for *confine.* Close doors and windows to confine the fire. Turn off oxygen or electrical items used in the general area of the fire.
- *E*—for *extinguish.* Use a fire extinguisher on a small fire that has not spread to a larger area.

Clear equipment from all normal and emergency exits. *Do not use elevators if there is a fire.*

See *Promoting Safety and Comfort: What To Do During a Fire.*

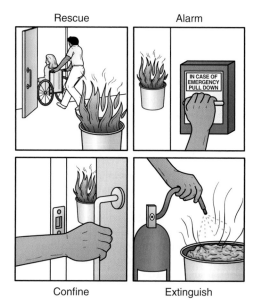

FIGURE 13-20 During a fire, remember *RACE: Rescue, Alarm, Confine, Extinguish.*

PROMOTING SAFETY AND COMFORT

What To Do During a Fire

Safety

Touch doors before opening them. Do not open a hot door. Use another exit from the room or building. If your clothing is on fire, do not run. Drop to the floor or ground. Cover your face. Roll to smother flames. If another person's clothing is on fire, get the person to the floor or ground. Roll the person or cover the person with a blanket, bedspread, or coat to smother the flames.

For smoke, cover your nose and mouth with a damp cloth. Do the same for patients, residents, visitors, and other staff. Have everyone crawl to the nearest exit.

Do the following if you cannot exit the building because of flames or smoke.
- Call 911 or the fire department. Tell the operator where you are. Give exact information: agency name and address or the home care patient's name, address, phone number, and where you are in the building or home.
- Cover your nose and mouth with a damp cloth. Do the same for patients, residents, visitors, and other staff.
- Move away from the fire. Go to a room with a window. Close the room door. Stuff wet towels, blankets, sheets, or bedspreads at the bottom of the door.
- Open the window.
- Hang something from the window (towel, sheet, blanket, clothing). This helps firefighters find you.

Using a Fire Extinguisher. Different extinguishers are used for different kinds of fires.

- Oil and grease fires
- Electrical fires
- Paper and wood fires

A general procedure for using a fire extinguisher follows. See procedure: *Using a Fire Extinguisher.*

Using a Fire Extinguisher

PROCEDURE

1 Pull the fire alarm.
2 Get the nearest fire extinguisher.
3 Carry it upright.
4 Take it to the fire.

5 Follow the word *PASS.*
  a P—for *pull the safety pin* (Fig. 13-21, *A*). This unlocks the handle.
  b A—for *aim low* (Fig. 13-21, *B*). Direct the hose or nozzle at the base of the fire. Do not try to spray the tops of the flames.
  c S—for *squeeze the lever* (Fig. 13-21, *C*). Squeeze or push down on the lever, handle, or button to start the stream. Release the lever, handle, or button to stop the stream.
  d S—for *sweep back and forth* (Fig. 13-21, *D*). Sweep the stream back and forth (side to side) at the base of the fire.

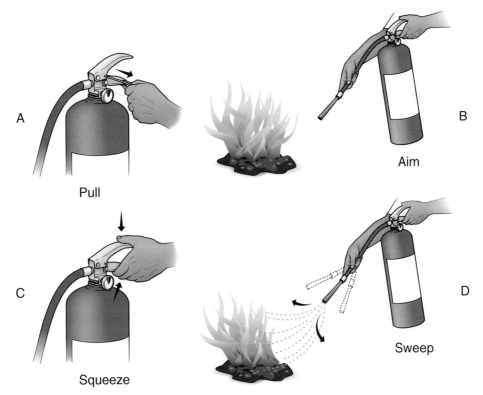

A
Pull

Aim
B

C
Squeeze

Sweep
D

FIGURE 13-21 Using a fire extinguisher. **A,** *Pull* the safety pin. **B,** *Aim* the hose at the base of the fire. **C,** *Squeeze* the top handle down. **D,** *Sweep* back and forth.

Evacuating. Agencies have evacuation procedures. Patients and residents closest to the fire go out first. Those who can walk are given blankets to wrap around themselves. A staff member takes them to a safe place. Figures 13-22 and 13-23 show how to rescue persons who cannot walk. Once firefighters arrive, they direct rescue efforts.

Elopement

The Centers for Medicare & Medicaid Services (CMS) requires that an agency's emergency preparedness plan address elopement. *Elopement is when a patient or resident leaves the agency without staff knowledge.* The person who leaves a safe setting is at risk for many dangers. Heat or cold exposure, dehydration, drowning, and being struck by a vehicle are examples.

The agency must:
- Identify persons at risk for elopement.
- Monitor and supervise persons at risk.
- Address elopement in the person's care plan.
- Have a plan to find a missing patient or resident.

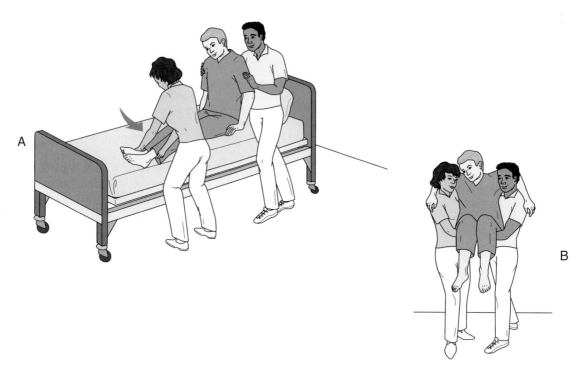

FIGURE 13-22 Swing-carry technique. **A,** Assist the person to a sitting position. A co-worker grasps the person's ankles as you both turn the person so he sits on the side of the bed. **B,** Pull the person's arm over your shoulder. With 1 arm, reach across the person's back to your co-worker's shoulder. Reach under the person's knees and grasp your co-worker's arm. Your co-worker does the same.

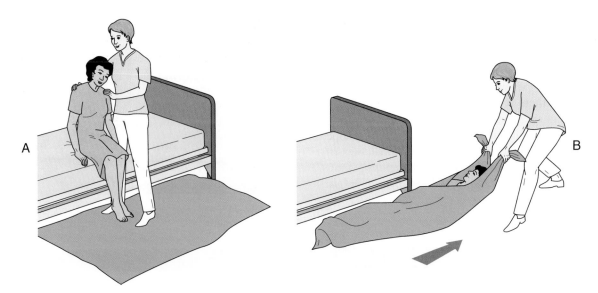

FIGURE 13-23 One-rescuer carry. **A,** Spread a blanket on the floor. Make sure the blanket will extend beyond the person's head. Assist the person to sit on the side of the bed. Grasp the person under the arms and cross your hands over her chest. Lower the person to the floor by sliding her down 1 of your legs. **B,** Wrap the blanket around the person. Grasp the blanket over the head area. Pull the person to a safe area.

WORKPLACE VIOLENCE

Workplace violence is violent acts (including assault or threat of assault) directed toward persons at work or while on duty. It includes:
- Murders
- Beatings, stabbings, and shootings
- Rapes and sexual assaults
- Use of weapons—firearms, bombs, knives, and so on
- Kidnapping
- Robbery
- Threats—obscene phone calls; threatening oral, written, or body language; and harassment of any nature (being followed, sworn at, or shouted at)
- Terrorism

Violence can occur anywhere in a health care setting. Common settings are mental health units, emergency rooms, waiting rooms, and nursing centers. The nursing team is at risk. Staff have the most contact with patients, residents, and visitors.

In the *Guidelines for Preventing Workplace Violence for Healthcare and Social Service Workers,* OSHA has identified these risk factors.
- Working with persons who have a history of violence, who abuse drugs or alcohol, are gang members, or are related to patients and residents
- Transporting patients and residents
- Working alone in an agency or a person's home
- Working in a setting where a staff member cannot see or escape from danger or a violent situation
- Poorly lit hallways, rooms, parking lots, and other areas
- Lacking a way to communicate an emergency situation
- Patients and residents and their families and friends have firearms, knives, and other weapons
- Working in areas with high crime rates
- Lacking policies and training to recognize and manage hostile and assaultive behaviors from patients, residents, visitors, and staff
- Low staff levels during meal times and visiting hours
- High staff turn-over rates
- Not enough security and mental health staff
- Long waits for patients or residents
- Over-crowded and uncomfortable waiting rooms
- Visitors being able to go anywhere in the agency
- A sense that violence is tolerated and that victims cannot contact the police or press charges

OSHA has guidelines for preventing workplace violence. Work-site hazards are identified. Prevention measures are followed. Also, staff receive safety and health training. You need to:
- Follow your agency's workplace violence prevention programs.
- Follow safety and security measures.
- Voice safety and security concerns.
- Report suspicious persons right away.
- Report violent incidents promptly and accurately.
- Serve on committees that review workplace violence.
- Attend training programs to recognize and manage agitation, assaultive behavior, and criminal intent.

Box 13-10 has some safety measures to prevent or control workplace violence. Box 13-11 lists personal safety practices. Follow them all the time. Complete an incident report for workplace violence.

Restraints may be ordered if persons are a threat to themselves or others (Chapter 15). Persons with mental health disorders are supervised as they move about in the agency. Aggressive and agitated persons are treated in open areas. Privacy and confidentiality are maintained. Security officers deal with agitated, aggressive, or disruptive persons.

See *Focus on Long-Term Care and Home Care: Workplace Violence*, p. 186.

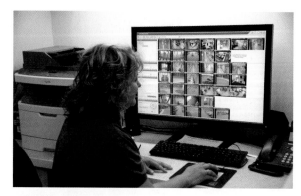

FIGURE 13-24 People entering and leaving the agency are monitored on a closed-circuit TV.

BOX 13-10 Workplace Violence—Safety Measures

Agitated or Aggressive Persons
- Stand away from the person. Judge the length of the person's arms and legs. Stand far enough away that the person cannot hit or kick you.
- Stand close to the door. Do not become trapped in the room.
- Identify items in the room that can be used as weapons. Move away from such objects. Vases, phones, radios, music players, letter openers, paper weights, and belts are examples.
- Know where to find and how to use panic buttons, call lights, alarms, closed-circuit monitors, pagers, personal alarms, and other security devices.
- Keep your hands free.
- Stay calm. Talk to the person in a calm manner. Do not raise your voice or argue, scold, or interrupt the person.
- Be aware of your body language. Do not point a finger or glare at the person. Do not put your hands on your hips.
- Do not touch the person.
- Tell the person that you will get the nurse to speak to him or her.
- Leave the room as soon as you can. Make sure the person is safe.
- Tell the nurse and security officer about the matter at once. Report items in the room that can be used as weapons.

Safety Devices
- Alarm systems, paging systems, closed-circuit video monitors (inside and outside), panic buttons, hand-held alarms, phones, 2-way radios, and phone systems are installed (Fig. 13-24). These systems have a direct line to security staff or the police.
- Staff wear personal alarm devices.
- Metal detectors are at entrances to identify guns, knives, or other weapons.
- Curved mirrors are in hallways and hard-to-see areas.
- Bullet-resistant, shatter-proof glass is at nurses' stations.
- Doors have glass panels.
- Door alarms remain on.
- Staff do not share security codes with anyone.

Weapons
- Jewelry and scarves are not worn. They can be used as weapons. For example, a person can grab earrings and bracelets. Or a person can strangle someone with a necklace or scarf.
- Long hair is worn up and off the collar (Chapter 6). A person can pull long hair and cause head injuries.
- Keys, scissors, pens, or other items that can serve as weapons are not visible.

Weapons—cont'd
- Pictures, vases, and other items that can serve as weapons are few in number.
- Tools or items left by maintenance staff or visitors are removed if they can serve as weapons.

Family and Visitors
- Visitors sign in and receive a pass to access patient and resident areas.
- Visiting hours and policies are enforced.
- A list of "restricted visitors" is made for patients and residents with a history of violence or who are victims of violence.
- Waiting rooms and lounges are comfortable and reduce stress.
- Family and visitors are informed in a timely manner.

Building Safety and Security
- Un-used doors are locked.
- Bright lights are inside and outside buildings.
- Broken lights, windows, and door locks are replaced or repaired.
- Staff restrooms lock and prevent access to visitors.
- Access to the pharmacy and drug storage areas is controlled.
- Furniture is placed for a clear exit route. This includes furniture in patient and resident rooms and in therapy areas, dining rooms, and lounges.
- Furniture and other items are secured so they cannot be used as weapons.
- Keys are always attended and secure.

Staff Safety Measures
- Staff receive an update about a person's violent history or an incident.
- Staff are not alone when caring for persons with agitated or aggressive behaviors.
- Staff wear ID badges that prove employment. IDs do not have last names or addresses.
- Staff use a "buddy system" when using elevators, stairways, restrooms, and low traffic areas.
- Uniforms fit well. Tight uniforms limit running. An attacker can grab loose uniforms.
- Shoes have good soles. Shoes that cause slipping limit running.
- Staff do not wear expensive jewelry or carry large sums of money.
- Vehicles are locked and in good repair.
- Security escort services are used for walking to vehicles, bus stops, or train stations.
- Staff have a "safe room" for emergencies.

BOX 13-11	Personal Safety

General Measures

- Know the area where you are going. Ask questions about the area.
- Make a "dry run" of the area. Know the way in advance. The shortest way is not always the safest.
- Let someone know where you are at all times. Tell someone when you leave and when you arrive at your destination. If you do not call when expected, the person knows something is wrong.
- Make it known that you do not carry drugs, needles, or syringes.
- Do not wear expensive jewelry or carry large amounts of money or valuables. Leave them at home. If someone wants what you have, give it. The only thing of value is you.
- Carry wallets, purses, and backpacks safely.
  - Men—Carry wallets in an inside coat pocket or side pant pocket. Never carry wallets in the rear pocket.
  - Women—Keep a firm grip on a purse. Keep it close to your body. A purse that zips closed is best.
  - Backpacks—Keep the backpack zipped and secure with a padlock.
- Do not display money or other targets of theft. Phones and other hand-held electronic devices are examples.
- Keep your phone in your hand but not visible to others. Clutch it in your closed hand.
- Keep your phone charged.
- Carry a whistle or shriek alarm.
- Avoid ATMs (automated teller machines) at night.
- Be careful when getting on elevators and when entering stairways.
- Do not approach a stranger or someone acting in a strange way. Report the matter at once.

Home Settings

- Keep doors and windows to the home locked at all times. This includes doors into the garage or the door from the garage into the house.
- Do not open doors to strangers. Ask for identification.
- Do not let a stranger into the home to use a phone or bathroom. Offer to call the police if the person needs help.
- Do not give personal information to callers or people at the door.

Car Safety

- Have plenty of gas in your car.
- Keep your car in good working order.
- Keep these in your car—local map, flashlight with working batteries, flares, a fire extinguisher, first aid kit.
- Raise the hood and use the flares if the car breaks down. Stay in the car. Call the police if you have a phone. If someone stops by to help, ask the person to call the police.
- Lock your car. Sometimes you may want to leave it unlocked. If you need to get in the car fast, you do not want to fumble with keys. Use your judgment. Do not leave anything in the car if you leave it unlocked.
- Have your car key ready so you can get into the car quickly. Do not fumble for keys on the way to or at the car.
- Check under the car as you approach it. A person hiding under the car can grab your ankle or leg. Leave at once if someone is under the car. The person under the car may be working with someone who is waiting to attack you while you are being held or injured at the leg or ankle.

Car Safety—cont'd

- Check the back seat before getting into the car. Make sure no one is in the car. Leave at once if someone is in the car.
- Lock car doors when you get in the car. Keep windows rolled up.
- Do not open the car door or window to talk to a person approaching your car.
- Do not get out of the car to remove something from the windshield.
- Keep purses, backpacks, and other valuables under the seat or near your side. Do not leave them on the seat. They are easy targets for smash-and-grab robbers.
- Do not hitchhike or pick up hitchhikers.
- Practice safety at a gas pump.
  - Take your wallet or purse with you to the pump. If you must keep your wallet, purse, or backpack in the car, keep all windows up and lock all doors. Keep your wallet, purse, and belongings out-of-sight. Called "sliders" by police, thieves can open the car door (or reach in a window) away from where you are standing and grab purses and other valuables.
  - Keep the car key in your hand. Newer cars with "smart keys" only need to sense that the key is in the car. The car can simply be started with a foot on the brake and pushing the "start" button.
  - Protect children in the car. Lock all doors and keep the door closest to you open.

Parking Your Car

- Check for places to park. Choose a well-lit area. In a parking garage, park near entrances, exits, and on the lower level. Try to get close to the attendant if possible. The closest space to your destination is not always the safest for parking.
- Park so you can leave quickly and easily. Park at street corners so no one can park in front of you. In parking lots, back in. You see more from the front windshield than from the back window.

Walking

- Do not wear headphones or earbuds. You cannot hear cars, buses, trains, and people around you.
- Use well-lit and busy streets. Avoid vacant lots, alleys, wooded areas, and construction sites. The shortest way is not always the safest.
- Walk near the curb. Stay away from doorways, shrubs, and bushes.
- Carry a phone. Know your location, and keep phone calls simple.
- Switch directions or cross the street if you think someone is following you. If the person follows you, move quickly to an open store, restaurant, or other public place. Ask for help. If nearby, go to a police or fire station.

Public Transportation

- Carry money for bus, train, or taxi fares. Have money in your pocket to avoid fumbling with a purse or wallet.
- Stand with others and near the ticket booth.
- Sit near the driver or conductor.
- Keep your phone in your hand.

Continued

BOX 13-11   Personal Safety—cont'd

If You Are Threatened or Attacked

- Scream as loud and as long as you can. Keep screaming. Men and women should scream.
- Yell "FIRE," not "help." Most people will respond to "FIRE."
- Use your car keys or house key as a weapon. Hold them in your strong hand. Have 1 key extended (Fig. 13-25). Hold the key firmly. If you are attacked, go for the person's face. Slash the person's face with the key. Do not use poking motions. Do not try for a certain target because you might miss.

If You Are Threatened or Attacked—cont'd

- Remember, you have 2 arms, 2 hands, 2 feet, and 2 knees. You can attack from more than 1 direction at once. Do not be shy—your attacker will not be. Push, pull, yank, and so on. You can attack a man's or woman's genitals.
- Use your thumbs as weapons. Go for the eyes and push hard.
- Carry a travel size can of aerosol hair spray. Go for the face.

FOCUS ON LONG-TERM CARE AND HOME CARE

Workplace Violence

Home Care

More measures are needed for home safety.

- Follow log-in and log-out procedures. Contact the agency when you arrive at the home, when you are leaving, and when you arrive at your next destination (another patient's home, the agency, your own home, or other destination).
- Have tracking applications on your phone and car.
- Know how to use the agency's paging system and a personal panic button.
- Keep your phone with you and on.
- Know at least 2 exit routes out of the home.
- Make sure the device you carry for supplies and equipment has a working lock.
- Always keep doors locked.
- Do not let strangers into the home or building.
- Do not give information over the phone (Chapter 8).
- Do not let any stranger know that you are with a child or an older, ill, or disabled person.

Child abuse, elder abuse, intimate partner violence, and workplace violence can occur in home settings. If you feel uncomfortable or threatened, tell the nurse. Give as much information as you can. Failing to report the matter does not help you or the patient. Follow agency policy for what to do if you are threatened or feel threatened. You may need to leave the home, ask for back-up help from the agency, or call the police.

The following can threaten your safety. Report these and other threats to the nurse.

- Sexual abuse or harassment by the patient or any person in the home—husband, wife, sister, brother, boyfriend, girlfriend, son, daughter, family, friends. See Chapter 5.
- Hitting, kicking, slapping, spitting, biting, scratching, pinching, pushing, or other attacks by the patient or anyone in the home.
- Attacks or threatened attacks with a weapon—knife, gun, bat, rope, tool (hammer, screwdriver, and so on), razor, scissors, spray, pot, pan, cane, chair, and so on.
- Denial of meal breaks, water, bathroom use, toilet paper, or hand-washing facilities.
- Denial of adequate sleeping conditions for a live-in situation.
- Poor heating or ventilation.
- Name calling, obscene language, or racial or cultural slurs.
- Exposure to unsafe conditions—blocked fire escapes, broken stairways, hoarding, pest infestations, and so on.

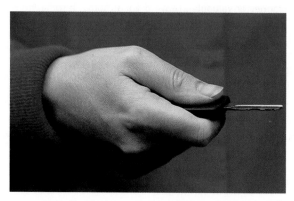

FIGURE 13-25 A key can be used as a weapon.

RISK MANAGEMENT

Risk management involves identifying and controlling risks and safety hazards affecting the agency. The intent is to:

- Protect all in the agency—patients, residents, visitors, and staff.
- Protect agency property from harm or danger.
- Protect the person's valuables.
- Prevent accidents and injuries.

Risk management deals with these and other safety issues.

- Accident and fire prevention
- Negligence and malpractice
- Abuse
- Workplace violence
- Federal and state requirements

Risk managers look for patterns and trends in incidents, complaints (patients, residents, staff, visitors), and accident and injury investigations. Unsafe situations are corrected. Procedure and training changes are made as needed.

Color-Coded Wristbands

Color-coded wristbands promote the person's safety and prevent harm. They quickly communicate an alert or warning (Fig. 13-26). The type of alert is printed on the band. The printing is useful in dim lighting and for persons who are color blind. These colors are common.

- Red—for an "allergy alert." Red is a warning to "stop." A red wristband warns of allergies to food, drugs, treatment supplies such as tape or latex gloves, dust, plants, grass, and so on. Allergies are not listed on the wristband.
- Yellow—for a "fall risk." Yellow implies "caution." Yellow wristbands are used for persons with a history of falls. Or they are used for persons at risk for falls because of dizziness, balance problems, confusion, and so on.
- Purple—for a "Do Not Resuscitate" (DNR) order. See Chapter 59.

Some agencies have colors for other alerts. For example, pink is for a "limb alert." This means that an arm or leg is not used for blood pressure measurements, blood draws, or intravenous infusions. To safely use color-coded wristbands:

- Know the colors used in your agency. Colors may vary among agencies.
- Check the care plan and your assignment sheet when you see a color-coded wristband. You need to know the reason for the wristband and the care measures needed. Ask the nurse if you have questions.
- Do not confuse "social cause" bands with your agency's color-coded wristbands. "Live Strong" is an example.
- Check for wristbands on persons transferred from another agency. That agency may use different colors. Or the meanings may differ from those in your agency. The nurse needs to remove wristbands from another agency.
- Tell the nurse if you think a person needs a color-coded wristband.

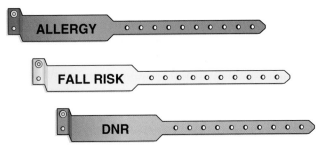

FIGURE 13-26 Color-coded wristbands. The alert is printed on the band.

Personal Belongings

The person's belongings must be kept safe. Often they are sent home with the family. A personal belongings list is completed. Each item is listed and described. The staff member and the person sign the completed list.

A valuables envelope is used for jewelry and money. Each jewelry item is listed and described on the envelope. Describe what you see. For example, describe a ring as having a white stone with 4 prongs in a yellow setting. Do not assume the stone is a diamond in a gold setting. For valuables:

- Count money with the person.
- Put money and each jewelry item in the envelope. Have the person watch. Seal and sign the envelope like a personal belongings list.
- Give the envelope to the nurse. Have a witness. The nurse takes it to the safe or sends it home with the family.

Dentures, eyeglasses, hearing aids, watches, some jewelry, radios and music players, computers, and other electronic devices are kept at the bedside. Items kept at the bedside are listed in the person's record. Some people keep money for newspapers and personal items. The amount kept is noted in the person's record.

See *Focus on Long-Term Care and Home Care: Personal Belongings.*

Reporting Incidents

An *incident is any event that has harmed or could harm a patient, resident, visitor, or staff member.* This includes:

- Accidents involving patients, residents, visitors, or staff.
- Errors in care—giving the wrong care, giving care to the wrong person, not giving care.
- Broken or lost items owned by the person. Dentures, hearing aids, and eyeglasses are examples.
- Lost money or clothing.
- Hazardous chemical incidents.
- Workplace violence incidents.

Report accidents and errors at once. Complete an *incident report* as soon as possible. Incident reports are reviewed by a risk management committee. The committee looks for patterns and trends in accidents or errors. For example, are falls occurring on the same shift and on the same unit? Are lost or missing items reported on the same shift or same unit? Are residents injured on the same shift or same unit? There may be new policies and procedures to prevent future incidents.

FOCUS ON LONG-TERM CARE AND HOME CARE

Personal Belongings

Long-Term Care

Clothing and shoes are labeled with the person's name. So are other items brought from home. Follow center procedures to label items.

FOCUS ON **PRIDE**

The Person, Family, and Yourself

P ersonal and Professional Responsibility

Always do your best to give safe care. When errors or accidents happen, take responsibility. Be accountable. Complete an incident report. Incident reports are used to improve systems and promote safety. Take pride in doing the right thing by honest reporting.

R ights and Respect

Respect for others' well-being affects your actions. If you value the person's safety, you will perform safety measures. For example, you will:

- Identify the person before giving care.
- Cut food into small pieces.
- Observe for swallowing problems and signs of choking.
- Use equipment correctly.
- Know what to do during a fire or disaster.
- Report concerns and incidents.

I ndependence and Social Interaction

Children and older persons are at increased risk for injury. Children often try to show independence before they are able to judge safety. Older persons often cannot do things they used to do. To promote safety:

- Know who you need to protect.
- Practice safety measures to prevent accidents and injuries.
- Respect the desire of older persons to maintain independence. Let them do as much as they safely can. Kindly communicate safety limits.

D elegation and Teamwork

Personal safety practices protect you and co-workers. Work as a team for the safety of all staff arriving and leaving the agency.

- Wait for a person finishing work a few minutes late.
- Walk with others to and from the parking area.
- Walk in well-lit areas at night.
- Do not leave the parking area until your co-workers are safely in their vehicles. Have them do the same for you.
- Offer to call security escort services for a co-worker going to a different location. For example, a person is walking to a bus stop.

E thics and Laws

Persons with developmental and intellectual disabilities (Chapter 54), young children, and older persons are at risk for choking. The following case shows what can occur when safety measures are neglected.

A 32-year-old man had an intellectual disability and epilepsy (a seizure disorder). He was a patient at a developmental center since the age of 25.

According to the facts reported in the court case, the following occurred.

- *He had a dinner of braised beef and noodles. The pieces of beef were about ½ inch wide and ¾ inch long.*
- *While eating, he stood up, coughed out his milk, reached for his throat, and collapsed.*
- *Efforts were made to revive him.*
- *He was transported to the hospital where he died a short while later.*

The lawsuit claimed negligence because:

- *His swallowing was affected by the dosage of a drug.*
- *He was not given a soft diet.*
- *He was not properly supervised at meal time.*

In the Court's opinion, negligent care resulted in the patient's death.

(B. Szydelko v The Department of Mental Health of the State of Illinois, 1984.)

You can help prevent choking. Know who is at risk. Ask the nurse or check the care plan. Monitor those persons closely. Check that they have the right diet. See Chapter 30 for more precautions.

FOCUS ON **PRIDE**: *Application*

As a student or new nursing assistant, it is normal to have fears of causing harm. What concerns do you have? How will you overcome your fears?

REVIEW QUESTIONS

Circle the BEST answer.

1 Safety measures are meant to prevent accidents and injuries while
  a Protecting rights
  b Limiting mobility
  c Limiting independence
  d Saving staff time

2 Which is *safe?*
  a Not wearing needed eyeglasses
  b Hearing problems
  c Memory problems
  d Oriented to person, time, and place

3 A person in a coma
  a Has suffered an electrical shock
  b Has dementia
  c Is unaware of surroundings
  d Has stopped breathing

4 A person with dementia
  a Has problems with thinking and reasoning
  b Is not aware of his or her surroundings
  c Is paralyzed
  d Has suffered an electrical shock

5 A person with quadriplegia is paralyzed
  a From the waist down
  b From the neck down
  c On the right side of the body
  d On the left side of the body

6 To identify a person, you
  a Call the person by name
  b Ask the person his or her name
  c Compare information on the ID bracelet against your assignment sheet
  d Ask both roommates their names

7 To prevent burns
  a Keep smoking materials at the person's bedside
  b Pour hot liquids near a person
  c Turn on hot water first
  d Check water temperature before the person enters the shower

8 Which prevents poisoning?
  a Keeping harmful products in low storage areas
  b Keeping harmful products in their original containers
  c Removing product labels
  d Storing harmful products near food

9 Which signals a poison?
  a The "Mr. Yuk" sticker
  b OSHA
  c RACE
  d PASS

10 Who is most at risk for lead poisoning?
  a An adult who works in health care
  b A teenager who plays paintball
  c A toddler who lives in a house built in 1970
  d An older woman who knits as a hobby

11 A home has lead-based plumbing. You should
  a Use hot tap water for cooking and drinking
  b Use hot tap water to make baby formula
  c Let cold water run for 1 to 2 minutes before using it for cooking
  d Be alert for signs of carbon monoxide poisoning

12 Which can cause suffocation?
  a Checking for loose teeth or dentures
  b Using electrical items that are in good repair
  c Cutting food into small, bite-sized pieces
  d Using restraints

13 The most common cause of choking in adults is
  a A loose denture
  b Meat
  c Marbles
  d Candy

14 If severe airway obstruction occurs, the person usually
  a Clutches at the throat
  b Can speak, cough, and breathe
  c Is calm
  d Has a seizure

15 These statements are about FBAO. Which is *true?*
  a A person is coughing forcefully. Give abdominal thrusts.
  b A person is pregnant. Give abdominal thrusts.
  c Injuries can occur from abdominal or chest thrusts.
  d Unconscious persons cannot choke.

16 Before using a new resident's electric shaver
  a Fill the sink with water
  b The maintenance staff must check the device
  c Check the SDS
  d Get an extension cord

17 You are using electrical equipment. Which measure is *unsafe?*
  a Following the manufacturer's instructions
  b Keeping electrical items away from water and spills
  c Pulling on the cord to remove a plug from an outlet
  d Turning off electrical items after using them

18 Which is *unsafe?*
  a A chair's weight capacity exceeds the person's weight.
  b A person's weight exceeds a wheelchair's weight capacity.
  c A person who cannot walk uses a wheelchair.
  d A person who cannot sit up is transported by stretcher.

19 You spilled a hazardous chemical. You should
  a Follow the instructions on the safety data sheet
  b Cover the spill and go tell the nurse
  c Wipe up the spill with paper towels
  d Leave the spill for housekeeping

20 The fire alarm sounds. Which action is *correct?*
  a Leave oxygen on.
  b Use elevators.
  c Open doors and windows.
  d Move residents to a safe place.

Continued

REVIEW QUESTIONS—cont'd

21 Your clothing is on fire. What should you do *first*?
   a Run to get help.
   b Call 911.
   c Use a fire extinguisher.
   d Drop to the floor and roll to smother the flames.

22 You work in a nursing center. In a severe weather alert, you should
   a Take cover
   b Follow the center's emergency preparedness plan
   c Make sure your family is safe
   d Pull the fire alarm

23 A person is agitated and aggressive. Which is *unsafe*?
   a Standing away from the person
   b Standing close to the door
   c Using touch to show you care
   d Talking to the person without raising your voice

24 Risk managers
   a Look for patterns or trends in accidents and errors
   b Prevent legal problems when injuries occur
   c Are only responsible for staff safety
   d Are the same as surveyors

25 You see a color-coded wristband. You should
   a Read the wristband for special instructions or care measures
   b Ask the person what it means
   c Check your assignment sheet and the person's care plan
   d Remove the wristband when the risk is no longer present

26 You work the night shift. Which is *safe*?
   a Parking in a dimly-lit area
   b Walking to your car alone
   c Finding your keys after getting to the car
   d Checking under the car and in your back seat

27 A resident brought a computer from home. To prevent property loss
   a Send the item home with the family
   b Label the item with the person's name
   c Put the item in a safe
   d Use a wheelchair pouch for the item

28 You gave a person the wrong treatment. Which is *true*?
   a Report the error at the end of the shift.
   b Take action only if the person was injured.
   c You are guilty of negligence.
   d You must complete an incident report.

Answers to Chapter 13 questions are on p. 885.

FOCUS ON **PRACTICE**
Problem Solving

A person begins to cough loudly during a meal. The person can speak a few words. You hear wheezing between breaths. What do you do? The person is suddenly unable to cough, speak, or breathe. What do you do?

Preventing Falls

OBJECTIVES

- Define the key terms and key abbreviations in this chapter.
- Identify the causes and risk factors for falls.
- Describe the safety measures that prevent falls.
- Explain how to use bed and chair alarms safely.
- Explain how to use bed rails safely.
- Explain the purpose of hand rails and grab bars.

- Explain how to use wheel locks safely.
- Describe how to use transfer/gait belts.
- Explain how to help the person who is falling.
- Perform the procedures described in this chapter.
- Explain how to promote PRIDE in the person, the family, and yourself.

KEY TERMS

bed rail A device that serves as a guard or barrier along the side of the bed; side rail
gait belt See "transfer belt"

position change alarm Any physical or electronic device that monitors a person's movement and alerts staff of movement
transfer belt A device applied around the waist and used to support a person who is unsteady or disabled; gait belt

KEY ABBREVIATIONS

CDC Centers for Disease Control and Prevention
CMS Centers for Medicare & Medicaid Services

ID Identification

The risk of falling increases with age. Persons older than 65 years are at risk. A history of falls increases the risk of falling again. Falls are the most common accidents in nursing centers.

According to the Centers for Disease Control and Prevention (CDC):

- Each year, over ¼ of adults age 65 and older fall.
- Falls are the main cause of injuries and injury-related deaths in older adults.
- Falls can cause serious injuries. Head injuries and fractures of the wrist, arm, ankle, and hip are examples.
- Fear of falling affects quality of life. The person may limit daily and social activities. Depression, feelings of helplessness, and social isolation can result. Less active, the person becomes weaker with an increased risk of falling.

See *Focus on Surveys: Preventing Falls*.

FOCUS ON **SURVEYS**

Preventing Falls

The Centers for Medicare & Medicaid Services (CMS) defines a *fall* as:

- Unintentionally coming to rest on the ground, floor, or other lower level. Force, such as being pushed, was not involved.
- When a person loses balance and would have fallen if staff did not act to prevent the fall.
- When a person is found on the floor unless matters suggest otherwise.
- When a person falls but is not injured. A fall without injury is still a fall.
  The survey team will observe and interview staff about:
- Fall risk factors described in this chapter.
- The hazards described in this chapter and in Chapter 13.
- Safety measures to prevent falls.
- The safe use of bed rails, hand rails and grab bars, and wheel locks.
- The safe use of adaptive (assistive) devices. Canes, walkers, and transfer/gait belts (p. 198) are examples.
- Safe transfer (Chapter 20) and ambulation (Chapter 34) procedures.
- Answering call lights promptly.
- Following the person's care plan and meeting care needs.

CAUSES AND RISK FACTORS FOR FALLS

Most falls are caused by many risk factors. The more risk factors present, the greater the risk of falling. The accident risk factors described in Chapter 13 can lead to falls. The problems listed in Box 14-1 increase a person's risk of falling.

See *Focus on Long-Term Care and Home Care: Causes and Risk Factors for Falls.*

See *Teamwork and Time Management: Causes and Risk Factors for Falls.*

BOX 14-1	Fall Risk Factors

Care Setting
- Bed height: too low or too high
- Care equipment: IV (intravenous) poles, drainage tubes and bags, and others
- Floors: cluttered, wet, slippery, or uneven
- Furniture out-of-place
- Lighting: poor or glares
- No hand rails or grab bars
- Restraint use
- Setting: new, strange, and unfamiliar
- Throw rugs or other tripping hazards
- Wet and slippery bathtubs and showers
- Wheelchairs, walkers, canes, and crutches: improper use or fit

The Person
- Age: over 65 years
- Alcohol: over-use
- Balance problems
- Blood pressure: low or high
- Confusion; disorientation
- Depression
- Dizziness or light-headedness; dizziness on standing
- Drug side effects
  - Confusion and disorientation
  - Coordination: poor
  - Diarrhea
  - Dizziness
  - Drowsiness
  - Fainting
  - Low blood pressure when standing or sitting
  - Unsteadiness
  - Urination: frequent
- Elimination: incontinence (urinary or fecal), frequency, urgency, urinating at night (*nocturia*)
- Falls: history of; fear of falling
- Foot problems; foot pain
- Gait: unsteady
- Joint pain and stiffness
- Judgment: poor
- Memory problems
- Mobility: impaired
- Pain
- Reaction time: slow
- Shoes that fit poorly; no shoes or shoes without slip-resistant surfaces
- Sleep problems
- Vision problems
- Weakness; leg weakness

FOCUS ON LONG-TERM CARE AND HOME CARE

Causes and Risk Factors for Falls

Long-Term Care

Nursing center residents are at increased risk for falls. Weakness and walking problems are common causes. Care setting hazards are other causes—poor lighting, wet floors, incorrect bed height. Other risk factors are transfer problems (Chapter 20), shoes that fit poorly, and improper use or fit of wheelchairs, walkers, canes, and other devices. See Box 14-1.

Home Care

In the home, many factors increase fall risks. Hazards include:
- Cluttered rooms, stairways, and hallways
- Objects on the floor and stairways—wires, cords, shoes, books, magazines, blankets, and so on
- Throw rugs
- Pets
- Flooring problems—loose tiles and floor boards, raised linoleum, frayed carpet
- Wet floors and slippery bathtub or shower floors
- Ice or snow on driveways, steps, and sidewalks
- Loose or missing hand rails and grab bars (p. 197)
- Poor lighting
- No footwear or unsafe footwear—slippers, shoes without slip-resistant surfaces, and shoes with long shoelaces
- Adaptive (assistive) devices that need repair—walkers, canes, wheelchairs
- Having to climb or reach for objects

TEAMWORK AND TIME MANAGEMENT

Causes and Risk Factors for Falls

The health team must protect the person. If you see something unsafe, tell the nurse at once. Do not assume the nurse knows or that the matter is being corrected.

Answer call lights promptly. This includes the call lights of patients and residents assigned to co-workers.

During shift changes, staff are busy going off and coming on duty. Confusion can occur about who gives care and answers call lights. Falls can result. Know your role during shift changes. Nursing staff must work together to prevent falls.

FALL PREVENTION PROGRAMS

Agencies have fall prevention programs. The measures in Box 14-2 are part of the program and the person's care plan. Many measures also apply to home settings. The care plan also lists measures for the person's risk factors.

Common sense and simple safety measures can prevent many falls. The health team works with the person and family to reduce fall risks. The goal is to prevent falls without decreasing quality of life.

See *Focus on Communication: Fall Prevention Programs*, p. 194.

See *Focus on Long-Term Care and Home Care: Fall Prevention Programs*, p. 194.

See *Promoting Safety and Comfort: Fall Prevention Programs*, p. 194.

BOX 14-2	Preventing Falls

Basic Needs
- Fluid needs are met.
- Eyeglasses and hearing aids are worn as needed. Reading glasses are not worn when up and about.
- Tasks are explained before and while performing them.
- Help is given with elimination needs. Assist the person to the bathroom or with the bedpan, urinal, or commode.
- The bedpan, urinal, or commode is kept within reach if the person can use the device without help.
- A warm drink, soft lights, or a back massage is used to calm the person who is agitated.
- Barriers are used to prevent wandering (Fig. 14-1, p. 194).
- The person is properly positioned in bed or a chair or wheelchair. Use pillows, wedge pads, seats, or other positioning devices as the nurse and care plan direct (Chapter 18).
- Correct procedures and equipment are used for transfers (Chapter 20). Follow the care plan.
- The person is involved in meaningful activities.
- Exercise programs are followed. They help improve balance, strength, walking, and physical function.

Bathrooms and Shower/Tub Rooms
- Tubs and showers have slip-resistant surfaces or slip-resistant bath mats.
- The person uses grab bars (safety bars) in bathrooms and showers (p. 197).
- Shower chairs are used (Chapter 24).
- Safety measures for tub baths and showers are followed (Chapter 24).

Floors, Stairs, and Hallways
- Carpeting (if used) is wall-to-wall or tacked down.
- Scatter, area, and throw rugs are not used.
- Floor covers are 1 color. Bold designs can cause dizziness in older persons.
- Floors have non-glare, slip-resistant surfaces.
- Non-skid wax is used on hardwood, tiled, or linoleum floors.
- Slip-resistant strips are on the floor next to the bed and in the bathroom. They are intact.
- Loose floor boards and tiles are reported. So are frayed rugs and carpets.
- Floors and stairs are free of clutter, cords, and other items that can cause tripping.
- Floors are free of spills. Wipe up spills at once. Put a WET FLOOR sign by the wet area.
- Floors are free of excess furniture and equipment.
- Electrical and extension cords are out of the way. This includes power strips.

Floors, Stairs, and Hallways—cont'd
- Equipment and supplies are kept on 1 side of the hallway.
- Hand rails (p. 197) are on both sides of stairs and hallways.
- The person uses hand rails when walking or using stairs.

Furniture
- Furniture is placed for easy movement.
- Furniture is kept in place. It is not re-arranged.
- Chairs have armrests. Armrests give support when standing or sitting.
- A phone, lamp, and personal belongings are within reach.

Beds and Other Equipment
- The bed is at the correct height for the person. Follow the care plan. The bed is raised for bedside care. Then it is lowered to a safe and comfortable level for the person. The distance from the bed to the floor is reduced if the person falls or gets out of bed.
- Bed rails (p. 196) are used according to the care plan.
- A mattress, special mat, or floor cushion is on the floor by the bed (Fig. 14-2, p. 195). This reduces the chance of injury if the person falls or gets out of bed.
- Wheelchairs, walkers, canes, and crutches fit properly. They are in good repair. Another person's equipment is not used.
- Crutches, canes, and walkers have slip-resistant tips.
- Wheelchair and stretcher safety is followed (Chapter 20).
- Wheel locks on beds (p. 197), wheelchairs, stretchers, commodes, and shower chairs are in working order. Wheels are locked for transfers.
- Linens are checked for sharp objects and for the person's property (dentures, eyeglasses, hearing aids, and so on).

Lighting
- Rooms, hallways, and stairways have good lighting. So do bathrooms and shower/tub rooms.
- Light switches are within reach and easy to find.
- Light switches are at the top and bottom of stairways.
- Night-lights are in bedrooms, hallways, and bathrooms.

Shoes and Clothing
- Slip-resistant footwear is worn. Socks, bedroom slippers, and long shoelaces are avoided.
- Shoes fit well. They do not slip up and down on the feet. All shoelaces and straps are fastened.
- Clothing fits properly. Clothing is not loose or dragging on the floor.
- Belts are tied or secured in place.

Continued

| BOX 14-2 | Preventing Falls—cont'd |

Call Lights and Alarms
- The person is taught how to use the call light (Chapter 21).
- The call light is always within the person's reach. This includes when sitting in the chair or on the commode and when in the bathroom and shower/tub room.
- The person is asked to use the call light when help is needed.
  - To get out of bed or a chair or return to bed
  - To walk
  - To get to or from the bathroom
  - To get on or off the toilet, bedpan, or commode
  - To stand to use the urinal
- Call lights are answered promptly. The person may need help right away. He or she may not wait for help.
- Bed, chair, door, floor mat, and belt alarms are used as directed in the care plan. They sense when the person tries to get up, get out of bed, or open a door. See "Position Change Alarms."
- Alarms are responded to at once.

Observation
- The person is checked often. This may be every 15 minutes or as required by the care plan. Careful and frequent observation is important.
- Frequent checks are made on persons with poor judgment or memory. This may be every 15 minutes or as required by the care plan.

Observation—cont'd
- Persons at risk for falls are close to the nurses' station.
- Family and friends are asked to visit during busy times. Meal times and shift changes are examples. They are also asked to visit during the evening and night shifts.
- Sitters, companions, or volunteers are provided to stay with the person.

Other
- Color-coded alerts warn of a fall risk. Yellow is common for a fall alert. Besides wristbands (Chapter 13), some agencies also use color-coded blankets, slip-resistant footwear, socks, and magnets or stickers on room doors.
- Caution is used when turning corners, entering corridor intersections, and going through doors. You could injure a person coming from the other direction.
- Pull (do not push) wheelchairs, stretchers, carts, and other wheeled equipment through doorways. You lead the way and can see where you are going.
- A safety check is made of the room after visitors leave. (See the inside of the back cover.) They may have lowered a bed rail, moved a call light, or moved a walker out of reach. Or they may have brought an item that could harm the person.

FOCUS ON COMMUNICATION

Fall Prevention Programs

A person can fall when reaching for needed items. The person reaches too far and falls. Or the person tries to get up without help. To prevent falls, ask the person:
- "What things would you like near you?"
- "Can I move this closer to you?"
- "Can you reach the call light?"
- "Can you reach your cane?" (Walker and wheelchair are other examples.)
- "Do you need to use the bathroom?"
- "Do you need anything else before I leave the room?"

FOCUS ON LONG-TERM CARE AND HOME CARE

Fall Prevention Programs

Home Care

People of all ages fall in home settings. Older persons are at risk. Simple changes can prevent falls (Chapter 12). So can some of the measures in Box 14-2. For example:
- Place furniture to allow clear walking paths.
- Remove throw and area rugs.
- Keep objects off the floor and stairs.
- Use night-lights in bedrooms, hallways, and bathrooms.
- Place a lamp by the bed if bedroom lights are hard to reach.
- Keep often-used items within easy reach. In kitchens, move items to lower shelves.
- Place slip-resistant bath mats or self-stick strips in showers and tubs.

PROMOTING SAFETY AND COMFORT

Fall Prevention Programs

Safety
Some people have vision problems. Besides the measures in Box 14-2, other safety measures are needed to prevent falls. See Chapter 46.

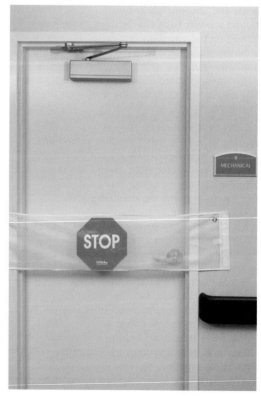

FIGURE 14-1 Barriers are used to prevent wandering.

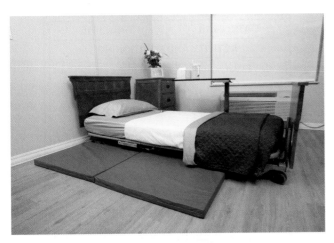

FIGURE 14-2 Floor cushion.

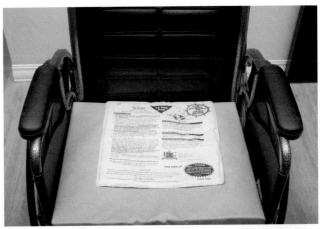

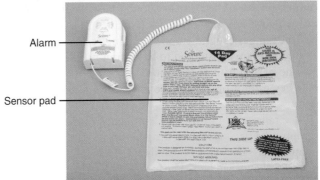

Alarm

Sensor pad

FIGURE 14-3 A position change alarm. This alarm has a sensor pad. The alarm sounds when the person moves off of the pad.

Position Change Alarms

The CMS describes a *position change alarm as any physical or electronic device that monitors a person's movement and alerts staff of movement.* Types include:

- Chair and bed sensor pads (Fig. 14-3)
- Bedside alarm mats
- Alarms clipped to clothing
- Seat-belt alarms
- Wireless motion sensors

To alert staff, the device makes a sound—alarm, beep, chime, music, and so on. Some play a recorded message. For example: "Please do not get up. Sit down and use your call light for help."

Position change alarms do not include door and elevator alarms that monitor wandering.

To use position change alarms safely:

- Follow the manufacturer's instructions.
- Mount the alarm securely out of the person's reach.
- Place the alarm at least 2 feet away from the person's ear. Alarms are loud.
- Test the alarm before leaving the person. If the device does not work, stay with the person. Call for the nurse.
- Respond to alarms at once.

For an alarm with a cord that attaches (clips) to clothing:

- Attach the clip securely out of the person's reach. The clip is at the back near the shoulder. Check that clothing is not frayed or torn.
- Check the cord. The cord should allow movement for comfort but be short enough to sound if the person moves from the safe area. The cord must not be tangled in bed rails, linens, chair parts, and so on.

Alarms do not replace close observation. Persons at risk for falls are checked often. Careful and frequent observation is important.

See *Promoting Safety and Comfort: Position Change Alarms.*

PROMOTING SAFETY AND COMFORT

Position Change Alarms

Safety

When position change alarms are used:

- Patterns and routines are monitored. For example, do alarms sound at certain times? Before or after meals, at bedtime, or when needing the bathroom are examples.
- Enough supervision is provided for the person's needs.
- Staff must respond to an alarm at once. False alarms are common. As a result, staff do not always respond or do not respond promptly. This increases the risk for falls.

Comfort

Alarms that limit freedom of movement may be considered a restraint (Chapter 15). For example, a person avoids moving because the alarm disrupts staff and other patients or residents. Alarms can cause:

- Embarrassment
- Loss of dignity
- Decreased mobility
- Incontinence
- Sleep problems from the sound of the alarm or fear of moving in bed
- Confusion, fear, agitation, anxiety, or irritation when the alarm sounds

Bed Rails

A *bed rail* (side rail) *is a device that serves as a guard or barrier along the side of the bed.* Bed rails are on both sides of the bed. They are raised and lowered (Fig. 14-4). They lock in place with levers, latches, or buttons. Bed rails are quarter (¼), half (½), three quarters (¾), or the full length of the bed. When half-length rails are used, each side has 1 or 2 rails (see Fig. 14-4).

The nurse and the care plan tell you when to raise bed rails. They are needed by persons who are unconscious or sedated with drugs. Some confused or disoriented people need them. When bed rails are needed, keep them up at all times except when giving bedside care.

Bed rails present hazards. When raised, the person cannot get out of bed. He or she can fall if trying to climb over them. *Entrapment* is a risk (Chapter 21). That is, the person can get caught, trapped, entangled, or strangled.

Bed rails are considered to be restraints (Chapter 15) if:

* The person cannot get out of bed.
* They cannot or will not be lowered to allow the person to leave the bed.

Bed rails cannot be used unless needed to treat a medical symptom. They must be in the person's best interest. Some people feel safer with bed rails up. Others use them for position changes in bed. The person or legal representative must give written consent for raised bed rails. The need for bed rails is carefully noted in the person's medical record and care plan.

The procedures in this book include bed rails. This helps you learn to use them correctly. The nurse, the care plan, and your assignment sheet tell you who uses bed rails. If a person does not use them, omit the "raise bed rails" and "lower bed rails" steps.

Check the person often. Tell the nurse that you checked the person. If allowed to chart, record when you checked the person and your observations (Fig. 14-5).

See *Focus on Children and Older Persons: Bed Rails.*
See *Focus on Long-Term Care and Home Care: Bed Rails.*
See *Promoting Safety and Comfort: Bed Rails.*

DATE: 06/16	TIME: 1415
ACTIVITY AND POSITIONING	

☐ Ambulate	☐ Chair
☐ Self	☒ Bed
☒ Assist of 1	☒ Right side
☐ Assist of 2	☐ Left side
☐ Mechanical lift	☐ Back

Turned Mr. Adams from his back to his right side. Placed pillows under his head, against his back, and under his left leg. He stated he was comfortable with needed items in reach (water mug, phone, tissues, urinal, call light). I told him that I will check on him every 15 minutes and to use the call light if he needs anything.

SAFETY	
☐ Gait belt	☒ Belongings in reach
☐ Slip-resistant shoes	☒ Bed rails raised
☒ Call light in reach	☐ Bed rails lowered
☒ Bed in low position	☐ Bed/chair alarm

FIGURE 14-5 Charting sample.

FOCUS ON **CHILDREN AND OLDER PERSONS**

Bed Rails

Children

Drop-side cribs do not meet current federal safety standards. Cribs manufactured since June 2011 meet safety standards that ban a drop-side rail. Older cribs may not meet current safety standards. Medical cribs with drop sides are allowed in hospitals. See Chapter 56 and Appendix D for more information about crib safety.

For toddlers and older children, rails placed on beds may cause entrapment (Chapter 21). Rails must fit the child's bed and be installed according to the manufacturer's instructions.

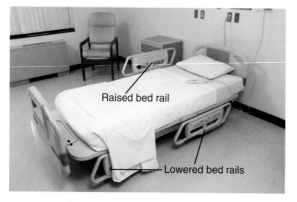

FIGURE 14-4 Bed rails. A far bed rail is raised. The near bed rails are lowered.

FOCUS ON **LONG-TERM CARE AND HOME CARE**

Bed Rails

Long-Term Care

Not all nursing center residents use bed rails. The person's personal choice and condition determine their use. You need to know who does and does not use bed rails. Consult the nurse and the person's care plan.

Home Care

Some home care patients use bed rails. The same risks and safety measures apply. Check the safety of bed rails installed by the family. Look for loose or poor-fitting rails. Tell the nurse if you suspect a problem.

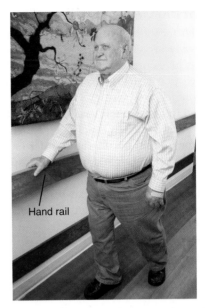

FIGURE 14-6 Hand rails provide support when walking.

Hand Rails and Grab Bars

Hand rails are in hallways and stairways (Fig. 14-6). They give support to persons who are weak or unsteady when walking.

Grab bars (safety bars) are in bathrooms and in shower/tub rooms (Fig. 14-7). They provide support to sit down or get up from a toilet. They also are used when standing in the shower and to get in and out of the shower or tub.

Wheel Locks

Bed wheels let the bed move easily. Wheels have locks to prevent the bed from moving (Fig. 14-8). Wheels are locked at all times except when moving the bed. Make sure bed wheels are locked:

- When giving bedside care
- When you transfer a person to and from bed

Wheelchair and stretcher wheels also are locked during transfers (Chapter 20). You or the person can be injured if the bed, wheelchair, or stretcher moves.

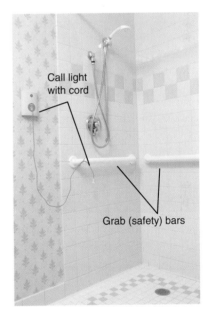

FIGURE 14-7 Grab bars (safety bars) in a shower.

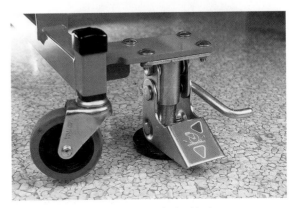

FIGURE 14-8 Bed wheel lock.

TRANSFER/GAIT BELTS

A *transfer belt (gait belt) is a device applied around the waist and used to support a person who is unsteady or disabled* (Fig. 14-9). It helps prevent falls and injuries.

- When used to transfer a person (Chapter 20), it is called a *transfer belt*.
- When used to help a person walk, it is called a *gait belt*.

The belt goes around the waist. Grasp the belt from underneath for support during the transfer or to assist the person to walk. If the belt has handles, grasp the belt by the handles (Fig. 14-10).

The standard-sized transfer/gait belt fits waist sizes up to 51 inches. Bariatric-sized belts fit waist sizes up to 71 inches. The nurse and care plan tell you what size to use. If the person's waist size is greater than 71 inches, follow the nurse's directions and the care plan.

See *Promoting Safety and Comfort: Transfer/Gait Belts.*
See procedure: *Using a Transfer/Gait Belt.*

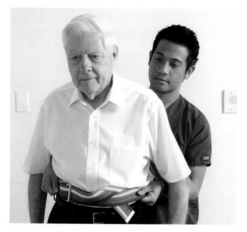

FIGURE 14-9 Transfer/gait belt. The buckle is off-center. Excess strap is tucked into the belt. The nursing assistant grasps the belt from underneath.

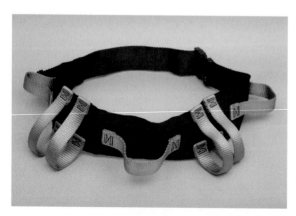

FIGURE 14-10 A transfer/gait belt with handles.

PROMOTING SAFETY AND COMFORT
Transfer/Gait Belts

Safety

Transfer/gait belts are routinely used in nursing centers. If the person needs help, a belt is required. For safe use, always follow the manufacturer's instructions.

Do not use a broken or soiled belt. Before use, check the belt for damage.

- Broken stitches or parts
- Torn, cut, or frayed material
- Broken or cracked buckles
- A buckle that does not hold securely

Some transfer/gait belts have a quick release buckle (Fig. 14-11). Position the buckle at the back where the person cannot reach or release it. Injury could result if the buckle is released.

Do not leave excess strap dangling. Tuck the excess strap into the belt (see Fig. 14-9).

Remove the belt after the procedure. Do not leave the person alone while wearing a transfer/gait belt. The belt is not used as a seat belt or to position a person in a chair or on a toilet or commode.

Using a transfer/gait belt is unsafe for some persons. The belt could cause pressure or rub against care equipment. Check with the nurse and the care plan before using a transfer/gait belt if the person has:

- An ostomy—colostomy, ileostomy, urostomy (Chapters 29 and 51)
- A gastrostomy tube (Chapter 32)
- Chronic obstructive pulmonary disease (Chapter 49)
- An abdominal or chest wound, incision, or drainage tube
- Monitoring equipment
- A hernia (Part of an organ protrudes or projects through an opening in a muscle wall. Hernias often involve a loop of bowel or the stomach.)
- Other conditions or equipment involving the chest or abdomen

Comfort

A transfer/gait belt is always applied over clothing—never over bare skin. Also, it is applied around the waist and under the breasts. Breasts must not be caught under the belt. The belt buckle is never positioned over the person's spine.

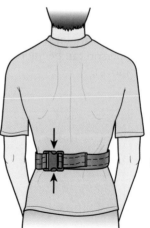

To release the buckle:
1 Press the buttons on both sides of the buckle together.
2 Pull the buckle apart.

FIGURE 14-11 A transfer/gait belt with a quick release buckle. The buckle is positioned off-center at the back.

Using a Transfer/Gait Belt

QUALITY OF LIFE

- Knock before entering the person's room.
- Address the person by name.
- Introduce yourself by name and title.

- Explain the procedure before starting and during the procedure.
- Protect the person's rights during the procedure.
- Handle the person gently during the procedure.

PRE-PROCEDURE

1 See *Promoting Safety and Comfort: Transfer/Gait Belts.*
2 Practice hand hygiene.
3 Obtain a transfer/gait belt of the correct type and size.

4 Identify the person. Check the identification (ID) bracelet against the assignment sheet. Use 2 identifiers (Chapter 13). Also call the person by name.
5 Provide for privacy.

PROCEDURE

6 Assist the person to a sitting position.
7 Apply the belt. Hold the belt by the buckle. Wrap the belt around the person's waist over clothing. Do not apply it over bare skin.
  a *For a belt with a metal buckle:*
    1) Insert the belt's metal tip into the buckle. Pass the belt through the side with the teeth first (Fig. 14-12, *A*).
    2) Bring the belt tip across the front of the buckle. Insert the tip through the buckle's smooth side (Fig. 14-12, *B*).
  b *For a belt with a quick release buckle,* push the belt ends together to secure the buckle.
8 Tighten the belt so it is snug. It should not cause discomfort or impair breathing. You should be able to slide your open, flat hand under the belt. Ask about the person's comfort. If the belt is too loose or too tight, adjust the belt as needed.

9 Make sure that the person's breasts are not caught under the belt.
10 Place the buckle off-center in the front (Fig. 14-12, *C*) or off-center in the back (see Fig. 14-11) for the person's comfort. A quick release buckle is in the back out of the person's reach. The buckle is not over the spine.
11 Tuck any excess strap into the belt (see Fig. 14-12, *C*).
12 Complete the transfer (Chapter 20) or ambulation procedure (Chapter 34). Grasp the belt from underneath with 2 hands (see Fig. 14-9). Or grasp the belt by the handles.

POST-PROCEDURE

13 Remove the belt after the procedure in step 12. The person is not left alone wearing the belt.
  a *For a belt with a metal buckle:*
    1) Bring the belt strap back through the buckle's smooth side.
    2) Pull the belt through the side with the teeth.
  b *For a belt with a quick release buckle,* push inward on the quick release buttons (see Fig. 14-11).
  c Remove the belt from the person's waist. Do not drag the belt across the waist.

14 Provide for comfort. (See the inside of the back cover.)
15 Place the call light and other needed items within reach.
16 Unscreen the person.
17 Complete a safety check of the room. (See the inside of the back cover.)
18 Return the transfer/gait belt to its proper place.
19 Practice hand hygiene.
20 Report and record your observations.

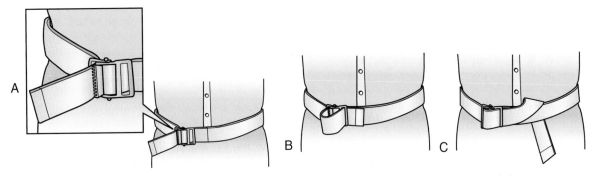

FIGURE 14-12 Applying a transfer/gait belt at the waist. **A,** The belt is inserted into the buckle. The belt goes through the side with the teeth first. **B,** The belt is inserted into the buckle's smooth side. **C,** The buckle is off-center in the front. Excess strap is tucked into the belt.

THE FALLING PERSON

A person may start to fall when standing or walking. The person may be weak, light-headed, or dizzy. Fainting may occur. Falling may be caused by slipping or sliding on spills, waxed floors, throw rugs, or improper shoes. See p. 192 for the causes and risk factors for falls.

Do not try to prevent the fall. You could injure yourself and the person while twisting and straining to prevent the fall. You could lose your balance and you both could fall. Head, wrist, arm, hip, knee, and back injuries could occur.

If a person starts to fall, bring the person close to your body. Ease him or her to the floor. This lets you control the direction of the fall. You can also protect the person's head. Do not let the person move or get up before the nurse checks for injuries. Reassure the person and explain that the nurse will check for injuries before the person is helped up.

If you find a person on the floor, do not move the person. Stay with the person and call for the nurse.

An incident report is completed after all falls (Chapter 13). The nurse may have you help with the report.

See *Focus on Children and Older Persons: The Falling Person.*

See *Promoting Safety and Comfort: The Falling Person.*

See procedure: *Helping the Falling Person.*

FOCUS ON CHILDREN AND OLDER PERSONS

The Falling Person

Older Persons

Some older persons are confused. A confused person may not understand why you do not want him or her to move or get up after a fall. Forcing a person not to move may injure the person and you. You may need to let the person move for his or her safety and your own. Never use force to hold a person down. Stay calm and protect the person from injury. Talk to the person in a quiet, soothing voice. Call for help.

PROMOTING SAFETY AND COMFORT

The Falling Person

Safety

If a bariatric person starts to fall, there is little that you can do. For the person's safety and yours:
* *Do not* use the procedure: *Helping the Falling Person.*
* Move items that could cause injury out of the way. Do so as fast as possible.
* Try to protect the person's head from striking the floor, equipment, or other objects.
* Call for the nurse at once. Stay with the person.
* Assist the health team to return the person to bed.

Helping the Falling Person

PROCEDURE

1 Stand behind the person with your feet apart. Keep your back straight.
2 Bring the person close to your body as fast as possible (Fig. 14-13, *A*). Use the transfer/gait belt. Or wrap your arms around the person's waist. If necessary, hold the person under the arms.
3 Move your leg so the person's buttocks rest on it (Fig. 14-13, *B*). Move your leg that is near the person.

4 Lower the person to the floor. The person slides down your leg to the floor (Fig. 14-13, *C*). Bend at your hips and knees as you lower the person.
5 Call for a nurse to check the person. Stay with the person.
6 Help the nurse return the person to bed. Ask other staff to help if needed.

POST-PROCEDURE

7 Provide for comfort. (See the inside of the back cover.)
8 Place the call light and other needed items within reach.
9 Raise or lower bed rails. Follow the care plan.
10 Complete a safety check of the room. (See the inside of the back cover.)
11 Practice hand hygiene.

12 Report and record the following.
  * How the fall occurred
  * How far the person walked
  * If the person was standing or walking
  * How activity was tolerated before the fall
  * Complaints before the fall
  * How much help the person needed while walking
13 Complete an incident report (Chapter 13).

A   B   C

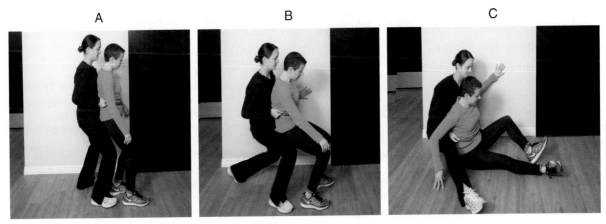

FIGURE 14-13 Helping the falling person. **A,** The falling person is supported with the gait belt. **B,** The person's buttocks rest on the nursing assistant's leg. **C,** The person is eased to the floor.

MOVING THE PERSON FROM THE FLOOR

After a fall, the nurse will assess the person for injuries. Special procedures are used to move a person with severe injuries. Assist as the nurse directs.

If there are no injuries or minor injuries, follow the nurse's directions to move the person from the floor. The Occupational Safety and Health Administration (OSHA) recommends minimal manual lifting or not lifting when possible. A mechanical lift (Chapter 20) may be used (Fig. 14-14). The lift must reach the floor.

If the person can stand alone, the nurse has staff stand by as the person stands up. Or a transfer/gait belt is used to assist the person.

If a manual lift is required, protect yourself from injury.

- Use good body mechanics (Chapter 18).
- Roll the person onto his or her side and position an assist device (Chapter 19). A blanket or drawsheet (Chapter 22) are examples. Avoid reaching across the person.
- Have at least 2 staff members on each side of the person. The larger the person, the more staff needed.
- Bend your knees, not your back. Do not twist.
- For the lift:
  1 Kneel on 1 knee.
  2 Grasp the blanket, drawsheet, or other device.
  3 Lift smoothly with your legs as you stand. Stand together on the "count of 3." Do not bend your back.

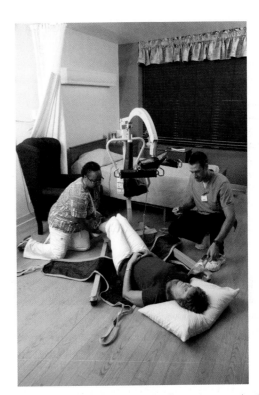

FIGURE 14-14 Moving the person from the floor using a mechanical lift.

FOCUS ON **PRIDE**

The Person, Family, and Yourself

Personal and Professional Responsibility

Safety measures can take time. Resist the urge to take short cuts. Take the time to:

- Find and use adaptive (assistive) devices.
- Put slip-resistant footwear on the person.
- Raise or lower the bed and bed rails as needed.
- Lock wheels on beds, stretchers, and wheelchairs.
- Ask for help.

Take time for safety. Take pride in doing the right thing.

Rights and Respect

Fear of falling does not make a person feel safe. Before moving a person, explain what you will do and what he or she needs to do. Also give step-by-step instructions. Good communication supports the person's right to safety and security.

Independence and Social Interaction

Some people feel that safety devices limit independence. Using a transfer/gait belt is an example. Listen to the person's concerns. Kindly explain the reason for the safety device. If the person still refuses, tell the nurse. Do not be talked out of a safety measure or using a safety device. Safety is always a priority.

Delegation and Teamwork

Helping co-workers is part of teamwork. Communication is needed for safety. To help a co-worker's patient or resident, you must know:

- Is the person at risk for falls?
- Is the person weak? Can he or she bear weight?
- Are there activity limits?
- How many staff are needed for the task?
- Are adaptive (assistive) devices needed? A cane, transfer belt, wheelchair, and walker are examples.
- Is other equipment needed? A mechanical lift (Chapter 20) is an example.

Ethics and Laws

Failing to prevent falls can result in legal action. The following is a real case in which the nursing staff neglected to use safety measures to prevent a fall.

A patient fell and injured her right shoulder 6 days after knee surgery. The patient claimed that the nursing staff did not follow orders to assist with walking to and from the bathroom. According to the patient:

- *She asked for help to raise herself from a commode to a standing position.*
- *She was not given assistance.*
- *She fell when the commode (with wheels) shifted while she tried to stand.*

According to the hospital's lawyers, the staff did not use a transfer belt. Failure to use the belt violated hospital policy. The case settled for $25,000.

(N. Martinez and M. Martinez v St. Catherine's Hospital, Sentry Insurance and Wisconsin Patient Compensation Fund, 1998, Wisconsin.)

FOCUS ON **PRIDE**: *Application*

A person is embarrassed about needing a transfer/gait belt and walker. How will you promote safety and dignity? What if the person refuses to use the devices?

REVIEW QUESTIONS

Circle the BEST answer.

1 These statements are about falls. Which is *true*?
   a Most are caused by many risk factors.
   b Serious injuries are unlikely.
   c Falling indoors is not common.
   d Nursing center residents are at decreased risk.

2 Which person has the lowest risk of falls?
   a A 75-year-old with confusion
   b A 68-year-old with a history of falls
   c A 60-year-old with a hearing aid
   d An 80-year-old with urinary incontinence

3 A person's care plan includes fall prevention measures. Which should you question?
   a Assist with elimination needs.
   b Keep phone, lamp, and TV controls within reach.
   c Check the person every 2 hours.
   d Complete a safety check after visitors leave the room.

4 You observe the following in the person's room. Which is *unsafe*?
   a The lamp cord is by the chair.
   b The chair has armrests.
   c The night-light is on.
   d The bed is in a low position.

5 You note the following after a person is dressed. Which is *safe*?
   a Pant cuffs are dragging on the floor.
   b The person is wearing slip-resistant shoes.
   c The belt is not fastened.
   d The shirt is too big.

6 A resident's chair alarm goes off. What should you do?
   a Find the resident's nursing assistant.
   b Tell the nurse.
   c Assist the resident.
   d Wait for someone to respond to the alarm.

REVIEW QUESTIONS—cont'd

7 To help prevent falls, you need to report
  a Equipment and supplies being on 1 side of the hallway
  b A floor cushion beside the bed
  c A co-worker pulling a wheelchair through a doorway
  d Clutter on stairways

8 Bed rails are used
  a When you think they are needed
  b According to the care plan
  c When the bed is raised
  d To support persons who are weak or unsteady

9 Before transferring a person to bed, you must
  a Raise the bed rails
  b Get a grab bar
  c Lock the bed wheels
  d Remove the person's shoes

10 A transfer/gait belt is applied
  a To the skin
  b Over clothing at the waist
  c Over the breasts
  d Under the robe

11 To safely use a transfer/gait belt, you must
  a Follow the manufacturer's instructions
  b Be able to slide a closed fist under the belt
  c Leave the belt on if the person is left alone
  d Position the buckle over the person's spine

12 You apply a transfer/gait belt. What should you do with the excess strap?
  a Cut it off.
  b Wrap it around the person's waist.
  c Tuck it into the belt.
  d Let it dangle.

13 A person starts to fall. Your *first* action is to
  a Try to prevent the fall
  b Call for help
  c Bring the person close to your body as fast as possible
  d Lower the person to the floor

14 When a bariatric person falls, you should
  a Try to stop the fall
  b Try to protect the person's head
  c Quickly pull the person close to you
  d Do nothing

15 You found a person lying on the floor. What should you do?
  a Lock the bed wheels.
  b Help the person back to bed.
  c Apply a transfer belt.
  d Call for the nurse.

Answers to Chapter 14 questions are on p. 885.

FOCUS ON **PRACTICE**
Problem Solving

You are assisting a resident in the bathroom. The resident is not to be left alone while in the bathroom. You hear a chair alarm sound in the hallway outside the door. What will you do?

15

Restraint Alternatives and Restraints

OBJECTIVES

- Define the key terms and key abbreviations in this chapter.
- Describe the purpose of restraints.
- Identify the risk factors related to restraint use.
- Identify restraint alternatives.
- Explain the legal aspects of restraint use.

- Explain how to use restraints safely.
- Perform the procedure described in this chapter.
- Explain how to promote PRIDE in the person, the family, and yourself.

KEY TERMS

chemical restraint Any drug used for discipline or convenience and not required to treat medical symptoms

convenience Any action taken to control or manage a person's behavior that requires less effort by the staff; the action is not in the person's best interest

discipline Any action taken by the agency to punish or penalize a patient or resident

enabler A device that limits freedom of movement but is used to promote independence, comfort, or safety

freedom of movement Any change in place or position of the body or any part of the body that the person can control

medical symptom An indication or characteristic of a physical or psychological condition

physical restraint Any manual method or physical or mechanical device, material, or equipment attached to or near the person's body that he or she cannot remove easily and that restricts freedom of movement or normal access to one's body

remove easily The manual method, device, material, or equipment used to restrain the person that can be removed intentionally by the person in the same manner it was applied by the staff

KEY ABBREVIATIONS

CMS	Centers for Medicare & Medicaid Services	ROM	Range-of-motion
FDA	Food and Drug Administration	TJC	The Joint Commission
ID	Identification		

Chapters 13 and 14 have many safety measures. Some persons need extra protection. They may present dangers to themselves or others (including staff).

The Centers for Medicare & Medicaid Services (CMS) has rules for restraint use. CMS rules protect the person's right to be free from restraint. Restraints may be used for a brief time to treat a medical symptom that would require restraint use or for the immediate physical safety of the person or others. Restraints may be used when less restrictive measures fail to protect the person or others. They must be discontinued as soon as possible.

The CMS uses these terms.

- *Physical restraint—any manual method or physical or mechanical device, material, or equipment attached to or near the person's body that he or she cannot remove easily and that restricts freedom of movement or normal access to one's body.*

- *Chemical restraint—any drug used for discipline or convenience and not required to treat medical symptoms.* The drug or dosage is not a standard treatment for the person's condition.
- *Freedom of movement—any change in place or position of the body or any part of the body that the person can control.*
- *Convenience—any action taken to control or manage a person's behavior that requires less effort by the staff; the action is not in the person's best interest.*
- *Discipline—any action taken by the agency to punish or penalize a patient or resident.*
- *Remove easily—the manual method, device, material, or equipment used to restrain the person that can be removed intentionally by the person in the same manner it was applied by the staff.* For example, the person can put bed rails down, untie a knot, or open a buckle.

HISTORY OF RESTRAINT USE

Restraints were once used to *prevent* falls. However, there is no evidence that restraints prevent falls. Injuries are more serious from falls in restrained persons than in those not restrained.

Restraints also were used to prevent wandering or interfering with treatment. They were often used for confusion, poor judgment, or behavior problems. Older persons were restrained more often than younger persons were. Restraints were viewed as safety measures. However, they can cause serious harm, even death. See "Risks From Restraint Use" on p. 207.

Besides the CMS, the Food and Drug Administration (FDA), state agencies, and The Joint Commission (TJC—an accrediting agency) have restraint guidelines. They do not forbid restraint use. *All other appropriate alternatives must be considered or tried first.*

Every agency has policies and procedures for restraints. They include identifying persons at risk for harm, harmful behaviors, restraint alternatives, and proper restraint use. Staff training is required.

RESTRAINT ALTERNATIVES

Often there are causes and reasons for harmful behaviors. Knowing and treating the cause can prevent restraint use. The nurse tries to learn what the behavior means.

- Is the person in pain, ill, or injured?
- Is the person short of breath? Do cells have enough oxygen (Chapter 43)?
- Is the person afraid in a new setting?
- Does the person need to use the bathroom?
- Is clothing or a wound dressing (Chapter 40) tight or causing discomfort?
- Is the person uncomfortable?
- Are body fluids, secretions, or excretions causing skin irritation?
- Is the person too hot or too cold? Hungry or thirsty?
- What are the person's life-long habits?
- Does the person have problems communicating?
- Is the person seeing, hearing, or feeling things that are not real (Chapters 52 and 53)?
- Is the person confused or disoriented (Chapter 53)?
- Are drugs causing the behaviors?

Restraint alternatives are identified in the care plan (Box 15-1). Restraint alternatives may not protect the person. The doctor may need to order restraints.

BOX 15-1	Restraint Alternatives

Physical Needs

- Life-long habits and routines are in the care plan. For example, showers before breakfast; reads in the bathroom; walks outside before lunch; watches TV after lunch.
- Pillows, wedge cushions, and posture and positioning devices are used.
- Food, fluid, hygiene, and elimination needs are met.
- The bedpan, urinal, or commode is within reach.
- Back massages are given.
- A calm, quiet setting is provided.
- Exercise programs are provided.
- Outdoor time is planned for nice weather.
- Furniture meets the person's needs—lower bed, reclining chair, rocking chair, chair or wheelchair with lap-top tray (Fig. 15-1, p. 206).
- Observations and visits are made at least every 15 minutes or more often. Follow the care plan.
- The person's room is close to the nurses' station.
- Lighting meets the person's needs and preferences.
- Staff assignments are consistent.
- Sleep is not interrupted.
- Noise levels are reduced.

Safety and Security Needs

- The call light is within reach. The person is reminded to use the call light.
- Call lights are answered promptly.
- The person wanders in safe areas.
- All staff are aware of persons who tend to wander. This includes staff in other departments.
- Knob guards are used on doors.

Safety and Security Needs—cont'd

- Falls and injuries are prevented (Chapter 14).
  - Padded hip protectors are worn under clothing (Fig. 15-2, p. 206).
  - The bed is lowered close to the floor. A soft mat or floor cushion is next to the bed.
  - Bolsters or roll guards are used. These padded devices are placed along the sides of the bed to prevent rolling out of bed.
- Bed, chair, and door alarms are used.
- Walls and furniture corners are padded.
- Procedures and care measures are explained.
- Frequent explanations are given about equipment or devices.
- Confused persons are oriented to person, time, and place. (To *orient* means *to remind the person of his or her name and the date, time, and setting.*) Calendars and clocks are provided. See Chapter 53.

Love, Belonging, and Self-Esteem Needs

- Diversion is provided—TV, videos, music, games, relaxation, and so on.
- The person watches videos of family and friends and of their visits.
- Time is spent in supervised areas (dining room, lounge, by the nurses' station).
- Family, friends, and volunteers visit.
- The person has companions or sitters.
- Time is spent with the person.
- Extra time is spent with a person who is restless.
- Reminiscing is done with the person.
- The person does jobs or tasks he or she consents to.

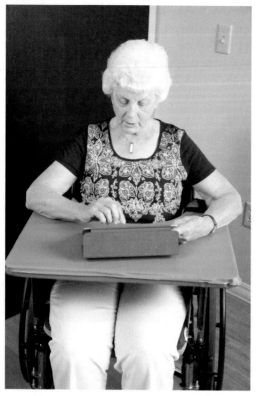

FIGURE 15-1 This lap-top tray is a restraint alternative. It is a restraint when used to prevent freedom of movement.

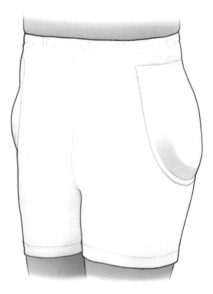

FIGURE 15-2 Hip protector.

SAFE RESTRAINT USE

Restraints can cause serious injury and death. They are not used to discipline a person or for staff convenience. Restraints are used only when necessary to treat a *medical symptom—an indication or characteristic of a physical or psychological condition.* Symptoms may be physical, emotional, or behavioral. Sometimes restraints are needed to protect the person or others. That is, a person may have violent or aggressive behaviors that are harmful to self or others or that are threatening to others.

See *Focus on Surveys: Safe Restraint Use.*

See *Promoting Safety and Comfort: Safe Restraint Use.*

Physical and Chemical Restraints

A *physical restraint* includes these points.

- May be any manual method, physical or mechanical device, material, or equipment.
- Is attached to or next to the person's body.
- Cannot be removed easily by the person.
- Restricts freedom of movement or normal access to one's body.

Physical restraints are applied to the chest, waist, elbows, wrists, hands, or ankles. They confine the person to a bed or chair. Or they prevent movement of a body part. Some furniture or barriers also prevent freedom of movement.

- A device used with a chair that the person cannot remove easily. The device prevents the person from rising. Tables, bars, lap trays, lap cushions, and belts are examples (see Fig. 15-1).
- Any chair that prevents the person from rising.
- Any bed or chair placed so close to the wall that the person cannot get out of the bed or chair.
- Bed rails (Chapter 14) that prevent the person from getting out of bed. They cannot or will not be lowered to allow the person to leave the bed.
- Tucking in or using Velcro (or other device) to hold a sheet, fabric, or clothing so tightly that freedom of movement is restricted.

Drugs or drug dosages are *chemical restraints* if they:

- Control behavior or restrict movement.
- Are not standard treatment for the person's condition.

Drugs cannot be used for discipline or staff convenience. They cannot be used if they affect physical or mental function.

Some drugs can help persons who are confused, disoriented, anxious, agitated, or aggressive. The doctor may order drugs to control such behaviors. The drugs should not make the person sleepy and unable to function at his or her highest level.

Enablers. An *enabler is a device that limits freedom of movement but is used to promote independence, comfort, or safety.* Some devices can be restraints or enablers. When the person can easily remove the device and it helps the person function, it is an enabler. For example:

- A chair or wheelchair with a lap-top tray for meals, writing, and so on (see Fig. 15-1). The tray is an enabler. If used to limit freedom of movement, the tray is a restraint.
- A person wants raised bed rails. They are used to move in bed and to prevent falling out of bed. The bed rails are enablers, not restraints.

Risks From Restraint Use

Box 15-2 lists the risks from restraints. Injuries can occur as the person tries to get free of the restraint. Injuries also occur from using the wrong restraint, applying it wrong, or keeping it on too long. Cuts, bruises, and fractures are common. *The most serious risk is death from strangulation.*

Restraints are medical devices. The *Safe Medical Devices Act* applies if a restraint causes illness, injury, or death. Also, the CMS requires the reporting of any death that occurs:

- While a person is in a restraint.
- Within 24 hours after a restraint was removed.
- Within 1 week after a restraint was removed. This applies if the restraint may have contributed directly or indirectly to the person's death.

See *Promoting Safety and Comfort: Risks From Restraint Use.*

BOX 15-2 | **Risks From Restraint Use**

- Constipation
- Contractures
- Cuts and bruises
- Decline in physical function (ability to walk and muscle problems are examples)
- Dehydration
- Falls
- Fractures
- Head trauma
- Incontinence
- Infections: pneumonia and urinary tract
- Nerve injuries
- Pressure injuries
- Social problems and mental health disorders: agitation, anger, delirium, depression, loss of dignity, embarrassment and humiliation, mistrust, loss of self-respect, reduced social contact, withdrawal
- Strangulation

PROMOTING SAFETY AND COMFORT

Risks From Restraint Use

Safety

If you find a person strangling from a restraint:

- Release the restraint. Or cut the strap if you have scissors in your pocket or within reach.
- Shout for help and for a nurse as you are releasing the restraint.
- Stay with the person. Follow the guidelines for cardiopulmonary resuscitation (CPR) and rescue breathing (Chapter 58). Follow agency policy. Assist the nurse as directed.

Laws, Rules, and Guidelines

Federal and state laws and rules for restraint use are followed. So are accrediting agency (TJC) guidelines. They are part of the agency's policies and procedures for restraint use.

- *Restraints must protect the person.* Restraints do not replace properly supervising and observing the person. A restrained person requires more staff time for care, supervision, and observation. When used, the restraint must be the best safety measure for the person. Restraints are not used to punish or penalize uncooperative persons.
- *A doctor's order is required.* The doctor gives the reason for the restraint, what body part to restrain, what to use, and how long to use it. This information is on the care plan and your assignment sheet. In an emergency, the nurse can decide to apply restraints before getting a doctor's order.
- *The least restrictive method is used.* It allows the greatest amount of movement or body access possible. Some restraints attach to the person's body and to a non-movable object—bed frame or chair frame. Vest, jacket, ankle, wrist, hand, and some belt restraints are examples. They restrict freedom of movement or body access. Other restraints are near but not attached to the person's body (bed rails or wedge cushions). They do not totally restrict freedom of movement. They allow access to certain body parts.
- *Restraints are used only after other measures fail to protect the person* (see Box 15-1). Some people can harm themselves or others. Safety measures must protect the person and prevent harm to others. Many fall prevention measures are restraint alternatives (Chapter 14).
- *Unnecessary restraint is false imprisonment* (Chapter 5). You must understand the reason for the restraint and its risks. If not, politely ask about its use. An unneeded restraint may lead to false imprisonment charges.
- *Informed consent is required.* The person must understand the reason for the restraint and possible risks. The person is told how the restraint will help medical treatment. If the person cannot give consent, his or her legal representative is given the information. Consent is needed before a restraint can be used. The doctor or nurse provides needed information and obtains consent.

See *Focus on Communication: Laws, Rules, and Guidelines.*

Safety Guidelines

The restrained person must be kept safe (Box 15-3). Also remember these key points.

- *Observe for increased confusion and agitation.* Whether confused or alert, people are aware of restricted movements. They may try to get out of the restraint or struggle to pull at it. Some restrained persons beg others to free or to help release them. These behaviors often are viewed as signs of confusion. Confusion can increase because of not understanding what is happening. Provide repeated explanations and reassurance. Spending time with them has a calming effect.
- *Protect the person's quality of life.* Restraints are used only for a brief time. The care plan must show how to reduce restraint use. You must meet the person's physical, emotional, and social needs. Visit with the person and explain the reason for the restraint.
- *Follow the manufacturer's instructions to safely apply and secure the restraint.* Tight restraints affect circulation and breathing. The person must be comfortable and able to move the restrained part to a limited and safe extent. Restraints must be applied and secured properly.
- *Apply restraints with enough help to protect the person and staff from injury.* Sometimes restraints must be applied quickly. Combative and agitated people can hurt themselves and the staff when restraints are applied. Enough staff members are needed to complete the task safely and quickly.
- *Observe the person at least every 15 minutes or as often as directed by the nurse and the care plan.* Restraints are dangerous. Injuries and deaths can result from improper restraint use and poor observation. Prevent complications. Breathing and circulation problems are examples. Constant observation may be required for persons:
  - Who are aggressive, combative, or agitated.
  - At risk for aspiration—breathing food, fluid, vomitus, or an object into the lungs (Chapter 30). Persons who are supine (lying down) and unable to sit up are examples.
  - At risk for suicide (Chapter 52).
- *Remove or release the restraint, re-position the person, and meet basic needs at least every 2 hours. Or do so as often as noted in the care plan.* See Box 15-3.

See *Teamwork and Time Management: Safety Guidelines.*
See *Focus on Communication: Safety Guidelines,* p. 210.

Text continued on p. 213.

FOCUS ON COMMUNICATION

Laws, Rules, and Guidelines

You may not know the reason for a restraint. If so, politely ask the nurse why it is needed. For example:
- "Why does Mr. Reed need a restraint?"
- "Why did the doctor order a restraint for Ms. Porter?"

TEAMWORK AND TIME MANAGEMENT

Safety Guidelines

Make sure you know who is restrained on your unit. When you walk past the person or the person's room, check if the person is safe and comfortable. Answer the person's call light promptly.

BOX 15-3 **Safety Guidelines for Using Restraints**

Before Applying Restraints

- Do not use sheets, towels, tape, rope, straps, bandages, Velcro, or other items to restrain a person.
- Apply a restraint only after learning about its proper use.
- Demonstrate correct application of the restraint before applying it.
- Use the correct restraint and size. Small restraints are tight. They cause discomfort and agitation and restrict breathing and circulation. Strangulation is a risk from big or loose restraints.
- Use only restraints that have the manufacturer's instructions and warning labels.
  - Read the warning labels. Note the front and back of the restraint.
  - Follow the instructions. Some restraints are safe for bed, chair, and wheelchair use. Others are used only with certain equipment.
- Use intact restraints.
  - Look for broken stitches, tears, cuts, or frayed fabric or straps.
  - Look for missing or loose buckles, locks, hooks, loops, or straps or other damage. The restraint must hold securely.
- Test zippers, buckles, locks, hooks, loops, and other closures. The device must fasten securely.
- Do not alter or repair a restraint.
- Do not use soiled or damaged restraints. Have the nurse inspect a damaged product.
- Do not use a restraint near a fire, a flame, smoking materials, or other heat source.

Applying Restraints

- Follow agency policies and procedures and the manufacturer's instructions.
- Do not use a restraint to position a person:
  - On a toilet.
  - On furniture that does not allow for correct application.
  - In a vehicle. The restraint is not a seat belt.
  - In a home setting. Federal law restricts some restraints for use only in health care agencies.
- Position the person in good alignment before applying the restraint (Chapter 18). When in a chair, position the person so the hips are well to the back of the chair.
- Pad bony areas and the skin as directed by the nurse. This prevents pressure and injury from the restraint.
- Follow the manufacturer's instructions. A restraint applied wrong or backward may cause serious injury or death. Death may occur from suffocation or strangulation.
  - *Vest restraint*—The "V" neck is in front (Fig. 15-3, p. 210).
  - *Jacket restraint*—The opening is in the back.
  - *Belt restraint when in a chair*—Apply the restraint at a 45-degree angle over the thighs (Fig. 15-4, p. 210).
- Do not criss-cross straps in the back unless required by the manufacturer's instructions (Fig. 15-5, p. 211). Straps may loosen when the person moves and cause serious injury.
- Secure restraints according to the manufacturer's instructions. Quick release buckles (Fig. 15-6, p. 211) or quick release knots (Fig. 15-7, p. 211) are used. Both are easy to release in an emergency.
- Secure straps out of the person's reach.
- Leave 1 to 2 inches of slack in the straps if directed to do so by the nurse. This allows some movement of the part.

Applying Restraints—cont'd

- Secure the restraint to the movable part of the bed frame (Fig. 15-8, p. 212). The restraint will not tighten or loosen when the head or foot of the bed is raised or lowered. For chairs, secure straps under the seat of the wheelchair or chair (Fig. 15-9, p. 212).
- Check for snugness after applying the restraint. The restraint should be snug but allow some movement of the restrained part. Follow the manufacturer's instructions. For example:
  - *If applied to the chest or waist*—Make sure the person can breathe easily. A flat hand should slide between the restraint and the person's body (Fig. 15-10, p. 212). Check with the nurse if you have very small or very large hands. Small or large hands could cause a tight or loose restraint.
  - *For limb holders and mitt restraints*—You should be able to slide 1 finger under the device. Check with the nurse if you have very small or very large fingers. Small or large fingers could cause a tight or loose restraint.
- Make sure that straps cannot tighten, loosen, slip, slide, or cause too much slack. The straps can change if pulled on by the person. Changing the bed or seat (or cushion) position can also change the straps. Injury or death can result from:
  - Tight straps that can impair breathing and cause suffocation.
  - Loose straps that allow the person to get free of the restraint.
  - Loose straps that allow the person to slip or slide off the bed or chair. The person can become suspended in the restraint (Figs. 15-11 and 15-12, p. 212). Chest compression and suffocation can result from strangulation.
- Never secure restraints to the bed rails. The person may be able to reach bed rails to release knots or buckles. Also, injury is likely when raising or lowering bed rails.
- Use bed rail covers or gap protectors as instructed by the nurse (Fig. 15-13, p. 212). The person can become trapped or suspended (see Fig. 15-11) between:
  - The bars of a bed rail
  - The space between half-length (split) bed rails
  - The bed rail and mattress
  - The head-board or foot-board and mattress

After Applying Restraints

- Keep bed rails up when using a vest, jacket, or belt restraint. Also use bed rail covers or gap protectors. Otherwise the person could fall off the bed and strangle on the restraint. Or the person can get caught between half-length bed rails.
- Do not use back cushions when a person is restrained in a chair. If the cushion moves out of place, slack occurs in the straps. Strangulation is a risk if the person slides forward or down from the extra slack.
- Do not cover the person with a sheet, blanket, bedspread, or other covering. The restraint must be within plain view at all times.
- Check the person at least every 15 minutes for safety, comfort, and signs of injury. Or check the person more often as directed by the nurse and the care plan.
- Monitor persons in the supine (back-lying) position constantly. Aspiration is a great risk if vomiting occurs (Chapter 30). Call for the nurse at once.

Continued

BOX 15-3	Safety Guidelines for Using Restraints—cont'd

After Applying Restraints—cont'd

- Check the person's circulation at least every 15 minutes or more often as directed by the nurse and the care plan.
  - *For limb holders or mitt restraints*—You should feel a pulse at a pulse site below the restraint. Fingers or toes should be warm and pink. Tell the nurse at once if:
    - *You cannot feel a pulse.*
    - *Fingers or toes are cold, pale, or blue in color.*
    - *The person complains of pain, numbness, or tingling in the restrained part.*
    - *The skin is red or damaged.*
  - *For a belt, jacket, or vest restraint*—The person should be able to breathe easily. Also check the position of the restraint, especially in the front and back.
- Keep scissors in your pocket. In an emergency such as strangulation, cutting the tie may be faster than releasing a knot or buckle. Never leave scissors where the person can reach them. Make sure the person cannot reach the scissors in your pocket.

After Applying Restraints—cont'd

- Remove or release the restraint and re-position the person every 2 hours or more often as noted in the care plan. The restraint is removed or released for at least 10 minutes. Meet the person's basic needs.
  - Measure vital signs.
  - Meet elimination needs.
  - Offer food and fluids.
  - Meet hygiene needs.
  - Give skin care.
  - Perform range-of-motion (ROM) exercises or help the person walk. Follow the care plan.
  - Provide for physical and emotional comfort. (See the inside of the back cover.)
- Keep the call light and other needed items within the person's reach. Record that this was done.
- Complete a safety check before leaving the room. (See the inside of the back cover.)
- Report to the nurse every time you checked the person and removed or released the restraint. Report your observations and the care given. Follow agency policy for recording. See "Reporting and Recording," p. 213.

FOCUS ON COMMUNICATION

Safety Guidelines

Restraints can increase confusion. Remind the person of the reason for the restraint and to call for help when it is needed. Do so as often as needed. For example:

- "Your doctor ordered this restraint so you don't hurt yourself. If you need to get up, please call for help. I'll check on you every 15 minutes. Other staff will check on you too."
- "How does the restraint feel? Is it too tight? Is it too loose?"

- "Please put your call light on. I want to make sure that you can reach and use it with the restraint on."
- "Please call for help right away if the restraint is too tight."
- "Please call for help right away if you feel pain in your fingers or hands. Also call for me if you feel numbness or tingling."
- "Please call for help right away if you are having problems breathing."
- "Please use your call light if you need anything."

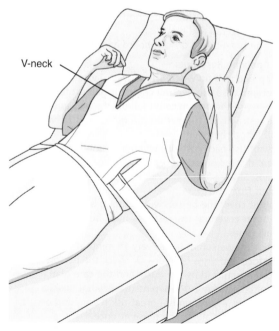

FIGURE 15-3 Vest restraint. The "V" neck is in front.

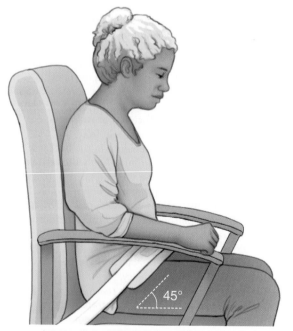

FIGURE 15-4 The belt restraint is at a 45-degree angle over the thighs.

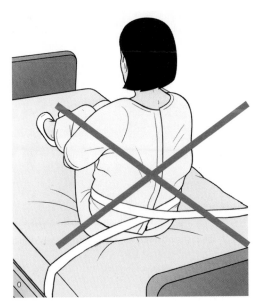

FIGURE 15-5 Never criss-cross vest or jacket straps in the back.

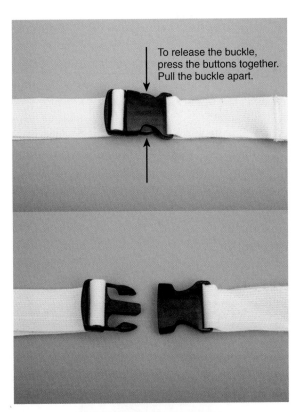

FIGURE 15-6 Quick release buckle.

To release the buckle, press the buttons together. Pull the buckle apart.

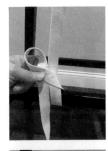

1 Wrap the strap around an area out of the person's reach—a moveable part of the bed frame or below the chair or wheelchair seat.

Cross the loose end over the front of the strap.

Make a loop.

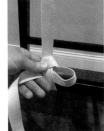

2 Pass the loop through the area where the strap crosses.

Pull to tighten.

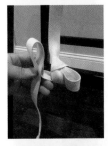

3 Make a second loop with the loose end.

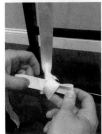

4 Pass the second loop through the first loop.

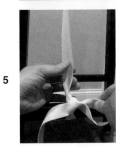

5 Pull to tighten.

Check that the strap is secure.

To untie, pull the loose end.

FIGURE 15-7 Quick release knot.

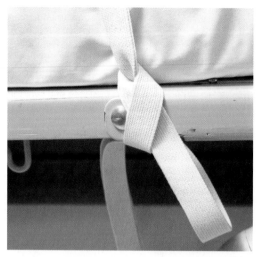

FIGURE 15-8 The restraint is secured to the movable part of the bed frame.

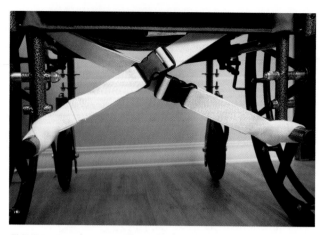

FIGURE 15-9 The restraint straps are secured to the wheelchair frame.

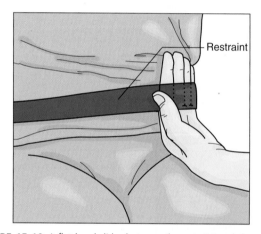

FIGURE 15-10 A flat hand slides between the restraint and the person.

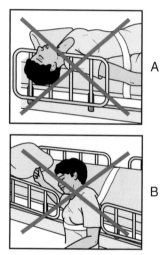

FIGURE 15-11 A, A person can get suspended and caught between bed rail bars. B, The person can get suspended and caught between half-length bed rails.

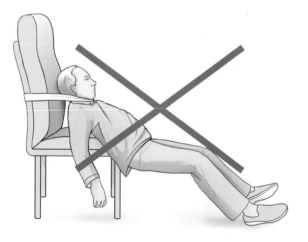

FIGURE 15-12 Strangulation can result if the person slides forward or down because of extra slack in the restraint.

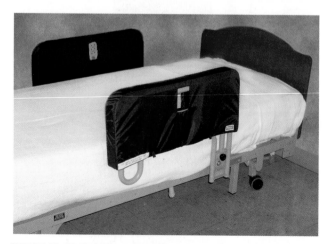

FIGURE 15-13 Bed rail protector. (From Perry AG, Potter PA, Ostendorf WR: *Clinical nursing skills & techniques,* ed 9, St Louis, 2018, Elsevier.)

Reporting and Recording

Restraint information is recorded in the person's medical record (Fig. 15-14). If you apply restraints or care for a restrained person, report and record:

- The type of restraint applied
- The body part or parts restrained
- Safety measures taken (for example, bed rails padded and up, call light within reach)
- The time you applied the restraint
- The time you removed or released the restraint and for how long
- The person's vital signs
- The care given when the restraint was removed and for how long
- Skin color and condition
- Condition of the extremities
- The pulse felt in the restrained part
- Changes in the person's behavior
  Report the following complaints at once.
- Difficulty breathing
- Pain, numbness, or tingling in the restrained part
- Discomfort
- A tight restraint

Applying Restraints

Restraints are made of cloth or leather. Cloth restraints (soft restraints) are mitts, belts, straps, jackets, and vests. They are applied to the wrists, hands, waist, and chest. Leather restraints are applied to the wrists and ankles. Sometimes leather restraints are applied to 5 points: wrists (2), ankles (2), and to the thighs, pelvis, or chest (1). Leather restraints are used for extreme agitation and combativeness.

Limb Holders. Limb holders limit arm or leg movement (Fig. 15-15, p. 214). They may be applied to the wrists when the person:

- Is at risk for pulling out tubes used for life-saving treatment (intravenous [IV] infusion, feeding tube).
- Is at risk for pulling at devices that monitor vital signs.
- Scratches at, pulls at, picks at, or peels the skin, a wound, or a dressing. This can damage the skin or the wound.

Limb holders may be applied to the ankles to limit leg movement.

Mitt Restraints. Hands are placed in mitt restraints. They prevent finger use. They allow hand, wrist, and arm movements. They have the same purpose as wrist restraints. Most mitts are padded (Fig. 15-16, p. 214).

RESTRAINT MONITORING

Restraint Type and Location

☐ Limb holder		☒ Mitt		☐ Elbow splint	
☐ Right wrist	☐ Right ankle	☒ Right wrist		☐ Right arm	
☐ Left wrist	☐ Left ankle	☒ Left wrist		☐ Left arm	

☐ Belt	☐ Vest	☐ Jacket	☐ Other:

Care Measures

☒ Restraints released/removed	☒ Food/fluid needs met	☒ Comfort measures
Duration: 15 minutes	☒ ROM/exercise/activity	☒ Skin care
☒ Restraints re-applied	☒ Urinary/bowel elimination	☒ Hygiene
☐ Measures refused	☒ Positioning	☐ Other:
Notified nurse: E. Scott, RN	☒ Call light and needed items in reach	

Vital Signs

Temp 98.4 °F	Pulse 70	R 14	BP 116 / 72 mmHg	Pain 0 /10

Circulation Observations (Normal in blue)

Color: ☒ Pink ☐ Pale ☐ Cyanotic (bluish)	**Tell the nurse at once if any observations are abnormal.**
Temperature: ☐ Hot ☒ Warm ☐ Cool ☐ Cold	
Sensation: ☒ Good sensation ☐ Numbness/tingling ☐ No sensation	Notified nurse:
Movement: ☒ Able to move extremities ☐ Unable to move extremities	
Pulses: ☒ Pulses present in all extremities ☐ Pulse faint/absent in any extremity	

Behavior Observations

☒ Alert	☐ Agitated	☐ Restless	☐ Drowsy
☒ Calm/cooperative	☐ Aggressive	☐ Confused	☐ Sleeping

FIGURE 15-14 Charting sample.

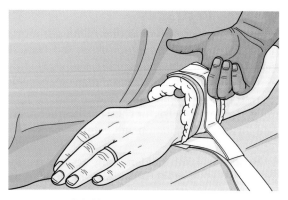

FIGURE 15-15 Limb holder. The soft part is toward the skin. Note that 1 finger fits between the holder and the wrist.

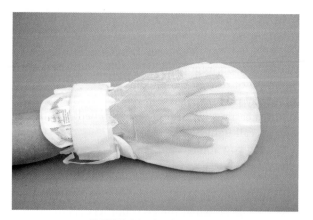

FIGURE 15-16 Mitt restraint.

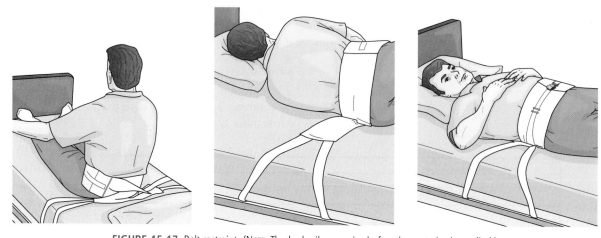

FIGURE 15-17 Belt restraint. (NOTE: The bed rails are raised after the restraint is applied.)

Belt Restraints. Belt restraints (Fig. 15-17) may be used for persons at risk for injuries from falls. The person cannot get out of bed or out of a chair. However, the person can turn from side to side or sit up in bed.

The belt is applied around the waist and secured to the bed or chair (lap belt). It is applied over a garment. The person can release the quick release type. It is less restrictive than those that only staff can release.

Vest Restraints and Jacket Restraints. Vest and jacket restraints are applied to the chest. They have the same purpose as belt restraints. The person cannot turn in bed or get out of a chair.

A jacket restraint is applied with the opening in the back. For a vest restraint, the "V" neck is in front. If needed, the vest crosses in the front (Fig. 15-18). The restraint is always applied over a garment. (NOTE: The straps of vest and jacket restraints cross in the front. A vest or jacket restraint may have positioning slots in the back [Fig. 15-19]. If so, criss-cross straps following the manufacturer's instructions.)

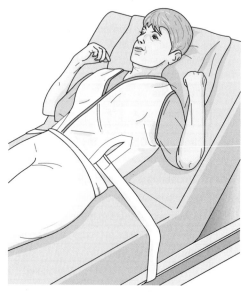

FIGURE 15-18 This vest restraint criss-crosses in front. (NOTE: The bed rails are raised after the restraint is applied.)

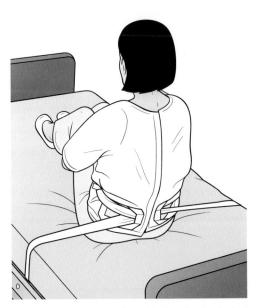

FIGURE 15-19 Jacket restraint with positioning slots in the back. (NOTE: The bed rails are raised after the restraint is applied.)

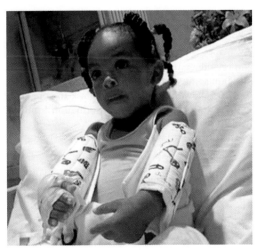

FIGURE 15-20 Elbow splints. (From Hockenberry MJ, Wilson D, Rodgers CC: *Wong's nursing care of infants and children*, ed 11, St Louis, 2019, Elsevier.)

Vest and jacket restraints have life-threatening risks if the person slides down in the bed or chair. Death can occur from strangulation. If caught in the restraint, it can become so tight that the person's chest cannot expand to inhale air. The person quickly suffocates and dies. Correct application is critical. You are advised to only assist the nurse in applying them. The nurse should have full responsibility for applying a vest or jacket restraint.

See *Focus on Communication: Applying Restraints.*
See *Focus on Children and Older Persons: Applying Restraints.*
See *Delegation Guidelines: Applying Restraints*, p. 216.
See *Promoting Safety and Comfort: Applying Restraints*, p. 216.
See procedure: *Applying Restraints*, p. 217.

FOCUS ON **COMMUNICATION**

Applying Restraints

If you do not know how to apply a certain restraint, do not do so. Ask the nurse to show you the correct way. You can say: "I've never applied this restraint before. Would you please show me how and then watch me apply it?" Thank the nurse for helping you.

Explain to the person what you are going to do. Then tell the person what you are doing step-by-step. Always check for safety and comfort. You can ask: "How does the restraint feel? Is it too tight? Is it too loose?"

Place the call light within reach. Make sure the person can use it with the restraint on. Remind the person to call if uncomfortable or if anything is needed.

FOCUS ON **CHILDREN AND OLDER PERSONS**

Applying Restraints

Children
Elbow splints limit arm movements. They prevent infants and children from bending their elbows (Fig. 15-20). They prevent scratching and touching incisions or pulling out tubes. Both arms are restrained to achieve the desired effect.

Older Persons
Restraints may increase confusion and agitation in persons with dementia. They do not understand what is happening. They may resist your efforts to apply a restraint. They may try to get free from the restraint. Serious injury and death are risks.

See *Promoting Safety and Comfort: Applying Restraints*, p. 216.

DELEGATION GUIDELINES

Applying Restraints

Applying restraints may be considered a nursing responsibility (Chapter 4) in some agencies. You may assist the nurse or the nurse may be allowed to delegate the task to you. Before applying a restraint, you need this information from the nurse and the care plan.

- Why the doctor ordered the restraint.
- What type and size to use.
- Where to apply the restraint.
- How to safely apply the restraint. Have the nurse show you how to apply it. Then show correct application back to the nurse.
- How to correctly position the person.
- What bony areas to pad and how to pad them.
- If bed rail covers or gap protectors are needed.
- If bed rails are up or down.
- What special equipment is needed.
- If the person needs to be checked more often than every 15 minutes. If yes, how often?
- When to apply and release the restraint.
- What observations to report and record. See "Reporting and Recording," p. 213.
- When to report observations.
- What patient or resident concerns to report at once.

PROMOTING SAFETY AND COMFORT

Applying Restraints

Safety

Restraints can cause serious harm, even death. Always follow the manufacturer's instructions for the restraint ordered. Instructions for 1 restraint may not apply to another. Also, the manufacturer may have instructions for applying restraints on persons who are agitated.

Never use force. Ask a co-worker to help if a person is confused and agitated. Report problems to the nurse at once.

Check the person at least every 15 minutes or more often as directed by the nurse and the care plan. Make sure the call light is within reach. Ask the person to use the call light at the first sign of problems or discomfort.

Never use a restraint as a seat belt in a car or other vehicle.

Mitt Restraints

Mitt restraints prevent finger use. Often they are not secured to the bed or chair. Therefore the person can raise the mitt to his or her mouth. Observe the person closely so that he or she does not:

- Use the teeth to remove or damage the device.
- Ingest any mitt material.

Persons with mitt restraints may be able to walk about. Falls are a risk. Practice safety measures to prevent falls (Chapter 14).

Belt, Vest, and Jacket Restraints

When a belt, vest, or jacket restraint is used, monitor the person so that he or she cannot:

- Slide forward or down in the chair or bed and become suspended or entrapped.
- Fall off the chair or mattress and become suspended or entrapped.

Comfort

Restraints limit movement. This affects position changes and reaching needed items. Position the person in good alignment before applying a restraint (Chapter 18). Make sure needed items are within reach—call light, water mug, tissues, phone, bed controls, and so on.

Applying Restraints

QUALITY OF LIFE

- Knock before entering the person's room.
- Address the person by name.
- Introduce yourself by name and title.

- Explain the procedure before starting and during the procedure.
- Protect the person's rights during the procedure.
- Handle the person gently during the procedure.

PRE-PROCEDURE

1 Follow *Delegation Guidelines: Applying Restraints.* See *Promoting Safety and Comfort:*
   a *Safe Restraint Use,* p. 206
   b *Applying Restraints*
2 Collect the following as instructed by the nurse.
   - Correct type and size of restraint
   - Padding for skin and bony areas
   - Bed rail pads or gap protectors (if needed)

3 Practice hand hygiene.
4 Identify the person. Check the ID (identification) bracelet against the assignment sheet. Use 2 identifiers (Chapter 13). Also call the person by name.
5 Provide for privacy.

PROCEDURE

6 Position the person for comfort and good alignment.
7 Put the bed rail pads or gap protectors (if needed) on the bed for the person in bed. Follow the manufacturer's instructions.
8 Pad bony areas. Follow the nurse's instructions and the care plan.
9 Read and follow the manufacturer's instructions. Note the front and back of the restraint.
10 *For limb holders to the wrists:*
   a Place the soft or foam part toward the skin.
   b Secure the holder so it is snug but not tight. Make sure you can slide 1 finger under the holder (see Fig. 15-15). Adjust the straps if the holder is too loose or too tight. Check for snugness again.
   c Secure the straps to the movable part of the bed frame out of the person's reach. Use the buckle or a quick release knot.
   d Repeat step 10, a–c for the other wrist.
11 *For mitt restraints:*
   a Clean and dry the person's hands.
   b Insert the person's hand into the restraint with the palm down.
   c Wrap the wrist strap around the smallest part of the wrist. Secure the strap with the hook-and-loop or other closure.
   d Secure the restraint to the bed if directed to do so. Secure the straps to the movable part of the bed frame out of the person's reach. Use the buckle or a quick release knot.
   e Check for snugness. Slide 1 finger between the restraint and the wrist. Adjust the straps if the restraint is too loose or too tight. Check for snugness again.
   f Repeat step 11, b–e for the other hand.

12 *For a belt restraint:*
   a Assist the person to a sitting position.
   b Apply the restraint.
   c Remove wrinkles or creases from the front and back.
   d Bring the ties through the slots in the belt.
   e Position the straps at a 45-degree angle between the wheelchair seat and sides (see Fig. 15-4). If in bed, help the person lie down.
   f Make sure the person is comfortable and in good alignment.
   g Secure the straps to the movable part of the bed frame. Use the buckle or a quick release knot. The buckle or knot is out of the person's reach. For a wheelchair, criss-cross and secure the straps as in Figure 15-9.
   h Check for snugness. Slide an open hand between the restraint and the person. Adjust the restraint if it is too loose or too tight. Check for snugness again.
13 *For a vest restraint:*
   a Assist the person to a sitting position. If in a wheelchair:
      1) The person is as far back in the wheelchair as possible.
      2) The buttocks are against the chair back.
   b Apply the restraint. The "V" neck is in the front.
   c Bring the straps through the slots if the vest criss-crosses (see Fig 15-18).
   d Make sure side seams are under the arms. Remove wrinkles in the front and back. Close the zipper if the device opens in the back. Or fasten with other closures.
   e Position the straps at a 45-degree angle between the wheelchair seat and sides. If in bed, help the person lie down.
   f Make sure the person is comfortable and in good alignment.
   g Secure the straps to the movable part of the bed frame at waist level. Use the buckle or a quick release knot. The buckle or knot is out of the person's reach. For a wheelchair, criss-cross and secure the straps as in Figure 15-9.
   h Check for snugness. Slide an open hand between the restraint and the person. Adjust the restraint if it is too loose or too tight. Check for snugness again.

Continued

Applying Restraints—cont'd

PROCEDURE—cont'd

14 *For a jacket restraint:*
a Assist the person to a sitting position. If in a wheelchair:
1) The person is as far back in the wheelchair as possible.
2) The buttocks are against the chair back.
b Apply the restraint. The jacket opening goes in the back.
c Make sure the side seams are under the arms. Remove wrinkles in the front and back.
d Close the back with the zipper or other closures.
e Position the straps at a 45-degree angle between the wheelchair seat and sides. If in bed, help the person lie down.
f Make sure the person is comfortable and in good alignment.
g Secure the straps to the movable part of the bed frame at waist level. Use the buckle or a quick release knot. The buckle or knot is out of the person's reach. For a wheelchair, criss-cross and secure the straps as in Figure 15-9.
h Check for snugness. Slide an open hand between the restraint and the person. Adjust the restraint if it is too loose or too tight. Check for snugness again.

15 *For elbow splints:*
a Release the adjustment straps (hook-and-loop).
b Place the buckles toward the person.
c Wrap a splint over 1 arm. The splint is centered over the elbow. The opening is toward the inside of the arm.
d Secure the splint following the manufacturer's instructions. Use the clips provided by the manufacturer if securing the splint to a sleeve.
e Check for snugness. Follow the manufacturer's instructions. Adjust the splint if it is too loose or too tight. Check for snugness again.
f Repeat step 15, a–e for the other arm.

POST-PROCEDURE

16 Position the person as the nurse directs.
17 Provide for comfort. (See the inside of the back cover.)
18 Place the call light and other needed items within the person's reach.
19 Raise or lower bed rails. Follow the care plan and the manufacturer's instructions for the restraint.
20 Unscreen the person.
21 Complete a safety check of the room. (See the inside of the back cover.)
22 Practice hand hygiene.
23 Check the person and the restraint at least every 15 minutes or more often as directed by the nurse and the care plan. Report and record your observations.
a *For wrist holders, mitt restraints, or elbow splints:* check the pulse, color, and temperature of the restrained parts.
b *For a vest, jacket, or belt restraint:* check the person's breathing. Make sure the restraint is properly positioned in the front and back. *Release the restraint and call for the nurse at once if the person is not breathing or is having problems breathing.*

24 Do the following at least every 2 hours for at least 10 minutes.
a Remove or release the restraint.
b Measure vital signs.
c Re-position the person.
d Meet food, fluid, hygiene, and elimination needs.
e Give skin care.
f Perform ROM exercises or help the person walk. Follow the care plan.
g Provide for physical and emotional comfort. (See the inside of the back cover.)
h Re-apply the restraint.
25 Complete a safety check of the room. (See the inside of the back cover.)
26 Practice hand hygiene.
27 Report and record your observations and the care given.

FOCUS ON **PRIDE**

The Person, Family, and Yourself

Personal and Professional Responsibility

Restraints have many risks. See Box 15-2. Therefore restraint use brings many responsibilities. You must:

- Promote safety and comfort.
- Apply the restraint properly.
- Observe the person closely.
- Meet basic needs.
- Report any concerns to the nurse.

Rights and Respect

You may be asked to assist with restraint alternatives (see Box 15-1). Make a true effort. Be honest. Do not tell the nurse you tried if you did not. Do your best to allow the person the right to freedom from restraint.

Independence and Social Interaction

All restraints limit movement. Independence is restricted. To promote independence:

- Keep the call light within reach at all times. Make sure the person can use it. Tell the person to signal for you if anything is needed. Answer the call light and meet the person's needs promptly.
- Keep needed items within reach. This is most important with restraints that allow hand and arm use. Belt, vest, and jacket restraints and elbow splints are examples.
- Allow choice. For example, let the person choose what to eat and drink when you release the restraint and meet needs.
- Let the person do as much as is safely possible.

Personal choice and freedom of movement promote independence, dignity, and self-esteem. Provide care that gives restrained persons the independence they deserve.

Delegation and Teamwork

Care conferences are held to meet the person's safety needs. Your input has value. Share your observations and ideas. For example, a person does not try to get out of a chair when looking at photos or reading a book. You share this with the team for the person's care plan.

Ethics and Laws

Imagine the following.

- You need to use the bathroom. Your arms are restrained. You cannot get up or use your call light. You soil yourself with urine.
- You are uncomfortable. You have a vest restraint. You cannot move or turn in bed.
- You are thirsty. Your wrists are restrained. You cannot reach the water mug.
- You hear the fire alarm. You have on a restraint. You cannot get up to move to a safe place. You must wait to be rescued.

What would you do? Would you calmly lie or sit there? Would you try to get free from the restraint? Would you yell for help? Would the staff think that you are uncomfortable? Or would they think that you are agitated and uncooperative? Would you feel angry, embarrassed, or humiliated?

Ethics deals with how others are treated. Treat the person like you would want to be treated—with kindness, caring, respect, and dignity.

FOCUS ON **PRIDE**: *Application*

Describe 3 scenarios involving behavior that is dangerous or that interferes with treatment. List ideas for managing the behavior without using restraints.

REVIEW QUESTIONS

*Circle **T** if the statement is TRUE or **F** if it is FALSE.*

1 T F Restraint alternatives fail to protect a person. You can apply a restraint.

2 T F A restraint restricts a person's freedom of movement.

3 T F Some drugs are restraints.

4 T F Restraints can be used for staff convenience.

5 T F A device is a restraint only if it is attached to the person's body.

6 T F Bed rails are restraints if they cannot be lowered. The person cannot leave the bed.

7 T F Restraints are used only for a person's specific medical symptom.

8 T F Unnecessary restraint is false imprisonment.

9 T F You can apply restraints when you think they are needed.

10 T F You can use a vest restraint to position a person on the toilet.

11 T F Restraints are removed or released at least every 2 hours.

12 T F Restraints are tied to bed rails.

13 T F Wrist holders are used to prevent falls.

14 T F The "V" neck on a vest restraint is in front.

15 T F Bed rails are left down when a vest restraint is used.

Circle the BEST answer.

16 Which is a restraint alternative?
   a Positioning the person's chair close to the wall
   b Raising all bed rails
   c Giving a drug that restricts movement
   d Padding walls and corners of furniture

17 Physical restraints
   a Can be removed easily by the person
   b Are not allowed by the CMS
   c Require a doctor's order
   d Are safer than chemical restraints

Continued

REVIEW QUESTIONS—cont'd

18 The following can occur from restraints. Which is the *most* serious?
   a Fractures
   b Strangulation
   c Pressure injuries
   d Urinary tract infections

19 A belt restraint is applied to a person in bed. Where are the straps secured?
   a To the bed rails
   b To the head-board
   c To the movable part of the bed frame
   d To the foot-board

20 A person has a restraint. You check the person and the position of the restraint at least every
   a 15 minutes
   b 30 minutes
   c Hour
   d 3 hours

21 A person has mitt restraints. Which will you report to the nurse at once?
   a The hands are clean, warm, and dry.
   b The person has numbness in the hands.
   c You removed the restraints for 10 minutes.
   d You felt a pulse in both arms.

22 When applying restraints, you should
   a Know when to apply and release them
   b Use force if the person is agitated
   c Allow plenty of slack in the straps
   d Apply a restraint you have not used before

23 A person has a vest restraint. To check for snugness, slide
   a A fist between the vest and the person
   b 1 finger between the vest and the person
   c An open hand between the vest and the person
   d 2 fingers between the vest and the person

24 The correct way to apply any restraint is to follow the
   a Nurse's directions
   b Doctor's orders
   c Care plan
   d Manufacturer's instructions

Answers to Chapter 15 questions are on p. 885.

FOCUS ON PRACTICE

Problem Solving

A person uses a wheelchair and often tries to get up without help. What are some alternatives to restraints that may be tried? If a restraint is needed, how will you provide for the person's basic needs?

Preventing Infection

OBJECTIVES

- Define the key terms and key abbreviations in this chapter.
- Identify what microbes need to live and grow.
- List the signs and symptoms of infection.
- Explain the chain of infection.
- Describe healthcare-associated infections and the persons at risk.
- Describe the principles of medical asepsis.
- Explain the rules of hand hygiene.
- Explain how to care for equipment and supplies.
- Describe disinfection and sterilization methods.
- Explain the Bloodborne Pathogen Standard.
- Explain the principles of surgical asepsis.
- Perform the procedures described in this chapter.
- Explain how to promote PRIDE in the person, the family, and yourself.

KEY TERMS

antibiotic A drug that kills certain microbes that cause infection

antisepsis The processes, procedures, and chemical treatments that kill microbes or prevent them from causing an infection; *anti* means *against* and *sepsis* means *infection*

asepsis The absence *(a)* of disease-producing microbes; *sepsis* means *infection*

carrier A human or animal that is a reservoir for microbes but does not develop the infection

clean technique See "medical asepsis"

contamination The process of becoming unclean

cross-contamination Passing microbes from 1 person to another by contaminated hands, equipment, or supplies

disinfectant A liquid chemical that can kill many or all pathogens except spores

disinfection The process of killing pathogens

healthcare-associated infection (HAI) An infection that develops in a person cared for in any setting where health care is given; the infection is related to receiving health care

immunity Protection against a certain disease

infection A disease state resulting from the invasion and growth of microbes in the body

infection control Practices and procedures that prevent the spread of infection

medical asepsis Practices used to reduce the number of microbes and prevent their spread from 1 person or place to another person or place; clean technique

microbe See "microorganism"

microorganism A small *(micro)* living thing *(organism)* seen only with a microscope; microbe

non-pathogen A microbe that does not usually cause an infection

normal flora Microbes that live and grow in a certain area

pathogen A microbe that is harmful and can cause an infection

spore A bacterium protected by a hard shell

sterile The absence of *all* microbes

sterile field A work area free of *all* pathogens and non-pathogens (including spores)

sterile technique See "surgical asepsis"

sterilization The process of destroying *all* microbes

surgical asepsis The practices used to remove *all* microbes; sterile technique

vaccination Giving a vaccine to produce immunity against an infectious disease

vaccine A preparation containing dead or weakened microbes

vector A carrier (animal, insect) that transmits disease

vehicle Any substance that transmits microbes

KEY ABBREVIATIONS

AIDS	Acquired immunodeficiency syndrome		HIV	Human immunodeficiency virus
C. diff	Clostridioides difficile; Clostridium difficile		MDRO	Multidrug-resistant organism
cm	Centimeter		MRSA	Methicillin-resistant Staphylococcus aureus
EPA	Environmental Protection Agency		OPIM	Other potentially infectious materials
GI	Gastro-intestinal		OSHA	Occupational Safety and Health Administration
HAI	Healthcare-associated infection		PPE	Personal protective equipment
HBV	Hepatitis B virus		VRE	Vancomycin-resistant Enterococci

An *infection is a disease state resulting from the invasion and growth of microbes in the body.* Infection is a major safety and health hazard. Minor infections are short-term. Some infections are serious and can cause death. Infants, older persons, and disabled persons are at risk. Certain *practices and procedures prevent the spread of infection (infection control).* The goal is to protect patients, residents, visitors, and staff from infection.

This chapter includes measures of antisepsis. *Antisepsis is the processes, procedures, and chemical treatments that kill microbes or prevent them from causing an infection.* (Anti *means* against. Sepsis *means* infection.)

MICROORGANISMS

A *microorganism (microbe) is a small* (micro) *living thing* (organism) *seen only with a microscope.* Commonly called *germs*, microbes are everywhere—mouth, nose, respiratory tract, stomach, and intestines. They are on the skin and in the air, soil, water, and food. They are on animals, clothing, and furniture.

Microbes that are harmful and can cause infections are called **pathogens. Non-pathogens** *are microbes that do not usually cause an infection.*

Types of Microbes

There are 5 types of microbes.
- *Bacteria*—1-celled organisms that multiply rapidly. They can cause an infection in any body system.
- *Fungi*—plant-like organisms that live on other plants or animals. Mushrooms, yeasts, and mold are common fungi. Fungi can infect the mouth, vagina, skin, feet, and other body areas.
- *Protozoa*—1-celled animals. They can infect the blood, brain, intestines, and other body areas.
- *Rickettsiae*—found in fleas, lice, ticks, and other insects. They are spread to humans by insect bites. Rocky Mountain spotted fever is an example. The person has fever, chills, headache, and rash.
- *Viruses*—grow in living cells. They cause many diseases including the common cold, herpes, acquired immunodeficiency syndrome (AIDS), and hepatitis.

Requirements of Microbes

Microbes need a reservoir to live and grow. The *reservoir* (host) is the place where a microbe lives and grows. People, plants, animals, the soil, food, and water are common reservoirs. Microbes need *water* and *nourishment* from the reservoir. Most need *oxygen* to live. A *warm* and *dark* environment is needed. Most grow best at body temperature. They are destroyed by heat and light.

Normal Flora

Normal flora are microbes that live and grow in a certain area. Certain microbes are in the respiratory tract, in the intestines, and on the skin. They are non-pathogens when in or on a natural reservoir. When a non-pathogen is transmitted from its natural site to another site or host, it becomes a pathogen. For example, *Escherichia coli (E. coli)* is normally in the colon. If it enters the urinary system, it can cause an infection.

Multidrug-Resistant Organisms

Multidrug-resistant organisms (MDROs) are microbes that can resist the effects of antibiotics. *Antibiotics are drugs that kill certain microbes that cause infections.* Some microbes can change their structures, making them harder to kill. They can live in the presence of antibiotics. Therefore the infections they cause are hard to treat.

MDROs are caused by prescribing antibiotics when not needed (over-prescribing). Not taking antibiotics for the days prescribed is another cause. Common MDROs are:
- *Methicillin-resistant Staphylococcus aureus (MRSA). Staphylococcus aureus* ("staph") is found in the nose and on the skin. MRSA is resistant to antibiotics often used for "staph" infections. MRSA can cause serious wound and bloodstream infections and pneumonia.
- *Vancomycin-resistant Enterococci (VRE). Enterococcus* is found in the intestines and in feces. It can be transmitted to others by contaminated hands, toilet seats, care equipment, and other items that the hands touch. When not in the intestines, enterococci can cause urinary tract, wound, pelvic, and other infections. Enterococci resistant to vancomycin (an antibiotic) are called *vancomycin-resistant Enterococci* (VRE).

INFECTION

A *local infection* is in a body part. A *systemic infection* involves the whole body. *(Systemic* means *entire.)* The person has some or all of the signs and symptoms listed in Box 16-1.

See *Focus on Children and Older Persons: Infection.*

See *Focus on Surveys: Infection.*

BOX 16-1 **Infection—Signs and Symptoms**

- *Fever* (elevated body temperature)
- Pulse and respirations: increased
- Chills
- Pain, tenderness, or limited use of a body part
- Fatigue and loss of energy
- Appetite: loss of *(anorexia)*
- Nausea and vomiting
- Diarrhea
- Rash
- Sores on mucous membranes
- Redness and swelling of a body part
- Discharge or drainage from the infected area
- Heat or warmth in a body part
- Headache
- Muscle aches
- Joint pain
- Confusion

FOCUS ON CHILDREN AND OLDER PERSONS

Infection

Older Persons

The immune system protects the body from disease and infection (Chapter 10). Changes occur in this system with aging making older persons at risk for infection.

An older person may not show the signs and symptoms in Box 16-1. The person may have a slight fever or no fever at all. Redness and swelling may be very slight. The person may not complain of pain. Confusion and delirium may occur (Chapter 53).

An infection can be life-threatening before the older person shows signs and symptoms. Report minor behavior or condition changes at once.

Healing takes longer in older persons. Therefore an infection can prolong rehabilitation. Independence and quality of life are affected.

FOCUS ON SURVEYS

Infection

Infection control practices are a focus of surveys. You may be asked about the signs and symptoms of infection.
- What you do when you observe them
- Who do you tell

The Chain of Infection

The chain of infection (Fig. 16-1) involves a:
- Source—A pathogen.
- Reservoir—The pathogen needs a place to grow and multiply. A *carrier is a human or animal that is a reservoir for microbes but does not develop the infection.* Carriers can pass pathogens to others. A *vector is a carrier (animal, insect) that transmits disease.* Common vectors are:
  - Dogs—carry rabies
  - Mosquitoes—carry malaria
  - Ticks—carry Rocky Mountain spotted fever
  - Mites—cause scabies (Chapter 25)
- Portal of exit—The pathogen needs a way to leave the reservoir. Exits are the respiratory, gastro-intestinal (GI), urinary, and reproductive tracts; breaks in the skin; and blood.
- Method of transmission—The pathogen is *transmitted* to another host (Fig. 16-2, p. 224). A *vehicle is any substance that transmits microbes.*
- Portal of entry—The pathogen enters the body. Portals of entry and exit are the same—the respiratory, GI, urinary, and reproductive tracts; breaks in the skin; and blood.
- Susceptible host—The transmitted microbe needs a host where it can grow and multiply. Susceptible hosts are at risk for infection.

Susceptible Hosts. Susceptible hosts include persons who:
- Are very young or who are older.
- Are ill.
- Were exposed to the pathogen.
- Do not follow practices to prevent infection.

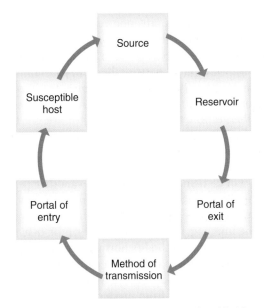

FIGURE 16-1 The chain of infection. (Redrawn and modified from Potter PA, Perry AG, Stockert PA, Hall AM: *Fundamentals of nursing,* ed 9, St Louis, 2017, Elsevier.)

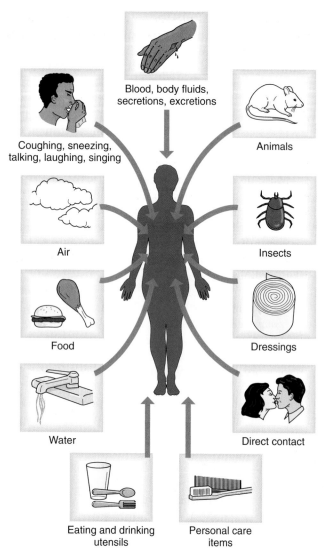

FIGURE 16-2 Methods of transmitting microbes.

Healthcare-Associated Infections

A *healthcare-associated infection (HAI) is an infection that develops in a person cared for in any setting where health care is given* (Box 16-2). *The infection is related to receiving health care.* Hospitals, nursing centers, clinics, and home care settings are examples. HAIs also are called nosocomial infections. (*Nosocomial* comes from the Greek word for *hospital.*)

HAIs are caused by normal flora. Or they are caused by microbes from other sources. For example, *E. coli* is normally in the colon and feces. Poor wiping after bowel movements can cause *E. coli* to enter the urinary system. With poor hand-washing, *E. coli* spreads to any body part, thing, or person the hands touch.

Microbes can enter the body from care equipment and supplies. Such items must be free of microbes. Staff can transfer microbes from 1 person to another and from themselves to others. Common sites for HAIs are:

* The urinary system
* The respiratory system
* Wounds and surgical sites
* The bloodstream

Patients and residents are weak from disease or injury. Some have wounds or open skin areas. Infants and older persons have a hard time fighting infections. The health team must prevent infection by:

* Medical asepsis. This includes hand hygiene.
* Surgical asepsis, p. 236.
* Standard Precautions, Chapter 17.
* Transmission-Based Precautions, Chapter 17.
* The Bloodborne Pathogen Standard, p. 233.

See *Focus on Long-Term Care and Home Care: Healthcare-Associated Infections.*

The ability to resist infection relates to age, nutrition, stress, fatigue, and health. Drugs, disease, and injury also are factors. Severe infection can be deadly for:

* *Burn patients.* Burns destroy the skin, providing a portal of entry for microbes. Microbes are from the person's normal flora (p. 222), the health care setting, and the health team. MRSA and VRE are great concerns. Burns affect the immune system (Chapter 10) and the ability to fight infection.
* *Transplant patients.* A *transplant* involves transferring an organ or tissue from 1 person to another person or from 1 body part to another body part. Kidney, liver, heart, lung, bone, and skin transplants are examples. To the immune system, the new organ or tissue is a foreign object. The body's normal immune response is to attack (reject) the new organ or tissue. Drugs are given to prevent rejection. They suppress (prevent) the immune system from producing antibodies. Antibodies are needed to fight infection.
* *Chemotherapy patients.* Some chemotherapy drugs given to treat cancer affect the production of white blood cells (WBCs). WBCs are needed to fight infection.

BOX 16-2	**Healthcare-Associated Infections—Examples**

* *Clostridioides difficile* (also known as *Clostridium difficile* or *C. diff*)—Chapter 29
* Gastro-intestinal infections
* Hepatitis A, B, and C—Chapter 50
* Human immunodeficiency virus—Chapter 47
* Influenza—Chapter 49
* Methicillin-resistant *Staphylococcus aureus*—p. 222
* Tuberculosis—Chapter 49
* Vancomycin-resistant *Enterococci*—p. 222

Modified from Centers for Disease Control and Prevention: Healthcare-associated infections (HAI): diseases and organisms in healthcare settings, Atlanta, page reviewed October 7, 2019.

ASEPSIS

Asepsis is the absence (a) *of disease-producing microbes.* (*Sepsis means* infection.) Microbes are everywhere. Measures are needed to achieve asepsis. *Medical asepsis (clean technique) is the practices used to:*

- *Reduce the number of microbes.*
- *Prevent microbes from spreading from 1 person or place to another person or place.*

Microbes cannot be present during surgery or on instruments inserted into the body. Open wounds (cuts, burns, incisions) require the absence of microbes. They are portals of entry for microbes. *Surgical asepsis (sterile technique) is the practices used to remove all microbes. Sterile means the absence of all microbes*—pathogens and non-pathogens. *Sterilization is the process of destroying all microbes* (pathogens and non-pathogens).

Contamination is the process of becoming unclean. In medical asepsis, an item or area is *clean* when it is free of pathogens. The item or area is *contaminated* when pathogens are present. A *sterile* item or area is *contaminated* when pathogens or non-pathogens are present. *Cross-contamination is passing microbes from 1 person to another by contaminated hands, equipment, or supplies* (Fig. 16-3). Medical asepsis and surgical asepsis (p. 236) prevent cross-contamination.

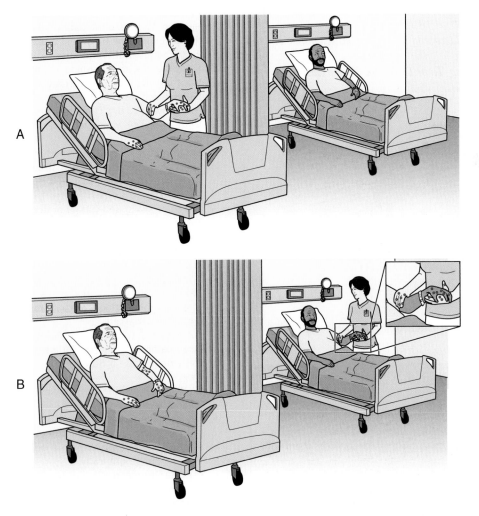

FIGURE 16-3 Cross-contamination. **A,** Microbes on the person's skin are transmitted to the nursing assistant's hands. **B,** The nursing assistant's contaminated hands transmit microbes from 1 person to another.

Common Aseptic Practices

Aseptic practices break the chain of infection. To prevent the spread of microbes, wash your hands:

- After elimination.
- After changing tampons or sanitary pads.
- After contact with your own or another person's blood, body fluids, secretions, or excretions. This includes saliva, vomitus, urine, feces (stools), vaginal discharge, mucus, semen, wound drainage, pus, and respiratory secretions.
- After coughing, sneezing, or blowing your nose.
- Before and after handling, preparing, or eating food.
- After smoking.

Also do the following.

- Provide all persons with their own linens and personal care items.
- Cover your nose and mouth when coughing, sneezing, or blowing your nose. If without tissues, cough or sneeze into your upper arm (Fig. 16-4). Do not cough or sneeze into your hands.
- Bathe, wash hair, and brush your teeth regularly.
- Wash fruit and raw vegetables before eating or serving them.
- Wash cooking and eating utensils with soap and water after use.

See *Focus on Children and Older Persons: Common Aseptic Practices.*

See *Focus on Long-Term Care and Home Care: Common Aseptic Practices.*

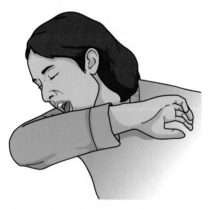

FIGURE 16-4 Sneezing into the upper arm.

Hand Hygiene

Hand hygiene is the easiest and most important way to prevent the spread of microbes and infection. You use your hands for almost everything. They are easily contaminated. They can spread microbes to other persons or items (see Fig. 16-3). *Practice hand hygiene before and after giving care.* See Box 16-3 for the rules of hand hygiene.

See *Focus on Surveys: Hand Hygiene.*

See *Promoting Safety and Comfort: Hand Hygiene.*

See procedure: *Hand-Washing,* p. 229.

See procedure: *Using an Alcohol-Based Hand Sanitizer,* p. 229.

Text continued on p. 230.

BOX 16-3	**Rules of Hand Hygiene**

- Wash your hands (with soap and water):
  - When they are visibly dirty or soiled with blood, body fluids, secretions, or excretions
  - Before eating and after using a restroom
  - After known or suspected exposure to *C. diff* (p. 224 and Chapter 29) or to persons with infectious diarrhea
  - If exposure to the anthrax spore is suspected or proven
  - If an alcohol-based hand sanitizer is not available
- Use an alcohol-based hand sanitizer for hand hygiene if your hands are not visibly soiled.
  - Before direct contact with a person.
  - After contact with the person's intact skin. After taking a pulse or blood pressure or after moving a person are examples.
  - After contact with body fluids or excretions, mucous membranes, non-intact skin, and wound dressings if hands are not visibly soiled.
  - When moving from a contaminated body site to a clean body site.
  - After contact with items in the person's care setting.
  - After removing gloves.
- Follow these rules for washing your hands with soap and water. See procedure: *Hand-Washing*, p. 229.
  - Wash your hands under warm running water. Do not use hot water.
  - Stand away from the sink. Do not let your hands, body, or uniform touch the sink. The sink is contaminated. See Figure 16-5, p. 228.
  - Do not touch the inside of the sink at any time.
  - Keep your hands and forearms lower than your elbows. If you hold your hands and forearms up, dirty water runs from your hands to your forearms and elbows. Those areas become contaminated.
- Rub your palms together (Fig. 16-6, p. 228) and interlace your fingers (Fig. 16-7, p. 228) to work up a good lather. The rubbing action helps remove microbes and dirt.
- Pay attention to areas often missed during hand-washing—thumbs, knuckles, sides of the hands, little fingers, and under the nails.
- Clean fingernails by rubbing the fingertips against your palms (Fig. 16-8, p. 228).
- Use a nail file or orangewood stick to clean under fingernails (Fig. 16-9, p. 228). Microbes grow easily under the fingernails.
- Wash your hands for at least 15 to 20 seconds. Wash longer if they are dirty or soiled with blood, body fluids, secretions, or excretions. Use your judgment and follow agency policy.
- Use clean, dry paper towels to dry your hands.
- Dry your hands starting at the fingertips. Work up to your forearms (Fig. 16-10, p. 228). You will dry the cleanest area first.
- Use a clean, dry paper towel for each faucet to turn the water off (Fig. 16-11, p. 229). Faucets are contaminated. The paper towels prevent you from contaminating your clean hands.
- Follow these rules when decontaminating your hands with an alcohol-based hand sanitizer. See procedure: *Using an Alcohol-Based Hand Sanitizer*, p. 229 and Figure 16-12, p. 230.
  - Apply the product to the palm of 1 hand. Follow the manufacturer's instructions for the amount to use.
  - Rub your hands together.
  - Cover all surfaces of your hands and fingers.
  - Continue rubbing your hands together until your hands are dry.
- Apply hand lotion or cream after hand hygiene. This prevents the skin from chapping and drying. Skin breaks can occur in chapped and dry skin. Skin breaks are portals of entry for microbes.

Modified from Centers for Disease Control and Prevention: Guidelines for hand hygiene in health-care settings, Morbidity and Mortality Weekly, *Report 51 (RR-16), October 2002.*

FOCUS ON **SURVEYS**

Hand Hygiene

Hand hygiene is a focus of surveys. A surveyor may:

- Observe you washing your hands or using an alcohol-based hand sanitizer according to agency policy.
- Observe if you practice hand hygiene:
  - After each direct patient or resident contact
  - Before and after all procedures
  - After removing gloves
  - When entering or leaving the room of a person on Transmission-Based Precautions (Chapter 17)
- Ask you questions about:
  - When you should wash your hands
  - When you can use an alcohol-based hand sanitizer

PROMOTING SAFETY AND COMFORT

Hand Hygiene

Safety

Hand hygiene is very important. You use your hands for almost every task. They can pick up microbes from a person, place, or thing. Your hands transfer them to other people, places, or things. Always practice hand hygiene before and after giving care.

Comfort

You will practice hand hygiene frequently during your shift. Hand lotions and hand creams help prevent chapping and dry skin. Use an agency-approved lotion or cream.

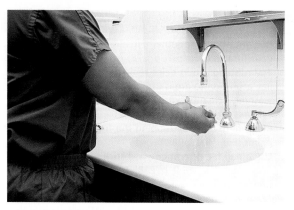

FIGURE 16-5 The uniform does not touch the sink. Hands are lower than the elbows. Hands do not touch the inside of the sink.

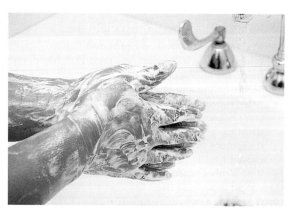

FIGURE 16-6 The palms are rubbed together to work up a good lather.

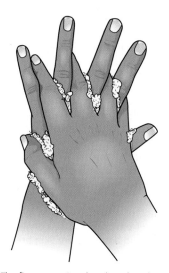

FIGURE 16-7 The fingers are interlaced to clean between the fingers.

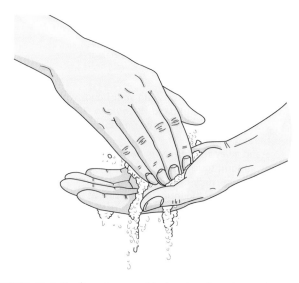

FIGURE 16-8 The fingertips are rubbed against the palms to clean under the fingernails.

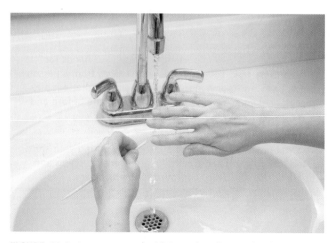

FIGURE 16-9 An orangewood stick is used to clean under the fingernails.

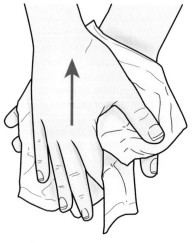

FIGURE 16-10 Hands are dried starting at the fingertips and working up to the forearms.

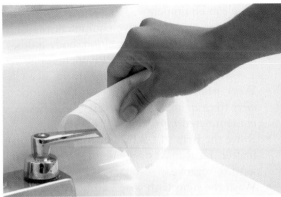
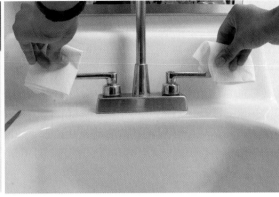

FIGURE 16-11 A paper towel is used to turn off each faucet.

Hand-Washing
PROCEDURE

1 See *Promoting Safety and Comfort: Hand Hygiene,* p. 227.
2 Make sure you have soap, paper towels, an orangewood stick or nail file, and a wastebasket. Collect missing items.
3 Push your watch up your arm 4 to 5 inches. Push long uniform sleeves up too.
4 Stand away from the sink so your clothes do not touch the sink (see Fig. 16-5). Stand so the soap and faucet are easy to reach. Do not touch the inside of the sink at any time.
5 Turn on and adjust the water until it feels warm.
6 Wet your wrists and hands. Keep your hands lower than your elbows. Be sure to wet the area 3 to 4 inches above your wrists.
7 Apply about 1 teaspoon of soap to your hands.
8 Rub your palms together and interlace your fingers to work up a good lather (see Fig. 16-6). Lather your wrists, hands, and fingers. Keep your hands lower than your elbows. This step should last at least 15 to 20 seconds.
9 Wash each hand and wrist thoroughly. Clean the back of your fingers and between your fingers (see Fig. 16-7).

10 Clean under the fingernails. Rub your fingertips against your palms (see Fig. 16-8).
11 Clean under the fingernails with a nail file or orangewood stick (see Fig. 16-9). Do this for the first hand-washing of the day and when your hands are highly soiled.
12 Rinse your wrists, hands, and fingers well. Water flows from above the wrists to your fingertips.
13 Repeat steps 7 through 12, if needed.
14 Dry your fingers, hands, and wrists with clean, dry paper towels. Pat dry starting at your fingertips (see Fig. 16-10).
15 Discard the paper towels into the wastebasket.
16 Turn off faucets with clean, dry paper towels. This prevents you from contaminating your hands (see Fig. 16-11). Use a clean paper towel for each faucet. Or use knee or foot controls to turn off the faucet.
17 Discard the paper towels into the wastebasket.

Using an Alcohol-Based Hand Sanitizer
PROCEDURE

1 See *Promoting Safety and Comfort: Hand Hygiene,* p. 227.
2 Apply a palmful of an alcohol-based hand sanitizer into a cupped hand (see Fig. 16-12, *A*).
3 Rub your palms together (see Fig. 16-12, *B*).
4 Rub the palm of 1 hand over the back of the other (see Fig. 16-12, *C*). Do the same for the other hand.
5 Rub your palms together with your fingers interlaced (see Fig. 16-12, *D*).

6 Interlock your fingers as in Figure 16-12, *E*. Rub your fingers back and forth.
7 Rub the thumb of 1 hand in the palm of the other (see Fig. 16-12, *F*). Do the same for the other thumb.
8 Rub the fingers of 1 hand into the palm of the other hand (see Fig. 16-12, *G*). Use a circular motion. Do the same for the fingers of the other hand.
9 Continue rubbing your hands until they are dry.

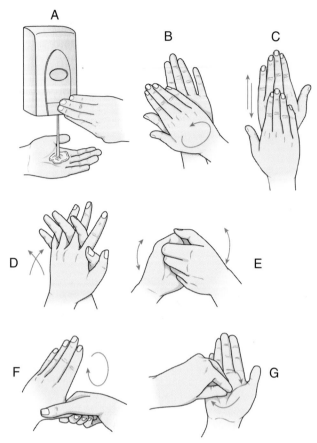

FIGURE 16-12 Using an alcohol-based hand sanitizer. **A,** A palmful of an alcohol-based hand sanitizer is applied into a cupped hand. **B,** The palms are rubbed together. **C,** The palm of 1 hand is rubbed over the back of the other. **D,** The palms are rubbed together with the fingers interlaced. **E,** The fingers are interlocked and rubbed back and forth. **F,** The thumb of 1 hand is rubbed in the palm of the other. **G,** The fingers of 1 hand are rubbed into the palm of the other hand with circular motions.

Supplies and Equipment

Disposable supplies and equipment help prevent the spread of infection. Discard single-use items after use. A person uses multi-use items many times. They include plastic bedpans, urinals, wash basins, and water mugs. Label multi-use items with the person's name and room and bed number. Do not "borrow" them for another person.

Non-disposable items are cleaned and then disinfected. Then they are sterilized usually by the supply department.

Cleaning. Cleaning reduces the number of microbes present. It also removes organic matter such as food and blood, body fluids, secretions, and excretions. *Organic matter* comes from living plants and animals and will decay.

To clean equipment:

- Wear personal protective equipment (PPE) to clean items contaminated with blood, body fluids, secretions, or excretions. PPE includes gloves, a mask, a gown, and goggles or a face shield. See Chapter 17.
- Work from *clean* to *dirty* areas. If you work from a *dirty* to *clean* area, the *clean* area becomes contaminated *(dirty)*.
- Rinse the item in cold water to remove organic matter. Heat makes organic matter thick, sticky, and hard to remove.
- Wash the item with soap and hot water.
- Scrub thoroughly. Use a brush if necessary.
- Rinse the item in warm water. Dry the item.
- Disinfect the item. Or have it sterilized.
- Disinfect equipment and the sink used for cleaning.
- Discard PPE.
- Practice hand hygiene.

Agencies usually have *clean* and *dirty* utility rooms. Equipment is cleaned in the *dirty* utility room. Then it is disinfected or sterilized in the *clean* utility room.

Disinfection. *Disinfection is the process of killing pathogens.* Spores are not destroyed. *Spores are bacteria protected by a hard shell.* Spores are killed by very high temperatures.

Disinfectants are used for cleaning. A *disinfectant is a liquid chemical that can kill many or all pathogens except spores.* Disinfectants are used to clean counters, tubs, showers, and re-usable items. Such items include:

- Blood pressure cuffs
- Commodes and bedpans
- Shower chairs
- Wheelchairs and stretchers
- Furniture

    See *Focus on Long-Term Care and Home Care: Disinfection.*
    See *Promoting Safety and Comfort: Disinfection.*

Sterilization. Sterilizing destroys all non-pathogens, pathogens, and spores. Very high temperatures are used. Heat destroys microbes.

Boiling water, radiation, liquid or gas chemicals, dry heat, and *steam under pressure* are sterilization methods. An autoclave (Fig. 16-13) is a pressure steam sterilizer. Glass, surgical items, and metal items are autoclaved. High temperatures destroy plastic and rubber items. They are not autoclaved.

    See *Focus on Long-Term Care and Home Care: Sterilization.*

Other Aseptic Measures

Hand hygiene, cleaning, disinfection, and sterilization are important aseptic measures. So are the measures listed in Box 16-4. They are useful in home and health care settings and in every-day life.

FOCUS ON LONG-TERM CARE AND HOME CARE

Disinfection

Home Care

Detergent and hot water are used to clean cooking, eating, and drinking utensils and linens. Household disinfectants are used for surfaces—floors, toilets, tubs, and showers. Use the products the family prefers or as the nurse instructs.

White vinegar and water is a good, cheap disinfectant. You can use it to clean bedpans, urinals, commodes, toilets, mirrors, bathroom tiles, and so on. Recipes for vinegar solutions vary. Ask the nurse how much vinegar and water to use. The following is common. To make a vinegar solution:

* Mix ½ cup of white vinegar with ½ gallon (8 cups) of water.
* Label the container as a "vinegar solution: ½ cup white vinegar, ½ gallon (8 cups) water."
* Write the date, time, and your name on the label.

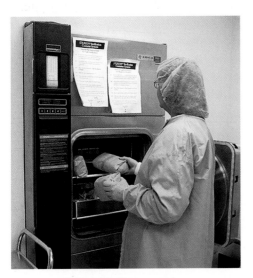

FIGURE 16-13 An autoclave.

PROMOTING SAFETY AND COMFORT

Disinfection

Safety

Disinfectants can burn and irritate the skin. Wear utility gloves or rubber household gloves to prevent skin irritation. These gloves are waterproof. Do not wear disposable gloves.

Some disinfectants have special measures for use and storage. Check the safety data sheet (SDS) before handling a disinfectant. See Chapter 13.

FOCUS ON LONG-TERM CARE AND HOME CARE

Sterilization

Home Care

You can use boiling water to sterilize items in the home. Methods vary. The following is an example.

1 Use a pot big enough to hold the items.
2 Wash the items with soap and hot water.
3 Fill the pot with cold water. Completely cover all items with water.
4 Bring the water to a full boil.
5 Boil the items for 10 minutes. Add 1 minute for each 1000 feet of elevation. For example, if the home is 2000 feet above sea level, boil items for 2 more minutes for a total of 12 minutes.
6 Turn off the heat.
7 Use tongs to remove the hot items to a clean towel. Remove items 1 at a time.
8 Let the items air-dry.
9 Put the items away as the family prefers or as the nurse instructs.

Many people use dishwashers for baby bottles. However, many dishwashers do not get hot enough to sterilize items.

BOX 16-4	**Aseptic Measures**

Controlling Reservoirs (Hosts—You or the Person)

* Provide for hygiene needs (Chapters 23 and 24).
* Wash contaminated areas with soap and water. Feces (stools), urine, blood, body fluids, secretions, and excretions can contain microbes.
* Use leak-proof plastic bags for soiled tissues, linens, and other items.
* Keep tables, counters, wheelchair trays, and other surfaces clean and dry.
* Label bottles with the person's name and the date the bottle was opened.
* Keep bottles and fluid containers tightly capped or covered.
* Keep drainage containers below the drainage site (Chapters 28 and 40).
* Empty drainage containers and dispose of drainage following agency policy. Usually drainage containers are emptied every shift. The nurse may have you empty them more often.

Controlling Portals of Exit

* Cover your nose and mouth to cough or sneeze.
* Provide the person with tissues to use when coughing or sneezing.
* Wear PPE as needed (Chapter 17).

Controlling Transmission

* Provide all persons with their own personal care equipment. This includes wash basins, bedpans, urinals, commodes, and eating and drinking utensils.
* Do not take equipment from 1 person's room to use for another person. Even if un-used, do not take the item from 1 room to another.
* Hold equipment and linens away from your uniform (Fig. 16-14, p. 232).
* Practice hand hygiene. See Box 16-3.

Continued

BOX 16-4	Aseptic Measures—cont'd

Controlling Transmission—cont'd

- Assist the person with hand-washing.
  - Before and after eating
  - After elimination
  - After changing tampons, sanitary napkins, or other personal hygiene products
  - After contact with blood, body fluids, secretions, or excretions
- Prevent dust movement. Do not shake linens or equipment. Use a damp cloth for dusting.
- Clean from *clean* to *dirty* areas. This prevents soiling a clean area.
- Clean away from your body. Do not dust, brush, or wipe toward yourself. Otherwise you transmit microbes to your skin, hair, and clothing.
- Flush urine and stools down the toilet. Avoid splatters and splashes.
- Pour contaminated liquids directly into sinks or toilets. Avoid splashing onto other areas.
- Do not sit on the person's bed or chair. You will pick up microbes and transfer them to other surfaces that you sit on.
- Do not use items on the floor. The floor is contaminated.
- Follow agency disinfection procedures to clean:
  - Tubs, showers, and shower chairs after each use
  - Bedpans, urinals, and commodes after each use
- Report pests—ants, spiders, mice, and so on.

Controlling Portals of Entry

- Provide good skin care and oral hygiene (Chapters 23 and 24). This promotes intact skin and mucous membranes.
- Protect the skin from injury.
  - Do not let the person lie on tubes or other items.
  - Make sure linens are dry and wrinkle-free (Chapter 22).
  - Turn and re-position the person as directed by the nurse and care plan (Chapters 18 and 19).
- Assist with or clean the genital area after elimination. (See "Perineal Care" in Chapter 24.) Wipe and clean from the urethra (cleanest area) to the rectum (dirtiest area). This helps prevent urinary tract infections.
- Make sure drainage tubes are properly connected. This prevents microbes from entering the drainage system.

Protecting the Susceptible Host

- Follow the care plan to meet nutrition and fluid needs (Chapters 30, 31, and 32). This helps prevent infection.
- Assist with deep-breathing and coughing exercises as directed (Chapter 43). This helps prevent respiratory infections.

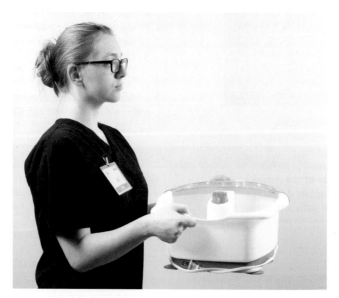

FIGURE 16-14 Hold equipment away from your uniform.

BLOODBORNE PATHOGEN STANDARD

The human immunodeficiency virus (HIV) and the hepatitis B virus (HBV) are major health concerns (Chapters 47 and 50). The *Bloodborne Pathogen Standard* protects the health team from exposure to these viruses. It is a regulation of the Occupational Safety and Health Administration (OSHA). See Box 16-5 for some terms used in the standard and prevention measures.

Found in the blood, HIV and HBV are bloodborne pathogens. They exit the body through blood. They are spread to others by blood and other potentially infectious materials (OPIM) (see Box 16-5).

See *Focus on Surveys: Bloodborne Pathogen Standard (Laundry)*, p. 234.

See *Focus on Long-Term Care and Home Care: Bloodborne Pathogen Standard (Regulated Waste)*, p. 234.

See *Promoting Safety and Comfort: Bloodborne Pathogen Standard*, p. 235.

BOX 16-5	Bloodborne Pathogen Standard—Terms and Prevention Measures

Blood. Human blood, human blood components, and products made from human blood.

Bloodborne pathogens. Pathogens present in human blood that can cause disease in humans. They include HBV and HIV.

Contaminated. The presence or anticipated presence of blood or OPIM on an item or surface.

Contaminated laundry. Laundry soiled with blood or OPIM or that may contain sharps.
- Handle it as little as possible.
- Wear gloves or other needed PPE.
- Bag contaminated laundry where it is used.
- Mark laundry bags or containers with the *BIOHAZARD* symbol (Chapter 17) for laundry sent off-site.
- Place wet, contaminated laundry in leak-proof containers before transport. The containers are color-coded in red or have the *BIOHAZARD* symbol.

Contaminated sharps. Any contaminated object that can open the skin—needles, scalpels, broken glass, and so on.

Decontamination. The use of physical or chemical means to remove, inactivate, or destroy bloodborne pathogens on a surface or item. Contaminated equipment and work surfaces are cleaned and decontaminated with a proper disinfectant.
- Upon completing tasks
- At once for obvious contamination
- At the end of your work shift when surfaces became contaminated since the last cleaning

Engineering controls. Controls that isolate or remove the bloodborne pathogen hazard from the workplace (sharps disposal containers, self-sheathing needles). For broken glass:
- Use a brush and dustpan or tongs to clean up broken glass.
- Do not pick up broken glass with your hands, not even with gloves.
- Discard broken glass into a puncture-resistant container.

Exposure incident. Eye, mouth, other mucous membrane, non-intact skin, or parenteral contact with blood or OPIM that results from an employee's duties.

Occupational exposure. Reasonably anticipated skin, eye, mucous membrane, or parenteral contact with blood or OPIM that may result from an employee's duties.

Other potentially infectious materials (OPIM). They include:
- Human body fluids—semen, vaginal secretions, cerebrospinal fluid, synovial fluid, pleural fluid, pericardial fluid, peritoneal fluid, amniotic fluid, saliva in dental procedures, body fluid that is visibly contaminated with blood, and all body fluids when it is difficult or impossible to differentiate between them
- Any tissue or organ (other than intact skin) from a human (living or dead)
- HIV-containing cell or tissue cultures, organ cultures, and HIV- or HBV-containing culture medium or other solutions

Parenteral. Piercing mucous membranes or the skin through needle-sticks, human bites, cuts, abrasions, and so on.

Personal protective equipment (PPE). The clothing or equipment worn by staff for protection against a hazard. This includes gloves, goggles, face shields, masks, laboratory coats, gowns, shoe covers, and surgical caps. Blood or OPIM must not pass through them. They protect your clothes, under-garments, skin, eyes, mouth, and hair. PPE is free to staff. OSHA requires these measures.
- Remove PPE before leaving the work area.
- Remove PPE when it becomes contaminated.
- Place used PPE in marked areas or containers when being stored, washed, decontaminated, or discarded.
- Wear gloves for contact with blood or OPIM.
- Wear gloves to handle or touch contaminated items or surfaces.
- Replace worn, punctured, or contaminated gloves.
- Do not wash or decontaminate disposable gloves for re-use.
- Discard utility gloves that show signs of cracking, peeling, tearing, or puncturing. Utility gloves are decontaminated for re-use if the process will not ruin them.

Regulated waste. Closable, puncture-resistant, leak-proof containers color-coded in red with the *BIOHAZARD* symbol (Chapter 17) are used for:
- Liquid or semi-liquid blood or OPIM
- Items contaminated with blood or OPIM
- Items caked with blood or OPIM
- Contaminated sharps

Continued

| BOX 16-5 | Bloodborne Pathogen Standard—Terms and Prevention Measures—cont'd |

Source individual. Any person (living or dead) whose blood or OPIM may be a source of exposure to staff. Examples include but are not limited to:

- Hospital and clinic patients
- Clients in agencies for the intellectually and developmentally disabled
- Trauma victims
- Clients of drug and alcohol treatment agencies
- Hospice and nursing center residents
- Human remains
- Persons who donate or sell blood or blood components

Work practice controls. Controls that reduce the likelihood of exposure by limiting splatters, splashes, and sprays. Producing droplets also is avoided.

- Do not eat, drink, smoke, apply cosmetics or lip balm, or handle contact lenses in areas of exposure.
- Do not store food or drinks where blood or OPIM are kept.
- Practice hand hygiene after removing gloves.
- Wash hands as soon as possible after skin contact with blood or OPIM.
- Do not re-cap, bend, or remove needles by hand. Use a mechanical means (forceps) or a 1-handed method.
- Do not shear or break needles.
- Discard needles and sharp instruments (such as razors) in containers that are closable, puncture-resistant, and leak-proof. Containers are color-coded in red and have the *BIOHAZARD* symbol. Containers must be upright and not allowed to over-fill.

FOCUS ON SURVEYS

Bloodborne Pathogen Standard: Laundry

Surveyors will observe how staff handle, store, process, and transport linens. For example, do staff:

- Handle linens in a way to prevent exposure of urine or stools?
- Handle linens in a way to prevent the spread of infection?
- Handle linens according to agency policies and procedures?
- Store and transport linens properly?

FOCUS ON LONG-TERM CARE AND HOME CARE

Bloodborne Pathogen Standard: Regulated Waste

Home Care

Dressings, gloves, and other items are used in home care. So are syringes, needles, and sharps (such as razors). The patient or family may use syringes and needles. You may use safety razors for shaving (Chapter 25) and lancets for blood glucose testing (Chapter 38). Proper disposal:

- Protects neighbors, children, pets, janitors, housekeepers, sanitation workers, and sewage treatment workers from injury and infection. HIV, AIDS, and hepatitis B and C are risks.
- Prevents needle sharing and re-using sharps.
- Protects the environment.

According to the Environmental Protection Agency (EPA) and the Food and Drug Administration (FDA):

- Do not throw loose needles, syringes, or sharps into the trash or into a recycling bin.
- Do not flush needles, syringes, or sharps down the toilet.
- Do not put needles, syringes, or sharps in recycling containers for bottles, plastics, and paper.
- Properly store used needles, syringes, and sharps. Put them in a commercial or household sharps container right after use (Fig. 16-15). A household container can be a hard plastic, puncture-resistant container with a screw-on lid. Detergent bottles with screw-on lids are examples. Secure the lid in place with heavy tape for added protection. See Figure 16-15, *B.*
  - Label the container with "Do Not Recycle" or "SHARPS" label.
  - Put sharps in the container point-first.
  - Do not use soda cans or bottles, milk cartons, glass bottles, coffee cans, aluminum cans, or other containers that are not puncture-resistant.
  - Keep storage containers where children cannot reach them.

For sharps container disposal, the nurse and care plan tell you what to use at the person's address. The EPA describes these disposal options.

- *Drop-off collection sites.* Sharps containers are taken to a collection site. Hospitals, doctors' offices, clinics, pharmacies, health departments, and police and fire stations are examples. So are medical waste facilities.
- *Household hazardous waste collection sites.* Sharps containers are placed in sharps collection bins at a collection site.
- *Residential special waste pick-up services.* Used sharps are placed in a special recycling-type container. The container is placed outside the home for special waste handlers. Programs have regular pick-up times or require a call for pick-up.
- *Mail-back programs.* Used sharps are placed in special containers and mailed to a collection site. U.S. Postal Service procedures are followed. The program works well for rural areas.
- *Syringe-exchange programs.* Used needles and syringes are exchanged for new ones. The agency operating the program disposes of used ones.
- *Home needle destruction devices.* Such devices clip, melt, or burn the needle. The syringe and destroyed needle are placed in the trash.

Dressings, gloves, soiled bed protectors, and other care items also need proper disposal.

- Place them in plastic bags.
- Close the bags securely.
- Label each bag with a "Do Not Recycle" label.
- Place the bags in a trash can with a lid.
- Make sure animals cannot get into the trash can. Trash scents can attract animals.

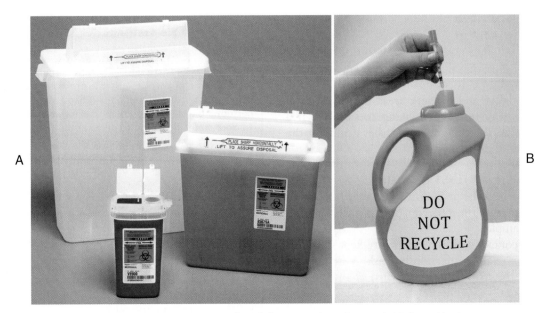

FIGURE 16-15 Sharps containers. **A,** FDA-cleared sharps containers. **B,** Household disposable sharps container labeled with "Do Not Recycle." The needle with syringe is inserted "point first." (A from Warekois RS, Robinson R: *Phlebotomy worktext and procedures manual*, ed 4, St Louis, 2016, Elsevier.)

PROMOTING SAFETY AND COMFORT

Bloodborne Pathogen Standard

Safety

The agency identifies staff at risk for exposure to blood or OPIM. All caregivers and laundry, supply, and housekeeping staffs are at risk. Staff at risk receive free training upon employment and yearly. Training is also done for new or changed tasks involving exposure to bloodborne pathogens.

Training includes:

- The causes, signs, and symptoms of bloodborne diseases
- How bloodborne pathogens are spread
- The tasks that might cause exposure
- The use and limits of safe work practices and PPE
- Information about the hepatitis B vaccination
- Who to contact and what to do in an emergency
- Information on reporting an exposure incident, post-exposure evaluation, and follow-up

The hepatitis B vaccine produces immunity against hepatitis B. *Immunity means that a person has protection against a certain disease.* He or she will not get the disease. A *vaccination involves giving a vaccine to produce immunity against an infectious disease. A **vaccine** is a preparation containing dead or weakened microbes.* The hepatitis B vaccination involves 3 injections (shots). Injection 2 is given 1 month after the first. Injection 3 is given at least 4 months after the first one. The vaccination can be given before or after HBV exposure.

The agency must offer the hepatitis B vaccination after you are trained about the vaccine and within 10 days of your first working day. The agency pays for it. You can refuse the vaccination. If so, you must sign a statement refusing the vaccine. You can have the vaccination at a later time if you want.

Exposure Incidents

An *exposure incident* is any eye, mouth, other mucous membrane, non-intact skin, or parenteral contact with blood or OPIM. *Parenteral* means *piercing the mucous membranes or the skin.* Causes include needle-sticks, human bites, cuts, and abrasions.

Report exposure incidents at once. Medical evaluation, follow-up, and testing are free. Your blood is tested for HIV and HBV. If you refuse testing, the blood sample is kept for at least 90 days. Testing is done later if you desire.

Confidentiality is important. You are told about any medical conditions that may need treatment. You receive a written opinion within 15 days after the evaluation is complete.

The *source individual* is the person whose blood or body fluids are the source of an exposure incident. His or her blood is tested for HIV or HBV. The agency informs you about laws affecting the source's identity and test results.

SURGICAL ASEPSIS

Surgical asepsis (sterile technique) is the practices used to remove all microbes. Sterile means the absence of all microbes. Surgical asepsis is required any time the skin or sterile tissues are entered.

Surgery and labor and delivery areas require surgical asepsis. So do many tests and nursing procedures. If a break occurs in sterile technique, microbes can enter the body. Infection is a risk.

Assisting With Sterile Procedures

You can assist with sterile procedures. You may be allowed to perform certain sterile procedures. A sterile dressing change is an example.

All items in contact with the person are kept sterile. If an item is contaminated, infection is a risk. A sterile field is needed. A *sterile field is a work area free of all pathogens and non-pathogens (including spores)*. See Figure 16-16. Box 16-6 lists the principles and practices of surgical asepsis. Follow them for a sterile field.

See *Delegation Guidelines: Assisting With Sterile Procedures.*

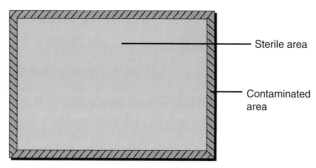

FIGURE 16-16 A sterile field. A 1-inch (2.5 cm) margin around the sterile field is considered contaminated. The shading and slash marks show that the 1-inch (2.5 cm) margin is contaminated.

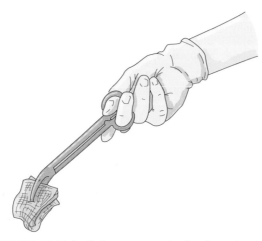

FIGURE 16-17 Sterile forceps are used to handle sterile items.

BOX 16-6	Surgical Asepsis—Principles and Practices

- A sterile item can touch only another sterile item.
  - If a sterile item touches a clean item, the sterile item is contaminated.
  - If a clean item touches a sterile item, the sterile item is contaminated.
  - A sterile package is contaminated if open, torn, punctured, wet, or moist.
  - A sterile package is contaminated when the expiration date has passed.
  - Place only sterile items on a sterile field.
  - Use sterile gloves or sterile forceps to handle other sterile items (Fig. 16-17).
  - Consider any item to be contaminated if not sure of its sterility.
  - Do not use contaminated items. They are discarded or re-sterilized.
- A sterile field or sterile items are always kept within your vision and above your waist.
  - If you cannot see an item, it is contaminated.
  - If the item is below your waist, it is contaminated.
  - Keep sterile-gloved hands above your waist and in your sight.
  - Do not leave a sterile field unattended.
  - Do not turn your back on a sterile field.
- Airborne microbes can contaminate sterile items or a sterile field.
  - Prevent drafts. Close the door and avoid extra movements. Ask other staff in the room to avoid extra movements.
  - Avoid coughing, sneezing, talking, or laughing over a sterile field. Turn your head away from the sterile field if you must talk.
  - Wear a mask if you need to talk during the procedure.
  - Do not perform or assist with sterile procedures if you have a respiratory infection.
  - Do not reach over a sterile field.
- Fluid flows downward, in the direction of gravity.
  - Hold wet items down (see Fig. 16-17). If held up, fluid flows down into a contaminated area.
- The sterile field is kept dry, unless the area below it is sterile.
  - The sterile field is contaminated if it gets wet and the area below it is not sterile.
  - Avoid spilling and splashing when pouring sterile fluids into sterile containers.
- The edges of a sterile field are contaminated.
  - A 1-inch (2.5 centimeter [cm]) margin around the sterile field is considered contaminated (see Fig. 16-16).
  - Place all sterile items inside the 1-inch (2.5 cm) margin of the sterile field.
  - Items outside the 1-inch (2.5 cm) margin are contaminated.
- Honesty is essential to sterile technique.
  - Be honest if you contaminate an item or sterile field, even if other staff are not present.
  - Remove the contaminated item and correct the matter. If necessary, start over with sterile supplies.
  - Report the contamination to the nurse.

Sterile Gloving

Before donning (putting on) sterile gloves, the sterile field is set up. After sterile gloves are on, you can handle sterile items within the sterile field. Do not touch anything outside the sterile field.

Sterile gloves are single-use. They come in many sizes to fit snugly. The insides are powdered for ease in donning gloves. The right and left gloves are marked on the package.

See *Promoting Safety and Comfort: Sterile Gloving*.

See procedure: *Sterile Gloving*, p. 238.

PROMOTING SAFETY AND COMFORT

Sterile Gloving

Safety

Always keep sterile gloved hands above your waist and within your vision. Touch only items within the sterile field. If you contaminate the gloves, remove them. Tell the nurse what happened. Practice hand hygiene and put on a new pair. Replace gloves that are torn, cut, or punctured.

Comfort

If you, the nurse, or the person contaminates your gloves, they must be removed. This means leaving the bedside for another pair. Care is delayed. The person's comfort is affected if the care is painful or involves an uncomfortable position. When collecting supplies, get an extra pair of gloves. The gloves are in the room if the first pair is contaminated. Care can continue with little delay.

Sterile Gloving

PROCEDURE

1 Follow *Delegation Guidelines: Assisting With Sterile Procedures*, p. 236. See *Promoting Safety and Comfort: Sterile Gloving*, p. 237.
2 Practice hand hygiene.
3 Inspect the package of sterile gloves for sterility.
  a Check the expiration date.
  b See if the package is dry.
  c Check for tears, holes, punctures, and watermarks.
4 Create a work surface with enough room.
  a Arrange the work surface at waist level and within your vision.
  b Clean and dry the work surface.
  c Do not reach over or turn your back on the work surface.
5 Open the package. Grasp the flaps. Gently peel them back.
6 Remove the inner package. Place it on your work surface.
7 Note the labels on the inner package—*left, right, up,* and *down.*
8 Arrange the inner package for left, right, up, and down. Left glove is on your left; right glove is on your right. Cuffs are near you; fingers point away from you.
9 Grasp the folded edges of the inner package. Use the thumb and index finger of each hand.
10 Fold back the inner package to expose the gloves (Fig. 16-18, *A*). Do not touch or otherwise contaminate the inside package or the gloves. The inside of the inner package is a sterile field.
11 Note that each glove has a cuff about 2 to 3 inches wide. The cuffs and insides of the gloves are *not sterile.*

12 Put on the right glove if you are right-handed. Put on the left glove if you are left-handed.
  a Pick up the glove with your other hand. Use your thumb and index and middle fingers (Fig. 16-18, *B*).
  b Touch only the cuff and inside of the glove.
  c Turn the hand to be gloved palm side up.
  d Lift the cuff up. Slide your fingers and hand into the glove (Fig. 16-18, *C*).
  e Pull the glove up over your hand. If some fingers get stuck, leave them that way until the other glove is on. *Do not use your ungloved hand to straighten the glove. Do not let the outside of the glove touch any non-sterile surface.*
  f Leave the cuff turned down.
13 Put on the other glove. Use your gloved hand.
  a Reach under the cuff of the second glove. Use the 4 fingers of your gloved hand (Fig. 16-18, *D*). Keep your gloved thumb close to your gloved palm.
  b Put on the second glove (Fig. 16-18, *E*). Your gloved hand cannot touch the cuff or any surface. Hold the thumb of your first gloved hand away from the second gloved palm.
14 Adjust each glove with the other hand. The gloves should be smooth and comfortable (Fig. 16-18, *F*).
15 Slide your fingers under the cuffs to pull them up (Fig. 16-18, *G*).
16 Touch only sterile items.
17 Remove and discard the gloves. See Chapter 17.
18 Practice hand hygiene.

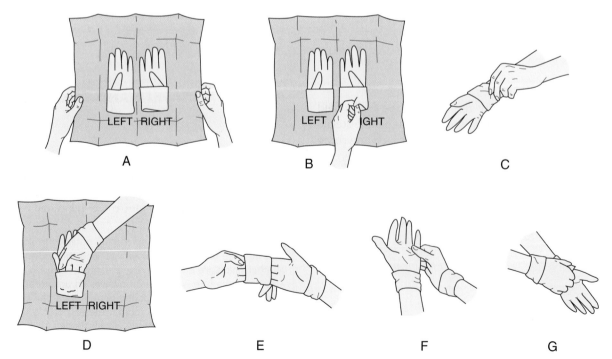

FIGURE 16-18 Sterile gloving. **A,** Open the inner wrapper to expose the gloves. **B,** Pick up the glove at the cuff with your thumb and index and middle fingers. **C,** Slide your fingers and hand into the glove. **D,** Reach under the cuff of the other glove with your fingers. **E,** Pull on the second glove. **F,** Adjust each glove for comfort. **G,** Slide your fingers under the cuff to pull them up.

FOCUS ON **PRIDE**

The Person, Family, and Yourself

P ersonal and Professional Responsibility

Your actions affect the person's risk for infection. You are responsible for following the guidelines in this chapter. Practice good hand hygiene before and after giving care. Follow the rules of hand hygiene.

R ights and Respect

The health team must prevent the spread of microbes and infection. Even one careless act can spread microbes. This affects the person's health and safety. Be very careful about your work. Take pride in providing care that protects the person from infection. Infection can seriously affect quality of life.

I ndependence and Social Interaction

Patients and residents often cannot perform their usual hygiene measures. Hand hygiene is an example. Ask patients and residents if they would like to wash their hands. Ask them often and assist as needed. When independence is limited, protect the person, yourself, and others by promoting hand hygiene.

D elegation and Teamwork

Before making delegation decisions, the nurse considers the person's needs and risks. If delegated care of persons at increased risk for infection, you must:

- Practice medical asepsis at all times. Practice surgical asepsis when assisting with sterile procedures.
- Practice hand hygiene.
- Follow the Bloodborne Pathogen Standard at all times.
- Follow Standard Precautions and any Transmission-Based Precautions ordered for the person. See Chapter 17.
- Wear PPE as directed by the nurse.
- Follow the person's care plan.
- Report any signs or symptoms of infection at once.
- Provide good oral hygiene and skin care (Chapters 23 and 24).
- Tell the nurse if you have any sign or symptom of an infection.

E thics and Laws

The following is a real case showing how failure to follow infection control procedures led to patient harm.

A patient, Mr. Helman, had hip surgery (August 1) following a car accident in which he suffered many injuries. His roommate, Mr. Hagerup, had a back injury that caused paralysis from the waist down. The men shared a room for about 2 weeks.

Eight days after Mr. Helman's hip surgery (August 9), Mr. Hagerup complained of a boil under his right arm. (Author note: A boil is a local skin infection. The infection causes a painful red bump. When opened, purulent drainage comes from the boil. Purulent drainage is thick and green, yellow, or brown in color.) The boil was treated with hot compresses. On August 10, there was purulent drainage from the boil. On the same day, a drainage specimen was sent to the laboratory. On August 13, the laboratory report showed the boil drainage contained a type of staphylococcus. Mr. Hagerup was moved at once to an isolation room.

Between August 10 and August 13, the nursing team cared for Mr. Helman and Mr. Hagerup. They "moved from one patient to the other, changed sheets, gave sponge baths, changed dressings, administered back rubs...[and] carried out the necessary hospital routine for the care of the two men. They did not observe sterile techniques...[to be used] when infection is suspected; they did not wash their hands or leave the room between administering to the patients."

On August 13, Mr. Helman's surgical wound opened and drained a large amount of purulent drainage. Laboratory tests showed the drainage contained the same microbe found in Mr. Hagerup's wound. Mr. Helman's wound infection destroyed bone, tissue, and ligaments. He had another surgery on October 28. His hip was fused in a "nearly immovable position." (To fuse means to unite 2 or more bones together.) He was discharged from the hospital on March 14. He needed home care and doctor's care.

In a lawsuit against the hospital, the jury returned a verdict in favor of Mr. Helman. The hospital appealed the verdict. The court hearing the appeal upheld the verdict in favor of Mr. Helman.

(G. E. Helman et al. v Sacred Heart Hospital, Washington, 1963.)

FOCUS ON **PRIDE**: *Application*

Consider your every-day actions. How do they affect infection control? Give some examples. Identify areas to improve. How might your attitude affect how you prevent infection at work?

REVIEW QUESTIONS

Circle T if the statement is TRUE or F if it is FALSE.

1 T F   Microbes are pathogens in their natural sites.

2 T F   A pathogen can cause an infection.

3 T F   An infection results when microbes invade and grow in the body.

4 T F   An item is sterile if non-pathogens are present.

5 T F   You hold your hands and forearms up during hand-washing.

6 T F   A towel falls to the floor. The towel is contaminated.

7 T F   Un-used items in the person's room are used for another person.

8 T F   A person received the hepatitis B vaccine. The person will develop the disease.

9 T F   You can flush household sharps down the toilet.

10 T F   You can throw household sharps in the trash.

11 T F   The 1-inch edge around a sterile field is considered contaminated.

12 T F   The inside and cuffs of sterile gloves are not sterile.

Circle the BEST answer.

13 Which area is *best* for a pathogen to live and grow?
a A cold and wet area
b A warm and dark area
c A hot and bright area
d A dry area without oxygen

14 Which is a sign of infection?
a A bruise
b Redness in a body part
c Warm, dry, and intact skin
d A bleeding wound

15 To control a portal of exit
a Cover the mouth and nose when coughing
b Position drainage containers above the drainage site
c Clean the genital area from the rectum to the urethra
d Leave an open wound uncovered

16 Preventing healthcare-associated infections involves
a Sterilizing all care items
b Over-prescribing antibiotics
c Hand hygiene before and after giving care
d Avoiding vaccinations

17 You have blood on your hand. What should you do?
a Wash your hands with soap and water.
b Use an alcohol-based hand sanitizer.
c Rinse your hands.
d Wash your hands with a disinfectant.

18 You move from a contaminated body site to a clean body site. Your hands are not visibly soiled. What should you do?
a Disinfect your gloves.
b Practice hand hygiene.
c Rinse your hands.
d Continue care without hand hygiene.

19 To use an alcohol-based hand sanitizer correctly
a Wash your hands before applying the hand sanitizer
b Rinse your hands after applying the hand sanitizer
c Rub the product only on the palms of your hands
d Rub your hands together until they are dry

20 When cleaning equipment
a Rinse the item in hot water before cleaning
b Wash the item with soap and cold water
c Use a brush if necessary
d Work from dirty to clean areas

21 The Bloodborne Pathogen Standard involves microbes spread through
a Blood and OPIM
b Only blood
c Droplets
d Close contact

22 According to the Bloodborne Pathogen Standard, you should
a Practice hand hygiene after removing gloves
b Discard a used razor in a wastebasket
c Tell the nurse about exposure to blood before washing your hands
d Refuse the hepatitis B vaccine

23 You were exposed to a bloodborne pathogen. Which is *true*?
a You do not have to report the exposure.
b You pay for required tests.
c You can refuse HIV and HBV testing.
d The source individual can refuse testing.

24 These statements are about surgical asepsis. Which is *true*?
a If a sterile item touches a clean item, the sterile item is clean.
b Wet sterile items are held up.
c A torn sterile package is still sterile.
d If you cannot see an item, it is considered contaminated.

25 You have on sterile gloves. You can touch
a Anything on your work surface
b Anything on the sterile field
c Anything below your waist
d Any part of your uniform

Answers to Chapter 16 questions are on p. 886.

FOCUS ON **PRACTICE**
Problem Solving

Two residents share a room. You make both beds without practicing hand hygiene between beds. Why is this a problem? When should you practice hand hygiene? Can you use an alcohol-based hand sanitizer? When must you use soap and water?

Isolation Precautions

OBJECTIVES

- Explain why isolation precautions are used.
- Explain the difference between *clean* and *dirty*.
- Explain the purpose of Standard Precautions.
- Describe how to follow Standard Precautions.
- Explain the purpose of Transmission-Based Precautions.
- Describe 3 types of Transmission-Based Precautions.
- Describe the rules for Transmission-Based Precautions.
- Explain how to use personal protective equipment.
- Identify the order for donning and removing personal protective equipment.

- Describe how to bag and double-bag items.
- Describe how to collect specimens when Transmission-Based Precautions are used.
- Describe how to transport a person who needs Transmission-Based Precautions.
- Explain how to meet the needs of the person when Transmission-Based Precautions are used.
- Perform the procedures described in this chapter.
- Explain how to promote PRIDE in the person, the family, and yourself.

KEY TERMS

biohazardous waste Items contaminated with blood, body fluids, secretions, or excretions; *bio* means *life* and *hazardous* means *dangerous* or *harmful*

communicable disease A disease caused by a pathogen that spreads easily; contagious disease

contagious disease See "communicable disease"

personal protective equipment (PPE) The clothing or equipment worn by the staff for protection against a hazard

KEY ABBREVIATIONS

CDC	Centers for Disease Control and Prevention	**PPE**	Personal protective equipment
OPIM	Other potentially infectious materials	**TB**	Tuberculosis

Blood, body fluids, secretions, and excretions can transmit pathogens. Sometimes barriers are needed to keep pathogens in a certain area—usually the person's room. This requires isolation precautions.

The *Guidelines for Isolation Precautions: Preventing Transmission of Infectious Agents in Healthcare Settings 2007* is followed. This is a guideline of the Centers for Disease Control and Prevention (CDC). Isolation precautions prevent the spread of *communicable diseases (contagious diseases). They are diseases caused by pathogens that spread easily.*

Isolation precautions are based on *clean* and *dirty*. *Clean* areas or objects have no pathogens. They are not contaminated or *dirty*. *Dirty* areas or objects are contaminated with pathogens. If a *clean* area or object has contact with something dirty, the clean area or object is now *dirty*. *Clean* and *dirty* also depend on how the pathogen is spread.

The CDC guideline has 2 tiers of precautions.
- Standard Precautions
- Transmission-Based Precautions (p. 243)

STANDARD PRECAUTIONS

Standard Precautions (Box 17-1, p. 242):
- Reduce the risk of spreading pathogens.
- Reduce the risk of spreading known and unknown infections. *Standard Precautions are used for all persons whenever care is given.* They prevent the spread of infection from:
  - Blood.
  - All body fluids, secretions, and excretions (except sweat) even if blood is not visible. Sweat is not known to spread infection.
  - Non-intact skin (skin with open breaks).
  - Mucous membranes.

BOX 17-1   Standard Precautions

Hand Hygiene
- Follow the rules for hand hygiene. See Chapter 16.
- Touch surfaces close to the person only when necessary. This prevents contaminating clean hands from room or care setting surfaces. It also prevents transmitting pathogens from contaminated hands to other surfaces.
- Do not wear fake nails or nail extenders for contact with persons at risk for infection or other adverse outcomes. (NOTE: Follow agency policy about wearing non-natural nails [fake nails, nail extenders, and so on]. Non-natural nails are not allowed in some agencies.)

Personal Protective Equipment (PPE) (p. 245)
- Wear PPE when contact with blood or body fluids is likely.
- Do not contaminate your clothing or skin when removing PPE.
- Remove and discard PPE before leaving the person's room or care setting.

Gloves (p. 246)
- Wear gloves when contact with the following is likely.
  - Blood
  - Potentially infectious materials (body fluids, secretions, and excretions are examples)
  - Mucous membranes
  - Non-intact skin
  - Skin that may be contaminated (for example, from urine or stools)
- Wear gloves that fit and are needed for the task.
  - Wear disposable gloves for direct care.
  - Wear disposable gloves or utility gloves to clean equipment or care settings.
- Remove gloves after contact with:
  - The person
  - The person's care setting
  - Equipment used in the person's care or other care equipment
- Remove gloves after contact with a person and before going to another person. Do not wear the same pair of gloves for the care of more than 1 person.
- Do not wash gloves for re-use.
- Change gloves during care if your hands will move from a contaminated body site to a clean body site.

Gowns (p. 245)
- Wear a gown to protect your skin and clothing when contact with blood, body fluids, secretions, or excretions is likely.
- Wear a gown for direct contact with a person who has uncontained secretions or excretions.
- Remove the gown and perform hand hygiene before leaving the person's room or care setting.
- Do not re-use gowns, even for repeat contact with the same person.

Mouth, Nose, and Eye Protection (pp. 245–246)
- Wear PPE—masks, goggles, face shields, or a combination of each—for procedures and tasks that are likely to cause splashes and sprays of blood, body fluids, secretions, and excretions.
- Wear the correct PPE for the procedure or task.
- Wear gloves, a gown, and 1 of the following for procedures or tasks likely to cause sprays of respiratory secretions.
  - A face shield that fully covers the front and sides of the face
  - A mask with attached shield
  - A mask and goggles

Respiratory Hygiene/Cough Etiquette
- Instruct persons with respiratory symptoms to:
  - Cover the nose and mouth to cough or sneeze.
  - Use tissues to contain respiratory secretions.
  - Dispose of tissues in the nearest no-touch waste container.
  - Perform hand hygiene after contact with respiratory secretions.
- Provide visitors with masks according to agency policy.

Care Equipment
- Wear the correct PPE to handle:
  - Care equipment that is visibly soiled with blood, body fluids, secretions, or excretions
  - Care equipment that may have been in contact with blood, body fluids, secretions, or excretions
- Remove organic material before disinfection and sterilization procedures. Follow agency policy for using cleaning agents.

Care of the Environment
- Follow agency procedures to clean and maintain surfaces. Care setting surfaces and care equipment are examples. Surfaces near the person may need frequent cleaning and maintenance—door knobs, bed rails, over-bed tables, walker and cane handles, toilet surfaces and areas, and so on.
- Follow agency procedures to clean and disinfect multi-use electronic equipment. This includes:
  - Items used by patients and residents
  - Items used to give care
  - Mobile devices that are moved in and out of patient or resident rooms
- Follow these rules for children's toys. This includes toys in waiting areas.
  - Select toys that are easy to clean and disinfect.
  - Do not allow stuffed, furry toys if they will be shared.
  - Clean and disinfect large stationary toys (for example, climbing equipment) at least weekly and when visibly soiled.
  - Rinse toys with water after disinfection if they are likely to be mouthed by children. Or wash them in a dishwasher.
  - Clean and disinfect a toy at once when it needs cleaning. Or store the toy in a labeled container away from toys that are clean and ready for use.

Textiles and Laundry
- Handle used textiles and fabrics (linens) with minimum agitation. This prevents contamination of air, surfaces, and other persons.

Worker Safety
- Protect yourself and others from exposure to bloodborne pathogens. This includes handling needles and other sharps. See "Bloodborne Pathogen Standard" in Chapter 16.
- Use a mouthpiece, resuscitation bag, or other ventilation device for resuscitation to prevent contact with the person's mouth and oral secretions. See Chapter 58.

Patient or Resident Placement
- A private room is preferred if the person is at risk for transmitting the infection to others.
- Follow the nurse's directions if a private room is not available.

Modified from Siegel JD, Rhinehart E, Jackson M, Chiarello L, and the Healthcare Infection Control Practices Advisory Committee: Guideline for isolation precautions: preventing transmission of infectious agents in healthcare settings 2007, *Atlanta, page reviewed July 22, 2019, Centers for Disease Control and Prevention.*

TRANSMISSION-BASED PRECAUTIONS

Some infections require Transmission-Based Precautions. They are commonly called "isolation precautions." Transmission-Based Precautions require wearing PPE—gloves, gown, mask, goggles, or face shield. Needed PPE depends on how the infection is spread.

Disposable (single-use) equipment is used when possible. Or dedicated equipment is kept in the room. *Dedicated equipment* is only used for 1 person. For example, a thermometer and blood pressure equipment are kept in the room. The equipment is not removed for use on another person. Equipment that must be shared is disinfected after use. A mechanical lift (Chapter 20) is an example.

The nurse may have you help set up an isolation room. Follow agency procedures. The following are common.
- PPE is in a cart or cabinet outside the room (Fig. 17-1). Re-stock supplies as needed.
- A sign is placed outside the room to alert staff and visitors to use PPE.
- A wastebasket and linen cart are inside the room. Color-coded or biohazard bags (p. 251) are used.
- Dedicated equipment, leak-proof plastic bags, and a disinfectant are supplied.

Removing linens, trash, and equipment from the room may require double-bagging (p. 251). Follow agency procedures to collect specimens and transport persons.

The 3 types of Transmission-Based Precautions are described in Box 17-2. Agency policies may differ from those in this text. The rules in Box 17-3 (p. 244) are a guide for giving safe care when using Transmission-Based Precautions.

See *Focus on Communication: Transmission-Based Precautions*, p. 244.

See *Focus on Surveys: Transmission-Based Precautions*, p. 245.

See *Delegation Guidelines: Transmission-Based Precautions*, p. 245.

See *Promoting Safety and Comfort: Transmission-Based Precautions*, p. 245.

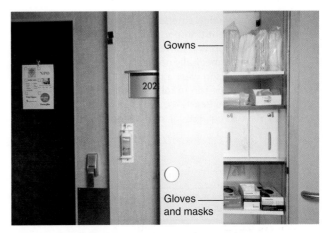

FIGURE 17-1 PPE is outside the person's room.

BOX 17-2	Transmission-Based Precautions

Contact Precautions
- Used for persons with known or suspected infections or conditions that increase the risk of contact (touch) transmission.
- Patient or resident placement:
  - A single room is preferred.
  - If a room is shared with another person not infected with the same agent:
    - Keep the persons separated—more than 3 feet apart.
    - Keep the privacy curtain between the beds closed.
    - Change PPE and practice hand hygiene between contact with persons in the same room. Do so regardless of whether 1 or both persons are on contact precautions.
- Gloves:
  - Don (put on) gloves upon entering the person's room or care setting.
  - Wear gloves to touch the person's intact skin.
  - Wear gloves to touch surfaces or items near the person.

Contact Precautions—cont'd
- Gown:
  - Wear a gown when clothing may have direct contact with the person.
  - Wear a gown when contact is likely with surfaces or equipment near the person.
  - Don the gown upon entering the person's room.
  - Remove the gown and practice hand hygiene before leaving the person's room.
  - Make sure your clothing and skin do not touch potentially contaminated surfaces after removing the gown.
- Patient or resident transport:
  - Limit transport and movement of the person outside of the room to medically-necessary purposes.
  - Cover the infected area of the person's body.
  - Remove and discard contaminated PPE and practice hand hygiene before transporting the person.
  - Don clean PPE to handle the person at the transport destination.
- Care equipment:
  - Follow Standard Precautions.
  - Use disposable equipment when possible. If possible, leave non-disposable equipment in the person's room.
  - Clean and disinfect non-disposable and multiple-use equipment before use on another person.

Continued

BOX 17-2   Transmission-Based Precautions—cont'd

Droplet Precautions

- Used for persons known or suspected to be infected with pathogens transmitted by respiratory droplets. Such droplets come from coughing, sneezing, or talking.
- Patient or resident placement:
  - A single room is preferred.
  - If a room is shared with another person who is not infected with the same agent:
    - Keep the persons separated—more than 3 feet apart.
    - Keep the privacy curtain between the beds closed.
    - Change PPE and practice hand hygiene between contact with persons in the same room. Do so regardless of whether 1 or both persons are on droplet precautions.
- PPE:
  - Don a mask upon entering the person's room.
- Patient or resident transport:
  - Limit transport and movement of the person outside of the room to medically-necessary purposes.
  - Have the person wear a mask.
  - Instruct the person to follow Respiratory Hygiene/Cough Etiquette (see Box 17-1).
  - No mask is required for staff transporting the person.

Airborne Precautions

- Used for persons known or suspected to be infected with pathogens transmitted person-to-person by the airborne route. Tuberculosis (TB), measles, chicken pox, smallpox, and shingles are examples.
- The person is placed in an airborne infection isolation room (AIIR). If not available, the person is transferred to an agency with an AIIR. The room door is kept closed except when someone enters or leaves the room.
- Staff susceptible to the infection do not enter the room. This is if immune staff members are available.
- PPE:
  - An agency-approved respirator is worn on entering the room or home of a person with suspected or confirmed TB or smallpox.
  - Agency policy is followed for respiratory protection for measles, chicken pox, or shingles.
- Patient or resident transport:
  - Limit transport and movement of the person outside of the room to medically-necessary purposes.
  - Have the person wear a surgical mask.
  - Instruct the person to follow Respiratory Hygiene/Cough Etiquette (see Box 17-1).
  - Cover skin lesions infected with the microbe.
  - No mask or respirator is required for staff transporting the person if the person is wearing a mask and skin lesions are covered.

Modified from Siegel JD, Rhinehart E, Jackson M, Chiarello L, and the Healthcare Infection Control Practices Advisory Committee: Guideline for isolation precautions: preventing transmission of infectious agents in healthcare settings 2007, Atlanta, page reviewed July 22, 2019, Centers for Disease Control and Prevention.

BOX 17-3   Rules for Transmission-Based Precautions

- Tell the nurse if you have any cuts, open skin areas, a sore throat, vomiting, or diarrhea.
- Collect all needed items before entering the room.
- Do not touch your hair, nose, mouth, eyes, or other body parts.
- Do not touch any clean area or object if your hands are contaminated.
- Wash your hands with soap and water if they are visibly dirty or contaminated with blood, body fluids, secretions, or excretions.
- Place clean items on paper towels.
- Do not shake linens.
- Use paper towels to turn faucets on and off.
- Use a paper towel to open the door to the person's room. Discard it after use.
- Do not contaminate equipment and supplies. Floors are contaminated. So is any object on the floor or that falls to the floor.
- Clean floors with mops wetted with a disinfectant solution. Floor dust is contaminated.
- Prevent drafts. Drafts can carry some microbes in the air.
- Use paper towels to handle contaminated items.
- Remove items from the room in leak-proof plastic bags.
- Double-bag items if the outside of the bag is or can be contaminated (p. 251).
- Follow agency procedures to remove and transport re-usable and disposable items. For meal trays:
  - Place re-usable dishes, drinking vessels, eating utensils, and trays in a leak-proof plastic bag. A co-worker is outside the room with the bag. You place contaminated items in the bag. Items are returned to the food service (dietary) department.
  - Discard disposable dishes, drinking vessels, eating utensils, and trays in the waste container in the person's room.

FOCUS ON COMMUNICATION

Transmission-Based Precautions

The health team and visitors must know what PPE to use. Signs are a common way to communicate the type of precaution and the needed PPE. Signs are posted at the person's doorway. In long-term care settings, signs may instruct visitors to see the nurse before entering the person's room.

Visitors may ask why PPE is needed. Some visitors ignore signs or requests to wear PPE. To communicate with the person and visitors about PPE, you can politely say:

- "Your visitors will need to wear a gown and gloves while in your room."

- "Please wear this mask. It is our policy to protect you, your family member, and others."
  Tell the nurse if the person or visitors have more questions. Also tell the nurse if someone refuses to wear PPE.

Others on the health team may not wear needed PPE. Remind the person about needing PPE. Offer to get the person PPE. For example, you can say:

- "I'll get you the mask that you need."
- "Here are gloves and a gown you need."
  Be polite. Tell the nurse if the person refuses.

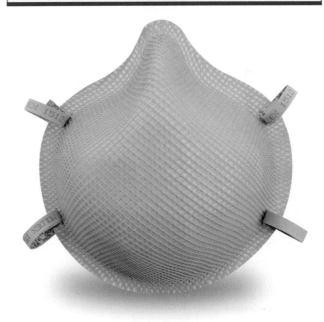

FIGURE 17-2 A respirator. (© Moldex.)

Personal Protective Equipment

Personal protective equipment (PPE) is the clothing or equipment worn by the staff for protection against a hazard. PPE prevents the spread of microbes. The PPE needed depends on tasks, procedures, care measures, and the type of Transmission-Based Precautions used. Sometimes only gloves are needed. The nurse tells you when a gown, goggles or a face shield, and a mask are needed.

See *Teamwork and Time Management: Personal Protective Equipment.*

Gowns. Gowns protect your clothes and body from contact with blood, body fluids, secretions, and excretions. They also protect against splashes and sprays. Gowns are worn with gloves and with other PPE as needed.

A gown must completely cover your body front from the neck to the knees. The long sleeves have tight cuffs. Opening in the back, the gown is tied at the neck and waist. The gown front and sleeves are considered *contaminated.*

Gowns are used once. A wet gown is contaminated. Hold water basins and wet items out away from the gown. Avoid contact with wet surfaces. Remove a wet gown and put on a dry one. Discard disposable gowns after use.

Masks and Respirators. You wear disposable masks:
- To prevent contact with infectious materials from the person. Respiratory secretions and splashes or sprays of blood or body fluids are examples.
- To protect the person from infectious agents carried in your mouth or nose during sterile procedures.

A wet or moist mask is *contaminated.* Breathing can cause masks to become wet or moist. Apply a new mask when contamination occurs.

A mask fits snugly over your nose and mouth. Practice hand hygiene before putting on a mask. To remove a mask, touch only the ties or the elastic bands. The front of the mask is contaminated.

Agency-approved respirators (Fig. 17-2) are worn when caring for persons with smallpox or TB and other airborne infections. See Chapter 49 for more information about persons with TB.

Goggles and Face Shields. Goggles protect your eyes from splashing or spraying of blood, body fluids, secretions, and excretions. Face shields can protect your eyes and other areas of the face. Splashes and sprays can occur when you give care, clean items, or dispose of fluids.

The front (outside) of goggles or a face shield is *contaminated*. The headband, ties, or ear-pieces used to secure the device are *clean*. Use them to remove the device after hand hygiene when they are safe to touch with bare hands. Lift the ties or ear-pieces from the back when removing the device.

Discard disposable goggles or face shields after use. Re-usable eyewear is cleaned before re-use. It is washed with soap and water. Then a disinfectant is used.

See *Promoting Safety and Comfort: Goggles and Face Shields.*

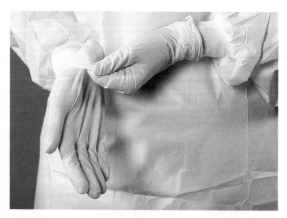

FIGURE 17-3 The gloves cover the gown cuffs.

PROMOTING SAFETY AND COMFORT

Goggles and Face Shields

Safety
Eyeglasses and contact lenses do not provide eye protection. The face shield must fit over eyeglasses with minimal gaps.

Gloves. A natural barrier, the skin prevents microbes from entering the body. Small skin breaks on the hands and fingers are common and may be hard to see. Disposable gloves provide a barrier. They protect:

- You from the person's pathogens
- The person from microbes on your hands

Wear gloves when you will have contact with blood, body fluids, secretions, excretions, mucous membranes, non-intact skin, or other potentially infectious materials (OPIM). See Chapter 16 for OPIM. Also wear gloves when contact is likely with contaminated items or surfaces.

Wearing gloves is the most common measure for Standard Precautions and Transmission-Based Precautions. When using gloves:

- Consider the outside of gloves to be *contaminated.*
- Apply to dry hands. Gloves are easier to put on dry hands.
- Do not tear gloves when putting them on. Carelessness, long fingernails, and rings can tear gloves. Blood, body fluids, secretions, excretions, or OPIM can enter the glove through a tear. This contaminates your hand.
- Remove and discard torn, cut, or punctured gloves at once. Practice hand hygiene. Then put on a new pair.
- Apply a new pair for every person.
- Wear gloves once. Discard them after use.
- Put on new gloves just before touching mucous membranes or non-intact skin.
- Put on new gloves when gloves become contaminated with blood, body fluids, secretions, excretions, or OPIM. A task may require more than 1 pair of gloves.
- Change gloves when moving from a contaminated body site to a clean body site.

- Change gloves when touching portable computer keyboards or other equipment that is moved from room to room.
- Put on gloves last when worn with other PPE.
- Make sure gloves cover your wrists. If you wear a gown, gloves cover the cuffs (Fig. 17-3).
- Remove gloves so the inside part is on the outside. The inside is *clean.*
- Practice hand hygiene after removing gloves.
See *Promoting Safety and Comfort: Gloves.*

PROMOTING SAFETY AND COMFORT

Gloves

Safety
No special method is needed to put on non-sterile gloves. To remove gloves, see procedure: *Donning and Removing Personal Protective Equipment*, p. 250.

Some gloves are made of latex (a rubber product). Latex allergies can cause skin rashes. Difficulty breathing and shock are more serious problems. Report skin rashes, breathing problems, and symptoms of shock (Chapter 58) to the nurse at once.

You may have a latex allergy. Some patients and residents are allergic to latex. This is noted on the care plan and your assignment sheet. Latex-free gloves are worn for latex allergies.

Comfort
Gloves are needed when contact with blood, body fluids, secretions, excretions, mucous membranes, or non-intact skin is likely. Gloves are not needed when such contact is not likely. Back massages and brushing and combing hair are examples if the skin is intact. To reduce exposure to latex, wear gloves only when needed.

Donning and Removing PPE. The PPE worn depends on the type of precautions needed. According to the CDC's isolation guidelines, gloves are always worn with gowns. Sometimes other PPE is needed when gowns are worn.

See *Promoting Safety and Comfort: Donning and Removing PPE.*

See procedure: *Donning and Removing Personal Protective Equipment*, p. 250.

Text continued on p. 251.

PROMOTING SAFETY AND COMFORT

Donning and Removing PPE

Safety

According to the CDC, PPE is donned and removed in the following order.

- Donning PPE (Fig. 17-4, *A*):
  1. Gown
  2. Mask or respirator
  3. Eyewear (goggles or face shield)
  4. Gloves
- Removing PPE (removed at the doorway before leaving the person's room):
  - Method 1 (Fig. 17-4, *B*, p. 248)
    1. Gloves
    2. Eyewear (goggles or face shield)
    3. Gown
    4. Mask or respirator (a respirator is removed after leaving the person's room and closing the door)

- Method 2 (Fig. 17-4, *C*, p. 249)
  1. Gown and gloves
  2. Eyewear (goggles or face shield)
  3. Mask or respirator (a respirator is removed after leaving the person's room and closing the door)

Practice hand hygiene after removing PPE. Practice hand hygiene between steps if your hands become contaminated. Then practice hand hygiene again after removing all PPE.

NOTE: *Some state competency tests require hand hygiene after removing each PPE item. And some states use a different order for donning and removing PPE. Follow the procedures used in your state and agency.*

Some severe and deadly infections require additional PPE—full face shield, helmet, or headpiece; coveralls with socks or special gowns; double gloving; boot or shoe covers; and aprons. Special training is needed to care for such patients and for donning and removing the PPE.

SEQUENCE FOR PUTTING ON PERSONAL PROTECTIVE EQUIPMENT (PPE)

The type of PPE used will vary based on the level of precautions required, such as standard and contact, droplet or airborne infection isolation precautions. The procedure for putting on and removing PPE should be tailored to the specific type of PPE.

1. GOWN

- Fully cover torso from neck to knees, arms to end of wrists, and wrap around the back
- Fasten in back of neck and waist

2. MASK OR RESPIRATOR

- Secure ties or elastic bands at middle of head and neck
- Fit flexible band to nose bridge
- Fit snug to face and below chin
- Fit-check respirator

3. GOGGLES OR FACE SHIELD

- Place over face and eyes and adjust to fit

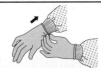

4. GLOVES

- Extend to cover wrist of isolation gown

A

USE SAFE WORK PRACTICES TO PROTECT YOURSELF AND LIMIT THE SPREAD OF CONTAMINATION

- Keep hands away from face
- Limit surfaces touched
- Change gloves when torn or heavily contaminated
- Perform hand hygiene

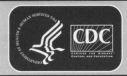

CS250672-E

FIGURE 17-4 A, Donning PPE. (From Centers for Disease Control and Prevention, Department of Health and Human Services.)

Continued

HOW TO SAFELY REMOVE PERSONAL PROTECTIVE EQUIPMENT (PPE) EXAMPLE 1

There are a variety of ways to safely remove PPE without contaminating your clothing, skin, or mucous membranes with potentially infectious materials. Here is one example. **Remove all PPE before exiting the patient room** except a respirator, if worn. Remove the respirator **after** leaving the patient room and closing the door. Remove PPE in the following sequence:

1. GLOVES

- Outside of gloves are contaminated!
- If your hands get contaminated during glove removal, immediately wash your hands or use an alcohol-based hand sanitizer
- Using a gloved hand, grasp the palm area of the other gloved hand and peel off first glove
- Hold removed glove in gloved hand
- Slide fingers of ungloved hand under remaining glove at wrist and peel off second glove over first glove
- Discard gloves in a waste container

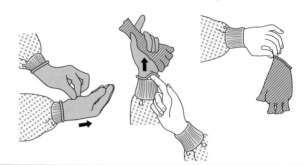

2. GOGGLES OR FACE SHIELD

- Outside of goggles or face shield are contaminated!
- If your hands get contaminated during goggle or face shield removal, immediately wash your hands or use an alcohol-based hand sanitizer
- Remove goggles or face shield from the back by lifting head band or ear pieces
- If the item is reusable, place in designated receptacle for reprocessing. Otherwise, discard in a waste container

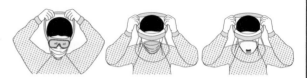

3. GOWN

B

- Gown front and sleeves are contaminated!
- If your hands get contaminated during gown removal, immediately wash your hands or use an alcohol-based hand sanitizer
- Unfasten gown ties, taking care that sleeves don't contact your body when reaching for ties
- Pull gown away from neck and shoulders, touching inside of gown only
- Turn gown inside out
- Fold or roll into a bundle and discard in a waste container

4. MASK OR RESPIRATOR

- Front of mask/respirator is contaminated — DO NOT TOUCH!
- If your hands get contaminated during mask/respirator removal, immediately wash your hands or use an alcohol-based hand sanitizer
- Grasp bottom ties or elastics of the mask/respirator, then the ones at the top, and remove without touching the front
- Discard in a waste container

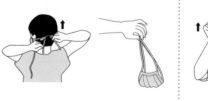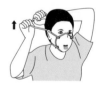

5. WASH HANDS OR USE AN ALCOHOL-BASED HAND SANITIZER IMMEDIATELY AFTER REMOVING ALL PPE

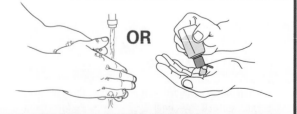

OR

PERFORM HAND HYGIENE BETWEEN STEPS IF HANDS BECOME CONTAMINATED AND IMMEDIATELY AFTER REMOVING ALL PPE

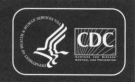

CS250672-E

FIGURE 17-4, cont'd B, Method 1: Removing PPE.

HOW TO SAFELY REMOVE PERSONAL PROTECTIVE EQUIPMENT (PPE) EXAMPLE 2

Here is another way to safely remove PPE without contaminating your clothing, skin, or mucous membranes with potentially infectious materials. **Remove all PPE before exiting the patient room** except a respirator, if worn. Remove the respirator **after** leaving the patient room and closing the door. Remove PPE in the following sequence:

1. GOWN AND GLOVES

- Gown front and sleeves and the outside of gloves are contaminated!
- If your hands get contaminated during gown or glove removal, immediately wash your hands or use an alcohol-based hand sanitizer
- Grasp the gown in the front and pull away from your body so that the ties break, touching outside of gown only with gloved hands
- While removing the gown, fold or roll the gown inside-out into a bundle
- As you are removing the gown, peel off your gloves at the same time, only touching the inside of the gloves and gown with your bare hands. Place the gown and gloves into a waste container

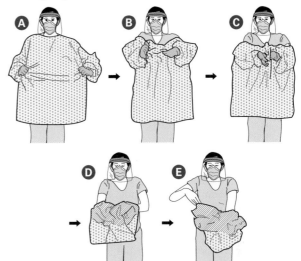

2. GOGGLES OR FACE SHIELD

- Outside of goggles or face shield are contaminated!
- If your hands get contaminated during goggle or face shield removal, immediately wash your hands or use an alcohol-based hand sanitizer
- Remove goggles or face shield from the back by lifting head band and without touching the front of the goggles or face shield
- If the item is reusable, place in designated receptacle for reprocessing. Otherwise, discard in a waste container

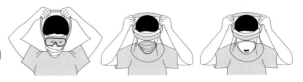

3. MASK OR RESPIRATOR

- Front of mask/respirator is contaminated — DO NOT TOUCH!
- If your hands get contaminated during mask/respirator removal, immediately wash your hands or use an alcohol-based hand sanitizer
- Grasp bottom ties or elastics of the mask/respirator, then the ones at the top, and remove without touching the front
- Discard in a waste container

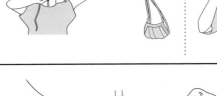

4. WASH HANDS OR USE AN ALCOHOL-BASED HAND SANITIZER IMMEDIATELY AFTER REMOVING ALL PPE

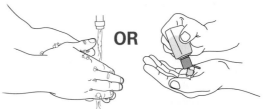

PERFORM HAND HYGIENE BETWEEN STEPS IF HANDS BECOME CONTAMINATED AND IMMEDIATELY AFTER REMOVING ALL PPE

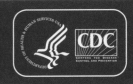

CS250672-E

FIGURE 17-4, cont'd C, Method 2: Removing PPE.

Donning and Removing Personal Protective Equipment

PROCEDURE

1 Follow *Delegation Guidelines: Transmission-Based Precautions*, p. 245. See *Promoting Safety and Comfort:*
   a *Transmission-Based Precautions*, p. 245
   b *Goggles and Face Shields*, p. 246
   c *Gloves*, p. 246
   d *Donning and Removing PPE*, p. 247
2 Remove your watch and all jewelry.
3 Roll up uniform sleeves.
4 Practice hand hygiene.
5 Put on a gown (see Fig. 17-4, *A*).
   a Hold a clean gown out in front of you.
   b Unfold the gown. Face the back of the gown. Do not shake it.
   c Put your hands and arms through the sleeves.
   d Make sure the gown covers you from your neck to your knees. It must cover your arms to the end of your wrists.
   e Tie the strings at the back of the neck.
   f Over-lap the back of the gown. Make sure it covers your uniform. The gown should be snug, not loose.
   g Tie the waist strings. Tie them at the back or the side. Do not tie them in front.
6 Put on a mask or respirator (see Fig. 17-4, *A*).
   a Pick up a mask by its upper ties. Do not touch the part that will cover your face.
   b Place the mask over your nose and mouth (Fig. 17-5, *A*).
   c Place the upper strings above your ears. Tie them at the back in the middle of your head (Fig. 17-5, *B*).
   d Tie the lower strings at the back of your neck (Fig. 17-5, *C*). The lower part of the mask is under your chin.
   e Pinch the metal band around your nose. The top of the mask must be snug over your nose. If you wear eyeglasses, the mask must be snug under the bottom of the eyeglasses.
   f Make sure the mask is snug over your face and under your chin.
7 Put on goggles or a face shield (if needed and if not part of the mask) (see Fig. 17-4, *A*).
   a Place the device over your face and eyes.
   b Adjust the device to fit.
8 Put on gloves. Make sure the gloves cover the wrists of the gown.
9 Provide care.
10 Remove and discard the PPE. Practice hand hygiene between each step if your hands become contaminated.
   a *Method 1: Gloves, goggles or face shield, gown, mask or respirator* (see Fig. 17-4, *B*)
      1) Remove and discard the gloves.
         a) Make sure that glove touches only glove.
         b) Grasp a glove at the palm (Fig. 17-6, *A*). Grasp it on the outside.
         c) Pull the glove down over your hand so it is inside-out (Fig. 17-6, *B*).
         d) Hold the removed glove with your other gloved hand.
         e) Reach inside the other glove. Use the first 2 fingers of the ungloved hand (Fig. 17-6, *C*).
         f) Pull the glove down inside-out over your hand and the other glove (Fig. 17-6, *D*).
         g) Discard the gloves.

      2) Remove and discard the goggles or face shield if worn.
         a) Lift the headband or ear-pieces from the back. Do not touch the front of the device.
         b) Discard the device. If re-usable, follow agency policy.
      3) Remove and discard the gown. Do not touch the outside of the gown.
         a) Untie the neck and then the waist strings.
         b) Pull the gown down and away from your neck and shoulders. Only touch the inside of the gown.
         c) Turn the gown inside-out as it is removed. Hold it at the inside shoulder seams and bring your hands together.
         d) Fold or roll up the gown away from you. Keep it inside-out. Do not let the gown touch the floor.
         e) Discard the gown.
      4) Remove and discard the mask if worn. (NOTE: Remove a respirator after leaving the room and closing the door.)
         a) Untie the lower strings of the mask.
         b) Untie the top strings.
         c) Hold the top strings. Remove the mask without touching the front of the mask.
         d) Discard the mask.
   b *Method 2: Gown and gloves, goggles or face shield, mask or respirator* (see Fig. 17-4, *C*).
      1) Remove and discard the gown and gloves.
         a) Grasp the gown in front with your gloved hands. Pull away from your body so the ties break. Only touch the outside of the gown.
         b) Fold or roll the gown inside-out into a bundle while removing the gown. Keep it inside-out. Do not let the gown touch the floor.
         c) Peel off your gloves as you remove the gown. Only touch the inside of the gloves and gown with your bare hands.
         d) Discard the gown and gloves.
      2) Remove and discard the goggles or face shield.
         a) Lift the headband or ear-pieces from the back. Do not touch the front of the device.
         b) Discard the device. If re-usable, follow agency policy.
      3) Remove and discard the mask if worn. (NOTE: Remove a respirator after leaving the room and closing the door.)
         a) Untie the lower strings of the mask.
         b) Untie the top strings.
         c) Hold the top strings. Remove the mask without touching the front of the mask.
         d) Discard the mask.
11 Practice hand hygiene after removing all PPE.

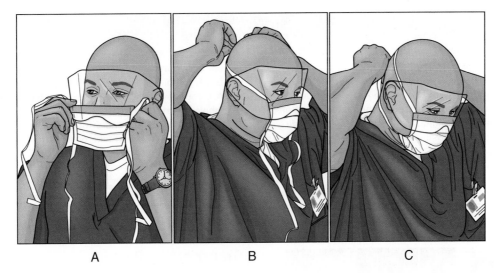

FIGURE 17-5 Donning a mask. (NOTE: The mask has a face shield.) **A,** The mask covers the nose and mouth. **B,** Upper strings are tied at the back of the head. **C,** Lower strings are tied at the back of the neck.

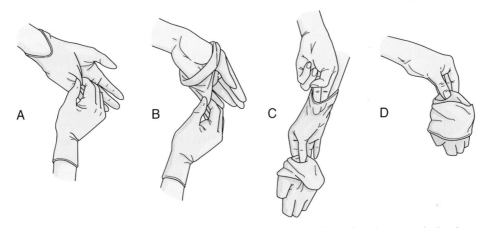

FIGURE 17-6 Removing gloves. **A,** Grasp the glove at the palm. **B,** Pull the glove down over the hand. The glove is inside-out. **C,** Insert the fingers of the ungloved hand inside the other glove. **D,** Pull the glove down and over the other hand and glove. The glove is inside-out.

Bagging Items

Contaminated items are bagged for removal from the person's room. Leak-proof plastic bags are used. They have the *BIOHAZARD* symbol (Fig. 17-7). ***Biohazardous waste** is items contaminated with blood, body fluids, secretions, or excretions.* (Bio *means* life. Hazardous *means* dangerous *or* harmful.)

Bag and transport linens following agency policy. Laundry bags with contaminated linens and laundry need a *BIOHAZARD* symbol. Melt-away bags dissolve in hot water. Once soiled linens are bagged, no one needs to handle them. Do not over-fill the bag. Tie the bag securely. Then place it in a laundry hamper lined with a biohazard plastic bag.

Trash is placed in a container labeled with the *BIOHAZARD* symbol. Follow agency policy for bagging and transporting trash, equipment, and supplies.

Usually 1 bag is needed. Double-bagging involves 2 bags. Double-bagging is needed if the outside of the bag is wet, soiled, or may be contaminated.

See procedure: *Double-Bagging,* p. 252.

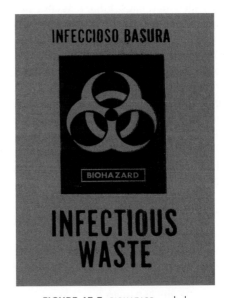

FIGURE 17-7 *BIOHAZARD* symbol.

Double-Bagging

PROCEDURE

1 Ask a co-worker to help you. He or she stands outside the doorway. You are in the room.
2 Place soiled linens, laundry, re-usable items, disposable supplies, and trash in the right containers. Containers are lined with leak-proof biohazard bags. These are the *dirty (contaminated)* bags.
3 Seal the *dirty* bag securely.
4 Ask your co-worker to make a wide cuff on a *clean* bag. It is held wide open. The cuff protects the hands from contamination (Fig. 17-8, *A*).

5 Place the *dirty* bag into the *clean* bag (Fig. 17-8, *B*). Do not touch the outside of the *clean* bag.
6 Ask your co-worker to seal the *clean* bag. Have the bag labeled with the *BIOHAZARD* symbol.
7 Repeat steps 3, 4, 5, and 6 for other *dirty* bags.
8 Ask your co-worker to take or send the bags to the appropriate department for disposal, disinfection, or sterilization.

A 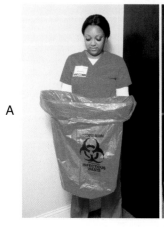 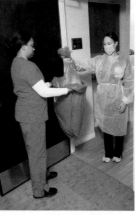 B

FIGURE 17-8 Double-bagging. **A,** A cuff is made on a clean bag. **B,** One nursing assistant is in the room by the doorway. The other is outside the doorway. The *dirty* bag is placed inside the *clean* bag.

Collecting Specimens. Blood, body fluids, secretions, and excretions often require laboratory testing (Chapter 38). Specimens are transported to the laboratory in biohazard specimen bags. Follow agency procedures to collect, store, and transport specimens when a person is on Transmission-Based Precautions. Remember to:

- Label the specimen container and biohazard specimen bag. Apply warning labels according to agency policy.
- Wear gloves and other PPE as required.
- Avoid contaminating the outside of the specimen container and the outside of the biohazard bag. The following method is common.
- Leave the biohazard bag outside the room.
- Place the specimen container on a paper towel inside the room.
- Collect the specimen (Chapter 38). Do not contaminate the outside of the container. Secure the lid.
- Remove and discard PPE. Practice hand hygiene.
- Use a paper towel to pick up the container. Place the specimen in the biohazard bag. Do not contaminate the outside of the specimen bag.
- Discard the paper towel.
- Practice hand hygiene.

Transporting Persons

Persons on Transmission-Based Precautions usually do not leave their rooms. Sometimes they go to other areas for treatments or tests that cannot be done in the person's room.

Transport procedures vary among agencies. Some require transport by bed. This prevents contaminating wheelchairs and stretchers. Others use wheelchairs and stretchers.

A safe transport protects others from the infection. Follow agency procedures and these guidelines for the Transmission-Based Precautions being used.

- Alert staff in the receiving area that the person requires isolation precautions. Advise of the type of precaution and the PPE needed.
- Have the person wear a clean gown or pajamas.
- Have the person wear needed PPE. Follow the care plan and the nurse's instructions.
- Provide needed barriers. Examples include:
  - Providing tissues and a leak-proof bag for respiratory secretions. Used tissues are placed in the bag.
  - Covering skin lesions or infected or draining areas.
- Wear PPE as required.
- Place an extra layer of sheets and absorbent pads on the stretcher or wheelchair. This protects against draining body fluids.
- Do not let others on the elevator. This reduces exposure to infection.
- Disinfect the stretcher or wheelchair after use.

Meeting Basic Needs

The person has love, belonging, and self-esteem needs. Often they are unmet during Transmission-Based Precautions. Visitors and staff might avoid the person. Applying PPE takes extra effort before entering the room. Some are not sure what they can touch. They may fear getting the disease.

The person may feel lonely, unwanted, rejected, dirty, and undesirable. The person knows the disease can be spread to others. Without intending to, visitors and staff can make the person feel ashamed and guilty for having a contagious disease.

See *Focus on Communication: Meeting Basic Needs*.

See *Focus on Children and Older Persons: Meeting Basic Needs*.

FOCUS ON COMMUNICATION

Meeting Basic Needs

The nurse explains the need for Transmission-Based Precautions and PPE to the person, visitors, you, and other staff. Ask questions to make sure you understand the need and what to do.

How you communicate with the person is important. Some questions or statements can make the person feel dirty or ashamed. Be careful what you say. For example, do not say:
- "How did you get that?"
- "What were you doing?"
- "I'm afraid to touch you."
- "Don't breathe on me."

Always treat the person with respect, kindness, and dignity.

FOCUS ON CHILDREN AND OLDER PERSONS

Meeting Basic Needs

Children

Goggles, face shields, masks, and gowns may scare infants and children. Parents and staff look different. Gloves and gowns prevent skin-to-skin contact with parents. Because of likely contamination, toys and comfort items (blankets, stuffed animals) may be kept from the child. This increases the child's distress.

The nurse prepares the child and family for isolation. Simple explanations are given to the child. Depending on age, the nurse may give the child a mask and goggles or face shield to touch and play with.

Children need to see the faces of people entering the room. Let the child see your face before putting on a mask, goggles, or a face shield. Say "hello" to the child from the doorway and state your name.

Older Persons

Persons with poor vision need to know who you are. Let them see your face before you put on a mask, goggles, or a face shield. State your name at the doorway and explain what you need to do. Then put on PPE.

Some older persons have dementia. PPE may increase confusion and cause fear and agitation. These measures can help.
- Let the person see your face before putting on PPE.
- Tell the person who you are and what you need to do.
- Use a calm, soothing voice.
- Do not rush the person.
- Use touch to reassure the person.
- Follow the care plan and the nurse's instructions for other measures to help the person.
- Report signs of increased confusion or behavior changes.

FOCUS ON PRIDE

The Person, Family, and Yourself

P ersonal and Professional Responsibility

Standard Precautions and Transmission-Based Precautions are important for the person's safety and yours. You can easily contaminate your gloves and supplies.

Do not use a contaminated item. Be honest with yourself and responsible. Take pride in providing care that prevents the spread of infection.

R ights and Respect

Caring for persons who need Transmission-Based Precautions can be a challenge. Extra time and effort are needed to apply and remove PPE and clean equipment used in the room. You may feel frustrated.

The person must not feel like a burden. The person deserves the same kindness and respect you give others. You must:
- Watch your verbal and nonverbal communication (Chapter 7).
- Avoid complaining.
- Practice good teamwork and time management.
- Tell the nurse if you are feeling overwhelmed.

I ndependence and Social Interaction

The person on Transmission-Based Precautions may feel isolated and lonely. To help the person:
- Remember that the pathogen is undesirable, not the person.
- Treat the person with respect, kindness, and dignity.
- Provide newspapers, magazines, books, a current TV guide, and other reading matter.
- Provide hobby materials if possible.
- Place a clock in the room.
- Suggest that the person call family and friends.
- Plan your work so you can stay to visit with the person.
- Say "hello" from the doorway often.

Remember, items brought into the person' s room become contaminated. Disinfect or discard the items according to agency policy.

Continued

FOCUS ON **PRIDE**—cont'd

The Person, Family, and Yourself

D elegation and Teamwork

You may be involved in the care of a person who requires Transmission-Based Precautions. Review the precaution with the nurse. Make sure you understand the type of precaution ordered and necessary safety measures.

If you need help, ask your co-workers to assist. In turn, assist your co-workers when they need help.

E thics and Laws

The CDC's isolation guideline is aimed at reducing the number of healthcare-associated infections (Chapter 16). Surveyors (Chapter 1) will observe how staff follow the guideline. You are ethically responsible for following the guideline. Doing so protects the person, staff, and visitors.

FOCUS ON **PRIDE**: *Application*

Explain the emotional and social effects of Transmission-Based Precautions. How can you help meet these needs?

REVIEW QUESTIONS

Circle the BEST answer.

1 Isolation precautions
   a Treat communicable diseases
   b Destroy pathogens
   c Keep pathogens within a certain area
   d Destroy all microbes

2 Which statement about Standard Precautions is *true?*
   a They are used for all persons.
   b The 3 types are contact, droplet, and airborne.
   c They are used only in hospitals.
   d They require a doctor's order.

3 What PPE is needed to serve a meal tray to a patient requiring contact precautions?
   a A gown and gloves
   b A gown, mask, and gloves
   c A gown, mask, goggles, and gloves
   d None

4 A patient requires droplet precautions. There is 1 mask left outside room. You should
   a Not use the mask
   b Use the mask and return it for re-use
   c Use the mask and re-stock the masks
   d Wait until a co-worker re-stocks the masks to give care

5 A resident requires Transmission-Based Precautions. You can
   a Use linens that fall on the floor
   b Touch your hair and face in the person's room
   c Use a leak-proof plastic bag to remove a meal tray from the room
   d Keep PPE on when leaving the room to get supplies

6 A mask
   a Is removed before other PPE is removed
   b Is clean on the inside
   c Is contaminated when moist
   d Should fit loosely for breathing

7 To use PPE correctly
   a Never change gloves in the person's room
   b Tie a gown's waist strings in front
   c Don gloves first when applying PPE
   d Apply new PPE for each person

8 Which task requires gloves?
   a Measuring blood pressure
   b Giving a back massage
   c Providing denture care
   d Moving the person up in bed

9 Goggles or a face shield is worn
   a When using Standard Precautions
   b When splashing body fluids is likely
   c If you have an eye infection
   d When assisting with sterile procedures

10 A specimen is needed from a patient on Transmission-Based Precautions. Which contaminates the specimen container?
   a Handling the container with a paper towel
   b Placing the container on a paper towel in the bathroom
   c Spilling the specimen on the outside of the container
   d Placing the container in a biohazard bag

Answers to Chapter 17 questions are on p. 886.

FOCUS ON PRACTICE

Problem Solving

A nurse enters the room of a person who requires contact precautions. The nurse is not wearing PPE. You need help to move the person in bed. Will you ask the nurse to help? What PPE is needed? What precautions are needed upon entering and leaving the room and while in the room?

Body Mechanics

OBJECTIVES

- Define the key terms and key abbreviations in this chapter.
- Explain the purpose and rules of body mechanics.
- Identify the risk factors for work-related injuries.
- Identify the activities at high risk for work-related injuries, including back injuries.

- Identify the causes, signs, and symptoms of back injuries.
- Explain how to prevent work-related injuries.
- Position persons in the basic bed positions and in a chair.
- Explain how to promote PRIDE in the person, the family, and yourself.

KEY TERMS

base of support The area on which an object rests
body alignment The way the head, trunk, arms, and legs align with one another; posture
body mechanics Using the body in an efficient and careful way
dorsal recumbent position The back-lying or supine position
ergonomics The science of designing a job to fit the worker; *ergo* means *work*, *nomos* means *law*
Fowler's position A semi-sitting position; the head of the bed is raised between 45 and 60 degrees
lateral position The person lies on 1 side or the other; side-lying position

musculo-skeletal disorders (MSDs) Injuries and disorders of the muscles, tendons, ligaments, joints, and cartilage
posture See "body alignment"
prone position The person lies on the abdomen with the head turned to 1 side
semi-prone side position See "Sims' position"
side-lying position See "lateral position"
Sims' position A left side-lying position in which the upper leg (right leg) is sharply flexed so it is not on the lower leg (left leg) and the lower arm (left arm) is behind the person; semi-prone side position
supine position The back-lying or dorsal recumbent position

KEY ABBREVIATIONS

MSD   Musculo-skeletal disorder

OSHA   Occupational Safety and Health Administration

Body mechanics *means using the body in an efficient and careful way.* It involves good posture, balance, and using your strongest and largest muscles for work. Fatigue, muscle strain, and injury can result from the incorrect use and positioning of the body during activity or rest.

Focus on the person's and your own body mechanics. Good body mechanics reduce the risk of injury.

See *Body Structure and Function Review: The Musculo-Skeletal System*, p. 256. For greater detail, see Chapter 10.

BODY STRUCTURE AND FUNCTION REVIEW

The Musculo-Skeletal System

The *musculo-skeletal system:*
- Provides the framework for the body.
- Lets the body move.
- Protects internal organs.
- Gives the body shape.

Bones

Bones are hard, rigid structures. Bones:
- Bear the body's weight—leg bones.
- Allow skill and ease in movement—bones in the wrists, fingers, ankles, and toes.
- Protect the organs—ribs, skull, pelvic bones, and shoulder blades.
- Allow various degrees of movement and flexibility—vertebrae in the spinal column.

Joints

A *joint* is the point at which 2 or more bones meet. Joints allow movement. There are 3 major types of joints (Fig. 18-1).
- A *ball-and-socket joint* allows movement in all directions. The rounded end of 1 bone fits into the hollow end of another bone. Hip and shoulder joints are ball-and-socket joints.
- A *hinge joint* allows movement in 1 direction. The elbow is a hinge joint.
- A *pivot joint* allows turning from side to side. A pivot joint connects the skull to the spine.

Some joints do not move. They connect the bones of the skull.

Muscles

The human body has more than 500 *muscles* (Fig. 18-2). Some muscles are *voluntary.* They are consciously controlled. *Skeletal muscles* attached to bones are voluntary. Arm and leg muscles are examples. Other muscles are *involuntary.* They work automatically. Muscles in the stomach, intestines, and blood vessels are examples. *Cardiac muscle* in the heart is involuntary. The cardiac muscle pumps blood throughout the body.

Muscles move body parts and maintain posture. When muscles contract, they use energy. Heat is produced.

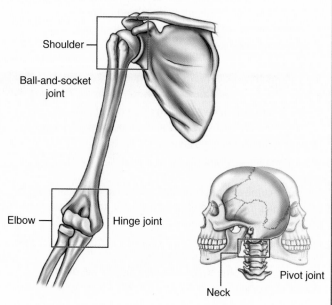

FIGURE 18-1 Types of joints. (Modified from Herlihy B: *The human body in health and illness,* ed 6, St Louis, 2018, Elsevier.)

PRINCIPLES OF BODY MECHANICS

Body alignment (posture) is the way the head, trunk, arms, and legs align with one another. Good alignment lets the body move and function with strength and efficiency. Standing, sitting, and lying down require good alignment.

Base of support is the area on which an object rests. A good base of support is needed for balance (Fig. 18-3). When standing, your feet are your base of support. Stand with your feet apart for a wider base of support and more balance.

The strongest and largest muscles are in the shoulders, upper arms, hips, and thighs. Use these muscles to handle and move persons and heavy objects. Otherwise, you place strain and exertion on the smaller and weaker muscles. This causes fatigue and injury. *Back injuries are a major risk.* For good body mechanics:
- Bend your knees and squat to lift a heavy object (Fig. 18-4). Do not bend from your waist. Bending from the waist places strain on small back muscles.
- Hold items close to your body and base of support (see Fig. 18-4). This involves upper arm and shoulder muscles. Holding objects away from the body places strain on small muscles in the lower arms.

BODY STRUCTURE AND FUNCTION REVIEW—cont'd

The Musculo-Skeletal System

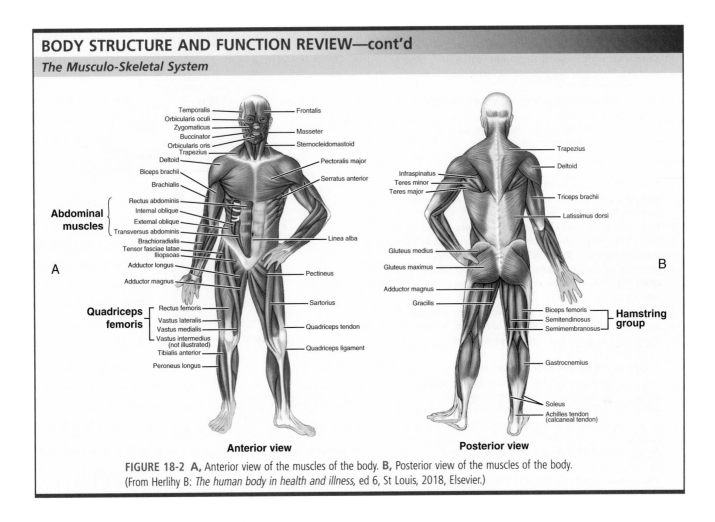

FIGURE 18-2 A, Anterior view of the muscles of the body. **B,** Posterior view of the muscles of the body.
(From Herlihy B: *The human body in health and illness,* ed 6, St Louis, 2018, Elsevier.)

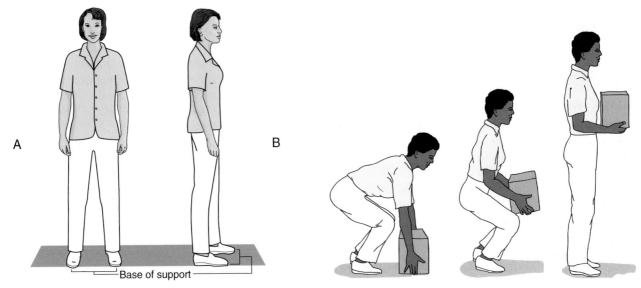

FIGURE 18-3 A, Anterior (front) view of an adult in good body alignment. The feet are apart for a wide base of support. **B,** Lateral (side) view of an adult with good posture and alignment.

FIGURE 18-4 Picking up a box using good body mechanics.

BOX 18-1	Rules for Body Mechanics

- Keep your body in good alignment with a wide base of support. Your feet are at least 12 inches apart or shoulder-width apart.
- Use an upright working posture. Bend your legs. Do not bend your back.
- Use the stronger and larger muscles in your shoulders, upper arms, thighs, and hips.
- Keep objects close to your body to lift, move, or carry them (see Fig. 18-4).
- Avoid unnecessary bending and reaching. Raise the bed and over-bed table to waist level or to a comfortable working height.
- Face your work area. This prevents unnecessary twisting.
- Push, slide, or pull heavy objects when you can rather than lifting them. Pushing is easier than pulling.
- Widen your base of support to push or pull. Move your front leg forward when pushing. Move your rear leg back when pulling (Fig. 18-5).
- Use both hands and arms to lift, move, or carry objects.
- Turn your whole body to change direction. Do not twist.
- Work with smooth and even movements. Avoid sudden or jerky motions.
- Do not lean over a person to give care.
- *Get help from a co-worker to move persons or heavy objects. Do not lift or move them by yourself.*
- Bend your hips and knees to lift heavy objects from the floor (see Fig. 18-4). Straighten your back as the object reaches thigh level. Your leg and thigh muscles work to raise the item off the floor and to waist level.
- Do not lift objects higher than chest level. Do not lift above your shoulders. Use a step stool or ladder to reach an object higher than chest level.

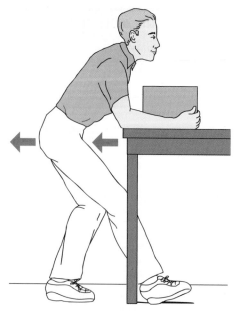

FIGURE 18-5 Move your rear leg back when pulling.

Rules for Body Mechanics

All activities require good body mechanics. You must safely and efficiently handle and move persons and heavy objects. Follow the rules in Box 18-1.

WORK-RELATED INJURIES

Musculo-skeletal disorders (MSDs) are injuries and disorders of the muscles, tendons, ligaments, joints, and cartilage. They can be caused or made worse by the work setting. They can involve the nervous system. The arms and back are often affected. So are the hands, fingers, neck, wrists, legs, and shoulders. MSDs can develop slowly over weeks, months, and years. Or they can occur from 1 event. Pain, numbness, tingling, stiff joints, difficulty moving, and muscle loss can occur. Sometimes there is paralysis.

Early signs and symptoms include pain, limited joint movement, or swelling. Time off work is often needed. Disabilities can result.

MSD Risk Factors

The Occupational Safety and Health Administration (OSHA) has identified MSD risk factors. An MSD is more likely if risk factors are combined. For example, a task involves both force and repeating actions.

- *Force*—the amount of physical effort needed for a task. Lifting or transferring heavy persons, preventing falls, and sudden motions are examples.
- *Repeating action*—doing the same motion or series of motions often or continually. Re-positioning persons and transfers to and from beds, chairs, and commodes without adequate rest breaks are examples.
- *Awkward postures*—assuming positions that place stress on the body. Examples are reaching above shoulder height, kneeling, squatting, leaning over a bed, bending, or twisting the torso while lifting.
- *Heavy lifting*—manually lifting people who cannot move themselves.

According to the U.S. Department of Labor, nursing assistants are at great risk. The tasks listed in Box 18-2 are known to be high risk for MSDs.

| BOX 18-2 | Musculo-Skeletal Disorders—Risk Factors |

- Transfers—to and from beds, chairs, wheelchairs, toilets, stretchers, and bathtubs
- Trying to stop a person from falling
- Picking up a person from the floor to the bed
- Lifting alone
- Lifting persons who are confused or uncooperative
- Lifting persons who cannot support their own weight
- Lifting heavy persons
- Weighing a person
- Moving a person up in bed
- Re-positioning a person in a bed or in a chair
- Changing an incontinence product
- Making beds
- Dressing and undressing a person
- Feeding a person in bed
- Giving a bed bath
- Applying anti-embolism stockings
- Prolonged holding of a body part for care measures—arm, leg, abdomen, skin fold

PROMOTING SAFETY AND COMFORT

Back Injuries

Safety
The activities listed in Box 18-2 are related to back injuries in nursing centers. Use good body mechanics to protect yourself from injury. Get help and avoid lifting and bending the back when possible.

PROMOTING SAFETY AND COMFORT

Preventing MSDs

Safety
Injuries commonly occur from manually lifting, transferring, and re-positioning persons. Proper body mechanics alone do not reduce MSDs. Policies and procedures that minimize manual lifting must be followed to prevent injuries. Use assist devices and mechanical lifts (Chapters 19 and 20) when possible.

Back Injuries. Back injuries are major threats. Back injuries can occur from repeated activities or from 1 event. Signs and symptoms include:
- Pain when trying to assume a normal posture
- Decreased mobility
- Pain when standing or rising from a seated position
These and other factors can lead to back disorders.
- Reaching while lifting
- Poor posture when sitting or standing
- Staying in 1 position too long
- Poor body mechanics when lifting, pushing, pulling, or carrying objects
- Poor physical condition—not having the strength or endurance to perform tasks without strain
- Repeated lifting of awkward items, equipment, or persons
- Shifting weight when a person loses balance or strength while moving
- Twisting or bending while lifting or to perform a task
- Maintaining a bent posture such as leaning over a bed
- Reaching over raised bed rails
- Working in a confined, crowded, or cluttered area (rooms, bathrooms, hallways)
- Fatigue
- Poor footing, such as on slippery floors
- Lifting with forceful movement

Follow the rules and safety measures in this chapter to prevent back injuries. Be very careful during tasks associated with back injuries.

See *Promoting Safety and Comfort: Back Injuries.*

Preventing MSDs

The work setting must be free of hazards that cause or may cause death or serious physical harm to staff. The employer must make reasonable attempts to prevent or reduce the hazard.

Ergonomics is the science of designing a job to fit the worker. (Ergo *means* work. Nomos *means* law.) It involves changing the task, work station, equipment, and tools to help reduce stress on the worker's body. The goal is to eliminate a serious work-related MSD.

Always report a work-related injury as soon as possible. Early attention can prevent the problem from becoming worse. Also, injuries are often less serious and less costly to treat with early attention.

To prevent work-related MSDs, follow the rules in Box 18-1 and Box 18-3, p. 260.

See *Promoting Safety and Comfort: Preventing MSDs.*

BOX 18-3   Preventing Work-Related Injuries

General Guidelines

- Wear shoes with good traction. Avoid shoes with worn-down soles or sides. Good traction helps prevent slips or falls.
- Use assist equipment and devices (Chapters 19 and 20) when possible instead of lifting and moving the person manually. Follow the care plan.
- Get help from other staff. The nurse and care plan tell you the number of staff needed for a task.
- Plan and prepare for the task. For example, know what equipment is needed, where to place chairs or wheelchairs, and what side of the bed to work on.
- Schedule harder tasks early in your shift.
- Balance lighter and harder tasks. Plan to complete a lighter task after a harder one.
- Lock (brake) bed wheels and wheelchair or stretcher wheels.
- Tell the person how to help. Give clear, simple instructions. Give the person time to respond.
- Do not hold or grab the person under the underarms.
- Do not let the person hold or grasp you around your neck.

Manual Lifting

- Minimize or eliminate manual lifting when possible.
- Stand with good posture. Keep your back straight.
- Bend your legs, not your back.
- Use the large muscles in your legs to do the work.
- Face the person.
- Do not twist or turn. Pick up your feet and pivot your whole body in the direction of the move.
- Keep what you are moving close to you.
- Move the person toward you, not away from you.
- Use a wide, balanced base of support. Stand with 1 foot slightly ahead of the other.
- Use smooth, even movements. Avoid jerking movements.
- Lift on the "count of 3" when lifting with others. Everyone lifts at the same time.

Moving the Person in Bed (Chapter 19)

- Adjust the bed height to a safe and comfortable level for you.
- Lower the bed rail.
- Work on the side where the person will be closest to you.
- Place equipment or other items close to you at waist level or at a comfortable working height.
- Use friction-reducing devices—drawsheets, turning pads, large re-usable waterproof under-pads, slide sheets (Chapters 19 and 20).

Transfer/Gait Belts (Chapter 14)

- Keep the person as close to you as possible.
- Avoid bending your back, reaching, or twisting for these and other nursing tasks:
  - Applying or removing a transfer/gait belt
  - Lowering the person to the chair, bed, toilet, or floor
  - Helping the person walk
- Use a gentle rocking motion to help the person stand. The rocking motion gives strength and force as you help the person stand.

Stand and Pivot Transfers (Chapter 20)

- Use assist devices as directed. Follow the care plan.
- Use a transfer belt as directed. The nurse may have you use a transfer belt with handles. See Chapter 14.
- Plan the transfer so the person's strong side moves first.
- Lower the bed so the person can place his or her feet on the floor.
- Get the person close to the edge of the bed or the chair. Ask the person to lean forward as he or she stands.
- Block the person's weak leg with your legs or knees. If the position is awkward:
  - Use a transfer belt with handles.
  - Straddle your legs around the person's weak leg.
- Keep your feet at least shoulder-width apart.
- Bend your legs. Do not bend your back.
- Use a gentle rocking motion to help the person stand. The rocking motion gives strength and force as you help the person stand.
- Pivot with your feet to turn.

Lateral Transfers (Chapter 20)

- Position surfaces close to each other.
- Adjust surfaces to about waist height or to a comfortable working height. Do 1 of the following as directed by the nurse and care plan.
  - Adjust the surfaces to the same level.
  - Adjust the receiving surface so it is slightly lower (about $\frac{1}{2}$ inch) than the surface the person is on. This allows the use of gravity. For example, for a bed to stretcher transfer, the stretcher surface is lower than the bed.
- Lower bed rails and stretcher side rails.
- Use friction-reducing devices.
- Get a good hand-hold. Roll up drawsheets, turning pads, large re-usable waterproof under-pads, and slide sheets. Or use assist devices with handles.
- Kneel on the bed or stretcher. This prevents extended reaches and bending your back.
- Have staff on both sides of the bed or the other surface. Move the person on the "count of 3." Use a smooth, push-pull motion. Do not reach across the person.

Transporting the Person and Equipment

- Push, do not pull.
- Keep the load close to your body.
- Use an upright posture.
- Push with your whole body, not just your arms.
- Move down the center of the hallway. This helps avoid collisions.
- Watch out for door handles and high thresholds on floors. These can cause abrupt stops.

Transferring the Person From the Floor

- See Chapter 14.

Modified from Cal/OSHA: A back injury prevention guide for health care providers, Sacramento, Calif, 1997, Author; and Occupational Safety and Health Administration: Guidelines for nursing homes: ergonomics for the prevention of musculoskeletal disorders, *Washington, DC, revised March 2009, Author.*

POSITIONING THE PERSON

The person must be positioned correctly at all times. Regular position changes and good alignment promote comfort and well-being. Breathing is easier. Circulation is promoted. Pressure injuries and contractures are prevented. A *contracture* is the lack of joint mobility caused by the abnormal shortening of a muscle (Chapter 34).

Many patients and residents are able to move and turn when in bed or a chair. Some need reminding or help to adjust their positions. Others depend entirely on the nursing team for position changes.

Whether in bed or chair, the person is re-positioned at least every 2 hours or more often. Follow the nurse's instructions and the care plan. To safely position a person:

- Use good body mechanics.
- Ask a co-worker to help you if needed.
- Explain the procedure to the person.
- Provide for privacy.
- Be gentle when moving the person.
- Use pillows as directed by the nurse for support and alignment.
- Provide for comfort after positioning. (See the inside of the back cover.)
- Place the call light and other needed items within reach after positioning.
- Complete a safety check before leaving the room. (See the inside of the back cover.)

See *Focus on Communication: Positioning the Person.*
See *Delegation Guidelines: Positioning the Person.*
See *Promoting Safety and Comfort: Positioning the Person.*

FOCUS ON **COMMUNICATION**

Positioning the Person

Moving can be painful. Some older persons have painful joints. Pain is common after surgery or injury. Avoid causing pain when positioning the person. Explain what you will do before and during the procedure. Move the person slowly and gently. Give the person time to tell you if a movement is painful. Make sure the person is comfortable. You can say:

- "Am I hurting you?"
- "Please tell me if I'm moving you too fast."
- "Please tell me if you feel pain or discomfort."
- "Do you need a pillow adjusted?"
- "Are you comfortable?"
- "How can I help make you more comfortable?"

DELEGATION GUIDELINES

Positioning the Person

Many routine nursing tasks involve positioning and re-positioning. When delegated such tasks, you need this information from the nurse and the care plan.

- Position or positioning limits ordered by the doctor
- How often to turn and re-position the person
- How many staff members need to help you
- What assist devices to use (Chapters 19 and 20)
- What skin care measures to perform (Chapter 24)
- What range-of-motion exercises to perform (Chapter 34)
- Where to place pillows
- What positioning devices are needed and how to use them (Chapter 34)
- What observations to report and record
- When to report observations
- What patient and resident concerns to report at once

PROMOTING SAFETY AND COMFORT

Positioning the Person

Safety

Pressure injuries (Chapter 41) are serious threats from lying or sitting too long in 1 place. Wet, soiled, and wrinkled linens are other causes. When you re-position a person, make sure linens are clean, dry, and wrinkle-free. Change or straighten linens as needed.

Contractures can develop from staying in 1 position too long (Chapter 34). Re-positioning, exercise, and activity help prevent contractures.

Comfort

Pillows and positioning devices support body parts and provide good alignment. This promotes comfort. Place pillows and positioning devices as directed by the nurse and the care plan.

Older persons may have limited range of motion in their necks. Usually the prone and Sims' positions (pp. 263 and 264) are not comfortable for them. Check with the nurse before positioning an older person in the prone or Sims' position.

Fowler's Positions

Fowler's position is a semi-sitting position. The head of the bed is raised between 45 and 60 degrees (Fig. 18-6). The knees may be slightly elevated. Other forms of Fowler's position include:

- *Semi-Fowler's position*—the head of the bed is raised 30 degrees (Chapter 21). Some agencies define semi-Fowler's position as the head of the bed is raised 30 degrees and the knee portion is raised 15 degrees.
- *High-Fowler's position*—the head of the bed is raised 60 to 90 degrees (Chapter 21).

For good alignment:

- The spine is straight.
- The head is supported with a small pillow.
- The arms are supported with pillows.

The nurse may have you place small pillows under the lower back, thighs, and ankles. Persons with heart and respiratory disorders usually breathe easier in Fowler's position.

See *Focus on Math: Fowler's Positions.*

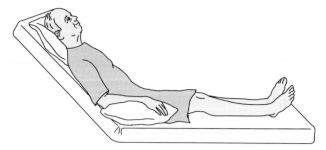

FIGURE 18-6 Fowler's position.

FOCUS ON MATH

Fowler's Positions

When 2 lines meet, an angle is formed. Angles are measured in degrees (°). Degrees range from 0 to 360. With bed positions, you need a basic understanding of angle measurements between 0° and 90°.

To estimate the angle:
1 Use the bed frame and the head of the bed as the 2 lines.
2 Estimate the angle from the bed frame to the head of the bed. See Figure 18-7.

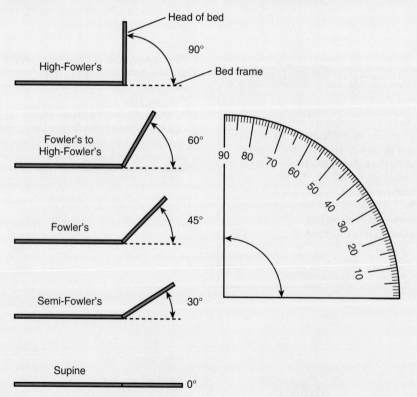

FIGURE 18-7 Measuring bed angles. The angle is measured from the bed frame to the back of the head of the bed. As the head of the bed rises, the angle increases.

Supine Position

The *supine position (dorsal recumbent position) is the back-lying position* (Fig. 18-8).

* The bed is flat.
* The head and shoulders are supported on a pillow.
* Arms and hands are at the sides. You can support the arms with regular pillows. Or you can support the hands on small pillows with the palms down.

The nurse may have you place a folded or rolled towel under the lower back and a small pillow under the thighs. A pillow under the lower legs lifts the heels off of the bed. This prevents the heels from rubbing on the sheets.

Prone Position

In the *prone position, the person lies on the abdomen with the head turned to 1 side.*

* The bed is flat.
* Small pillows are under the head, abdomen, and lower legs (Fig. 18-9).
* Arms are flexed at the elbows with the hands near the head.

You also can position a person with the feet hanging over the end of the mattress (Fig. 18-10). A pillow is not needed under the feet.

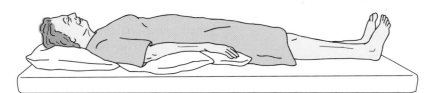

FIGURE 18-8 Supine position.

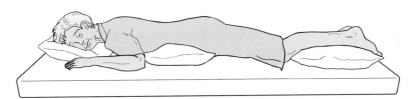

FIGURE 18-9 Prone position.

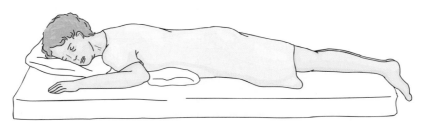

FIGURE 18-10 Prone position with the feet hanging over the edge of the mattress.

Lateral Position

In the *lateral position (side-lying position)*, *the person lies on 1 side or the other* (Fig. 18-11).

- The bed is flat.
- A pillow is under the head and neck.
- The upper leg is in front of the lower leg. (The nurse may ask you to position the upper leg behind the lower leg, not on top of it.)
- The ankle, upper leg, and thigh are supported with pillows.
- A small pillow is against the person's back. The person rolls back against the pillow so that his or her back is at a 45-degree angle with the mattress.
- A small pillow is under the upper hand and arm.

Sims' Position

The *Sims' position (semi-prone side position) is a left side-lying position. The upper leg (right leg) is sharply flexed so it is not on the lower leg (left leg). The lower arm (left arm) is behind the person* (Fig. 18-12).

- The bed is flat.
- A pillow is under the person's head and shoulder.
- The upper leg (right leg) is supported with a pillow.
- A pillow is under the upper arm (right arm) and hand (right hand).

Chair Position

Persons who sit in chairs must hold their upper bodies and heads erect. If not, poor alignment results. For good alignment:

- The person's back and buttocks are against the back of the chair.
- Feet are flat on the floor or wheelchair footplates. Never leave feet unsupported.
- Backs of the knees and calves are slightly away from the edge of the seat (Fig. 18-13).

The nurse may have you put a small pillow between the person's lower back and the chair. This supports the lower back. *Remember, a pillow is not used behind the back if restraints are used* (Chapter 15).

Paralyzed arms are supported. Pillows or elevated arm-rests are used. Some persons have positioners (Fig. 18-14). Ask the nurse about their correct use. The nurse may have you position the wrists at a slight upward angle.

Some people need postural supports if they cannot keep their upper bodies erect. Postural supports promote good alignment. The health team selects the best product for the person's needs. Safety, dignity, and function are considered.

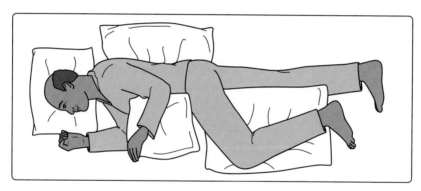

FIGURE 18-11 Lateral position.

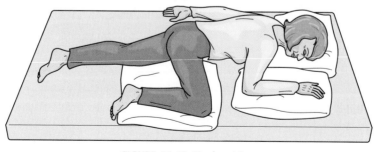

FIGURE 18-12 Sims' position.

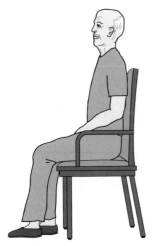

FIGURE 18-13 Chair position.

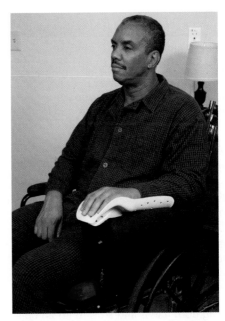

FIGURE 18-14 Elevated armrest and positioner.

FOCUS ON **PRIDE**

The Person, Family, and Yourself

Personal and Professional Responsibility

You make decisions daily about protecting yourself.

- Do you bend at the waist or the hips and knees to lift objects?
- Do you reach or use a step stool to get high objects?
- Do you exercise for strength and endurance?
- Do you raise the bed when giving bedside care?
- Do you move a person alone or get help?

Your decisions affect the safety of yourself and others. Use good judgment at home and in the workplace. Protect yourself from harm.

Rights and Respect

OSHA requires a safe work setting. You have the right to ask employers about safety plans to reduce your risk of injury. Ask about training programs related to body mechanics, safe handling of persons, and workplace hazards. Know and follow agency procedures to report problems.

Independence and Social Interaction

Talk with the person while positioning him or her. Ask what he or she prefers. Doing so promotes comfort, independence, and social interaction.

Delegation and Teamwork

Know which tasks increase your risk for injury. Use caution when doing them. Get help when needed.

Thinking that injuries happen only to others is dangerous. Anyone can be injured. Your safety is important. Take pride in working carefully.

Ethics and Laws

Failure to move and position the person correctly places the person at risk. For example, a person develops a pressure injury after being slumped in a chair for 3 hours. Or a person is injured from being moved without enough help. You must give care in a way that maintains or improves quality of life, health, and safety.

FOCUS ON **PRIDE**: *Application*

What changes will you make in your daily life to protect yourself from injury? How do you plan to protect yourself in the workplace?

REVIEW QUESTIONS

Circle the BEST answer.

1 Good body mechanics involve
   a Having an upright posture
   b Having a narrow base of support
   c Using the muscles in the back and lower arms
   d Lifting a heavy object alone

2 Good alignment means
   a The area on which an object rests
   b Having the head, trunk, arms, and legs aligned with one another
   c Using muscles, tendons, ligaments, and joints correctly
   d The back-lying or supine position

3 Which action shows poor body mechanics?
   a Holding an object close to your body
   b Facing the direction you are working to prevent twisting
   c Leaning over a raised bed rail to give care
   d Using both hands and arms to lift an object

4 You need to move a large chair in a resident's room. You should
   a Push or slide the chair
   b Lift and carry the chair
   c Ask the nurse to move the chair for you
   d Pull the chair using quick, jerking motions

5 The purpose of ergonomics is to
   a Reduce stress on the worker's body
   b Safely position the person
   c Promote quality of life
   d Use good body mechanics

6 Risk of MSDs decreases with
   a Repeating actions
   b Awkward postures
   c Avoiding manual lifting when possible
   d Greater force

7 Which statement about back injuries is *true*?
   a Back injuries cannot be prevented.
   b Pain when assuming normal posture is a symptom.
   c Nursing center staff are at low risk.
   d Bending to change bed linens does not cause back injuries.

8 Which statement about positioning is *true*?
   a Re-positioning prevents pressure injuries and contractures.
   b Circulation is not affected by positioning.
   c Position changes are avoided if moving causes pain.
   d Persons in chairs are re-positioned less often than those in bed.

9 You position a resident in the lateral position. Where do you place the call light?
   a At the foot of the bed
   b At the head of the bed
   c Behind the person
   d Within the person's reach

10 Patients and residents are re-positioned at least every
   a 15 minutes
   b 30 minutes
   c 2 hours
   d 3 hours

11 The back-lying position is called
   a Fowler's position
   b The supine position
   c The lateral position
   d Sims' position

12 For Fowler's position
   a The bed is flat
   b The head of the bed is raised 45 to 60 degrees
   c The person's head is turned to 1 side
   d The feet hang over the edge of the mattress

13 A pillow is placed against the person's back in
   a A chair while restraints are used
   b The prone position
   c The lateral position
   d Sims' position

14 When in a chair, the person's feet
   a Must be flat on the floor
   b Are positioned on footplates
   c Dangle
   d Are positioned on pillows

Answers to Chapter 18 questions are on p. 886.

FOCUS ON PRACTICE

Problem Solving

To complete tasks quickly, you do not raise the bed to a comfortable working level. You move persons alone instead of getting help. You lean over the bed instead of moving to the other side. Why do these actions put you at increased risk for injury?

You now have back pain. Your walking is affected. How does this affect your work and daily life? How could you have avoided this problem?

Moving the Person

OBJECTIVES

- Define the key terms and key abbreviation in this chapter.
- Identify comfort and safety measures for moving the person.
- Explain how to prevent work-related injuries when moving persons.
- Identify the delegation information needed before moving the person.
- Perform the procedures described in this chapter.
- Explain how to promote PRIDE in the person, the family, and yourself.

KEY TERMS

bed mobility How a person moves to and from a lying position, turns from side to side, and re-positions in a bed or other sleeping furniture
friction The rubbing of 1 surface against another

logrolling Turning the person as a unit, in alignment, with 1 motion
shearing When the skin sticks to a surface while muscles slide in the direction the body is moving

KEY ABBREVIATION

ID Identification

You will move persons often. You assist with bed mobility. *Bed mobility is how a person moves to and from a lying position, turns from side to side, and re-positions in a bed or other sleeping furniture.* You also position persons in chairs and wheelchairs. You must work carefully to protect yourself and the person from injury.

See *Focus on Communication: Moving the Person.*

See *Delegation Guidelines: Moving the Person,* p. 268.

See *Promoting Safety and Comfort: Moving the Person,* p. 268.

FOCUS ON COMMUNICATION

Moving the Person

Moving can be painful after an injury or surgery. Many older persons have painful joints. Provide for comfort and avoid causing pain. You can say:
- "Please tell me when you feel pain or discomfort."
- "Do you need a pillow adjusted?"
- "Are you comfortable?"
- "How can I make you more comfortable?"

Before beginning a procedure, tell the person what you and your co-workers will do. Also explain what the person needs to do. Just before the move, remind the person what will happen.

The procedures in this chapter have you move the person on the "count of 3." Staff smoothly move the person at the same time. One co-worker leads by counting. Decide who will count before the move. Be sure the person and staff know who is leading and what to do. You can say:

We will help you move up in bed. I will count "1, 2, 3." When I say "3," push against the bed with your feet and pull up with the trapeze. We will help you move when I say "3."

DELEGATION GUIDELINES

Moving the Person

Moving procedures are routine nursing tasks. Many tasks involve moving persons. Before moving a person, you need this information from the nurse and the care plan.

- The person's height and weight.
- How much help the person needs. These terms may be used.
  - *Independent*—moves without help.
  - *Supervision*—moves without help but needs supervision or cues. To *cue* means *to remind the person what to do.*
  - *Limited assistance*—staff guide (but do not lift) the arms or legs. The person moves on his or her own.
  - *Extensive assistance*—staff provide weight-bearing support to help the person move.
  - *Total dependence*—staff move the person.
- The person's physical abilities. Does the person have strength in his or her arms and legs?
- If the person has a weak side. If yes, which side?
- If the person has problems that increase the risk of injury. Weakness, dizziness, confusion, hearing or vision problems, recent surgery, and fragile skin are examples.
- The person's ability to follow directions.
- Possible behavior problems. Combative, agitated, uncooperative, and unpredictable behaviors are examples.
- The number of staff needed to complete the task safely.
- Any doctor's orders for moving the person.
- What procedure to use.
- What equipment to use.
- What observations to report and record:
  - Who helped you with the move
  - How much help the person needed
  - How the person tolerated the move
  - How you positioned the person
  - Complaints of pain or discomfort
- When to report observations.
- What patient or resident concerns to report at once.

PROMOTING SAFETY AND COMFORT

Moving the Person

Safety

Many older persons have fragile bones and joints. To prevent injuries:

- Follow the rules of body mechanics (Chapter 18).
- Always have help to move the person.
- Move the person carefully.
- Keep the person in good alignment during and after the procedure.
- Make sure the face, nose, and mouth are not blocked by a pillow or other device.

Comfort

To promote mental comfort when moving the person:

- Explain what you will do and how the person can help. Be courteous. Treat the person with dignity.
- Screen and cover the person for privacy.

Keep the person in good alignment. Use pillows and other positioning devices to position the person as directed by the nurse and the care plan. If a pillow is allowed under the person's head, position it under the head and shoulders.

PREVENTING WORK-RELATED INJURIES

Moving procedures involve lifting, awkward postures, and repeated motions. These increase your risk for injury. You must prevent work-related injuries during moving procedures. See Chapter 18.

Good body mechanics alone will not prevent injury. The Occupational Safety and Health Administration (OSHA) recommends:

- Minimizing manual lifting in all cases
- Eliminating manual lifting when possible

Each person is different. Careful planning is needed to move the person safely. You must know about the person's physical abilities and the number of staff needed. The number of staff depends on the person's height, weight, cognitive function, and physical abilities. The nurse and care plan tell you what procedure to use and the equipment needed. Always follow the manufacturer's instructions. Ask for training to use equipment and devices safely.

See *Focus on Children and Older Persons: Preventing Work-Related Injuries.*

See *Teamwork and Time Management: Preventing Work-Related Injuries.*

See *Promoting Safety and Comfort: Preventing Work-Related Injuries.*

FOCUS ON CHILDREN AND OLDER PERSONS

Preventing Work-Related Injuries

Older Persons

Persons with dementia may not understand what you are doing. They may resist your efforts. The person may shout, grab you, or try to hit you. Always have a co-worker help you. Do not force the person. The person's care plan has measures for safe care. For example:

- Proceed slowly.
- Use a calm, pleasant voice.
- Distract the person. For example, let the person hold a washcloth or other soft object. This helps distract the person and keeps the hands busy.

Tell the nurse at once if you have problems moving the person.

TEAMWORK AND TIME MANAGEMENT

Preventing Work-Related Injuries

Patients and residents are moved, turned, and re-positioned often. These procedures are best done by at least 2 staff members.

Friendships are common among co-workers. And some working relationships are better than others. Do not just ask for help from or give help to friends or those with whom you work well. Include all co-workers. This includes new staff and those from other units.

PROTECTING THE SKIN

Protect the person's skin during moving procedures. Friction and shearing injure the skin. Both cause infection and pressure injuries (Chapter 41).

- *Friction is the rubbing of 1 surface against another.* When moved in bed, the person's skin rubs against the sheet.
- *Shearing is when the skin sticks to a surface while muscles slide in the direction the body is moving* (Fig. 19-1). It occurs when the person slides down in bed or is moved in bed.

To reduce friction and shearing when moving the person in bed:
- Roll the person.
- Use friction-reducing devices. Such devices include a lift sheet (turning sheet). Drawsheets (Chapter 22) serve as lift sheets (turning sheets). Turning pads (Fig. 19-2, p. 270), large re-usable waterproof under-pads (Chapter 22), and slide sheets (p. 274) are other friction-reducing devices.

See *Focus on Children and Older Persons: Protecting the Skin.*

See *Focus on Surveys: Protecting the Skin.*

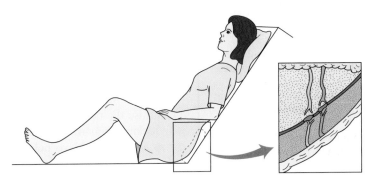

FIGURE 19-1 Shearing. When the head of the bed is raised to a sitting position, skin on the buttocks stays in place. However, internal structures move forward as the person slides down in bed. This pinches the skin between the mattress and the hip bones.

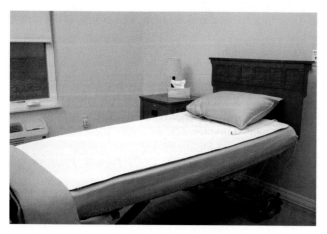

FIGURE 19-2 Turning pad.

MOVING PERSONS IN BED

Some persons can move and turn in bed. Others need help from at least 1 person. Those who are weak, unconscious, paralyzed, or in casts need help. Sometimes 2 or 3 people or a mechanical lift (Chapter 20) is needed. Follow the guidelines in Box 19-1 to lift or move persons in bed.

See *Focus on Communication: Moving Persons in Bed.*

See *Delegation Guidelines: Moving Persons in Bed.*

Raising the Person's Head and Shoulders

Sometimes you raise the person's head and shoulders to give care. Moving the pillow requires this procedure. You can raise the person's head and shoulders easily and safely by locking arms with the person. *Do not pull on the person's arm or shoulder.* Have help with older persons and with those who are heavy or hard to move. This protects the person and you from injury.

See procedure: *Raising the Person's Head and Shoulders.*

Raising the Person's Head and Shoulders

QUALITY OF LIFE

- Knock before entering the person's room.
- Address the person by name.
- Introduce yourself by name and title.

- Explain the procedure before starting and during the procedure.
- Protect the person's rights during the procedure.
- Handle the person gently during the procedure.

PRE-PROCEDURE

1 Follow *Delegation Guidelines:*
   a *Moving the Person*, p. 268
   b *Moving Persons in Bed*
   See *Promoting Safety and Comfort:*
   a *Moving the Person*, p. 268
   b *Preventing Work-Related Injuries*, p. 269
2 Decide if you will work alone (Fig. 19-3) or if you will ask a co-worker to assist (Fig. 19-4, p. 272). Ask a co-worker to assist if needed.

3 Practice hand hygiene.
4 Identify the person. Check the ID (identification) bracelet against the assignment sheet. Use 2 identifiers (Chapter 13). Also call the person by name.
5 Provide for privacy.
6 Lock (brake) the bed wheels.
7 Raise the bed for body mechanics. Bed rails are up if used.

PROCEDURE

8 Have your co-worker stand on the other side of the bed. Lower the bed rails if up.
9 Ask the person to put the near arm behind your near arm and shoulder. His or her hand rests on top of your shoulder. If you are standing on the right side, the person's right hand rests on your right shoulder (see Fig. 19-3, *A*). The person does the same with your co-worker. The person's left hand rests on your co-worker's left shoulder (see Fig. 19-4, *A*).
10 Put your arm nearest to the person under his or her arm. Your hand is on the person's shoulder. Your co-worker does the same.

11 Put your free arm under the person's neck and shoulders (see Fig. 19-3, *B*). Your co-worker does the same (see Fig. 19-4, *B*). Support the neck.
12 Help the person rise to a sitting or semi-sitting position on the "count of 3" (see Figs. 19-3, *C* and 19-4, *C*).
13 Use the arm and hand that supported the person's neck and shoulders to give care (see Fig. 19-3, *D*). Your co-worker supports the person (see Fig. 19-4, *D*).
14 Help the person lie down. Provide support with your locked arm. Support the person's neck and shoulders with your other arm. Your co-worker does the same.

POST-PROCEDURE

15 Provide for comfort. (See the inside of the back cover.)
16 Place the call light and other needed items within reach.
17 Lower the bed to a safe and comfortable level. Follow the care plan.
18 Raise or lower bed rails. Follow the care plan.

19 Unscreen the person.
20 Complete a safety check of the room. (See the inside of the back cover.)
21 Practice hand hygiene.
22 Report and record your observations.

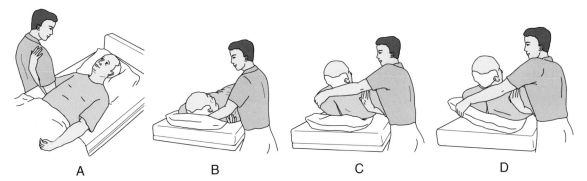

A   B   C   D

FIGURE 19-3 Raising the person's head and shoulders by locking arms with the person. **A,** The person's near arm is behind the nursing assistant's near arm and shoulder. **B,** The nursing assistant's far arm is under the person's neck and shoulders. The near arm is under the person's near arm. **C,** The person is raised to a semi-sitting position by locking arms. **D,** The nursing assistant lifts the pillow while the person is in a semi-sitting position.

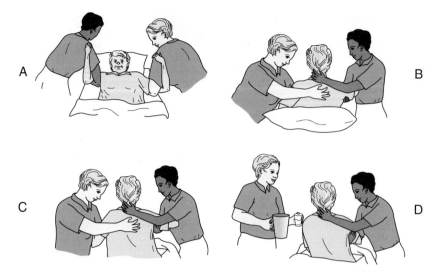

FIGURE 19-4 Raising the person's head and shoulders with a co-worker. **A,** Two nursing assistants lock arms with the person. **B,** The nursing assistants each have an arm under the person's head and neck. **C,** The nursing assistants raise the person to a semi-sitting position. **D,** One nursing assistant supports the person. The other gives care.

Moving the Person Up in Bed

When the head of the bed is raised, it is easy to slide down toward the middle and foot of the bed (Fig. 19-5). You move the person up in bed for good alignment and comfort.

You can sometimes move light-weight adults up in bed alone if they assist using a trapeze. However, it is best done with help and an assist device (p. 274). For heavy, weak, and older persons, 2 or more staff members are needed. Always protect the person and yourself from injury.

See *Promoting Safety and Comfort: Moving the Person Up in Bed.*

See procedure: *Moving the Person Up in Bed.*

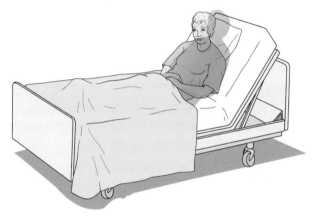

FIGURE 19-5 A person in poor alignment after sliding down in bed.

PROMOTING SAFETY AND COMFORT

Moving the Person Up in Bed

Safety

Do not let the person's head hit the head-board when moving up in bed. If the person can be without a pillow, place it upright against the head-board.

This procedure is best done with at least 2 staff members. Work from the side of the bed. *Do not pull the person from the head of the bed.* Use assist devices as directed by the nurse and the care plan. Ask any questions before you begin the procedure.

Perform the procedure alone only if all of the following conditions are met.

- The person is small in size.
- The person can follow directions.
- The person can assist with much of the moving.
- The person uses a trapeze.
- The person can push against the mattress with the feet.
- The nurse says it is safe to do so.
- You are comfortable doing so.

Moving the Person Up in Bed

QUALITY OF LIFE

- Knock before entering the person's room.
- Address the person by name.
- Introduce yourself by name and title.

- Explain the procedure before starting and during the procedure.
- Protect the person's rights during the procedure.
- Handle the person gently during the procedure.

PRE-PROCEDURE

1 Follow *Delegation Guidelines:*
 a *Moving the Person,* p. 268
 b *Moving Persons in Bed,* p. 270
 See *Promoting Safety and Comfort:*
 a *Moving the Person,* p. 268
 b *Preventing Work-Related Injuries,* p. 269
 c *Moving the Person Up in Bed*
2 Ask a co-worker to help you.

3 Practice hand hygiene.
4 Identify the person. Check the ID bracelet against the assignment sheet. Use 2 identifiers (Chapter 13). Also call the person by name.
5 Provide for privacy.
6 Lock (brake) the bed wheels.
7 Raise the bed for body mechanics. Bed rails are up if used.

PROCEDURE

8 Lower the head of the bed to a level appropriate for the person. It is as flat as possible.
9 Stand on 1 side of the bed. Your co-worker stands on the other side.
10 Lower the bed rails if up.
11 Remove pillows as directed by the nurse. Place a pillow upright against the head-board if the person can be without it.
12 Stand with a wide base of support. Point the foot near the head of the bed toward the head of the bed. Face the head of the bed.
13 Bend your hips and knees. Keep your back straight.

14 Place 1 arm under the person's shoulder and 1 arm under the thighs. Your co-worker does the same. Grasp each other's forearms (Fig. 19-6).
15 Ask the person to grasp the trapeze.
16 Have the person flex both knees.
17 Explain that:
 a You will count "1, 2, 3."
 b The move will be on "3."
 c On "3," the person pushes against the bed with the feet if able. And the person pulls up with the trapeze.
18 Move the person to the head of the bed on the "count of 3." Shift your weight from your rear leg to your front leg (see Fig. 19-6). Your co-worker does the same.
19 Repeat steps 12 through 18 if necessary.

POST-PROCEDURE

20 Put the pillow under the person's head and shoulders. Straighten linens.
21 Position the person in good alignment. Raise the head of the bed to a level appropriate for the person.
22 Provide for comfort. (See the inside of the back cover.)
23 Place the call light and other needed items within reach.
24 Lower the bed to a safe and comfortable level. Follow the care plan.

25 Raise or lower bed rails. Follow the care plan.
26 Unscreen the person.
27 Complete a safety check of the room. (See the inside of the back cover.)
28 Practice hand hygiene.
29 Report and record your observations.

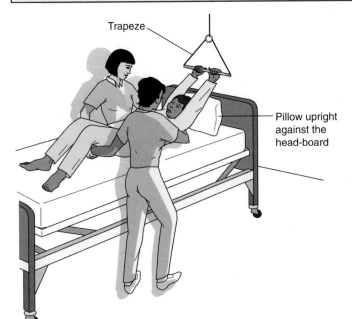

Trapeze

Pillow upright against the head-board

FIGURE 19-6 A person is moved up in bed by 2 nursing assistants. Each has 1 arm under the person's shoulders and the other under the thighs. Arms are locked under the person. The person grasps the trapeze and flexes the knees. The nursing assistants shift their weight from the rear leg to the front leg to move the person up in bed.

Moving the Person Up in Bed With an Assist Device

You use assist devices to move some persons up in bed. Assist devices include a drawsheet (lift sheet, turning sheet), flat sheet folded in half, turning pad, slide sheet (Fig. 19-7), and large re-usable waterproof under-pad. With these devices, the person is moved more evenly. And shearing and friction are reduced.

To position the device, you must turn the person. See procedure: *Turning and Re-Positioning the Person*, p. 278. You and at least 1 co-worker:

1 Turn the person to 1 side.
2 Place the device on the bed. Open and fan-fold the device toward the person. The device is positioned from the head to above the knees or lower.
3 Tell the person that he or she will roll over a "bump." Assure the person that he or she will not fall.
4 Turn the person to the other side. The person rolls over the device.
5 Pull the device tightly. Smooth any wrinkles.
6 Roll the person onto his or her back. The person is lying on the device.

At least 2 staff members are needed to move a person with an assist device. The procedure on the next page is used:

* Following the guidelines for moving persons in bed (see Box 19-1)
* For persons recovering from spinal cord surgery or spinal cord injuries
* For older persons

See *Promoting Safety and Comfort: Moving the Person Up in Bed With an Assist Device*.

See procedure: *Moving the Person Up in Bed With an Assist Device*.

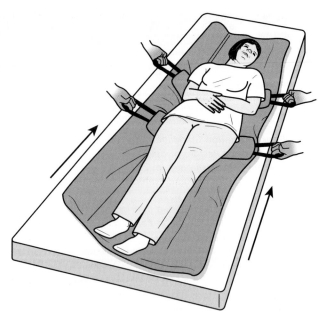

FIGURE 19-7 Slide sheet.

PROMOTING SAFETY AND COMFORT
Moving the Person Up in Bed With an Assist Device

Safety

Disposable, single-use under-pads are not strong enough to hold the person's weight during the move. Re-usable under-pads are stronger. Ask the nurse if the person's under-pad is safe as an assist device. For safety, the under-pad must:

* Be strong enough to support the person's weight.
* Be long enough to extend from under the person's head to above the knees or lower.
* Be wide enough for you and other staff to get a firm grip.

After using a slide sheet, remove it. If left in place, the person can slide down in bed or off the bed.

For persons with bariatric needs, the care plan may include:

* Using a friction-reducing device or bariatric lift and:
  * At least 2 staff members if the person can assist with the move.
  * At least 3 staff members if the person cannot assist with the move.
* Positioning the bed in Trendelenburg's position (Chapter 21). In this position, the head of the bed is lowered and the foot of the bed is raised. Gravity is used to pull the person up in bed. The position is used only if tolerated by the person and allowed by the doctor.
* Leaving the friction-reducing device under the person. The device is covered with a drawsheet. Leaving the device in place reduces the risk of injuries from placing and removing the device.

Moving the Person Up in Bed With an Assist Device

QUALITY OF LIFE

- Knock before entering the person's room.
- Address the person by name.
- Introduce yourself by name and title.

- Explain the procedure before starting and during the procedure.
- Protect the person's rights during the procedure.
- Handle the person gently during the procedure.

PRE-PROCEDURE

1 Follow *Delegation Guidelines:*
   a *Moving the Person,* p. 268
   b *Moving Persons in Bed,* p. 270
   See *Promoting Safety and Comfort:*
   a *Moving the Person,* p. 268
   b *Preventing Work-Related Injuries,* p. 269
   c *Moving the Person Up in Bed,* p. 272
   d *Moving the Person Up in Bed With an Assist Device*
2 Ask a co-worker to help you.

3 Obtain the needed assist device.
4 Practice hand hygiene.
5 Identify the person. Check the ID bracelet against the assignment sheet. Use 2 identifiers (Chapter 13). Also call the person by name.
6 Provide for privacy.
7 Lock (brake) the bed wheels.
8 Raise the bed for body mechanics. Bed rails are up if used.

PROCEDURE

9 Lower the head of the bed to a level appropriate for the person. It is as flat as possible.
10 Stand on 1 side of the bed. Your co-worker stands on the other side.
11 Lower the bed rails if up.
12 Remove pillows as directed by the nurse. Place a pillow upright against the head-board if the person can be without it.
13 Position the assist device.
14 Stand with a wide base of support. Point the foot near the head of the bed toward the head of the bed. Face the head of the bed.

15 Roll the sides of the assist device up close to the person. (NOTE: Omit this step if the device has handles.)
16 Grasp the rolled-up assist device firmly near the person's shoulders and hips (Fig. 19-8). Or grasp it by the handles. Support the head.
17 Bend your hips and knees.
18 Move the person up in bed on the "count of 3." Shift your weight from your rear leg to your front leg.
19 Repeat steps 14 through 18 if necessary.
20 Unroll the assist device. (NOTE: Omit this step if the device has handles.) Turn the person to remove the slide sheet if used.

POST-PROCEDURE

21 Put the pillow under the person's head and shoulders. Straighten linens.
22 Position the person in good alignment. Raise the head of the bed to a level appropriate for the person.
23 Provide for comfort. (See the inside of the back cover.)
24 Place the call light and other needed items within reach.
25 Lower the bed to a safe and comfortable level. Follow the care plan.

26 Raise or lower bed rails. Follow the care plan.
27 Unscreen the person.
28 Complete a safety check of the room. (See the inside of the back cover.)
29 Practice hand hygiene.
30 Report and record your observations.

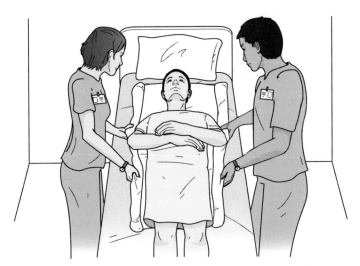

FIGURE 19-8 A drawsheet is used to move the person up in bed. It extends from the person's head to above the knees. Rolled close to the person, the drawsheet is held near the shoulders and hips.

Moving the Person to the Side of the Bed

Re-positioning and care procedures require moving the person to the side of the bed. Move the person to the side of the bed before turning. Otherwise, after turning, the person lies on the side of the bed—not in the middle.

Sometimes you have to reach over the person. During a bed bath is an example. You reach less if the person is near you.

In 1 method, the person is moved in segments (Fig. 19-9). Sometimes you can do this alone if the person is small in size. With at least 1 co-worker, use a mechanical lift (Chapter 20) or an assist device.

- Following the guidelines for moving persons in bed (see Box 19-1)
- For older persons
- For persons with arthritis
- For persons recovering from spinal cord injuries or surgeries

Assist devices for this procedure include a drawsheet (lift sheet, turning sheet), flat sheet folded in half, turning pad, slide sheet, and large re-usable waterproof under-pad. An assist device helps prevent pain and skin damage and injury to the bones, joints, and spinal cord.

See *Promoting Safety and Comfort: Moving the Person to the Side of the Bed.*

See procedure: *Moving the Person to the Side of the Bed.*

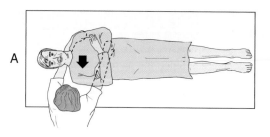
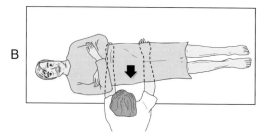
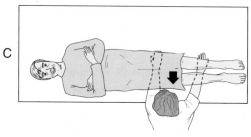

FIGURE 19-9 Moving the person to the side of the bed in segments. **A,** The upper part of the body is moved. **B,** The lower part of the body is moved. **C,** The legs and feet are moved.

PROMOTING SAFETY AND COMFORT
Moving the Person to the Side of the Bed

Safety
The person is moved to the side of the bed for tasks such as re-positioning, bedmaking, and bathing. Use the method and equipment that are best for the person. The nurse and the care plan tell you which method to use. The wrong method could cause serious injury.

To use an assist device, you need help from at least 1 co-worker. Depending on the person's size, more staff members may be needed.

Safety—cont'd
To use a slide sheet, place it under the person (p. 274). After moving the person, remove the device.

To move the person in segments, move the person toward you, not away from you. This helps protect you from injury.

Comfort
After moving the person to the side of the bed, position the pillow correctly. It should be under the person's head and shoulders.

Moving the Person to the Side of the Bed

QUALITY OF LIFE

- Knock before entering the person's room.
- Address the person by name.
- Introduce yourself by name and title.

- Explain the procedure before starting and during the procedure.
- Protect the person's rights during the procedure.
- Handle the person gently during the procedure.

PRE-PROCEDURE

1 Follow *Delegation Guidelines:*
   a *Moving the Person, p. 268*
   b *Moving Persons in Bed, p. 270*
   See *Promoting Safety and Comfort:*
   a *Moving the Person, p. 268*
   b *Preventing Work-Related Injuries, p. 269*
   c *Moving the Person to the Side of the Bed*
2 Ask 1 or 2 co-workers to help you if using an assist device.

3 Obtain a drawsheet.
4 Practice hand hygiene.
5 Identify the person. Check the ID bracelet against the assignment sheet. Use 2 identifiers (Chapter 13). Also call the person by name.
6 Provide for privacy.
7 Lock (brake) the bed wheels.
8 Raise the bed for body mechanics. Bed rails are up if used.

PROCEDURE

9 Lower the head of the bed to a level appropriate for the person. It is as flat as possible.
10 Stand on the side of the bed to which you will move the person.
11 Lower the bed rail near you if bed rails are used. (Both bed rails are lowered for step 16.)
12 Remove pillows as directed by the nurse.
13 Cross the person's arms over the chest.
14 Stand with your feet about 12 inches apart. One foot is in front of the other. Flex your knees.
15 *Method 1—moving the person in segments:*
   a Place your arm under the person's neck and shoulders. Grasp the far shoulder.
   b Place your other arm under the mid-back.
   c Move the upper part of the person's body toward you. Rock backward and shift your weight to your rear leg (see Fig. 19-9, *A*).
   d Place 1 arm under the person's waist and 1 under the thighs.
   e Rock backward to move the lower part of the person toward you (see Fig. 19-9, *B*).
   f Repeat the procedure for the legs and feet (see Fig. 19-9, *C*). Your arms should be under the person's thighs and calves.

16 *Method 2—moving the person with a drawsheet:*
   a Position the drawsheet.
   b Roll up the drawsheet close to the person (see Fig. 19-8).
   c Grasp the rolled-up drawsheet near the person's shoulders and hips. Your co-worker does the same. Support the person's head.
   d Rock backward on the "count of 3," moving the person toward you. Your co-worker rocks backward slightly and then forward toward you while keeping the arms straight.
   e Unroll the drawsheet. Remove any wrinkles.

POST-PROCEDURE

17 Put the pillow under the person's head and shoulders. Straighten linens.
18 Position the person in good alignment.
19 Provide for comfort. (See the inside of the back cover.)
20 Place the call light and other needed items within reach.
21 Lower the bed to a safe and comfortable level. Follow the care plan.

22 Raise or lower bed rails. Follow the care plan.
23 Unscreen the person.
24 Complete a safety check of the room. (See the inside of the back cover.)
25 Practice hand hygiene.
26 Report and record your observations.

⬛ TURNING PERSONS

Turning persons onto their sides helps prevent complications from bed rest (Chapter 34). Procedures and care measures often require the side-lying position. You also turn the person to position and to remove friction-reducing devices.

You turn the person toward you or away from you. The direction depends on the person's condition and the situation.

Many older persons have arthritis in their spines, hips, and knees. Less painful, logrolling (p. 280) is preferred for turning these persons.

See *Delegation Guidelines: Turning Persons.*
See *Promoting Safety and Comfort: Turning Persons.*
See procedure: *Turning and Re-Positioning the Person.*

DELEGATION GUIDELINES

Turning Persons

Before turning and re-positioning a person, you need this information from the nurse and the care plan.

- How much help the person needs
- The number of staff needed for safety
- The person's comfort level and painful body parts
- Which procedure to use
- What assist devices to use
- What supportive devices to use for positioning (Chapter 34)
- Where to place pillows
- What observations to report and record and those to report at once. (See *Delegation Guidelines: Moving the Person*, p. 268.)

PROMOTING SAFETY AND COMFORT

Turning Persons

Safety

Use good body mechanics to turn a person in bed. See Chapter 18.

Position the person in good alignment. This helps prevent musculo-skeletal injuries, skin breakdown, and pressure injuries.

Do not turn a person away from you with the far bed rail down. Raise the bed rail on the side near you. Then go to the other side of the bed. Lower the bed rail if up. Turn the person toward you.

Comfort

After turning, position the person in good alignment. Use pillows as directed to support the person in the side-lying position (Chapter 18). Make sure the person's face, nose, and mouth are not covered by a pillow or other device.

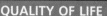

⬛ Turning and Re-Positioning the Person

QUALITY OF LIFE

- Knock before entering the person's room.
- Address the person by name.
- Introduce yourself by name and title.

- Explain the procedure before starting and during the procedure.
- Protect the person's rights during the procedure.
- Handle the person gently during the procedure.

PRE-PROCEDURE

1 Follow *Delegation Guidelines:*
   a *Moving the Person*, p. 268
   b *Moving Persons in Bed*, p. 270
   c *Turning Persons*
   See *Promoting Safety and Comfort:*
   a *Moving the Person*, p. 268
   b *Preventing Work-Related Injuries*, p. 269
   c *Moving the Person to the Side of the Bed*, p. 276
   d *Turning Persons*

2 Practice hand hygiene.
3 Identify the person. Check the ID bracelet against the assignment sheet. Use 2 identifiers (Chapter 13). Also call the person by name.
4 Provide for privacy.
5 Lock (brake) the bed wheels.
6 Raise the bed for body mechanics. Bed rails are up if used.

Turning and Re-Positioning the Person—cont'd

PROCEDURE

7 Lower the head of the bed to a level appropriate for the person. It is as flat as possible.

8 Stand on the side of the bed opposite to where you will turn the person.

9 Lower the bed rail.

10 Move the person to the side near you. See procedure: *Moving the Person to the Side of the Bed,* p. 277.

11 Cross the person's arms over the chest. Cross the leg near you over the far leg.

12 *Turning the person away from you:*
  a Stand with a wide base of support. Flex the knees.
  b Place 1 hand on the person's shoulder. Place the other on the hip near you.
  c Roll the person gently away from you toward the raised bed rail (Fig. 19-10, *A*).
  d Shift your weight from your rear leg to your front leg.

13 *Turning the person toward you:*
  a Raise the bed rail.
  b Go to the other side of the bed. Lower the bed rail.
  c Stand with a wide base of support. Flex your knees.
  d Place 1 hand on the person's shoulder. Place the other on the far hip.
  e Pull the person toward you gently (Fig. 19-10, *B*).

14 Position the person. Follow the nurse's directions and the care plan. The following are common.
  a Place a pillow under the head and neck.
  b Adjust the shoulder. The person should not be on an arm.
  c Place a small pillow under the upper hand and arm.
  d Position a pillow against the back.
  e Flex the upper knee. Position the upper leg in front of the lower leg.
  f Support the upper leg and thigh on pillows. Make sure the ankle is supported.

POST-PROCEDURE

15 Provide for comfort. (See the inside of the back cover.)

16 Place the call light and other needed items within reach.

17 Lower the bed to a safe and comfortable level. Follow the care plan.

18 Raise or lower bed rails. Follow the care plan.

19 Unscreen the person.

20 Complete a safety check of the room. (See the inside of the back cover.)

21 Practice hand hygiene.

22 Report and record your observations.

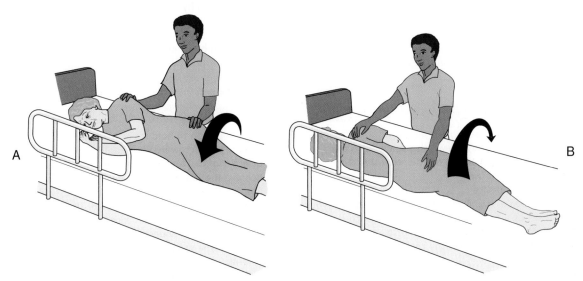

FIGURE 19-10 Turning the person. **A,** Turning the person away from you. **B,** Turning the person toward you. (*NOTE: Non-standard bed rails are used to show positioning.*)

Logrolling

Logrolling is turning the person as a unit, in alignment, with 1 motion. The head, neck, and spine are kept straight. The procedure is used to turn:

- Older persons with arthritic spines or knees.
- Persons recovering from hip fractures.
- Persons with spinal cord injuries.
- Persons recovering from spinal cord surgery.
  See *Promoting Safety and Comfort: Logrolling.*
  See procedure: *Logrolling the Person.*

PROMOTING SAFETY AND COMFORT

Logrolling

Safety

For logrolling, 2 or 3 staff members are needed. If the person is tall or heavy, 3 are needed. Sometimes you use an assist device—drawsheet (lift sheet, turning sheet), turning pad, large re-usable waterproof under-pad, slide sheet.

After spinal cord injury or surgery, the nurse tells you what to do step-by-step. Assist the nurse as directed.

Comfort

After spinal cord injury or surgery, the doctor orders positioning limits. Follow the nurse's directions and the care plan to position the person and use pillows.

Logrolling the Person

QUALITY OF LIFE

- Knock before entering the person's room.
- Address the person by name.
- Introduce yourself by name and title.

- Explain the procedure before starting and during the procedure.
- Protect the person's rights during the procedure.
- Handle the person gently during the procedure.

PRE-PROCEDURE

1 Follow *Delegation Guidelines:*
   a *Moving the Person*, p. 268
   b *Moving Persons in Bed*, p. 270
   c *Turning Persons*, p. 278
   See *Promoting Safety and Comfort:*
   a *Moving the Person*, p. 268
   b *Preventing Work-Related Injuries*, p. 269
   c *Turning Persons*, p. 278
   d *Logrolling*

2 Ask a co-worker to help you.
3 Obtain the needed assist device.
4 Practice hand hygiene.
5 Identify the person. Check the ID bracelet against the assignment sheet. Use 2 identifiers (Chapter 13). Also call the person by name.
6 Provide for privacy.
7 Lock (brake) the bed wheels.
8 Raise the bed for body mechanics. Bed rails are up if used.

PROCEDURE

9 Make sure the bed is flat.
10 Stand on the side opposite to which you will turn the person. Your co-worker stands on the other side.
11 Lower the bed rails if used.
12 Position the assist device.
13 Move the person as a unit to the side of the bed near you. Use the assist device. (If the person has a spinal cord injury or had spinal cord surgery, assist the nurse as directed.)
14 Place the person's arms across the chest. Place a pillow between the knees.
15 Raise the bed rail if used.
16 Go to the other side.
17 Stand near the shoulders and chest. Your co-worker stands near the hips and thighs.
18 Stand with a wide base of support. One foot is in front of the other.

19 Ask the person to hold his or her body rigid.
20 Roll the person toward you (Fig. 19-11, *A*). Or use the assist device (Fig. 19-11, *B*). Turn the person as a unit.
21 Remove the slide sheet (if used).
22 Position the person in good alignment. Use pillows as directed by the nurse and care plan. The following are common (unless the spinal cord is involved).
   a Place a pillow under the head and neck if allowed.
   b Adjust the shoulder. The person should not be on an arm.
   c Place a small pillow under the upper hand and arm.
   d Position a pillow against the back.
   e Flex the upper knee. Position the upper leg in front of the lower leg.
   f Support the upper leg and thigh on pillows. Make sure the ankle is supported.

POST-PROCEDURE

23 Provide for comfort. (See the inside of the back cover.)
24 Place the call light and other needed items within reach.
25 Lower the bed to a safe and comfortable level. Follow the care plan.
26 Raise or lower bed rails. Follow the care plan.

27 Unscreen the person.
28 Complete a safety check of the room. (See the inside of the back cover.)
29 Practice hand hygiene.
30 Report and record your observations.

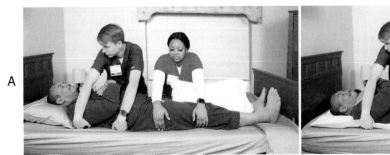
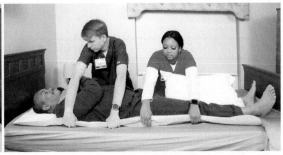

FIGURE 19-11 Logrolling. **A,** A pillow is between the person's legs. The arms are crossed on the chest. The person is on the far side of the bed. The person is turned as a unit. **B,** The assist device is used to logroll the person.

SITTING ON THE SIDE OF THE BED (DANGLING)

You will assist patients and residents to sit on the side of the bed *(dangle)*. The procedure is part of some tasks—assisting the person to stand, transferring from bed to chair, partial bath, and others. Patients and residents may become dizzy or faint when getting out of bed too fast. They may need to sit on the side of the bed for 1 to 5 minutes before walking or transferring. Or activity may increase in stages—bed rest, to dangling, to sitting in a chair, and then to walking. This is common after surgery.

While dangling the legs, the person coughs and deep breathes. He or she moves the legs back and forth in circles. This stimulates circulation.

Persons with balance and coordination problems need support. If dizziness or fainting occurs, lay the person down. Tell the nurse at once.

See *Focus on Children and Older Persons: Dangling.*

See *Delegation Guidelines: Dangling.*

See *Promoting Safety and Comfort: Dangling,* p. 282.

See procedure: *Sitting on the Side of the Bed (Dangling),* p. 283.

Text continued on p. 284.

FOCUS ON **CHILDREN AND OLDER PERSONS**

Dangling

Older Persons
Older persons may have circulatory changes. They may become dizzy or faint when getting up too fast. Let them sit on the side of the bed for a few minutes before standing.

DELEGATION GUIDELINES

Dangling

The nurse may ask you to help a person sit on the side of the bed. Before the dangling procedure, you need this information from the nurse and the care plan.

- Areas of weakness. For example, if the arms are weak, the person cannot hold on to the mattress for support. If the left side is weak, turn the person onto the stronger right side. The person uses the right arm to help move from the lying to sitting position.
- The amount of help the person needs.
- If you need a co-worker to help you.
- If the bed is raised or in a low position. If the person will walk or transfer to a chair, the bed is in a low position safe for a transfer (Chapter 20).
- How long the person needs to sit on the side of the bed.
- What exercises are to be done while dangling.
  - Range-of-motion exercises (Chapter 34)
  - Deep-breathing and coughing exercises (Chapter 43)
- What observations to report and record (Fig. 19-12, p. 282):
  - Pulse and respiratory rates (Chapter 33)
  - Pale or bluish skin color *(cyanosis)*
  - Complaints of dizziness, light-headedness, or difficulty breathing
  - How long the person dangled
  - The observations listed in *Delegation Guidelines: Moving the Person,* p. 268
- When to report observations.
- What patient or resident concerns to report at once.

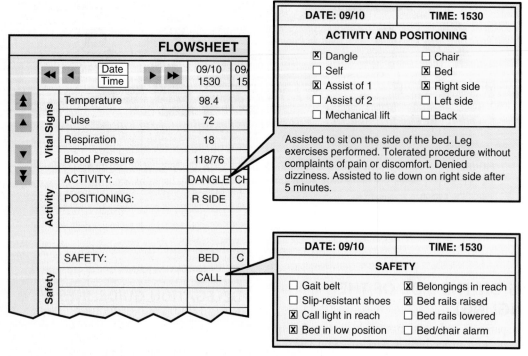

FIGURE 19-12 Charting sample—sitting on the side of the bed (dangling).

PROMOTING SAFETY AND COMFORT

Dangling

Safety

Sitting and balance problems can occur after illness, injury, surgery, and bed rest. Some disabilities affect sitting and balance. Support the person who is sitting on the side of the bed. Have a co-worker help you. This protects the person from falling and other injuries.

As the person sits on the side of the bed, you observe the person. Lay the person down and tell the nurse at once if the person:

- Is dizzy or light-headed.
- Has an abnormal pulse or respirations.
- Has difficulty breathing.
- Has pale or bluish skin.
  Do not leave the person alone. Provide support at all times.

Comfort

Provide for warmth during the procedure. Help the person put on a robe. Or cover the shoulders and back with a bath blanket.

The person may want to perform hygiene measures while sitting on the side of the bed. Oral hygiene and washing the face and hands are examples. These measures are refreshing and stimulate circulation. Follow the nurse's directions and the care plan.

Sitting on the Side of the Bed (Dangling)

QUALITY OF LIFE

- Knock before entering the person's room.
- Address the person by name.
- Introduce yourself by name and title.

- Explain the procedure before starting and during the procedure.
- Protect the person's rights during the procedure.
- Handle the person gently during the procedure.

PRE-PROCEDURE

1 Follow *Delegation Guidelines:*
  a *Moving the Person,* p. 268
  b *Dangling,* p. 281
  See *Promoting Safety and Comfort:*
  a *Moving the Person,* p. 268
  b *Preventing Work-Related Injuries,* p. 269
  c *Dangling*
2 Ask a co-worker to help you.
3 Practice hand hygiene.

4 Identify the person. Check the ID bracelet against the assignment sheet. Use 2 identifiers (Chapter 13). Also call the person by name.
5 Provide for privacy.
6 Decide which side of the bed to use.
7 Move furniture to provide moving space.
8 Lock (brake) the bed wheels.
9 Raise the bed for body mechanics. Bed rails are up if used.

PROCEDURE

10 Lower the bed rail if up.
11 Position the person in a side-lying position facing you. The person lies on the strong side.
12 Raise the head of the bed to a sitting position.
13 Stand by the person's hips. Face the foot of the bed.
14 Stand with your feet apart. The foot near the head of the bed is in front of the other foot.
15 Slide 1 arm under the person's neck and shoulders. Grasp the far shoulder. Place your other hand over the thighs near the knees (Fig. 19-13, *A*).
16 Pivot toward the foot of the bed while moving the person's legs and feet over the side of the bed. As the legs go over the edge of the mattress, the trunk is upright (Fig. 19-13, *B*).
17 Have the person hold on to the edge of the mattress. This supports the person in the sitting position. If possible, raise a half-length bed rail (on the person's strong side) for the person to grasp. Have your co-worker support the person at all times.

18 Check the person's condition.
  • Ask how the person feels. Ask if the person feels dizzy or light-headed.
  • Check the pulse and respirations.
  • Check for difficulty breathing.
  • Note if the skin is pale or bluish in color *(cyanosis).*
19 Reverse the procedure to return the person to bed. (Or prepare the person to walk or for a transfer to a chair or wheelchair. Lower the bed to a safe and comfortable level. The person's feet are flat on the floor.)
20 Lower the head of the bed after the person returns to bed. Help him or her move to the center of the bed.
21 Position the person in good alignment.

POST-PROCEDURE

22 Provide for comfort. (See the inside of the back cover.)
23 Place the call light and other needed items within reach.
24 Lower the bed to a safe and comfortable level. Follow the care plan.
25 Raise or lower bed rails. Follow the care plan.
26 Return furniture to its proper place.

27 Unscreen the person.
28 Complete a safety check of the room. (See the inside of the back cover.)
29 Practice hand hygiene.
30 Report and record your observations.

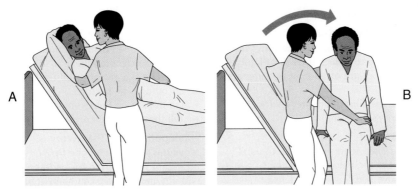

FIGURE 19-13 Helping the person sit on the side of the bed. **A,** The person's shoulders and thighs are supported. **B,** The person sits upright as the legs and feet are moved over the edge of the bed.

RE-POSITIONING IN A CHAIR OR WHEELCHAIR

The person can slide down in a chair or wheelchair. For good alignment and safety, the person's back and buttocks must be against the back of the chair.

If the person cannot help with re-positioning, use a mechanical lift (Chapter 20). Follow the nurse's directions and the care plan for the best way to re-position a person in a chair or wheelchair. *Do not pull the person from behind the chair or wheelchair.*

If the person's chair reclines:

1 Ask a co-worker to help you.
2 Lock (brake) the wheels.
3 Recline the chair.
4 Position a friction-reducing device (drawsheet or slide sheet) under the person.
5 Grasp the device (Fig. 19-14).
6 Use the device to move the person up. See procedure: *Moving the Person Up in Bed With an Assist Device,* p. 275. Then remove the slide sheet.

Use the following method if the person is alert and cooperative. The person must be able to follow directions. And the person must have the strength to help.

1 Lock (brake) the wheelchair wheels. Remove or swing front rigging out of the way. See Chapter 20 for wheelchair safety.
2 Position the person's feet flat on the floor.
3 Apply a transfer belt (Chapter 14).
4 Position the person's arms on the armrests.
5 Stand in front of the person. Block his or her knees and feet with your knees and feet.
6 Grasp the transfer belt on each side while the person leans forward.
7 Ask the person to push with his or her feet and arms on the "count of 3."
8 Move the person back into the chair on the "count of 3" as the person pushes with his or her feet and arms (Fig. 19-15).
9 Remove the transfer belt.

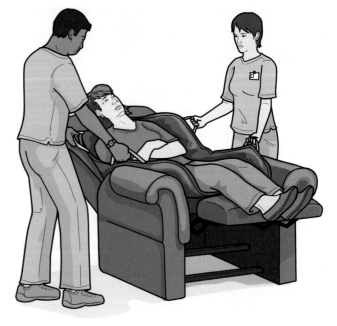

FIGURE 19-14 Re-positioning in a reclining chair.

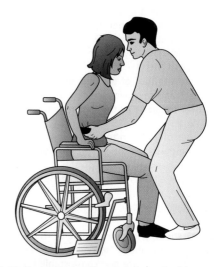

FIGURE 19-15 Re-positioning the person in a wheelchair. A transfer belt is used to move the person to the back of the chair.

FOCUS ON **PRIDE**

The Person, Family, and Yourself

Personal and Professional Responsibility

Many agencies have safe handling programs. Some states have safe handling laws. The goals are to reduce the risk of injury and improve quality of care. Programs often limit or eliminate manual lifting.

Ask employers about safe handling programs. Ask how you can be involved in your agency's program.

Rights and Respect

How would you feel if these statements were made to you?
• "You're too heavy. I need to get help to move you."
• "I'll get hurt if I try to move you."

What you say affects the person's self-esteem. Choose your words carefully. Show respect in what you say.

Independence and Social Interaction

Persons who need help moving may feel embarrassed or helpless. To promote independence and self-esteem:
• Focus on the person's abilities.
• Encourage the person.
• Let the person help as much as safely possible.
• Tell the person when you notice even small improvements.

Delegation and Teamwork

Moving is safer when done by 2 or more workers. This is very important when caring for bariatric persons. Moving a person without enough help can harm you, your co-workers, and the person. Work as a team to protect yourself and others from injury.

FOCUS ON **P R I D E** — cont'd

The Person, Family, and Yourself

E thics and Laws

The following is a real lawsuit filed against a hospital.

A patient had a history of shoulder injuries and surgeries. A nurse positioned the patient in a sitting position. The patient testified that she had immediate pain and heard a popping sound in her arm. The patient sued the hospital for a shoulder injury. In her lawsuit, the patient claimed that:

- *A large sign warned the staff not to touch her arms. The sign was posted by her husband.*
- *The nurse was negligent for not reading the sign and the patient's chart.*
  The hospital claimed that:
- *There was no sign.*
- *The nurse did not pull on the patient's arm.*
- *The patient caused her own injury.*
  The jury found in favor of the hospital.
  (T. Rosen v Verdugo Hills Hospital, California, 1999.)

The hospital did not have to pay damages (Chapter 5). But the lawsuit cost time, money, effort, and stress for all involved.

Always be careful. Follow delegation guidelines, the care plan, and the nurse's instructions. Also listen to the person. Ask the nurse if you are unsure how to safely move a person. Do not put yourself in a position where you may be at fault.

FOCUS ON **PRIDE**: *Application*

Most moving procedures require a team effort. How well do you work with others? What can you improve?

REVIEW QUESTIONS

Circle the BEST answer.

1 You move the person on the "count of 3" to
   a Save time
   b Distract the person from the move
   c Move the person smoothly
   d Move the person slowly

2 Good body mechanics alone will prevent injury when moving persons.
   a True
   b False

3 Before moving a person, you must know what the person is able to do.
   a True
   b False

4 Drawsheets and slide sheets are used to
   a Remove shearing
   b Reduce friction
   c Promote independence
   d Improve posture

5 To protect the person's skin when moving in bed
   a Roll the person
   b Slide the person
   c Move the mattress
   d Use a transfer belt

6 When moving persons in bed
   a The nurse tells you how to position them
   b You decide which procedure to use
   c Bed rails are used at all times
   d 3 workers are needed for safety

7 A resident with dementia needs to be moved up in bed. You should
   a Wait until the person is asleep
   b Avoid rushing
   c Move the person alone
   d Continue if the person resists the move

8 As an assist device, a drawsheet is placed so that it
   a Covers the person's body
   b Extends from the mid-back to mid-thigh level
   c Is under the head to the above the knees
   d Covers the entire mattress

9 A person needs to be moved up in bed. The person is partially able to assist. You should
   a Stand by for safety but not assist
   b Move the person up in bed by yourself
   c Tell the person not to assist to avoid injury
   d Ask for help and get a friction-reducing device

10 Before turning a person onto his or her side, you
   a Move the person to the middle of the bed
   b Move the person to the side of the bed
   c Raise the head of the bed
   d Position pillows for comfort

11 A patient with a spinal cord injury is turned with
   a The logrolling procedure
   b A transfer belt
   c A mechanical lift
   d A pillow under the head and neck

12 To assist with dangling, you need to know
   a If a transfer belt is needed
   b Where to position pillows
   c If a mechanical lift is needed
   d Which side is stronger

13 To protect the person's rights during dangling
   a Leave the room as the person dangles
   b Perform the procedure alone
   c Ask the person what procedure to use
   d Close the privacy curtain

14 A person is able to help move. To re-position the person in a wheelchair
   a Pull the person from behind
   b Unlock the wheelchair wheels
   c Position the person's feet flat on the floor
   d Position the person's arms across the chest

Answers to Chapter 19 questions are on p. 886.

FOCUS ON **PRACTICE**

Problem Solving

A person with right-sided weakness needs to sit on the side of the bed (dangle). Which side of the bed is best—right, left, or either? Why? The person becomes pale and dizzy while dangling. What will you do?

Transferring the Person

OBJECTIVES

- Define the key terms and key abbreviation in this chapter.
- Explain how to prevent work-related injuries during transfers.
- Identify the delegation information needed to transfer a person.
- Identify comfort and safety measures for transferring the person.
- Explain wheelchair and stretcher safety.
- Perform the procedures described in this chapter.
- Explain how to promote PRIDE in the person, the family, and yourself.

KEY TERMS

lateral transfer When a person moves between 2 horizontal surfaces

pivot To turn one's body from a set standing position

transfer How a person moves to and from a surface

KEY ABBREVIATION

ID   Identification

Patients and residents move to and from surfaces such as beds, chairs, wheelchairs, shower chairs, commodes, toilets, and stretchers. A *transfer is how a person moves to and from a surface.* The amount of help needed and the method used vary with the person's abilities. You will assist with transfers often.

Rules for body mechanics and the safety measures for preventing work-related injuries apply to transfers (Chapter 18). So do the rules for moving persons (Chapter 19). Protect yourself and the person from injury. Use your body and transfer devices and equipment correctly.

See *Focus on Communication: Transferring the Person.*

See *Teamwork and Time Management: Transferring the Person.*

See *Delegation Guidelines: Transferring the Person.*

See *Promoting Safety and Comfort: Transferring the Person,* p. 288.

FOCUS ON COMMUNICATION

Transferring the Person

Transfers can be painful for older persons and for many persons after injury or surgery. Ask about comfort. Remind the person to tell you about discomfort.

- "Please tell me if you feel pain or discomfort."
- "Tell me to stop if you feel pain."

Before any transfer, tell the person what you and your co-workers will do. Also explain what the person needs to do. Give step-by-step instructions during the procedure.

The procedures in this chapter explain how to transfer on the "count of 3." You and the person or you and your co-workers move at the same time. For example:

I will help you transfer to the chair. I will count "1, 2, 3." When I say "3," push on the mattress with your hands and stand. I will steady you with the transfer belt as you stand. You will turn so your legs touch the seat's edge. Grab the chair's armrests. I will help you sit.

TEAMWORK AND TIME MANAGEMENT

Transferring the Person

Some agencies have "lift teams" that perform most transfer procedures. They use assist equipment and do not manually lift a person unless necessary.

The nurse tells the lift team of scheduled procedures. The team is called by pager, phone, or other device for unscheduled transfers.

Follow agency procedures to check or add to the lift team's schedule. If the person is on the schedule, check to make sure that the procedure was done. Unscheduled or unexpected events can cause delays. Thank the team for the work they do. Their work protects patients, residents, and you from injury.

Some transfer devices are used by other staff members. Mechanical lifts (p. 300) are examples. After using a shared device, return it to the storage area. Do not leave the device in a person's room or other area. Co-workers should not have to search for a device.

You may need help from 1 or 2 co-workers for a safe transfer. Politely ask co-workers to help you. Tell them what time you need the help and for how long. This helps them plan their own work. Thank your co-workers for helping you. Willingly help them when asked.

DELEGATION GUIDELINES

Transferring the Person

Transfer procedures are routine nursing tasks. They include:
- Stand and pivot transfers (p. 291)
- Lateral transfers (p. 298)
- Transfers using a mechanical lift (p. 300)

Before transferring a person, you need information from the nurse and care plan.

All Transfers
- What procedure to use.
  - *Transferring the Person to a Chair or Wheelchair,* p. 292
  - *Transferring the Person From a Chair or Wheelchair to Bed,* p. 295
  - *Transferring the Person To and From the Toilet,* p. 296
  - *Moving the Person to a Stretcher,* p. 299
  - *Transferring the Person Using a Stand-Assist Mechanical Lift,* p. 302
  - *Transferring the Person Using a Full-Sling Mechanical Lift,* p. 304
- The person's weight and height.
- How much help the person needs. These terms may be used.
  - *Independent*—the person transfers without help.
  - *Supervision*—the person transfers without help but needs supervision or cues.
  - *Limited assistance*—staff guide (but do not lift) the arms or legs. The person transfers on his or her own.
  - *Extensive assistance*—staff or a mechanical lift provides weight-bearing support to help the person transfer.
  - *Total dependence*—staff transfer the person with a mechanical lift.
- The person's physical abilities.
  - Can the person sit up, stand up, or walk without help?
  - Does the person have strength in the arms and legs?
- If the person has a weak side. If yes, which side?
- If the person has problems that increase the risk of injury. Dizziness, confusion, hearing or vision problems, recent surgery, and fragile skin are examples.
- The person's ability to follow directions.
- If behavior problems are likely. Combative, agitated, uncooperative, and unpredictable behaviors are examples.
- The number of staff needed for a safe transfer.
- What equipment to use.

Stand and Pivot Transfers
- What equipment to use—transfer belt, wheelchair, stand-assist device (p. 291), positioning devices, wheelchair cushion, bed or chair alarm, and so on.
- Areas of weakness. For example, if the arms are weak, the person cannot hold on to the mattress for support. If the left side is weak, he or she gets out of bed on the stronger right side. The person uses the right arm to help move.

Lateral Transfers
- What friction-reducing device to use—drawsheet (lift sheet, turning sheet), turning pad, large re-usable waterproof under-pad, slide sheet, or other lateral sliding aid (lateral transfer device).

Mechanical Lifts
- What lift to use—stand-assist mechanical lift or full-sling mechanical lift.
- The lift's weight limit. Do not exceed the lift's weight limit.
- If you need to apply an abdominal binder. For the person with bariatric needs, an abdominal binder may be used if the abdomen is in the way. See Chapter 40.
- What type and size sling to use.
- If a padded, unpadded, or mesh sling is needed.

Reporting and Recording
- What observations to report and record:
  - The amount of help needed to transfer the person
  - How the person helped with the procedure
  - How the person tolerated the transfer
  - How you positioned the person
  - The person's pulse, respirations, and blood pressure if asked to measure them before, during, or after the procedure
  - Complaints of dizziness, pain, discomfort, difficulty breathing, weakness, or fatigue
  - Who helped you with the transfer
- When to report observations.
- What patient or resident concerns to report at once.

PROMOTING SAFETY AND COMFORT

Transferring the Person

Safety

To prevent injuries to fragile bones and joints:

- Follow the rules of body mechanics and the safety measures for preventing work-related injuries (Chapter 18).
- Have help to transfer the person.
- Use assist devices as directed by the nurse and the care plan. Wheelchair, walker or cane (Chapter 34), and transfer belt (Chapter 14) are examples.
- Transfer the person carefully and in good alignment.

Decide how to transfer the person before you begin. Ask needed staff to help. Arrange the room to allow enough space for a safe transfer. Correctly place the chair, wheelchair, or other device. Also plan to protect drainage tubes or containers connected to the person.

Raise or lower the bed to a safe and comfortable level for the transfer. If the person will stand, the feet must be flat on the floor. For lateral transfers the bed is at a safe working height for staff.

Comfort

To promote mental comfort:

- Explain what you will do and how the person can help.
- Screen and cover the person for privacy.
- Reassure the person that mechanical lifts (p. 300) are safe. To promote physical comfort:
- Keep the person in good alignment.
- Do not pull on any part of the person's body.
- Raise the head of the bed as soon as possible. Lying flat for too long can cause discomfort and trouble breathing.
- Use pillows and other positioning devices as directed by the nurse and the care plan.

WHEELCHAIR AND STRETCHER SAFETY

Wheelchairs are useful for people who cannot walk or who have severe problems walking (Fig. 20-1). Wheelchairs are moved by:

- The person using the hand rims or the feet.
- The person using hand, chin, mouth, or other controls on a motorized wheelchair.
- Another person using the hand grips/push handles. Stretchers are used to transport persons who:
- Cannot sit up
- Must stay in a lying position
- Are seriously ill

The stretcher is covered with a folded flat sheet, fitted stretcher sheet, or bath blanket. A pillow and extra blankets are on hand. If the nurse allows, raise the head of the stretcher to a Fowler's or semi-Fowler's position (Chapter 18) for comfort.

Follow the safety measures in Box 20-1 to use wheelchairs and stretchers. The person can fall from the wheelchair or stretcher. Or the person can fall during transfers to and from the wheelchair or stretcher.

Remember to use good body mechanics for wheelchair and stretcher transfers and transport (Chapter 18). Also follow the safety measures to prevent equipment accidents (Chapter 13).

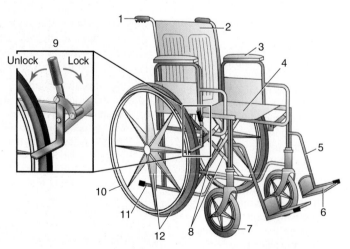

1 Hand grip/push handle	7 Caster
2 Back upholstery	8 Crossbrace
3 Armrest	9 Wheel lock/brake
4 Seat upholstery	10 Wheel and hand rim
5 Front rigging	11 Tipping lever
6 Footplate	12 Tire and wheel spokes

FIGURE 20-1 Parts of a wheelchair.

| BOX 20-1 | **Wheelchair and Stretcher Safety** |

Wheelchair Safety

Maintenance

- Check that you can lock and unlock the wheel locks (brakes).
- Check for flat or loose tires. A wheel lock (brake) will not work on a flat or loose tire.
- Make sure wheel spokes are intact. Damaged, broken, or loose spokes can interfere with moving the wheelchair or locking (braking) the wheels.
- Make sure the casters point forward. This keeps the wheelchair balanced and stable.
- Clean the wheelchair according to agency policy.
- Follow the safety measures to prevent equipment accidents (Chapter 13).

Transfers

- Lock (brake) both wheels before you transfer a person to or from the wheelchair (see Fig. 20-1). Make sure bed wheels are locked.
- Remove the near armrest (if removable) for lateral transfers to and from the bed, toilet, commode, tub, or car (p. 298). Leave the armrests in place if the person will push off of them to stand.
- Remove or swing front rigging out of the way for transfers to and from the wheelchair (Fig. 20-2, p. 290). Raise the footplates.
- Position the person's feet on the footplates. The feet must not touch or drag on the floor when the chair is moving.
- Do not let the person stand on the footplates.
- Do not let the footplates fall back onto the person's legs.
- Provide needed wheelchair accessories—safety belt, pouch, tray, lap-board, cushion.

Transport

- Use good body mechanics (Chapter 18).
- Follow the care plan for the number of staff needed for a safe transport. This depends on:
  - The person's weight
  - If the person is cooperative
  - If the wheelchair is motorized
- Push the chair forward to transport the person. Do not pull the chair backward unless going through a doorway or down a steep ramp or incline.

Wheelchair Safety—cont'd

Transport—cont'd

- Move wheelchairs up and down ramps and curbs safely (Figs. 20-3 and 20-4, p. 290).
  - Going up a ramp: push the wheelchair front-first.
  - Going down a ramp: face the back of the wheelchair. Roll it backward looking behind when moving the wheelchair.
  - Going up a curb:
    - Position the wheelchair so the front casters are at the curb.
    - Tilt the wheelchair back so the front casters are above the curb.
    - Push the wheelchair forward until you can set the wheelchair down over the curb.
    - Push the rear wheels up over the curb.
  - Going down a curb:
    - Turn the wheelchair so the rear wheels are at the curb.
    - Lower the rear wheels down the curb.
    - Lower the front casters down the curb.
- Follow the care plan for keeping the wheels locked (braked) when not moving the wheelchair. Locking (braking) the wheels prevents the chair from moving if the person moves to or from the chair. (Locking the wheelchair may be viewed as a restraint. See Chapter 15.)

Stretcher Safety

- Have 2 or more co-workers help you transfer the person to or from the stretcher.
- Lock (brake) the stretcher wheels before the transfer.
- Fasten the safety straps when the person is properly positioned on the stretcher.
- Follow the care plan for the number of staff needed for a safe transport. As many as 4 staff members may be needed. This depends on:
  - The person's weight
  - If the person is cooperative
- Raise the side rails. Keep them up during the transport.
- Make sure the person's arms, hands, legs, and feet do not dangle through the side rail bars.
- Stand at the head of the stretcher. Your co-worker stands at the foot of the stretcher.
- Move the stretcher feet first (Fig. 20-5, p. 291). The staff member at the head of the stretcher watches the person's breathing and color during the transport.
- Do not leave the person alone.

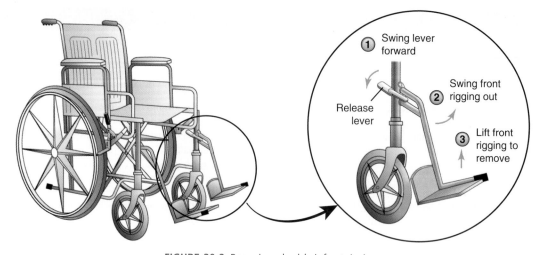

FIGURE 20-2 Removing wheelchair front rigging.

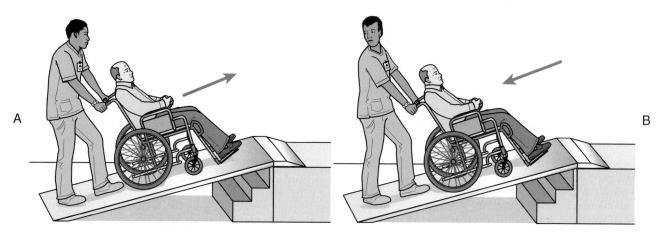

FIGURE 20-3 A, Moving a wheelchair up a ramp. **B,** Moving a wheelchair down a ramp.

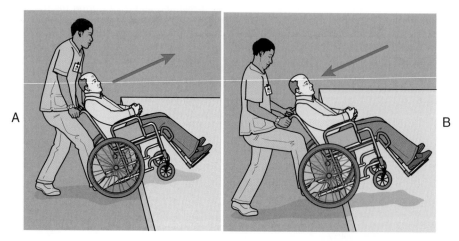

FIGURE 20-4 A, Moving a wheelchair up a curb. **B,** Moving a wheelchair down a curb.

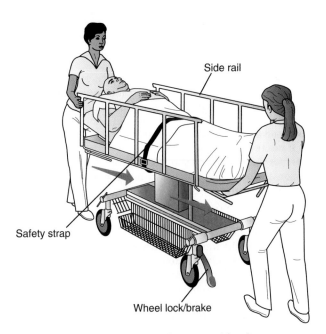

Side rail

Safety strap

Wheel lock/brake

FIGURE 20-5 The stretcher is moved feet first.

Safety

The person wears slip-resistant footwear for stand and pivot transfers. Such footwear helps prevent slipping, sliding, and falls. Tie shoelaces securely. Otherwise the person can trip and fall.

Long gowns and robes can cause the person to trip and fall. Also avoid robes with long ties.

Lock (brake) bed and wheelchair wheels and wheels on other devices. This prevents the bed and the device from moving during the transfer. Otherwise, the person can fall. You also are at risk for injury.

The person must not put his or her arms around your neck. Otherwise the person can pull you forward or cause you to lose balance. Neck, back, and other injuries are possible. To stand, the person pushes off the mattress or the chair or wheelchair armrests. Or the person uses a bed rail or stand-assist device (Fig. 20-6). Follow the care plan and the nurse's directions.

Comfort

After the transfer, position the person in good alignment. Place the call light and other needed items within reach.

STAND AND PIVOT TRANSFERS

Some persons can stand and pivot. *Pivot means to turn one's body from a set standing position.* A stand and pivot transfer is used if:

- The legs are strong enough to bear some or all of the person's weight.
- The person can cooperate and follow directions.
- The person can assist with the transfer.
  See *Delegation Guidelines: Transferring the Person*, p. 287.
  See *Promoting Safety and Comfort: Stand and Pivot Transfers.*

Transfer Belts

Transfer belts (gait belts) are discussed in Chapter 14. They are used to:

- Support patients and residents during transfers.
- Re-position persons in chairs and wheelchairs (Chapter 19).
- Assist with ambulation (Chapter 34).
  Wider belts have padded handles. They are easier to grip and allow better control should the person fall.

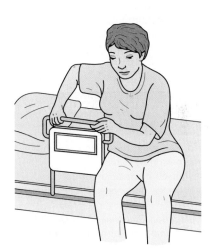

FIGURE 20-6 Stand-assist bed attachment.

Bed to Chair or Wheelchair Transfers

Safety is important for chair and wheelchair transfers. Help the person out of bed on his or her strong side. If the left side is weak and the right side is strong, get the person out of bed on the right side. The strong side moves first. It pulls the weaker side along. Transfers from the weak side are awkward and unsafe.

The chair or wheelchair is placed beside the bed at the head or foot of the bed. The armrest almost touches the bed.

- If at the head of the bed, the seat faces the foot of the bed.
- If at the foot of the bed, the seat faces the head of the bed.

See *Focus on Surveys: Bed to Chair or Wheelchair Transfers.*

See *Promoting Safety and Comfort: Bed to Chair or Wheelchair Transfers.*

See procedure: *Transferring the Person to a Chair or Wheelchair.*

FOCUS ON SURVEYS

Bed to Chair or Wheelchair Transfers

Agencies must ensure that nursing assistants can safely perform the skills needed for safe care. Surveyors will observe how nursing assistants function. One skill of focus is transferring a person from the bed to a wheelchair.

PROMOTING SAFETY AND COMFORT

Bed to Chair or Wheelchair Transfers

Safety

The chair or wheelchair must support the person's weight. The number of staff needed depends on the person's abilities, condition, and size (weight and height). Sometimes you need a mechanical lift (p. 300).

If not using a mechanical lift, use a transfer belt. It is safer for the person and you. Putting your arms around the person and grasping the shoulder blades is another method. This can cause the person discomfort and be stressful for you. Use this method only if the nurse and care plan direct and you are comfortable doing so.

Bed and wheelchair wheels are locked (braked) for a safe transfer. After the transfer, the wheelchair wheels are unlocked (brakes released) to position the chair as the person prefers. Then lock (brake) the wheels or keep them unlocked according to the care plan. Locked wheels may be viewed as restraints if the person cannot unlock them to move the wheelchair (Chapter 15). However, falls and other injuries are risks if the person tries to stand when the wheels are unlocked.

Comfort

Most wheelchairs and bedside chairs have vinyl seats and backs. Vinyl holds body heat. The person becomes warm and perspires (sweats) more. If the nurse allows, cover the back and seat with a folded bath blanket. This increases comfort.

Some people have wheelchair cushions or positioning devices. Ask the nurse how to use and place the devices. Also follow the manufacturer's instructions.

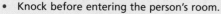 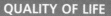

Transferring the Person to a Chair or Wheelchair

QUALITY OF LIFE

- Knock before entering the person's room.
- Address the person by name.
- Introduce yourself by name and title.

- Explain the procedure before starting and during the procedure.
- Protect the person's rights during the procedure.
- Handle the person gently during the procedure.

PRE-PROCEDURE

1 Follow *Delegation Guidelines: Transferring the Person,* p. 287. See *Promoting Safety and Comfort:*
   a *Transfer/Gait Belts,* Chapter 14
   b *Transferring the Person,* p. 288
   c *Stand and Pivot Transfers,* p. 291
   d *Bed to Chair or Wheelchair Transfers*
2 Collect the following.
   - Wheelchair or arm chair
   - Bath blanket
   - Lap blanket (if used)
   - Robe and slip-resistant footwear
   - Paper or sheet
   - Transfer belt (if needed)
   - Seat cushion (if needed)

3 Practice hand hygiene.
4 Identify the person. Check the identification (ID) bracelet against the assignment sheet. Use 2 identifiers (Chapter 13). Also call the person by name.
5 Provide for privacy.
6 Decide which side of the bed to use. Move furniture for a safe transfer.

Transferring the Person to a Chair or Wheelchair—cont'd

PROCEDURE

7 Raise the wheelchair footplates. Remove or swing front rigging out of the way if possible. Position the chair or wheelchair beside the bed on the person's strong side.
  a If at the head of the bed, it faces the foot of the bed.
  b If at the foot of the bed, it faces the head of the bed.
  c The armrest almost touches the bed.

8 Place a folded bath blanket or cushion on the seat (if needed).

9 Lock (brake) the wheelchair wheels. Make sure bed wheels are locked.

10 Fan-fold top linens to the foot of the bed.

11 Place the paper or sheet under the person's feet. (This protects linens from footwear.) Put footwear on the person.

12 Lower the bed to a safe and comfortable level for the person. Follow the care plan.

13 Help the person sit on the side of the bed (Chapter 19). Feet must be flat on the floor.

14 Help the person put on a robe.

15 Apply the transfer belt if needed (Chapter 14). It is applied at the waist over clothing.

16 *Method 1—using a transfer belt:*
  a Stand in front of the person.
  b Have the person hold on to the mattress.
  c Make sure the feet are flat on the floor.
  d Have the person lean forward.
  e Grasp the transfer belt at each side. Grasp the handles or grasp the belt from underneath. Hands are in an upward position (upward grasp). See Chapter 14.
  f Prevent the person from sliding or falling. Do 1 of the following.
    1) Brace your knees against the person's knees (Fig. 20-7, p. 294). Block his or her feet with your feet.
    2) Use the knee and foot of 1 leg to block the person's weak leg or foot. Place your other foot slightly behind you for balance.
    3) Straddle your legs around the weak leg.
  g Explain the following.
    1) You will count "1, 2, 3."
    2) The move will be on "3."
    3) On "3," the person pushes down on the mattress and stands.
  h Ask the person to push down on the mattress and stand on the "count of 3." Assist the person to a standing position as you straighten your knees (Fig. 20-8, *A*, p. 294).

17 *Method 2—no transfer belt:* (NOTE: Use this method only if directed by the nurse and the care plan and you are comfortable doing so.)
  a Follow steps 16, a–c.
  b Place your hands under the person's arms. Your hands are around the shoulder blades (Fig. 20-8, *B*, p. 294).
  c Have the person lean forward.
  d Prevent the person from sliding or falling. Do 1 of the following.
    1) Brace your knees against the person's knees. Block his or her feet with your feet.
    2) Use the knee and foot of 1 leg to block the person's weak leg or foot. Place your other foot slightly behind you for balance.
    3) Straddle your legs around the weak leg.
  e Explain the "count of 3." See step 16, g.
  f Ask the person to push down on the mattress and to stand on the "count of 3." Assist the person to a standing position as you straighten your knees.

18 Support the person in the standing position. Hold the transfer belt or keep your hands around the shoulder blades. Continue to prevent the person from sliding or falling.

19 Help the person pivot (turn) so he or she can grasp the far arm of the chair or wheelchair (Fig. 20-9, p. 294). The legs will touch the edge of the seat.

20 Continue to help the person pivot (turn) until the other armrest is grasped.

21 Lower him or her into the chair or wheelchair as you bend your hips and knees. The person leans forward and bends the elbows and knees (Fig. 20-10, p. 294).

22 Make sure the hips are to the back of the seat. Position the person in good alignment.

23 Attach the wheelchair front rigging. Position the person's feet on the footplates.

24 Cover the person's lap and legs with a lap blanket (if used). Keep the blanket off the floor and the wheels.

25 Remove the transfer belt if used.

26 Position the chair as the person prefers. Lock (brake) the wheelchair wheels according to the care plan.

POST-PROCEDURE

27 Provide for comfort. (See the inside of the back cover.)

28 Place the call light and other needed items within reach.

29 Unscreen the person.

30 Complete a safety check of the room. (See the inside of the back cover.)

31 Practice hand hygiene.

32 Report and record your observations.

33 See procedure: *Transferring the Person From a Chair or Wheelchair to Bed* (p. 295) to return the person to bed.

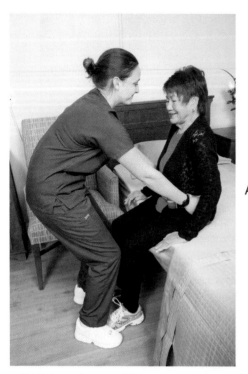

FIGURE 20-7 The person's knees are blocked by the nursing assistant's knees.

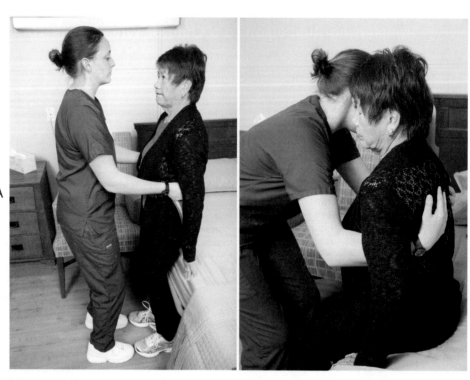

FIGURE 20-8 The person is assisted to a standing position. **A,** Method 1—with a transfer belt. The person is supported with the transfer belt. **B,** Method 2—without a transfer belt. The hands are under the person's arms and around the shoulder blades.

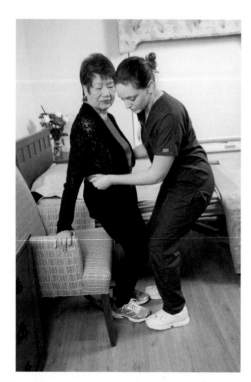

FIGURE 20-9 The person is supported as she grasps the far arm of the chair.

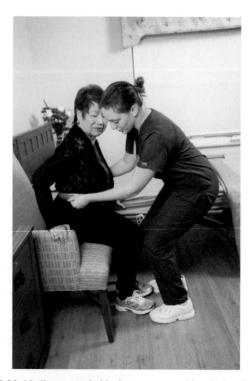

FIGURE 20-10 The person holds the armrests and bends the elbows and knees while being lowered into the chair.

Chair or Wheelchair to Bed Transfers

Chair or wheelchair to bed transfers have the same rules as bed to chair transfers. If the person is weak on 1 side, transfer the person so that the strong side moves first. Position the person so the strong side is near the bed. The strong side moves first. You may have to move the chair or wheelchair.

For example, a resident's right side is weak. The left side is strong. To transfer out of bed, the chair was on the left side of the bed. The left side (strong side) moved first. Now you will transfer the resident back to bed. With the chair on the left side of the bed, the resident's weak right side is near the bed. Moving the weak side first is not safe. Move the chair to the other side of the bed or turn the chair around. The resident's stronger left side will be near the bed. The stronger side moves first for a safe transfer.

See procedure: *Transferring the Person From a Chair or Wheelchair to Bed.*

Transferring the Person From a Chair or Wheelchair to Bed

QUALITY OF LIFE

- Knock before entering the person's room.
- Address the person by name.
- Introduce yourself by name and title.

- Explain the procedure before starting and during the procedure.
- Protect the person's rights during the procedure.
- Handle the person gently during the procedure.

PRE-PROCEDURE

1 Follow *Delegation Guidelines: Transferring the Person,* p. 287. See *Promoting Safety and Comfort:*
   a *Transfer/Gait Belts* (Chapter 14)
   b *Transferring the Person,* p. 288
   c *Stand and Pivot Transfers,* p. 291
   d *Bed to Chair or Wheelchair Transfers,* p. 292

2 Collect a transfer belt if needed.
3 Practice hand hygiene.
4 Identify the person. Check the ID bracelet against the assignment sheet. Use 2 identifiers (Chapter 13). Also call the person by name.
5 Provide for privacy.

PROCEDURE

6 Move furniture for moving space.
7 Raise the head of the bed to a sitting position. Lower the bed to a safe and comfortable level for the person. Follow the care plan. When the person transfers to the bed, the feet must be flat on the floor when sitting on the side of the bed.
8 Move the call light to the person's strong side when in bed.
9 Position the chair or wheelchair so the person's strong side is next to the bed (Fig. 20-11, p. 296). Have a co-worker help you if necessary.
10 Lock (brake) the wheelchair and bed wheels.
11 Remove and fold the lap blanket.
12 Remove the person's feet from the footplates. Raise the footplates. Remove or swing front rigging out of the way. Put slip-resistant footwear on the person if not already done.
13 Apply the transfer belt if needed.
14 Make sure the person's feet are flat on the floor.
15 Stand in front of the person.
16 Have the person hold on to the armrests. (If the nurse directs you to do so, place your arms under the person's arms. Your hands are around the shoulder blades.)
17 Have the person lean forward.
18 Grasp the transfer belt on each side if using it. Grasp underneath the belt. Hands are in an upward position (upward grasp).

19 Prevent the person from sliding or falling. Do 1 of the following.
   a Brace your knees against the person's knees. Block his or her feet with your feet.
   b Use the knee and foot of 1 leg to block the person's weak leg or foot. Place your other foot slightly behind you for balance.
   c Straddle your legs around the weak leg.
20 Explain the "count of 3." See procedure: *Transferring the Person to a Chair or Wheelchair,* p. 292.
21 Ask the person to push down on the armrests on the "count of 3." Assist the person into a standing position as you straighten your knees.
22 Support the person in the standing position. Hold the transfer belt or keep your hands around the shoulder blades. Continue to prevent the person from sliding or falling.
23 Help the person pivot (turn) to reach the edge of the mattress. The legs will touch the mattress.
24 Continue to help the person pivot (turn) until he or she reaches the mattress with both hands.
25 Lower him or her onto the bed as you bend your hips and knees. The person leans forward and bends the elbows and knees.
26 Remove the transfer belt.
27 Remove the robe and footwear.
28 Help the person lie down.

POST-PROCEDURE

29 Provide for comfort. (See the inside of the back cover.)
30 Place the call light and other needed items within reach.
31 Raise or lower bed rails. Follow the care plan.
32 Arrange furniture to meet the person's needs.
33 Unscreen the person.

34 Complete a safety check of the room. (See the inside of the back cover.)
35 Practice hand hygiene.
36 Report and record your observations.

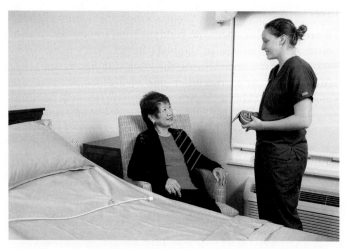

FIGURE 20-11 The chair is positioned so the person's strong side is near the bed. (Note: The "weak" side is indicated by slash marks.)

Transferring the Person To and From the Toilet

Using the bathroom for elimination promotes privacy, dignity, self-esteem, and independence. However, bathrooms are often small. There is little room for you or a wheelchair. Therefore transfers with wheelchairs and toilets are often hard. Falls and work-related injuries are risks.

The following procedure can be used if the person can stand and pivot from the wheelchair to the toilet. A transfer board (p. 298) or mechanical lift (p. 300) may be needed.

See *Promoting Safety and Comfort: Transferring the Person To and From the Toilet.*

See procedure: *Transferring the Person To and From the Toilet.*

Transferring the Person To and From the Toilet

QUALITY OF LIFE

- Knock before entering the person's room.
- Address the person by name.
- Introduce yourself by name and title.

- Explain the procedure before starting and during the procedure.
- Protect the person's rights during the procedure.
- Handle the person gently during the procedure.

PRE-PROCEDURE

1 Follow *Delegation Guidelines: Transferring the Person,* p. 287. See *Promoting Safety and Comfort:*
   a *Transfer/Gait Belts* (Chapter 14)
   b *Transferring the Person,* p. 288
   c *Stand and Pivot Transfers,* p. 291
   d *Bed to Chair or Wheelchair Transfers,* p. 292
   e *Transferring the Person To and From the Toilet*

2 Practice hand hygiene.

Transferring the Person To and From the Toilet—cont'd

PROCEDURE

3 Put slip-resistant footwear on the person.

4 Position the wheelchair next to the toilet if there is enough room (Fig. 20-12, *A*). Or position the chair at a right angle (90-degree angle) to the toilet (Fig. 20-12, *B*). (See *Focus on Math: Fowler's Positions* in Chapter 18.) It is best to have the person's strong side near the toilet.

5 Lock (brake) the wheelchair wheels.

6 Raise the footplates. Remove or swing front rigging out of the way.

7 Apply the transfer belt.

8 Help the person unfasten clothing.

9 Use the transfer belt to help the person stand and pivot (turn) to the toilet. See procedure: *Transferring the Person From a Chair or Wheelchair to Bed,* p. 295. The person uses the grab bars to pivot (turn) to the toilet.

10 Support the person with the transfer belt while he or she lowers clothing. Or have the person hold on to the grab bars for support. Lower the person's clothing.

11 Use the transfer belt to lower the person onto the toilet seat. Check for proper positioning on the toilet.

12 Remove the transfer belt.

13 Tell the person you will stay nearby. Remind the person to use the call light or call for you when help is needed. Stay with the person if required by the care plan.

14 Close the bathroom door for privacy.

15 Stay near the bathroom. Complete other tasks in the person's room. Check on the person every 5 minutes.

16 Knock on the bathroom door when the person calls for you.

17 Help with wiping, perineal care (Chapter 24), flushing, and hand-washing as needed. Wear gloves and practice hand hygiene after removing the gloves.

18 Apply the transfer belt.

19 Use the transfer belt to help the person stand.

20 Help the person raise and secure clothing.

21 Use the transfer belt to transfer the person to the wheelchair. See procedure: *Transferring the Person to a Chair or Wheelchair,* p. 292.

22 Make sure the person's buttocks are to the back of the seat. Position the person in good alignment.

23 Position the feet on the footplates.

24 Remove the transfer belt.

25 Cover the lap and legs with a lap blanket. Keep the blanket off the floor and wheels.

26 Position the chair as the person prefers. Lock (brake) the wheelchair wheels according to the care plan.

POST-PROCEDURE

27 Provide for comfort. (See the inside of the back cover.)

28 Place the call light and other needed items within reach.

29 Unscreen the person.

30 Complete a safety check of the room. (See the inside of the back cover.)

31 Practice hand hygiene.

32 Report and record your observations.

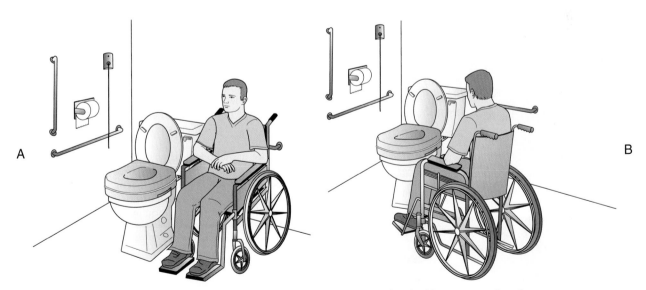

A   B

FIGURE 20-12 Wheelchair positions for a transfer to the toilet. **A,** The wheelchair is next to the toilet. **B,** The wheelchair is placed at a right angle (90-degree angle) to the toilet.

LATERAL TRANSFERS

A *lateral transfer moves a person between 2 horizontal surfaces.* The person slides from 1 surface to the other. A transfer from a bed to a stretcher is an example. A transfer from bed to a shower trolley (Chapter 24) is another example.

Lateral Transfer Devices

Friction and shearing injure the skin (Chapter 19). Infection and pressure injuries can result (Chapter 41). Friction-reducing devices protect the skin during lateral transfers. They also protect staff from injury.

Devices include:

- Lift sheet, turning sheet, or drawsheet (Chapters 19 and 22)
- Turning pad (Chapter 19)
- Large re-usable waterproof under-pad (Chapter 22)
- Slide sheet or other lateral sliding aid (lateral transfer device) (Fig. 20-13)

A transfer board (sliding board) (Fig. 20-14) may be used for seated lateral transfers if:

- The person has upper body strength.
- The person has good sitting balance.
- There is enough room to position the 2 surfaces close together.

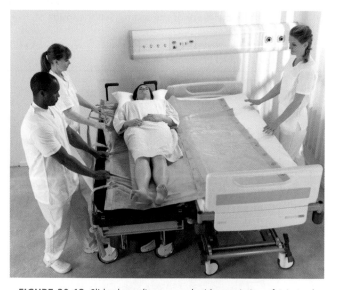

FIGURE 20-13 Slide sheet. (Image used with permission of Arjo Inc.)

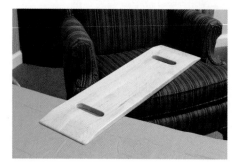

FIGURE 20-14 Transfer board (sliding board) for seated transfers to and from surfaces.

Moving the Person to a Stretcher

A friction-reducing device is used for transfers to and from stretchers. At least 2 or 3 staff are needed for a safe transfer.

- *If the person weighs less than 200 pounds*—a friction-reducing device or lateral sliding aid (lateral transfer device) is used.
- *If the person weighs more than 200 pounds*—a lateral sliding aid (lateral transfer device), mechanical ceiling lift (p. 300), or other device is used as directed. At least 3 staff members are needed.

For persons with bariatric needs, the nurse and care plan may direct staff to:

- Use a bariatric stretcher. Check for an "EC" (expanded capacity) or BARIATRIC label and the weight limit.
- Position the stretcher so it is $\frac{1}{2}$ inch lower than the bed.
- Use a lateral transfer device, bariatric ceiling lift (p. 300), or other device as directed.
- Transfer the person from his or her strong side.
- Apply an abdominal binder if the person's abdomen is in the way. See Chapter 40.

See *Promoting Safety and Comfort: Moving the Person to a Stretcher.*

See procedure: *Moving the Person to a Stretcher.*

PROMOTING SAFETY AND COMFORT

Moving the Person to a Stretcher

Safety

Protect yourself and the person from injury.

- Make sure you know how to use the device. Follow the manufacturer's instructions.
- Position the stretcher and bed surfaces as close as possible to each other.
- Avoid extended reaches and bending your back. You may need to kneel on the bed or stretcher.
- Follow the rules for stretcher safety (see Box 20-1).
- Make sure the bed and stretcher wheels are locked (braked).
- Practice good body mechanics and follow the guidelines for preventing work-related injuries (Chapter 18).
- Keep the person in good alignment.
- Make sure you have enough help.
- Hold the person securely. You must not drop the person.

Moving the Person to a Stretcher

QUALITY OF LIFE

- Knock before entering the person's room.
- Address the person by name.
- Introduce yourself by name and title.

- Explain the procedure before starting and during the procedure.
- Protect the person's rights during the procedure.
- Handle the person gently during the procedure.

PRE-PROCEDURE

1 Follow *Delegation Guidelines: Transferring the Person*, p. 287. See *Promoting Safety and Comfort:*
  a *Transferring the Person*, p. 288
  b *Moving the Person to a Stretcher*
2 Ask 1 or 2 staff members to help you.
3 Collect the following.
  - Stretcher covered with a sheet or bath blanket
  - Bath blanket
  - Pillow(s) if needed
  - Drawsheet, slide sheet, or other lateral transfer device

4 Practice hand hygiene.
5 Identify the person. Check the ID bracelet against the assignment sheet. Use 2 identifiers (Chapter 13). Also call the person by name.
6 Provide for privacy.
7 Raise the bed and stretcher for body mechanics.

PROCEDURE

8 Position yourself and co-workers.
  a 1 or 2 workers stand on the side of the bed where the stretcher will be.
  b 1 worker stands on the other side of the bed.
9 Lower the head of the bed. It is as flat as possible.
10 Lower the bed rails if used.
11 Cover the person with a bath blanket. Fan-fold top linens to the foot of the bed.
12 Position the assist device. Or loosen the drawsheet on each side.
13 Use the assist device to move the person to the side of the bed. This is the side where the stretcher will be.
14 Protect the person from falling. Hold the far arm and leg.

15 Have your co-workers position the stretcher next to the bed. They stand beside the stretcher (Fig. 20-15, *A*).
16 Lock (brake) the bed and stretcher wheels.
17 Grasp the assist device (Fig. 20-15, *B*).
18 Transfer the person to the stretcher on the "count of 3." Center the person on the stretcher.
19 Place a pillow or pillows under the person's head and shoulders if allowed. Raise the head of the stretcher if allowed.
20 Cover the person. Provide for comfort.
21 Fasten the safety straps. Raise the side rails.
22 Unlock the stretcher wheels (release the brakes). Transport the person.

POST-PROCEDURE

23 Practice hand hygiene.
24 Report and record:
  - The time of the transport
  - Where the person was transported to
  - Who went with him or her
  - How the transfer was tolerated

25 Reverse the procedure to return the person to bed.

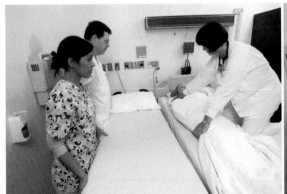
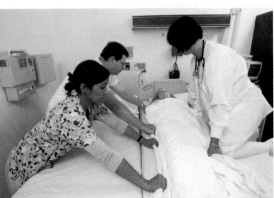

A B

FIGURE 20-15 Transferring the person to a stretcher. **A,** The stretcher is against the bed and is held in place. **B,** A drawsheet is used to transfer the person from the bed to a stretcher.

MECHANICAL LIFTS

Mechanical lifts are used for transfers to and from beds, chairs, wheelchairs, stretchers, tubs, shower chairs, toilets, commodes, whirlpools, or vehicles. They are used for persons who:

- Need weight-bearing support to transfer
- Cannot assist with transfers
- Are too heavy for staff to move

There are manual, battery-operated, and electric lifts. Two types are common.

- Stand-assist lifts (Fig. 20-16, *A* and Fig. 20-17, *A*)—for persons who require some help with transfers and can:
  - Bear some weight.
  - Follow directions.
  - Sit on the side of the bed with or without help.
  - Bend the hips, knees, and ankles.
- Full-sling mechanical lifts (Fig. 20-16, *B* and Fig. 20-17, *B*)—for persons who:
  - Cannot assist with transfers.
  - Are partially able or unable to bear weight.
  - Are heavy.
  - Have physical limits preventing other types of transfers.

Some lifts are mounted on the ceiling. Your agency may have floor or ceiling-mounted bariatric lifts (Fig. 20-18).

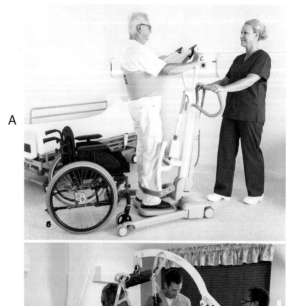

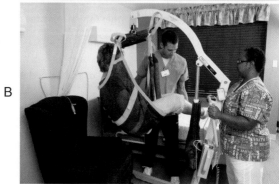

FIGURE 20-16 A, A stand-assist lift supports the upper body. **B,** A full-sling mechanical lift supports the entire body. (Part A used with permission of Arjo Inc.)

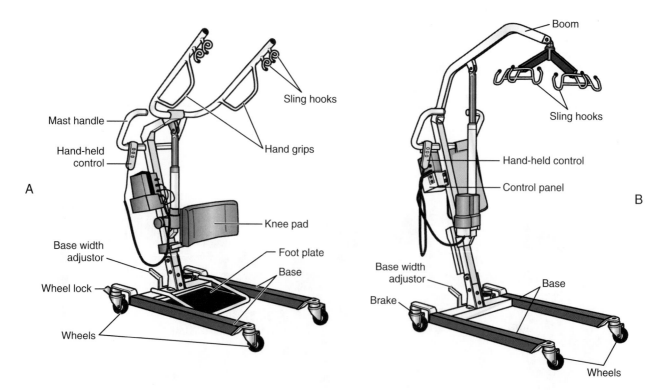

Stand-assist mechanical lift

Full-sling mechanical lift

FIGURE 20-17 Mechanical lifts. **A,** Parts of a stand-assist lift. **B,** Parts of a full-sling mechanical lift.

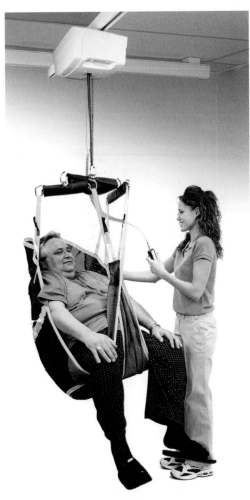

FIGURE 20-18 Bariatric ceiling lift. (Courtesy MedCare Products, Burnsville, Minn.)

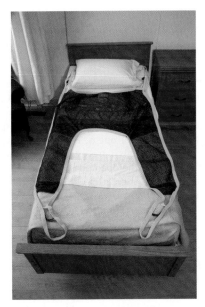

FIGURE 20-19 A full-sling.

Slings

The sling used depends on the lift type and the person's size, condition, and care needs. Slings are padded, unpadded, or made of mesh. Stand-assist slings support the upper body (see Fig. 20-16, *A*). Full-slings support the entire body (see Fig. 20-16, *B*). There are many types of full-slings.

- *Standard full-sling*—for normal transfers (Fig. 20-19).
- *Bathing sling*—for transfers from the bed or chair into a bathtub. Depending on the manufacturer's instructions, the sling may be left in place and attached to the lift during the bath.
- *Toileting sling*—the sling bottom is open. Each person has his or her own toileting sling.
- *Amputee sling*—for the person who has had both legs amputated.
- *Bariatric sling*—for use with a bariatric lift. There are also bariatric bathing and toileting slings. The nurse may have you leave the sling under the person when seated for short periods or at all times. If left in place, the person is not turned from side-to-side to place and remove the sling for each transfer. This reduces the risk of injury to the person and staff.

The nurse and care plan tell you what type and size sling to use. Follow agency policy and the manufacturer's instructions for using and washing contaminated slings. A sling is contaminated if it:

- Has any visible sign of blood, body fluids, secretions, or excretions.
- Is used on a person's bare skin.
- Is used to bathe a person.

Using a Mechanical Lift

Before using a lift:

- You must be trained in its use.
- It must work.
- The sling, straps, and hooks or chains must be in good repair.
- The person's weight must not exceed the lift's capacity.
- You need enough help. At least 2 staff members are needed for most lifts. Follow agency policy and the person's care plan.

There are different types of mechanical lifts. Always follow the manufacturer's instructions. The procedures that follow are used as a guide.

See *Promoting Safety and Comfort: Using a Mechanical Lift*, p. 302.

See procedure: *Transferring the Person Using a Stand-Assist Mechanical Lift*, p. 302.

See procedure: *Transferring the Person Using a Full-Sling Mechanical Lift*, p. 304.

PROMOTING SAFETY AND COMFORT
Using a Mechanical Lift

Safety

Always follow the manufacturer's instructions. Knowing how to use 1 lift does not mean that you know how to use others. If you have not used a certain lift before, ask for training. Ask the nurse to help you until you are comfortable using the lift.

The lift's base widens or opens. The base closes to fit under the bed and move through narrow areas. The lift is most stable with the base in the open position. Lock the base in the wide or open position when lifting, lowering, and moving when possible. If you must narrow the base, do so briefly. Return the base to the wide or open position as soon as possible.

For many lifts, the wheels are unlocked during lifting and lowering. This allows the lift to stabilize (become steady). For some stand-assist lifts, the wheels are locked (braked) when lifting and lowering. Follow the manufacturer's instructions for when to lock (brake) the lift's wheels. Bed and wheelchair wheels must be locked (braked).

Mechanical lifts must work correctly. Battery-powered lifts must have well-charged batteries. Tell the nurse when a lift needs repair or does not work properly.

Safety—cont'd

For persons with bariatric needs:
- Make sure the receiving surface (bed, chair, wheelchair, stretcher, and so on) has expanded capacity for the person's weight.
- Use a chair or wheelchair with arms that you can remove or lower.

One or 2 staff members are needed for a stand-assist mechanical lift. Follow the manufacturer's instructions and agency policy. Two staff members are needed to safely use a full-sling mechanical lift. Federal guidelines require that at least 1 staff member be 18 years of age or older.

Comfort

The person is lifted up and off the bed or chair. Falling is a common fear. For mental comfort, always explain the procedure before you begin. Also show the person how the lift works.

Transferring the Person Using a Stand-Assist Mechanical Lift

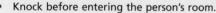

QUALITY OF LIFE

- Knock before entering the person's room.
- Address the person by name.
- Introduce yourself by name and title.

- Explain the procedure before starting and during the procedure.
- Protect the person's rights during the procedure.
- Handle the person gently during the procedure.

PRE-PROCEDURE

1 Follow *Delegation Guidelines: Transferring the Person*, p. 287. See *Promoting Safety and Comfort:*
  a *Transferring the Person*, p. 288
  b *Using a Mechanical Lift*
2 Ask a co-worker to help you (if needed).
3 Collect the following:
- Stand-assist mechanical lift and sling
- Arm chair or wheelchair
- Slip-resistant footwear
- Bath blanket or cushion
- Lap blanket (if used)

4 Practice hand hygiene.
5 Identify the person. Check the ID bracelet against the assignment sheet. Use 2 identifiers (Chapter 13). Also call the person by name.
6 Provide for privacy.

PROCEDURE

7 Place the chair (wheelchair) at the head of the bed. It is even with the head-board and about 1 foot away from the bed. Lock (brake) the wheelchair wheels. Place a folded bath blanket or cushion in the seat if needed.
8 Assist the person to a seated position on the side of the bed. See procedure: *Sitting on the Side of the Bed (Dangling)* in Chapter 19. The person's feet are flat on the floor. Bed wheels are locked.
9 Put footwear on the person.

10 Apply the sling.
  a Position the sling at the lower back.
  b Bring the straps around to the front of the chest. The straps are positioned under the arms.
  c Secure the waist belt around the person's waist. Adjust the belt so it is snug but not tight.
11 Position the lift in front of the person.
12 Widen the lift's base.
13 Lock (brake) the lift's wheels.

Transferring the Person Using a Stand-Assist Mechanical Lift—cont'd

PROCEDURE—cont'd

14 Have the person place the feet on the footplate and the knees against the knee pad. Assist as needed. If the lift has a knee strap, secure the strap around the legs. Adjust the strap so it is snug but not tight.

15 Attach the sling to the sling hooks.

16 Have the person grasp the lift's hand grips.

17 Unlock the lift's wheels (release the brakes).

18 Raise the person slightly off the bed. Check that the sling is secure, the feet are on the footplate, and the knees are against the knee pad (Fig. 20-20, *A*). If not, lower the person and correct the problem.

19 Raise the lift until the person is clear of the bed (Fig. 20-20, *B*). Or raise the person to a standing position (Fig. 20-20, *C*). Follow the care plan.

20 Adjust the base's width to move from the bed to the chair (wheelchair) if needed. Keep the base in the wide or open position as much as possible.

21 Move the lift to the chair (wheelchair). The person's back is toward the seat.

22 Lower the person into the chair (wheelchair). Guide the person into the seat. See Figure 20-20, *D and E*.

23 Lock (brake) the lift's wheels.

24 Unhook the sling from the sling hooks.

25 Unbuckle the waist belt. Remove the sling.

26 Unlock the lift's wheels (release the brakes).

27 Have the person lift the feet off of the footplate. Assist as needed. Move the lift. Position the feet flat on the floor or on the wheelchair footplates.

28 Cover the lap and legs with a lap blanket (if used). Keep it off the floor.

POST-PROCEDURE

29 Provide for comfort. (See the inside of the back cover.)

30 Place the call light and other needed items within reach.

31 Unscreen the person.

32 Complete a safety check of the room. (See the inside of the back cover.)

33 Practice hand hygiene.

34 Report and record your observations.

35 Reverse the procedure to return the person to bed.

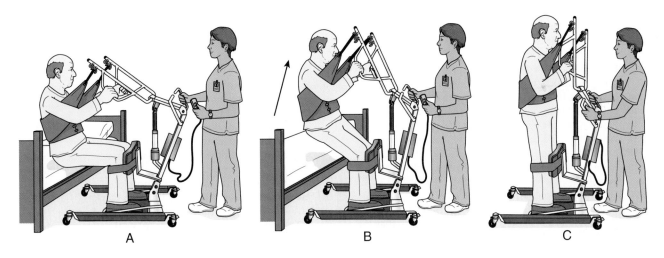

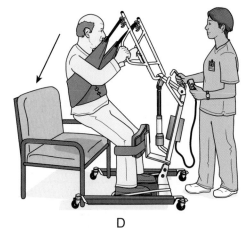

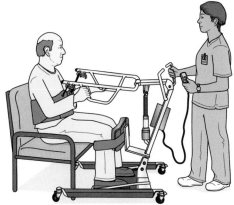

FIGURE 20-20 Using a stand-assist lift. **A,** The sling is around the person's lower back. The straps are under the arms. The waist belt is secure. Feet are on the footplate. The person holds the hand grips. **B,** The lift is raised. **C,** The person is in a standing position. **D,** The person is lowered into the chair. **E,** The person is seated. The back is against the back of the chair.

Transferring the Person Using a Full-Sling Mechanical Lift

QUALITY OF LIFE

- Knock before entering the person's room.
- Address the person by name.
- Introduce yourself by name and title.

- Explain the procedure before starting and during the procedure.
- Protect the person's rights during the procedure.
- Handle the person gently during the procedure.

PRE-PROCEDURE

1 Follow *Delegation Guidelines: Transferring the Person,* p. 287. See *Promoting Safety and Comfort:*
  a Transferring the Person, p. 288
  b Using a Mechanical Lift, p. 302
2 Ask a co-worker to help you.
3 Collect the following.
  - Full-sling mechanical lift and sling
  - Arm chair or wheelchair
  - Slip-resistant footwear
  - Bath blanket or cushion
  - Lap blanket (if used)
4 Practice hand hygiene.

5 Identify the person. Check the ID bracelet against the assignment sheet. Use 2 identifiers (Chapter 13). Also call the person by name.
6 Provide for privacy.
7 Raise the bed for body mechanics. Bed rails are up if used.

PROCEDURE

8 Lower the head of the bed to a level appropriate for the person. It is as flat as possible.
9 Stand on 1 side of the bed. Your co-worker stands on the other side.
10 Lower the bed rails if up. Lock (brake) the bed wheels.
11 Center the sling under the person (Fig. 20-21, *A*). To position the sling, turn the person from side to side (Chapter 19). Follow the manufacturer's instructions to position the sling.
12 Position the person in the semi-Fowler's position.
13 Place the chair (wheelchair) at the head of the bed. It is even with the head-board and about 1 foot away from the bed. Place a folded bath blanket or cushion in the seat if needed. Lock (brake) the wheelchair wheels.
14 Lower the bed so it is level with the chair.
15 Raise the lift to position it over the person.
16 Position the lift over the person (Fig. 20-21, *B*).
17 Widen the lift's base. Lock (brake) the lift wheels.
18 Attach the sling to the sling hooks (Fig. 20-21, *C*).
19 Raise the head of the bed to a comfortable level for the person.
20 Cross the person's arms over the chest.
21 Unlock the lift's wheels (release the brakes).
22 Raise the person slightly from the bed. Check that the sling is secure. If not, lower the person and correct the problem.

23 Raise the lift until the person and sling are free of the bed (Fig. 20-21, *D*).
24 Have your co-worker support the person's legs as you move the lift and the person away from the bed (Fig. 20-21, *E*).
25 Adjust the base's width to move from the bed to the chair (wheelchair) if needed. Keep the base in the wide or open position as much as possible.
26 Position the lift so the person's back is toward the chair (wheelchair).
27 Adjust the position of the chair (wheelchair) as needed to lower the person into it. Lock (brake) the wheelchair wheels.
28 Lower the person into the chair (wheelchair). Guide the person into the seat (Fig. 20-21, *F*).
29 Lock (brake) the lift wheels.
30 Unhook the sling. Unlock the lift's wheels (release the brakes). Move the lift away from the person. Remove the sling from under the person unless otherwise indicated.
31 Put footwear on the person. Position the feet flat on the floor or on the wheelchair footplates.
32 Cover the lap and legs with a lap blanket (if used). Keep it off the floor and wheels.
33 Position the chair (wheelchair) as the person prefers. Lock (brake) the wheelchair wheels according to the care plan.

POST-PROCEDURE

34 Provide for comfort. (See the inside of the back cover.)
35 Place the call light and other needed items within reach.
36 Unscreen the person.
37 Complete a safety check of the room. (See the inside of the back cover.)

38 Practice hand hygiene.
39 Report and record your observations.
40 Reverse the procedure to return the person to bed.

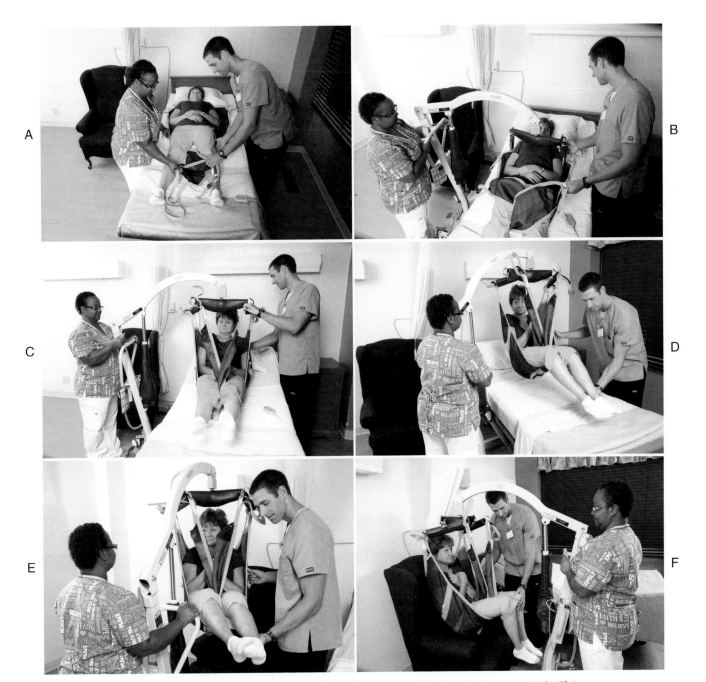

FIGURE 20-21 Using a full-sling mechanical lift. **A,** The sling is positioned under the person. **B,** The lift is over the person. **C,** The sling is attached to the lift. **D,** The lift is raised until the sling and person are off the bed. **E,** The legs are supported. The person and lift are moved away from the bed. **F,** The person is guided into a chair.

FOCUS ON **PRIDE**

The Person, Family, and Yourself

Personal and Professional Responsibility

Take time to plan and prepare for a transfer. Gather needed items. Organize the room and equipment. Remember to:

- Position the chair, wheelchair, stretcher, and so on for a safe transfer. Lock (brake) wheels.
- Remove wheelchair front rigging or swing it out of the way. Raise the footplates.
- Adjust the bed to a safe and comfortable height.
- Make sure a mechanical lift is charged.
- Move furniture or clutter out of the way.

Rights and Respect

Respect privacy during transfers. Close privacy curtains, doors, and window coverings. Properly cover the person.

Independence and Social Interaction

How you speak to the person makes a difference. To give directions:

- Speak slowly and clearly.
- Talk loudly enough for the person to hear you.
- Speak calmly and kindly. Never yell at or insult the person.
- Face the person and use eye contact when possible.
- Give 1 direction at a time.
- Repeat directions as needed. Be patient.
- Ask if the person has questions before proceeding.
  Your speech and tone must convey dignity. Show you value the person through respectful interactions.

Delegation and Teamwork

You need help to transfer a person. Your co-workers are busy. Do you ask for help? Or do you try to move the person alone? Never be afraid to ask for help. Ask politely and say thank you. Work as a team for the person's safety and to protect yourself and others from injury.

Ethics and Laws

The right way to transfer is not always the quickest way. Do not pull on the person's clothing or arm, underarm, or other body part. Choose to give care correctly. Take pride in giving care in a way that prevents harm and promotes comfort and safety.

FOCUS ON **PRIDE**: *Application*

Explaining procedures improves with practice. Practice explaining a transfer from the bed to a chair using:

- A stand and pivot transfer
- A stand-assist mechanical lift
- A full-sling mechanical lift

REVIEW QUESTIONS

Circle the BEST answer.

1 To promote comfort during a transfer
   a Pull the person to a standing position
   b Explain the procedure
   c Let the person choose the procedure
   d Open the privacy curtain

2 For a safe transfer to a chair
   a Tell the person to grasp you around your neck
   b Hold the person under the underarms
   c Manually lift the person
   d Move furniture and equipment as needed

3 You are preparing to transfer a person. Which statement promotes comfort?
   a "I'll move you quickly so it doesn't hurt."
   b "I'll leave the door open. This will not take long."
   c "Please tell me to stop if you feel pain."
   d "I'm nervous. I don't want to drop you."

4 A person uses a wheelchair. Which measure is *unsafe*?
   a The wheels are locked (braked) for transfers.
   b The chair is pulled backward for transport.
   c The feet are positioned on the footplates.
   d The casters point forward.

5 To use a stretcher safely
   a Unlock the wheels (release the brakes) for transfers to and from the stretcher
   b Fasten the safety straps
   c Lower the side rails during a transport
   d Move the stretcher head first

6 A stand and pivot transfer is *unsafe* for a person who
   a Is hard of hearing but can follow directions
   b Can bear some weight with the legs
   c Is confused and combative
   d Uses a transfer belt

7 To transfer the person to bed, a chair, or the wheelchair
   a The strong side moves first
   b The weak side moves first
   c Pillows are used for support
   d The transfer belt is removed

8 Which is *unsafe* for a stand and pivot transfer to a wheelchair?
   a The wheelchair's front rigging is removed.
   b The person's feet are flat on the floor.
   c The person is wearing slip-resistant footwear.
   d The wheelchair is behind you.

9 To transfer a person from a wheelchair to a toilet
   a Position the wheelchair facing the toilet
   b Remove the transfer belt when lowering clothing
   c Tell the person to hold on to the towel bar for support
   d Lock (brake) the wheelchair wheels

10 Which can be used for a lateral transfer from a bed to a stretcher?
   a Transfer belt
   b Slide sheet
   c Stand-assist mechanical lift
   d Trapeze

11 When using a mechanical lift
   a Position the lift on the person's strong side
   b Collect a sling, battery, and transfer belt
   c Compare the person's weight to the lift's weight limit
   d Allow the person to control the lift

12 For a safe transfer with a full-sling mechanical lift, at least
   a 1 worker is needed
   b 2 workers are needed
   c 3 workers are needed
   d 4 workers are needed

13 You are using a stand-assist mechanical lift. Which is *unsafe*?
   a The person is holding the lift's hand grips.
   b The person's feet are on the footplate.
   c The lift's base is narrow when lifting.
   d The person's knees are against the knee pad.

14 After a transfer, which should you do *first*?
   a Place the call light within reach.
   b Return the mechanical lift to the storage area.
   c Record the procedure.
   d Report to the nurse.

Answers to Chapter 20 questions are on p. 886.

FOCUS ON **PRACTICE**

Problem Solving

A resident needs to go to the bathroom right away. A full-sling mechanical lift is used for a safe transfer. You do not see another staff member nearby to help. What will you do?

The Person's Unit

OBJECTIVES

- Define the key terms and key abbreviations in this chapter.
- Explain how to maintain the person's unit.
- Describe the CMS requirements for resident rooms.
- Describe how to control the person's setting for his or her comfort.
- Describe the basic bed positions.
- Identify the 7 hospital bed system entrapment zones.
- Identify the persons at risk for bed entrapment.

- Explain how to use the furniture and equipment in the person's unit.
- Describe how a bathroom is equipped for the person's use.
- Describe how to promote safety, privacy, and comfort in the person's unit.
- Explain how to promote PRIDE in the person, the family, and yourself.

KEY TERMS

entrapment Getting caught, trapped, or entangled in spaces created by the bed rails, the mattress, the bed frame, the head-board, or the foot-board

Fowler's position A semi-sitting position; the head of the bed is raised between 45 and 60 degrees

full visual privacy Having the means to be completely free from public view while in bed

high-Fowler's position A semi-sitting position; the head of the bed is raised 60 to 90 degrees

hospital bed system The bed frame and its parts—mattress, bed rails, head- and foot-boards, and bed attachments

person's unit The space, furniture, and equipment used by the person in the agency

reverse Trendelenburg's position The head of the bed is raised and the foot of the bed is lowered

semi-Fowler's position The head of the bed is raised 30 degrees; or the head of the bed is raised 30 degrees and the knee portion is raised 15 degrees

Trendelenburg's position The head of the bed is lowered and the foot of the bed is raised

KEY ABBREVIATIONS

CMS	Centers for Medicare & Medicaid Services	IV	Intravenous
F	Fahrenheit		

The *person's unit* is the space, furniture, and equipment used by the person in the agency (Fig. 21-1). The person's unit is designed for comfort, safety, and privacy.

A private room is for 1 person. Semi-private rooms have 2, 3, or 4 units.

The person's unit is kept clean, neat, safe, and comfortable. See Box 21-1.

See *Focus on Long-Term Care and Home Care: The Person's Unit.*

FOCUS ON LONG-TERM CARE AND HOME CARE

The Person's Unit

Long-Term Care

The Centers for Medicare & Medicaid Services (CMS) has requirements for resident rooms. See Box 21-2. Resident units must be as personal and home-like as possible. Residents can bring and use some furniture and personal items from home. This promotes dignity and self-esteem.

As space allows, the person chooses where to place personal items. However, a resident cannot take or use another person's space. Doing so violates the other person's rights.

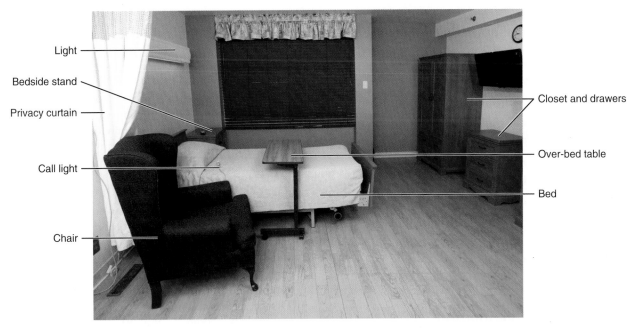

Light

Bedside stand

Privacy curtain

Call light

Chair

Closet and drawers

Over-bed table

Bed

FIGURE 21-1 Furniture and equipment in a resident's unit.

BOX 21-1	Maintaining the Person's Unit

- Keep the following within the person's reach. Arrange them as the person prefers.
  - Call light (p. 318). *The call light is within reach at all times.*
  - Over-bed table and bedside stand.
  - Phone, TV, bed, and light controls.
  - Tissues.
  - Other items as requested.
- Meet the needs of persons who cannot use the call system (p. 318).
- Adjust lighting, temperature, and ventilation for the person's comfort.
- Handle equipment carefully to prevent noise.
- Explain the causes of strange noises.
- Prevent odors. See p. 310.
- Use room deodorizers according to agency policy.
- Empty wastebaskets at least daily and when full. In some agencies, they are emptied every shift.
- Respect the person's belongings. An item may not be important to you. Yet even a scrap of paper can have great meaning to the person.
- Do not discard any items belonging to the person.
- Do not move furniture or the person's belongings. Persons with poor vision rely on memory or feel to find items.
- Straighten bed linens and towels as often as needed.
- Complete a safety check before leaving the room. (See the inside of the back cover.)

BOX 21-2	CMS Requirements for Resident Rooms

- Rooms are designed for 1 to 4 persons.
- Rooms have a direct access to an exit hallway.
- Rooms are designed or equipped for full visual privacy—ceiling-suspended privacy curtain that extends around the bed or movable screens, window coverings, and doors.
- Rooms have at least 1 window to the outside.
- Each person has closet space with racks and shelves.
- Toilet facilities are in the room or nearby (including bathing facilities).
- Rooms, bathrooms, and bathing areas have a call system.
- The person has a bed of proper height and size.
- The person has a clean, comfortable mattress.
- Bed and bath linens (towels and washcloths) are clean, dry, and in good condition.
- Bed linens are correct for the weather and climate.
- The room has furniture for clothing, personal items, and a chair for visitors.
- There is space for wheelchair or walker use.
- Rooms, drawers, and shelves are clean and orderly.
- Room temperature levels are between 71°F (Fahrenheit) and 81°F.
- Ventilation, humidity, and odor levels are acceptable.
- Non-smoking areas are identified.
- Sound levels are comfortable.
- Lighting is adequate and comfortable with little glare.
- The room is free of pests and rodents.
- Hand rails are in good repair.
- The person's setting is free of clutter.
- Personal supplies and items are correctly labeled and stored.
- Items are within reach for use in bed or the bathroom.
- The person has a raised toilet seat (if needed).

COMFORT

Age, illness, and activity affect comfort. So do temperature, ventilation, noise, odors, and lighting. These factors are controlled to meet the person's needs.

See *Focus on Communication: Comfort.*

FOCUS ON COMMUNICATION

Comfort

What is comfortable for 1 person may not be for another. Ask about the person's comfort. You can say:
- "How is the temperature? Is it too hot or too cold?"
- "Is the noise level okay?"
- "Please let me know if you notice any bad odors."
- "How is the lighting? Is it too bright or too dark?"
- "Are you comfortable?"

Temperature and Ventilation

Most healthy people are comfortable with room temperatures between 68°F and 74°F. This range may be too hot or too cold for others. Persons who are older or ill may need higher temperatures for comfort. The CMS requires that nursing centers maintain a temperature of 71°F to 81°F.

Less active persons may not like cool areas. They need warm clothing and warm room temperatures.

Stale room air and lingering odors affect comfort and rest. Ventilation systems provide fresh air and move room air, causing drafts. Infants, older persons, and those who are ill are sensitive to drafts.

To protect patients and residents from cool areas and drafts:
- Have them wear enough of the correct clothing.
- Offer lap coverings (blankets, afghans, throws) to those in chairs and wheelchairs to cover the legs.
- Provide enough blankets for warmth.
- Cover them with bath blankets when giving care.
- Move them from drafty areas.

See *Focus on Children and Older Persons: Temperature and Ventilation.*

FOCUS ON CHILDREN AND OLDER PERSONS

Temperature and Ventilation

Older Persons
Poor circulation and loss of the skin's fatty tissue layer occur with aging. Therefore older persons are sensitive to cold (Chapter 12). They may wear extra clothing for warmth. Many wear sweaters or jackets in warm weather. Respect the person's wishes and choices.

Odors

Odors occur in health care settings and in home care. Bowel movements and urine have embarrassing odors. So do draining wounds and vomitus. Body, breath, and smoke odors may offend others.

Some people are very sensitive to odors. They may become nauseated. Good nursing care, ventilation, and housekeeping practices help prevent odors. To reduce odors:
- Empty, clean, and disinfect bedpans, urinals, commodes, and kidney basins promptly.
- Make sure toilets are flushed.
- Check incontinent persons often (Chapters 27 and 29).
- Clean persons who are wet or soiled from urine, feces (stools), vomitus, or wound drainage.
- Change wet or soiled linens and clothing promptly.
- Follow agency policy for where to place wet or soiled linens and clothing.
- Keep laundry containers closed.
- Dispose of incontinence and ostomy products promptly (Chapters 27 and 29).
- Provide good hygiene to prevent body and breath odors (Chapters 23 and 24).
- Use room deodorizers as needed and allowed by agency policy. Do not use sprays around persons with breathing problems. Ask the nurse if you are unsure.

Smoke odors present special problems. If you smoke, follow the agency's policy. Practice hand-washing after smoking, after handling smoking materials, and before giving care. Pay attention to your uniform, hair, and breath because of smoke odors.

Noise

According to the CMS, a "comfortable" sound level:
- Does not interfere with a person's hearing.
- Promotes privacy when privacy is desired.
- Allows the person to take part in social activities.

Common health care sounds can be disturbing. Examples include:
- Clanging and clattering equipment, dishes, and meal trays
- Loud voices, TVs, music, and so on
- Ringing phones
- Intercom systems and call lights
- Equipment or wheels needing repair or oil
- Cleaning and housekeeping equipment

People want to know the cause and meaning of new sounds. This relates to safety and security needs. Some sounds seem dangerous, frightening, or irritating. Patients and residents may become upset, anxious, and uncomfortable. What is noise to 1 person may not be noise to another. For example, some people enjoy loud music. It disturbs others.

Health care agencies are designed to reduce noise. Window and floor coverings absorb noise. Plastic items make less noise than metal equipment (bedpans, urinals, wash basins). To decrease noise levels:

- Control your voice.
- Handle equipment carefully.
- Keep equipment in good working order.
- Answer phones, call lights, and intercoms promptly.
  See *Focus on Communication: Noise.*
  See *Focus on Children and Older Persons: Noise.*
  See *Focus on Surveys: Noise.*

FOCUS ON **COMMUNICATION**

Noise

All staff must try to reduce noise. To reduce noise:

- Do not talk loudly in the hallways or nurses' station. Loud talking and laughter in hallways and at the nurses' station are common. Patients and residents may think that the staff are talking and laughing about them.
- Ask others to speak more softly if necessary. Ask politely.
- Avoid unnecessary conversation. Be professional. Do not discuss inappropriate topics at work. Others may overhear and become offended.

FOCUS ON **CHILDREN AND OLDER PERSONS**

Noise

Older Persons

Persons with dementia do not understand what is happening around them. Common, every-day sounds may disturb them. For example, a person may not understand the sound of a ringing phone. He or she may have an extreme reaction to the sound (Chapter 53). The reaction may be more severe at night. This is likely if the sound startles or suddenly awakens the person. A dark, strange room can make the problem worse.

FOCUS ON **SURVEYS**

Noise

Surveyors will observe for comfortable sound levels.

- Do background noises affect the person's ability to be heard or take part in activities?
- Do staff raise their voices to be heard?
- Are sound levels comfortable in the evening and during the night?
- Is the intercom volume too loud?
  Do your best to decrease noise and provide comfortable sound levels.

Lighting

Safe and comfortable lighting:

- Lessens glares.
- Lets the person control the brightness, location, and direction of light.
- Lets visually impaired persons maintain or increase independent functioning.

Glares, shadows, and dull lighting can cause falls, headaches, and eyestrain. A bright room is cheerful. Dim light is better for relaxing and rest.

Adjust window coverings and lighting to meet the person's needs. The over-bed and ceiling lights provide soft, medium, or bright lighting.

Persons with poor vision need bright light. This is very important at meal time and when moving about in the room and agency. Bright lighting also helps the staff perform procedures.

Always keep light controls within the person's reach. This protects the right to personal choice.

See *Focus on Children and Older Persons: Lighting.*

FOCUS ON **CHILDREN AND OLDER PERSONS**

Lighting

Older Persons

Persons with dementia may have agitated or aggressive behaviors at times. Lighting control can be helpful. Soft, non-glare lights are relaxing. Bright lighting lets the person see more clearly. This may improve orientation.

ROOM FURNITURE AND EQUIPMENT

Rooms are furnished and equipped for safety and to meet basic needs—comfort, sleep, elimination, nutrition, hygiene, and activity. There is equipment to communicate with staff, family, and friends. The right to privacy is considered.

The Bed

Beds have electrical or manual controls. Beds are raised to give care and to reduce bending and reaching. A low position lets the person get out of bed with ease (Fig. 21-2, p. 312). The head and foot of the bed are flat or raised varying degrees.

Electric beds are common. Controls are on a side panel, bed rail, or the foot-board (Fig. 21-3, *A*, p. 312). Some controls are hand-held devices (Fig. 21-3, *B*, p. 312). Patients and residents are taught to use the controls safely. They are warned not to raise the bed to the high position or to adjust the bed to harmful positions. They are told of position limits or restrictions.

Manual beds have cranks at the foot of the bed (Fig. 21-4, p. 312). Pull the cranks up for use. Keep them down at all other times. Cranks in the "up" position are safety hazards. Anyone walking past may bump into them.

See *Focus on Long-Term Care and Home Care: The Bed*, p. 313.

See *Promoting Safety and Comfort: The Bed*, p. 313.

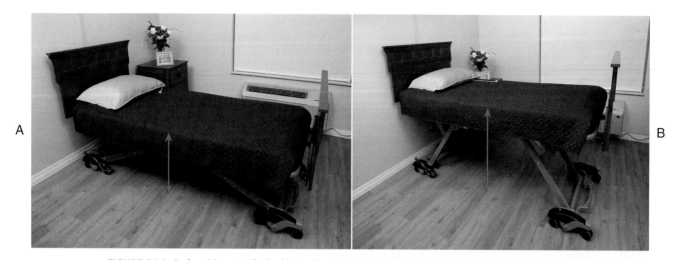

FIGURE 21-2 Bed positions. **A,** The bed is in a low horizontal position. **B,** The bed is in the highest horizontal position.

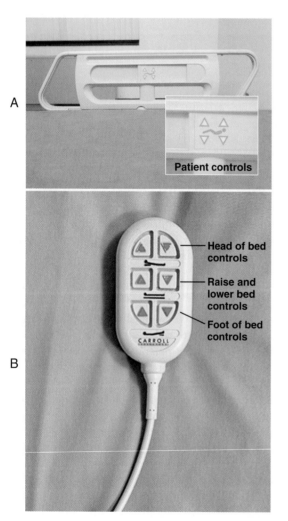

FIGURE 21-3 Electric bed controls. **A,** Electric bed controls on the bed rail. **B,** Hand-held bed control.

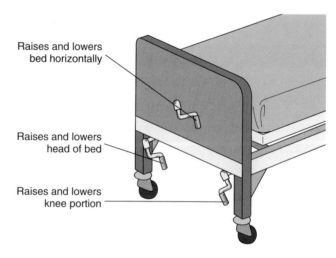

FIGURE 21-4 Manually operated bed.

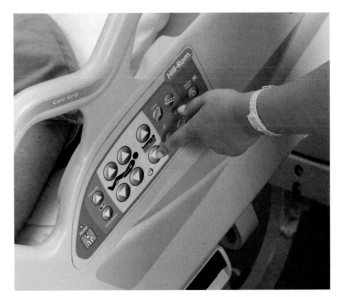

FIGURE 21-6 Controls for staff use are on the outer part of the rail. (Courtesy © Hill-Rom Services, Inc. Reprinted with permission. All rights reserved.)

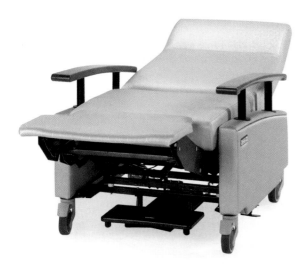

FIGURE 21-5 A medical (patient) recliner. (Courtesy © Hill-Rom Services, Inc. Reprinted with permission. All rights reserved.)

Bed Positions. There are 6 basic bed positions.

* *Flat* is a common sleeping position. The position is used for cervical traction and for some spinal cord surgeries and injuries (Chapter 48).
* *Fowler's position is a semi-sitting position. The head of the bed is raised between 45 and 60 degrees* (Fig. 21-7, p. 314). See Chapter 18.
* *High-Fowler's position is a semi-sitting position. The head of the bed is raised 60 to 90 degrees* (Fig. 21-8, p. 314).
* *Semi-Fowler's position means the head of the bed is raised 30 degrees* (Fig. 21-9, p. 314). Some agencies define semi-Fowler's position as when *the head of the bed is raised 30 degrees and the knee portion is raised 15 degrees.* This position is comfortable and prevents sliding down in bed. However, raising the knee portion can interfere with circulation in the legs. Know the definition used by your agency. Also check with the nurse before using semi-Fowler's position.
* *Trendelenburg's position means the head of the bed is lowered and the foot of the bed is raised* (Fig. 21-10, p. 314). A doctor orders the position. The bed frame is tilted. Or blocks are placed under the bed legs at the foot of the bed.
* *Reverse Trendelenburg's position means the head of the bed is raised and the foot of the bed is lowered* (Fig. 21-11, p. 314). A doctor orders this position. The bed frame is tilted. Or blocks are placed under the bed legs at the head of the bed.

See *Focus on Long-Term Care and Home Care: Bed Positions,* p. 314.

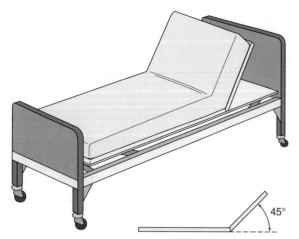

FIGURE 21-7 Fowler's position. In Fowler's position, the head of the bed is raised 45 to 60 degrees. The head of this bed is raised 45 degrees.

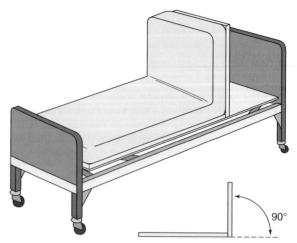

FIGURE 21-8 High-Fowler's position. In high-Fowler's position, the head of the bed is raised 60 to 90 degrees. The head of this bed is raised 90 degrees.

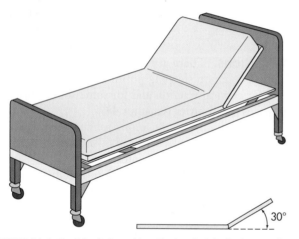

FIGURE 21-9 Semi-Fowler's position. The head of the bed is raised 30 degrees.

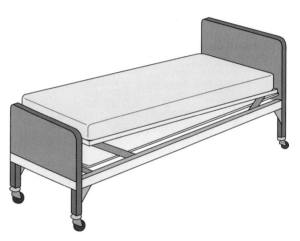

FIGURE 21-10 Trendelenburg's position. The head of the bed is lowered and the foot of the bed is raised.

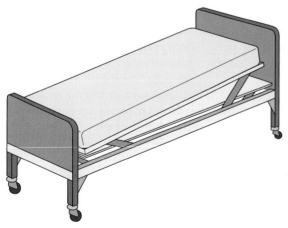

FIGURE 21-11 Reverse Trendelenburg's position. The head of the bed is raised and the foot of the bed is lowered.

FOCUS ON LONG-TERM CARE AND HOME CARE

Bed Positions

Home Care

Backrests are used with regular beds for Fowler's and semi-Fowler's positions (Fig. 21-12). Large, sturdy sofa pillows can be used. Check the head-board to make sure it is sturdy. It needs to provide support when the person leans against the backrest.

Bed Safety. Bed safety involves the *hospital bed system—the bed frame and its parts. The parts include the mattress, bed rails, head- and foot-boards, and bed attachments.*

Hospital bed systems have 7 entrapment zones (Fig. 21-13). ***Entrapment*** *means getting caught, trapped, or entangled in spaces created by the bed rails, the mattress, the bed frame, the head-board, or the foot-board.* Head, neck, or chest entrapment can cause serious injuries and death. Arm and leg entrapment also can occur. Persons at greatest risk:

- Are older.
- Are frail.
- Are confused or disoriented.
- Are restless.
- Have uncontrolled body movements.
- Have poor muscle control.
- Are small in size.
- Are restrained (Chapter 15).

Always check for entrapment. If a person is caught, trapped, or entangled in the bed or any of its parts, try to release the person. Also call for the nurse at once.

See *Focus on Children and Older Persons: Bed Safety,* p. 316.

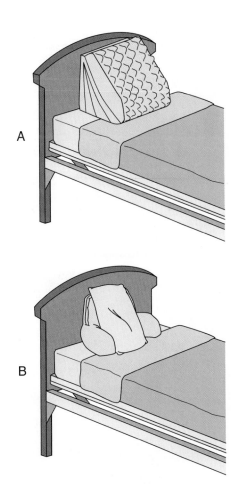

FIGURE 21-12 Backrests for regular beds. **A,** Wedge pillow. **B,** Study pillow (dorm pillow) with armrests. A pillow provides added support.

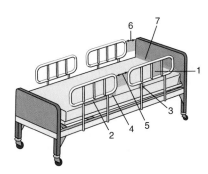

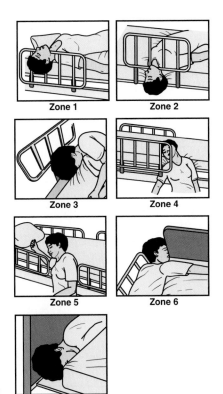

Zone 1: Within the rail

Zone 2: Between the top of the compressed mattress and the bottom of the rail, between the supports

Zone 3: Between the rail and the mattress

Zone 4: Between the top of the compressed mattress and the bottom of the rail, at the end of the rail

Zone 5: Between the split bed rails

Zone 6: Between the end of the rail and the side edge of the head-board or foot-board

Zone 7: Between the head-board or foot-board and the mattress end

FIGURE 21-13 Hospital bed system entrapment zones. (Redrawn from Food and Drug Administration: *Hospital bed system dimensional and assessment guidance to reduce entrapment,* March 10, 2006, content current as of August 23, 2018.)

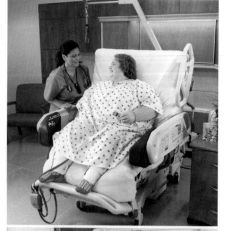

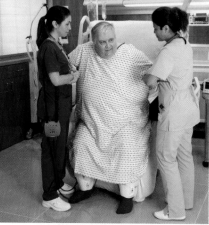

Bariatric Beds. Bariatric beds may have these and other features.

- A wide frame with a weight capacity from 500 to 1000 pounds. Some frames adjust for the person's height. For example, the bed length is shortened so the person's feet touch the foot-board. The person does not slide down in bed. Or the frame is made longer for a taller person.
- A chair position. The bed can become a chair without moving the person (Fig. 21-14, *A*). The foot-board becomes a footrest.
- Front and side egress positions. *Egress* means to *go out* or *leave*. Moving the foot-board out of the way allows a lying to sitting to standing position (Fig. 21-14, *B*). Or the person can get out of bed on the side.
- Power transport to move the bed. The person is not transferred to a stretcher for transport to other areas.
- A pressure-relief surface to prevent pressure injuries. The surface allows turning the person for care measures.
- A trapeze for the person to re-position himself or herself.
- A built-in scale.

  Bariatric beds vary depending on the model. Follow the manufacturer's instructions for safe use.

  See *Focus on Communication: Bariatric Beds.*

FIGURE 21-14 A, Bariatric bed converted to a chair. **B,** The bariatric bed allows the person to get out of bed from the chair position. (Courtesy © Hill-Rom Services, Inc. Reprinted with permission. All rights reserved.)

FOCUS ON **COMMUNICATION**

Bariatric Beds

Many persons who are obese are often disrespected. They have been insulted and judged by others. Low self-esteem and emotional problems can result. Such persons may be sensitive to comments about their weight or size.

Consider if a comment may offend the person. For example, do not say: "The nurse is getting a bed big enough for you." Instead, you can say: "The nurse is getting a bed that will be comfortable for you."

Be aware of your verbal and nonverbal communication. Your words and actions must show dignity and respect.

The Over-Bed Table

The over-bed table (Fig. 21-15) is moved over the bed by sliding the base under the bed. The table is raised or lowered for bed or chair use. Use the handle, crank, or lever to adjust table height. Some over-bed tables have a vanity area with a mirror and storage for beauty, hair care, shaving, or other personal items.

The person uses the over-bed table for meals, writing, reading, and other activities. The nursing team uses the over-bed table as a work area. Place only clean and sterile items on the table. Never place bedpans, urinals, or soiled linens on the over-bed table. Clean the table after use as a work surface. Also clean it before serving meal trays and after removing them.

The Bedside Stand

By the bed, the bedside stand is used for personal items and personal care equipment. It has a top drawer and a lower cabinet with shelves or drawers (Fig. 21-16).

- Stand top—used for tissues, clock, photos, phone, flowers, cards, and so on.
- Top drawer—used for eyeglass case, books, kidney basin (shaped like a kidney) with oral hygiene items.
- Middle drawer or shelf—stores the wash basin with personal care items (soap, lotion, washcloth and towels, and so on).
- Bottom drawer or lower shelf—stores the bedpan, urinal, and toilet paper.

Place only clean and sterile items on the bedside stand. Never place bedpans, urinals, or soiled linens on the top. Clean the bedside stand after use as a work surface.

Chairs

The person's unit has at least 1 chair (see Fig. 21-1). It must be comfortable, sturdy, and not move or tip during transfers. The person should be able to get in and out of the chair with ease. It should not be too low or too soft. Bariatric chairs are wider and have expanded capacity. Nursing center residents may bring chairs from home.

Privacy Curtains

The privacy curtain (see Fig. 21-1) can be pulled around the bed to provide privacy. *Always pull the curtain completely around the bed before giving care.*

Privacy curtains do not block sounds or voices. Others in the room can hear sounds or talking behind the curtain.

See *Focus on Long-Term Care and Home Care: Privacy Curtains.*

FOCUS ON LONG-TERM CARE AND HOME CARE

Privacy Curtains

Long-Term Care
According to the CMS, each person has the right to full visual privacy. *Full visual privacy is having the means to be completely free from public view while in bed.* The privacy curtain helps provide full visual privacy.

Home Care
Portable screens or room dividers help provide privacy in the home setting (Fig. 21-17, p. 318). Decorator styles provide color and are pleasant to look at.

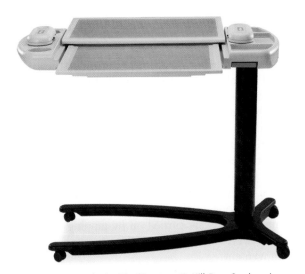

FIGURE 21-15 Over-bed table. (Courtesy © Hill-Rom Services, Inc. Reprinted with permission. All rights reserved.)

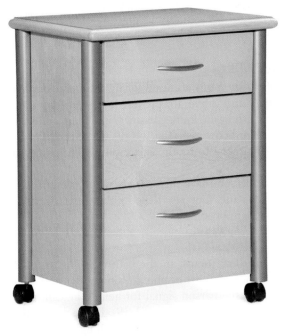

FIGURE 21-16 A bedside stand. (Courtesy © Hill-Rom Services, Inc. Reprinted with permission. All rights reserved.)

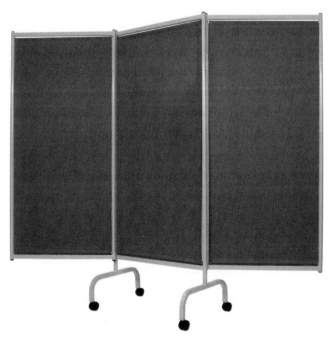

FIGURE 21-17 A portable screen provides privacy in the home. (Copyright Medicus Health.)

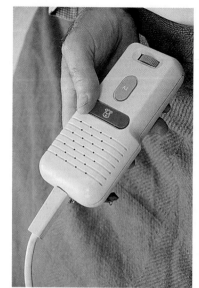

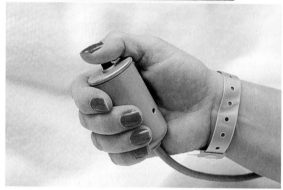

FIGURE 21-19 The call light. The call light button is pressed when help is needed. (NOTE: There are different types of call lights.)

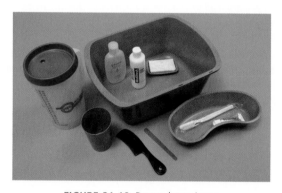

FIGURE 21-18 Personal care items.

Personal Care Items

Personal care items are used for hygiene and elimination. A bedpan and urinal are provided. The agency also provides a wash basin, kidney basin, water mug, and soap and soap dish or body wash (Fig. 21-18). Some provide powder, lotion, toothbrush, toothpaste, mouthwash, tissues, and a comb.

Some persons have their own oral and personal hygiene equipment and supplies. Respect the person's choices in personal care products.

The Call System

When in their rooms, in the bathroom, or in a bathing area, the person must be able to contact the staff. The call system lets the person signal for help. The call light is at the end of a long cord (Fig. 21-19). It attaches to the bed or chair with a clip. (See p. 320 for call lights in bathrooms and shower and tub rooms.) *Always keep the call light within the person's reach—in the room, bathroom, and shower or tub room.*

To get help, the person presses a button on the call light device. The call light connects to a light above the room door (Fig. 21-20). The call light also connects to a computer, light panel, or intercom system at the nurses' station. These tell the staff that the person needs help.

An intercom system lets the staff talk with the person from the nurses' station. The person states what is needed. Hard of hearing persons may have problems using an intercom. Remember confidentiality. When using an intercom, persons nearby can over-hear what is said.

Some call lights are turned on by tapping with a hand or fist (Fig. 21-21). They are useful for persons with limited hand movement.

Some people cannot use call lights. Examples are persons who are confused or in a coma. The care plan lists special communication measures. Check these persons often. Make sure their needs are met.

See *Focus on Communication: The Call System.*

See *Focus on Long-Term Care and Home Care: The Call System.*

See *Teamwork and Time Management: The Call System.*

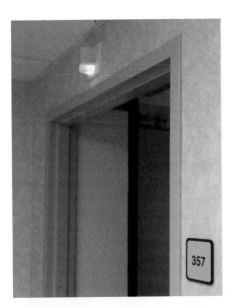

FIGURE 21-20 Light above the room door.

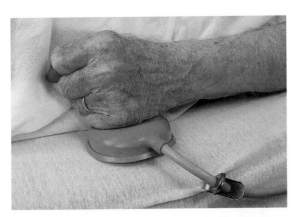

FIGURE 21-21 Call light for a person with limited hand movement.

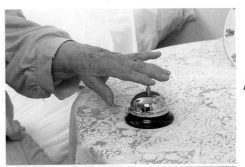

A

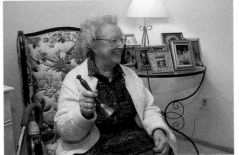

B

FIGURE 21-22 **A**, Tap bell. **B**, Dinner bell.

FOCUS ON LONG-TERM CARE AND HOME CARE

The Call System

Home Care

Some home care patients stay in bed or in a certain part of the home. They need a way to call for help. Tap bells, dinner bells, baby monitors, and other devices are useful (Fig. 21-22). Or you can give the person a small can with a few coins inside. Children's toys with bells, horns, and whistles may be useful.

FOCUS ON COMMUNICATION

The Call System

You will answer call lights for patients and residents not assigned to you. To promote quality of life and safe care, you can say:

- "My name is Chris Hines. I'm a nursing assistant. How can I help you?"
- "I need to check your care plan before bringing you more salt. I'll be right back. Is there anything else I can do before I leave?"
- "I can take your meal tray. I'll tell your nursing assistant what you ate."
- "Do you use the bathroom or the bedpan?"

Sometimes patients and residents signal for help often. Do not delay in meeting their needs. Never take call lights away from them. This is not safe. Avoid statements that make a person feel like a burden. For example, do not say:

- "I just helped you to the bathroom. Can't you wait?"
- "I was just in your room. What do you want now?"

Do not discourage the person from asking for help. The person may try to do something alone. This could cause injury. Tell the nurse. Your co-workers can help you meet the person's needs.

TEAMWORK AND TIME MANAGEMENT

The Call System

A person may use a call light for help when you are with another person. The same may happen to other staff. If staff answer call lights for each other, lights are answered promptly. Patients and residents receive quality care. Everyone is responsible for answering call lights even if not assigned to the person.

Call System Safety. The phrase "call light" refers to the call system. You must:

- Keep the call light within the person's reach. Even if the person cannot use the call light, keep it within reach for use by visitors and staff. They may need to call for help.
- Place the call light on the person's strong side.
- Remind the person to signal when help is needed.
- Answer call lights promptly. For example, the person may have an urgent elimination need. Prompt bathroom use prevents embarrassing problems. You also help prevent infection, skin breakdown, pressure injuries, and falls.
- Answer bathroom and shower or tub room call lights at once.

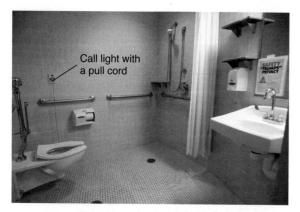

FIGURE 21-23 Bathroom in a person's room.

Call light with a pull cord

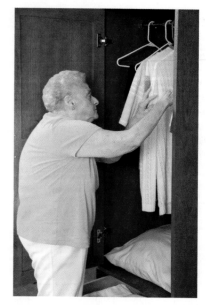

FIGURE 21-24 The resident can reach items in her closet.

The Bathroom

A toilet, sink, call system, and mirror are standard equipment in bathrooms (Fig. 21-23). Some bathrooms have showers.

Grab bars (safety bars) are by the toilet for getting on and off the toilet. Some bathrooms have higher toilets or raised toilet seats. They make wheelchair transfers easier and are helpful for persons with joint problems.

Towel racks, toilet paper, soap, paper towel dispenser, and a wastebasket are in the bathroom. They are within the person's reach.

The call light is a button or pull cord next to the toilet. The bathroom call light flashes red above the room door and at the nurses' station. To alert staff of bathroom use, the sound at the nurses' station is different from room call lights. Someone must respond at once when a person needs help in the bathroom.

Closet and Drawer Space

Closet and drawer space are provided (see Fig. 21-1). The CMS requires that nursing centers provide each person with closet space with shelves and a clothes rack (Fig. 21-24). The person must be able to reach and have free access to the closet and its contents.

Sometimes people hoard things—drugs, napkins, straws, food, sugar, salt, pepper, and so on. Hoarding causes safety and health risks (Chapter 13). The staff can inspect a person's closet or drawers if hoarding is suspected. The person is told of the inspection. He or she is present when it takes place.

See *Promoting Safety and Comfort: Closet and Drawer Space.*

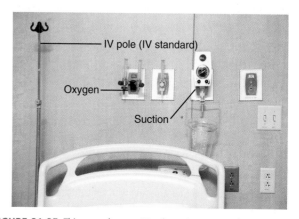

FIGURE 21-25 This room has an IV pole and oxygen and suction outlets.

IV pole (IV standard)

Oxygen

Suction

Other Equipment

Many agencies furnish rooms with a TV, radio, and clock for comfort and relaxation. Rooms may have phones, a computer, and Internet access.

Blood pressure equipment may be mounted on walls. There also are wall outlets for oxygen and suction (Fig. 21-25). Oxygen equipment and portable suction equipment are common in nursing centers and home care settings. For intravenous (IV) infusions, an IV pole (IV standard) is used to hang IV bags or feeding bags (Chapter 32).

PROMOTING SAFETY AND COMFORT

Closet and Drawer Space

Safety

The person's property is in closets and drawers. You need the person's permission to open or search such spaces.

The nurse may ask you to inspect a person's closet, drawers, or personal items. If so, the person must be present. Also have a co-worker with you as a witness. This protects you if the person claims that something was stolen or damaged.

FOCUS ON **PRIDE**

The Person, Family, and Yourself

Personal and Professional Responsibility

Reducing noise requires cooperation from all staff. It is not your responsibility alone. But you can help. Do your part to reduce noise. Politely remind others to speak softly if needed. Take pride in providing patients and residents with a quiet and comfortable setting.

Rights and Respect

Some nursing center residents bring personal items from home. Photos, TVs, radios, books, religious items, and plants are examples. A chair, footstool, lamp, and small table are often allowed.

Allow personal choice when arranging items. Make sure the person's choices:
- Are safe.
- Will not cause falls or other accidents.
- Do not interfere with the rights of others.

The center is the person's home. A home-like setting is important for quality of life.

Independence and Social Interaction

People want to be independent. Often accidents and injuries occur when the person tries to get needed items. The person has to reach too far and falls. Or he or she tries to get up without help.

To promote independence and safety:
- Keep needed personal items within reach.
- Place adaptive (assistive) devices nearby. Walkers and canes are examples.
- Place the call light within the person's reach. Answer call lights and tend to the person's needs promptly.

Delegation and Teamwork

Some nursing units check on the person at regular times. For example, every hour staff ask about needs, positioning, comfort, and needed personal items. Needs are met and the person is reminded that staff will return in 1 hour. Nursing staff sign a form each time. The person uses the call light for urgent needs.

If your unit uses this practice:
- Be prompt. Check on the person at the correct time.
- Be honest. Do not sign the form if you did not check on the person. Also, do not sign the form early.
- Have a good attitude. Do not complain. Reasons for the practice may be to improve care, decrease call light use, or help nurses with time management.

Ethics and Laws

This chapter focused on how the person's setting affects comfort and well-being. You are a part of that setting. You must help the person feel safe, secure, and comfortable. The following is an example of a nursing assistant who failed to do so.

A certified nursing assistant (CNA) worked at a nursing home in Arizona. In February 2002, she was counseled about her poor attendance and negative outbursts. In August 2002, it was noted that she gave poor care.
- *Residents were not turned and/or briefs were not changed every 2 hours according to facility policy.*
- *She continued to have negative outbursts.*

Ethics and Laws—cont'd

Later, it was reported to the Arizona State Board of Nursing that she abused a resident by failure to provide care and not meet his needs.
- *The resident was described as alert, paralyzed, on a ventilator for chronic respiratory failure, and totally dependent for all needs.*
- *The CNA was in his room many times during the night. She did not provide the care he requested.*
- *The CNA placed his call light out of reach. He used his head to use the call light for assistance.*

In November 2003, the CNA was terminated for resident abuse. The CNA was hired by another agency in December 2003. She worked there until March 2004. On March 17 she was counseled for:
- *Telling a resident that if she did not speak English she should back go to her country*
- *Being rough, rude, and verbally abusive to residents*
- *Refusing to work on a nursing unit "because all patients stink"*
- *Being critical and judgmental with new staff*
- *Leaving a resident to "pee in their britches" rather than helping him to the bathroom*

Her employment was terminated on March 19, 2004.

In January 2004, the Arizona State Board of Nursing sent the CNA a questionnaire. It was returned to the Board as undeliverable. The CNA failed to notify the Board of an address change within the 30 days required by law.

The Board revoked the CNA's certificate for unprofessional conduct. She violated the following aspects of the state's Nurse Practice Act.
- *Conduct or practice that is or might be harmful or dangerous to the health of a patient or the public*
- *Failing to follow an employer's policies and procedures designed to safeguard the client*
- *Failing to respect client rights and dignity*
- *Neglecting or abusing a client physically, verbally, or financially*
- *Practice in any other manner that gives the Board reasonable cause to believe that the health of a client or the public may be harmed*
- *Failing to notify the Board in writing within 30 days of any address change*

(Arizona State Board of Nursing, 2006.)

Always provide care in a way that promotes the person's comfort, safety, and quality of life. Bad conduct reduces quality of care and can result in job loss and loss of certification (license, registration).

FOCUS ON **PRIDE**: *Application*

What makes your living space comfortable and personal? How would this change if you lived in a nursing center? What would change in a hospital setting? Why is it important to provide privacy, safety, and comfort to persons in health care settings?

REVIEW QUESTIONS

Circle T if the statement is TRUE or F if it is FALSE.

1 T F The person's unit is considered private.

2 T F You should explain the cause of strange noises.

3 T F You can adjust the person's room temperature for your comfort.

4 T F Persons with dementia may have extreme reactions to strange sounds.

5 T F The privacy curtain prevents others from hearing conversations.

6 T F Soft, dim lighting is relaxing.

7 T F The call light is placed on the person's strong side.

8 T F The over-bed table and bedside stand should be within the person's reach.

9 T F You can look through a person's closet and drawers.

10 T F The person must be able to reach items in the closet.

Circle the BEST answer.

11 To maintain the person's unit
   a Throw away items that do not look important
   b Remove cards from the bedside stand
   c Place personal items as you choose
   d Straighten bed linens as needed

12 Which temperature range is required by the CMS?
   a 61°F to 68°F
   b 68°F to 74°F
   c 71°F to 81°F
   d 76°F to 82°F

13 To protect a person from drafts
   a Adjust the room temperature to 70°F
   b Provide a bath blanket during a bed bath
   c Dress the person in light-weight clothing
   d Position the person near a fan

14 To prevent odors
   a Place flowers in the room
   b Empty commodes at the end of your shift
   c Keep laundry containers open
   d Clean persons who are wet or soiled

15 To control noise
   a Answer phones after the third ring
   b Use the intercom system when possible
   c Handle equipment carefully
   d Talk with others in the hallway

16 Beds are raised horizontally to
   a Prevent bending and reaching when giving care
   b Promote the person's comfort
   c Raise the head of the bed
   d Lock the bed in position

17 The head of the bed is raised 30 degrees. This is called
   a Fowler's position
   b Semi-Fowler's position
   c Trendelenburg's position
   d Reverse Trendelenburg's position

18 Bed safety involves
   a Monitoring older and confused persons closely for entrapment
   b Removing the entrapment zones from the bed
   c Leaving the bed in the raised position
   d Restraining persons at risk for entrapment

19 Which statement about hospital bed system entrapment is *true*?
   a Bed rails present the only risk for entrapment.
   b Serious injury and death can occur.
   c A person must be small in size for entrapment to occur.
   d There are 3 entrapment zones.

20 The over-bed table is *not* used
   a For eating
   b As a working surface
   c For the urinal
   d To store shaving items

21 The bedpan is stored
   a In the closet
   b In the bedside stand
   c On the over-bed table
   d Under the bed

22 Call lights are answered
   a When you have time
   b At the end of your shift
   c Promptly
   d When you are near the person's room

Answers to Chapter 21 questions are on p. 886.

FOCUS ON **PRACTICE**

Problem Solving

Since your shift began, an hour ago, a resident has called for help 10 times. You just left the room and are helping another resident. The call light is used again. What do you do?

   The resident uses the call light more often at night, after family visits, and when not checked on regularly. How might this information be helpful for the nurse in care planning?

Bedmaking

- Define the key terms and key abbreviation in this chapter.
- Describe open, closed, occupied, and surgical beds.
- Explain when to change bed linens.
- Explain how to use drawsheets.
- Handle linens following the rules of medical asepsis.
- Perform the procedures described in this chapter.
- Explain how to promote PRIDE in the person, the family, and yourself.

KEY TERMS

cotton drawsheet A drawsheet made of cotton; it helps keep the mattress and bottom linens clean

drawsheet A small sheet placed over the middle of the bottom sheet

padded waterproof drawsheet A drawsheet made of an absorbent top and waterproof bottom used to protect the mattress and bottom linens from dampness and soiling

KEY ABBREVIATION

ID   Identification

Beds are made every day. Clean, dry, and wrinkle-free beds:

- Promote comfort.
- Prevent skin breakdown.
- Prevent pressure injuries (Chapter 41).

Beds are usually made in the morning after baths. Or they are made while the person is in the shower, up in the chair, or out of the room. To keep beds neat and clean:

- Change linens when they are wet, soiled, or damp.
- Straighten linens when loose or wrinkled and at bedtime.
- Check for and remove food and crumbs after meals and snacks.
- Check linens for dentures, eyeglasses, hearing aids, sharp objects, and other items.
- Follow Standard Precautions and the Bloodborne Pathogen Standard. Contact with blood, body fluids, secretions, or excretions is likely.

TYPES OF BEDS

Beds are made in these ways.

- A *closed bed* is not in use. Top linens are not folded back (Fig. 22-1, p. 324). The bed is ready for a new patient or resident. In nursing centers, closed beds are made for residents who are up during the day.
- An *open bed* is ready for use. Top linens are fan-folded to the foot of the bed so the person can get into bed. A closed bed becomes an open bed by fan-folding back the top linens (Fig. 22-2, p. 324).
- An *occupied bed* is made with the person in it (Fig. 22-3, p. 324).
- A *surgical bed* is made to transfer a person from a stretcher to bed (Fig. 22-4, p. 324). This includes an ambulance stretcher.

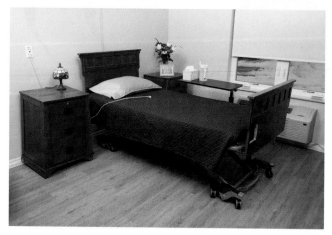

FIGURE 22-1 Closed bed.

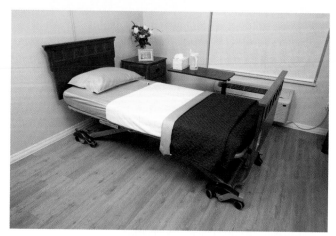

FIGURE 22-2 Open bed. Top linens are fan-folded to the foot of the bed.

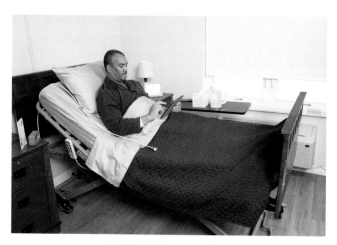

FIGURE 22-3 Occupied bed.

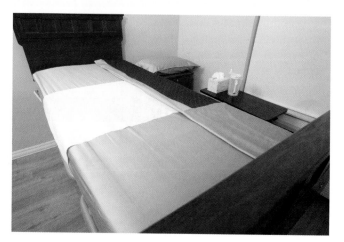

FIGURE 22-4 Surgical bed.

LINENS

When handling linens and making beds, practice medical asepsis. Your uniform is considered *dirty*. Always hold linens away from your body and uniform. Never shake linens. Shaking them spreads microbes. Place clean linens on a clean surface. Never put clean or used linens on the floor.

Collect needed linens. If the person has 2 pillows, get 2 pillowcases. The person may need extra blankets for warmth. Do not collect unneeded linens. Once in the person's room, extra linens are considered contaminated. You cannot use them for another person.

Collect linens in the order of use. That way you avoid fumbling with linens for the piece you need. Linens stay neat and clean in your stack. Bed linens are used in the following order.

- Mattress pad (if needed)
- Bottom sheet (flat or fitted)
- Cotton or padded waterproof drawsheet (if needed)
- Waterproof under-pad (if needed)
- Top sheet
- Blanket
- Bedspread
- Pillowcase(s)

When collecting linens for bedmaking, it is common to collect linens for personal hygiene. You may need to collect:

- Bath towel(s)
- Hand towel(s)
- Washcloth(s)
- Gown or pajamas
- Bath blanket

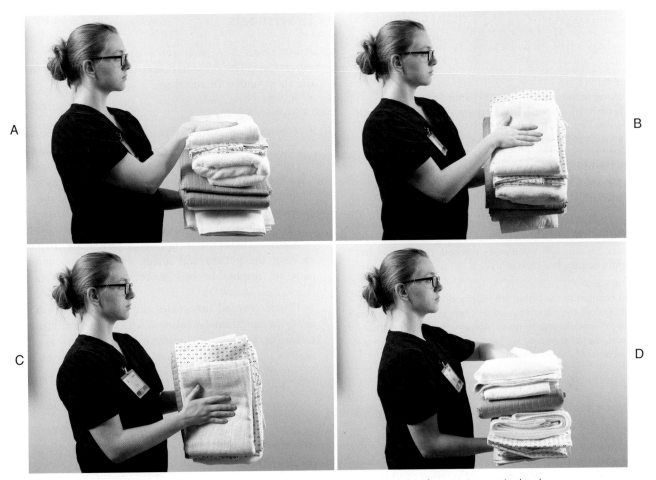

FIGURE 22-5 Collecting linens. Linens are held away from the body and uniform. **A,** One arm is placed over the top of the stack of linens. **B, C, and D,** The stack of linens is turned onto the other arm.

Use 1 arm to hold the linens. Use your other hand to pick them up. The first item to use is at the bottom of the stack. To get it on top, place your arm over the stack. Then turn the stack over onto the other arm (Fig. 22-5). The first item to use is now on top. Place the clean linens on a clean surface.

Remove used linens 1 piece at a time. Roll each piece away from you (Fig. 22-6). Roll linens so the soiled side is inside the roll and away from you. Discard each piece into a laundry bag.

In hospitals, top and bottom sheets, the drawsheet, the waterproof under-pad (if used), and pillowcases are usually changed daily. If still clean, the mattress pad, blanket, and bedspread are re-used for the same person.

Linens are not re-used if soiled, wet, or wrinkled. Change wet, damp, or soiled linens right away. Wear gloves and follow Standard Precautions and the Blood-borne Pathogen Standard.

See *Focus on Long-Term Care and Home Care: Linens*, p. 326.

See *Focus on Surveys: Linens*, p. 326.

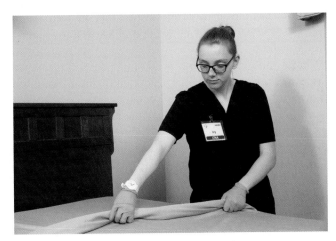

FIGURE 22-6 Roll used linens away from you.

Linens

Long-Term Care

In nursing centers, linens are not changed every day. A complete linen change is usually done on the person's bath or shower day. This may be 1 or 2 times a week. Linens are always changed if wet, damp, soiled, or very wrinkled.

Some residents bring linens from home. Use them to make the bed. The person's property, the linens must be labeled with the person's name. This prevents loss or confusion with another person's property.

Some centers have colored or printed linens. Let the person choose what color to use. Also let him or her decide how many pillows or blankets to use. If possible, the person chooses the time when you make the bed. The resident has the right to personal choice.

Home Care

Linen changes in the home are usually done 1 or 2 times a week. Follow the person's routine. Change linens more often if the person asks you to do so. Always change linens that are wet, damp, soiled, or very wrinkled. Contact the nurse if the person refuses a linen change.

Linens

Linens may contain microbes and blood, body fluids, secretions, or excretions. You must help prevent and control the spread of infection. Surveyors will observe:
- How you transport linens.
- If you practice hand hygiene after handling soiled or used linens.
- If you double-bag linens (Chapter 17) when the outside of the laundry bag is visibly contaminated or wet.
- If you bag contaminated linens where they are used. The person's room and the shower room are examples.

Drawsheets

A *drawsheet is a small sheet placed over the middle of the bottom sheet.* The drawsheet may have tuck tails for tucking the sheet under the mattress.
- A *cotton drawsheet is made of cotton. It helps keep the mattress and bottom linens clean* (Fig. 22-7, *A*).
- A *padded waterproof drawsheet is a drawsheet made of an absorbent top and waterproof bottom* (Fig. 22-7, *B*). *It protects the mattress and bottom linens from dampness and soiling.* The waterproof side is placed down, away from the person. The absorbent top is up, toward the person. Disposable waterproof drawsheets are discarded when wet, soiled, or wrinkled.

Many agencies use incontinence products (Chapter 27) to keep the person and linens dry. Waterproof under-pads or disposable bed protectors also are common (Fig. 22-7, *C and D*).

Plastic-covered mattresses can cause discomfort from heavy perspiration (sweating). A drawsheet reduces heat retention and absorbs moisture. Drawsheets are often used as assist devices to move and transfer persons in bed (Chapters 19 and 20). If used as an assist device, do not tuck the drawsheet in at the sides.

See *Focus on Long-Term Care and Home Care: Drawsheets.*

Drawsheets

Home Care

A flat sheet folded in half can serve as a cotton drawsheet. A twin-sized sheet is easier to use for this purpose. The nurse tells you what to use.

Medical supply stores and many drugstores sell waterproof drawsheets and waterproof under-pads. The nurse discusses the need for these items with the person and family.

Plastic mattress protectors do not protect bottom linens (cotton drawsheet, bottom sheet, and mattress pad). Some home care patients and families place plastic under the drawsheet. If so, tell the nurse. The nurse can assess what is safe for the person.

Do not use plastic trash bags or dry-cleaning bags. They are not strong enough to protect the linens and mattress. They slide easily and move out of place. Suffocation is a risk if the bag covers the person's nose and mouth.

MAKING BEDS

Safety and medical asepsis are important for bedmaking. Follow the rules in Box 22-1.

See *Focus on Long-Term Care and Home Care: Making Beds.*

See *Teamwork and Time Management: Making Beds,* p. 328.

See *Delegation Guidelines: Making Beds,* p. 328.

See *Promoting Safety and Comfort: Making Beds,* p. 328.

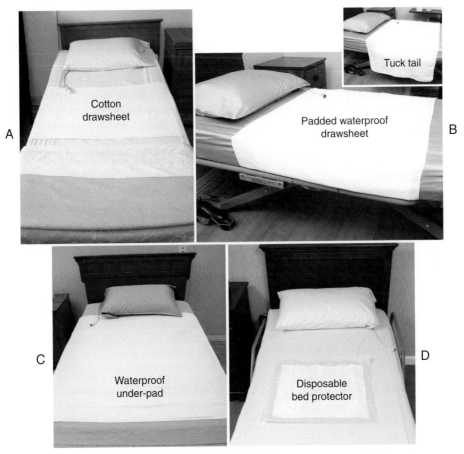

FIGURE 22-7 A, Cotton drawsheet. **B**, Padded waterproof drawsheet. **C**, Waterproof under-pad. **D**, Disposable bed protector.

BOX 22-1	**Rules for Bedmaking**

- Use good body mechanics at all times (Chapter 18).
- Follow the rules in Chapters 19 and 20 to safely move and transfer the person.
- Follow Standard Precautions and the Bloodborne Pathogen Standard.
- Practice hand hygiene before handling clean linens.
- Bring only needed linens to the person's room. You cannot use extra linens for another person. Extra linens are considered contaminated. Put them with the used laundry.
- Place clean linens on a clean surface. Use the bedside chair, over-bed table, or bedside stand. Place a clean barrier (towel, paper towel, disposable bed protector) between the clean surface and the linens if required by agency policy.
- Do not use torn or frayed linens.
- Never shake linens. Shaking spreads microbes.
- Hold linens away from your body and uniform. Do not let used or clean linens touch your uniform.
- Never put used linens on the floor or on clean linens. Follow agency policy for used linens.
- Bag used linens in the room where they are used. Use *BIOHAZARD* labels as needed (Chapter 17). Do not carry used linens un-bagged outside of the person's room.
- Keep bottom linens tucked in and wrinkle-free.
- Straighten and tighten loose sheets, blankets, and bedspreads as needed.
- Make as much of 1 side of the bed as possible before going to the other side. This saves time and energy.
- Change wet, damp, or soiled linens right away.

FOCUS ON **LONG-TERM CARE AND HOME CARE**

Making Beds

Home Care

Some home care patients have hospital beds. Others have twin-, regular-, queen-, and king-sized beds. Water beds, sofa sleepers, cots, and recliners are common. Make the bed (or sleeping surface) as the person wishes. Follow the rules in Box 22-1. If the person's wishes are not safe, tell the nurse.

You may have laundry responsibilities. Wash linens when soiling is fresh to help prevent staining. Urine, feces (stools), vomit, and blood can stain linens. Follow these guidelines.

- Wear gloves. Linens may contain blood, body fluids, secretions, or excretions.
- Rinse the item in cold water to remove the substance.
- Treat the stain. The person may use a stain-removing agent. Read and follow the manufacturer's instructions. Or follow the nurse's directions.
- Wash and dry linens as the person prefers.

TEAMWORK AND TIME MANAGEMENT

Making Beds

Making beds with a co-worker is faster, easier, and safer for patients, residents, you, and your co-worker. Make 1 side of the bed while your co-worker makes the other. Always thank your co-worker for helping you. Also help your co-worker make beds when asked to do so.

DELEGATION GUIDELINES

Making Beds

Bedmaking is a routine nursing task. Before making a bed, you need this information from the nurse and the care plan.

- What bed to make—closed, open, occupied, or surgical.
- If a cotton drawsheet, padded waterproof drawsheet, waterproof under-pad, or incontinence product is needed.
- If the person uses bed rails.
- The person's treatment, therapy, and activity schedules. For example, change a person's linens after a treatment. Or make a person's bed while he or she is in physical therapy.
- Position restrictions or the person's movement or activity limits.
- How to position the person and the positioning devices needed.
- If the bed needs to be locked into a certain position (Chapter 21).
- When to report observations.
- What patient or resident concerns to report at once.

PROMOTING SAFETY AND COMFORT

Making Beds

Safety

You need to raise the bed for body mechanics. The bed also is as flat as possible. Return the bed to the correct position when you are done. Lock the bed in position if ordered.

Bed wheels are locked (braked) during bedmaking. You may need to move the bed to avoid reaching. Unlock the wheels (release the brakes) to move the bed. Then lock (brake) the wheels.

Wear gloves to remove linens from the bed. Also follow other aspects of Standard Precautions and the Bloodborne Pathogen Standard. Linens may contain blood, body fluids, secretions, or excretions.

After making a bed, lower the bed to the correct level for the person. Follow the care plan. Raise or lower bed rails according to the care plan.

Comfort

For an occupied bed, cover the person with a bath blanket before removing the top sheet. Do not leave the person uncovered. The bath blanket provides warmth and privacy.

Adjust the pillow as needed during the procedure. After the procedure, position the person as directed by the nurse and the care plan. Always make sure linens are dry, straight, and wrinkle-free.

The Closed Bed

Closed beds are made for:

- Nursing center residents and home care patients who are up for most or all of the day. Top linens are folded back at bedtime. Clean linens are used as needed.
- New patients and residents. The bed is made after the bed system (Chapter 21) is cleaned and disinfected. Clean linens are needed for the entire bed.
  See procedure: *Making a Closed Bed.*

Text continued on p. 332.

Making a Closed Bed

QUALITY OF LIFE

- Knock before entering the person's room.
- Address the person by name.
- Introduce yourself by name and title.

- Explain the procedure before starting and during the procedure.
- Protect the person's rights during the procedure.
- Handle the person gently during the procedure.

PRE-PROCEDURE

1. Follow *Delegation Guidelines: Making Beds.* See *Promoting Safety and Comfort: Making Beds.*
2. Practice hand hygiene.
3. Collect clean linens.
   - Mattress pad (if needed)
   - Bottom sheet (flat sheet or fitted sheet)
   - Cotton drawsheet or padded waterproof drawsheet (if needed)
   - Waterproof under-pad (if needed)
   - Top sheet
   - Blanket
   - Bedspread
   - A pillowcase for each pillow

   - Bath towel
   - Hand towel
   - Washcloth
   - Gown or pajamas
   - Bath blanket
   - Gloves
   - Laundry bag
   - Towel, paper towels, or disposable bed protector (as a barrier for clean linens)

4. Place linens on a clean surface. First place the barrier between the clean surface and clean linens if required by agency policy.
5. Raise the bed for body mechanics. Bed rails are down.

Making a Closed Bed—cont'd

PROCEDURE

6 Put on the gloves.
7 Remove linens. Roll each piece away from you. Place each piece in a laundry bag. (NOTE: Discard the incontinence product, disposable bed protector, and disposable drawsheet in the trash. Do not put them in the laundry bag.)
8 Clean the bed frame and mattress (if this is your job).
9 Remove and discard the gloves. Practice hand hygiene.
10 Move the mattress to the head of the bed.
11 Put the mattress pad on the mattress. It is even with the top of the mattress.
12 Place the bottom sheet on the mattress pad (Fig. 22-8, p. 330). Unfold it length-wise. Place the center crease in the middle of the bed. For a flat sheet:
    a Place the lower edge even with the bottom of the mattress.
    b Place the large hem at the top and the small hem at the bottom.
    c Face hem-stitching downward, away from the person.
13 Open the sheet. Fan-fold it to the other side of the bed (Fig. 22-9, p. 330).
14 Tuck the corners of a fitted sheet over the mattress at the top and then foot of the bed. For a flat sheet, tuck the top of the sheet under the mattress. The sheet is tight and smooth.
15 Make a mitered corner at the top if using a flat sheet (Fig. 22-10, p. 330).
16 Place the cotton drawsheet or padded waterproof drawsheet on the bed. It is in the middle of the mattress.
    a Open and fan-fold the drawsheet to the other side of the bed.
    b Tuck the drawsheet under the mattress.
17 Go to the other side of the bed.
18 Miter the top corner of the flat bottom sheet.
19 Pull the bottom sheet tight so there are no wrinkles. Tuck in the sheet.
20 Pull the drawsheet tight so there are no wrinkles. (Fig. 22-11, p. 331).
21 *If using a waterproof under-pad,* place the waterproof under-pad on the bed. It is in the middle of the mattress. See Figure 22-7, C.
22 Go to the other side of the bed.

23 Put the top sheet on the bed.
    a Unfold it length-wise with the center crease in the middle.
    b Place the large hem even with the top of the mattress.
    c Open and fan-fold the sheet to the other side.
    d Face hem-stitching outward, away from the person.
    e Do not tuck the bottom in yet.
    f Never tuck top linens in on the sides.
24 Place the blanket on the bed.
    a Unfold it with the center crease in the middle.
    b Put the upper hem about 6 to 8 inches from the top of the mattress.
    c Open and fan-fold the blanket to the other side.
    d If steps 30 and 31 are not done, turn the top sheet down over the blanket. Hem-stitching is down, away from the person.
25 Place the bedspread on the bed.
    a Unfold it with the center crease in the middle.
    b Place the upper hem even with the top of the mattress.
    c Open and fan-fold the bedspread to the other side.
    d Make sure the bedspread facing the door is even. It covers all top linens.
26 Tuck in top linens together at the foot of the bed so they are smooth and tight. Make a mitered corner. Leave the side of the top linens untucked.
27 Go to the other side.
28 Straighten all top linens. Work from the head of the bed to the foot.
29 Tuck in top linens together at the foot of the bed. Make a mitered corner. Leave the top linens untucked at the sides.
30 Turn the top hem of the bedspread under the blanket to form a cuff (Fig. 22-12, p. 331).
31 Turn the top sheet down over the bedspread. Hem-stitching is down. (Steps 30 and 31 are not done in some agencies. The bedspread covers the pillow. If so, tuck the bedspread under the pillow.)
32 Put the pillowcase on the pillow (Figs. 22-13 and 22-14, p. 331). The zipper, tag, or seam end of the pillow is inserted into the pillowcase first. Fold extra material under the pillow at the open end of the pillowcase.
33 Place the pillow on the bed. The open end of the pillowcase is away from the door. The pillowcase seam is toward the head of the bed.

POST-PROCEDURE

34 Provide for comfort. (See the inside of the back cover.) NOTE: Omit this step if the bed is prepared for a new patient or resident.
35 Attach the call light to the bed. Or place it within the person's reach.
36 Lower the bed to a safe and comfortable level. Follow the care plan. The bed wheels are locked (braked).

37 Put the towels, washcloth, gown or pajamas, and bath blanket in the bedside stand.
38 Complete a safety check of the room. (See the inside of the back cover.)
39 Follow agency policy for used linens.
40 Practice hand hygiene.

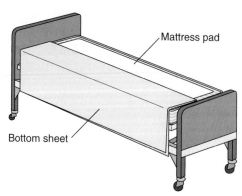

FIGURE 22-8 A flat bottom sheet is on the bed with the center crease in the middle. The lower edge of the sheet is even with the bottom of the mattress.

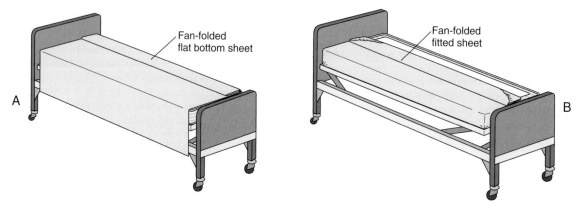

FIGURE 22-9 A, The flat bottom sheet is fan-folded to the other side of the bed. **B,** A fitted sheet is on the bed with the center crease in the middle.

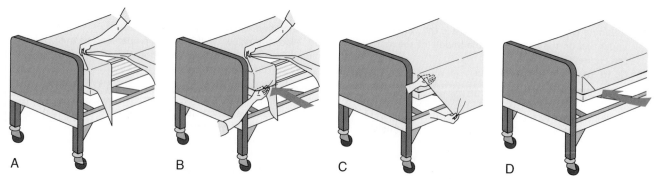

FIGURE 22-10 Making a mitered corner. **A,** The flat bottom sheet is tucked under the mattress at the head of the bed. The side of the sheet is raised onto the mattress. **B,** The remaining portion of the sheet is tucked under the mattress. **C,** The raised portion of the sheet is brought off the mattress. **D,** The entire side of the sheet is tucked under the mattress.

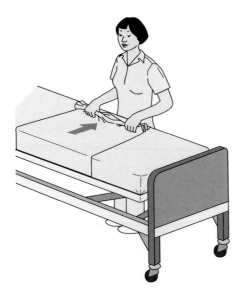

FIGURE 22-11 The drawsheet is pulled tight to remove wrinkles.

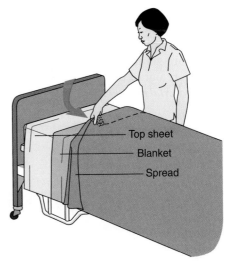

Top sheet
Blanket
Spread

FIGURE 22-12 The top hem of the bedspread is turned under the top hem of the blanket to make a cuff.

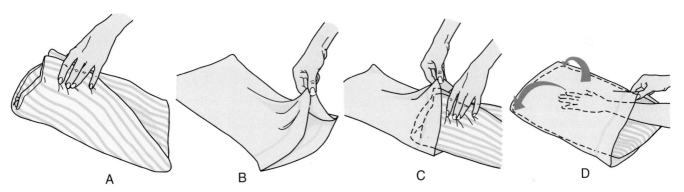

A   B   C   D

FIGURE 22-13 Putting a pillowcase on a pillow. **A,** Grasp the corners of the pillow at the zipper, tag, or seam end of the pillow and form a "V" with the pillow. **B,** Open the pillowcase with your free hand. **C,** Guide the "V" end of the pillow into the pillowcase. **D,** Let the "V" end of the pillow fall into the corners of the pillowcase.

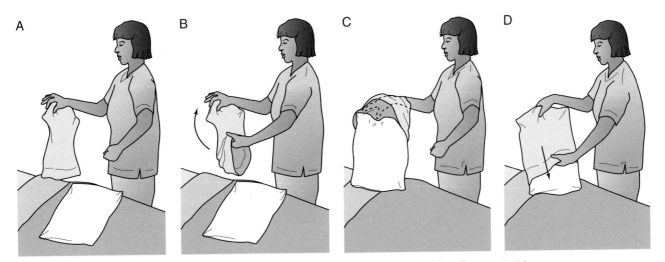

A   B   C   D

FIGURE 22-14 Putting a pillowcase on a pillow. **A,** Grasp the closed end of the pillowcase. **B,** Using your other hand, gather up the pillowcase. **C,** The pillowcase should cover your hand holding the closed end. Grasp the pillow with the hand covered by the pillowcase. **D,** Pull the pillowcase down over the pillow with your other hand.

The Open Bed

A closed bed becomes an open bed by fan-folding back the top linens. The person can get into bed with ease. Make this bed for:

- Newly admitted persons arriving by wheelchair
- Persons who are getting ready for bed
- Persons who are out of bed for a short time
  See procedure: *Making an Open Bed.*

The Occupied Bed

You make an occupied bed when the person stays in bed. Keep the person in good alignment. Follow restrictions or limits in the person's movement or position.

Explain each step to the person before it is done. This is important even if the person cannot respond or is in a coma.

See *Focus on Communication: The Occupied Bed.*
See *Promoting Safety and Comfort: The Occupied Bed.*
See procedure: *Making an Occupied Bed.*

Making an Open Bed

QUALITY OF LIFE

- Knock before entering the person's room.
- Address the person by name.
- Introduce yourself by name and title.

- Explain the procedure before starting and during the procedure.
- Protect the person's rights during the procedure.
- Handle the person gently during the procedure.

PROCEDURE

1 Follow *Delegation Guidelines: Making Beds,* p. 328. See *Promoting Safety and Comfort: Making Beds,* p. 328.
2 Practice hand hygiene.
3 Collect linens for a closed bed (p. 328).

4 Make a closed bed. (See procedure: *Making a Closed Bed,* p. 328.)
5 Fan-fold top linens to the foot of the bed (see Fig. 22-2).

POST-PROCEDURE

6 Place the call light and other needed items within reach.
7 Lower the bed to a safe and comfortable level for the person. Follow the care plan.
8 Put the towels, washcloth, gown or pajamas, and bath blanket in the bedside stand.

9 Provide for comfort. (See the inside of the back cover.)
10 Complete a safety check of the room. (See the inside of the back cover.)
11 Follow agency policy for used linens.
12 Practice hand hygiene.

FOCUS ON COMMUNICATION

The Occupied Bed

After making an occupied bed, ask about the person's comfort.
- "Are you comfortable?"
- "How can I make you more comfortable?"
- "Are you warm enough?"
- "Do you feel any creases or wrinkles?"
- "Can I adjust your pillow?"
  After making the bed, thank the person for cooperating.

PROMOTING SAFETY AND COMFORT

The Occupied Bed

Safety
The person lies on 1 side and then the other. Protect the person from falling out of bed. If bed rails are used, the far bed rail is up. If bed rails are not used, have a co-worker help you. You work on 1 side of the bed. Your co-worker is on the other side to help turn and position the person and prevent falling.

Comfort
For an occupied bed, you tuck used bottom linens under the person. Then you put clean linens on the bed. These are tucked under the used linens. The tucked linens create a "bump" in the middle of the bed. To make the other side, the person rolls over the "bump" to the other side of the bed. For comfort, make the "bump" as low as possible. Do this by fan-folding used and clean bottom linens neatly and flatly. Do not let the person's body touch the exposed surface of the mattress.

Making an Occupied Bed

QUALITY OF LIFE

- Knock before entering the person's room.
- Address the person by name.
- Introduce yourself by name and title.

- Explain the procedure before starting and during the procedure.
- Protect the person's rights during the procedure.
- Handle the person gently during the procedure.

PRE-PROCEDURE

1 Follow *Delegation Guidelines: Making Beds,* p. 328. See *Promoting Safety and Comfort:*
   a *Making Beds,* p. 328
   b *The Occupied Bed*
2 Practice hand hygiene.
3 Collect the following.
   - Gloves
   - Laundry bag
   - Clean linens (see procedure: *Making a Closed Bed,* p. 328)
   - Towel, paper towels, or disposable bed protector (as a barrier for clean linens)

4 Place linens on a clean surface. First place the barrier between the clean surface and clean linens if required by agency policy.
5 Identify the person. Check the ID (identification) bracelet against the assignment sheet. Use 2 identifiers (Chapter 13). Also call the person by name.
6 Provide for privacy.
7 Remove the call light.
8 Raise the bed for body mechanics. Bed rails are up if used. Bed wheels are locked (braked).
9 Lower the head of the bed. It is as flat as possible.

PROCEDURE

10 Practice hand hygiene. Put on gloves.
11 Loosen top linens at the foot of the bed.
12 Lower the bed rail near you if up.
13 Fold and remove the bedspread (Fig. 22-15, p. 334). Do the same for the blanket. Place each over the chair.
14 Cover the person with a bath blanket from the bedside stand.
   a Unfold the bath blanket over the top sheet.
   b Have the person hold the bath blanket. If he or she cannot, tuck the top part under the person's shoulders.
   c Grasp the top sheet under the bath blanket at the shoulders. Bring the sheet down toward the foot of the bed. Remove the sheet from under the blanket (Fig. 22-16, p. 335).
15 Position the person on his or her side facing away from you. Adjust the pillow for comfort.
16 Loosen bottom linens from the head to the foot of the bed.
17 Fan-fold bottom linens 1 at a time toward the person. Start with the drawsheet (Fig. 22-17, p. 335). If re-using the mattress pad, do not fan-fold it.
18 Remove and discard the gloves. Practice hand hygiene. Put on clean gloves.
19 Place a clean mattress pad on the bed. Unfold it length-wise with the center crease in the middle. Fan-fold the top part toward the person. If re-using the mattress pad, straighten and smooth any wrinkles.
20 Place the bottom sheet on the mattress pad. Hem-stitching is away from the person. Unfold the sheet with the crease in the middle. For a flat sheet, the small hem is even with the bottom of the mattress. Fan-fold the top part toward the person.
21 Tuck fitted sheet corners over the mattress. For a flat sheet, make a mitered corner at the head of the bed. Tuck the sheet under the mattress from the head to the foot of the bed.

22 *If using a drawsheet* (Fig. 22-18, p. 335):
   a Place the cotton drawsheet or padded waterproof drawsheet on the bed. It is in the middle of the mattress.
   b Open the drawsheet.
   c Fan-fold it toward the person.
   d Tuck in excess fabric.
23 *If using a waterproof under-pad:*
   a Place the waterproof under-pad on the bed. It is in the middle of the mattress.
   b Fan-fold it toward the person.
24 Explain to the person that he or she will roll over a "bump." Assure the person that he or she will not fall.
25 Help the person turn to the other side. Adjust the pillow for comfort.
26 Raise the bed rail. Go to the other side and lower the bed rail.
27 Loosen bottom linens. Remove 1 piece at a time. Place each piece in the laundry bag. (NOTE: Discard the disposable bed protector, incontinence product, and disposable drawsheet in the trash. Do not put them in the laundry bag.)
28 Remove and discard the gloves. Practice hand hygiene.
29 Straighten and smooth the mattress pad.
30 Pull the clean bottom sheet toward you. Tuck fitted sheet corners over the mattress. For a flat sheet, make a mitered corner at the top. Tuck the sheet under the mattress from the head to the foot of the bed.
31 Pull the drawsheet tightly toward you and tuck it in.
32 Position the person supine in the center of the bed. Adjust the pillow for comfort.
33 Put the top sheet on the bed. Unfold it length-wise with the crease in the middle. The large hem is even with the top of the mattress. Hem-stitching is on the outside.
34 Have the person hold the top sheet so you can remove the bath blanket. Or tuck the top sheet under the person's shoulders. Remove the bath blanket. Place it in the laundry bag.

Continued

Making an Occupied Bed—cont'd

PROCEDURE—cont'd

35 Unfold the blanket on the bed. The crease is in the middle and it covers the person. The upper hem is 6 to 8 inches from the top of the mattress.

36 Unfold the bedspread on the bed. The center crease is in the middle and it covers the person. The top hem is even with the mattress top.

37 Turn the top hem of the bedspread under the blanket to make a cuff.

38 Bring the top sheet down over the bedspread to form a cuff.

39 Go to the foot of the bed.

40 Make a 2-inch toe pleat across the foot of the bed (Fig. 22-19). The pleat (fold) is about 6 to 8 inches from the foot of the bed. The pleat prevents pressure on the toes from top linens.

41 Lift the mattress corner with 1 arm. Tuck all top linens under the bottom of the mattress. Avoid removing the toe pleat. Make a mitered corner. Leave the side of the top linens untucked.

42 Raise the bed rail. Go to the other side and lower the bed rail.

43 Straighten and smooth top linens.

44 Tuck all top linens under the bottom of the mattress. Make a mitered corner. Leave the side of the top linens untucked.

45 Change the pillowcase(s).

POST-PROCEDURE

46 Provide for comfort. (See the inside of the back cover.)

47 Place the call light and other needed items within reach.

48 Lower the bed to a safe and comfortable level. Follow the care plan. The bed wheels are locked (braked).

49 Raise or lower bed rails. Follow the care plan.

50 Put the clean towels, washcloth, gown or pajamas, and bath blanket in the bedside stand.

51 Unscreen the person.

52 Complete a safety check of the room. (See the inside of the back cover.)

53 Follow agency policy for used linens.

54 Practice hand hygiene.

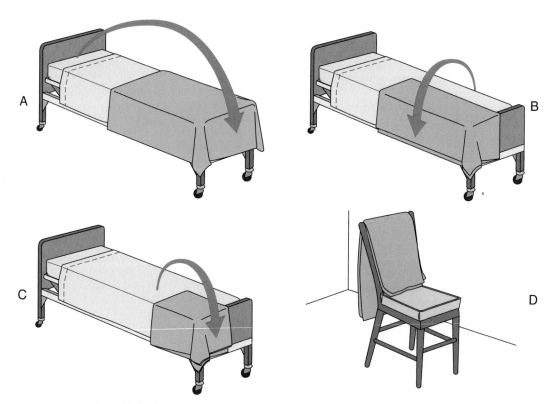

FIGURE 22-15 Folding linens for re-use. **A,** Fold the top edge of the bedspread down to the bottom edge. **B,** Fold the bedspread from the far side of the bed to the near side. **C,** Fold the top edge of the bedspread down to the bottom edge again. **D,** Place the folded bedspread over the back of the chair.

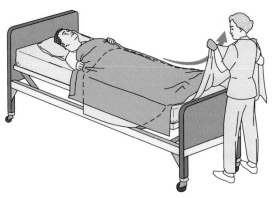

FIGURE 22-16 The person holds on to the bath blanket. The top sheet is removed from under the bath blanket. (Note: Bed rails are used according to the care plan.)

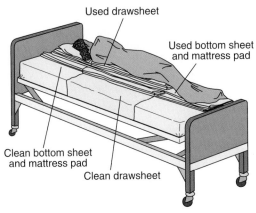

FIGURE 22-18 A clean bottom sheet and drawsheet are on the bed with both fan-folded and tucked under the person. (Note: Bed rails are used according to the care plan.)

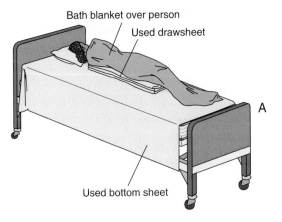

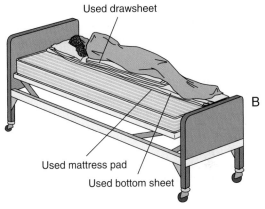

FIGURE 22-17 **A,** The used drawsheet is fan-folded and tucked under the person. **B,** All used bottom linens are tucked under the person. (Note: Bed rails are used according to the care plan.)

The Surgical Bed

The surgical bed also is called a *recovery bed* or *post-operative bed.* Top linens are folded to the side to transfer the person from a stretcher to the bed. These beds are made for persons:

* Returning to their rooms from surgery. A complete linen change is needed.
* Who arrive at the agency by ambulance. A complete linen change is needed if the person:
  * Is a new patient or resident.
  * Is returning to the agency from the hospital.
* Who go by stretcher to treatment or therapy areas. A complete linen change is not needed.
* Using portable tubs (Chapter 24). Because of bathing, a complete linen change is needed.

See *Promoting Safety and Comfort: The Surgical Bed.*
See procedure: *Making a Surgical Bed,* p. 336.

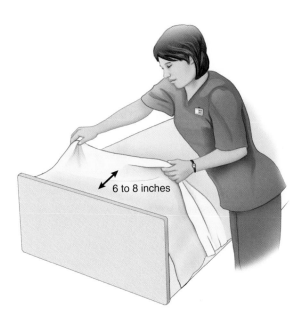

FIGURE 22-19 Making a toe pleat. Pull up on the top linens. Make a 2-inch pleat (fold) across the foot of the bed. The pleat is 6 to 8 inches from the foot of the bed.

PROMOTING SAFETY AND COMFORT

The Surgical Bed

Safety

See Chapter 20 for stretcher safety rules and the procedure: *Moving the Person to a Stretcher.* After the transfer, lower the bed to a safe and comfortable level for the person. Bed wheels are locked (braked). Raise or lower bed rails according to the care plan.

Making a Surgical Bed

PRE-PROCEDURE

1 Follow *Delegation Guidelines: Making Beds,* p. 328. See *Promoting Safety and Comfort:*
   a *Making Beds,* p. 328
   b *The Surgical Bed,* p. 335
2 Practice hand hygiene.
3 Collect the following.
   • Clean linens (see procedure: *Making a Closed Bed,* p. 328)
   • Gloves
   • Laundry bag
   • Equipment requested by the nurse
   • Towel, paper towels, or disposable bed protector (as a barrier for clean linens)

4 Place linens on a clean surface. First place the barrier between the clean surface and clean linens if required by agency policy.
5 Remove the call light.
6 Raise the bed for body mechanics.

PROCEDURE

7 Remove and place all linens in the laundry bag. Wear gloves. Practice hand hygiene after removing and discarding them.
8 Make a closed bed (see procedure: *Making a Closed Bed,* p. 328). Do not tuck top linens under the mattress.
9 Fold all top linens at the foot of the bed back onto the bed. The fold is even with the edge of the mattress (Fig. 22-20, *A*).

10 Know on which side of the bed the stretcher will be placed. Fan-fold linens length-wise to the other side of the bed (Fig. 22-20, *B*).
11 Put a pillowcase on each pillow.
12 Place the pillow(s) on a clean surface.

POST-PROCEDURE

13 Leave the bed in its highest position.
14 Leave both bed rails down.
15 Put the clean towels, washcloth, gown or pajamas, and bath blanket in the bedside stand.
16 Move furniture away from the bed. Allow room for the stretcher and the staff.

17 Do not attach the call light to the bed.
18 Complete a safety check of the room. (See the inside of the back cover.)
19 Follow agency policy for used linens.
20 Practice hand hygiene.

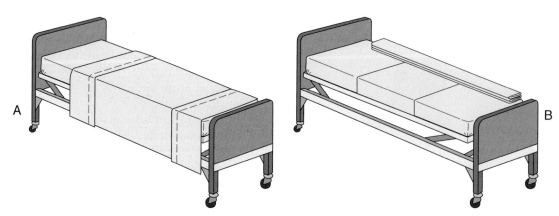

FIGURE 22-20 Surgical bed. **A,** The bottom of the top linens is folded back onto the bed. The fold is even with the bottom edge of the mattress. **B,** Top linens are fan-folded length-wise to the side of the bed.

FOCUS ON **PRIDE**
The Person, Family, and Yourself

Personal and Professional Responsibility

You are responsible for providing a neat and orderly setting. The bed must be clean and well made. If the person stays in bed, straighten and tighten linens as needed. These actions promote comfort and quality of life.

Rights and Respect

Nursing center residents often bring bedspreads, blankets, quilts, and so on from home. The items have meaning and value. For example, a resident uses an afghan at night. Made by his wife, the sight and smell of the afghan remind him of his wife and home.

Protect personal items from loss and damage. Handle the person's belongings with care and respect.

Independence and Social Interaction

Allow personal choice when possible. What is best for you may not be best for the person. Consider the person's preferences when planning your day and managing your time. The more choices are allowed, the greater the person's sense of control and independence.

Delegation and Teamwork

Some agencies have laundry containers in each room. Others have laundry carts in the hallways. Some agencies have a room for used linens. Others have laundry chutes.

When handling used linens:

- Wear gloves.
- Follow agency policy for used linens.
- Do not over-fill the laundry bag or container.
- Work as a team. Some units assign a person to empty linen containers. Linens must not over-flow carts. If you see a full cart, empty it. The person assigned the task may be busy.
- Clean up after yourself. If you fill a cart, empty it. If you place an item in a cart that will cause an odor, empty the cart.
- Place used linens in the correct location. If chutes are used, use the correct chute. Other chutes may be for trash.

Ethics and Laws

Always treat patients and residents with dignity, care, and kindness. In the following real event, the nurse ignored these values.

On August 2, 1990, a patient had back surgery. She was on complete bed rest until August 4 when the doctor ordered "increase activity up as tolerated with assist." According to the court case, the following occurred between the patient and a nurse.

- *On August 5 the patient woke up when the nurse bumped into her bed. The nurse told the patient that she had to get up and have her bed made. Despite pleas to stay in bed, the nurse said that she [the nurse] had to make the bed.*
- *The nurse pulled the patient by her arm. The patient pleaded to be left alone. The patient said that it hurt to have her arm pulled that way. The nurse let go of the patient's arm. The patient lay down in bed.*
- *The nurse pulled the patient's feet off the bed. In extreme pain, the patient "started to yell, to plead with the nurse not to do what she was doing and told her that it hurt."*
- *The nurse insisted that the patient had to get up. The nurse insisted that she had to make the bed. The nurse forced the patient into a standing position. The patient, in pain, told the nurse that she was going to "throw up or faint."*
- *The nurse shoved the patient "into a straight back chair using her hands to press down hard on the [patient's] shoulders."*
- *In extreme pain, the patient pleaded with the nurse and said that she was going to faint.*
- *The nurse then forced the patient's head between her knees down to her lap. The patient felt extreme pain in the middle of her back.*
- *The nurse raised the patient's back. In extreme pain, the patient could not get up when she had to do so. The patient continued to plead to be put back to bed.*
- *The nurse again told the patient that she had to make the bed. The nurse "ripped the sheet off the bed and used it to tie [the patient] to the chair with a knot towards the back."*
- *The patient "tried to reach forward to push the nurse's call button ... [The nurse] kicked and pushed the table away and out of the [patient's] grasp." The patient said that she wanted to call a nurse.*
- *The nurse left the room for 10 minutes. "She came back and made the bed with a laboratory technician." After making the bed, they put the patient back in bed. The patient was crying.*

The Appellate Court of Illinois, in reviewing the case, said the "negligence here was ... grossly apparent ..." The case was sent back to the trial court for a full trial.

(R. Prairie v University of Chicago Hospitals, 1998.)

If you see a person being mistreated and abused, take action. Get help. Protect the person.

FOCUS ON **PRIDE**: *Application*

Do you make your bed at home every day? If yes, why? If no, why? Explain why the look and feel of the bed can affect the person's comfort and safety.

REVIEW QUESTIONS

Circle T if the statement is TRUE or F if it is FALSE.

1 T F In nursing centers, complete linen changes are required for closed beds and surgical beds.

2 T F In home care, complete linen changes are done daily.

3 T F Hem-stitching faces away from the person.

4 T F To remove crumbs from the bed, you shake linens in the air.

5 T F The upper hem of the bedspread is even with the top of the mattress.

6 T F Top linens are fan-folded to the foot of the bed for an open bed.

7 T F A cotton drawsheet is used with a padded waterproof drawsheet.

8 T F Residents can bring bed coverings from home.

Circle the BEST answer.

9 To transfer a person from a stretcher to the bed, you make
   a A closed bed
   b An open bed
   c An occupied bed
   d A surgical bed

10 When handling linens
   a Put used linens on the floor
   b Hold linens away from your body and uniform
   c Shake linens to unfold them
   d Take extra linens to another person's room

11 For a resident out of bed most of the day, you make
   a A closed bed
   b An open bed
   c An occupied bed
   d A surgical bed

12 A complete linen change is done when
   a The drawsheet is wet
   b The bed is made for a new person
   c The person will transfer from a stretcher to a bed
   d Linens are loose or wrinkled

13 After making a closed bed
   a Unlock the bed wheels (release the brakes)
   b Leave the bed in the high position
   c Leave used linens in the room
   d Attach the call light to the bed

14 When making an occupied bed
   a Explain that the person will roll over a "bump" of linens
   b Wear the same gloves throughout the procedure
   c Lower the far bed rail if working alone
   d Fan-fold top linens to the foot of the bed

15 A surgical bed is kept
   a In Fowler's position
   b In the lowest position
   c In the highest position
   d In the supine position

Answers to Chapter 22 questions are on p. 886.

FOCUS ON PRACTICE

Problem Solving

You need to give a person a bath in bed (Chapter 24). The person must remain in bed. Which type of bed will you make? Will you change linens or give the bath first? While changing linens, when will you apply and remove gloves and practice hand hygiene?

Oral Hygiene

OBJECTIVES

- Define the key terms and key abbreviations in this chapter.
- Explain the purposes of oral hygiene.
- Explain why flossing is important.
- Describe the safety measures for giving mouth care to unconscious persons.

- Explain how to care for dentures.
- Identify the observations related to oral hygiene.
- Perform the procedures described in this chapter.
- Explain how to promote PRIDE in the person, the family, and yourself.

KEY TERMS

aspiration Breathing fluid, food, vomitus, or an object into the lungs
denture A removable replacement for missing teeth
hygiene The cleanliness practices that promote health and prevent disease
mouth care See "oral hygiene"

oral hygiene The practices that promote healthy tissues and structures of the mouth; mouth care
plaque A thin film that sticks to the teeth; it contains saliva, microbes, and other substances
tartar Hardened plaque

KEY ABBREVIATIONS

ADA   American Dental Association

ID   Identification

The teeth and mucous membranes of the mouth must be kept clean and intact. Otherwise teeth can decay and microbes can enter the body.

Illness, disease, and some drugs often cause:

- A bad taste in the mouth.
- A whitish coating in the mouth and on the tongue.
- Redness and swelling in the mouth and on the tongue.
- Dry mouth. Dry mouth is common from oxygen, smoking, decreased fluid intake, and anxiety.

See *Body Structure and Function Review: The Teeth and Gums.* For greater detail, see Chapter 10.

BODY STRUCTURE AND FUNCTION REVIEW

The Teeth and Gums

The *teeth* cut, chop, and grind food into small bits for digestion and swallowing.

With age, *primary teeth* (baby teeth) are replaced with *permanent teeth* (adult teeth). Normally, adults have 32 permanent teeth.

A tooth has 3 main parts: the *crown, neck,* and *root* (Fig. 23-1). The crown is the outer part. It is covered by enamel. The neck is surrounded by *gums (gingivae).* The root fits into the bone of the lower or upper jaw.

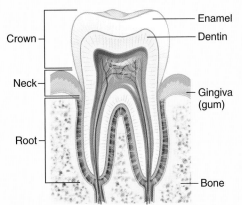

FIGURE 23-1 Parts of the tooth.

PURPOSE OF ORAL HYGIENE

Hygiene involves the cleanliness practices that promote health and prevent disease. **Oral hygiene (mouth care)** *relates to the practices that promote healthy tissues and structures of the mouth.* Oral hygiene:

- Keeps the mouth and teeth clean.
- Prevents mouth odors and infections.
- Increases comfort.
- Makes food taste better.
- Reduces the risk for *cavities (dental caries)* and *periodontal disease.*

Periodontal disease *(gum disease, pyorrhea)* is an inflammation of tissues around the teeth. Plaque and tartar build up from poor oral hygiene. **Plaque** *is a thin film that sticks to the teeth. It contains saliva, microbes, and other substances.* Plaque causes tooth decay *(cavities). Hardened plaque is called* **tartar.** Tartar builds up at the gum line near the neck of the tooth. Tartar buildup causes periodontal disease. The gums are red and swollen and bleed easily. Bone is destroyed and teeth loosen. Tooth loss is common.

The nurse assesses the person's need for mouth care. So may the speech-language pathologist and the dietitian.

See *Focus on Children and Older Persons: Purpose of Oral Hygiene.*

See *Delegation Guidelines: Purpose of Oral Hygiene.*

See *Promoting Safety and Comfort: Purpose of Oral Hygiene.*

FOCUS ON **CHILDREN AND OLDER PERSONS**

Purpose of Oral Hygiene

Children

Infants and young children need mouth care to remove food and bacteria. This helps prevent early childhood tooth decay *(baby bottle tooth decay, early childhood caries).* Common in the upper and lower front teeth, it can occur in all teeth (Fig. 23-2). Prolonged teeth exposure to liquids containing sugar is the usual cause. Breast-milk, milk, formula, fruit juice, and other sweetened drinks contain sugar. Sugar coats the teeth. Bacteria in the mouth use sugars in such drinks for nourishment. The bacteria produce acids that cause tooth decay.

For early childhood oral hygiene, see Box 23-1.

BOX 23-1   Oral Hygiene—Early Childhood

Preventing Tooth Decay

- Breast-feeding is preferred. Breast-milk keeps the baby's mouth healthy.
- Bottle-feeding:
  - Fill baby bottles only with milk, breast-milk, or formula.
  - Do not fill baby bottles with sugar water, juice, punch, soft drinks, or other liquids high in sugar.
  - Do not put the baby to bed with a bottle. Babies should finish a bottle before bedtime sleep or a nap.
  - Stop using baby bottles when the child is 12 to 14 months old.
  - Do not let the baby walk around with a bottle of milk, juice, or liquids high in sugar.
- Teach the baby how to drink from a cup around 6 months of age. The child should drink from a cup by 12 months of age.
- Avoid sharing saliva with the baby. Cleaning a baby's spoon or pacifier in your mouth passes your saliva to the baby. Cavity-causing bacteria could be in your mouth.
- Pacifiers:
  - Do not dip a pacifier in sugar, honey, or anything sweet.
  - Do not let a baby suck on a pacifier all the time.

Care of Gums and Teeth

- Wipe the baby's gums after each feeding. Use a gauze pad or washcloth that is clean and damp.
- Start brushing when the first tooth erupts. *(Erupt means to break through and become visible.)*
- Use fluoride toothpaste (Fig. 23-3):
  - Until age 3—use a smear (the size of a grain of rice) of fluoride toothpaste and a child-sized toothbrush.
  - Ages 3 to 6—use a pea-sized amount of fluoride toothpaste.
- Brush gently.
- Supervise brushing until the child can spit out toothpaste. This is usually until age 6 or 7.
- Have a brushing routine for the child. For example, you and the child brush together at the same time.
- See "Flossing."
- Consult a dentist about when to schedule the baby's first dental visit. Do so after the first tooth erupts.

Modified from National Institutes of Health: Tooth decay—early childhood, Bethesda, Md., page updated October 2, 2019, and American Dental Association: Mouth healthy™: baby bottle tooth decay, 2019.

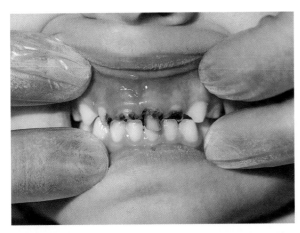

FIGURE 23-2 Baby bottle tooth decay. (From Eisen D, Lynch DP: *The mouth: diagnosis and treatment*, St Louis, 1998, Mosby.)

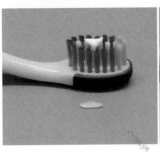

A   B

FIGURE 23-3 Toothpaste amounts in early childhood. **A,** A smear of toothpaste (the size of a grain of rice) is used until age 3. **B,** A pea-sized amount is used from ages 3 to 6. (ADA content –Toothpaste Amount image in early childhood; depicting pea sized. Copyright © 2011 American Dental Association. All rights reserved. Reprinted with permission.)

DELEGATION GUIDELINES
Purpose of Oral Hygiene

Oral hygiene procedures are routine nursing tasks. To assist with oral hygiene, you need this information from the nurse and the care plan.
- The type of oral hygiene to give. See procedures:
  - *Assisting the Person to Brush and Floss the Teeth,* p. 342
  - *Brushing and Flossing the Person's Teeth,* p. 343
  - *Providing Mouth Care for the Unconscious Person,* p. 345
  - *Providing Denture Care,* p. 347
- If flossing is needed.
- What cleaning agent and equipment to use.
- If you apply lubricant to the lips. If yes, what lubricant to use.
- How often to give oral hygiene.
- How much help the person needs.
- What observations to report and record:
  - Dry, cracked, swollen, or blistered lips
  - Mouth or breath odor
  - Redness, swelling, irritation, sores, or white patches in the mouth or on the tongue
  - Bleeding, swelling, or redness of the gums
  - Loose teeth
  - Rough, sharp, or chipped areas on dentures
- When to report observations.
- What patient or resident concerns to report at once.

PROMOTING SAFETY AND COMFORT
Purpose of Oral Hygiene

Safety
Follow Standard Precautions and the Bloodborne Pathogen Standard. You may have contact with the person's mucous membranes. Gums may bleed during mouth care. Also, the mouth has many microbes. Pathogens spread through sexual contact may be in the mouths of some persons.

Brush gently and carefully. Brushing hard can cause the gums to bleed. Inserting the toothbrush too far can stimulate the gag reflex.

NOTE: A task may require more than 1 pair of gloves. Change gloves as needed. Use careful judgment. Remember to practice hand hygiene after removing gloves.

Comfort
Assist with oral hygiene after sleep, after meals, and at bedtime. Many people practice oral hygiene before meals. Some persons need mouth care every 2 hours or more often.

FOCUS ON CHILDREN AND OLDER PERSONS
Flossing

Children
The ADA recommends that flossing start when 2 baby teeth touch. You need to floss for babies, toddlers, and pre-schoolers. You may need to remind and supervise older children when flossing.

FLOSSING

Floss is a soft thread for cleaning between the teeth. Flossing helps prevent periodontal disease and cavities by:
- Removing plaque from areas brushing cannot reach
- Removing food from between the teeth

The American Dental Association (ADA) recommends flossing at least once a day. Flossing can be done before or after brushing. The person can choose the best time for thorough flossing—in the morning, after a meal, at bedtime, or when convenient. You need to floss for persons who cannot do so themselves.

See *Focus on Children and Older Persons: Flossing.*

EQUIPMENT

A toothbrush, toothpaste, floss, and mouthwash are needed. A toothbrush with soft bristles is best.

Sponge swabs are used for sore, tender mouths and for unconscious persons. Use sponge swabs with care. Make sure the foam pad is tight on the stick. The person could choke on the foam pad if it comes off.

You also need a kidney basin, water cup, straw, tissues, towels, and gloves. Many persons bring oral hygiene equipment from home. Electronic toothbrushes are common.

BRUSHING AND FLOSSING TEETH

Many people can perform oral hygiene. Others need help gathering and setting up oral hygiene equipment. You perform oral hygiene for persons who:

- Are very weak.
- Cannot move or use their arms.
- Are too confused to brush their teeth.

See procedure: *Assisting the Person to Brush and Floss the Teeth*.

See procedure: *Brushing and Flossing the Person's Teeth*.

Assisting the Person to Brush and Floss the Teeth

QUALITY OF LIFE

- Knock before entering the person's room.
- Address the person by name.
- Introduce yourself by name and title.

- Explain the procedure before starting and during the procedure.
- Protect the person's rights during the procedure.
- Handle the person gently during the procedure.

PRE-PROCEDURE

1 Follow *Delegation Guidelines: Purpose of Oral Hygiene*, p. 341. See *Promoting Safety and Comfort: Purpose of Oral Hygiene*, p. 341.
2 Practice hand hygiene.
3 Collect the following.
   - Toothbrush with soft bristles
   - Toothpaste
   - Mouthwash (or solution noted on the care plan)
   - Floss (if used)
   - Water cup with cool water
   - Straw
   - Kidney basin
   - Hand towel
   - Paper towels
   - Gloves

4 Place the paper towels on the over-bed table. Arrange items on top of them.
5 Identify the person. Check the ID (identification) bracelet against the assignment sheet. Use 2 identifiers (Chapter 13). Also call the person by name.
6 Provide for privacy.
7 Lower the bed rail near you if up.

PROCEDURE

8 Position the person for oral hygiene.
9 Place the towel over the chest. This protects garments and linens from spills.
10 Adjust the over-bed table in front of the person.

11 Let the person perform oral hygiene. This includes brushing the teeth and tongue, rinsing the mouth, flossing, and using mouthwash or other solution.
12 Remove the towel when the person is done.
13 Move the over-bed table as the person prefers.

POST-PROCEDURE

14 Assist with hand hygiene.
15 Provide for comfort. (See the inside of the back cover.)
16 Place the call light and other needed items within reach.
17 Raise or lower bed rails. Follow the care plan.
18 Rinse the toothbrush. Clean, rinse, and dry equipment. Use clean, dry paper towels for drying. Return the toothbrush and equipment to their proper place. Wear gloves.
19 Wipe the over-bed table with paper towels. Discard the paper towels.

20 Unscreen the person.
21 Complete a safety check of the room. (See the inside of the back cover.)
22 Follow agency policy for used linens.
23 Remove and discard the gloves. Practice hand hygiene.
24 Report and record your observations.

Brushing and Flossing the Person's Teeth

QUALITY OF LIFE

- Knock before entering the person's room.
- Address the person by name.
- Introduce yourself by name and title.

- Explain the procedure before starting and during the procedure.
- Protect the person's rights during the procedure.
- Handle the person gently during the procedure.

PRE-PROCEDURE

1 Follow *Delegation Guidelines: Purpose of Oral Hygiene,* p. 341. See *Promoting Safety and Comfort: Purpose of Oral Hygiene,* p. 341.
2 Practice hand hygiene.
3 Collect the following.
   - Toothbrush with soft bristles
   - Toothpaste
   - Mouthwash (or solution noted on the care plan)
   - Floss (if used)
   - Water cup with cool water
   - Straw
   - Kidney basin
   - Hand towel
   - Paper towels
   - Gloves

4 Place the paper towels on the over-bed table. Arrange items on top of them.
5 Identify the person. Check the ID bracelet against the assignment sheet. Use 2 identifiers (Chapter 13). Also call the person by name.
6 Provide for privacy.
7 Raise the bed for body mechanics. Bed rails are up if used.

PROCEDURE

8 Lower the bed rail near you if up.
9 Assist the person to a sitting position or to a side-lying position near you. (NOTE: Some state competency tests require that the person is at a 75- to 90-degree angle.)
10 Place the towel across the chest.
11 Adjust the over-bed table so you can reach it with ease.
12 Practice hand hygiene. Put on the gloves.
13 Hold the toothbrush over the kidney basin. Pour some water over the brush.
14 Apply toothpaste to the toothbrush.
15 Brush the teeth gently (Fig. 23-4, p. 344). Brush the inner, outer, and chewing surfaces of upper and lower teeth.
16 Brush the tongue gently. Also gently brush the roof of the mouth, inside of the cheeks, and gums.
17 Let the person rinse the mouth with water. Hold the kidney basin under the chin (Fig. 23-5, p. 344). Repeat this step as needed.

18 Floss the person's teeth (optional). See Figure 23-6, p. 344.
   a Break off an 18-inch piece of floss from the dispenser.
   b Wrap the floss around the middle fingers of each hand (see Fig. 23-6, *A*).
   c Stretch the floss with your thumbs. Hold the floss between your thumbs and index fingers.
   d Start at the back side of the upper back tooth on the right side. Work around to the left side.
   e Rub gently against the side of the tooth. Use up-and-down motions (see Fig. 23-6, *B*). Do not jerk or snap the floss against the tooth or into the gums.
   f Curve the floss into a "C" shape against the tooth at the gum line. Rub the side of the tooth with the floss from the gum line to the crown. Use up-and-down motions.
   g Move to a new section of floss after every second tooth. Remember to floss the back side of the last tooth.
   h Floss the lower teeth. Start on the right side. Work around to the left side. Remember to floss the back side of the last tooth.
   i Discard the floss.
19 Let the person use mouthwash or other solution. Hold the kidney basin under the chin.
20 Wipe the person's mouth. Remove the towel.
21 Remove and discard the gloves. Practice hand hygiene.

POST-PROCEDURE

22 Assist with hand hygiene.
23 Provide for comfort. (See the inside of the back cover.)
24 Place the call light and other needed items within reach.
25 Lower the bed to a safe and comfortable level. Follow the care plan.
26 Raise or lower bed rails. Follow the care plan.
27 Rinse the toothbrush. Clean, rinse, and dry equipment. Use clean, dry paper towels for drying. Return the toothbrush and equipment to their proper place. Wear gloves.

28 Wipe off the over-bed table with paper towels. Discard the paper towels.
29 Unscreen the person.
30 Complete a safety check of the room. (See the inside of the back cover.)
31 Follow agency policy for used linens.
32 Remove and discard the gloves. Practice hand hygiene.
33 Report and record your observations.

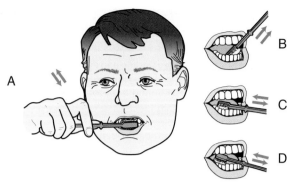

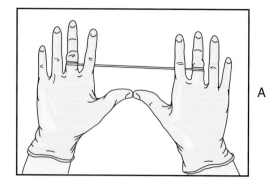

FIGURE 23-4 Brushing teeth. **A,** The brush is held at a 45-degree angle to the gums. Teeth are brushed with short strokes. **B,** The brush is at a 45-degree angle against the inside of the front teeth. Teeth are brushed from the gum to the crown of the tooth with short strokes. **C,** The brush is held horizontally against the inner surfaces of the teeth. The teeth are brushed back and forth. **D,** The brush is positioned on the chewing surfaces of the teeth. The teeth are brushed back and forth.

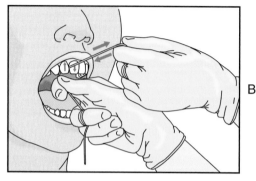

FIGURE 23-6 Flossing. **A,** Floss is wrapped around the middle fingers. **B,** Floss is moved in up-and-down motions between the teeth. Floss is moved up and down from the gum line to the crown.

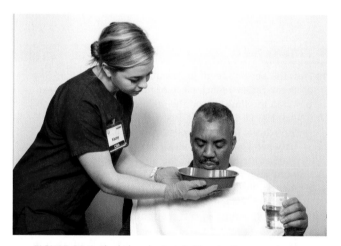

FIGURE 23-5 The kidney basin is held under the person's chin.

Mouth Care for the Unconscious Person

Unconscious (comatose) persons cannot eat or drink. Some breathe with their mouths open. Many receive oxygen. These factors cause mouth dryness. They also cause crusting on the tongue and mucous membranes. Oral hygiene keeps the mouth clean and moist. It also helps prevent infection.

The care plan states what cleaning agent to use. Apply the cleaning agent with sponge swabs. To prevent the lips from cracking, apply a lubricant (check the care plan) after cleaning.

Unconscious persons usually cannot swallow. Protect them from choking and aspiration. *Aspiration is breathing fluid, food, vomitus, or an object into the lungs.* It can cause pneumonia and death. To prevent aspiration:

* Position the person on 1 side with the head turned well to the side (Fig. 23-7). In this position, excess fluid can run out of the mouth.
* Use a small amount of fluid to clean the mouth.
* Do not insert dentures. Unconscious persons do not wear dentures.

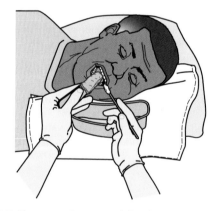

FIGURE 23-7 The unconscious person's head is turned well to the side to prevent aspiration. A plastic tongue depressor keeps the mouth open while cleaning the mouth with swabs.

Keep the person's mouth open with a plastic tongue depressor (Fig. 23-8). Do not use your fingers. The person can bite down on them. The bite breaks the skin, allowing microbes to enter the body. Infection is a risk.

Mouth care is given at least every 2 hours. Follow the nurse's directions and the care plan.

See *Focus on Communication: Mouth Care for the Unconscious Person.*

See *Promoting Safety and Comfort: Mouth Care for the Unconscious Person.*

See procedure: *Providing Mouth Care for the Unconscious Person.*

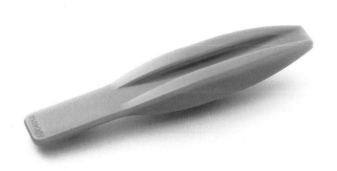

FIGURE 23-8 Plastic tongue depressor. (© American Diagnostic Corp, 2017.)

FOCUS ON **COMMUNICATION**
Mouth Care for the Unconscious Person

Unconscious persons cannot speak or respond to you. However, some can hear. Always assume that unconscious persons can hear. Explain what you are doing step-by-step. Also, tell the person when you are done, when you are leaving, and when you will return.

PROMOTING SAFETY AND COMFORT
Mouth Care for the Unconscious Person

Safety

Use sponge swabs with care. Make sure the sponge pad is tight on the stick. The person could aspirate or choke on the sponge if it comes off the stick.

Comfort

Unconscious persons are re-positioned at least every 2 hours. Combine mouth care with skin care, re-positioning, and other comfort measures.

Providing Mouth Care for the Unconscious Person

QUALITY OF LIFE

- Knock before entering the person's room.
- Address the person by name.
- Introduce yourself by name and title.

- Explain the procedure before starting and during the procedure.
- Protect the person's rights during the procedure.
- Handle the person gently during the procedure.

PRE-PROCEDURE

1. Follow *Delegation Guidelines: Purpose of Oral Hygiene*, p. 341. See *Promoting Safety and Comfort:*
   a. *Purpose of Oral Hygiene*, p. 341
   b. *Mouth Care for the Unconscious Person*
2. Practice hand hygiene.
3. Collect the following.
   - Cleaning agent (check the care plan)
   - Sponge swabs
   - Plastic tongue depressor
   - Water cup with cool water
   - Hand towel
   - Kidney basin
   - Lip lubricant (check the care plan)
   - Paper towels
   - Gloves
4. Place the paper towels on the over-bed table. Arrange items on top of them.
5. Identify the person. Check the ID bracelet against the assignment sheet. Use 2 identifiers (Chapter 13). Also call the person by name.
6. Provide for privacy.
7. Raise the bed for body mechanics. Bed rails are up if used.

PROCEDURE

8. Lower the bed rail near you.
9. Position the person in a side-lying position near you. Turn his or her head well to the side.
10. Place the towel under the person's face and along the chest. This protects the person and bed.
11. Put on the gloves.
12. Place the kidney basin under the chin.
13. Separate the upper and lower teeth. Use the plastic tongue depressor. Be gentle. Never use force. If you have problems, ask the nurse for help.
14. Moisten the sponge swabs with the cleaning agent. Squeeze out excess cleaning agent.
15. Clean the mouth.
    a. Clean the chewing and inner surfaces of the teeth.
    b. Clean the gums and outer surfaces of the teeth.
    c. Swab the roof of the mouth, inside of the cheeks, and the lips.
    d. Swab the tongue.
    e. Moisten and squeeze out a clean swab. Swab the mouth to rinse.
    f. Place used swabs in the kidney basin.
16. Remove the kidney basin and supplies.
17. Wipe the person's mouth. Remove the towel.
18. Apply lubricant to the lips.
19. Remove and discard the gloves. Practice hand hygiene.

Continued

Providing Mouth Care for the Unconscious Person—cont'd

POST-PROCEDURE

20 Provide for comfort. (See the inside of the back cover.)
21 Place the call light and other needed items within reach.
22 Lower the bed to a safe and comfortable level. Follow the care plan.
23 Raise or lower bed rails. Follow the care plan.
24 Clean, rinse, dry, and return equipment to its proper place. Use clean, dry paper towels for drying. Discard disposable items. (Wear gloves.)
25 Wipe off the over-bed table with paper towels. Discard the paper towels.

26 Unscreen the person.
27 Complete a safety check of the room. (See the inside of the back cover.)
28 Tell the person that you are leaving the room. Tell him or her when you will return.
29 Follow agency policy for used linens.
30 Remove and discard the gloves. Practice hand hygiene.
31 Report and record your observations.

Denture Care

A *denture is a removable replacement for missing teeth* (Fig. 23-9). Tooth loss occurs from gum disease, tooth decay, or injury. Often called *false teeth*, complete and partial dentures are common.

- *Complete (full) dentures.* Dentures replace all of the upper or lower teeth.
- *Partial dentures.* The person has some teeth. The partial denture replaces the missing teeth.

Mouth care is given and dentures cleaned as often as natural teeth. Dentures are slippery when wet. They easily break or chip if dropped onto a hard surface (floor, sink, counter). Hold them firmly when removing or inserting them. During cleaning, firmly hold them over a sink filled half-way with water. Line the sink with a towel. This prevents the dentures from falling onto a hard surface.

For cleaning, you need a denture cleaner, denture cup (see Fig. 23-9), and denture brush or toothbrush. Use only denture cleaning products to avoid damaging dentures.

The manufacturer's instructions tell how to use the cleaning agent and what water temperature to use. Hot water causes warping—dentures lose their shape. When not worn, store them in a denture cup with cool or warm water or a denture soaking solution. Otherwise they can dry out and warp.

Dentures are usually removed at bedtime. They are soaked over-night in a denture cleaning solution or water. Rinse the dentures before they are inserted.

Some people do not wear their dentures. Others wear them only for eating. Remind patients and residents not to wrap dentures in tissues or napkins. Otherwise, they are easily discarded.

If able, the person cleans the dentures. You clean dentures for persons who cannot do so.

See *Promoting Safety and Comfort: Denture Care.*
See procedure: *Providing Denture Care.*

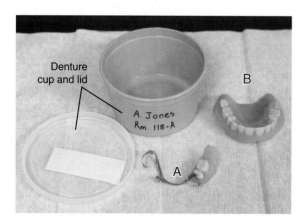

FIGURE 23-9 Dentures and a denture cup. **A,** Partial denture. **B,** Complete (full) denture.

PROMOTING SAFETY AND COMFORT

Denture Care

Safety

The person's property, dentures are costly. Handle them very carefully. Label the denture cup and lid with the person's name and room and bed number (see Fig. 23-9). Report lost or damaged dentures at once.

Never carry dentures in your hands. Always use a denture cup or kidney basin. You could easily drop the dentures if holding them.

Dentures are rinsed under running water. Do not rinse dentures in the water used to fill the sink. Do not place dentures in the sink. The sink is contaminated.

Comfort

Persons with partial dentures have some teeth. They need to brush and floss natural teeth. See procedure: *Assisting the Person to Brush and Floss the Teeth,* p. 342. Or see procedure: *Brushing and Flossing the Person's Teeth,* p. 343.

A denture adhesive may be used to hold dentures in place and keep food out of the inner part of the denture. The product (paste, cream, powder, pad, or strip) is applied to clean dentures. Follow the manufacturer's instructions for how to apply and the amount to use. When cleaning dentures, gently brush to remove the adhesive. Adhesives are not used to fix dentures that fit poorly. Tell the nurse if dentures are loose.

Providing Denture Care

QUALITY OF LIFE

- Knock before entering the person's room.
- Address the person by name.
- Introduce yourself by name and title.

- Explain the procedure before starting and during the procedure.
- Protect the person's rights during the procedure.
- Handle the person gently during the procedure.

PRE-PROCEDURE

1 Follow *Delegation Guidelines: Purpose of Oral Hygiene*, p. 341. See *Promoting Safety and Comfort:*
  a Purpose of Oral Hygiene, p. 341
  b Denture Care
2 Practice hand hygiene.
3 Collect the following.
- Denture brush or toothbrush (for cleaning dentures)
- Denture cup and lid labeled with the person's name and room and bed number
- Denture cleaning agent
- Denture adhesive as noted in the care plan (if needed)
- Mouthwash (or other noted solution)
- Kidney basin
- 2 hand towels
- Gauze squares
- Paper towels
- Gloves

4 Place the paper towels on the over-bed table. Arrange items on top of them.
5 Identify the person. Check the ID bracelet against the assignment sheet. Use 2 identifiers (Chapter 13). Also call the person by name.
6 Provide for privacy.

PROCEDURE

7 Line the bottom of the sink with a towel. Do not use paper towels. Fill the sink half-way with water.
8 Raise the bed for body mechanics.
9 Lower the bed rail near you if up.
10 Practice hand hygiene. Put on the gloves.
11 Place a towel over the person's chest.
12 Have the person remove the dentures. Carefully place them in the kidney basin.
13 Remove the dentures if the person cannot do so. Use gauze squares for a good grip on the slippery dentures.
  a Grasp the upper denture with your thumb and index finger (Fig. 23-10, p. 348). Move it up and down slightly to break the seal. Gently remove the denture. Place it in the kidney basin.
  b Grasp and remove the lower denture with your thumb and index finger. Turn it slightly and lift it out of the person's mouth. Place it in the kidney basin.
14 Follow the care plan for raising bed rails.
15 Take the kidney basin, denture cup and lid, denture brush, and denture cleaning agent to the sink.
16 Rinse the denture cup and lid.
17 Rinse each denture under cool or warm running water. Follow agency policy for water temperature.
18 Return dentures to the kidney basin.
19 Apply the denture cleaning agent to the brush.
20 Brush each denture as in Figure 23-11, p. 348. Brush the inner, outer, and chewing surfaces and all surfaces that touch the gums.

21 Rinse the dentures under running water. Use warm or cool water as directed by the cleaning agent manufacturer.
22 Place dentures in the denture cup. Cover the dentures with cool or warm water. Follow agency policy for water temperature. Close the lid tightly.
23 Clean the kidney basin.
24 Take the denture cup and kidney basin to the over-bed table. Lower the bed rail if up.
25 Have the person use mouthwash (or noted solution). Hold the kidney basin under the chin.
26 Apply denture adhesive if used. Follow the manufacturer's instructions for how to apply and the amount to use.
27 Have the person insert the dentures. Insert them if the person cannot.
  a Hold the upper denture firmly with your thumb and index finger. Raise the upper lip with the other hand. Insert the denture. Gently press on the denture with your index finger to make sure it is in place.
  b Hold the lower denture with your thumb and index finger. Pull the lower lip down slightly. Insert the denture. Gently press down on it to make sure it is in place.
28 Place the denture cup with the dentures in the top drawer of the bedside stand if the dentures are not worn. The dentures must be in water or in a denture soaking solution. Make sure the lid is on tight.
29 Wipe the person's mouth. Remove the towel.
30 Remove and discard the gloves. Practice hand hygiene.

Continued

Providing Denture Care—cont'd

POST-PROCEDURE

31 Assist with hand hygiene.
32 Provide for comfort. (See the inside of the back cover.)
33 Place the call light and other needed items within reach.
34 Lower the bed to a safe and comfortable level. Follow the care plan.
35 Raise or lower bed rails. Follow the care plan.
36 Remove the towel from the sink. Drain the sink.
37 Rinse the brushes. Empty and rinse the denture cup. Clean, rinse, and dry equipment. Use clean, dry paper towels for drying. Return the brushes and equipment to their proper place. Discard disposable items. Wear gloves for this step.

38 Wipe off the over-bed table with paper towels. Discard the paper towels.
39 Unscreen the person.
40 Complete a safety check of the room. (See the inside of the back cover.)
41 Follow agency policy for used linens.
42 Remove and discard the gloves. Practice hand hygiene.
43 Report and record your observations.

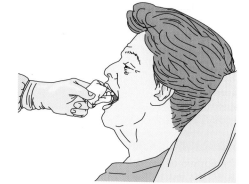

FIGURE 23-10 Remove the upper denture by grasping it with the thumb and index finger of 1 hand. Use a piece of gauze to grasp the denture.

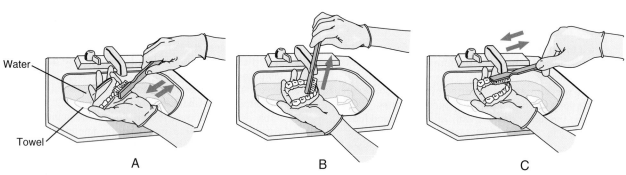

Water

Towel

A   B   C

FIGURE 23-11 Cleaning dentures. **A,** Brush the outer surfaces of the denture with back-and-forth motions. (Note that the denture is held over the sink. The sink is lined with a towel and filled half-way with water.) **B,** Position the brush vertically to clean the inner surfaces of the denture. Use upward strokes. **C,** Brush the chewing surfaces with back-and-forth motions.

REPORTING AND RECORDING

You make many observations while assisting with oral hygiene.

- Dry, cracked, swollen, or blistered lips
- Mouth or breath odor
- Redness, swelling, irritation, sores, or white patches in the mouth or on the tongue
- Bleeding, swelling, or redness of the gums
- Loose teeth
- Rough, sharp, or chipped areas on dentures

Report and record your observations and the oral hygiene given (Fig. 23-12). If not recorded, it is assumed that oral hygiene was not given. This can cause serious legal problems. Tell the nurse if the person refuses oral hygiene or if it was not given for another reason.

ORAL HYGIENE

Observations

Lips	Gums	Mouth and tongue
☒ Dry, cracked	☐ Bleeding	☐ Mouth or breath odor
☐ Swelling	☐ Swelling	☐ Swelling
☐ Blisters	☐ Redness	☐ Redness
☐ Pain	☐ Pain or irritation	☐ Pain or irritation
☐ Other: _____	☐ Other: _____	☐ Sores
		☐ White patches

Teeth
☒ Pain
☐ Loose teeth
☐ Other: _____

Dentures
☐ Rough or sharp area(s)
☐ Chipped area(s)
☐ Loose denture(s)

☐ Other: _____

Nurse notified: M. Rhodes, RN

Care Measures

Oral hygiene
☒ Teeth brushed
☒ Mouth structures brushed (tongue, roof of mouth, inside of cheeks, gums)
☒ Teeth flossed
☐ Mouth structures cleaned with sponge swabs
☒ Lip lubricant applied

Denture care
☐ Upper denture
☐ Lower denture
☐ Denture(s) cleaned
☐ Adhesive applied
☐ Denture(s) placed in mouth
☐ Denture(s) soaked in cleaning solution

FIGURE 23-12 Charting sample.

FOCUS ON PRIDE

The Person, Family, and Yourself

Personal and Professional Responsibility

Good oral hygiene helps prevent cavities, periodontal disease, and tooth loss. It also helps prevent breath odors that can be offensive to patients and residents. You have a personal and professional responsibility to practice thorough brushing and flossing.

Rights and Respect

Many people do not like being seen without their dentures. The person has the right to privacy. Allow privacy when the person cleans dentures. If you clean dentures, return them to the person as quickly as possible.

Independence and Social Interaction

Poor oral hygiene can affect appearance and cause breath odors. When self-esteem is affected, the person may avoid social contact with others. Follow the care plan to meet the person's social needs.

Delegation and Teamwork

After meals, you will remove food trays from patient and resident rooms or assist residents from dining rooms. You will do so for persons assigned to you and to your co-workers. Always check food trays and place settings for dentures. Some persons remove them after meals or wrap them in napkins after eating. Costly to replace, such dentures are easily discarded by the staff.

Ethics and Laws

Illness, drugs, oxygen, and other factors can dry the mucous membranes of the mouth. Some people like to brush their teeth at different times throughout the day and before and after meals. Doing so keeps the mouth feeling fresh, moist, and clean.

Thorough oral hygiene takes time. Follow the person's preferences for when and how often to assist with oral hygiene. Do not neglect oral hygiene.

FOCUS ON PRIDE: Application

What are your oral hygiene practices? How do you feel after performing oral hygiene? How can you improve your practices?

REVIEW QUESTIONS

Circle T if the statement is TRUE and F if it is FALSE.

1   T   F   A toothbrush with hard bristles is used for oral hygiene.

2   T   F   A baby's teeth are flossed when 2 teeth touch.

3   T   F   Unconscious persons are supine for mouth care.

4   T   F   You use your fingers to keep the unconscious person's mouth open for oral hygiene.

5   T   F   The upper denture is in the sink while cleaning the lower denture.

6   T   F   A person has a partial denture. Natural teeth are brushed.

Circle the BEST answer.

7   You perform oral hygiene to
   a   Prevent aspiration
   b   Remove excess oils and perspiration
   c   Prevent mouth odors and infection
   d   Remove cavities

8   A person should floss
   a   Every morning
   b   Before meals
   c   Before brushing
   d   At least once a day

9   When cleaning dentures
   a   Rinse the dentures in the water in the sink
   b   Carry the dentures in your hands
   c   Line the sink with a towel
   d   Rinse the dentures in hot water

10   Which must you report to the nurse?
   a   Clean dentures
   b   Moist and intact lips
   c   Bleeding gums
   d   Food between the teeth

Answers to Chapter 23 questions are on p. 886.

FOCUS ON PRACTICE

Problem Solving

Two residents share a bathroom. You are gathering supplies for oral care. Two toothbrushes and toothpaste are in the bathroom. The items are not labeled. What will you do? How can you be sure that residents use their own equipment?

Daily Hygiene and Bathing

OBJECTIVES

- Define the key terms and key abbreviations in this chapter.
- Explain why daily hygiene and bathing are important.
- Describe the care given before and after breakfast, after lunch, and in the evening.
- Describe the rules for bathing.
- Identify safety measures for tub baths and showers.

- Explain the purposes of perineal care.
- Identify the observations to report and record related to daily hygiene and bathing.
- Perform the procedures described in this chapter.
- Explain how to promote PRIDE in the person, the family, and yourself.

KEY TERMS

AM care See "early morning care"
circumcised The fold of skin (foreskin) covering the glans of the penis was surgically removed
diaphoresis Profuse (excessive) sweating
early morning care Routine care given before breakfast; AM care
evening care Care given in the evening at bedtime; PM care

morning care Care given after breakfast; hygiene measures are more thorough at this time
pericare See "perineal care"
perineal care Cleaning the genital and anal areas; pericare
PM care See "evening care"
uncircumcised Foreskin covers the head of the penis

KEY ABBREVIATIONS

C   Centigrade
F   Fahrenheit

ID   Identification

Daily hygiene and bathing practices promote comfort, safety, and health. The skin is the body's first line of defense against disease. Intact skin prevents microbes from entering the body and causing an infection. Besides cleansing, hygiene measures prevent body and breath odors, are relaxing, and increase circulation.

Culture and personal choice affect hygiene. (See *Caring About Culture: Daily Hygiene and Bathing*, p. 352.) Bathing type and time preferences vary—shower or tub bath; morning, bedtime, before or after work, and so on. Bathing frequency also varies—daily, weekly, 1 or 2 times a week, 1 or 2 times a day. Some illnesses and dry skin may limit bathing to every 2 or 3 days. Some people do not have water for bathing. Others cannot afford soap, deodorant, shampoo, or other hygiene products.

Many factors affect daily hygiene needs—perspiration (sweating), elimination, vomiting, drainage from wounds or body openings, bed rest, and activity. Illness and aging can affect self-care abilities. Some people need help with hygiene. The nurse uses the nursing process to meet the person's needs. Follow the nurse's directions and the care plan.

See *Body Structure and Function Review: The Skin*, p. 352. For greater detail, see Chapter 10.

See *Focus on Communication: Daily Hygiene and Bathing*, p. 352.

See *Focus on Children and Older Persons: Daily Hygiene and Bathing*, p. 353.

See *Promoting Safety and Comfort: Daily Hygiene and Bathing*, p. 353.

✿ CARING ABOUT CULTURE

Daily Hygiene and Bathing

Personal hygiene is very important to *East Indian Hindus*. For religious duty, at least 1 bath a day is required. Some believe bathing after a meal is harmful. Another belief is that a cold bath prevents a blood disease. Some believe that eye injuries can occur if bath water is too hot. Hot water can be added to cold water. However, cold water is not added to hot water for a bath. After bathing, the body is carefully dried with a towel.

(NOTE: Each person is unique. A person may not follow all of the beliefs and practices of his or her culture. Follow the care plan.)

From Giger JN: Transcultural nursing: assessment and intervention, *ed 6, St Louis, 2013, Mosby.*

FOCUS ON COMMUNICATION

Daily Hygiene and Bathing

During hygiene and bathing procedures, the person must be warm enough. You can ask:
- "Is the water warm enough?" "Is it too hot?" "Is it too cold?"
- "Are you warm enough?"
- "Do you need another bath blanket?"
- "Is the water starting to cool?"
- "Is the room warm enough?"

BODY STRUCTURE AND FUNCTION REVIEW

The Skin

The *skin* is the body's natural covering. There are 2 skin layers (Fig. 24-1).
- The *epidermis* is the outer layer. Living cells die, flake off, and are replaced by new living cells. Living cells of the epidermis contain *pigment* that gives skin its color. This layer has no blood vessels and few nerve endings.
- The *dermis* is the inner layer. It is made up of connective tissue. Blood vessels, nerves, sweat glands, oil glands, and hair roots are found in the dermis.

Sweat glands (sudoriferous glands) help regulate body temperature. Sweat is secreted through pores in the skin. The body is cooled as sweat evaporates. *Oil glands (sebaceous glands)* secrete an oily substance near the hair shafts. The oil helps to keep the hair and skin soft and shiny.

The skin has many functions.
- Provides the body's protective covering.
- Prevents microbes and other substances from entering the body.
- Prevents excess amounts of water from leaving the body.
- Protects organs from injury.
- Contains nerve endings that sense pleasant and unpleasant stimulation. They sense cold, pain, touch, and pressure to protect the body from injury.
- Helps regulate body temperature. Blood vessels *dilate* (widen) when the temperature outside the body is high. More blood is brought to the body surface for cooling during evaporation. When blood vessels *constrict* (narrow), the body retains heat. This is because less blood reaches the skin.
- Stores fat and water.

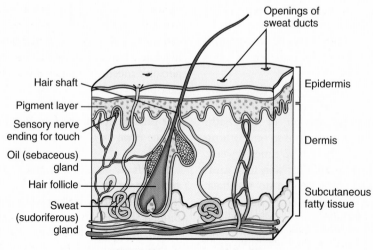

FIGURE 24-1 Structures of the skin.

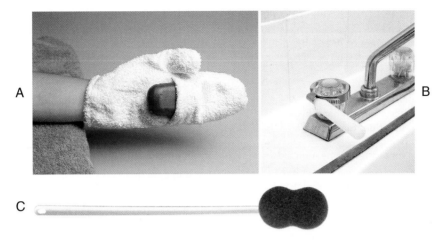

FIGURE 24-2 Adaptive (assistive) devices for hygiene. **A,** The wash mitt holds a bar of soap. **B,** A tap turner makes round knobs easy to turn. **C,** A long-handled sponge is used for hard-to-reach body parts. (Courtesy ElderStore, Alpharetta, Ga.)

FOCUS ON **CHILDREN AND OLDER PERSONS**

Daily Hygiene and Bathing

Older Persons
Some older persons resist hygiene efforts. Illness, disability, dementia, and personal choice are common reasons. Follow the care plan. Also see Chapter 53.

Bending and reaching are hard for older and disabled persons. Some have weak hand grips. They cannot hold soap or a washcloth. Adaptive (assistive) devices for hygiene promote independence (Fig. 24-2). Let the person do as much as safely possible.

PROMOTING SAFETY AND COMFORT

Daily Hygiene and Bathing

Safety
Hygiene and bathing measures often involve exposing and touching private areas—breasts, perineum, rectum. Sexual abuse has occurred in health care settings. The person may feel threatened or actually be abused. He or she needs to call for help. Keep the call light within the person's reach at all times. And always act in a professional manner.

You make observations while assisting with daily hygiene and bathing. The *Delegation Guidelines* in this chapter list the observations to report and record. Also report the following at once.

- Bleeding
- Signs of skin breakdown
- Discharge from the vagina, urinary tract, or rectum
- Unusual odors
- Changes from prior observations

NOTE: A task may require more than 1 pair of gloves. Change gloves as needed. Use careful judgment. Remember to practice hand hygiene after removing gloves.

DAILY HYGIENE

Most people have hygiene routines and habits. For example, teeth are brushed and the face and hands washed after sleep. These and other hygiene measures are common before and after meals and at bedtime.

Infants and young children need help with hygiene. So do some weak and disabled persons. Routine care is given during the day and evening (Box 24-1, p. 354).

- *Early morning care (AM care)—routine care given before breakfast.*
- *Morning care—care given after breakfast. Hygiene measures are more thorough at this time.*
- *Evening care (PM care)—care given in the evening at bedtime.*

You also assist with hygiene as needed. Always protect the right to privacy and to personal choice.

BATHING

Bathing cleans the skin and the genital and anal areas. Microbes, dead skin, perspiration, and excess oils are removed. A bath is refreshing and relaxing. Circulation is stimulated and body parts exercised. Observations are made and you have time to talk to the person.

Complete or partial bed baths, tub baths, or showers are given. The method depends on the person's condition, self-care abilities, and personal choice. In hospitals, bathing is common after breakfast. In nursing centers, bathing is usually before or after breakfast or after the evening meal. The person's choice of bath time is respected when possible.

The rules for bed baths, showers, and tub baths are listed in Box 24-2 (p. 354). Table 24-1 (p. 354) describes common skin care products.

See *Focus on Children and Older Persons: Bathing,* p. 355.
See *Delegation Guidelines: Bathing,* p. 356.
See *Promoting Safety and Comfort: Bathing,* p. 356.

Text continued on p. 357.

BOX 24-1   Daily Care

Before Breakfast (Early Morning Care or AM Care)
- Prepare for breakfast or morning tests.
- Assist with elimination.
- Clean incontinent persons.
- Change wet or soiled linens and garments.
- Assist with washing the face and with hand hygiene.
- Assist with oral hygiene. Insert dentures if worn.
- Assist with dressing and hair care.
- Assist with eyeglasses or contact lenses, hearing aids, and other needed devices.
- Position for breakfast—dining room, bedside chair, or in bed.
- Make beds and straighten units.

After Breakfast (Morning Care)
- Assist with elimination.
- Clean incontinent persons.
- Change wet or soiled linens and garments.
- Assist with washing the face, hand hygiene, oral hygiene, bathing, and perineal care.
- Provide back massages and other comfort measures.
- Assist with hair care, shaving, dressing, and undressing.
- Assist with range-of-motion exercises and ambulation.
- Clean eyeglasses.
- Make beds and straighten rooms.

Afternoon Care
- Prepare for naps, visitors, or activity programs.
- Assist with elimination.
- Clean incontinent persons.
- Change wet or soiled linens and garments.
- Assist with washing the face, hand hygiene, oral hygiene, and hair care.
- Assist with range-of-motion exercises and ambulation.
- Straighten beds and units.

Evening Care (PM Care)
- Prepare for sleep.
- Assist with elimination.
- Clean incontinent persons.
- Change wet or soiled linens and garments.
- Assist with washing the face and with hand hygiene.
- Assist with oral hygiene. Remove dentures if worn.
- Provide back massages and other comfort measures.
- Help with changing into sleepwear.
- Store eyeglasses or contact lenses, hearing aids, and other devices.
- Straighten beds and units.

BOX 24-2   Rules for Bathing

- Follow the care plan for bathing method and skin care products.
- Allow personal choice when possible.
- Follow Standard Precautions and the Bloodborne Pathogen Standard.
- Collect needed items before the procedure.
- Remove hearing aids before bathing. Water will damage hearing aids.
- Provide for privacy. Screen the person. Close doors and window coverings—drapes, shades, blinds, shutters, and so on.
- Assist with elimination. Bathing stimulates the need to urinate. Comfort and relaxation increase if the person urinates first.
- Cover the person for warmth and privacy.
- Reduce drafts. Close doors and windows.
- Protect the person from falling.
- Use good body mechanics at all times.
- Follow the rules to safely move and transfer the person (Chapters 19 and 20).
- Know what water temperature to use. See *Delegation Guidelines: Bathing*, p. 356.
- Keep bar soap in the soap dish between latherings. This prevents soapy water. It also prevents slipping and falls in showers and tubs.
- Wash from clean to dirty areas.
- Encourage the person to help as much as safely possible.
- Rinse the skin thoroughly. You must remove all soap.
- Pat dry the skin to avoid irritating or breaking the skin. Do not rub the skin.
- Dry well under the breasts, between skin folds, in the perineal area (p. 366), and between the toes.
- Bathe skin when urine or feces (stools) are present. This prevents skin breakdown and odors.

TABLE 24-1   Skin Care Products

Type	Purpose	Care Considerations
Bar soaps	• Clean the skin • Remove dirt, dead skin, skin oil, some microbes, and perspiration	• Can dry and irritate the skin. Easily injured, dry skin causes itching and discomfort. • Rinse the skin thoroughly to remove all soap. • Not needed for every bath. Plain water can clean the skin. • Plain water is often used for older persons with dry skin. • People with dry skin may use soaps with bath oils. • Not used for very dry skin.
Body washes and shower gels	• See "Bar soaps"	• Gentle on the skin. • May contain a moisturizer or skin softener. • Liquid. Not a solid like bar soap. • Rinse thoroughly.

TABLE 24-1	Skin Care Products—cont'd	
Type	Purpose	Care Considerations
No-rinse cleansers	• Clean the skin • Control odor • Moisturize	• Sprays and foams are common. • Apply to a damp or dry washcloth or the person's skin. Follow the manufacturer's instructions. Wash and pat dry. No rinsing is needed. • Perineal cleansers are for perineal care (p. 366).
Bath oils	• Keep the skin soft • Prevent dry skin	• Some soaps have bath oil. • Liquid bath oil can be added to bath water. • Bath oils make showers and tubs slippery. Practice safety measures to prevent falls.
Creams and lotions	• Protect the skin from the drying effect of air and evaporation	• Do not feel greasy but leave an oily film on the skin. • Lotion is applied to bony areas after bathing to prevent skin breakdown (back, elbows, knees, and heels). • Lotion is used for back massages (Chapter 35).
Powders	• Absorb moisture • Prevent friction when skin surfaces rub together	• May be applied under the breasts, under the arms, in the groin area (where a thigh and the abdomen meet), and between the toes. • Applied in a thin, even layer after drying the skin. • Excessive amounts cause caking and crusts that irritate the skin.
Deodorants	• Mask and control body odors	• Applied to the underarms. • Not applied to irritated skin. • Do not replace bathing.
Antiperspirants	• Reduce the amount of perspiration	• See "Deodorants."

FOCUS ON CHILDREN AND OLDER PERSONS

Bathing

Children
The care plan reflects the child's normal practices and needs during illness. Many older children enjoy showers. The nurse tells you how much help and supervision the child needs. Remember, independence and privacy are important to older children.

See "Bathing an Infant" in Chapter 56.

Older Persons
Aging and soap dry the skin. Dry skin is easily damaged. Therefore older persons need a complete bed bath, tub bath, or shower only twice a week. They have partial baths on the other days. Some bathe daily without soap. Thorough rinsing is needed for soap. Lotions and oils help soften the skin.

Bathing procedures can threaten persons with dementia. They do not understand what is happening or why. They may fear harm or danger. Confusion can increase. Some may resist care and become agitated and combative. They may shout at you and cry out for help. Remain calm, patient, and soothing.

The person may be calmer and less confused or agitated during a certain time of day. Bathing is scheduled for calm times. The nurse decides the best bathing procedure for the person.

The rules in Box 24-2 apply. The care plan also has measures to help the person through the bath. For example:
- Say "cleaned up" or "washed," rather than "shower" or "bath."
- Complete pre-procedure activities. Ready supplies and linens and have everything you need.
- Provide for warmth. Prevent drafts. Have extra towels and a robe nearby.
- Provide good lighting.
- Play soft music to help the person relax.
- Provide for safety.
  - Use a hand-held shower nozzle.
  - Have the person use a shower chair or shower bench.
  - Do not use bath oil. It can make the tub or shower slippery. And it may cause a urinary tract infection.
  - Do not leave the person alone in the tub or shower.
- Draw bath water ahead of time. Test the water temperature and adjust as needed.
- Tell the person what you are doing step-by-step. Use clear, simple words.
- Let the person help as much as possible. For example, give the person a washcloth. Ask him or her to wash the arms or let the person hold the washcloth if safe to do so.
- Put a towel over the shoulders or lap (tub bath or shower). This helps the person feel less exposed.
- Do not rush the person.
- Use a calm, pleasant voice.
- Distract the person if needed.
- Calm the person.
- Handle the person gently.
- Try a partial bath if a shower or tub bath agitates the person.
- Try the bath later if the person continues to resist care.

DELEGATION GUIDELINES

Bathing

Bathing procedures are routine nursing tasks. To assist with bathing, you need this information from the nurse and the care plan.

- What bath to give—complete bed bath, partial bath, tub bath, shower, towel bath, or bag bath.
- How much help the person needs.
- Activity or position limits.
- What water temperature to use. Bath water for bed baths cools rapidly. Heat is lost to the wash basin, over-bed table, washcloth, and your hands. Therefore water temperature for complete bed baths and partial bed baths is usually between 110°F and 115°F (Fahrenheit) (43.3°C and 46.1°C [centigrade]) for adults. Older persons have fragile skin. They need lower water temperatures.
- If you should clean under the toenails.
- What skin care products the person prefers.

- What observations to report and record:
  - The color of the skin, lips, nail beds, and sclera (whites of the eyes)
  - If the skin appears pale, gray-ish, yellow (jaundice—Chapter 50), or bluish (cyanotic)
  - The location and description of rashes
  - Skin texture—smooth, rough, scaly, flaky, dry, moist
  - Diaphoresis—profuse (excessive) sweating
  - Bruises or open skin areas
  - Pale, reddened, or discolored areas, particularly over bony parts
  - Drainage or bleeding from wounds or body openings
  - Swelling of the feet and legs
  - Corns or calluses on the feet
  - Skin temperature (cold, cool, warm, hot)
  - Complaints of pain or discomfort
- When to report observations.
- What patient or resident concerns to report at once.

PROMOTING SAFETY AND COMFORT

Bathing

Safety

Water: Hot water can burn the skin. Measure water temperature according to agency policy. If unsure if the water is too hot, ask the nurse to check it.

Falls and injuries: Protect the person from falls and other injuries. Practice the safety and comfort measures in Chapters 13, 14, and 35.

Body mechanics: Use good body mechanics to protect yourself from injury (Chapter 18). For the procedure that follows, you work on 1 side of the bed. To avoid straining and reaching, move the person to the side of the bed near you. Or wash 1 side of the body and then move to the other side to finish the bath. If room space allows, wash the side of the body near you (eyes and face, arm, hand, chest, abdomen, leg, foot). Then move the over-bed table with equipment and supplies to the other side of the bed. Finish the bath (arm, hand, leg, foot, back, and perineal care) on that side.

Powder: Apply powder with caution. Do not use powders near persons with respiratory disorders. Inhaling powder can irritate the airway and lungs. Before using powder, check with the nurse and the care plan. To safely apply powder:
- Turn away from the person.
- Sprinkle a small amount onto your hand or a cloth. Do not shake or sprinkle powder onto the person.
- Apply the powder in a thin layer.
- Make sure powder does not get on the floor. Powder is slippery and can cause falls.

Bedmaking: You will make the bed after the bath. Lower the bed to a safe and comfortable level for the person. For an occupied bed, raise or lower bed rails according to the care plan. Make sure the bed wheels are locked.

Safety—cont'd

Preventing infection: Protect the person and yourself from infection. During baths and bedmaking, contact with blood, body fluids, secretions, or excretions is likely. Follow Standard Precautions and the Bloodborne Pathogen Standard.

Bathing equipment: Bathing equipment must be clean. A wash basin is used for 1 person. Tubs and showers may be used by many persons. See p. 362 for "Tub Baths and Showers."

Foot care: Ask the nurse if you should clean under the person's toenails. The device used (orangewood stick or nail file) has a sharp tip that could injure the person. Foot injuries can be very serious for some persons. See Chapter 25.

Comfort

Elimination: Before bathing, let the person meet elimination needs (Chapters 27 and 29). Bathing stimulates the need to urinate. Comfort is greater with an empty bladder. Also bathing is not interrupted.

Oral hygiene: Oral hygiene is common before or after bathing. Allow personal choice and follow the care plan.

Warmth: Provide for warmth. Cover the person with a bath blanket. Protect the person from drafts. Make sure the water is warm enough. Cool water causes chilling.

Clothing and sleepwear: If the person prefers, remove clothing or sleepwear after washing the eyes, face, ears, and neck. Removing clothing or sleepwear at this time helps the person feel less exposed and provides more mental comfort with the bath.

Perineal care: If able, have the person wash the genital and anal areas. This promotes privacy and helps prevent embarrassment. See "Perineal Care," p. 366.

Persons With Bariatric Needs

Persons with bariatric needs may need help with hygiene. They may not be able to reach body parts. Skin folds are common. Good hygiene and skin care promote comfort and prevent pressure injuries and other skin problems.

The rules for bathing in Box 24-2 apply. Always follow the person's care plan for:

- How often to bathe the person.
- The bathing method—bed bath, shower, whirlpool.
- The number of staff needed.
- The equipment needed. A bariatric shower chair is an example.
- The cleaning agent to use. Harsh soaps that dry and irritate the skin are avoided.
- How often to clean under skin folds. Such care may be needed several times a day. The person may perspire heavily. Moisture can collect between skin folds, providing a place for microbes to live and grow. Skin irritation and a rash can occur (Fig. 24-3).

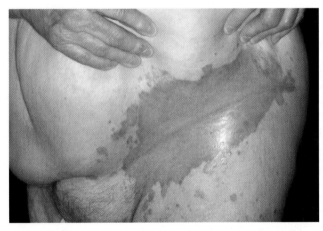

FIGURE 24-3 Rash in a skin fold. (From Habif TP: *Clinical dermatology: A color guide to diagnosis and therapy*, ed 6, Philadelphia, 2016, Elsevier.)

- How to dry under skin folds. The nurse may have you use a hand-held hair dryer on the "cool" setting.
- What product to place under skin folds. The nurse may have you place gauze or cotton-fabric under the folds. The material reduces friction and absorbs moisture.
- What skin care products to use and where to use them—powder, lotion, and so on.

See *Teamwork and Time Management: Persons With Bariatric Needs.*

TEAMWORK AND TIME MANAGEMENT
Persons With Bariatric Needs

Bathing bariatric persons requires teamwork and planning. You may need help to hold skin folds while you clean, dry, and apply skin care products. Or you need to turn or transfer the person. Ask your co-workers for help in advance. Plan a time that is best for the person, your co-workers, and you.

Also allow extra time for hygiene measures. Plan your work to avoid seeming rushed. The person must not feel like a burden. If unsure how much time to allow, ask others who have cared for the person. They can share about the time and help needed.

The Complete Bed Bath

For a complete bed bath, you wash the person's entire body in bed. Bed baths are usually needed by persons who are:

- Unconscious
- Paralyzed
- In casts or traction
- Weak from illness or surgery
- Unable to bathe themselves

A bed bath is new to some people. Some are embarrassed to have their bodies seen. Some fear exposure. Explain how you give the bath and provide for privacy.

See procedure: *Giving a Complete Bed Bath.*

Text continued on p. 360.

Giving a Complete Bed Bath

QUALITY OF LIFE

- Knock before entering the person's room.
- Address the person by name.
- Introduce yourself by name and title.

- Explain the procedure before starting and during the procedure.
- Protect the person's rights during the procedure.
- Handle the person gently during the procedure.

PRE-PROCEDURE

1 Follow *Delegation Guidelines: Bathing.* See *Promoting Safety and Comfort:*
  a *Daily Hygiene and Bathing,* p. 353
  b *Bathing*
2 Practice hand hygiene.

3 Identify the person. Check the ID (identification) bracelet against the assignment sheet. Use 2 identifiers (Chapter 13). Also call the person by name.
4 Collect clean linens. (See procedure: *Making a Closed Bed* in Chapter 22.) Place linens on a clean surface.

Continued

Giving a Complete Bed Bath—cont'd

PRE-PROCEDURE—cont'd

5 Collect the following.
  - Wash basin
  - Soap or body wash
  - Water thermometer
  - Orangewood stick or nail file
  - Washcloth (and at least 4 washcloths for perineal care, p. 366)
  - 2 bath towels and 2 hand towels
  - Bath blanket
  - Clothing or sleepwear
  - Lotion and powder
  - Deodorant or antiperspirant
  - Brush and comb
  - Other grooming items as requested
  - Paper towels
  - Gloves

6 Cover the over-bed table with paper towels. Arrange items on the over-bed table. Adjust the height as needed.

7 Provide for privacy.

8 Raise the bed for body mechanics. Bed rails are up if used. Lower the bed rail near you if up.

PROCEDURE

9 Practice hand hygiene. Put on gloves.

10 Remove clothing or sleepwear. Do not expose the person. Follow agency policy for used clothing or sleepwear.

11 Cover the person with a bath blanket. Remove top linens (see procedure: *Making an Occupied Bed* in Chapter 22).

12 Lower the head of the bed. It is as flat as possible. The person has a least 1 pillow.

13 Fill the wash basin ⅔ (two-thirds) full with water. Raise the bed rail before leaving the bedside. Follow the care plan for water temperature. Water temperature is usually 110°F to 115°F (43.3°C to 46.1°C) for adults. Measure water temperature. Use the water thermometer. Or dip your elbow or inner wrist into the basin to test the water.

14 Lower the bed rail near you if up.

15 Have the person check the water temperature. Adjust the water temperature as needed. Raise the bed rail before leaving the bedside. Lower it when you return.

16 Place the basin on the over-bed table.

17 Place a hand towel over the person's chest.

18 Make a mitt with the washcloth (Fig. 24-4). Use a mitt for the entire bath.

19 Have the person close the eyes. Wash the eyelids and around the eyes with water. Do not use soap.
  a Clean the far eye. Gently wipe from the inner to the outer aspect of the eye with a corner of the mitt (Fig. 24-5).
  b Clean around the eye near you. Use a clean part of the washcloth for each stroke.

20 Apply soap or body wash to the washcloth if the person prefers for washing the face.

21 Wash the face and ears. Use soap or the body wash to wash the neck. Rinse all areas and pat dry with the towel on the chest.

22 Help the person move to the side of the bed near you.

23 Expose the far arm. Place a bath towel length-wise under the arm. Apply soap or body wash to the washcloth.

24 Support the arm with your palm under the person's elbow. His or her forearm rests on your forearm.

25 Wash the arm, shoulder, and underarm. Use long, firm strokes (Fig. 24-6). Rinse and pat dry.

26 Place the basin on the towel. Put the person's hand into the water (Fig. 24-7). Wash the hand well. Clean under the fingernails with an orangewood stick or nail file.

27 Have the person exercise the hand and fingers.

28 Remove the basin. Dry the hand well. Cover the arm with the bath blanket.

29 Repeat steps 23 to 28 for the near arm.

30 Place a bath towel over the chest cross-wise. Hold the towel in place. Pull the bath blanket from under the towel to the waist. Apply soap or body wash to the washcloth.

31 Lift the towel slightly and wash the chest (Fig. 24-8, p. 360). Do not expose the person. Rinse and pat dry, especially under the breasts.

32 Move the towel length-wise over the chest and abdomen. Do not expose the person. Pull the bath blanket down to the pubic area. Apply soap or body wash to the washcloth.

33 Lift the towel slightly and wash the abdomen (Fig. 24-9, p. 360). Rinse and pat dry.

34 Pull the bath blanket up to the shoulders. Cover both arms. Remove the towel.

35 Change soapy or cool water. Measure bath water temperature as in step 13. If bed rails are used, raise the bed rail near you before leaving the bedside. Lower it when you return.

36 Uncover the far leg. Do not expose the genital area. Place a towel length-wise under the foot and leg. Apply soap or body wash to a washcloth.

37 Bend the knee and support the leg with your arm. Wash it with long, firm strokes. Rinse and pat dry.

38 Place the basin on the towel near the foot.

39 Lift the leg slightly. Slide the basin under the foot.

40 Place the foot in the basin (Fig. 24-10, p. 360). Use an orangewood stick or nail file to clean under the toenails if instructed to do so. If the person cannot bend the knees:
  a Wash the foot with soap or body wash. Carefully separate the toes. Rinse and pat dry.
  b Clean under the toenails with an orangewood stick or nail file if directed to do so.

41 Remove the basin. Dry the leg and foot. Apply lotion to the foot if directed by the nurse and care plan. Do not apply lotion between the toes. Cover the leg with the bath blanket. Remove the towel.

42 Repeat steps 36 to 41 for the near leg.

43 Change the water. Measure water temperature as in step 13. Raise the bed rail near you before leaving the bedside. Lower it when you return.

44 Turn the person onto the side away from you. The person is covered with the bath blanket.

45 Uncover the back and buttocks. Do not expose the person. Place a towel length-wise on the bed along the back. Apply soap or body wash to a washcloth.

46 Wash the back. Work from the back of the neck to the lower end of the buttocks. Use long, firm, continuous strokes (Fig. 24-11, p. 360). Rinse and dry well.

47 Turn the person onto his or her back.

Giving a Complete Bed Bath—cont'd

PROCEDURE—cont'd

48 Change water for perineal care (p. 366). See step 14 in procedure: *Giving Female Perineal Care* (p. 367) for water temperature. (Some state competency tests also require changing gloves and hand hygiene at this time.) Raise the bed rail near you before leaving the bedside. Lower it when you return.

49 Have the person perform perineal care if able. Provide perineal care if the person cannot do so. At least 4 washcloths are used. (Practice hand hygiene and wear gloves for perineal care.)

50 Remove and discard the gloves. Practice hand hygiene.

51 Give a back massage (Chapter 35).

52 Apply lotion, powder, and deodorant or antiperspirant as requested. See *Promoting Safety and Comfort: Bathing*, p. 356.

53 Put clean garments on the person (Chapter 26).

54 Comb and brush the person's hair (Chapter 25).

55 Make the bed.

POST-PROCEDURE

56 Provide for comfort. (See the inside of the back cover.)

57 Place the call light and other needed items within reach.

58 Lower the bed to a safe and comfortable level. Follow the care plan.

59 Raise or lower bed rails. Follow the care plan.

60 Put on clean gloves.

61 Empty, clean, rinse, and dry the wash basin. Use clean, dry paper towels for drying. Return the basin and other supplies to their proper place.

62 Wipe off the over-bed table with paper towels. Discard the paper towels.

63 Unscreen the person.

64 Complete a safety check of the room. (See the inside of the back cover.)

65 Follow agency policy for used linens.

66 Remove and discard the gloves. Practice hand hygiene.

67 Report and record your observations.

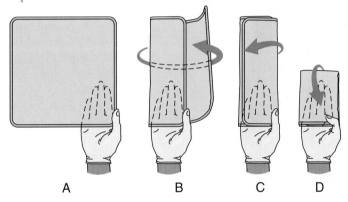

FIGURE 24-4 Making a mitted washcloth. **A,** Grasp the near side of the washcloth with your thumb. **B,** Bring the washcloth around and behind your hand. **C,** Fold the side of the washcloth over your palm as you grasp it with your thumb. **D,** Fold the top of the washcloth down and tuck it under next to your palm.

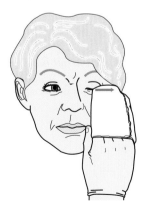

FIGURE 24-5 Wash the eyes with a mitted washcloth. Wipe from the inner to the outer aspect of the eye.

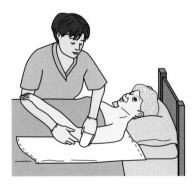

FIGURE 24-6 The arm is washed with firm, long strokes using a mitted washcloth. (NOTE: Bed rails are used according to the care plan.)

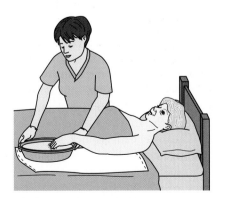

FIGURE 24-7 The hand is washed by placing the wash basin on the bed. (NOTE: Bed rails are used according to the care plan.)

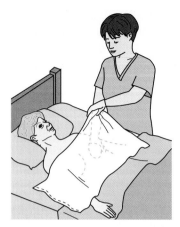

FIGURE 24-8 The breasts are not exposed during the bath. A bath towel is placed horizontally over the chest area. The towel is lifted slightly to reach under and wash the breasts and chest. (NOTE: Bed rails are used according to the care plan.)

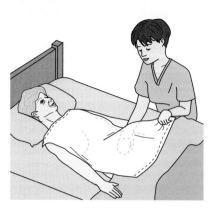

FIGURE 24-9 The bath towel is turned so that it is vertical to cover the breasts and abdomen. The towel is lifted slightly to bathe the abdomen. The bath blanket covers the pubic area. (NOTE: Bed rails are used according to the care plan.)

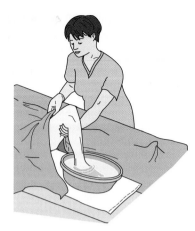

FIGURE 24-10 The foot is washed by placing it in the wash basin on the bed. (NOTE: Bed rails are used according to the care plan.)

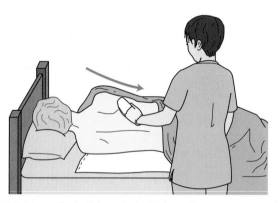

FIGURE 24-11 The back is washed with long, firm, continuous strokes. Note that the person is in a side-lying position. A towel is placed length-wise on the bed to protect the linens from water. (NOTE: Bed rails are used according to the care plan.)

Towel Baths

For a towel bath, an over-sized towel covers the person from the neck to the feet. The towel is wet with a solution of water and cleaning, skin-softening, and drying agents. The drying agent lets the skin dry fast. No rinsing is needed. The nurse and care plan tell you when to give a towel bath. To give a towel bath, follow agency policy.

The towel bath is quick, soothing, and relaxing. Persons with dementia often respond well to towel baths.

Bag Baths

Bag baths are commercially prepared. The plastic bag has 8 to 10 washcloths moistened with a cleansing agent. No rinsing is needed. To give a bag bath:

- Follow the manufacturer's instructions to warm the washcloths.
- Use a new washcloth for each body part.
- Let the skin air-dry. You do not need towels.
- Discard the washcloths following agency policy. Do not flush them down the toilet.

The Partial Bath

For a *partial bath*, the face, hands, underarms, back, buttocks, and perineal area are washed. Bathing prevents odors and discomfort in those areas. Some persons can wash in bed, at the bedside, or at the sink. Assist as needed. Most need help washing the back. You give partial baths to persons who cannot bathe themselves.

The rules for bathing apply (see Box 24-2). So do the complete bed bath considerations.

See procedure: *Assisting With the Partial Bath.*

Assisting With the Partial Bath

QUALITY OF LIFE

- Knock before entering the person's room.
- Address the person by name.
- Introduce yourself by name and title.

- Explain the procedure before starting and during the procedure.
- Protect the person's rights during the procedure.
- Handle the person gently during the procedure.

PRE-PROCEDURE

1 Follow *Delegation Guidelines: Bathing*, p. 356. See *Promoting Safety and Comfort:*
   a *Daily Hygiene and Bathing*, p. 353
   b *Bathing*, p. 356

2 Follow steps 2 through 7 in procedure: *Giving a Complete Bed Bath*, p. 357.

PROCEDURE

3 Make sure the bed is in a low position.
4 Practice hand hygiene. Put on gloves.
5 Cover the person with a bath blanket. Remove top linens.
6 Fill the wash basin ⅔ (two-thirds) full with water. Water temperature is usually 110°F to 115°F (43.3°C to 46.1°C) or as directed by the nurse. Measure water temperature with the water thermometer. Or test bath water by dipping your elbow or inner wrist into the basin.
7 Have the person check the water temperature. Adjust the water temperature as needed.
8 Place the basin on the over-bed table.
9 Position the person in Fowler's position or sitting at the bedside.
10 Adjust the over-bed table so the person can reach the basin and supplies.
11 Help the person undress. Use the bath blanket for privacy and warmth.
12 Have the person wash easy-to-reach body parts (Fig. 24-12). Explain that you will wash the back and areas the person cannot reach.
13 Place the call light within reach. Have the person signal when help is needed or bathing is complete.

14 Remove and discard the gloves. Practice hand hygiene. Then leave the room.
15 Return when the call light is on. Knock before entering. Practice hand hygiene.
16 Change the bath water. Measure bath water temperature as in step 6.
17 Raise the bed for body mechanics. The far bed rail is up if used.
18 Ask what was washed. Put on gloves. Wash and dry areas the person could not reach. The face, hands, underarms, back, buttocks, and perineal area are washed for the partial bath.
19 Remove and discard the gloves. Practice hand hygiene.
20 Give a back massage (Chapter 35).
21 Apply lotion, powder, and deodorant or antiperspirant as requested.
22 Assist with clean garments, hair care, and other grooming needs.
23 Make the bed.

POST-PROCEDURE

24 Provide for comfort. (See the inside of the back cover.)
25 Place the call light and other needed items within reach.
26 Lower the bed to a safe and comfortable level. Follow the care plan.
27 Raise or lower bed rails. Follow the care plan.
28 Put on clean gloves.
29 Empty, clean, rinse, and dry the wash basin. Use clean, dry paper towels for drying. Return the basin and supplies to their proper place.

30 Wipe off the over-bed table with the paper towels. Discard the paper towels.
31 Unscreen the person.
32 Complete a safety check of the room. (See the inside of the back cover.)
33 Follow agency policy for used linens.
34 Remove and discard the gloves. Practice hand hygiene.
35 Report and record your observations.

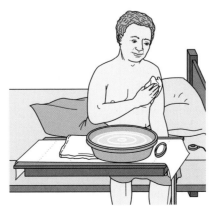

FIGURE 24-12 The person is bathing himself while sitting on the side of the bed. Needed equipment is within reach.

Tub Baths and Showers

Some people like tub baths. Others like showers. Falls, burns, and chilling from water are risks. Safety is important (Box 24-3). The measures in Box 24-2 also apply. Also follow the nurse's directions and the care plan.

BOX 24-3 Tub Bath and Shower Safety

Tub Baths and Showers

- Clean, disinfect, and dry the tub or shower before and after use. Dry the tub or shower room floor.
- Make sure hand rails, grab bars (safety bars), hydraulic lifts, and other safety aids are in working order.
- Place a bath mat in the tub or on the shower floor. This is not needed if there are slip-resistant strips or a slip-resistant surface.
- Provide for warmth and privacy. This includes during transport to and from the tub or shower room.
- Place the call light and other needed items within reach. Show how to use the call light.
- Have the person use grab bars (safety bars) to get in and out of the tub or shower.
- Follow the safety measures and transfer procedures for wheelchairs when using wheeled shower chairs. See Chapter 20.
- Know what water temperature to use (usually 105°F/40.5°C).
- Turn cold water on first, then hot water. Turn hot water off first, then cold water.
- Keep bar soap in the soap dish between latherings. This helps prevent slipping and falls in tubs and showers. It also prevents soapy tub water.
- Avoid bath oils. They make tub and shower surfaces slippery.
- Do not leave weak or unsteady persons unattended.
- Stay within hearing distance if the person can be left alone. Wait outside the door or shower curtain. You must be nearby if the person calls for you or has an accident.

Tub Baths

- Fill the tub before the person gets into it. For a tub with a side entry door, fill the tub with the person in it. Follow the manufacturer's instructions.
- Monitor water temperature as the tub fills.
- Use the digital display or a water thermometer to measure water temperature.
- Have the person check the water temperature. Adjust as needed.
- Drain the tub before the person gets out of the tub.

Showers

- Adjust water temperature to prevent chilling and burns.
- Use the digital display when checking water temperature.
- Have the person check the water temperature. Adjust as needed.
- Direct water away from the person when adjusting water temperature and pressure.
- Keep the water spray directed toward the person during the shower. This provides for warmth.
- Do not direct water spray toward the face. This can frighten the person.
- Turn off the shower before the person gets out of the shower.

Tub Baths

Tub baths are relaxing. However, a tub bath can make a person feel faint, weak, or tired. These are great risks for persons who were on bed rest. A tub bath lasts no longer than 20 minutes.

To get in and out of the tub, the person may use:

- A tub with a side entry door (Fig. 24-13).
- Bathing lift. The device transports and lifts the person into the tub (Fig. 24-14).
- Mechanical lift (Chapter 20).

Whirlpool tubs have a cleansing action. You wash the upper body. Carefully wash under the breasts and between skin folds. Also wash the perineal area. Pat dry the person with towels after the bath.

Showers

Some people can stand during a shower. Grab bars (safety bars) are used for support. Showers have slip-resistant surfaces. If not, a bath mat is used. Weak or unsteady persons use:

- *Shower chairs.* Water drains through an opening (Fig. 24-15). You use the chair to transport the person to and from the shower. Lock (brake) the wheels during the shower to prevent the chair from moving.
- *Shower benches.* The person is seated for the shower (Fig. 24-16).
- *Shower stalls or cabinets.* The person walks into the device or is wheeled to the cabinet in a shower chair (Fig. 24-17). Use the hand-held nozzle for the shower.
- *Shower trolleys (portable tubs).* The person has a shower lying down (Fig. 24-18, p. 364). Lower the sides to transfer the person from the bed to the trolley. Then raise the side rails for transport to the tub or shower room. Use the hand-held nozzle for the shower.

Some shower rooms have 2 or more stations. Provide for privacy. Properly screen and cover the person. Also close doors and shower curtains.

See *Focus on Long-Term Care and Home Care: Tub Baths and Showers*, p. 364.

See *Teamwork and Time Management: Tub Baths and Showers*, p. 364.

See *Delegation Guidelines: Tub Baths and Showers*, p. 364.

See *Promoting Safety and Comfort: Tub Baths and Showers*, p. 364.

See procedure: *Assisting With a Tub Bath or Shower*, p. 365.

Text continued on p. 366.

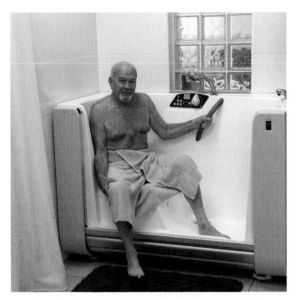

FIGURE 24-13 Tub with a side entry door. (Image used with permission of Arjo Inc.)

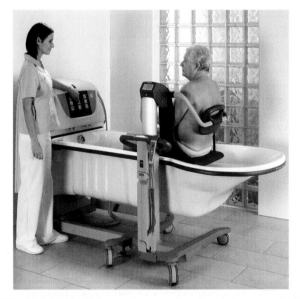

FIGURE 24-14 The lift lowers the person into the tub. (Image used with permission of Arjo Inc.)

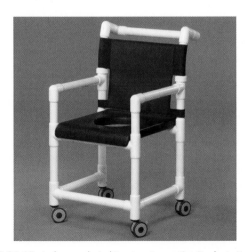

FIGURE 24-15 A shower chair. (Courtesy Innovative Products Unlimited, Niles, Mich.)

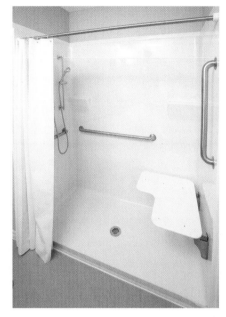

FIGURE 24-16 A shower bench.

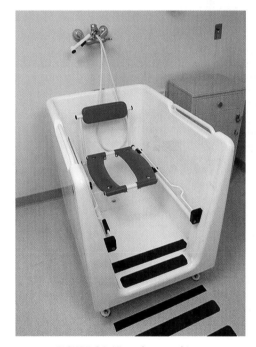

FIGURE 24-17 A shower cabinet.

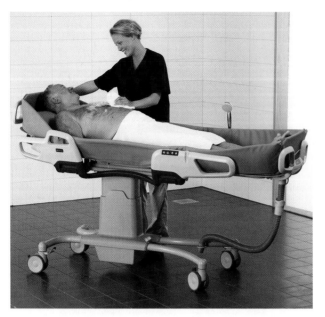

FIGURE 24-18 Shower trolley. The sides are lowered for transfers into and out of the trolley. (Image used with permission of Arjo Inc.)

FOCUS ON LONG-TERM CARE AND HOME CARE

Tub Baths and Showers

Home Care

Many homes have shower stalls or bathtub-shower units. To step into the tub or shower, have the person use the grab bars (safety bars). Help the person in and out of the tub or shower as needed.

The person may need a shower chair. The nurse helps the person and family find a safe chair for shower use.

The bathtub unit may not have a shower. A hand-held shower nozzle can be installed.

TEAMWORK AND TIME MANAGEMENT

Tub Baths and Showers

You need to reserve the tub or shower room and equipment for the person. Your co-workers do the same for their patients and residents.

Consider the needs of others. For example:
- You reserve the shower room from 0945 to 1030. Do your best to follow the schedule. Have the shower room clean and ready for the next person.
- You and a co-worker schedule a shower for the same time. Plan new times with your co-worker.

All bed linens are changed on the person's bath or shower day. Ask co-workers to make the bed while you assist with the tub bath or shower. Also ask them to straighten the person's unit. The person returns to a clean bed and unit. Return the favor when your co-workers are assisting with tub baths, showers, or other care measures.

Shower chairs are often shared. Clean, disinfect, and dry the chair after use. Return the shower chair to its proper place. Other staff know where to find it. Staff do not waste time looking for equipment.

DELEGATION GUIDELINES

Tub Baths and Showers

Before assisting with a tub bath or shower, you need this information from the nurse and the care plan:
- If the person takes a tub bath or shower
- What water temperature to use (usually 105°F/40.5°C)
- What equipment is needed—bathing lift, mechanical lift, shower chair, shower cabinet, shower trolley, and so on
- What size shower chair to use (if needed)—standard or bariatric
- How much help the person needs
- If the person can bathe himself or herself
- What observations to report and record:
  - Dizziness
  - Light-headedness
  - See *Delegation Guidelines: Bathing,* p. 356
- When to report observations
- What patient or resident concerns to report at once

PROMOTING SAFETY AND COMFORT

Tub Baths and Showers

Safety

Some persons are very weak. At least 2 staff are needed for safe tub baths and showers. If the person is heavy, 3 or more staff may be needed.

The person may use a tub with a side entry door, a shower chair, a shower trolley, or other device. Follow the manufacturer's instructions.

Protect the person from falls, chilling, and burns. Follow the safety measures in Chapters 13 and 14. Remember to measure water temperature.

Clean, disinfect, and dry the tub or shower before and after use. This prevents the spread of microbes and infection.

Comfort

Warmth and privacy promote comfort during tub baths and showers.
- Make sure the tub or shower room is warm.
- Provide for privacy. Close the room door, screen the person, and close window coverings.
- Make sure the water is warm enough for the person.
- Have the person remove clothing or robe and footwear just before getting into the tub or shower. Do not have the person exposed longer than necessary.
- Leave the room if the person can be left alone. Stay within hearing distance.

Assisting With a Tub Bath or Shower

QUALITY OF LIFE

- Knock before entering the person's room.
- Address the person by name.
- Introduce yourself by name and title.

- Explain the procedure before starting and during the procedure.
- Protect the person's rights during the procedure.
- Handle the person gently during the procedure.

PRE-PROCEDURE

1 Follow *Delegation Guidelines:*
   a *Bathing*, p. 356
   b *Tub Baths and Showers*
  See *Promoting Safety and Comfort:*
   a *Daily Hygiene and Bathing*, p. 353
   b *Bathing*, p. 356
   c *Tub Baths and Showers*
2 Reserve the tub or shower room.
3 Practice hand hygiene.
4 Identify the person. Check the ID bracelet against the assignment sheet. Use 2 identifiers (Chapter 13). Also call the person by name.

5 Collect the following.
- Washcloth and 2 bath towels
- Bath blanket
- Soap, shower gel, or body wash
- Water thermometer (for a tub bath)
- Clothing or sleepwear
- Grooming items as requested
- Robe and slip-resistant footwear
- Rubber bath mat if needed
- Disposable bath mat
- Gloves
- Wheelchair, shower chair, shower bench, and so on as needed

PROCEDURE

6 Place items in the tub or shower room. Use the space provided or a chair.
7 Clean, disinfect, and dry the tub or shower. Also dry the tub or shower room floor. Use clean, dry paper towels for drying. Wear gloves for this step. Practice hand hygiene after removing and discarding the gloves.
8 Place a rubber bath mat in the tub or on the shower floor. Do not block the drain.
9 Place the disposable bath mat on the floor in front of the tub or shower.
10 Put the OCCUPIED sign on the door.
11 Return to the person's room. Provide for privacy. Practice hand hygiene.
12 Help the person sit on the side of the bed.
13 Help the person put on a robe and slip-resistant footwear. Or the person can leave on clothing.
14 Assist or transport the person to the tub or shower room.
15 Have the person sit on a chair if he or she walked to the tub or shower room.
16 Provide for privacy.
17 *For a tub bath:*
   a Fill the tub half-way with warm water (usually 105°F/40.5°C). Follow the care plan for water temperature.
   b Measure water temperature. Use the water thermometer or check the digital display.
   c Have the person check the water temperature. Adjust the water temperature as needed.
18 *For a shower:*
   a Turn on the shower.
   b Adjust water temperature and pressure. Check the digital display. Water temperature is usually 105°F/40.5°C.
   c Have the person check the water temperature. Adjust the water temperature as needed.
19 Help the person undress and remove footwear.

20 Help the person into the tub or shower. Position the shower chair and lock (brake) the wheels.
21 Assist with washing as necessary. Wear gloves.
   a Wash the face, neck, arms, hands, chest, abdomen, legs, feet, back, and buttocks.
   b Provide perineal care if the person is not able. Wear clean gloves and use clean washcloths. Remove and discard gloves. Practice hand hygiene.
   c Follow the care plan and the person's preference for shampooing hair (Chapter 25). Assist with shampooing as needed.
22 Have the person use the call light when done or when help is needed. Remind the person that a tub bath lasts no longer than 20 minutes.
23 Place a towel across the chair.
24 Leave the room if the person can bathe alone. If not, stay in the room or nearby. Remove and discard the gloves and practice hand hygiene if you will leave the room.
25 Check the person at least every 5 minutes.
26 Return when the person signals for you. Knock before entering. Practice hand hygiene.
27 Turn off the shower or drain the tub. Cover the person with the bath blanket while the tub drains.
28 Help the person out of the shower or tub and onto the chair.
29 Help the person dry off. Pat gently. Dry well under the breasts, between skin folds, in the perineal area, and between the toes.
30 Apply lotion, powder, and deodorant or antiperspirant as requested.
31 Help the person dress and put on footwear.
32 Help the person return to the room. Provide for privacy.
33 Assist the person to a chair or into bed.
34 Provide a back massage if the person returns to bed (Chapter 35).
35 Assist with hair care and other grooming needs.

Continued

Assisting With a Tub Bath or Shower—cont'd

POST-PROCEDURE

36 Provide for comfort. (See the inside of the back cover.)
37 Place the call light and other needed items within reach.
38 Raise or lower bed rails. Follow the care plan.
39 Unscreen the person.
40 Complete a safety check of the room. (See the inside of the back cover.)

41 Clean, disinfect, and dry the tub or shower. Dry the tub or shower room floor. Use clean, dry paper towels for drying. Remove soiled linens. Wear gloves.
42 Discard disposable items. Put the UNOCCUPIED sign on the door. Return supplies to their proper place.
43 Follow agency policy for used linens.
44 Remove and discard the gloves. Practice hand hygiene.
45 Report and record your observations.

PERINEAL CARE

Perineal care (pericare) involves cleaning the genital and anal areas. These areas provide a warm, moist, and dark place for microbes to grow. Cleaning prevents infection and odors and promotes comfort.

Perineal care is done daily during the bath. It also is done when the area is soiled with urine or feces (stools). Perineal care is very important for persons who:

- Have urinary catheters (Chapter 28).
- Have had rectal or genital surgery.
- Are menstruating (Chapter 10).
- Are incontinent of urine or feces (stools) (Chapters 27 and 29).
- Are uncircumcised (Fig. 24-19). Being *circumcised means that the fold of skin (foreskin) covering the glans of the penis was surgically removed.* Being *uncircumcised means foreskin covers the head of the penis.*

The person does perineal care if able. Otherwise, the nursing staff does so. This procedure can embarrass the person and staff, especially when it involves the other gender.

Perineal and *perineum* are not common terms. Most people understand *privates, private parts, crotch, genitals,* or *the area between your legs.* Use terms the person understands and that sound professional. Do not use slang or vulgar terms.

Work from *front to back* or *top to bottom.* The urethral area (front or top) is the cleanest. The anal area (back or bottom) is the dirtiest. Therefore clean from the urethra to the anal area. This prevents spreading bacteria from the anal area to the vagina and urinary system.

The perineal area is delicate and easily injured. Use warm water, not hot. Use washcloths, towelettes, cotton balls,

or swabs according to agency policy. Rinse the area thoroughly. Pat dry after rinsing. This reduces moisture and promotes comfort.

See *Focus on Communication: Perineal Care.*
See *Delegation Guidelines: Perineal Care.*
See *Promoting Safety and Comfort: Perineal Care.*
See procedure: *Giving Female Perineal Care.*
See procedure: *Giving Male Perineal Care,* p. 370.

Text continued on p. 371.

FOCUS ON COMMUNICATION

Perineal Care

Talking to the person about perineal care may be difficult. You may be embarrassed. However, you must explain the procedure. You can say:

- "I'll give you some privacy to finish your bath. Can you reach everything you need? Please call for me if you need help. Here is your call light."
- "I'll give you time to finish your bath. Please wash your genital and rectal areas. Signal for me when you're done or need help."
- "Next I'll clean between your legs. I'll keep you covered with the bath blanket. I'll tell you before I touch you. Please tell me if you feel any pain or discomfort."
- "I'll clean your private parts now. Please let me know if you feel any pain or discomfort."

DELEGATION GUIDELINES

Perineal Care

Before giving perineal care, you need this information from the nurse and the care plan.

- When to give perineal care.
- What terms the person understands—perineum, privates, private parts, crotch, area between the legs, and so on.
- How much help the person needs.
- What water temperature to use—usually 105°F to 109°F (40.5°C to 42.7°C). Water in a basin cools rapidly.
- What cleaning agent to use.
- Any position restrictions or limits.
- What observations to report and record:
  - Odors
  - Redness, swelling, discharge, bleeding, or irritation
  - Complaints of pain, burning, or other discomfort
  - Signs of urinary or fecal incontinence
- When to report observations.
- What patient or resident concerns to report at once.

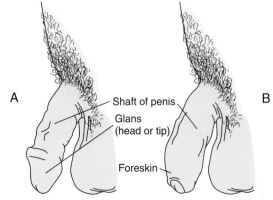

FIGURE 24-19 A, Circumcised male. **B,** Uncircumcised male.

A
Shaft of penis
Glans (head or tip)
Foreskin
B

PROMOTING SAFETY AND COMFORT

Perineal Care

Safety

Hot water can burn perineal tissues. To prevent burns, measure water temperature according to agency policy. If water seems too hot, ask the nurse to check it.

Protect yourself and the person from infection. Contact with blood, body fluids, secretions, or excretions is likely during perineal care. Follow Standard Precautions and the Bloodborne Pathogen Standard.

Persons who are incontinent need perineal care. Protect the person and dry garments and linens from wet or soiled items. Remove the wet or soiled incontinence product, garments, and linens. Then apply clean, dry ones. See Chapter 27.

Comfort

If you provide perineal care, explain how you protect privacy. Always act in a professional manner.

Perineal care involves touching the genital and anal areas. The person may prefer someone of the same gender for this care. Or the person may fear sexual assault. Always obtain the person's consent before providing perineal care. For mental comfort, the person may want a family member or another staff member present to witness the procedure. Ask if he or she wants someone present and that person's name. Also keep the call light within the person's reach. If feeling threatened, the person can call for help.

If able, the person performs perineal care. This promotes privacy and helps prevent embarrassment. You need to:

1. Provide clean water. See step 14 in procedure: *Giving Female Perineal Care*.
2. Adjust the over-bed table so the person can reach the wash basin, soap, and towels with ease.
3. Make sure the person understands what to do.
4. Place the call light and other needed items within reach. Have the person signal when finished.
5. Lower the bed to a safe and comfortable level. Follow the care plan.
6. Remove and discard the gloves. Practice hand hygiene.
7. Leave the room.
8. Answer the call light promptly. Knock before entering the room.
9. Raise the bed for body mechanics.
10. Practice hand hygiene. Put on gloves.
11. Make sure the person has cleaned thoroughly. Assist the person with hand hygiene.
12. Finish the bathing procedure.

Giving Female Perineal Care

QUALITY OF LIFE

- Knock before entering the person's room.
- Address the person by name.
- Introduce yourself by name and title.

- Explain the procedure before starting and during the procedure.
- Protect the person's rights during the procedure.
- Handle the person gently during the procedure.

PRE-PROCEDURE

1. Follow *Delegation Guidelines: Perineal Care*. See *Promoting Safety and Comfort*:
   a *Daily Hygiene and Bathing*, p. 353
   b *Perineal Care*
2. Practice hand hygiene.
3. Collect the following.
   - Soap, body wash, or other cleansing agent as directed
   - At least 4 washcloths
   - Bath towel
   - Bath blanket
   - Water thermometer
   - Wash basin
   - Waterproof under-pad
   - Gloves
   - Laundry bag
   - Paper towels

4. Cover the over-bed table with paper towels. Arrange items on top of them.
5. Identify the person. Check the ID bracelet against the assignment sheet. Use 2 identifiers (Chapter 13). Also call the person by name.
6. Provide for privacy.
7. Raise the bed for body mechanics. Bed rails are up if used.

Continued

Giving Female Perineal Care—cont'd

PROCEDURE

8 Lower the bed rail near you if up.
9 Practice hand hygiene. Put on gloves.
10 Cover the person with a bath blanket. Move top linens to the foot of the bed.
11 Position the person on the back.
12 Drape the person as in Figure 24-20.
13 Raise the bed rail if used.
14 Fill the wash basin. Water temperature is usually 105°F to 109°F (40.5°C to 42.7°C). Follow the care plan for water temperature. Measure water temperature according to agency policy.
15 Have the person check the water temperature. Adjust the water temperature as needed. Raise the bed rail before leaving the bedside. Lower it when you return.
16 Place the basin on the over-bed table.
17 Lower the bed rail if up.
18 Help the person flex the knees and spread the legs. Or help the person spread the legs as much as possible with the knees straight.
19 Fold the corner of the bath blanket between the legs onto the abdomen.
20 Place a waterproof under-pad under the buttocks. Remove any wet or soiled incontinence products.
21 Remove and discard the gloves. Practice hand hygiene. Put on clean gloves.
22 Wet the washcloths.
23 Squeeze out water from a washcloth. Make a mitted washcloth. Apply soap, body wash, or other cleansing agent. (Squeeze out water every time you change washcloths. Do not place used washcloths back in the basin. Put used washcloths in the laundry bag.)
24 Clean the perineum. Change washcloths as needed.
  a Separate the labia.
  b Clean 1 side of the labia. Clean downward from front to back (top to bottom) with 1 stroke (Fig. 24-21, *A*). Use 1 part of a washcloth.
  c Clean the other side of the labia. Clean downward from front to back (top to bottom) with 1 stroke (Fig. 24-21, *B*). Use a clean part of a washcloth.
  d Clean the vaginal area. Clean downward from front to back (top to bottom) with 1 stroke (Fig. 24-21, *C*). Use a clean part of a washcloth.

25 Rinse the perineum with a clean washcloth. Change washcloths as needed.
  a Separate the labia.
  b Rinse 1 side of the labia. Rinse downward from front to back (top to bottom) with 1 stroke. Use 1 part of a washcloth.
  c Rinse the other side of the labia. Rinse downward from front to back (top to bottom) with 1 stroke. Use a clean part of a washcloth.
  d Rinse the vaginal area. Rinse downward from front to back (top to bottom) with 1 stroke. Use a clean part of a washcloth.
26 Pat dry the perineal area with the towel. Dry from front to back (top to bottom).
27 Fold the blanket back between the legs.
28 Help the person lower the legs and turn onto the side away from you.
29 Apply soap, body wash, or other cleansing agent to a clean mitted washcloth.
30 Clean and rinse the rectal area.
  a Clean from the vagina to the anus with 1 stroke (Fig. 24-22). Use 1 part of the washcloth.
  b Repeat steps 29 and 30-a until the area is clean. Use a clean part of the washcloth for each stroke. Change washcloths as needed.
  c Rinse the rectal area with a clean washcloth. Rinse from the vagina to the anus. Repeat as necessary. Use a clean part of the washcloth for each stroke. Change washcloths as needed.
31 Pat dry the rectal area with the towel. Dry from the vagina to the anus.
32 Remove the waterproof under-pad.
33 Remove and discard the gloves. Practice hand hygiene. Put on clean gloves.
34 Provide clean and dry linens and incontinence products as needed.
35 Position the person for comfort.

POST-PROCEDURE

36 Cover the person. Remove the bath blanket.
37 Provide for comfort. (See the inside of the back cover.)
38 Place the call light and other needed items within reach.
39 Lower the bed to a safe and comfortable level. Follow the care plan.
40 Raise or lower bed rails. Follow the care plan.
41 Empty, clean, rinse, and dry the wash basin. Use clean, dry paper towels for drying.
42 Return the basin and supplies to their proper place.

43 Wipe off the over-bed table with the paper towels. Discard the paper towels.
44 Unscreen the person.
45 Complete a safety check of the room. (See the inside of the back cover.)
46 Follow agency policy for used linens.
47 Remove and discard the gloves. Practice hand hygiene.
48 Report and record your observations.

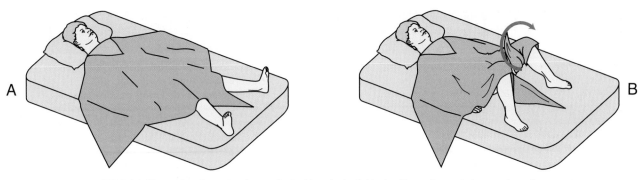

FIGURE 24-20 Draping for perineal care. **A,** Position the bath blanket like a diamond: 1 corner is at the neck, there is a corner at each side, and 1 corner is between the legs. **B,** Wrap the blanket around a leg by bringing the corner around the leg and over the top. Tuck the corner under the hip. Repeat for the other leg.

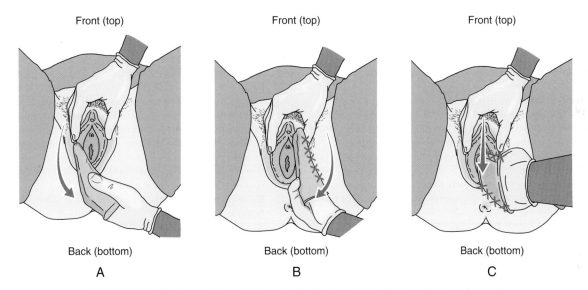

FIGURE 24-21 Cleaning the perineum. **A,** Separate the labia with 1 hand. Use a mitted washcloth to clean 1 side of the labia with a downward stroke. **B,** Clean the other side of the labia with a clean part of the washcloth. Use a downward stroke. **C,** Clean the vaginal area with a clean part of the washcloth. Use a downward stroke. (NOTE: Used areas of the washcloth are marked with Xs.)

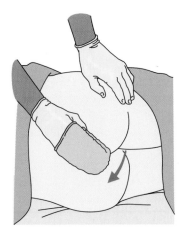

FIGURE 24-22 Clean the rectal area by wiping from the vagina to the anus. The side-lying position allows thorough cleaning of the anal area.

Giving Male Perineal Care

QUALITY OF LIFE

- Knock before entering the person's room.
- Address the person by name.
- Introduce yourself by name and title.

- Explain the procedure before starting and during the procedure.
- Protect the person's rights during the procedure.
- Handle the person gently during the procedure.

PROCEDURE

1 Follow steps 1 through 17 in procedure: *Giving Female Perineal Care,* p. 367. Drape the person as in Figure 24-20.
2 Fold the corner of the bath blanket between the legs onto the person's abdomen.
3 Place a waterproof under-pad under the buttocks. Remove any wet or soiled incontinence products.
4 Remove and discard the gloves. Practice hand hygiene. Put on clean gloves.
5 Wet the washcloths.
6 Squeeze out water from a washcloth. Make a mitted washcloth. Apply soap, body wash, or other cleansing agent. (Squeeze out water every time you change washcloths. Do not place used washcloths back in the basin. Put used washcloths in the laundry bag.)
7 Retract the foreskin if the person is uncircumcised (Fig. 24-23).
8 Grasp the penis.
9 Clean the tip. Use a circular motion. Start at the meatus and work outward (Fig. 24-24, *A*). Repeat as needed. Use a clean part of the washcloth each time.
10 Rinse the tip with another washcloth. Use the same circular motion.
11 Return the foreskin to its natural position after rinsing. After rinsing, dry under the foreskin if agency policy or the person's preference.

12 Clean the shaft of the penis. Use firm downward strokes (Fig. 24-24, *B*). Use a clean part of a washcloth for each stroke.
13 Rinse the shaft. Use the same downward motion as in step 12. Use a clean part of a washcloth for each stroke.
14 Help the person flex the knees and spread the legs. Or help the person spread the legs as much as possible with the knees straight.
15 Clean the scrotum. Use a clean part of a washcloth.
16 Rinse the scrotum. Use a clean part of a washcloth. Observe for redness and irritation of the skin folds.
17 Pat dry the penis and the scrotum. Use the towel.
18 Fold the bath blanket back between the legs.
19 Help the person lower the legs and turn onto the side away from you.
20 Clean the rectal area. Clean from the scrotum (front or top) to the anus (back or bottom). (See procedure: *Giving Female Perineal Care,* p. 367). Rinse and dry well.
21 Remove the waterproof under-pad.
22 Remove and discard the gloves. Practice hand hygiene. Put on clean gloves.
23 Provide clean and dry linens and incontinence products.
24 Position the person for comfort.
25 Follow steps 36 through 48 in procedure: *Giving Female Perineal Care,* p. 367.

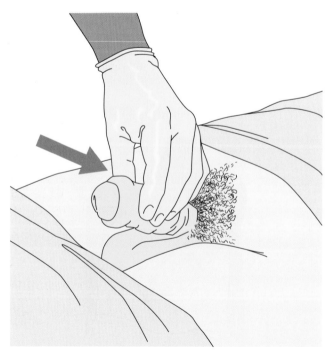

FIGURE 24-23 Pull back the foreskin of the uncircumcised male for perineal care. Return it to the normal position immediately after cleaning and rinsing.

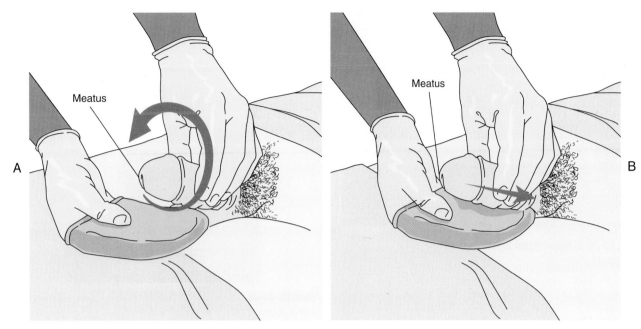

FIGURE 24-24 Cleaning the penis. **A,** Clean the tip with a circular motion starting at the meatus. **B,** Clean the shaft with downward strokes.

REPORTING AND RECORDING

You make many observations while assisting with daily hygiene and bathing. See Box 24-4 for a summary of the observations to report and record.

You must report and record the care given (Fig. 24-27, p. 372). If not recorded, it is assumed that care was not given. This can cause serious legal problems. Tell the nurse if the person refuses care or if care is not given for another reason.

BOX 24-4	Daily Hygiene and Bathing Observations

Report the Following at Once
- Bleeding
- Signs of skin breakdown
- Discharge from the vagina or urinary tract
- Unusual odors
- Changes from prior observations

Bathing
- The color of the skin, lips, nail beds, and sclera (whites of the eyes)
- If the skin appears pale, gray-ish, yellow (*jaundice*—Chapter 50), or bluish (*cyanotic*)
- The location and description of rashes
- Skin texture—smooth, rough, scaly, flaky, dry, moist
- *Diaphoresis*—profuse (excessive) sweating
- Bruises (Fig. 24-25, p. 372). or open skin areas
- Pale, reddened, or discolored areas, particularly over bony parts
- Drainage or bleeding from wounds or body coverings
- Swelling of the feet and legs (Fig. 24-26, p. 372).
- Corns or calluses on the feet (Chapter 40)
- Skin temperature (cold, cool, warm, hot)
- Complaints of pain or discomfort

Perineal Care
- Odors
- Redness, swelling, discharge, bleeding, or irritation
- Complaints of pain, burning, or other discomfort
- Signs of urinary or fecal incontinence

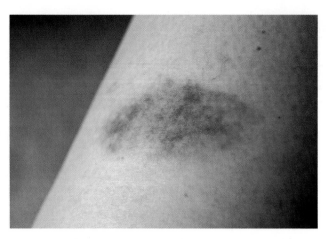

FIGURE 24-25 A bruise. Report bruising to the nurse. (Copyright © iStock.com/diephosi.)

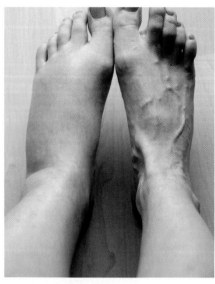

FIGURE 24-26 The left foot and leg are swollen. Report swelling to the nurse. (Copyright © iStock.com/vidka.)

SKIN CARE

Abnormal Skin Observations

Problems:
- ☐ Blister
- ☐ Non-intact skin (open skin)
- ☐ Bruise
- ☐ Bleeding
- ☐ Drainage/discharge
- ☐ Swelling
- ☒ Rash
- ☒ Itching
- ☐ Odor

Color:
- ☒ Redness
- ☐ Pallor (pale skin)
- ☐ Gray
- ☐ Cyanosis (blue skin)
- ☐ Jaundice (yellow skin)

Texture:
- ☐ Rough
- ☐ Scaly/flaky

Temperature:
- ☐ Cold
- ☐ Cool
- ☐ Hot

Moisture:
- ☐ Dry
- ☐ Moist
- ☐ Diaphoresis (sweating)

Nurse notified: J. Anderson, RN

☐ No new skin issues

Bathing

- ☐ Shower
- ☐ Tub bath
- ☒ Complete bed bath
- ☐ Partial bath
- ☐ Bag/towel bath
- ☒ Perineal care

Click to mark affected area(s).

Right   Left   Left   Right

FIGURE 24-27 Charting sample.

FOCUS ON PRIDE

The Person, Family, and Yourself

Personal and Professional Responsibility

Daily hygiene and bathing procedures are routine nursing tasks. They are important for the person's quality of life, health, and safety. Follow the care plan to meet the person's needs and preferences. Take pride in giving care that helps the person's over-all well-being.

Rights and Respect

Patients and residents have the right to choose schedules and routines. They also have the right to refuse care. Some persons refuse if it does not meet their preferences. For example:

- Preferring a bath, a person refuses a shower.
- A person prefers to bathe at night, not in the morning.
- A person prefers a certain nursing assistant for care. The person refuses care by others.

Refusing care for these reasons does not mean the person refuses to be clean. The person may accept if preferences are met. Tell the nurse of any refusal. Adjust as needed to respect the person's preferences.

Independence and Social Interaction

Bathing is a personal matter. Allow personal choice for bath time, products used, what to wear, and so on. Encourage self-care to the extent possible. Self-care promotes independence and improves self-esteem.

Delegation and Teamwork

Some agencies have commercial warmers for bath blankets. If a warmer is getting low, fill it. Otherwise, staff find an empty warmer. A co-worker has to fill it and wait for a blanket to heat up. Take pride in being a helpful and courteous team member.

Ethics and Laws

Always be careful. Harm can result from routine care measures. Follow the safety measures in this chapter at all times.

A patient (Mr. Genza) was paralyzed on his right side because of a stroke. He could not walk or talk. He could stand with difficulty. He died at age 51 from burns suffered during a shower.

A wrongful death suit was filed for what was claimed to be negligent care. According to the facts reported in the court case, the following occurred.

- *An attendant took the patient to the shower in a wheelchair.*
- *The attendant undressed the patient. The patient was placed on a chair and under running water in a shower.*
- *The attendant claimed that he tested the water.*
- *The shower room was supervised by an RN (registered nurse). The RN testified that an attendant was required to be present at all times while a paralyzed patient was receiving care.*
- *The attendant stated that he washed the patient's back and head. Then he went to attend to another patient 5 or 6 feet from the shower. A tub was between the attendant and Mr. Genza.*

- *When the attendant asked if he needed to get out of the shower, Mr. Genza indicated that he did not.*
- *Two minutes later, the attendant was getting another patient out of the tub. The attendant heard Mr. Genza shout and saw that the shower handle was moved from its original setting.*
- *Two days later, Mr. Genza died from burns.*
- *On the day of the accident, the hot water gauge read 171°F. It tested at 158°F to 159°F.*
- *An expert witness stated that 110°F is hot enough for shower room use.*
- *In the Court's opinion, the home was grossly negligent for:*
  - *Failing to provide the supervision needed by a helpless person*
  - *Providing water facilities that were dangerous and a threat to the lives of anyone using them*

(Mr. Lewinsky v State of Illinois, 1967.)

In another case, a daughter filed a complaint for the wrongful death of her mother. According to the complaint, on August 29, 1993, a nurse's aide ran water in a whirlpool bath for the nursing home resident. The nurse's aide tested the water with her bare arm and hand. She found the water satisfactory. The resident also tested the water by putting her foot into the water, which showed that the water was okay. Using a chair lift, the resident was transferred into the tub.

After the bath, the nurse's aide asked 2 co-workers to help her get the resident out of the tub. After getting her out, a co-worker noted a small spot on the resident's left hip. The resident had no burns on her body before the bath. However, redness of her extremities was noted over the next 30 minutes. Blisters began and continued to form.

The resident had second and third degree burns from her mid-back down over her buttocks, the perineal area, and lower extremities. (Author note: A first degree burn means the epidermis is damaged. A second degree burn involves the epidermis and part of the dermis. A third degree burn involves the epidermis and the entire dermis.) The resident was transferred to the hospital. She died on September 1, 1993.

The daughter sued the county, the nursing home and hospital, the nursing home administrator, hospital board members, and the nurse's aide. The trial court dismissed the case on a legal technicality. However, the Appellate Court reversed the dismissal by the trial court and returned the case to court for trial.

(D. Burton v Choctaw County Mississippi, Choctaw Hospital d/b/a Choctaw County Nursing Home, and others, 1997.)

FOCUS ON PRIDE: *Application*

The care measures in this chapter are private and personal. What concerns do you have about the procedures in this chapter? How will you stay calm and professional and ease the person's worries?

REVIEW QUESTIONS

Circle T if the statement is TRUE and F if it is FALSE.

1 T F   During evening care, you prepare the person for sleep.

2 T F   Bath oils cleanse the skin.

3 T F   Powders absorb moisture and prevent friction.

4 T F   Deodorants reduce the amount of perspiration.

5 T F   You need to report diaphoresis.

6 T F   To wash the eye, wash from the inner to the outer aspect.

7 T F   You ask when a co-worker needs the shower room. This shows good teamwork and time management.

8 T F   A tub bath lasts 30 minutes.

9 T F   Washcloths are rinsed and re-used during perineal care.

10 T F   Perineal care helps prevent infection.

11 T F   Foreskin is returned to its normal position after rinsing.

12 T F   Report bleeding to the nurse at once.

Circle the BEST answer.

13 A long-handled sponge
   a Can be shared by residents
   b Is not used for older persons
   c Promotes independence
   d Is used for a complete bed bath

14 When assisting with daily care, you
   a Clean an incontinent person as often as needed
   b Give early morning care after breakfast
   c Follow your own routines and habits
   d Change soiled linens in the afternoon

15 To apply powder
   a Turn the person toward you
   b Sprinkle a small amount onto your hand
   c Apply a thick layer of powder
   d Shake the powder onto the person

16 Soaps
   a Dry the skin
   b Replace skin oils
   c Soften the skin
   d Reduce perspiration

17 When bathing a person
   a Keep bar soap in the wash basin or tub
   b Wash from the dirtiest to the cleanest area
   c Assist with elimination after a bath
   d Rinse the skin well to remove all soap

18 Water for a complete bed bath is between
   a 100°F and 104°F
   b 105°F and 109°F
   c 110°F and 115°F
   d 120°F and 125°F

19 When drying the person
   a Dry well between skin folds
   b Rub the skin dry
   c Avoid drying between the toes
   d Allow the person to air dry

20 Which is helpful when showering a person with confusion?
   a Gather supplies after the person is in the shower.
   b Do not explain what you are doing.
   c Work quickly if the person resists.
   d Put a towel over the lap and shoulders.

21 When assisting with a shower in a shower room
   a Direct the water spray at the person's face
   b Allow a weak person to stand if you provide support
   c Go to the person's room to make the bed during the shower
   d Clean, disinfect, and dry the shower before and after use

22 Water temperature for perineal care is between
   a 100°F and 104°F
   b 105°F and 109°F
   c 110°F and 115°F
   d 120°F and 125°F

23 These statements are about perineal care. Which is *true?*
   a Do not explain the procedure to avoid embarrassment.
   b The person does perineal care if able.
   c Clean from the back (bottom) to the front (top).
   d Draping the person is not needed.

24 You see a rash under a breast during a bath. You should
   a Ask the nurse to observe the area
   b Scrub the skin
   c Apply lotion to the area
   d Avoid drying the skin

Answers to Chapter 24 questions are on p. 886.

FOCUS ON **PRACTICE**

Problem Solving

You are asked to help a nursing assistant give perineal care. The nursing assistant gathered 1 washcloth and no gloves for the procedure. What will you do?

Grooming

OBJECTIVES

- Define the key terms and key abbreviations in this chapter.
- Explain why grooming is important.
- Explain how to safely provide grooming measures—hair care, shaving, and nail and foot care.
- Perform the procedures described in this chapter.
- Explain how to promote PRIDE in the person, the family, and yourself.

KEY TERMS

alopecia Hair loss

anticoagulant A drug that prevents or slows down *(anti)* blood clotting *(coagulate)*

dandruff Excessive amounts of dry, white flakes from the scalp

hirsutism Excessive body hair

infestation Being in or on a host

lice See "pediculosis"

mite A very small spider-like organism

pediculosis Infestation with wingless insects that feed on blood; lice

pediculosis capitis Infestation of the scalp *(capitis)* with lice

pediculosis corporis Infestation of the body *(corporis)* with lice

pediculosis pubis Infestation of the pubic *(pubis)* hair with lice

scabies A skin disorder caused by a female mite

KEY ABBREVIATIONS

C   Centigrade
F   Fahrenheit

ID   Identification

Hair care, shaving, and nail and foot care prevent infection and promote comfort. Such measures affect love, belonging, and self-esteem needs.

For both men and women, hair care—head, facial, underarms, legs, and so on—are matters of personal choice. So is the care of hands and feet. Cultural requirements or preferences also influence grooming measures. Some want only clean hair. Others want a certain hair-style. Some want only clean hands. Others want polished nails. Men may shave and groom their beards. Likewise, women may shave their legs and underarms. Some women use hair removal methods for facial hair.

As with hygiene, the person performs grooming measures to the extent possible. This promotes independence and quality of life. The person may use adaptive (assistive) devices (Fig. 25-1).

See *Focus on Surveys: Grooming*, p. 376.

See *Teamwork and Time Management: Grooming*, p. 376.

NOTE: A task may require more than 1 pair of gloves. Change gloves as needed. Use careful judgment. Remember to practice hand hygiene after removing gloves.

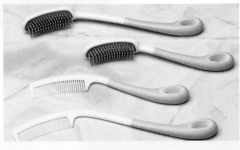

FIGURE 25-1 Long-handled combs and brushes for hair care (Courtesy North Coast Medical Inc., Morgan Hill, Calif.)

HAIR CARE

The look and feel of hair affect mental well-being. The nursing process reflects the person's culture, personal choice, skin and scalp conditions, health history, and self-care ability. You assist with hair care as needed.

See *Focus on Long-Term Care and Home Care: Hair Care.*

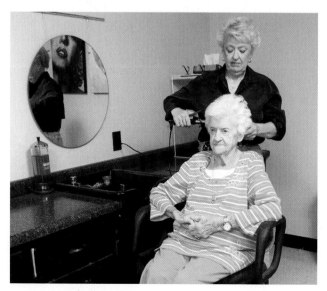

FIGURE 25-2 Beauty shop in a nursing center.

Skin and Scalp Conditions

Skin and scalp conditions include:

- *Alopecia—hair loss.* Hair loss may be complete or partial. Caused by heredity, male pattern baldness occurs with aging. Hair thins in some women with aging. Cancer treatments (radiation therapy to the head and chemotherapy) may cause alopecia in all age-groups. Skin disease, stress, poor nutrition, pregnancy, some drugs, and hormone changes are other causes. Except for hair loss from aging, hair usually grows back.
- *Hirsutism—excessive body hair.* It can occur in men, women, and children. Causes are heredity and abnormal amounts of male hormones.
- *Dandruff—excessive amounts of dry, white flakes from the scalp.* Itching is common. Sometimes eyebrows and ear canals are involved. Medicated shampoos may be ordered.
- *Pediculosis (lice)—infestation with wingless insects that feed on blood* (Fig. 25-3). *Infestation means being in or on a host.* Lice attach their eggs *(nits)* to hair shafts. Nits are oval and yellow to white in color. They hatch in about 1 week. After hatching, they bite the scalp or skin to feed on blood. About the size of a sesame seed, adult lice are tan to gray-ish white in color. Lice easily spread to others through clothing, head coverings, furniture, beds, towels, bed linens, sexual contact, combs, and brushes. Lice are treated with medicated shampoos, lotions, and creams specific for lice. Thorough bathing is needed. So is washing clothing and linens in hot water. Lice bites cause severe itching.
  - *Pediculosis capitis—infestation of the scalp* (capitis) *with lice.* It is commonly called "head lice."
  - *Pediculosis pubis—infestation of the pubic* (pubis) *hair with lice.* This form is also called "crabs."
  - *Pediculosis corporis—infestation of the body* (corporis) *with lice.*
- *Scabies—a skin disorder caused by a female mite* (Fig. 25-4). A *mite is a very small spider-like organism.* The female mite burrows into the skin and lays eggs. After hatching, the females produce more eggs. Infested with mites, the person has a rash and intense itching. Common sites are between the fingers, the wrists, underarms, thighs, and genital area. Other sites include the breasts, waist, and buttocks. Highly contagious, scabies is transmitted to others by close contact. Special creams are ordered to kill the mites. The person's room is cleaned. Clothing and linens are washed in hot water.

See *Focus on Communication: Skin and Scalp Conditions.*

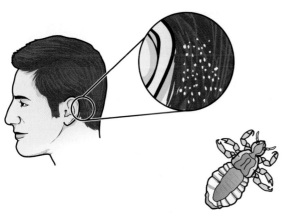

FIGURE 25-3 Head lice. (Redrawn from Medline Plus: *Head lice.* Bethesda, Md., National Institutes of Health.)

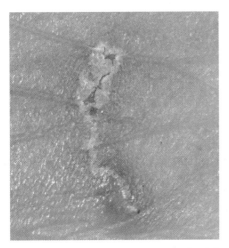

FIGURE 25-4 Scabies. (From Marks JG, Miller JJ: *Lookingbill & Marks' principles of dermatology,* ed 4, St Louis, 2006, Saunders.)

Brushing and Combing Hair

Brushing and combing hair are part of early morning care, morning care, and afternoon care (Chapter 24). Some people also do so before meals, before visitors arrive, and at bedtime.

Encourage patients and residents to do their own hair care. The person chooses how to brush, comb, and style hair. Assist as needed.

Brushing increases blood flow to the scalp. And it brings scalp oils along the hair shaft to help keep hair soft and shiny. To brush and comb hair, work from the scalp to the hair ends.

Daily brushing and combing prevent matted and tangled hair. So does braiding. You need the person's consent to braid hair. Report matted or tangled hair to the nurse. Brush through the matting and tangling from the hair ends to the scalp. *Never cut the person's hair.*

Special measures are needed for curly, coarse, and dry hair. For curly hair, use a wide-tooth comb. Start at the neckline. Working upward, lift and fluff hair outward. Continue to the forehead. To make combing easier, wet hair or apply hair care products as directed. Follow the care plan for coarse and dry hair.

The person's hair care practices and products are part of the care plan. Let the person guide hair care.

See *Caring About Culture: Brushing and Combing Hair.*

See *Focus on Children and Older Persons: Brushing and Combing Hair.*

See *Delegation Guidelines: Brushing and Combing Hair,* p. 378.

See *Promoting Safety and Comfort: Brushing and Combing Hair,* p. 378.

See procedure: *Brushing and Combing Hair,* p. 378.

Text continued on p. 380.

FOCUS ON COMMUNICATION

Skin and Scalp Conditions

Some skin or scalp conditions may alarm you. Remain professional. Do not say things that may embarrass the person.

Report an abnormal skin or scalp condition. Describe your observations. For example:

• "There are small red dots on Mr. Olson's right underarm. Would you please look at them?"
• "I saw some small white specks in Ms. Smith's hair. Would you please look at them before I wash her hair?"

CARING ABOUT CULTURE

Brushing and Combing Hair

Small braids (corn-rows) are common in some cultural groups. The braids are left intact for shampooing. To undo these braids, the nurse obtains the person's consent.

(NOTE: Each person is unique. A person may not follow all of the beliefs and practices of his or her culture. Follow the care plan.)

FOCUS ON CHILDREN AND OLDER PERSONS

Brushing and Combing Hair

Children
Hair-styles are important to older children and teenagers. Do not make judgments about hair-styles. Style hair in a way that pleases the child and parents. Do not style hair according to your standards or customs.

DELEGATION GUIDELINES
Brushing and Combing Hair

Brushing and combing hair are routine nursing tasks. To brush and comb hair, you need this information from the nurse and the care plan.

- How much help the person needs
- What to do for matted or tangled hair
- What to do for curly, coarse, or dry hair
- What hair care products to use
- The person's preferences and routine hair care measures
- What observations to report and record:
  - Scalp sores
  - Flaking
  - Itching
  - Rash
  - Hair falling out in patches; patches of hair loss
  - Very dry or very oily hair
  - Matted or tangled hair
  - The presence of nits or lice
    - Nits (lice eggs attached to hair shafts)—oval and yellow to white in color
    - Lice—about the size of a sesame seed and gray-ish white in color
    - Itching
    - Complaints of a tickling feeling or something moving in the hair
    - Irritability
    - Sores on the head or body caused by scratching
    - Rash
- When to report observations
- What patient or resident concerns to report at once

PROMOTING SAFETY AND COMFORT
Brushing and Combing Hair

Safety

Sharp brush bristles can injure the scalp. So can sharp or broken teeth on a comb. Report concerns about the person's brush or comb.

Wear gloves if the person has scalp sores, nits, lice, or other hair or scalp problems. Follow Standard Precautions and the Bloodborne Pathogen Standard.

Comfort

Protect garments from falling hair with a towel across the back and shoulders. For the person in bed, give hair care before changing linens and the pillowcase. If after a linen change, place a towel across the pillow to collect falling hair.

Brushing and Combing Hair

QUALITY OF LIFE

- Knock before entering the person's room.
- Address the person by name.
- Introduce yourself by name and title.

- Explain the procedure before starting and during the procedure.
- Protect the person's rights during the procedure.
- Handle the person gently during the procedure.

PRE-PROCEDURE

1. Follow *Delegation Guidelines: Brushing and Combing Hair.* See *Promoting Safety and Comfort: Brushing and Combing Hair.*
2. Practice hand hygiene.
3. Identify the person. Check the ID (identification) bracelet against the assignment sheet. Use 2 identifiers (Chapter 13). Also call the person by name.

4. Ask the person how to style hair.
5. Collect the following.
   - Comb and brush
   - Bath towel
   - Other hair care items as requested
6. Arrange items on the bedside stand.
7. Provide for privacy.

Brushing and Combing Hair—cont'd

PROCEDURE

8 Lower the bed rail if up.

9 Position the person.

  a *In a chair*—Help the person to the chair. The person puts on a robe and slip-resistant footwear when up.

  b *In bed*—Raise the bed for body mechanics. Bed rails are up if used. Lower the bed rail near you. Assist the person to a semi-Fowler's position if allowed.

10 Place a towel across the back and shoulders or across the pillow.

11 Have the person remove eyeglasses. Put them in the eyeglass case. Put the case inside the bedside stand.

12 *Hair that is not matted or tangled.*

  a Use the comb to part the hair.

    1) Part hair down the middle into 2 sides (Fig. 25-5, *A*).

    2) Divide 1 side into 2 smaller sections (Fig. 25-5, *B*).

  b Brush 1 of the small sections of hair. Start at the scalp and brush toward the hair ends (Fig. 25-6). Do the same for the other small section of hair. If the person prefers, brush long hair starting at the hair ends.

  c Repeat steps 12, a(2) and b for the other side.

13 *Matted or tangled hair.*

  a Take a small section of hair near the ends.

  b Comb or brush through to the hair ends.

  c Add small sections of hair as you work up to the scalp.

  d Comb or brush through each longer section to the hair ends.

14 Style the hair as the person prefers.

15 Remove the towel.

16 Have the person put on the eyeglasses.

POST-PROCEDURE

17 Provide for comfort. (See the inside of the back cover.)

18 Place the call light and other needed items within reach.

19 Lower the bed to a safe and comfortable level. Follow the care plan.

20 Raise or lower bed rails. Follow the care plan.

21 Remove hair from the brush or comb. Clean, rinse, dry, and return hair care items to their proper place. Use clean, dry paper towels for drying. Wear gloves for this step. Remove and discard the gloves. Practice hand hygiene.

22 Unscreen the person.

23 Complete a safety check of the room. (See the inside of the back cover.)

24 Follow agency policy for used linens.

25 Practice hand hygiene.

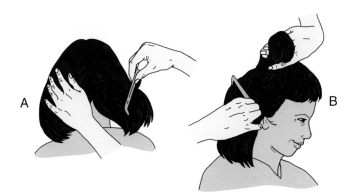

FIGURE 25-5 Part hair. **A,** Part hair down the middle. Divide it into 2 sides. **B,** Then part 1 side into 2 smaller sections.

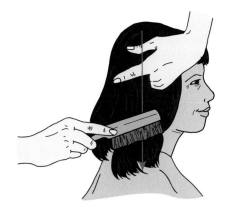

FIGURE 25-6 Brush hair by starting at the scalp. Brush down to the hair ends.

Shampooing

People shampoo 1, 2, or 3 times a week or daily. Frequency factors include hair and scalp condition, hair-style, and personal choice.

Shampoo method depends on the person's condition, safety factors, and personal choice. The nurse tells you what method to use.

- *Shampoo during the shower or tub bath.* Use a hand-held nozzle for persons in shower chairs or taking tub baths. Direct a spray of water at the hair.
- *Shampoo at the sink.* The person sits or lies facing away from the sink. A folded towel placed over the sink edge protects the neck. The person's head is tilted back over the sink edge or a shampoo tray is used (Fig. 25-7). Use a water pitcher or hand-held nozzle to wet and rinse the hair.
- *Shampoo in bed.* The person's head and shoulders are at the edge of the bed if possible. A shampoo basin under the head protects the linens and mattress from water. The device drains into a basin on a chair by the bed (Fig. 25-8). Use a water pitcher to wet and rinse the hair.

Commercial shampoo caps have a cleaning agent that does not need rinsing. Some caps also have a conditioner. To use a shampoo cap:

1 Warm the package following the manufacturer's instructions.
2 Check the temperature. The cap should be warm. Do not use a cap that is too hot.
3 Apply the cap to the person's head.
4 Massage the hair and scalp gently through the cap. Follow the manufacturer's instructions for how long to massage—usually 1 to 3 minutes. Longer hair may require more time.
5 Remove the cap. Do not rinse the hair. Dry the hair with a towel if needed.
6 Comb the hair.

Dry and style hair as soon as possible after the shampoo. Women may want hair curled or rolled up before drying. Check with the nurse before doing so.

See *Focus on Children and Older Persons: Shampooing.*

See *Focus on Long-Term Care and Home Care: Shampooing.*

See *Delegation Guidelines: Shampooing.*

See *Promoting Safety and Comfort: Shampooing.*

See procedure: *Shampooing the Person's Hair in Bed,* p. 382.

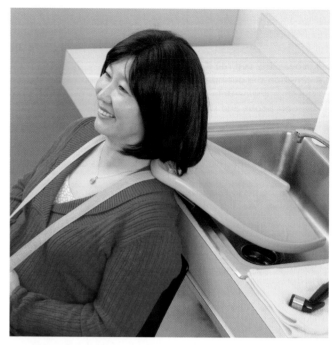

FIGURE 25-7 Shampooing at the sink with a shampoo tray. (Courtesy SP Ableware – Maddak, Wayne, N.J.)

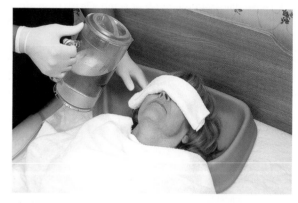

FIGURE 25-8 A shampoo basin is used for a shampoo in bed. Water drains into a collecting basin.

FOCUS ON CHILDREN AND OLDER PERSONS

Shampooing

Children

Oil gland secretion increases with puberty. Therefore adolescents tend to have oily hair. They may need to shampoo often.

Older Persons

Oil gland secretion decreases with aging. Therefore older persons have dry hair. They may shampoo less often than younger adults do.

FOCUS ON LONG-TERM CARE AND HOME CARE

Shampooing

Long-Term Care

Shampooing is usually done weekly on the person's bath or shower day. If hair is done by a hairdresser or barber, do not shampoo the hair. A shower cap is worn during the tub bath or shower.

DELEGATION GUIDELINES

Shampooing

Shampooing may be viewed as a routine nursing task in some agencies. To give a shampoo, you need this information from the nurse and the care plan.
- When to shampoo the person's hair
- What method to use
- What shampoo and conditioner to use
- How to use and store medicated products
- The person's position restrictions or limits
- What water temperature to use—usually 105°F (Fahrenheit) (40.5°C [centigrade])
- If hair is curled or rolled up before drying
- What observations to report and record:
  - *See Delegation Guidelines: Brushing and Combing Hair*, p. 378
  - How the person tolerated the procedure
- When to report observations
- What patient or resident concerns to report at once

PROMOTING SAFETY AND COMFORT

Shampooing

Safety

Remove hearing aids before shampooing. Water will damage hearing aids.

Wear gloves if the person has scalp sores, nits, lice, or other hair or scalp problems. Follow Standard Precautions and the Bloodborne Pathogen Standard.

Keep shampoo away from and out of the eyes. Have the person hold a washcloth over the eyes. To rinse, cup your hand at the person's forehead. This keeps soapy water from running down the forehead and into the eyes.

For a shampoo on a stretcher at a sink, see Chapter 20 for stretcher safety. For safe stretcher transfers, see procedure: *Moving the Person to a Stretcher* in Chapter 20. Lock (brake) the wheels and use the safety straps and side rails. Keep the far side rail raised during the procedure.

Some people shampoo themselves during a tub bath or shower. Place an extra towel and requested shampoo products within the person's reach. Assist as needed.

Comfort

For a shampoo during the tub bath or shower, the person tips the head back to keep shampoo and water out of the eyes. Support the back of the head with 1 hand. Shampoo with your other hand. Some persons cannot tip their heads back. They lean forward and hold a folded washcloth over the eyes. Support the forehead with 1 hand as you shampoo with the other. Make sure that the person can breathe easily.

Many people have limited range of motion in their necks. They are not shampooed at the sink or on a stretcher.

Shampooing the Person's Hair in Bed

QUALITY OF LIFE

- Knock before entering the person's room.
- Address the person by name.
- Introduce yourself by name and title.

- Explain the procedure before starting and during the procedure.
- Protect the person's rights during the procedure.
- Handle the person gently during the procedure.

PRE-PROCEDURE

1 Follow *Delegation Guidelines: Shampooing*, p. 381. See *Promoting Safety and Comfort: Shampooing*, p. 381.
2 Practice hand hygiene.
3 Collect the following.
   - 2 bath towels
   - Washcloth
   - Shampoo
   - Hair conditioner (if requested)
   - Water thermometer
   - Water pitcher
   - Shampoo basin
   - Collecting basin
   - Waterproof under-pad
   - Gloves (if needed)
   - Comb and brush
   - Hair dryer
4 Arrange items nearby. Place the collecting basin on a chair by the bed.
5 Identify the person. Check the ID bracelet against the assignment sheet. Use 2 identifiers (Chapter 13). Also call the person by name.
6 Provide for privacy.
7 Raise the bed for body mechanics. Bed rails are up if used.
8 Practice hand hygiene.

PROCEDURE

9 Lower the bed rail near you if up.
10 Cover the person's chest with a bath towel.
11 Brush and comb the hair to remove snarls and tangles.
12 Position the person for a shampoo in bed:
   a Lower the head of the bed and remove the pillow.
   b Place the waterproof under-pad and shampoo basin under the head and shoulders.
   c Support the head and neck with a folded towel if necessary.
13 Raise the bed rail if used.
14 Fill the water pitcher. Water temperature is usually 105°F (40.5°C). Test water temperature according to agency policy. Have the person check the water temperature. Adjust the water temperature as needed. Raise the bed rail before leaving the bedside.
15 Lower the bed rail near you if up.
16 Put on gloves (if needed).
17 Have the person hold a washcloth over the eyes. It should not cover the nose and mouth. (NOTE: A damp washcloth is easier to hold and will not slip. However, your agency may require a dry washcloth.)
18 Use the water pitcher to wet the hair. Ask the person about the water temperature and adjust as needed.
19 Apply a small amount of shampoo.
20 Work up a lather with both hands. Start at the hairline. Work toward the back of the head.
21 Massage the scalp with your fingertips. Do not scratch the scalp with your fingernails.
22 Rinse the hair until the water runs clear.
23 Repeat steps 19 through 22.
24 Apply conditioner. Follow directions on the container.
25 Squeeze water from the hair.
26 Cover the hair with a bath towel.
27 Remove the shampoo basin, collecting basin, and waterproof under-pad.
28 Dry the person's face with the towel on the chest.
29 Raise the head of the bed.
30 Rub the hair and scalp with the towel. Rub gently. Use the second towel if the first one is wet.
31 Comb the hair to remove snarls and tangles.
32 Dry and style hair.
33 Remove and discard the gloves (if used). Practice hand hygiene.

POST-PROCEDURE

34 Provide for comfort. (See the inside of the back cover.)
35 Place the call light and other needed items within reach.
36 Lower the bed to a safe and comfortable level. Follow the care plan.
37 Raise or lower bed rails. Follow the care plan.
38 Unscreen the person.
39 Complete a safety check of the room. (See the inside of the back cover.)
40 Clean the brush and comb. Clean, rinse, dry, and return equipment to its proper place. Use clean, dry paper towels for drying. Wear gloves for this step. Discard disposable items. Remove and discard the gloves.
41 Follow agency policy for used linens.
42 Practice hand hygiene.
43 Report and record your observations.

![icon] SHAVING

Shaving is common for facial hair and for leg and underarm hair. Other hair removal methods include waxing, hair removal products, plucking, and threading. See Box 25-1 for shaving rules.

Safety razors or electric shavers are used (Fig. 25-9). When using the person's or the agency's electric shaver, clean it before and after use. To brush out whiskers or hair, follow the manufacturer's instructions. Also follow agency procedures.

Safety razors (blade razors) have razor blades. They can cause nicks and cuts. Do not use safety razors on persons with healing problems or on those taking anticoagulant drugs. An *anticoagulant is a drug that prevents or slows down* (anti) *blood clotting* (coagulate). Bleeding occurs easily and is hard to stop. A nick or cut can cause serious bleeding. Electric shavers are used.

See *Focus on Children and Older Persons: Shaving.*

See *Delegation Guidelines: Shaving.*

See *Promoting Safety and Comfort: Shaving,* p. 384.

See procedure: *Shaving the Person's Face With a Safety Razor,* p. 384.

BOX 25-1	Rules for Shaving

- Use electric shavers for persons taking anticoagulant drugs. Never use safety razors.
- Protect bed linens. Place a towel under the part to be shaved. Or place a towel across the person's chest and shoulders to protect clothing.
- Soften facial hair before shaving. Apply a warm, moist washcloth or towel to the face for a few minutes. Then pat dry the face. Apply talcum powder if the person or the nurse asks that you do so.
- Lather the area with shaving cream or soap and water if using a safety razor.
- Encourage the person to do as much as safely possible.
- Hold the skin taut as needed.
- Shave in the correct direction.
  - *Shaving the face with a safety razor*—shave in the direction of hair growth.
  - *Shaving the underarms with a safety razor*—shave in the direction of hair growth.
  - *Shaving the legs with a safety razor*—shave up from the ankles. This is against hair growth.
  - *Using an electric shaver*—shave against the direction of hair growth. For a rotary-type shaver, move the shaver in small circles over the face. (NOTE: Some state competency tests require shaving in the direction of hair growth. Follow the manufacturer's instructions and the rules in your state and agency.)
- Do not cut, nick, or irritate the skin.
- Rinse the skin thoroughly.
- Apply direct pressure to nicks or cuts (Chapter 58).
- Report nicks, cuts, or irritation at once.

FOCUS ON **CHILDREN AND OLDER PERSONS**

Shaving

Older Persons

Older persons with wrinkled skin are at risk for nicks and cuts. Safety razors are not used for them or persons with dementia. Persons with dementia may not understand what you are doing. They may resist care and move suddenly. Serious nicks and cuts can occur. Use electric shavers for these persons.

DELEGATION GUIDELINES

Shaving

Facial shaving is a routine nursing task. Shaving beards and mustaches is not a routine nursing task. Nor is shaving legs and underarms.

To shave a person's face, you need this information from the nurse and the care plan.
- What shaver to use—electric or safety
- If the person takes anticoagulant drugs
- When to shave the person
- What facial hair to shave
- If there are tender or sensitive areas on the person's face
- What observations to report and record:
  - Nicks (report at once)
  - Cuts (report at once)
  - Bleeding (report at once)
  - Irritation
- When to report observations
- What patient or resident concerns to report at once

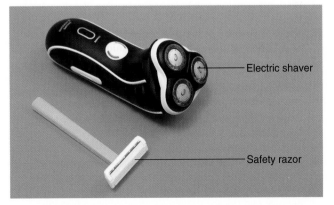

FIGURE 25-9 Electric shaver and safety razor.

Electric shaver

Safety razor

PROMOTING SAFETY AND COMFORT

Shaving

Safety

Safety razors are very sharp. Protect the person and yourself from nicks and cuts. Prevent contact with blood. For an electric shaver, follow safety measures for electrical equipment (Chapter 13).

Rinse the safety razor often during the procedure. Rinsing removes whiskers (or hair) and lather. Then wipe the razor. To protect yourself from cuts:

- Place several thicknesses of tissues or paper towels on the over-bed table. Do not hold them in your hand.
- Wipe the razor on the tissues or paper towels.

Follow Standard Precautions and the Bloodborne Pathogen Standard. Discard used razor blades and disposable shavers in the sharps container. Do not re-cap the razor.

Comfort

The neck area below the jaw may be tender and sensitive. Some electric shavers become very warm or hot during use. The heat can irritate the skin. Shave tender areas first while the shaver is cool. Then move to other areas of the face.

Some people apply lotion or after-shave to the skin after shaving. Lotion softens the skin. After-shave closes skin pores. To soften the skin and open pores, apply warmth before shaving (see Box 25-1).

Shaving the Person's Face With a Safety Razor

QUALITY OF LIFE

- Knock before entering the person's room.
- Address the person by name.
- Introduce yourself by name and title.

- Explain the procedure before starting and during the procedure.
- Protect the person's rights during the procedure.
- Handle the person gently during the procedure.

PRE-PROCEDURE

1 Follow *Delegation Guidelines: Shaving*, p. 383.
   See *Promoting Safety and Comfort: Shaving*.
2 Practice hand hygiene.
3 Collect the following.
   - Wash basin
   - Bath towel
   - Hand towel
   - Washcloth
   - Safety razor
   - Mirror
   - Shaving cream, soap, or lotion
   - Shaving brush
   - After-shave or lotion
   - Tissues or paper towels
   - Gloves
4 Arrange paper towels and supplies on the over-bed table.
5 Identify the person. Check the ID bracelet against the assignment sheet. Use 2 identifiers (Chapter 13). Also call the person by name.
6 Provide for privacy.
7 Raise the bed for body mechanics. Bed rails are up if used.

PROCEDURE

8 Fill the wash basin with warm water.
9 Place the basin on the over-bed table.
10 Lower the bed rail near you if up.
11 Practice hand hygiene. Put on gloves.
12 Assist the person to semi-Fowler's position if allowed or to the supine position.
13 Adjust lighting to clearly see the person's face.
14 Place the towel over the person's chest and shoulders.
15 Adjust the over-bed table for easy reach.
16 Tighten the razor blade to the shaver if necessary.
17 Wash the person's face. Do not dry.
18 Wet the washcloth or towel. Wring it out.
19 Apply the warm washcloth or towel to the face for a few minutes.

20 Apply shaving cream with your hands. (If needed, change gloves or wipe excess shaving cream from your gloves using a towel or paper towel.) Or use a shaving brush to apply lather.
21 Hold the skin taut with 1 hand.
22 Shave in the direction of hair growth. Use shorter strokes around the chin and lips (Fig. 25-10).
23 Rinse the razor often. Wipe it with tissues or paper towels.
24 Apply direct pressure to any bleeding areas (Chapter 58).
25 Wash off remaining shaving cream or soap. Pat dry with a towel.
26 Apply after-shave or lotion if requested. (If there are nicks or cuts, do not apply after-shave or lotion.)
27 Remove and discard the towel and gloves. Practice hand hygiene.

POST-PROCEDURE

28 Provide for comfort. (See the inside of the back cover.)
29 Place the call light and other needed items within reach.
30 Lower the bed to a safe and comfortable level. Follow the care plan.
31 Raise or lower bed rails. Follow the care plan.
32 Clean, rinse, dry, and return equipment and supplies to their proper place. Use clean, dry paper towels for drying. Discard the razor blade or disposable razor into the sharps container. Discard other disposable items. Wear gloves.

33 Wipe off the over-bed table with clean, dry paper towels. Discard the paper towels.
34 Unscreen the person.
35 Complete a safety check of the room. (See the inside of the back cover.)
36 Follow agency policy for used linens.
37 Remove and discard the gloves. Practice hand hygiene.
38 Report nicks, cuts, irritation, or bleeding to the nurse at once. Also report and record other observations.

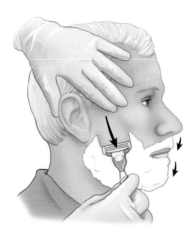

FIGURE 25-10 Shave the face in the direction of hair growth. Use long strokes on the larger areas of the face. Use short strokes around the chin and lips.

Caring for Mustaches and Beards

Mustaches and beards need daily care. Food and mouth and nose drainage can collect in the whiskers. Daily washing and combing are needed. Ask the person how to groom his mustache or beard. *Never shave or trim a mustache or beard.*

Shaving Legs and Underarms

Shaving legs and underarms varies among cultures. Some persons shave only the lower legs. Others shave to mid-thigh or the entire leg.

To shave legs and underarms:
- Follow the rules in Box 25-1.
- Collect shaving items with bath items.
- Shave after bathing while the skin is soft.
- Use soap and water, shaving cream, or lotion for the lather. Follow the care plan.
- Use the kidney basin to rinse the razor. Do not use bath water.

NAIL AND FOOT CARE

Nail and foot care prevents infection, injury, and odors. Hangnails, ingrown nails (nails that grow in at the side), and nails torn away from the skin cause skin breaks. Skin breaks are portals of entry for microbes. Long or broken nails can scratch the skin and snag clothing.

Dirty feet, socks, or stockings harbor microbes and cause odors. Shoes and socks provide a warm, moist place for microbes to grow. Injuries occur from stubbing toes, stepping on sharp objects, or being stepped on. Poorly fitting shoes cause blisters.

Poor circulation prolongs healing. Diabetes and vascular diseases cause poor circulation. Foot injuries or infections are very serious for older persons and those with circulatory disorders. Gangrene and amputation are serious complications (Chapter 48).

Nails are easier to clean and trim right after soaking or bathing. Use nail clippers to cut fingernails. *Never use scissors.* Use extreme caution to prevent damage to nearby tissues.

Trimming and clipping toenails can easily cause injuries. *Some agencies do not let nursing assistants cut or trim toenails. Follow agency policy.*

See *Teamwork and Time Management: Nail and Foot Care.*

See *Focus on Long-Term Care and Home Care: Nail and Foot Care.*

See *Delegation Guidelines: Nail and Foot Care,* p. 386.

See *Promoting Safety and Comfort: Nail and Foot Care,* p. 386.

See procedure: *Giving Nail and Foot Care,* p. 387.

TEAMWORK AND TIME MANAGEMENT

Nail and Foot Care

Use your time well when giving nail and foot care. The fingernails soak for 5 to 10 minutes. The feet soak for 15 to 20 minutes. Make the person's bed or straighten the person's unit during soak time. Or assist with brushing and combing hair. Check your assignment sheet for other ways to meet the person's needs.

FOCUS ON LONG-TERM CARE AND HOME CARE

Nail and Foot Care

Home Care

The feet soak during a tub bath. Or if able, the person can sit on the side of the tub to soak the feet. Make sure the person can step into and out of the tub. Or have the person use a shower bench to get in and out of the tub (Chapter 24). Otherwise, soak the feet in a basin or a whirlpool foot bath.

If comfortable for the person, he or she can soak the fingers in the sink. Or have the person sit at a table. Soak the fingers in a bowl or small basin.

Follow the care plan and the nurse's directions for how to position the person for nail and foot care.

DELEGATION GUIDELINES

Nail and Foot Care

The procedure that follows is a routine nursing task. Trimming and clipping toenails is a nursing responsibility that may be delegated to you in some agencies.

To give nail and foot care, you need this information from the nurse and the care plan.

- What water temperature to use
- How long to soak fingernails (usually 5 to 10 minutes)
- How long to soak feet (usually 15 to 20 minutes or less)
- If fingernails should be filed but not trimmed
- How to position the person
- What observations to report and record:
  - Dry, reddened, irritated, or callused areas
  - Breaks in the skin
  - Corns (Chapter 40) on top of and between the toes
  - Blisters
  - Very thick nails
  - Loose nails
- When to report observations
- What patient or resident concerns to report at once

PROMOTING SAFETY AND COMFORT

Nail and Foot Care

Safety

To cut fingernails, use nail clippers. Clip the fingernails straight across (Fig. 25-11). Then file the nails.

Some states and agencies do not let nursing assistants cut and trim toenails. A nurse or podiatrist (foot *[pod]* doctor) cuts toenails and provides foot care for the following persons. *You do not cut or trim the fingernails or toenails for persons who:*

- Have diabetes
- Have poor circulation
- Take drugs that affect blood clotting
- Have nail fungus, very thick nails, or ingrown nails (Chapter 40)

Check between the toes for cracks and sores. If not treated, a serious infection could occur.

The feet are easily burned. Persons with decreased sensation or circulatory problems may not feel hot temperatures.

After soaking, apply lotion or petroleum jelly to the feet if directed to do so. This can cause slippery feet. The person wears slip-resistant footwear before you transfer the person or let the person walk.

Breaks in the skin and bleeding can occur. Follow Standard Precautions and the Bloodborne Pathogen Standard.

Comfort

Sometimes you just trim the fingernails. Sometimes you just give foot care. To do both, the person sits at the over-bed table (Fig. 25-12). Provide for warmth and comfort.

Provide for your comfort during nail and foot care. Sit in front of the over-bed table to clean and trim fingernails. For foot care, rest the person's lower leg and foot on your lap. Or position the feet on the floor and kneel on the floor. Lay a towel across your lap or put a bath mat on the floor to protect your uniform. Use good body mechanics. Always support the person's foot and ankle during foot care.

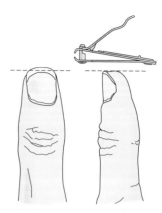

FIGURE 25-11 Clip fingernails straight across. Use nail clippers.

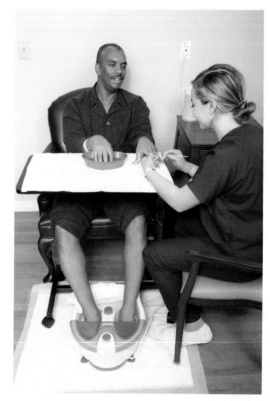

FIGURE 25-12 Nail and foot care. The feet soak in a whirlpool foot bath. The fingers soak in a kidney basin.

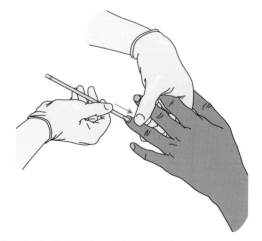

FIGURE 25-13 Push the cuticle back with an orangewood stick.

Giving Nail and Foot Care

QUALITY OF LIFE

- Knock before entering the person's room.
- Address the person by name.
- Introduce yourself by name and title.
- Explain the procedure before starting and during the procedure.
- Protect the person's rights during the procedure.
- Handle the person gently during the procedure.

PRE-PROCEDURE

1 Follow *Delegation Guidelines: Nail and Foot Care*. See *Promoting Safety and Comfort: Nail and Foot Care*.
2 Practice hand hygiene.
3 Collect the following.
   - Wash basin or whirlpool foot bath
   - Soap
   - Water thermometer
   - Bath towel
   - Hand towel
   - Washcloth
   - Kidney basin
   - Nail clippers
   - Orangewood stick
   - Emery board or nail file
   - Lotion for the hands
   - Lotion or petroleum jelly for the feet
   - Paper towels
   - Bath mat
   - Gloves
4 Arrange paper towels and other items on the over-bed table.
5 Identify the person. Check the ID bracelet against the assignment sheet. Use 2 identifiers (Chapter 13). Also call the person by name.
6 Provide for privacy.
7 Assist the person to the bedside chair. Remove footwear and socks or stockings. Place the call light and other needed items within reach.

PROCEDURE

8 Place the bath mat under the feet.
9 Fill the wash basin or whirlpool foot bath ⅔ (two-thirds) full with water. The nurse tells you what water temperature to use. (Measure water temperature with a water thermometer. Or test it by dipping your elbow or inner wrist into the basin. Follow agency policy.) Have the person check the water temperature and adjust as needed.
10 Place the basin or foot bath on the bath mat.
11 Put on gloves.
12 Help the person put his or her bare feet into the water. Both feet are covered by water.
13 Adjust the over-bed table in front of the person.
14 Fill the kidney basin ⅔ (two-thirds) full with water. See step 9 for water temperature.
15 Place the kidney basin on the over-bed table.
16 Place the person's fingers into the basin. Position the arms for comfort (see Fig. 25-12).
17 Let the fingers soak for 5 to 10 minutes. Let the feet soak for 15 to 20 minutes. Re-warm water as needed.
18 Remove the kidney basin.
19 Dry the hands and between the fingers thoroughly.
20 Clean under the fingernails with the orangewood stick. Wipe the orangewood stick with a towel after each nail.
21 Push cuticles back gently with the orangewood stick, towel, or washcloth (Fig. 25-13).
22 Clip fingernails straight across with the nail clippers (see Fig. 25-11).
23 File and shape nails with an emery board or nail file. Nails are smooth with no rough edges. Check each nail for smoothness. File as needed.
24 Apply lotion to the hands. Warm the lotion first. To warm lotion, rub some between your hands or hold the bottle under warm water.
25 Move the over-bed table to the side.
26 Remove and discard the gloves. Practice hand hygiene. Put on clean gloves. (NOTE: Some state competency tests require clean gloves for foot care.)
27 Lift a foot out of the water. Support the foot and ankle with 1 hand. With your other hand, wash the foot and between the toes with soap and a washcloth. Return the foot to the water to rinse the foot and between the toes.
28 Repeat step 27 for the other foot.
29 Remove the feet from the water. Dry thoroughly, especially between the toes. Support the foot and ankle as needed.
30 Apply lotion or petroleum jelly to the tops, soles, and heels of the feet. Do not apply between the toes. Warm lotion or petroleum jelly first (see step 24). Remove excess lotion or petroleum jelly with a towel. Support the foot and ankle as needed.
31 Remove and discard the gloves. Practice hand hygiene.
32 Help the person put on slip-resistant footwear.

POST-PROCEDURE

33 Provide for comfort. (See the inside of the back cover.)
34 Place the call light and other needed items within reach.
35 Raise or lower bed rails. Follow the care plan.
36 Clean, rinse, dry, and return equipment and supplies to their proper place. Use clean, dry paper towels for drying. Discard disposable items. Wear gloves and practice hand hygiene after removing them.
37 Unscreen the person.
38 Complete a safety check of the room. (See the inside of the back cover.)
39 Follow agency policy for used linens.
40 Remove and discard the gloves. Practice hand hygiene.
41 Report and record your observations.

FOCUS ON **PRIDE**

The Person, Family, and Yourself

P ersonal and Professional Responsibility

Grooming promotes comfort, self-esteem, and body image. Clean hair and nails help mental well-being. So does a clean-shaven face or a well-groomed beard or mustache.

Focus on your appearance. Patients, residents, and families notice when others are not well groomed. If not groomed well, they may question the quality of care you provide. Have a professional appearance.

R ights and Respect

Grooming preferences vary. You may not like the person's hair-style or personal care products. Do not judge the person by your standards or impose your choices on the person. Respect the right to choose. Assist with grooming in a way that improves the person's self-esteem.

I ndependence and Social Interaction

Some family members want to help with grooming. For example, they want to style the person's hair. Or they want to apply lotion to the person's hands and feet.

With the person's permission, allow family to assist with grooming as much as safely possible. This promotes social interaction. It also involves the family in the person's care.

D elegation and Teamwork

Grooming takes time. You, the person, the nurse, and other team members work together to plan and organize care. For example, a resident had a stroke. Breakfast is at 0800, speech therapy is at 0930, and family visits during lunch. The resident prefers to comb hair and shave after breakfast but before visitors arrive. You plan to assist the resident with grooming after breakfast and before speech therapy.

E thics and Laws

Patients and residents have the right to be free from mistreatment and restraint (Chapter 2). The following is a case where a nurse did not follow these ethical principles.

A nurse told a patient that she was going to cut his hair and trim his beard. The patient repeatedly stated that he did not want a haircut or his beard trimmed. The patient protested and resisted the nurse's actions. She continued her actions while 2 other staff members restrained the patient.

The patient reported the incident to his social worker. An internal investigation was conducted.

The nurse lost her job. The United States Court of Appeals agreed that the nurse's termination was warranted because of:

- *The nature and seriousness of the offense*
- *The restraint of the patient after he repeatedly objected* (L. Taylor v Department of Veterans Affairs, 2006.)

Never force a care measure on a person. If a person resists or refuses care, stop. Do not proceed. Politely ask the person for the reason. Tell the nurse. You, the nurse, and the person can discuss a solution.

FOCUS ON **PRIDE**: *Application*

The family may notice when grooming differs from usual. The family may tell you what they expect. Why are their comments important? How can you show that you value their input?

REVIEW QUESTIONS

Circle T if the statement is TRUE or F if it is FALSE.

1 T F Surveyors observe if residents are well groomed.

2 T F Shared grooming equipment is cleaned and returned to its proper place after use.

3 T F Scabies is contagious.

4 T F You can cut matted hair.

5 T F A hearing aid can be worn during shampooing.

6 T F Mustaches are trimmed weekly.

7 T F Feet are soaked for 25 to 30 minutes.

8 T F Fingernails are clipped straight across.

9 T F Gloves are worn for nail care.

10 T F A person has poor circulation in the legs and feet. You can trim the person's toenails.

Circle the BEST answer.

11 A person with alopecia has
   a Excessive body hair
   b Dry, white flakes from the scalp
   c An infestation with lice
   d Hair loss

12 Which should you report before giving hair care?
   a Braided hair
   b White specks in the hair
   c Dry hair
   d Dirty hair

13 Which prevents hair from matting and tangling?
   a Bed rest
   b Daily brushing and combing
   c Daily shampooing
   d Cutting hair

REVIEW QUESTIONS—cont'd

14 A person's hair is *not* matted or tangled. When brushing hair, start at
   a The forehead and brush backward
   b The hair ends
   c The scalp
   d The back of the neck and brush forward

15 Brushing keeps the hair
   a Soft and shiny
   b Clean
   c Free of lice
   d Long

16 A person requests a shampoo. You should
   a Shampoo hair during the person's shower
   b Shampoo hair at the sink
   c Shampoo the person in bed
   d Follow the care plan

17 To keep shampoo out of the eyes during a shower
   a Do not rinse the top of the head
   b Wipe off the shampoo with a washcloth
   c Have the person wear eyeglasses
   d Place a washcloth over the eyes and tip the head back

18 When shaving a person's face with a safety razor
   a Discard the razor in the wastebasket when done
   b Shave against the direction of hair growth
   c Hold the skin taut
   d Shave when the skin is dry

19 A person is nicked during shaving. Your *first* action is to
   a Wash your hands
   b Apply direct pressure
   c Tell the nurse
   d Apply a bandage

20 Fingernails are cut with
   a An emery board
   b Scissors
   c A nail file
   d Nail clippers

21 Fingernails are cleaned
   a Before soaking
   b After soaking
   c After trimming
   d After trimming toenails

22 When giving foot care
   a Dry well between the toes
   b Apply lotion between the toes
   c Do not wash between the toes
   d Do not use soap

Answers to Chapter 25 questions are on p. 886.

FOCUS ON PRACTICE

Problem Solving

A resident with dementia has long fingernails. Some are broken and have rough edges. As you begin nail care, the resident resists by pulling away and yelling at you. What do you do? Why is nail care important for this resident? How might you provide care safely?

OBJECTIVES

- Define the key terms and key abbreviations in this chapter.
- Identify when garments need to be changed.
- Explain the rules for dressing and undressing.
- Explain how to safely change a patient gown on a person with an IV.

- Perform the procedures described in this chapter.
- Explain how to promote PRIDE in the person, the family, and yourself.

KEY TERMS

affected side The side of the body with weakness from illness or injury; weak side
garment An item of clothing

unaffected side The side of the body opposite the affected side; strong side
under-garment An item of clothing worn next to the skin under clothing

KEY ABBREVIATIONS

ID Identification

IV Intravenous

Clothing affects comfort and body image. The ability to dress and undress oneself promotes dignity and independence. You will assist patients and residents with dressing needs.

See *Focus on Surveys: Dressing and Undressing.*

FOCUS ON SURVEYS

Dressing and Undressing

Surveyors will observe if residents:
- Are dressed in their own clothes.
- Are dressed in clothing of their choice.
- Are wearing the correct clothing for the time of day.

CHANGING GARMENTS

A *garment is an item of clothing.* Age, gender, culture, comfort, season, and personal preference affect garment choices. An *under-garment is an item of clothing worn next to the skin under clothing.* Bras, undershirts, underwear, underpants, panties, slips, briefs, and boxer shorts are examples. Incontinence products may be worn (Chapter 27).

Garments are often changed in the morning and at bedtime. They also are changed:
- After bathing
- When wet or soiled
- On admission and discharge

Hospital patients wear gowns (patient gowns) that open in the back. For some examinations and procedures, the opening is in front (Chapter 37). Nursing center residents wear street clothes during the day and sleepwear at bedtime.

See *Focus on Communication: Changing Garments.*
See *Focus on Long-Term Care and Home Care: Changing Garments.*

FOCUS ON COMMUNICATION

Changing Garments

When changing garments, promote personal choice and independence. You can ask:
- "What would you like to wear today?"
- "There's a concert today. Do you want to wear something special?"
- "Do you need help with your buttons?"
- "Would you like help with your zipper?"

There are many types of and names for under-garments. For example, a person may refer to underpants as "drawers," "skivvies," or "britches." Persons in cold climates may wear "long johns." Use terms the person uses and understands. Be respectful and professional.

Changing Garments

Long-Term Care

Personal choice is a resident right. Let the person choose
what to wear.

Resident clothing is labeled with the person's name in a
way that respects dignity. For example, labels are inside
clothing or shoes. Or a color-coded system is used. Know
your agency's policy. Residents must be dressed in their own
clothing.

Home Care

Patients often wear street clothes during the day. Or
sleepwear and robes are worn. The procedures that follow
apply to sleepwear, robes, and street clothes.

| BOX 26-1 | **Rules for Dressing and Undressing** |

- Provide for privacy. Do not expose the person.
- Encourage the person to do as much as possible.
- Let the person choose what to wear. Have the person
  choose the right under-garments.
- Make sure garments and footwear are the correct size.
- Remove clothing from the *unaffected side* (strong side)
  first.
- Put clothing on the *affected side* (weak side) first.
- Support the arm or leg to remove or put on a garment.
- Move and handle the body gently. Do not force a joint
  beyond its range of motion or to the point of pain. See
  Chapter 34.

Dressing and Undressing

Some persons dress and undress themselves. Others need
help. Allow the person to do as much as safely possible.
This promotes independence. Adaptive (assistive) devices
may be used (Fig. 26-1).

Health problems can cause weakness or affect function
on 1 side of the body. Stroke and hip fracture are examples
(Chapter 48). When assisting with dressing and undressing, you need to know about areas of weakness.

- The *affected side* (weak side) is the side of the body with
  weakness from illness or injury.
- The *unaffected side* (strong side) is the side of the body
  opposite the affected side.

To assist with dressing and undressing, follow the rules
in Box 26-1.

See *Focus on Children and Older Persons: Dressing and
Undressing*, p. 392.

See *Delegation Guidelines: Dressing and Undressing*,
p. 392.

See *Promoting Safety and Comfort: Dressing and
Undressing*, p. 392.

See procedure: *Undressing the Person*, p. 392.

See procedure: *Dressing the Person*, p. 395.

Text continued on p. 396.

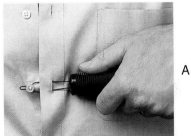

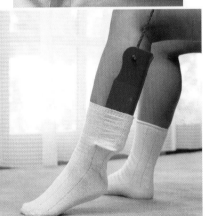

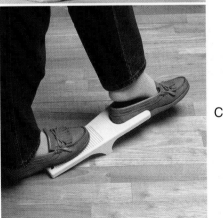

FIGURE 26-1 Dressing aids. **A,** A button hook to button and zip
clothing. **B,** A sock assist to pull on socks and stockings. **C,** A shoe
remover to take off shoes. (Courtesy North Coast Medical Inc., Morgan
Hill, Calif.)

FOCUS ON CHILDREN AND OLDER PERSONS

Dressing and Undressing

Older Persons

Persons with dementia often take longer to dress. Choosing clothing may be hard. Wearing the wrong clothing for the season and wearing clothes that do not match are common. Or they forget to put on a piece of clothing.

Allow the person to dress himself or herself to the extent possible. The Alzheimer's and Related Dementias Education and Referral Center (ADEAR) suggests the following.

- Try to assist with dressing at the same time each day. Dressing becomes part of the daily routine.
- Allow extra time. Do not rush the person.
- Let the person choose from 2 or 3 outfits. The family may buy several of the same outfit. Dressing is easier if the person insists on wearing the same thing.
- Choose comfortable, easy to get on and off clothes. Garments with elastic waistbands and Velcro closures are examples. There are no zippers, buttons, hooks, snaps, or other closures.
- Stack clothes in the order they are put on. The person sees 1 item at a time. For example, an under-garment is put on first. The item is on top of the stack.
- Give clear, simple, and step-by-step directions. Give the person 1 item at a time.

DELEGATION GUIDELINES

Dressing and Undressing

Changing garments is a routine nursing task. To assist with dressing and undressing, you need this information from the nurse and the care plan.

- How much help the person needs
- If the person has an affected side (weak side)
- If certain garments are needed
- What observations to report and record:
  - How much help was given
  - How the person tolerated the procedure
  - Complaints by the person
  - Changes in the person's behavior
- When to report observations
- What patient or resident concerns to report at once

PROMOTING SAFETY AND COMFORT

Dressing and Undressing

Safety

To assist with dressing and undressing in bed, you turn the person from side to side. If the person uses bed rails, raise the far bed rail. If bed rails are not used, ask a co-worker to help turn and position the person. This protects the person from falling.

Follow the safety measures for transfers (Chapter 20) and tub baths and showers (Chapter 24) when undressing and dressing in a tub or shower room. Follow the care plan for the transfer method and number of staff needed.
Remember:

- Slip-resistant footwear is worn for transfers.
- Be sure the floor is dry.
- Have the person use grab bars (safety bars) for support.
- Lock (brake) the wheels on a wheelchair and shower chair.
- Apply a transfer belt (gait belt) over clothing.

Undressing the Person

QUALITY OF LIFE

- Knock before entering the person's room.
- Address the person by name.
- Introduce yourself by name and title.

- Explain the procedure before starting and during the procedure.
- Protect the person's rights during the procedure.
- Handle the person gently during the procedure.

PRE-PROCEDURE

1 Follow *Delegation Guidelines: Dressing and Undressing.* See *Promoting Safety and Comfort: Dressing and Undressing.*
2 Ask a co-worker to help turn and position the person if needed.
3 Practice hand hygiene.
4 Collect a bath blanket and clothing requested by the person.

5 Identify the person. Check the ID (identification) bracelet against the assignment sheet. Use 2 identifiers (Chapter 13). Also call the person by name.
6 Provide for privacy.
7 Raise the bed for body mechanics. Bed rails are up if used.
8 Lower the bed rail on the person's affected (weak) side.
9 Position him or her supine.
10 Cover the person with a bath blanket. Fan-fold linens to the foot of the bed.

Undressing the Person—cont'd

PROCEDURE

11 Remove garments that open in back.
  a Raise the head and shoulders. Or turn the person onto the side away from you.
  b Undo buttons, zippers, ties, or snaps.
  c Bring the sides of the garment to the sides of the person (Fig. 26-2). For a side-lying position, tuck the far side of the garment under the person. Fold the near side onto the chest (Fig. 26-3).
  d Position the person supine.
  e Slide the garment off the shoulder on the unaffected (strong) side. Remove it from the arm (Fig. 26-4, p. 394).
  f Remove the garment from the affected (weak) side.

12 Remove garments that open in the front.
  a Undo buttons, zippers, ties, or snaps.
  b Slide the garment off the shoulder and arm on the unaffected (strong) side.
  c Help the person sit up or raise the head and shoulders. Bring the garment to the affected (weak) side (Fig. 26-5, p. 394).
  d Lower the head and shoulders. Remove the garment from the affected (weak) side.
  e If you cannot raise the head and shoulders:
    1) Turn the person toward you. Tuck the removed part of the garment under the person.
    2) Turn the person onto the side away from you.
    3) Pull the side of the garment out from under the person. Make sure he or she will not lie on it when supine.
    4) Return the person to the supine position.
    5) Remove the garment from the affected (weak) side.

13 Remove pullover garments.
  a Undo buttons, zippers, ties, or snaps.
  b Remove the garment from the unaffected (strong) side.
  c Raise the head and shoulders. Or turn the person onto the side away from you. Bring the garment up to the neck (Fig. 26-6, p. 394).
  d Bring the garment over the head.
  e Remove the garment from the affected (weak) side.
  f Position the person in the supine position.

14 Remove pants or slacks.
  a Remove footwear and socks.
  b Position the person supine.
  c Undo buttons, zippers, ties, snaps, or buckles.
  d Remove the belt.
  e Have the person lift the buttocks off the bed. Slide the pants down over the hips and buttocks (Fig. 26-7, p. 394). Have the person lower the hips and buttocks.
  f If the person cannot raise the hips off the bed:
    1) Turn the person toward you.
    2) Slide the pants off the hip and buttocks on the unaffected (strong) side (Fig. 26-8, p. 394).
    3) Turn the person away from you.
    4) Slide the pants off the hip and buttocks on the affected (weak) side (Fig. 26-9, p. 394).
  g Slide the pants down the legs and over the feet.

15 Dress the person. See procedure: *Dressing the Person,* p. 395.

POST-PROCEDURE

16 Provide for comfort. (See the inside of the back cover.)
17 Place the call light and other needed items within reach.
18 Lower the bed to a safe and comfortable level. Follow the care plan.
19 Raise or lower bed rails. Follow the care plan.
20 Unscreen the person.
21 Complete a safety check of the room. (See the inside of the back cover.)
22 Follow agency policy for removed clothing.
23 Practice hand hygiene.
24 Report and record your observations.

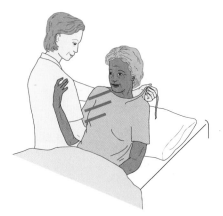

FIGURE 26-2 The sides of the garment are brought from the back to the sides of the person. (NOTE: *The affected [weak] side is indicated by slash marks.*)

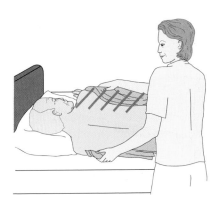

FIGURE 26-3 A garment that opens in the back is removed from the person in the side-lying position. The far side of the garment is tucked under the person. The near side is folded onto the person's chest. (NOTE: *The affected [weak] side is indicated by slash marks.*)

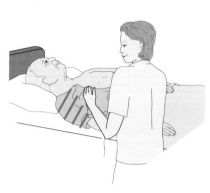

FIGURE 26-4 The garment is removed from the unaffected (strong) side first. (NOTE: *The affected [weak] side is indicated by slash marks.*)

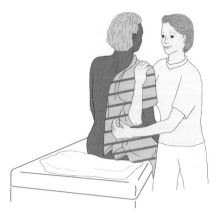

FIGURE 26-5 A front-opening garment is removed with the person's head and shoulders raised. The garment is removed from the unaffected (strong) side first. Then it is brought around the back to the affected (weak) side. (NOTE: *The affected [weak] side is indicated by slash marks.*)

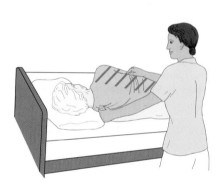

FIGURE 26-6 A pullover garment is removed from the unaffected (strong) side first. Then the garment is brought up to the person's neck so that it can be removed from the affected (weak) side. (NOTE: *The affected [weak] side is indicated by slash marks.*)

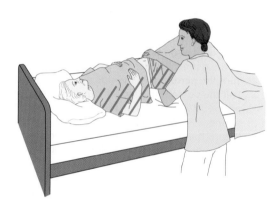

FIGURE 26-7 The person lifts the hips and buttocks to remove the pants. The pants are slid down over the hips and buttocks. (NOTE: *The affected [weak] side is indicated by slash marks.*)

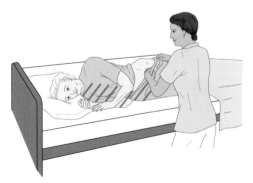

FIGURE 26-8 Pants are removed in the side-lying position. They are removed from the unaffected (strong) side first. They are slid over the hip and buttock. (NOTE: *The affected [weak] side is indicated by slash marks.*)

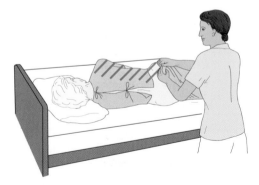

FIGURE 26-9 The person is turned onto the unaffected (strong) side. The pants are removed from the affected (weak) side. (NOTE: *The affected [weak] side is indicated by slash marks.*)

Dressing the Person

QUALITY OF LIFE

- Knock before entering the person's room.
- Address the person by name.
- Introduce yourself by name and title.

- Explain the procedure before starting and during the procedure.
- Protect the person's rights during the procedure.
- Handle the person gently during the procedure.

PRE-PROCEDURE

1 Follow *Delegation Guidelines: Dressing and Undressing,* p. 392. See *Promoting Safety and Comfort: Dressing and Undressing,* p. 392.
2 Ask a co-worker to help turn and position the person if needed.
3 Practice hand hygiene.
4 Ask what the person would like to wear.
5 Get a bath blanket and clothing requested by the person.
6 Identify the person. Check the ID bracelet against the assignment sheet. Use 2 identifiers (Chapter 13). Also call the person by name.

7 Provide for privacy.
8 Raise the bed for body mechanics. Bed rails are up if used.
9 Lower the bed rail (if up) on the person's affected (weak) side.
10 Position the person supine.
11 Cover the person with a bath blanket. Fan-fold linens to the foot of the bed.
12 Undress the person. See procedure: *Undressing the Person,* p. 392.

PROCEDURE

13 Put on garments that open in the back.
  a Slide the garment onto the arm and shoulder of the affected (weak) side.
  b Slide the garment onto the arm and shoulder of the unaffected (strong) side.
  c Raise the person's head and shoulders.
  d Bring the sides to the back.
  e If you cannot raise the person's head and shoulders:
    1) Turn the person toward you.
    2) Bring 1 side of the garment to the person's back (Fig. 26-10, *A,* p. 396).
    3) Turn the person away from you.
    4) Bring the other side to the person's back (Fig. 26-10, *B,* p. 396).
  f Fasten buttons, zippers, ties, snaps, or other closures.
  g Position the person supine.
14 Put on garments that open in the front.
  a Slide the garment onto the arm and shoulder on the affected (weak) side.
  b Raise the head and shoulders. Bring the side of the garment around to the back. Lower the person down. Slide the garment onto the arm and shoulder of the unaffected (strong) arm.
  c If the person cannot raise the head and shoulders:
    1) Turn the person away from you.
    2) Tuck the garment under him or her.
    3) Turn the person toward you.
    4) Pull the garment out from under him or her.
    5) Turn the person back to the supine position.
    6) Slide the garment over the arm and shoulder of the unaffected (strong) arm.
  d Fasten buttons, zippers, ties, snaps, or other closures.
15 Put on pullover garments.
  a Slide the arm and shoulder of the garment onto the affected (weak) side (Fig. 26-11, *A,* p. 396).
  b Raise the person's head and shoulders.

  c Bring the neck of the garment over the head.
  d Slide the arm and shoulder of the garment onto the unaffected (strong) side. Bring the garment down.
  e If the person cannot assume a semi-sitting position:
    1) Bring the neck of the garment over the head.
    2) Slide the arm and shoulder of the garment onto the unaffected (strong) side (Fig. 26-11, *B,* p. 396).
    3) Turn the person onto the unaffected (strong) side.
    4) Pull the garment down on the person's affected (weak) side.
    5) Turn the person onto the affected (weak) side.
    6) Pull the garment down on the person's unaffected (strong) side.
  f Position the person supine.
16 Put on pants or slacks:
  a Slide the pants over the feet and up the legs.
  b Have the person raise the hips and buttocks off the bed.
  c Bring the pants up over the buttock and hip on the affected (weak) side.
  d Pull the pants over the buttock and hip on the unaffected (strong) side.
  e If the person cannot raise the hips and buttocks:
    1) Turn the person onto the unaffected (strong) side.
    2) Pull the pants over the buttock and hip on the affected (weak) side.
    3) Turn the person onto the affected (weak) side.
    4) Pull the pants over the buttock and hip on the unaffected (strong) side.
    5) Position the person supine.
  f Fasten buttons, zippers, ties, snaps, a belt buckle, or other closures.
17 Put socks and slip-resistant footwear on the person. Socks are up all the way and smooth.
18 Help the person get out of bed. If the person stays in bed, cover the person. Remove the bath blanket.

POST-PROCEDURE

19 Provide for comfort. (See the inside of the back cover.)
20 Place the call light and other needed items within reach.
21 Lower the bed to a safe and comfortable level. Follow the care plan.
22 Raise or lower bed rails. Follow the care plan.
23 Unscreen the person.

24 Complete a safety check of the room. (See the inside of the back cover.)
25 Follow agency policy for removed clothing.
26 Practice hand hygiene.
27 Report and record your observations.

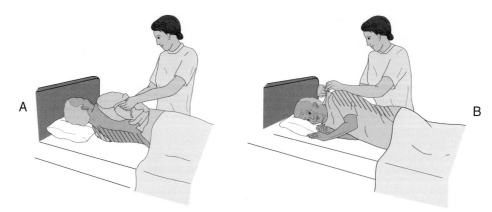

FIGURE 26-10 Applying garments that open in the back. **A,** The side-lying position can be used to put on garments that open in the back. Turn the person toward you after the garment is put on the arms. Bring the side of the garment to the person's back. **B,** Then turn the person away from you. Bring the other side of the garment to the back and fasten. (NOTE: *The affected [weak] side is indicated by slash marks.*)

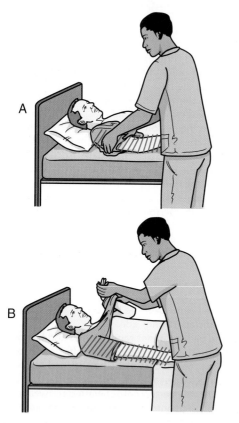

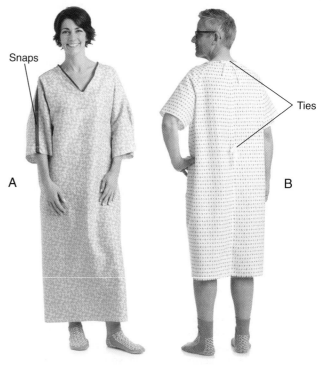

FIGURE 26-12 Patient gowns. **A,** IV therapy gown. Snaps on the sleeves allow for easy changing. **B,** Standard gown. This gown ties at the neck and back. (Courtesy Medline Industries, Inc. © Medline Industries, Inc. 2019.)

FIGURE 26-11 Applying pullover garments. **A,** Apply the garment to the affected (weak) side first. **B,** Bring the garment up over the head and slide it onto the unaffected (strong) side. (NOTE: *The affected [weak] side is indicated by slash marks.*)

Changing Patient Gowns

Patient gowns are designed for comfort and to allow treatment (Fig. 26-12).

- An *intravenous (IV) therapy gown* is used for IV therapy (Chapter 32). The gown opens along the sleeves and closes with ties, snaps, or Velcro.
- A *standard gown* does not open along the sleeves.

For injury or paralysis, remove the gown from the unaffected (strong) arm first. Support the affected (weak) arm while removing the gown. Put the clean gown on the affected (weak) arm first and then on the unaffected (strong) arm.

See *Delegation Guidelines: Changing Patient Gowns.*

See *Promoting Safety and Comfort: Changing Patient Gowns.*

See procedure: *Changing a Standard Patient Gown on a Person With an IV.*

DELEGATION GUIDELINES

Changing Patient Gowns

Changing a patient gown on a person without an IV is a routine nursing task. If the person has an IV but no IV pump (Fig. 26-13, p. 398), the task may be a delegated nursing responsibility. Before changing a gown on a person with an IV, you need this information from the nurse and the care plan.

- Which arm has the IV
- If the person has an IV pump (see *Promoting Safety and Comfort: Changing Patient Gowns*)

PROMOTING SAFETY AND COMFORT

Changing Patient Gowns

Safety

IV pumps control the *flow rate*—how fast fluid enters a vein (Chapter 32). You do not adjust controls on IV pumps. For an IV pump and a standard gown, do not use the following procedure. The nurse handles the arm with the IV.

To change a gown, you move the IV bag. Moving the IV bag can change the IV flow rate. Always ask the nurse to check the flow rate after you change a gown.

Do not disconnect or remove any part of the IV set-up.

Comfort

Some gowns tie at the upper back. The back and buttocks are exposed when the person stands. Cover the person for warmth and privacy. A robe or a second gown worn backwards will cover the back and buttocks. Other gowns over-lap in the back and tie at the side. These gowns provide more privacy. When tied at the side, uncomfortable bows and knots at the back are avoided.

Changing a Standard Patient Gown on a Person With an IV

QUALITY OF LIFE

- Knock before entering the person's room.
- Address the person by name.
- Introduce yourself by name and title.

- Explain the procedure before starting and during the procedure.
- Protect the person's rights during the procedure.
- Handle the person gently during the procedure.

PRE-PROCEDURE

1. Follow *Delegation Guidelines: Changing Patient Gowns.* See *Promoting Safety and Comfort: Changing Patient Gowns.*
2. Practice hand hygiene.
3. Get a clean gown and bath blanket.

4. Identify the person. Check the ID bracelet against the assignment sheet. Use 2 identifiers (Chapter 13). Also call the person by name.
5. Provide for privacy.
6. Raise the bed for body mechanics. Bed rails are up if used.

PROCEDURE

7. Lower the bed rail near you (if up).
8. Cover the person with the bath blanket. Fan-fold linens to the foot of the bed.
9. Untie the gown. Free parts that the person is lying on.
10. Remove the gown from the arm with *no IV.*
11. Gather up the sleeve of the arm *with the IV.* Slide it over the IV site and tubing. Remove the arm and hand from the sleeve (see Fig. 26-13, *A*).
12. Keep the sleeve gathered. Slide your arm along the tubing to the bag (see Fig. 26-13, *B*).
13. Remove the bag from the pole. Slide the bag and tubing through the sleeve (see Fig. 26-13, *C*). Do not pull on the tubing. Keep the bag above the person.

14. Hang the IV bag on the pole.
15. Gather the sleeve of the clean gown that will go on the arm with the IV.
16. Remove the bag from the pole. Slip the sleeve over the bag at the shoulder part of the gown (see Fig. 26-13, *D*). Hang the bag.
17. Slide the gathered sleeve over the tubing, hand, arm, and IV site. Then slide it onto the shoulder.
18. Put the other side of the gown on the person. Fasten the gown.
19. Cover the person. Remove the bath blanket.

POST-PROCEDURE

20. Provide for comfort. (See the inside of the back cover.)
21. Place the call light and other needed items within reach.
22. Lower the bed to a safe and comfortable level. Follow the care plan.
23. Raise or lower bed rails. Follow the care plan.
24. Unscreen the person.

25. Complete a safety check of the room. (See the inside of the back cover.)
26. Follow agency policy for used linens.
27. Practice hand hygiene.
28. Ask the nurse to check the flow rate.
29. Report and record your observations.

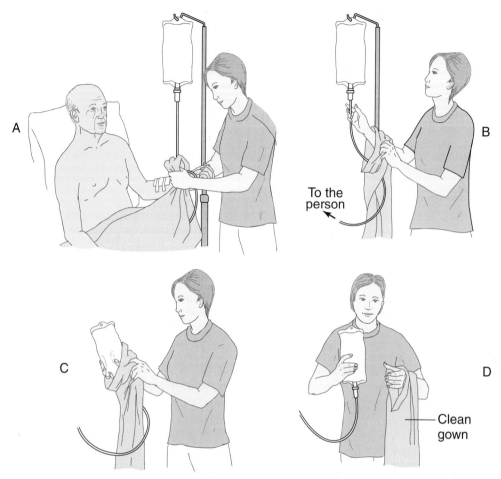

FIGURE 26-13 Changing a gown. **A,** Remove the gown from the arm with no IV. Gather up the sleeve on the arm with the IV. Slip it over the IV site and tubing and remove it from the arm and hand. **B,** Slip the gathered sleeve along the IV tubing to the bag. **C,** Remove the IV bag from the pole and pass it through the sleeve. **D,** Slip the gathered sleeve of the clean gown over the IV bag at the shoulder part of the gown.

FOCUS ON **PRIDE**

The Person, Family, and Yourself

Personal and Professional Responsibility
Care measures are not just tasks to be completed. Show that you value the person.
- Be pleasant. Talk with the person.
- Avoid seeming rushed. Let the person know that you have time for him or her.
- Do a good job. Be thorough and careful.
- Compliment the person after dressing.

Rights and Respect
Appearance affects self-esteem. Garments should be clean, not wrinkled, and comfortable. Matching clothes and clothes for the correct season are worn. If a garment does not fit well, change it. Dress the person in a way that promotes dignity and respect.

Independence and Social Interaction
Ask what clothing the person prefers. Ask about comfort and appearance. Personal choice promotes independence and quality of life.

Delegation and Teamwork
Some garments are worn as part of the person's treatment. Elastic stockings and binders or compression garments are examples (Chapters 39 and 40). You need more information from the nurse and the care plan before applying such garments.

Ethics and Laws
Special care measures are needed for persons with confusion or dementia who resist care (Chapter 53). Forcing care is wrong. Patience and problem solving are needed. A co-worker or family member may help with dressing. Or garments are changed at another time. Follow the person's routine and be kind and gentle.

FOCUS ON **PRIDE**: *Application*

How does clothing affect your self-image? How will you promote dignity and independence when assisting with dressing and undressing?

REVIEW QUESTIONS

Circle the BEST answer.

1 In long-term care
   a Patient gowns are worn
   b Sleepwear is worn during the day
   c Garments are changed every other day
   d Street clothes are worn during the day

2 For spilled coffee on a shirt, you should
   a Give the person a sweater to cover the spill
   b Dry the shirt with a towel
   c Change the shirt at bedtime
   d Change the shirt right away

3 Garments are removed
   a From the affected (weak) side first
   b From the unaffected (strong) side first
   c From either side first
   d In the same way they are applied

4 Garments are applied
   a To the affected (weak) side first
   b To the unaffected (strong) side first
   c To either side first
   d In the same way they are removed

5 When dressing
   a Support the arm or leg
   b Choose clothing for the person
   c Do as much for the person as possible
   d Move the person quickly

6 When dressing a person with dementia
   a Choose clothing with buttons
   b Give more than 1 direction at a time
   c Offer many clothing options
   d Follow the person's routine

7 An IV therapy gown
   a Opens at the sleeves
   b Does not have sleeves
   c Must be changed by the nurse
   d Provides less privacy than a standard gown

8 When changing the gown on a person with an IV
   a Keep the IV bag below the person's arm
   b Stop the IV pump to change the gown
   c Have the nurse check the flow rate afterward
   d Disconnect the IV to change the gown

Answers to Chapter 26 questions are on p. 886.

FOCUS ON PRACTICE

Problem Solving

Two residents share a room. After dressing the person you notice the shirt belongs to the resident's roommate. What will you do? How could this have been prevented?

Urinary Needs

OBJECTIVES

- Define the key terms and key abbreviations in this chapter.
- Describe the rules for normal urination.
- Describe normal urine.
- Identify the observations to report to the nurse.
- Describe urinary incontinence and the care required.

- Describe bladder training methods.
- Perform the procedures described in this chapter.
- Explain how to promote PRIDE in the person, the family, and yourself.

KEY TERMS

dysuria Painful or difficult *(dys)* urination *(uria)*; burning on urination

enuresis Involuntary loss or leakage of urine during sleep; bed-wetting

functional incontinence The person has bladder control but cannot use the toilet in time

groin Where a thigh and the abdomen meet

hematuria Blood *(hemat)* in the urine *(uria)*

mixed incontinence The combination of stress incontinence and urge incontinence

nocturia Frequent urination *(uria)* at night *(noc)*

oliguria Scant amount *(olig)* of urine *(uria)*; less than 500 mL in 24 hours

over-flow incontinence Small amounts of urine leak from a full bladder

polyuria Abnormally large amounts *(poly)* of urine *(uria)*

reflex incontinence Urine is lost at predictable intervals when a specific amount of urine is in the bladder

stress incontinence When urine leaks during exercise and certain movements that cause pressure on the bladder

transient incontinence Temporary or occasional incontinence that is reversed when the cause is treated

urge incontinence The loss of urine in response to a sudden, urgent need to void; the person cannot get to a toilet in time

urinary frequency Voiding at frequent intervals

urinary incontinence (UI) The involuntary loss or leakage of urine

urinary retention Not being able to completely empty the bladder

urinary urgency The need to void at once

urination The process of emptying urine from the bladder; voiding

voiding See "urination"

KEY ABBREVIATIONS

BM	Bowel movement
ID	Identification
mL	Milliliter

OAB	Over-active bladder
UI	Urinary incontinence
UTI	Urinary tract infection

Eliminating waste is a physical need. The digestive system rids the body of solid wastes. The lungs remove carbon dioxide. Sweat contains water and other substances. Blood contains waste products from body cells burning food for energy. The urinary system removes waste products from the blood. It also maintains water and electrolyte balance.

See *Body Structure and Function Review: The Urinary System.*

See *Teamwork and Time Management: Urinary Needs.*

See *Promoting Safety and Comfort: Urinary Needs.*

BODY STRUCTURE AND FUNCTION REVIEW

The Urinary System

The 2 *kidneys* (Fig. 27-1) lie in the upper abdomen against the back muscles on each side of the spine. Blood passes through the 2 kidneys. *Urine* is formed in the kidneys.

Urine consists of wastes and excess fluids filtered out of the blood. Urine flows through the 2 *ureters* to the urinary *bladder*. Urine is stored in the bladder. The *urethra* connects the bladder to the outside of the body. The opening at the end of the urethra is called the *meatus*. Urine passes from the body through the meatus. Urine is a clear, yellowish fluid.

See Chapter 10 for more information.

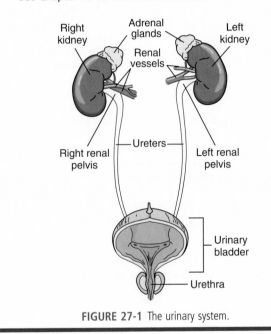

FIGURE 27-1 The urinary system.

TEAMWORK AND TIME MANAGEMENT

Urinary Needs

Urinary needs may be urgent. Answer call lights promptly. Also, answer call lights for co-workers. Otherwise incontinence may result (p. 410). The person is wet and embarrassed. Skin breakdown and infection are risks. Your co-worker has extra work—changing wet linens and garments. You like help when busy. So do your co-workers.

PROMOTING SAFETY AND COMFORT

Urinary Needs

Safety

Urinary elimination measures often involve exposing and touching private areas—the perineum and rectum. Sexual abuse has occurred in health care settings. The person may feel threatened or is actually being abused. He or she needs to call for help. Keep the call light within the person's reach at all times. Always act in a professional manner.

Urine may contain blood and microbes. Microbes can live and grow in bedpans, urinals, commodes, and urinary drainage bags (Chapter 28). Follow Standard Precautions and the Bloodborne Pathogen Standard to handle urinary devices and their contents. This includes incontinence products. Thoroughly clean and disinfect bedpans, urinals, and commodes after use. Remember to practice hand hygiene.

Each person is given his or her own bedpan or urinal. Some states and agencies require labeling the devices with the person's name and room and bed number. Equipment is not shared among patients and residents.

NOTE: A task may require more than 1 pair of gloves. Change gloves as needed. Use careful judgment. Remember to practice hand hygiene after removing gloves.

NORMAL URINATION

The healthy adult produces about 1500 mL (milliliters) or 3 pints of urine a day. Many factors affect urine production—age, disease, the amount and kinds of fluid ingested, salt, body temperature, perspiration (sweating), and some drugs. Some substances increase urine production—coffee, tea, alcohol, and some drugs. A diet high in salt and some drugs cause the body to retain water. When water is retained, less urine is produced.

Urination (voiding) means the process of emptying urine from the bladder. The amount of fluid intake, habits, and available toilet facilities affect frequency. So do activity, work, bladder problems, and illness. People usually void at bedtime, after sleep, and before meals. Some void more often. Voiding at night disturbs sleep.

See *Focus on Communication: Normal Urination*, p. 402.

See *Focus on Children and Older Persons: Normal Urination*, p. 402.

See *Delegation Guidelines: Normal Urination*, p. 402.

FOCUS ON COMMUNICATION

Normal Urination

Patients and residents may not use the terms "voiding" or "urinating." The person may not understand your words. Do not ask: "Do you need to void?" or "Do you need to urinate?" Instead, you can ask these questions.

- "Do you need to use the bathroom?"
- "Do you need the bedpan (urinal)?"
- "Do you need to pass urine?"
- "Do you need to pass water?"
- "Do you need to pee?"

The word "pee" may offend some persons. Choose words the person understands and uses. Follow the care plan.

FOCUS ON CHILDREN AND OLDER PERSONS

Normal Urination

Children

Infants produce 200 to 300 mL of urine a day. The amount increases as the baby grows older. An infant can have 6 to 20 wet diapers a day. Tell the nurse at once if an infant does not have a wet diaper for several hours. This signals dehydration. It is very serious in infants.

DELEGATION GUIDELINES

Normal Urination

Assisting patients and residents with bathroom, bedpan, urinal, and commode use are routine nursing tasks. Follow the rules in Box 27-1 and the person's care plan.

BOX 27-1 Rules for Normal Urination

- Practice medical asepsis.
- Follow Standard Precautions and the Bloodborne Pathogen Standard.
- Provide fluids as the nurse and care plan direct.
- Follow voiding routines and habits. Check with the nurse and the person's care plan.
- Help the person to the bathroom upon request. Or provide the bedpan, urinal, or commode. The need to void may be urgent.
- Help the person assume a normal position for voiding if possible. Women sit or squat. Men stand.
- Warm the bedpan or urinal if time permits. The need may be urgent.
- Cover the person for warmth and privacy.
- Provide for privacy. Pull the privacy curtain around the bed, close room and bathroom doors, and close window coverings.
- Leave the room if the person can be alone. Stay nearby if the person is weak, unsteady, or at risk for falling (Chapter 14). Do not leave persons with dementia alone (Chapter 53).
- Tell the person that running water in the sink, flushing the toilet, or playing music can mask voiding sounds. Voiding with others nearby embarrasses some people.
- Place the call light and toilet paper within reach.
- Allow enough time. Do not rush the person.
- Promote relaxation. Some people like to read.
- Run water in a sink if the person cannot start the urine stream. Or place the person's fingers in warm water.
- Provide perineal care as needed (Chapter 24).
- Assist with hand hygiene after voiding. Provide a wash basin, soap, washcloth, and towel. Some agencies provide hand-wipes.
- Assist the person with urinary needs at regular times. Some people are embarrassed or are too weak to ask for help.

Observations

Normal urine is pale yellow, straw-colored, or amber (Fig. 27-2). It is clear with no particles. A faint odor is normal. Observe urine for color, clarity, odor, amount (output), particles, and blood.

Red food dyes, beets, blackberries, and rhubarb cause red-colored urine. Carrots and sweet potatoes cause bright yellow urine. Brown urine may signal a liver disorder. Certain drugs change urine color. Asparagus causes a urine odor.

Ask the nurse to observe urine that looks or smells abnormal. Report the problems in Table 27-1. The nurse uses the information for the nursing process.

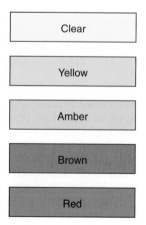

| Clear |
| Yellow |
| Amber |
| Brown |
| Red |

FIGURE 27-2 Color chart for urine.

Problem	Definition	Some Causes
TABLE 27-1	**Urinary Elimination Problems**	
Dysuria	Painful or difficult (dys) urination (uria); burning on urination	Urinary tract infection (UTI), trauma, urinary tract obstruction
Enuresis	Involuntary loss or leakage of urine during sleep; bed-wetting	Normal in early childhood (see p. 411 for causes in children), hormone imbalance, UTI, sleep apnea, diabetes, constipation, nervous system or urinary tract problems, caffeine use
Hematuria	Blood (hemat) in the urine (uria)	Kidney disease, UTI, trauma
Nocturia	Frequent urination (uria) at night (noc)	Excess fluid intake, kidney disease, prostate problems
Oliguria	Scant amount (olig) of urine (uria); less than 500 mL in 24 hours	Poor fluid intake, shock, burns, kidney disease, heart failure
Polyuria	Abnormally large amounts (poly) of urine (uria)	Drugs, excess fluid intake, diabetes, hormone imbalance
Urinary frequency	Voiding at frequent intervals	Excess fluid intake, UTI, pressure on the bladder, drugs
Urinary incontinence (UI)	The involuntary loss or leakage of urine	Trauma, disease, UTI, reproductive or urinary tract surgeries, aging, fecal impaction, constipation, not getting to the bathroom in time
Urinary retention	Not being able to completely empty the bladder	Prostate problems, nerve damage, UTI, drugs, surgery, kidney stones, constipation, trauma
Urinary urgency	The need to void at once	UTI, fear of incontinence, full bladder, stress

Bedpans

Bedpans are used when the person cannot be out of bed. Women use bedpans for voiding and bowel movements (BMs). Men use them for BMs.

The *standard bedpan* is shown in Figure 27-3, *A*. The wide rim goes under the buttocks. A *fracture pan* has a thin rim. It is only about ½-inch deep at one end (Fig. 27-3, *B*). The smaller end (flat end) goes under the buttocks (Fig. 27-4). Fracture pans are used:

- By persons with casts
- By persons in traction
- By persons with limited back motion
- By older persons with osteoporosis (fragile bones) or arthritis
- After spinal cord injury or surgery
- After a hip fracture or hip replacement surgery

Like a fracture pan, the small end (flat end) of a *bariatric bedpan* is placed under the buttocks (Fig. 27-5). Some have a weight capacity of 1200 pounds.

See *Delegation Guidelines: Bedpans*, p. 404.
See *Promoting Safety and Comfort: Bedpans*, p. 404.
See procedure: *Giving the Bedpan*, p. 404.

Text continued on p. 406.

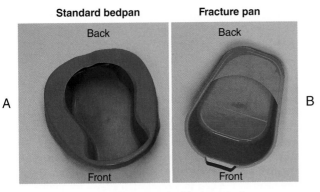

FIGURE 27-3 Bedpans. **A,** Standard bedpan. **B,** Fracture pan.

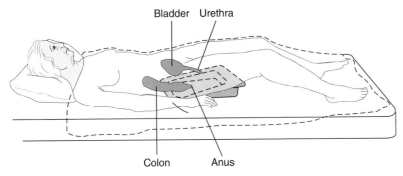

FIGURE 27-4 A person positioned on a fracture pan. The small end (flat end) is under the buttocks.

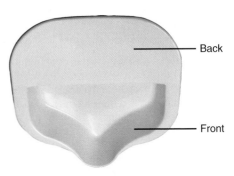

FIGURE 27-5 Bariatric bedpan. (Image courtesy AliMed, Inc., Dedham, Mass.)

DELEGATION GUIDELINES

Bedpans

To assist with a bedpan, you need this information from the nurse and the care plan.

- What bedpan to use—standard bedpan, fracture pan, bariatric bedpan
- Position or activity limits
- If you can leave the room or if you need to stay with the person
- If the nurse will observe the results before you flush the contents
- What observations to report and record:
  - Urine color, clarity, and odor
  - Amount
  - Presence of particles
  - Blood in the urine
  - Cloudy urine
  - Complaints of urgency, burning, dysuria, or other problems (see Table 27-1)
  - For bowel movements, see Chapter 29
- When to report observations
- What patient or resident concerns to report at once

PROMOTING SAFETY AND COMFORT

Bedpans

Safety

Remember to raise the bed as needed for good body mechanics. Lower the bed before leaving the room. Raise or lower the bed rails according to the care plan.

Comfort

Most bedpans are plastic. Made of stainless steel, metal bedpans are often cold. Warm metal bedpans with warm water and dry them before use. Use clean, dry paper towels for drying.

The person must not sit on a bedpan for a long time. Bedpans are uncomfortable. They can lead to pressure injuries (Chapter 41).

Giving the Bedpan

QUALITY OF LIFE

- Knock before entering the person's room.
- Address the person by name.
- Introduce yourself by name and title.

- Explain the procedure before starting and during the procedure.
- Protect the person's rights during the procedure.
- Handle the person gently during the procedure.

PRE-PROCEDURE

1 Follow *Delegation Guidelines:*
   a *Normal Urination,* p. 402
   b *Bedpans*
   See *Promoting Safety and Comfort:*
   a *Urinary Needs,* p. 401
   b *Bedpans*
2 Provide for privacy.
3 Practice hand hygiene.

4 Put on gloves.
5 Collect the following.
   - Bedpan
   - Bedpan cover (optional)
   - Toilet paper
   - Waterproof under-pad (if required by agency policy)
   - Bath blanket (optional)
6 Arrange equipment on the chair or bed.

PROCEDURE

7 Raise the bed for body mechanics (if the person's needs are not urgent). Lower the bed rail near you (if up).
8 Lower the head of the bed. Position the person supine. Or raise the head of the bed slightly for comfort.
9 Cover the person with a bath blanket if time allows. Fold the top linens and gown out of the way. Keep the lower body covered.
10 Have the person flex the knees and raise the buttocks. He or she pushes against the mattress with the feet.
11 Slide your hand under the lower back. Help raise the buttocks. If using a waterproof under-pad, place it under the buttocks.
12 Slide the bedpan under the person (Fig. 27-6). Make sure the bedpan is centered under the person.
13 If the person cannot assist in getting on the bedpan:
   a Place the waterproof under-pad under the buttocks if using one.
   b Turn the person onto the side away from you.
   c Place the bedpan firmly against the buttocks (Fig. 27-7).
   d Hold the bedpan securely. Turn the person onto his or her back.
   e Make sure the bedpan is centered under the person.

14 Cover the person.
15 Raise the head of the bed so the person is in a sitting position (Fowler's position) for a standard bedpan. Or raise the head of the bed to a comfortable level for the person. (NOTE: Some state competency tests require removing gloves and hand hygiene before raising the head of the bed.)
16 Make sure the person is correctly positioned on the bedpan (Fig. 27-8).
17 Raise the bed rail if used. Lower the bed.
18 Place the toilet paper and call light within reach. (NOTE: For some state competency tests you ask the person to use hand wipes for hand hygiene after wiping with toilet paper.)
19 Ask the person to signal when done or when help is needed. (Stay with the person if necessary. Be respectful. Provide as much privacy as possible.)
20 Remove and discard the gloves. Practice hand hygiene.
21 Leave the room and close the door.
22 Return when the person signals. Or check on the person every 5 minutes. Knock before entering.
23 Practice hand hygiene. Put on gloves.

Giving the Bedpan—cont'd

PROCEDURE—cont'd

24 Raise the bed for body mechanics. Lower the bed rail (if used) and lower the head of the bed.

25 Have the person raise the buttocks. Remove the bedpan. Or hold the bedpan and turn the person onto the side away from you.

26 Clean the genital area if the person cannot do so.
   a Clean from the meatus (front or top) to the anus (back or bottom) with toilet paper. Use fresh toilet paper for each wipe.
   b Provide perineal care if needed (Chapter 24).
   c Remove and discard the waterproof under-pad (if used).

27 Cover the bedpan. Take it to the bathroom. Raise the bed rail (if used) before leaving the bedside.

28 Note the color, amount (output), and character of urine or feces (stools). See "Measuring Intake and Output" in Chapter 31.

29 Empty the bedpan contents into the toilet and flush.

30 Rinse the bedpan. Pour the rinse into the toilet and flush.

31 Clean the bedpan with a disinfectant. Pour disinfectant into the toilet and flush. Dry the bedpan with clean, dry paper towels.

32 Return the bedpan to its proper place.

33 Remove and discard the gloves. Practice hand hygiene and put on clean gloves.

34 Help the person with hand hygiene.

35 Remove and discard the gloves. Practice hand hygiene.

36 Cover the person with the top linens. Remove the bath blanket (if used).

POST-PROCEDURE

37 Provide for comfort. (See the inside of the back cover.)

38 Place the call light and other needed items within reach.

39 Lower the bed to a safe and comfortable level. Follow the care plan.

40 Raise or lower bed rails. Follow the care plan.

41 Unscreen the person.

42 Complete a safety check of the room. (See the inside of the back cover.)

43 Follow agency policy for used linens.

44 Practice hand hygiene.

45 Report and record your observations.

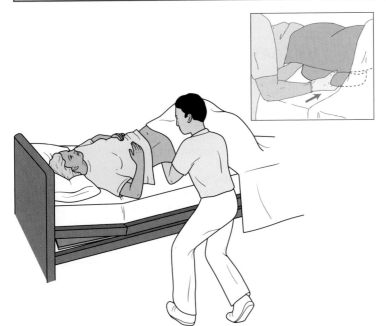

FIGURE 27-6 The person raises the buttocks off the bed with help. The bedpan is slid under the person.

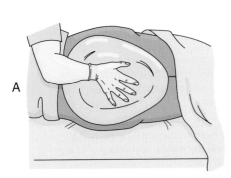

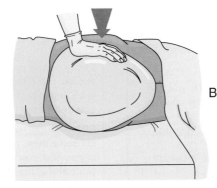

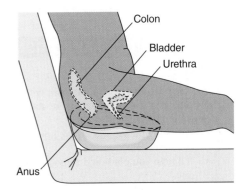

FIGURE 27-7 Giving a bedpan in the side-lying position. **A,** Position the person on the side away from you. Place the bedpan firmly against the buttocks. **B,** Push downward on the bedpan and toward the person.

FIGURE 27-8 The person is positioned on the bedpan so the urethra and anus are directly over the opening.

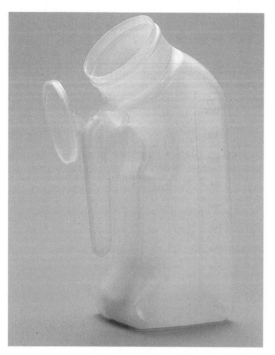

FIGURE 27-9 Male urinal.

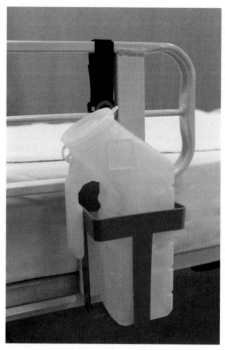

FIGURE 27-10 Urinal holder.

Urinals

Men use urinals to void (Fig. 27-9). Plastic urinals have caps and hook-type handles. Urinals are used when standing (preferred), sitting, or lying in bed. Some men need support when standing.

After voiding, the man closes the urinal cap. This prevents urine spills. He hangs the urinal on the bed rail or places it in a urinal holder attached to the bed rail, wheelchair, or walker (Fig. 27-10).

Remind men to use their call lights after using a urinal. The urinal needs to be emptied as soon as possible to prevent spills, slipping, and the growth of microbes. Also remind them not to place urinals on over-bed tables and bedside stands. Over-bed tables are used for eating and as a work surface. Bedside stands are used for personal items and supplies. These surfaces must not be contaminated with urine.

Some beds do not have bed rails. Follow agency policy for where to place urinals.

See *Focus on Communication: Urinals.*
See *Delegation Guidelines: Urinals.*
See *Promoting Safety and Comfort: Urinals.*
See procedure: *Giving the Urinal.*

FOCUS ON COMMUNICATION

Urinals

You may need to assist some men with urinals. Or you may need to stay with the person. For comfort, explain why you must help. You can say:

- "I'll help you use the urinal. I need to stay with you so you don't fall."
- "I'll help you place and remove the urinal so it doesn't spill."

DELEGATION GUIDELINES

Urinals

To assist with urinals, you need this information from the nurse and the care plan.

- How the urinal is used—standing, sitting, or lying in bed.
- If help is needed to place or hold the urinal.
- If the man needs support to stand. If yes, how many staff are needed.
- If you need to stay with the person.
- If the nurse needs to observe the urine.
- What observations to report and record (see *Delegation Guidelines: Bedpans,* p. 404).
- When to report observations.
- What patient or resident concerns to report at once.

PROMOTING SAFETY AND COMFORT

Urinals

Safety

Empty urinals promptly to prevent odors and the spread of microbes. A filled urinal spills easily, causing hazards. Also, it is an unpleasant sight and causes odors. Urinals are cleaned and disinfected like bedpans.

Comfort

For some men, you may need to place the penis in the urinal. This may embarrass the person and you. Act in a professional manner.

Giving the Urinal

QUALITY OF LIFE

- Knock before entering the person's room.
- Address the person by name.
- Introduce yourself by name and title.

- Explain the procedure before starting and during the procedure.
- Protect the person's rights during the procedure.
- Handle the person gently during the procedure.

PRE-PROCEDURE

1 Follow *Delegation Guidelines:*
  a *Normal Urination,* p. 402
  b *Urinals*
  See *Promoting Safety and Comfort:*
  a *Urinary Needs,* p. 401
  b *Urinals*
2 Provide for privacy.

3 Determine if the man will stand, sit, or lie in bed.
4 Practice hand hygiene.
5 Put on gloves.
6 Collect the following.
  - Urinal
  - Slip-resistant footwear for standing

PROCEDURE

7 *Standing to use the urinal* (Fig. 27-11 *A*):
  a Help him sit on the side of the bed.
  b Put slip-resistant footwear on him.
  c Help him stand. Provide support if he is unsteady.
  d Give him the urinal.
8 *Using the urinal in bed* (Fig. 27-11 *B*):
  a Give him the urinal.
  b Remind him to tilt the bottom down to prevent spills.
9 *Positioning the urinal (in bed or standing):*
  a Help the person stand (step 7) if he will stand.
  b Position the urinal.
  c Place the penis in the urinal if he cannot do so.
  d Cover him for privacy.
10 Place the call light within reach. Ask him to signal when done or when help is needed.
11 Provide for privacy.
12 Remove and discard the gloves. Practice hand hygiene.

13 Leave the room and close the door.
14 Return when he signals for you. Or check on him every 5 minutes. Knock before entering.
15 Practice hand hygiene. Put on gloves.
16 Close the urinal cap. Take it to the bathroom.
17 Note the color, amount (output), and clarity of urine.
18 Empty the urinal into the toilet and flush.
19 Rinse the urinal with cold water. Pour rinse into the toilet and flush.
20 Clean the urinal with a disinfectant. Pour disinfectant into the toilet and flush. Dry the urinal with clean, dry paper towels.
21 Return the urinal to its proper place.
22 Remove and discard the gloves. Practice hand hygiene and put on clean gloves.
23 Assist with hand hygiene.
24 Remove and discard the gloves. Practice hand hygiene.

POST-PROCEDURE

25 Provide for comfort. (See the inside of the back cover.)
26 Place the call light and other needed items within reach.
27 Raise or lower bed rails. Follow the care plan.
28 Unscreen him.

29 Complete a safety check of the room. (See the inside of the back cover.)
30 Follow agency policy for used linens.
31 Practice hand hygiene.
32 Report and record your observations.

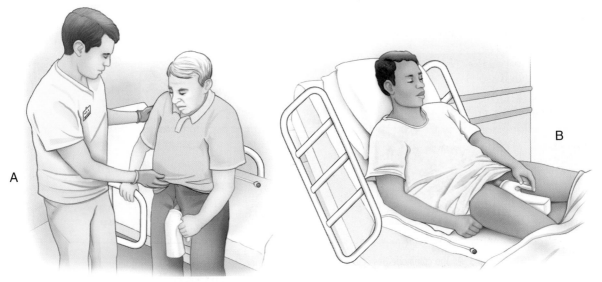

FIGURE 27-11 Using the male urinal. **A,** Standing. **B,** In bed.

Female Urinals. Female urinals are shaped to fit against a woman's body (Fig. 27-12). They can be used standing, sitting, or lying down (supine or lateral position). The device is positioned snugly under the urethra. The woman tilts her pelvis forward to the device when urinating. Proper positioning of the urinal is important to prevent leaking when voiding or removing the device.

Commodes

A commode (bedside commode) is a chair or wheelchair with an opening for a container (Fig. 27-13). Persons unable to walk to the bathroom often use commodes. The commode allows a normal position for elimination. The commode arms and back provide support and help prevent falls.

Some commodes, with the containers removed, are placed over toilets. The person uses the commode arms for support to sit and stand. And the commode serves as a higher toilet seat. If the commode has wheels, lock the wheels after properly positioning the commode over the toilet.

See *Delegation Guidelines: Commodes.*
See *Promoting Safety and Comfort: Commodes.*
See procedure: *Helping the Person to the Commode.*

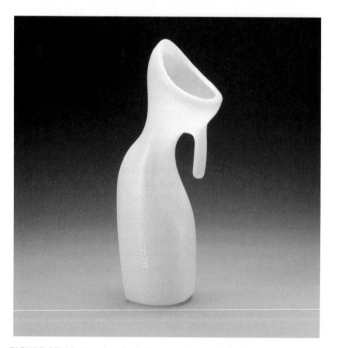

FIGURE 27-12 Female urinal. (Courtesy Viscot Medical, LLC, East Hanover, N.J.)

DELEGATION GUIDELINES

Commodes

You need this information from the nurse and care plan when assisting with commode use.
- If the commode is used at the bedside or over the toilet
- How much help the person needs
- If you can leave the room or if you need to stay with the person
- If the nurse needs to observe urine or BMs before you flush the contents
- What observations to report and record (see *Delegation Guidelines: Bedpans*, p. 404)
- When to report observations
- What patient or resident concerns to report at once

PROMOTING SAFETY AND COMFORT

Commodes

Safety
You will transfer the person to and from the commode. Practice safe transfer procedures (Chapter 20). Use the transfer belt and lock the wheels. Remove the transfer belt after the transfer. See "Transfer/Gait Belts" in Chapter 14.

Each person is given his or her own commode. The commode is not shared among patients and residents. When no longer needed, the commode is returned to the supply department for disinfection.

Comfort
After transfer to the commode, cover the person's lap and legs with a bath blanket. This promotes warmth and privacy.

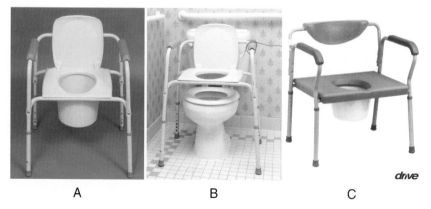

A   B   C

FIGURE 27-13 A, The commode has a toilet seat with a container. The container slides out from under the seat for emptying or to use the commode over the toilet. **B,** The container is removed. The commode chair is placed over the toilet. **C,** Bariatric commode. (**C,** Courtesy Medical Depot, Inc., Port Washington, N.Y.)

Helping the Person to the Commode

QUALITY OF LIFE

- Knock before entering the person's room.
- Address the person by name.
- Introduce yourself by name and title.

- Explain the procedure before starting and during the procedure.
- Protect the person's rights during the procedure.
- Handle the person gently during the procedure.

PRE-PROCEDURE

1 Follow *Delegation Guidelines:*
   a *Normal Urination,* p. 402
   b *Commodes*
   See *Promoting Safety and Comfort:*
   a *Urinary Needs,* p. 401
   b *Commodes*
2 Provide for privacy.
3 Practice hand hygiene.

4 Put on gloves.
5 Collect the following.
   - Commode
   - Toilet paper
   - Bath blanket
   - Transfer belt
   - Robe and slip-resistant footwear

PROCEDURE

6 Place the commode next to the bed.
7 Help the person sit on the side of the bed. Lower the bed rail if used.
8 Help the person put on a robe and slip-resistant footwear.
9 Apply the transfer belt.
10 Assist the person to the commode. Use the transfer belt.
11 Remove the transfer belt. Cover the person with a bath blanket for warmth.
12 Place the toilet paper and call light within reach.
13 Ask the person to signal when done or when help is needed. (Stay with the person if necessary. Be respectful. Provide as much privacy as possible.)
14 Remove and discard the gloves. Practice hand hygiene.
15 Leave the room. Close the door.
16 Return when the person signals. Or check on the person every 5 minutes. Knock before entering.
17 Practice hand hygiene. Put on the gloves.
18 Help the person clean the genital area as needed. Remove and discard the gloves. Practice hand hygiene.
19 Apply the transfer belt. Help the person back to bed using the transfer belt. Remove the transfer belt, robe, and footwear. Raise the bed rail if used.

20 Put on clean gloves. Remove and cover the commode container.
21 Take the container to the bathroom.
22 Observe urine and feces (stools) for color, amount (output), and character.
23 Empty the contents into the toilet and flush.
24 Rinse the container. Pour the rinse into the toilet and flush.
25 Clean and disinfect the container. Pour disinfectant into the toilet and flush. Dry the container with clean, dry paper towels.
26 Return the container to the commode. Close the lid. Clean other parts of the commode if necessary.
27 Return supplies to their proper place.
28 Remove and discard the gloves. Practice hand hygiene and put on clean gloves.
29 Assist with hand hygiene.
30 Remove and discard the gloves. Practice hand hygiene.

POST-PROCEDURE

31 Provide for comfort. (See the inside of the back cover.)
32 Place the call light and other needed items within reach.
33 Raise or lower bed rails. Follow the care plan.
34 Unscreen the person.
35 Complete a safety check of the room. (See the inside of the back cover.)

36 Follow agency policy for used linens.
37 Practice hand hygiene.
38 Report and record your observations.

URINARY INCONTINENCE

Urinary incontinence (UI) is the involuntary loss or leakage of urine. Older persons are at risk for UI because of urinary tract changes, medical and surgical conditions, and drug therapy. Incontinence is not a normal part of aging.

Types of Urinary Incontinence

UI may be temporary or permanent. See Box 27-2 for risk factors and causes. Some factors can be reversed. Others cannot. Common types of incontinence are:

- *Stress incontinence—urine leaks during exercise and certain movements that cause pressure on the bladder.* Urine loss is small. Often called *dribbling,* it occurs with laughing, sneezing, coughing, lifting, or other activities.
- *Urge incontinence—urine is lost in response to a sudden, urgent need to void. The person cannot get to a toilet in time.* Urinary frequency, urinary urgency, and night-time voiding are common.
- *Mixed incontinence—a combination of stress incontinence and urge incontinence.* Many older women have this type.
- *Over-flow incontinence—small amounts of urine leak from a full bladder.* The person feels like the bladder is not empty. The person dribbles and may have a weak urine stream.
- *Functional incontinence—the person has bladder control but cannot use the toilet in time.* Immobility, restraints, unanswered call lights, no call light within reach, and difficulty removing clothing are causes. Not knowing where to find the bathroom, confusion, and disorientation are other causes.
- *Reflex incontinence—urine is lost at predictable intervals when a specific amount of urine is in the bladder.* The person does not feel the need to void. Nervous system disorders and injuries are common causes.
- *Transient incontinence—temporary or occasional incontinence that is reversed when the cause is treated.* (*Transient* means *for a short time.*)

Managing Urinary Incontinence

The goals of managing UI are to:
- Prevent UTIs.
- Restore as much bladder function as possible.

UI is embarrassing and uncomfortable. Garments are wet and odors develop. Skin irritation, infection, and pressure injuries are risks. Falls are a risk from trying to get to the bathroom quickly. Pride, dignity, and self-esteem are affected. Social isolation, loss of independence, and depression are common. Quality of life suffers.

The person's care plan may include some of the measures in Box 27-3. *Good skin care and dry garments and linens are essential.* Promoting normal urinary elimination prevents incontinence in some people (see Box 27-1). Others need bladder training (p. 417). Sometimes catheters are needed (Chapter 28).

BOX 27-2	Urinary Incontinence—Risk Factors and Causes

Risk Factors
- Women—pregnancy, childbirth, menopause
- Men—prostate problems
- Age—bladder muscles lose strength; the bladder holds less urine
- Over-weight—pressure on the bladder increases
- Smoking—coughing increases pressure on the bladder; irritates the bladder leading to over-active bladder
- *Over-active bladder (OAB)*—a condition in which there is a nearly constant urge to urinate; the person usually does not leak urine but urge incontinence may develop
- Diabetes—nerve damage affects the bladder
- Kidney disease
- Immobility
- Restraint use
- Delays in voiding—see "Functional incontinence"
- Confusion and disorientation

Temporary Incontinence—Causes
- Alcohol and caffeine—increased urine production, stimulates the bladder leading to urge incontinence.
- Bladder irritation—some drinks and foods irritate the bladder. Sodas, tea, coffee, spicy foods, citrus fruits, and tomatoes are examples.
- Constipation or fecal impaction—irritates the nerves shared by the bladder and rectum. See Chapter 29.
- Delirium—see Chapter 53.
- Drug therapies.
- Increased fluid intake—urine production increases.
- Urinary tract infection (UTI)—irritates the bladder causing an urgent need to void.

Permanent Incontinence—Causes
- Aging changes
- Alzheimer's disease and other dementias (Chapter 53)
- Bladder cancer
- Bladder stones
- Hysterectomy—removal (*ectomy*) of the uterus (*hyster*) causing damage to the pelvic muscles
- Menopause
- Nervous system disorders (Chapter 48)
- Obstruction of the urinary tract
- Pregnancy and childbirth
- Prostate problems—prostatitis (inflammation [*itis*] of the prostate [*prostat*]), enlarged prostate, prostate cancer

---

UI is linked to abuse, mistreatment, and neglect. Frequent care is needed. The person may wet again right after skin care and changing wet garments and linens. Remember, the person does not choose to be incontinent. The person cannot control UI. Be patient. The person's needs are great. If feeling short-tempered, talk to the nurse. The person has the right to be free from abuse, mistreatment, and neglect. Kindness, empathy, understanding, and patience are needed.

See *Focus on Children and Older Persons: Managing Urinary Incontinence.*

See *Focus on Surveys: Managing Urinary Incontinence,* p. 412.

BOX 27-3	Urinary Incontinence—Nursing Measures

- Record the person's voidings:
  - Voiding times
    - Incontinent
    - Successful use of the toilet, bedpan, urinal, or commode
  - Amount voided (Chapter 31)
- Answer call lights promptly. The need to void may be urgent.
- Promote normal urinary elimination (see Box 27-1).
- Promote normal bowel elimination (Chapter 29).
- Assist with elimination after sleep, before and after meals, at bedtime, and when help is requested.
- Follow the person's bladder training program (p. 417).
- Provide a clear path to the bathroom.
- Have the person wear easy-to-remove clothing. UI can occur while dealing with buttons, zippers, other closures, and under-garments.
- Encourage pelvic muscle exercises as instructed by the nurse.
- Check the person often to make sure he or she is clean and dry.

- Help prevent UTIs.
  - Promote fluid intake as the nurse directs.
  - Have the person wear cotton underwear.
  - Keep the perineal area clean and dry.
  - Clean from front to back (top to bottom) during perineal care (Chapter 24).
- Decrease fluid intake at bedtime.
- Provide good skin care.
- Apply a barrier cream or moisturizer (cream, lotion, paste) to the skin or perineum as directed by the nurse. The application prevents irritation and skin damage.
- Provide dry garments and linens.
- Observe for signs of skin breakdown (Chapters 40 and 41).
- Use incontinence products as the nurse directs. Follow the manufacturer's instructions.
- Do not leave urinals in place to collect urine for persons who are incontinent.
- Keep the perineal area clean and dry (Chapter 24).
  - Protect the person and dry garments and linens from the wet incontinence product.
  - Remove wet incontinence products, garments, and linens.
  - Expose only the perineal area.
  - Use soap (or body wash) and water or a no-rinse incontinence cleanser (perineal rinse). Follow the care plan. For soap (or body wash) and water, use a safe and comfortable water temperature.
  - Dry the perineal area and buttocks.
  - Apply a clean, dry incontinence product and clean, dry garments and linens.
- Follow Standard Precautions and the Bloodborne Pathogen Standard.

FOCUS ON **CHILDREN AND OLDER PERSONS**

Managing Urinary Incontinence

Children
Wetting in younger children is normal. Most children achieve bladder control (dryness) around age 3. Day-time UI is usually diagnosed around 5 or 6 years of age and night-time UI around age 7.

Some health problems can cause UI in children.
- UTI
- Diabetes (Chapter 50)
- Kidney problems
- Nerve problems
- Constipation
- Urinary tract problems

Night-time UI *(enuresis, bed-wetting)* is more common than day-time UI. The exact cause is unknown but may involve more than 1 factor.
- Slower physical development. A small bladder holds less urine.
- Longer sleeping periods. More urine collects in the bladder over time.

- Producing more urine at night. The bladder over-fills.
- Not sensing a full bladder. The child does not wake up to void.
- Anxiety. Anxiety-causing events include abuse (physical or sexual), moving, starting at a new school, family events (a new baby, death, divorce).
- Family history of bed-wetting.

Besides health problems, causes of day-time UI include:
- Over-active bladder. The child has urgency, urge incontinence, or urinary frequency—voids 8 or more times a day and at least 2 times at night.
- Infrequent voiding. The child holds urine for a long time. The urge to void is ignored, letting the bladder over-fill and leak. UTIs can develop.
- Incomplete voiding. The child does not relax enough to allow the bladder to empty. UTIs can develop.

UI usually disappears as the child grows and develops. If needed, treatment may involve bladder training (p. 417), moisture alarms, and drug therapy.

Continued

FOCUS ON CHILDREN AND OLDER PERSONS—cont'd

Managing Urinary Incontinence—cont'd

Older Persons

Complications from incontinence pose serious problems for older persons. These include falls, pressure injuries, and UTIs. Hospital or long-term care stays are often necessary.

Persons with dementia may void in the wrong places. Trash cans, planters, heating vents, and closets are examples. Some persons throw incontinence products on the floor or in the toilet. Others resist staff efforts to stay clean and dry.

Provide safe care. The care plan may include measures recommended by the Alzheimer's Disease and Related Dementias Education and Referral Center (ADEAR).

- Remind the person to go to the bathroom every 2 to 3 hours during the day. Do not wait for the person to ask.
- Show the way or take the person to the bathroom.
- Keep pathways to the bathroom clear.
- Keep the bathroom clutter-free.
- Keep lights on in the pathway and bathroom.
- Have the person wear clothing and under-garments that are easy to remove.
- Post a big sign on the bathroom door that says "Toilet" or "Bathroom."

- Help the person in the bathroom.
- Observe for signs of needing to void. Restlessness and pulling at clothes are examples. Respond quickly.
- Stay calm when the person is incontinent. Reassure the person if he or she becomes upset.
- Report incontinence. Report the time, what the person was doing, and other observations. An incontinence pattern may emerge. If so, measures are planned to prevent the problem.
- Prevent incontinence during sleep. Limit the type and amount of fluids in the evening. Follow the care plan.
- Plan ahead for the person leaving the agency. Have the person wear easy-to-remove clothing. Pack extra clothing, incontinence products, and hygiene supplies. Know where to find restrooms.

You may need help keeping the person clean and dry. Ask your co-workers or the nurse for help.

Remember, everyone has the right to privacy and safe care. They also have the right to be treated with dignity.

FOCUS ON SURVEYS

Managing Urinary Incontinence

Surveyors observe how incontinence is prevented, improved, or managed. They observe if staff:
- Follow the person's care plan.
- Keep call lights within reach.
- Answer call lights promptly.
- Provide a clear pathway to the bathroom.
- Provide good lighting for voiding.
- Assist with bedpans, urinals, and commodes as needed.
- Assist the person to the bathroom as needed.
- Respond appropriately when incontinence occurs.
- Protect the person's dignity when incontinence occurs.
- Check incontinent persons often.
- Change wet incontinence products and clothing promptly.
- Prevent prolonged exposure of the skin to urine.
- Provide hygiene measures to prevent skin breakdown.

Applying Incontinence Products

Incontinence products help keep the person dry. They usually have 2 layers and a waterproof back. Fluid passes through the top layer. It is absorbed by the bottom layer. Products come in various sizes from small to bariatric.

Common incontinence products are shown in Figure 27-14. The nurse helps the person select products for his or her needs. To apply them, follow the manufacturer's instructions and agency procedures.

See *Focus on Communication: Applying Incontinence Products.*

See *Delegation Guidelines: Applying Incontinence Products.*

See *Promoting Safety and Comfort: Applying Incontinence Products.*

See procedure: *Applying Incontinence Products*, p. 414.

Text continued on p. 417.

FOCUS ON COMMUNICATION

Applying Incontinence Products

Incontinence products are often called "adult diapers." The word "diaper" may offend the person or lower self-esteem. Instead, say "brief," "pad," or "underwear." Some persons use the product's brand name. Use a term that promotes dignity and self-esteem.

DELEGATION GUIDELINES

Applying Incontinence Products

Changing incontinence products is a routine nursing task. To apply an incontinence product, you need this information from the nurse and the care plan.
- What product to use.
- What size to use.
- If a barrier cream is needed. If yes, what cream to use.
- What observations to report and record:
  - Complaints of pain, burning, irritation, or the need to void
  - Signs and symptoms of skin breakdown:
    - Redness, irritation, blisters
    - Complaints of pain, burning, tingling, or itching
  - The amount of urine—small, moderate, large
  - Urine color
  - Blood in the urine
  - Leakage
  - A poor product fit
- When to report observations.
- What patient or resident concerns to report at once.

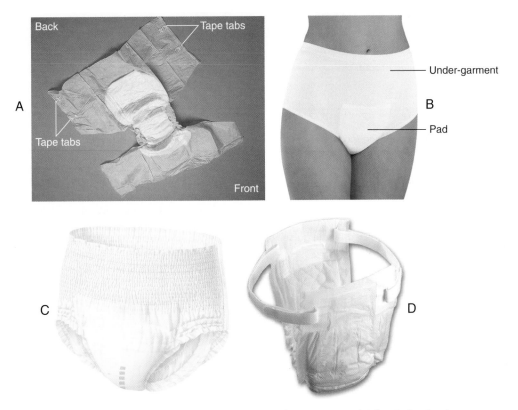

FIGURE 27-14 Disposable incontinence products. **A,** Complete incontinence brief. **B,** Pad and under-garment. **C,** Pull-on underwear. **D,** Belted under-garment. (**B,** Courtesy Hartmann USA, Inc., Rock Hill, S.C. **C,** Courtesy Hartmann Inc., Heidenheim, Germany. **D,** Courtesy Principle Business Enterprises, Dunbridge, Ohio.)

PROMOTING SAFETY AND COMFORT

Applying Incontinence Products

Safety

To safely apply an incontinence product, follow the manufacturer's instructions. The guidelines in Box 27-4 will help prevent:

- Leakage
- Skin irritation, skin damage, and pressure injuries
- Tearing of the product

    Remove the soiled incontinence product from front to back (top to bottom). Apply the new product from front to back (top to bottom). This prevents spreading bacteria from the anal area to the urinary system.

    Provide for safety if the person will stand for the procedure.

- Make sure the bed is in a low position that is safe and comfortable for the person.
- Lock (brake) the bed wheels.
- Have the person wear slip-resistant footwear.
- Provide something for the person to hold on to for balance and stability.

Comfort

For comfort, use the correct size. If the product is too large, urine can leak. If too small, the product will be too tight and uncomfortable.

BOX 27-4 | **Applying Incontinence Products**

- Follow the manufacturer's instructions.
- Use the correct size. The nurse tells you what size to use.
- Note the front and back of the product.
- Position the product correctly.
    - Center the product in the perineal area. For a male, the penis is downward.
    - Position the sides in the groin areas. The *groin is where a thigh and the abdomen meet.*
- Check for proper placement. The product should fit the shape of the body.
- Note the amount of urine (small, moderate, large). Also note how often you change the product. Large amounts of urine or diarrhea may require an extended-wear product (Chapter 29).
- Do not let the plastic backing touch the skin.
- Provide perineal care after each incontinent episode.
- Do not use the product as a turning or lift sheet.
- Attach the tabs correctly. Some products will tear if you try to unfasten the tape or change the tape's position.
    - Attach the lower tape first. Stretch the tape and attach it at a slightly upward angle. Do so for both sides.
    - Attach the upper tape after the lower tape is fastened. Stretch the tape and attach it in a horizontal manner. Do so for both sides.

Applying Incontinence Products

QUALITY OF LIFE

- Knock before entering the person's room.
- Address the person by name.
- Introduce yourself by name and title.

- Explain the procedure before starting and during the procedure.
- Protect the person's rights during the procedure.
- Handle the person gently during the procedure.

PRE-PROCEDURE

1 Follow *Delegation Guidelines: Applying Incontinence Products*, p. 412. See *Promoting Safety and Comfort:*
   a *Urinary Needs,* p. 401
   b *Applying Incontinence Products,* p. 413
2 Practice hand hygiene.
3 Collect the following.
   - Incontinence product as directed by the nurse
   - Barrier cream or moisturizer as directed by the nurse
   - Soap, body wash, or incontinence cleanser
   - Items for perineal care (Chapter 24)
   - Waterproof under-pad
   - Paper towels
   - Plastic trash bag
   - Gloves
   - Slip-resistant footwear if the person will stand

4 Cover the over-bed table with paper towels. Arrange items on top of them.
5 Identify the person. Check the ID (identification) bracelet against the assignment sheet. Use 2 identifiers (Chapter 13). Also call the person by name.
6 Mark the date, time, and your initials on the new product.
7 Provide for privacy.
8 Fill the wash basin. Water temperature is usually 105°F to 109°F (Fahrenheit) (40.5°C to 42.7°C [centigrade]). Measure water temperature according to agency policy. Have the person check the water temperature and adjust as needed.
9 Raise the bed for body mechanics (unless the person will stand). Bed rails are up if used.

PROCEDURE

10 Lower the head of the bed. The bed is as flat as possible.
11 Lower the bed rail near you if up.
12 Practice hand hygiene. Put on the gloves.
13 Cover the person with a bath blanket. Lower top linens to the foot of the bed. Lower the pants or slacks. (Omit this step if the person will stand. See step 16.)
14 *Applying an incontinence brief with the person in bed* (Fig. 27-15):
   a Place a waterproof under-pad under the buttocks.
   b Loosen the tabs on each side of the used brief.
   c Remove the used brief from front to back (top to bottom). Roll the product up with the soiled side inside. To do so, do 1 of the following.
      1) Have the person spread the legs. Roll the front of the product toward the back (bottom). Turn the person onto the side away from you. Remove the brief.
      2) Turn the person onto the side away from you. Remove the brief (see Fig. 27-15, *A*).
   d Observe the urine as you roll the product up. Estimate the amount of urine: small, moderate, large. Observe for urine color and blood.
   e Place the used brief in the trash bag. Tie or seal the bag and set it aside.
   f Perform perineal care (Chapter 24) wearing clean gloves. Apply the barrier cream or moisturizer.
   g Remove and discard the gloves. Practice hand hygiene. Put on clean gloves.
   h Open the new brief. Fold it in half length-wise along the center (see Fig. 27-15, *B*).
   i Insert the brief between the legs from front to back (top to bottom) (see Fig. 27-15, *C*).
   j Unfold and spread the back panel (see Fig. 27-15, *D*).
   k Center the brief in the perineal area.
   l Turn the person onto his or her back.
   m Unfold and spread the front panel. Provide a "cup" shape in the perineal area. For a man, position the penis downward.
   n Make sure the brief is positioned high in the groin folds. The brief fits the shape of the body.

   o Secure the brief (see Fig. 27-15, *E*).
      1) Pull the lower tape tab forward on the side near you. Attach it at a slightly upward angle. Do the same for the other side.
      2) Pull the upper tape tab forward on the side near you. Attach it in a horizontal manner. Do the same for the other side.
   p Smooth out all wrinkles and folds.
15 *Applying a pad and under-garment with the person in bed* (Fig. 27-16, p. 416):
   a Place a waterproof under-pad under the buttocks.
   b Turn the person onto the side away from you.
   c Pull the under-garment down. The waistband is over the knee (see Fig. 27-16, *A*).
   d Remove the used pad from front to back (top to bottom). Observe the urine as you roll the product up (see Fig. 27-16, *B*). Estimate the amount of urine in the used product: small, moderate, large. Observe for urine color and blood.
   e Place the used pad in the trash bag. Tie or seal the bag and set it aside.
   f Perform perineal care (Chapter 24) wearing clean gloves. Apply the barrier cream or moisturizer.
   g Remove and discard the gloves. Practice hand hygiene. Put on clean gloves.
   h Fold the new pad in half length-wise along the center (see Fig. 27-16, *C*).
   i Insert the pad between the legs from front to back (top to bottom) (see Fig. 27-16, *D*).
   j Unfold and spread the back panel (see Fig. 27-16, *E*).
   k Center the pad in the perineal area.
   l Pull the garment up at the back (see Fig. 27-16, *F*).
   m Turn the person onto his or her back.
   n Unfold and spread the front panel (see Fig. 27-16, *G*). For a man, position the penis downward.
   o Pull the garment up in front (see Fig. 27-16, *H*).
   p Adjust the pad and under-garment for a good fit.

Applying Incontinence Products—cont'd

PROCEDURE—cont'd

16 *Applying pull-on underwear with the person standing* (Fig. 27-17, p. 417):
   a Help the person stand. Remove the pants or slacks.
   b Tear the side seams of the used underwear (see Fig. 27-17, *A*).
   c Remove the underwear from front to back (top to bottom) (see Fig. 27-17, *B*). Observe the urine as you roll the underwear up. Estimate the amount of urine in the used product: small, moderate, large. Observe for urine color and blood.
   d Place the used underwear in the trash bag. Tie or seal the bag and set it aside.
   e Perform perineal care (Chapter 24) wearing clean gloves. Apply the barrier cream or moisturizer.

   f Remove and discard the gloves. Practice hand hygiene. Put on clean gloves.
   g Have the person sit on the side of the bed.
   h Slide the new underwear over the feet to past the knees (see Fig. 27-17, *C*).
   i Help the person stand.
   j Pull the underwear up (see Fig. 27-17, *D*).
   k Adjust as needed for a good fit.

17 Ask about comfort. Ask if the product feels too loose or too tight. Check for wrinkles or creases. Make sure the product does not rub or irritate the groin. Adjust the product as needed.

18 Remove and discard the gloves. Practice hand hygiene.

19 Raise or put on pants or slacks.

POST-PROCEDURE

20 Provide for comfort. (See the inside of the back cover.)
21 Place the call light and other needed items within reach.
22 Lower the bed to a safe and comfortable level. Follow the care plan.
23 Raise or lower bed rails. Follow the care plan.
24 Unscreen the person.
25 Practice hand hygiene. Put on clean gloves.
26 Clean, rinse, dry, and return the wash basin and other equipment. Use clean, dry paper towels for drying. Return items to their proper place.

27 Remove and discard the gloves. Practice hand hygiene.
28 Complete a safety check of the room. (See the inside of the back cover.)
29 Follow agency policy for used linens.
30 Practice hand hygiene.
31 Report and record your observations.

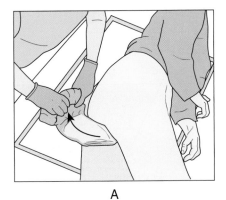

A

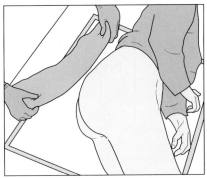

B

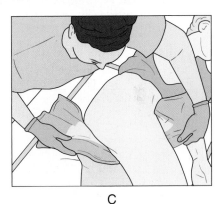

C

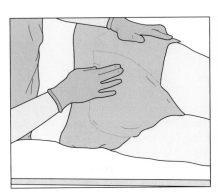

D

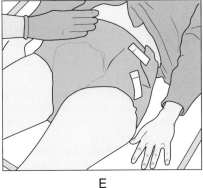

E

FIGURE 27-15 Applying an incontinence brief. **A,** The used brief is removed from front to back (top to bottom). **B,** The new brief is opened length-wise. **C,** The new brief is inserted length-wise between the legs from front to back (top to bottom). **D,** The back panel is spread open. **E,** The lower tape tab is attached at a slightly upward angle. The upper tape tab is attached in a horizontal manner.

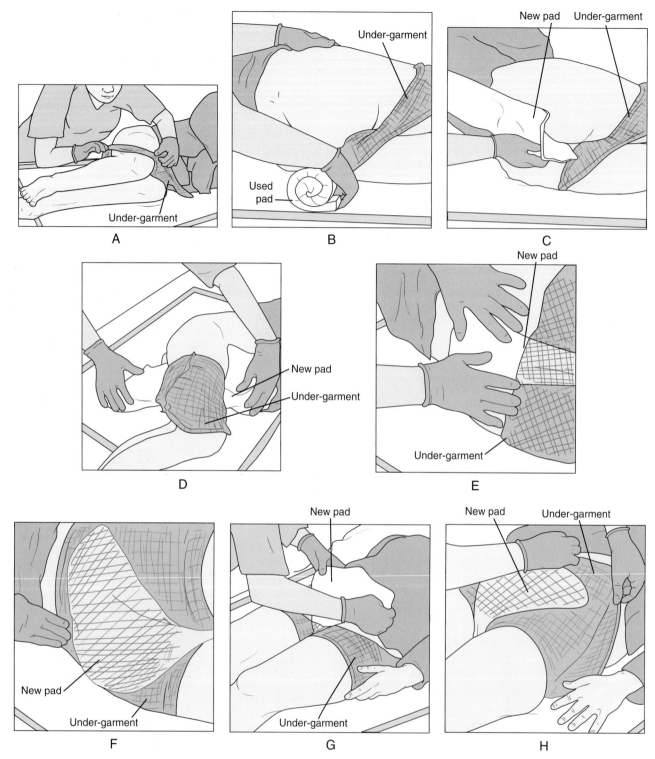

FIGURE 27-16 Applying a pad and under-garment. **A,** The under-garment is pulled down. The waistband is over the knee. **B,** The pad is rolled up as it is removed from front to back (top to bottom). **C,** The new pad is folded in half length-wise along the center. **D,** The pad is inserted between the legs from the front to back (top to bottom). **E,** The back panel is unfolded and spread out. **F,** The under-garment is pulled up at the back. **G,** The front panel is unfolded and spread open. **H,** The under-garment is pulled up in front.

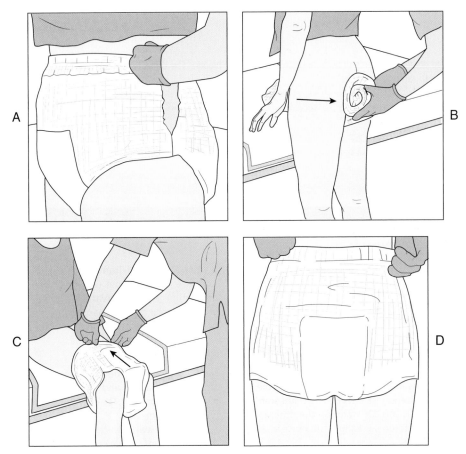

FIGURE 27-17 Applying pull-on underwear. **A,** The side seams are torn to remove the used underwear. **B,** The underwear is removed from front to back (top to bottom). **C,** The underwear is slid over the feet to past the knees. **D,** The underwear is pulled up.

BLADDER TRAINING

Bladder training may help with incontinence. Some persons need bladder training after catheter removal (Chapter 28). Control of urination is the goal. Bladder control promotes comfort and quality of life. It also increases self-esteem. Successful bladder training may take several weeks.

The rules for normal urination are followed (see Box 27-1). A normal position for voiding and privacy are important. The health team selects the best bladder training method for the person.

- *Bladder re-training (bladder rehabilitation).* The person needs to:
  - Resist or ignore the strong desire to urinate.
  - Postpone or delay voiding.
  - Urinate following a schedule rather than the urge to void.

The time between voidings increases as bladder re-training progresses.

- *Prompted voiding.* The person voids at scheduled times. The person learns to:
  - Recognize when the bladder is full.
  - Recognize the need to void.
  - Ask for help.
  - Respond when prompted to void.
- *Habit training/scheduled voiding.* Voiding is scheduled at regular times to match the person's voiding habits. This is usually every 2 to 4 hours while awake. The person does not delay or resist voiding.
- *Catheter clamping.* The catheter is clamped to prevent urine flow from the bladder (Chapter 28). See Figure 27-18, p. 418. It is usually clamped for 1 hour at first. Over time, it is clamped for 3 to 4 hours. Urine drains when the catheter is unclamped. After catheter removal, voiding is encouraged every 3 to 4 hours or according to the care plan.

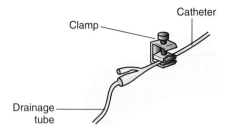

FIGURE 27-18 The clamped catheter prevents urine from draining out of the bladder. The clamp is applied to the catheter, not to the drainage tube.

FOCUS ON **PRIDE**

The Person, Family, and Yourself

Personal and Professional Responsibility

Some persons easily talk about urinary elimination. Others are shy or embarrassed. Note the person's verbal and nonverbal communication (Chapter 7). Watch for discomfort with words or topics. Be professional and speak with confidence. This puts the person at ease.

Rights and Respect

Illness, disease, and aging can affect voiding in private. Respect the right to privacy. Allow as much privacy as safely possible. If you must stay in the room, stand just outside the bathroom door in case the person needs you. Or stand on the other side of the privacy curtain if safe to do so. Follow the nurse's directions and the care plan.

Flush toilets and empty urinals, bedpans, and commodes promptly. The person has the right to a neat and clean setting. Do your best to promote comfort, dignity, and respect when assisting with elimination needs.

Independence and Social Interaction

Some persons can meet their own voiding needs. Others need some help but can be left alone to void. For persons needing some help, check on them often. Make sure the call light is within reach. Respond promptly.

Delegation and Teamwork

Accurate reporting and recording are important parts of delegation. See "Observations" on p. 402. Changes in urination may require changes in care. Report urinary problems and abnormal urine to the nurse. If unsure what to report or record, ask the nurse.

Ethics and Laws

Negligence occurs when a person does not act in a reasonable and careful manner and the person or the person's property is harmed (Chapter 5). The following is a real example of negligent care.

A patient was admitted to the hospital with a diagnosis of mild pneumonia. He was to be in the hospital for 24 to 48 hours. While in the hospital, he was left on the bedpan for 4 hours. Pressure injuries resulted. He died of pneumonia after 41 days in the hospital.

His family sued the hospital. The jury awarded the family $800,000.

(Estate of D. Roberts v William Beaumont Hospital, Mich., 2002.)

FOCUS ON **PRIDE**: *Application*

How does incontinence affect the person's dignity? How can it be prevented? Explain how your words and actions promote dignity when a person is incontinent.

REVIEW QUESTIONS

Circle the BEST answer.

1 Which is abnormal?
a Clear, amber urine
b Urine with a faint odor
c Cloudy urine with particles
d Urine output of 1500 mL in 24 hours

2 Which prevents normal elimination?
a Helping the person assume a normal position for voiding
b Providing privacy
c Helping the person to the bathroom as soon as requested
d Staying with the person who uses a bedpan

3 Which definition is *correct?*
a Dysuria means painful or difficult urination.
b Oliguria means a large amount of urine.
c Urinary retention means the need to void at once.
d Urinary incontinence means the inability to void.

4 The person using a standard bedpan is in
a Fowler's position
b The supine position
c The prone position
d The side-lying position

5 To use a fracture pan
a The person is in Fowler's position
b The smaller end (flat end) is under the buttocks
c The nurse must position the pan
d The pan can be left in place for a long time

6 After using the urinal, the person should
a Put it on the bedside stand
b Use the call light
c Put it on the over-bed table
d Empty it

7 A person is at risk for falling. What should you explain before commode use?
a "Do not use the armrests on the commode for support."
b "The wheels on the commode are unlocked for your safety."
c "I will leave the room while you use the commode."
d "I need to apply a transfer belt."

8 After a person uses a commode, you should
a Empty, clean, and disinfect the commode
b Return the commode to the supply area
c Get a new container
d Get a new commode

9 Urinary incontinence
a Is always permanent
b Requires bladder training
c Is a normal part of aging
d Requires good skin care

10 Which is a cause of functional incontinence?
a A nervous system disorder
b Sneezing
c Unanswered call light
d UTI

11 A resident with dementia is restless and pulling at the pants. What should you do first?
a Distract the person with an activity.
b Help the person to use the bathroom.
c Play calming music.
d Take the person for a walk.

12 When applying an incontinence product
a Let the plastic backing touch the person's skin
b Remove the old product from back to front
c Apply the new product from front to back
d Use the product to turn and position the person

13 The goal of bladder training is to
a Control the amount voided daily
b Promote voiding at times best for staff
c Allow the person to walk to the bathroom
d Gain control of urination

14 A person learns to ignore the urge to void. This type of bladder training is called
a Bladder re-training
b Prompted voiding
c Habit training
d Scheduled voiding

Answers to Chapter 27 questions are on p. 886.

FOCUS ON **PRACTICE**

Problem Solving

You assist a patient onto the commode. The person is unsteady and cannot be left alone. The person says: "I can't go if you stand here." What do you do? How will you provide privacy and safe care?

OBJECTIVES

- Define the key terms and key abbreviations in this chapter.
- Explain why urinary catheters are used.
- Describe 4 types of urinary catheters.
- Explain the purpose and rules for catheter care.
- Describe 2 urine drainage systems.
- Explain how to re-connect a catheter and drainage tubing.

- Explain how to remove an indwelling catheter.
- Explain how to apply a condom catheter.
- Perform the procedures described in this chapter.
- Explain how to promote PRIDE in the person, the family, and yourself.

KEY TERMS

catheter A tube used to drain or inject fluid through a body opening

catheterization The process of inserting a catheter

condom catheter A soft sheath that slides over the penis and is used to drain urine

Foley catheter See "indwelling catheter"

gravity A natural force that pulls things downward

indwelling catheter A catheter left in the bladder so urine drains constantly into a drainage bag; retention or Foley catheter

retention catheter See "indwelling catheter"

straight catheter A catheter that drains the bladder and then is removed

supra-pubic catheter A catheter surgically inserted into the bladder through an incision above *(supra)* the pubis bone *(pubic)*

KEY ABBREVIATIONS

BM	Bowel movement	IV	Intravenous
CAUTI	Catheter-associated urinary tract infection	mL	Milliliter
ID	Identification	UTI	Urinary tract infection

A *catheter is a tube used to drain or inject fluid through a body opening.* Inserted into the bladder, a urinary catheter drains urine. *Catheterization is the process of inserting a catheter.* With proper training, guidance, and assistance, some states and agencies let nursing assistants insert and remove urinary catheters.

See *Focus on Surveys: Urinary Catheters.*

See *Promoting Safety and Comfort: Urinary Catheters.*

FOCUS ON SURVEYS

Urinary Catheters

Surveys are done to check the quality of treatments and services. The surveyor may ask you about:

- Your training about handling catheters, catheter tubing, drainage bags, catheter care, urinary tract infections (UTIs), catheter-related injuries, dislodgment (moving out of place), and skin breakdown
- What observations to report, when to report them, and to whom you should report

Answer questions the best you can. If you do not know an answer, tell the surveyor who you would ask or where you would find the answer.

PROMOTING SAFETY AND COMFORT

Urinary Catheters

Safety

Urinary catheter procedures often involve exposing and touching the perineum. Sexual abuse has occurred in health care settings. The person may feel threatened or is actually being abused. He or she needs to call for help. Keep the call light within the person's reach at all times. Always act in a professional manner.

Urine may contain microbes and blood. Follow Standard Precautions and the Bloodborne Pathogen Standard for the procedures in this chapter.

NOTE: *A task may require more than 1 pair of gloves. Change gloves as needed. Use careful judgment. Remember to practice hand hygiene after removing gloves.*

CATHETERS

There are different types of catheters.

* A *straight catheter* *drains the bladder and then is removed.*
* An *indwelling catheter (retention* or *Foley catheter)* *is left in the bladder. Urine drains constantly into a drainage bag.* A balloon by the tip is inflated with sterile water after the catheter is inserted. The balloon prevents the catheter from coming out of the bladder (Fig. 28-1). Tubing connects the catheter to a urine drainage bag. See Figure 28-2 for parts of an indwelling catheter and urine drainage system.
* A *supra-pubic catheter* *is surgically inserted into the bladder through an incision above* (supra) *the pubis bone* (pubic). See Figure 28-3. Less common than the others, a supra-pubic catheter may be placed when the urethra is blocked or when a catheter is needed long-term.
* Used for men, a *condom catheter* is a soft sheath that slides over the penis. This type is not inserted into the bladder. See "Condom Catheters" on p. 432.
See *Delegation Guidelines: Catheters.*

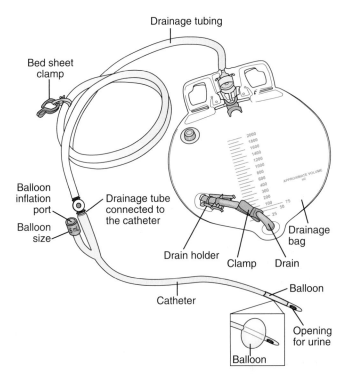

FIGURE 28-2 Parts of an indwelling catheter and urine drainage system.

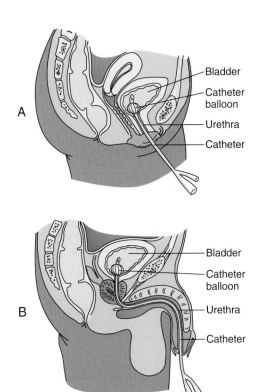

FIGURE 28-1 Indwelling catheter. **A,** Indwelling catheter in the female bladder. The inflated balloon at the tip prevents the catheter from slipping out through the urethra. **B,** Indwelling catheter with the balloon inflated in the male bladder.

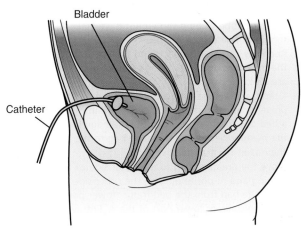

FIGURE 28-3 Supra-pubic catheter. (From Kostelnick C: *Mosby's textbook for long-term care nursing assistants,* ed 7, St Louis, 2015, Mosby.)

DELEGATION GUIDELINES
Catheters

Inserting and removing straight and indwelling catheters are nursing responsibilities. With proper training, guidance, and assistance, some states and agencies allow delegating the tasks to nursing assistants.

Inserting and removing supra-pubic catheters are not nursing responsibilities. The nurse cannot delegate the tasks to nursing assistants.

Purposes of Catheters

Catheters are used:

- To keep the bladder empty before, during, and after surgery. This reduces the risk of bladder injury during surgery. Also, urine amounts can be monitored. After surgery, a full bladder causes pressure on nearby organs. Such pressure can lead to pain or discomfort.
- To promote comfort. Some people are too weak or disabled to use the bedpan, urinal, commode, or toilet. Dying persons are examples. Catheters can promote comfort and prevent incontinence.
- To protect wounds and pressure injuries from contact with urine.
- For hourly urine output measurements.
- To collect sterile urine specimens.
- To measure the amount of urine in the bladder after the person voids (*residual urine*).

Catheters do not treat the cause of incontinence. They are a last resort for incontinence.

Catheter-Associated UTIs

The urinary system is sterile. Infection can occur if microbes enter. Catheters create a high risk for UTIs. A *catheter-associated urinary tract infection (CAUTI)* occurs when microbes enter the urinary tract through the catheter and cause an infection. Microbes travel up the catheter into the bladder and kidneys. CAUTIs can cause severe illness and death. Proper catheter care can reduce the risk of a CAUTI.

CATHETER CARE

You will care for persons with indwelling catheters. Follow the rules in Box 28-1 to promote safety and comfort.

See *Delegation Guidelines: Catheter Care*, p. 424.
See *Promoting Safety and Comfort: Catheter Care*, p. 424.
See procedure: *Giving Catheter Care*, p. 424.

Text continued on p. 426.

BOX 28-1	Indwelling Catheter Care

Preventing Infection

- Follow the rules of medical asepsis.
- Follow Standard Precautions and the Bloodborne Pathogen Standard.
- Encourage fluid intake as directed by the nurse and care plan.

The Drainage System

- Allow urine to flow freely through the catheter and drainage tube. Tubing should not have kinks. The person should not lie on the tubing.
- Keep the catheter connected to the drainage tube. Follow the measures on p. 426 if the catheter and drainage tube are disconnected.
- Keep the drainage tube and bag below the bladder. This prevents urine from flowing backward into the bladder. For a bed or chair transfer, keep the drainage bag lower than the bladder. Secure the drainage bag to the bed frame or chair after the transfer. See Figure 28-4.
- Move the drainage bag to the other side of the bed for turning and re-positioning on the other side.
- Hang the bag from the bed frame, lower part of the chair or wheelchair, or lower part of the IV (intravenous) pole.
- *Do not hang the drainage bag on a bed rail.* The bag is higher than the bladder when the bed rail is raised.
- Position tubing so it will not get tangled in the wheelchair wheels.
- Hold the bag lower than the bladder when the person walks.
- Do not let the drainage bag touch or rest on the floor. This can contaminate the system.
- Position drainage tubing in a straight line or coil it on the bed. Secure it to the bottom linens (Fig. 28-5). Follow the nurse's directions and agency policy. Use a clip, bed sheet clamp, or other device as the nurse directs. Tubing must not loop below the drainage bag.

The Catheter

- Secure the catheter as the nurse directs.
  - Females: to the thigh (see Fig. 28-5, *A*).
  - Males:
    - To the abdomen (see Fig. 28-5, *B*). This site may be used for long-term catheter use. The drainage bag remains below the bladder. Drainage is not affected.
    - To the thigh (see Fig. 28-5, *C*).

The Catheter—cont'd

- Use a tube holder, tape, leg band, or other device to secure the catheter to the thigh or abdomen (Fig. 28-6). The nurse tells you what to use. Securing the catheter prevents excess movement and friction at the insertion site (meatus). Catheter movement and friction can damage the meatus.
- Check for leaks. Check the connections to the drainage tube and the drainage bag. Report any leaks at once.
- Provide perineal care and catheter care according to the care plan—daily, twice a day, after bowel movements (BMs), or when vaginal discharge is present. (See procedure: *Giving Catheter Care*, p. 424.)

Measuring Urine (Output)

- Empty the drainage bag and measure urine:
  - At the end of the shift
  - To change to and from a leg bag and a standard drainage bag (p. 426)
  - When the bag is becoming full
  - Before measuring the person's weight (Chapter 36)
- Report an increase or decrease in urine amount.
- Provide a measuring container for each person. This prevents the spread of microbes from 1 person to another.
- Do not let the drain on the drainage bag touch any surface.
- See procedure: *Emptying a Urine Drainage Bag*, p. 428.

Observations

- Report complaints at once—pain, burning, the need to void, or irritation. Also report the color, clarity, and odor of urine and the presence of particles or blood.
- Observe for signs and symptoms of a UTI (Chapter 51). Report the following at once.
  - Fever.
  - Chills.
  - Flank pain or tenderness. The flank area is in the back between the ribs and the hip.
  - Change in the urine—blood, foul smell, particles, cloudiness, *oliguria* (scant amount of urine).
  - Change in mental or functional status—confusion, decreased appetite, falls, decreased activity, tiredness, and so on.
  - Urine leakage around the catheter.

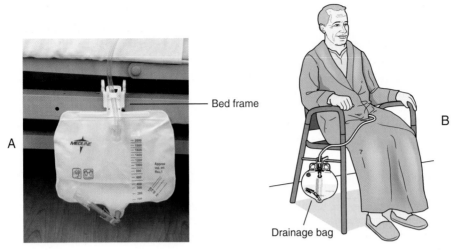

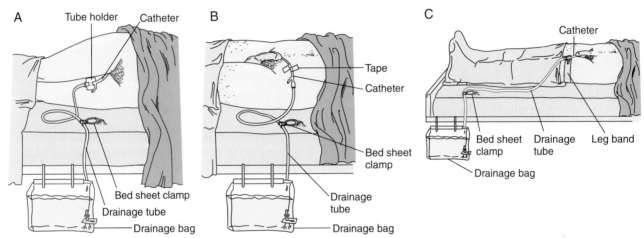

FIGURE 28-4 A, Urine drainage bag secured to the bed frame. **B,** Urine drainage bag secured to a chair.

FIGURE 28-5 Securing catheters. **A,** This catheter is secured to the woman's thigh with a tube holder. The drainage tube is coiled on the bed and secured to bottom linens with a bed sheet clamp. **B,** This catheter is secured to the man's abdomen with tape. Drainage tubing is secured to bottom linens with a bed sheet clamp. **C,** This catheter is secured to the man's thigh with a leg band. Drainage tubing is in a straight line and secured to bottom linens with a bed sheet clamp. The drainage bag is at the foot of the bed.

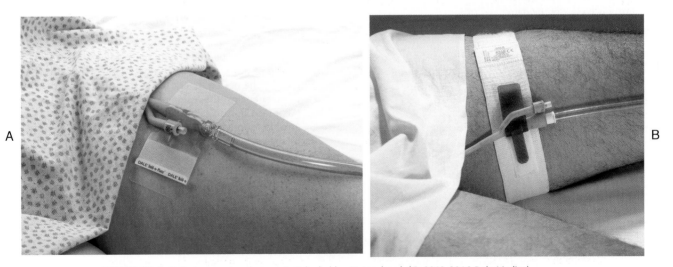

FIGURE 28-6 Catheter securing devices. **A,** Tube holder. **B,** Leg band. (© 2013-2016 Dale Medical Products, Inc. All rights reserved.)

DELEGATION GUIDELINES
Catheter Care

Catheter care is a routine nursing task. You need this information from the nurse and the care plan.

- When to give catheter care—daily, twice a day, after BMs, or because of vaginal discharge
- What water temperature to use for perineal care
- Where to secure the catheter—thigh or abdomen
- How to secure the catheter—tube holder, leg band, tape, or other device
- How to position the drainage tubing—straight line or coiled on the bed
- Where to secure the drainage tubing and hang the drainage bag—bed, chair, or wheelchair
- How to secure drainage tubing—clip, bed sheet clamp, or other device

- What observations to report and record:
  - Complaints of pain, burning, irritation, or the need to void (report at once)
  - Crusting, abnormal drainage, or secretions
  - The color, clarity, and odor of urine
  - Particles in the urine
  - Blood in the urine (report at once)
  - Cloudy urine
  - Urine leaking at the insertion site
  - Drainage system leaks
- When to report observations
- What patient or resident concerns to report at once

PROMOTING SAFETY AND COMFORT
Catheter Care

Safety

In some agencies, perineal care (Chapter 24) is sufficient hygiene for indwelling catheters. The procedure that follows is not used. Follow agency policy and the care plan when a person has a catheter.

When giving catheter care, clean, rinse, and dry the catheter from the meatus down at least 4 inches. Move in 1 direction (away from the meatus). If needed, repeat with a clean area of the washcloth or a clean washcloth.

Comfort

The catheter must not pull at the insertion site. This causes discomfort and irritation. Hold the catheter securely during catheter care. Then properly secure the catheter. Make sure the tubing is not under the person. Besides blocking urine flow, lying on the tubing is uncomfortable. It can also cause skin breakdown. To promote comfort, see Box 28-1.

Giving Catheter Care

QUALITY OF LIFE

- Knock before entering the person's room.
- Address the person by name.
- Introduce yourself by name and title.

- Explain the procedure before starting and during the procedure.
- Protect the person's rights during the procedure.
- Handle the person gently during the procedure.

PRE-PROCEDURE

1 Follow *Delegation Guidelines:*
   - *Perineal Care* (Chapter 24)
   - *Catheter Care*
   See *Promoting Safety and Comfort:*
   - *Perineal Care* (Chapter 24)
   - *Urinary Catheters*, p. 420
   - *Catheter Care*
2 Practice hand hygiene.
3 Collect the following.
   - Items for perineal care (Chapter 24)
   - Gloves
   - Bath blanket

4 Cover the over-bed table with paper towels. Arrange items on top of them.
5 Identify the person. Check the ID (identification) bracelet against the assignment sheet. Use 2 identifiers (Chapter 13). Also call the person by name.
6 Provide for privacy.
7 Fill the wash basin. Water temperature is about 105°F to 109°F (Fahrenheit) (40.5°C to 42.7°C [centigrade]). Measure water temperature according to agency policy. Have the person check the water temperature and adjust as needed.
8 Raise the bed for body mechanics. Bed rails are up if used.
9 Lower the bed rail near you if up.

Giving Catheter Care—cont'd

PROCEDURE

10 Practice hand hygiene. Put on the gloves. (NOTE: Some state competency tests require that gloves be applied after covering the person with the bath blanket.)
11 Cover the person with a bath blanket. Fan-fold top linens to the foot of the bed.
12 Position and drape the person for perineal care (Chapter 24).
13 Fold back the bath blanket to expose the perineal area.
14 Place the waterproof under-pad under the buttocks. To do so, have the person raise the buttocks off the bed. Or turn the person from side to side.
15 Check the drainage tubing. Make sure it is not kinked and that urine can flow freely.
16 Separate the labia (female). In an uncircumcised male, retract the foreskin (Chapter 24). Check for crusts, abnormal drainage, or secretions.
17 Give perineal care (Chapter 24). Keep the foreskin of the uncircumcised male retracted until step 25.
18 Apply soap, body wash, or other cleansing agent to a clean, wet washcloth.
19 Hold the catheter at the meatus. Do so for steps 20 through 24.
20 Wash around the catheter at the meatus. Use a circular motion. (NOTE: Complete this step if required by agency policy or your state's competency test.)
21 Clean the catheter from the meatus down the catheter at least 4 inches (Fig. 28-7). Clean downward, away from the meatus with 1 stroke. Do not tug or pull on the catheter. Repeat as needed with a clean area of the washcloth. Use a clean washcloth if needed.

22 Rinse around the catheter at the meatus with a clean washcloth. (NOTE: Complete this step if required by agency policy or your state's competency test.)
23 Rinse the catheter from the meatus down the catheter at least 4 inches. Rinse downward, away from the meatus with 1 stroke. Do not tug or pull on the catheter. Repeat as needed with a clean area of the washcloth. Use a clean washcloth if needed.
24 Pat dry the areas washed. Dry from the meatus down the catheter at least 4 inches. Do not tug or pull on the catheter.
25 Return the foreskin (uncircumcised male) to its natural position.
26 Pat dry the perineal area. Dry from front to back (top to bottom).
27 Secure the catheter. Position the tubing in a straight line or coiled on the bed. Follow the nurse's directions. Secure the tubing to the bottom linens (see Fig. 28-5).
28 Remove the waterproof under-pad.
29 Cover the person. Remove the bath blanket.
30 Remove and discard the gloves. Practice hand hygiene.

POST-PROCEDURE

31 Provide for comfort. (See the inside of the back cover.)
32 Place the call light and other needed items within reach.
33 Lower the bed to a safe and comfortable level. Follow the care plan.
34 Raise or lower bed rails. Follow the care plan.
35 Clean, rinse, dry, and return equipment to its proper place. Use clean, dry paper towels for drying. Discard disposable items. (Wear gloves for this step.)

36 Unscreen the person.
37 Complete a safety check of the room. (See the inside of the back cover.)
38 Follow agency policy for used linens.
39 Remove and discard the gloves. Practice hand hygiene.
40 Report and record your observations.

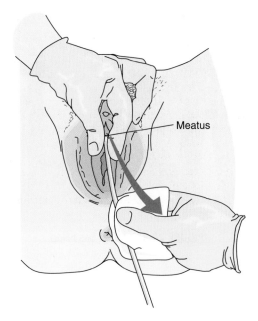

Meatus

FIGURE 28-7 Cleaning the catheter. Start at the meatus. Clean downward, away from the meatus. Clean at least 4 inches of the catheter.

URINE DRAINAGE SYSTEMS

A closed drainage system is used for indwelling catheters. Only urine should enter the system. See Box 28-1 to prevent infection and for proper care of the drainage system.

There are 2 types of urine drainage bags.

- *Standard drainage bags* usually hold at least 2000 mL (milliliters) of urine (see Fig. 28-4).
- *Leg bags* attach to the thigh or calf with elastic bands or Velcro. Leg bags hold less than 1000 mL of urine. Some people wear leg bags when up.

Drainage systems can become disconnected. If that happens, tell the nurse at once. Do not touch the ends of the catheter or tubing. Box 28-2 describes how to re-connect the catheter and tubing.

Leg bags are changed to standard drainage bags when the person is in bed. The drainage bags stay lower than bladder level. You need to open the closed drainage system. You must prevent microbes from entering the system.

See *Delegation Guidelines: Urine Drainage Systems.*
See *Promoting Safety and Comfort: Urine Drainage Systems.*
See procedure: *Changing a Leg Bag to a Standard Drainage Bag.*
See procedure: *Emptying a Urine Drainage Bag*, p. 428.

DELEGATION GUIDELINES

Urine Drainage Systems

Changing a drainage bag and emptying a urine drainage bag are routine nursing tasks. You need this information from the nurse and the care plan.

- When to empty the urine drainage bag
- If the person uses a leg bag
- What leg bag straps to use—elastic or Velcro
- When to switch a standard drainage bag and leg bag
- If you should clean or discard the drainage bag
- What observations to report and record:
  - The amount of urine measured (Chapter 31)
  - The color, clarity, and odor of urine
  - Particles in the urine
  - Blood in the urine
  - Cloudy urine
  - Complaints of pain, burning, irritation, or the need to urinate
  - Drainage system leaks
- When to report observations
- What patient or resident concerns to report at once

BOX 28-2 | Re-Connecting a Catheter and Drainage Tube

1. Practice hand hygiene. Put on gloves.
2. Wipe the end of the drainage tube with an antiseptic wipe.
3. Wipe the end of the catheter with another antiseptic wipe.
4. Do not put the ends down. Do not touch the ends after you clean them.
5. Connect the drainage tubing to the catheter.
6. Discard the wipes into a biohazard bag.
7. Remove the gloves. Practice hand hygiene.

PROMOTING SAFETY AND COMFORT

Urine Drainage Systems

Safety

Urine drains from the bladder through the catheter and into a drainage bag. Gravity allows urine to drain. *Gravity is a natural force that pulls things downward.* Always keep the drainage bag below bladder level. This allows urine to flow downward from the force of gravity.

For the procedure: *Changing a Leg Bag to a Standard Drainage Bag,* you will open sterile packages. You must keep sterile items free from contamination. Review "Surgical Asepsis" in Chapter 16.

Leg bags hold less urine than standard drainage bags. Check leg bags often. Empty the leg bag if it is becoming half full. Measure, report, and record the amount of urine.

Comfort

Urine in a drainage bag embarrasses some people. Visitors can see the urine. To promote mental comfort, have visitors sit on the side away from the drainage bag. Try to empty the bag before visitors arrive. Measure, report, and record the amount of urine.

Some agencies have drainage bag holders (Fig. 28-8). The drainage bag is placed inside the holder. The holder promotes privacy.

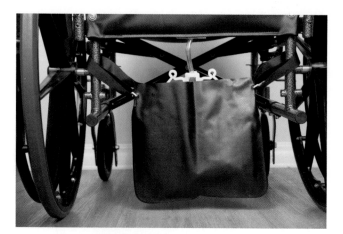

FIGURE 28-8 Drainage bag holder.

Changing a Leg Bag to a Standard Drainage Bag

QUALITY OF LIFE

- Knock before entering the person's room.
- Address the person by name.
- Introduce yourself by name and title.

- Explain the procedure before starting and during the procedure.
- Protect the person's rights during the procedure.
- Handle the person gently during the procedure.

PRE-PROCEDURE

1 Follow *Delegation Guidelines: Urine Drainage Systems*. See *Promoting Safety and Comfort:*
   - *Urinary Catheters*, p. 420
   - *Urine Drainage Systems*
2 Practice hand hygiene.
3 Collect the following.
   - Gloves
   - Standard drainage bag and tubing
   - Antiseptic wipes
   - Waterproof under-pad
   - Sterile cap and plug

- Catheter clamp
- Paper towels
- Bedpan and cover (optional)
- Bath blanket

4 Arrange paper towels and equipment on the over-bed table. Place the bedpan at the foot of the bed.
5 Identify the person. Check the ID bracelet against the assignment sheet. Use 2 identifiers (Chapter 13). Also call the person by name.
6 Provide for privacy.

PROCEDURE

7 Have the person sit on the side of the bed.
8 Practice hand hygiene. Put on the gloves.
9 Expose the catheter and leg bag.
10 Empty the drainage bag. See procedure: *Emptying a Urine Drainage Bag*, p. 428.
11 Clamp the catheter (Fig. 28-9, p. 428). This prevents urine from draining from the catheter into the drainage tubing.
12 Let urine drain from below the clamp into the drainage tubing. This empties the lower end of the catheter.
13 Help the person lie down.
14 Raise the bed rails if used. Raise the bed for body mechanics.
15 Lower the bed rail near you if up.
16 Cover the person with a bath blanket. Fan-fold top linens to the foot of the bed. Expose the catheter and leg bag.
17 Place the waterproof under-pad under the person's leg.
18 Open the antiseptic wipes. Set them on the paper towels.
19 Open the package with the sterile cap and plug. Set the package on the paper towels. Do not let anything touch the sterile cap or plug (Fig. 28-10, p. 428).
20 Open the package with the standard drainage bag and tubing.
21 Attach the standard drainage bag to the bed frame.
22 Disconnect the catheter from the drainage tubing. Do not let anything touch the ends.

23 Insert the sterile plug into the catheter end (Fig. 28-11, p. 428). Touch only the end of the plug. Do not touch the part that goes inside the catheter. (If you contaminate the end of the catheter, wipe the end with an antiseptic wipe. Do so before inserting the sterile plug.)
24 Place the sterile cap on the end of the leg bag drainage tube (see Fig. 28-11). (If you contaminate the tubing end, wipe the end with an antiseptic wipe. Do so before you put on the sterile cap.)
25 Remove the cap from the new standard drainage bag tubing.
26 Remove the sterile plug from the catheter.
27 Insert the end of the drainage tubing into the catheter.
28 Remove the clamp from the catheter.
29 Position drainage tubing in a straight line or coiled on the bed. Follow the nurse's directions. Secure the tubing to the bottom linens.
30 Remove the leg bag. Place it in the bedpan.
31 Remove and discard the waterproof under-pad.
32 Cover the person. Remove the bath blanket.
33 Take the bedpan to the bathroom.
34 Remove and discard the gloves. Practice hand hygiene.

POST-PROCEDURE

35 Provide for comfort. (See the inside of the back cover.)
36 Place the call light and other needed items within reach.
37 Lower the bed to a safe and comfortable level. Follow the care plan.
38 Raise or lower bed rails. Follow the care plan.
39 Unscreen the person.
40 Put on clean gloves. Discard disposable items.
41 Discard the drainage tubing and leg bag following agency policy. Or clean the bag following agency policy.
42 Clean and disinfect the bedpan. See procedure: *Giving the Bedpan* in Chapter 27.

43 Return the bedpan and other supplies to their proper place.
44 Remove and discard the gloves. Practice hand hygiene.
45 Complete a safety check of the room. (See the inside of the back cover.)
46 Follow agency policy for used linens.
47 Practice hand hygiene.
48 Report and record your observations.

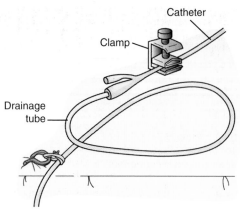

FIGURE 28-9 The clamped catheter prevents urine from draining out of the bladder. The clamp is applied directly to the catheter—not to the drainage tube.

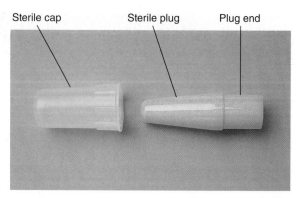

FIGURE 28-10 Sterile cap and catheter plug. The inside of the cap is sterile. Touch only the end of the plug.

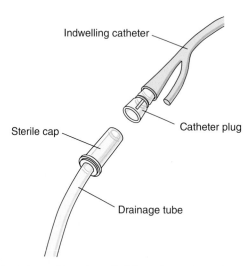

FIGURE 28-11 Sterile plug is inserted into the end of the catheter. The sterile cap is on the end of the drainage tube.

Emptying a Urine Drainage Bag

QUALITY OF LIFE

- Knock before entering the person's room.
- Address the person by name.
- Introduce yourself by name and title.

- Explain the procedure before starting and during the procedure.
- Protect the person's rights during the procedure.
- Handle the person gently during the procedure.

PRE-PROCEDURE

1 Follow *Delegation Guidelines: Urine Drainage Systems,* p. 426. See *Promoting Safety and Comfort:*
   - *Urinary Catheters,* p. 420
   - *Urine Drainage Systems,* p. 426
2 Collect the following.
   - Graduate (measuring container)
   - Gloves
   - Paper towels
   - Antiseptic wipes

3 Practice hand hygiene.
4 Identify the person. Check the ID bracelet against the assignment sheet. Use 2 identifiers (Chapter 13). Also call the person by name.
5 Provide for privacy.

Emptying a Urine Drainage Bag—cont'd

PROCEDURE

6 Put on the gloves.
7 Place a paper towel on the floor. Place the graduate on top of it.
8 Place the graduate under the drainage bag.
9 Open the clamp on the drain.
10 Let all urine drain into the graduate. The drain does not touch the graduate (Fig. 28-12).
11 Clean the end of the drain with an antiseptic wipe.
12 Clamp and position the drain in the holder (Fig. 28-13).
13 Measure urine. See procedure: *Measuring Intake and Output* in Chapter 31.

14 Remove and discard the paper towel.
15 Empty the graduate into the toilet and flush.
16 Rinse the graduate. Empty the rinse into the toilet and flush.
17 Clean, disinfect, and dry the graduate. Use clean, dry paper towels for drying.
18 Return the graduate to its proper place.
19 Remove and discard the gloves. Practice hand hygiene.
20 Record the time and amount of urine on the intake and output (I&O) record (Chapter 31).

POST-PROCEDURE

21 Provide for comfort. (See the inside of the back cover.)
22 Place the call light and other needed items within reach.
23 Unscreen the person.

24 Complete a safety check of the room. (See the inside of the back cover.)
25 Report and record the amount of urine and other observations.

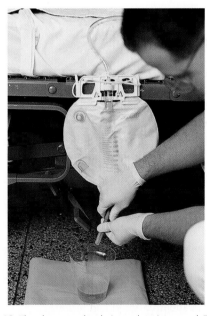

FIGURE 28-12 The clamp on the drainage bag is opened. The drain is directed into the graduate. The drain does not touch the inside of the graduate. (From Potter PA, Perry AG, Stockert PA, Hall AM: *Fundamentals of nursing,* ed 9, St Louis, 2017, Elsevier.)

Drainage tubing

Drainage bag

Holder   Clamp   Drain

FIGURE 28-13 The clamp is closed and positioned in the holder on the drainage bag.

REMOVING INDWELLING CATHETERS

An indwelling catheter has 2 lumens (passage-ways). Sterile water is injected through 1 lumen (balloon inflation port) to inflate the balloon (Fig. 28-14). The water is injected with a syringe. Urine drains from the bladder through the other lumen.

To remove the catheter, the balloon is deflated—the water is removed. You need a syringe large enough to hold all the water in the balloon. The nurse tells you what size syringe to use.

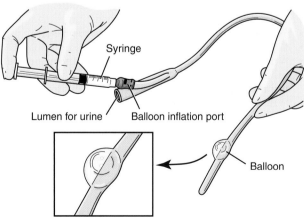

Syringe

Lumen for urine   Balloon inflation port

Balloon

FIGURE 28-14 The balloon of an indwelling catheter is inflated with water. A syringe is used to inject the water. A syringe also is used to remove the water.

The doctor orders catheter removal. The person may need bladder training first (Chapter 27). Dysuria and urinary frequency are common after removing catheters (Chapter 27).

See *Focus on Communication: Removing Indwelling Catheters.*
See *Focus on Math: Removing Indwelling Catheters.*
See *Delegation Guidelines: Removing Indwelling Catheters.*
See *Promoting Safety and Comfort: Removing Indwelling Catheters.*
See procedure: *Removing an Indwelling Catheter.*

FOCUS ON COMMUNICATION

Removing Indwelling Catheters

Explain the procedure to the person before starting and during the procedure. Also, tell the person about possible discomfort and when it might be felt. Have the person tell you at once if pain is felt or if you should stop. For example:

I'm going to remove your catheter. I will explain the procedure step-by-step. You may feel a little pressure or discomfort when I remove the tube. I will tell you before I remove it. Please tell me right away if you feel pain or if you need me to stop.

Ask the person to breathe out (exhale) when removing the catheter to distract the person and promote relaxation. Explain each step in a calm and professional way to reduce anxiety and provide comfort. Avoid seeming bossy or hurried. Politely tell the person what you will do and what he or she needs to do.

FOCUS ON MATH

Removing Indwelling Catheters

To remove indwelling catheters, you must know how to measure liquid using a syringe. Syringes are marked in milliliters (mL). An mL is a unit used to measure liquid. Read the syringe at the top of the plunger. See Figure 28-15.

The amount of water removed should equal the amount injected. The nurse tells you the amount used for balloon inflation. Subtract the amount removed from the amount injected. If there is a difference, tell the nurse before removing the catheter. For example:

- An indwelling catheter balloon is filled with 10 mL. You remove 7 mL. The difference is 3 mL. Do not remove the catheter. Call for the nurse.

$$10 \text{ mL} - 7 \text{ mL} = 3 \text{ mL}$$

- An indwelling catheter balloon is filled with 10 mL. You remove 10 mL. The difference is 0 mL. You can safely remove the catheter.

$$10 \text{ mL} - 10 \text{ mL} = 0 \text{ mL}$$

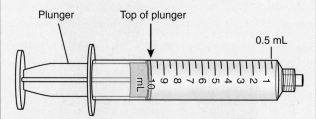

FIGURE 28-15 A syringe is read at the top of the plunger. This syringe measures 10 mL. Short lines mark 0.5 (one-half) mL measurements.

DELEGATION GUIDELINES

Removing Indwelling Catheters

Removing an indwelling catheter is a nursing responsibility. If the task is delegated to you, make sure that:
- Your state allows you to perform the procedure.
- The procedure is in your job description.
- You know how to use the supplies and equipment.
- You review the procedure with the nurse.
- A nurse is available to answer questions and to guide and assist you as needed.

If the above conditions are met, you need this information from the nurse.
- When to remove the catheter
- The amount of water used for balloon inflation
- Syringe size needed

- What observations to report and record:
  - Amount of water removed from the balloon
  - The amount of urine in the drainage bag
  - Color, clarity, and odor of urine
  - Particles in the urine
  - Blood in the urine
  - How the person tolerated the procedure
  - Complaints of pain, burning, irritation, or the need to void
  - Any other observations
- When to report observations
- What patient or resident concerns to report at once

PROMOTING SAFETY AND COMFORT

Removing Indwelling Catheters

Safety

The catheter package prescribes the amount of water needed to inflate the balloon. For proper inflation, the amount of water used is greater than the balloon size. See Figure 28-16.

Before removing the catheter, you must know the amount of water in the balloon. The nurse tells you the amount. You must remove all water from the balloon. If the balloon is filled with 10 mL, 10 mL must be removed. Otherwise, injury to the urethra is likely as the catheter is removed. Do not remove the catheter if water remains in the balloon. Call for the nurse at once.

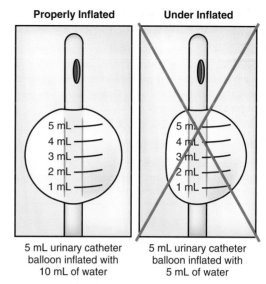

Properly Inflated   **Under Inflated**

5 mL urinary catheter balloon inflated with 10 mL of water

5 mL urinary catheter balloon inflated with 5 mL of water

FIGURE 28-16 The balloon must be inflated properly to avoid drainage and deflation problems. The balloon size marked on the catheter may not equal the amount of water in the balloon. The nurse tells you the amount of water in the balloon.

Removing an Indwelling Catheter

QUALITY OF LIFE

- Knock before entering the person's room.
- Address the person by name.
- Introduce yourself by name and title.

- Explain the procedure before starting and during the procedure.
- Protect the person's rights during the procedure.
- Handle the person gently during the procedure.

PRE-PROCEDURE

1 Follow *Delegation Guidelines: Removing Indwelling Catheters*. See *Promoting Safety and Comfort:*
   - *Urinary Catheters*, p. 420
   - *Removing Indwelling Catheters*
2 Practice hand hygiene.
3 Collect the following.
   - Disposable towel
   - Syringe in the size as directed by the nurse

   - Disposable bag
   - Gloves
   - Bath blanket
4 Identify the person. Check the ID bracelet against the assignment sheet. Use 2 identifiers (Chapter 13). Also call the person by name.
5 Provide for privacy.
6 Raise the bed for body mechanics. Bed rails are up if used.

PROCEDURE

7 Lower the bed rail near you if up.
8 Practice hand hygiene. Put on the gloves.
9 Position and drape the person as for perineal care (Chapter 24).
10 Cover the person with a bath blanket.
11 Check the size of the syringe. Know the amount of water in the balloon. Make sure the syringe is large enough to withdraw all the water from the balloon.
12 Remove the tube holder, leg band, or tape securing the catheter to the person.
13 Position the towel.
   a Female—between her legs
   b Male—over his thighs
14 Remove all of the water from the balloon. (NOTE: You must know how much water is in the balloon. For example, if the balloon is filled with 10 mL of water, you must remove 10 mL of water.)
   a Slide the syringe plunger up and down several times. This loosens the plunger.
   b Pull the plunger back to the 0.5 (one-half) mL mark.

c Attach the syringe to the catheter's balloon port gently. Use only enough force to get the syringe to stay in the port.
d Allow the water to drain into the syringe. Wait at least 30 seconds to allow the full amount to drain. Do not pull back on the plunger. Pressure in the balloon will force the plunger back and fill the syringe. If the water is draining slowly or not at all, call for the nurse. Do not remove the catheter if there is water in the balloon. The nurse may have you:
   1) Gently re-position the syringe in the port.
   2) Re-position the person.
   3) Pull back on the syringe gently and slowly. Forceful pulling can collapse the tube.
15 Pull the catheter straight out once all of the water is removed. Remove the catheter gently.
16 Discard the catheter into the bag.
17 Dry the perineal area with the towel. Discard the disposable towel in the bag.
18 Remove and discard the gloves. Practice hand hygiene.
19 Cover the person. Remove the bath blanket.

Continued

Removing an Indwelling Catheter—cont'd

POST-PROCEDURE

20 Provide for comfort. (See the inside of the back cover.)

21 Place the call light and other needed items within reach.

22 Lower the bed to a safe and comfortable level. Follow the care plan.

23 Raise or lower bed rails. Follow the care plan.

24 Unscreen the person.

25 Put on clean gloves. Discard disposable items. Discard the syringe according to agency policy.

26 Empty the drainage bag. See procedure: *Emptying a Urine Drainage Bag*, p. 428. Note the amount of urine.

27 Discard the drainage tubing and bag following agency policy.

28 Remove and discard the gloves. Practice hand hygiene.

29 Complete a safety check of the room. (See the inside of the back cover.)

30 Practice hand hygiene.

31 Report and record your observations.

CONDOM CATHETERS

Condom catheters are often used for incontinent men. They also are called *external catheters*, *Texas catheters*, and *urinary sheaths*. A *condom catheter is a soft sheath that slides over the penis and is used to drain urine.* Tubing connects the condom catheter to the drainage bag. Many men prefer leg bags (Fig. 28-17).

Condom catheters are changed daily after perineal care. To apply a condom catheter, follow the manufacturer's instructions. Thoroughly wash and dry the penis before applying the catheter.

Some condom catheters are self-adhering. Adhesive inside the catheter adheres to the penis. Non-adhering catheters are secured with elastic tape. Use the elastic tape packaged with the catheter. *Apply the tape in a spiral.* This allows blood flow to the penis. *Only use elastic tape. Adhesive tape and other tapes do not expand. Never use such tapes to secure condom catheters. Blood flow to the penis is cut off, injuring the penis.*

See *Delegation Guidelines: Condom Catheters.*
See *Promoting Safety and Comfort: Condom Catheters.*
See procedure: *Applying a Condom Catheter.*

DELEGATION GUIDELINES

Condom Catheters

Removing and applying a condom catheter is a nursing responsibility that may be safely delegated to you. In some states and agencies it is a routine nursing task.

Before removing and applying a condom catheter, you need this information from the nurse and the care plan.

*   What size to use—small, medium, or large
*   When to remove the catheter and apply a new one
*   If a leg bag or standard drainage bag is used
*   What leg bag straps to use—elastic or Velcro
*   What water temperature to use for perineal care
*   What observations to report and record:
    *   Reddened or open areas on the penis
    *   Swelling of the penis
    *   Color, clarity, and odor of urine
    *   Particles in the urine
    *   Blood in the urine
    *   Cloudy urine
*   When to report observations
*   What patient or resident concerns to report at once

PROMOTING SAFETY AND COMFORT

Condom Catheters

Safety

Do not apply a condom catheter if the penis is red, irritated, or shows signs of skin breakdown. Report your observations at once.

If you do not know how to use your agency's condom catheters, have the nurse show you the correct application. Then ask the nurse to observe you applying the catheter.

Blood must flow to the penis. If tape is needed, use the elastic tape packaged with the catheter. Apply it in a spiral.

Comfort

To apply a condom catheter, you need to touch and handle the penis. This can embarrass the man. Some men become sexually aroused. Act in a professional manner. Allow privacy if needed. Provide for safety and place the urinal within reach. Tell him when you will return or ask him to use the call light so you can finish the procedure. Knock before entering the room.

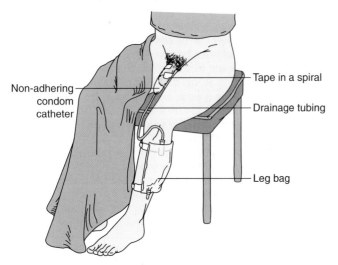

FIGURE 28-17 Condom catheter attached to a leg bag.

Non-adhering condom catheter

Tape in a spiral

Drainage tubing

Leg bag

Applying a Condom Catheter

QUALITY OF LIFE

- Knock before entering the person's room.
- Address the person by name.
- Introduce yourself by name and title.

- Explain the procedure before starting and during the procedure.
- Protect the person's rights during the procedure.
- Handle the person gently during the procedure.

PRE-PROCEDURE

1 Follow *Delegation Guidelines:*
- *Perineal Care* (Chapter 24)
- *Condom Catheters*
See *Promoting Safety and Comfort:*
- *Perineal Care* (Chapter 24)
- *Urinary Catheters,* p. 420
- *Condom Catheters*
2 Practice hand hygiene.
3 Collect the following.
- Condom catheter
- Elastic tape (if needed)
- Standard drainage bag or leg bag
- Cap for the drainage bag
- Basin of warm water (See procedure: *Giving Male Perineal Care* in Chapter 24.)

- Soap, body wash, or other cleansing agent
- Towel and washcloths
- Bath blanket
- Gloves
- Waterproof under-pad
- Paper towels

4 Cover the over-bed table with paper towels. Arrange items on top of them.
5 Identify the person. Check the ID bracelet against the assignment sheet. Use 2 identifiers (Chapter 13). Also call the person by name.
6 Provide for privacy.
7 Raise the bed for body mechanics. Bed rails are up if used.

PROCEDURE

8 Lower the bed rail near you if up.
9 Practice hand hygiene. Put on the gloves.
10 Cover the person with a bath blanket. Lower top linens to the knees.
11 Have the person raise his buttocks off the bed. Or turn him onto his side away from you.
12 Slide the waterproof under-pad under the buttocks.
13 Have him lower the buttocks. Or turn him onto his back.
14 Secure the standard drainage bag to the bed frame. Or have a leg bag ready. Close the drain.
15 Expose the genital area.
16 Remove the condom catheter.
- a Remove the tape (for the non-adhering type). Roll the sheath off the penis.
- b Disconnect the drainage tubing from the condom. Cap the drainage tube.
- c Discard the tape (if used) and condom.
17 Provide perineal care (Chapter 24). Observe the penis for reddened areas, skin breakdown, and irritation.
18 Remove and discard the gloves. Practice hand hygiene. Put on clean gloves.

19 Remove the protective backing from the condom. This exposes the adhesive strip.
20 Hold the penis firmly. Roll the condom onto the penis. Leave a 1-inch space between the penis and the end of the catheter (Fig. 28-18, p. 434).
21 Secure the condom.
- a *Self-adhering condom:* press the condom to the penis.
- b *Non-adhering condom secured with elastic tape:* apply elastic tape in a spiral. See Figure 28-18. Do not apply tape completely around the penis.
22 Make sure the penis tip does not touch the condom. Make sure the condom is not twisted.
23 Connect the condom to the drainage tubing. Secure excess tubing on the bed. Or attach a leg bag.
24 Remove the waterproof under-pad and gloves. Discard them. Practice hand hygiene.
25 Cover the person. Remove the bath blanket.

POST-PROCEDURE

26 Provide for comfort. (See the inside of the back cover.)
27 Place the call light and other needed items within reach.
28 Lower the bed to a safe and comfortable level. Follow the care plan.
29 Raise or lower bed rails. Follow the care plan.
30 Unscreen the person.
31 Practice hand hygiene. Put on clean gloves.
32 Measure and record the amount of urine in the bag. Clean or discard the drainage bag.

33 Clean, rinse, dry, and return the wash basin and other equipment. Use clean, dry paper towels for drying. Return items to their proper place.
34 Remove and discard the gloves. Practice hand hygiene.
35 Complete a safety check of the room. (See the inside of the back cover.)
36 Report and record your observations.

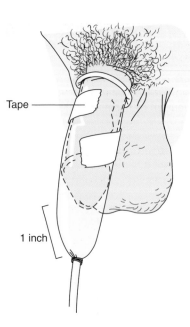

FIGURE 28-18 A non-adhering condom catheter applied to the penis. A 1-inch space is between the penis and the end of the catheter. Elastic tape is applied in a *spiral* to secure the condom catheter to the penis.

FOCUS ON **PRIDE**

The Person, Family, and Yourself

Personal and Professional Responsibility

With urinary catheters, the risk of UTIs is high. How you give care can decrease the risk of UTI. Do you:

- Prevent urine from flowing back into the bladder when moving the drainage bag?
- Use a clean area of the washcloth for each stroke during catheter care?
- Keep the drain from touching the graduate or other surface?
- Use a clean, separate graduate to empty each person's drainage bag?

Rights and Respect

Respect the right to privacy. For example, knock before entering a room. Before any procedure, explain how you will provide privacy. This is very important for procedures that involve exposing and touching private areas.

Independence and Social Interaction

Urinary catheters are short-term or long-term. Some persons manage their own catheters. The nurse teaches the person to provide catheter care. You:

- Give encouragement. Be kind, patient, and professional.
- Reinforce the nurse's instructions.
- Tell the nurse if the person has questions or if you think more teaching is needed.

Delegation and Teamwork

Tasks become more complex as more care equipment is needed. For example, you need to transfer a person from the chair to bed. The person has a urinary catheter. You must:

- Keep the catheter and drainage tube free of kinks.
- Keep the drainage bag below bladder level.
- Avoid resting the bag on the floor.
- Make sure the person is not lying on the drainage tube.

Ethics and Laws

With more training, some states and agencies allow nursing assistants to insert indwelling catheters. Follow state and agency rules. *Never* perform a task outside your role limits.

FOCUS ON **PRIDE**: *Application*

How might needing a urinary catheter affect the person mentally? How can you promote mental comfort?

REVIEW QUESTIONS

Circle the BEST answer.

1 Urinary catheters are used
- a To prevent urinary tract infections
- b To treat the cause of incontinence
- c To keep the bladder empty for surgery
- d For staff convenience with incontinent persons

2 A person has a catheter. Which is *safe?*
- a Keeping the drainage bag above the bladder level
- b Taping a leak at the connection site
- c Attaching the drainage bag to the bed rail
- d Removing a kink from the drainage tubing

3 A person has a catheter. Which is *correct?*
- a Report pain, burning, or irritation at once.
- b Allow the tubing to hang below the drainage bag.
- c Empty the drainage bag once daily.
- d Use the same graduate for all persons.

4 A person has a catheter. You are going to turn the person from the left to the right side. What should you do with the drainage bag?
- a Move it to the right side.
- b Keep it on the left side.
- c Hang it from an IV pole.
- d Remove it.

5 For a female, a catheter is secured to
- a The abdomen
- b The gown with a safety pin
- c The thigh with a tube holder
- d The bottom linens with a bed sheet clamp

6 For catheter care
- a Clean from the drainage tube connection up the catheter at least 4 inches
- b Clean from the meatus down the catheter at least 4 inches
- c Pull on the catheter to make sure it is secure
- d Clamp the catheter to prevent leaking

7 Which statement about drainage systems is *true?*
- a A leg bag holds about 2000 mL.
- b A standard drainage bag holds less than a leg bag.
- c A closed drainage system means the drain cannot be opened.
- d Microbes in the drainage system can cause a UTI.

8 A drainage system becomes disconnected. You need
- a A new drainage bag and paper towels
- b A sterile cap and catheter plug
- c Gloves and antiseptic wipes
- d A waterproof under-pad and a catheter clamp

9 When emptying a standard drainage bag
- a Do not let the drain touch the graduate
- b Gloves are not needed
- c Clamp the catheter
- d Clean the end of the catheter with an antiseptic wipe

10 You are going to remove a urinary catheter. You
- a Attach a needle to the syringe
- b Ask the nurse how much water is in the balloon
- c Tug on the catheter to see if it will come out
- d Use an antiseptic swab to clean the meatus

11 You are going to remove an indwelling catheter. The balloon is filled with 10 mL. You withdraw 6 mL. What should you do?
- a Call for the nurse.
- b Inject the water.
- c Pull the catheter out gently.
- d Cut the catheter.

12 For a condom catheter, you apply elastic tape
- a Completely around the penis
- b To the thigh
- c To the abdomen
- d In a spiral

Answers to Chapter 28 questions are on p. 886.

FOCUS ON **PRACTICE**

Problem Solving

A patient with a urinary catheter tells you: "I feel like I have to pee, and I feel pressure down there." The patient points to the lower abdomen. There is no urine in the drainage bag. Is this normal? What do you do?

OBJECTIVES

- Define the key terms and key abbreviations in this chapter.
- Describe normal defecation and the observations to report.
- Identify the factors affecting bowel elimination.
- Explain how to promote comfort and safety during bowel movements.
- Describe the common bowel problems.
- Describe bowel training.

- Explain the purpose of enemas.
- Describe the common enema solutions.
- Describe the rules for giving enemas.
- Describe how to care for a person with an ostomy.
- Perform the procedures described in this chapter.
- Explain how to promote PRIDE in the person, the family, and yourself.

KEY TERMS

colostomy A surgically created opening *(stomy)* between the colon *(colo)* and the body's surface

constipation The passage of a hard, dry stool

defecation The process of excreting feces from the rectum through the anus; a bowel movement

dehydration The excessive loss of water from tissues

diarrhea The frequent passage of liquid stools

enema The introduction of fluid into the rectum and lower colon

fecal impaction The prolonged retention and buildup of feces in the rectum

fecal incontinence The inability to control the passage of feces and flatus through the anus

feces The semi-solid mass of waste products in the colon that is expelled through the anus; stool or stools

flatulence The excessive formation of gas or air in the stomach and intestines

flatus Gas or air passed through the anus

ileostomy A surgically created opening *(stomy)* between the ileum (small intestine *[ileo]*) and the body's surface

ostomy A surgically created opening that connects an internal organ to the body's surface; see "colostomy" and "ileostomy"

peristalsis The alternating contraction and relaxation of intestinal muscles

stoma A surgically created opening seen on the body's surface; see "colostomy" and "ileostomy"

stool Excreted feces

suppository A cone-shaped, solid drug that is inserted into a body opening; it melts at body temperature

KEY ABBREVIATIONS

BM	Bowel movement	ID	Identification
C. diff	*Clostridioides difficile; Clostridium difficile*	IV	Intravenous
CMS	Centers for Medicare & Medicaid Services	mL	Milliliter
GI	Gastro-intestinal	SSE	Soapsuds enema

Bowel elimination is a basic physical need. Wastes are excreted from the gastro-intestinal (GI) system (Chapter 10). Normal bowel elimination is important. Problems easily occur. You assist patients and residents to meet bowel needs.

See *Body Structure and Function Review: The Gastro-Intestinal Tract.*

See *Delegation Guidelines: Bowel Needs.*

See *Promoting Safety and Comfort: Bowel Needs.*

BODY STRUCTURE AND FUNCTION REVIEW

The Gastro-Intestinal Tract

Bowel elimination is the excretion of wastes through the gastro-intestinal (GI) tract (Chapter 10). The digestive system (GI system) is shown in Figure 29-1. Food and fluids are normally taken in through the *mouth.* They are partially digested in the *stomach.* The partially digested food and fluids are called *chyme.*

Chyme passes from the stomach into the *small intestine (small bowel).* Further digestion and absorption of nutrients occur as the chyme passes through the small bowel. The chyme enters the *large intestine* (*large bowel* or *colon*) where fluid is absorbed. Chyme becomes less fluid and more solid in consistency. *Feces (stool or stools) refers to the semi-solid mass of waste products in the colon that is expelled through the anus.*

Feces move through the intestines by peristalsis. *Peristalsis is the alternating contraction and relaxation of intestinal muscles.* The feces move through the large intestine to the *rectum.* Feces are stored in the rectum and excreted from the body. *Defecation (bowel movement) is the process of excreting feces from the rectum through the anus. Stool refers to excreted feces.*

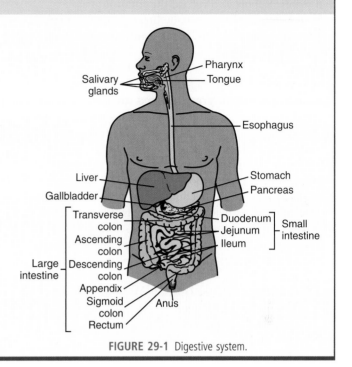

FIGURE 29-1 Digestive system.

DELEGATION GUIDELINES

Bowel Needs

The procedures in this chapter are not routine nursing tasks. They may be delegated nursing responsibilities in some states and agencies. Before performing a procedure, make sure that:

* Your state allows you to perform the procedure.
* The procedure is in your job description.
* You have the necessary education and training.
* You review the procedure with a nurse.
* A nurse is available to answer questions and to guide and assist you as needed.

PROMOTING SAFETY AND COMFORT

Bowel Needs

Safety

Assisting with bowel needs may involve exposing and touching the rectum, a private area. And you may have to give perineal care. Sexual abuse has occurred in health care settings. The person may feel threatened or is actually being abused. He or she needs to call for help. Always keep the call light within the person's reach. And always act in a professional manner.

Contact with stools is likely when assisting with bowel needs. Stools contain microbes and may contain blood. Follow Standard Precautions and the Bloodborne Pathogen Standard.

NOTE: A task may require more than 1 pair of gloves. Change gloves as needed. Use careful judgment. Remember to practice hand hygiene after removing gloves.

NORMAL BOWEL MOVEMENTS

Bowel movements (BMs) vary from person to person—daily, 2 to 3 times a day, every 2 to 3 days. Time of day also varies.

See *Focus on Children and Older Persons: Normal Bowel Movements.*

FOCUS ON **CHILDREN AND OLDER PERSONS**

Normal Bowel Movements

Children

Breast-fed infants have yellow stools that are thick liquid to very soft. Bottle-fed infants have yellowish-brown liquid stools or greenish-brown, pasty stools. Stool color and consistency change with solid foods.

Newborns usually have a BM with every feeding. Frequency changes as they grow older. Some infants have 2 or 3 BMs a day. Others have just 1.

Observations

Carefully observe stools. Ask the nurse to observe abnormal stools. Report and record the following.

- Color (Fig. 29-2)—normally brown. Beets, tomato juice or soup, red Jell-O, and foods with red food coloring can cause red-colored stools. Green vegetables can cause green stools. Diseases and infection can cause clay-colored or white, pale, orange-colored, or green-colored stools.
- Amount—small, medium, large. Liquid (watery) stools are measured in milliliters (mL). See "Intake and Output" in Chapter 31.
- Presence of mucus—usually none. Disease and infection can cause stools with mucus.
- Signs of bleeding—bleeding in the stomach and small intestine causes black or tarry stools. Bleeding in the lower colon and rectum causes red-colored stools.
- Odor—usually a normal odor caused by bacteria in the intestines. Certain foods and drugs can cause odors.
- Shape and consistency (Fig. 29-3)—normally soft, formed, moist, and shaped like the rectum.
- The time the person had a BM.
- Number and frequency of BMs.
- Complaints of pain or discomfort
  See *Focus on Communication: Observations.*

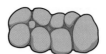
Formed with lumps

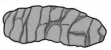
Formed with cracks

Smooth and soft

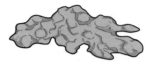
Small hard lumps

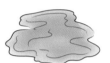
Small soft lumps

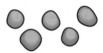
Loose and unformed

Watery

FIGURE 29-3 Stool shapes and consistencies.

FOCUS ON COMMUNICATION

Observations

Many patients and residents tend to their own bowel needs. However, information is needed for the person's record and the nursing process. To ask about BMs, you can say:

- "Did you have a BM today?"
- "Please tell me about your BM."
- "When did you have a BM?"
- "What was the amount?"
- "Were the stools soft or hard?"
- "Were the stools formed or loose?"
- "What was the color?"
- "Did you have any bleeding, pain, or problems having a BM?"
- "Did you pass any gas?"
- "Do you need to pass more gas?"
- "Do you need help cleaning yourself?"

For some people and children, *poop* is a common term for a BM. Follow the care plan for what word to use with the person.

Follow agency policy to report and record what the person said or what you observed. Use the agency's form to record BMs (Fig. 29-4). Or record in the person's chart. For example:

Resident reported a medium-sized, soft, formed, brown BM after breakfast today. Denied bleeding, pain, straining, or other problems. Resident performed perineal care.

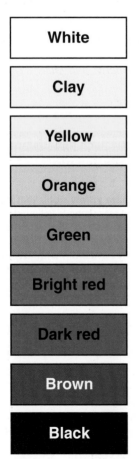

White

Clay

Yellow

Orange

Green

Bright red

Dark red

Brown

Black

FIGURE 29-2 Color chart for stools.

DATE: 01/21		TIME: 1015

BOWEL ELIMINATION: OBSERVATIONS

Shape & consistency	Color	Amount
☐ Watery	☐ White	☐ None
☐ Loose and unformed	☐ Clay	☐ Small
☐ Lumps	☐ Yellow	☒ Medium
☐ Small soft	☐ Orange	☐ Large
☐ Small hard	☐ Green	Volume:
☐ Smooth and soft	☐ Bright red	☐ mL
☒ Formed	☐ Dark red	**Pain**
☒ With cracks	☒ Brown	☒ No
☐ With lumps	☐ Black	☐ Yes
		Rating ☐ /10

Notes	Odor
Denied straining or other problems. Observed stools and reported observations to the nurse.	☒ Normal
	☐ Abnormal
	Flatus
	☒ Passing flatus
Nurse notified: C. Yung, RN	☐ No flatus

FIGURE 29-4 Bowel elimination record.

FACTORS AFFECTING BMs

These factors affect BM frequency, consistency, color, and odor. Normal, regular elimination is a goal of the nursing process.

- *Privacy.* Lack of privacy can prevent a BM despite the urge. Odors and sounds are embarrassing. Some people ignore the urge when people are present.
- *Habits.* After breakfast is a common time for BMs when eating stimulates peristalsis. Being relaxed, not tense, is helpful. To relax, some people drink a hot beverage, read, or take a walk.
- *Diet—high-fiber foods.* High-fiber foods leave a residue, creating bulk to prevent constipation (p. 440). Fruits, vegetables, and whole-grain cereals and breads are high in fiber. Intake of such foods may be poor. Digestion problems and chewing difficulties (loss of teeth, poorly fitting dentures) are causes. Bran may be added to cereal, prunes, or prune juice.
- *Diet—other foods.* Milk and milk products may cause constipation or diarrhea. Chocolate and other foods cause similar reactions. Spicy foods can irritate the intestines, causing frequent BMs or diarrhea. Gas-forming foods stimulate peristalsis, aiding BMs. Such foods include onions, beans, cabbage, cauliflower, radishes, and cucumbers.
- *Fluids.* Feces contain water. Stool consistency depends on how much water is absorbed by the colon. Feces harden and dry when large amounts of water are absorbed or from poor fluid intake or vomiting. Hard, dry feces move slowly through the colon, leading to constipation. Drinking 6 to 8 glasses of water daily promotes normal BMs. Warm fluids—coffee, tea, hot cider, warm water—increase peristalsis.
- *Activity.* Exercise and activity maintain muscle tone and stimulate peristalsis. Inactivity or bed rest may result from disease, surgery, injury, and aging. Constipation is a risk.

- *Drugs.* Drugs can cause or prevent constipation or diarrhea. Pain-relief drugs can slow peristalsis, causing constipation. Antibiotics (used to fight or prevent infections) often cause diarrhea. Diarrhea occurs when the antibiotics kill normal flora in the colon. Normal flora is needed to form feces. (See "Normal Flora" in Chapter 16.)
- *Disability.* Some people have a BM whenever feces enter the rectum. They have no control. A bowel training program is needed (p. 444).
- *Aging.* Age affects bowel elimination.

See *Focus on Children and Older Persons: Factors Affecting BMs.*

FOCUS ON CHILDREN AND OLDER PERSONS

Factors Affecting BMs

Children

Infants and toddlers cannot control BMs. They have a BM whenever feces enter the rectum. Bowel training is learned between 2 and 3 years of age.

Older Persons

Aging causes GI changes. Feces pass through the intestines more slowly. Constipation is a risk. Some older persons lose bowel control. Older persons are at risk for GI tumors and disorders.

Older persons may not completely empty the rectum. They often have a BM about 30 to 60 minutes after the first BM.

Many older persons are very concerned if they do not have a BM every day. The nurse instructs about normal elimination.

Safety and Comfort

The care plan has measures to meet bowel needs. It may involve diet, fluids, and exercise. The measures in Box 29-1 (p. 440) promote safety and comfort.

See *Focus on Communication: Safety and Comfort.*
See *Teamwork and Time Management: Safety and Comfort.*

FOCUS ON COMMUNICATION

Safety and Comfort

Odors and sounds are common with BMs. Control your verbal and nonverbal responses. Be professional. Do not laugh at or make fun of a person. Your words and actions must promote comfort, dignity, and self-esteem.

TEAMWORK AND TIME MANAGEMENT

Safety and Comfort

BM needs may be urgent. Answer call lights promptly. Also help co-workers answer call lights. Listen closely for bathroom call lights. The sound and light color are different from call lights in rooms. Respond at once. Do not leave patients and residents sitting on toilets, commodes, or bedpans. Do not leave them sitting or lying in stools.

BOX 29-1	Safety and Comfort—Bowel Needs

- Assist the person promptly. BM needs may be urgent.
- Follow Standard Precautions and the Bloodborne Pathogen Standard.
- Provide for privacy.
  - Ask visitors to leave the room.
  - Close doors, privacy curtains, and window coverings.
- Assist to the toilet or commode. Or provide the bedpan.
- Wheel the person into the bathroom on the commode if possible. This provides privacy. Remove the container and position the commode over the toilet. Then lock (brake) the commode wheels.
- Warm the bedpan (if used).
- Position the person in a sitting or squatting position.
- Cover the person for warmth and privacy.
- Allow enough time for a BM.
- Place the call light and toilet paper within reach.
- Leave the room if the person can be alone. Check on the person at least every 5 minutes.
- Stay nearby if the person is weak or unsteady.
- Provide perineal care.
- Dispose of stools promptly. This reduces odors and prevents the spread of microbes.
- Assist the person with hand hygiene after elimination.
- Follow the care plan for fecal incontinence.

COMMON PROBLEMS

Common problems include constipation, fecal impaction, diarrhea, fecal incontinence, and flatulence.

Constipation

Constipation is the passage of a hard, dry stool. Feces move slowly through the bowel. This allows more time for water absorption. The person strains to have a BM. Stools are large or marble-sized. Large stools cause pain as they pass through the anus. Common causes of constipation include:

- A low-fiber diet
- Ignoring the urge to have a BM
- Decreased fluid intake
- Inactivity
- Drugs
- Aging
- Certain diseases

Diet changes, fluids, and activity prevent or relieve constipation. The doctor may order 1 or more of the following.

- Stool softeners—drugs that soften feces. A BM is easier when feces are soft.
- Laxatives—drugs that promote bowel elimination. They increase the bulk of feces, soften feces, and lubricate the intestinal wall.
- Suppositories (p. 444).
- Enemas (p. 444).

Fecal Impaction

A *fecal impaction is the prolonged retention and buildup of feces in the rectum.* Feces are hard or putty-like. Fecal impaction results from un-relieved constipation. The person cannot have a BM. More water is absorbed from the already hard feces. Liquid feces pass around the hardened fecal mass in the rectum and seep from the anus.

Signs and symptoms of fecal impaction include:
- Trying many times to have a BM
- Abdominal discomfort
- Abdominal distention (swelling)
- Nausea
- Cramping
- Rectal pain
- Poor appetite (especially older persons)
- Confusion (especially older persons)
- Fever (especially older persons)

The nurse does a digital (finger) exam to check for an impaction. A lubricated, gloved finger is inserted into the rectum to feel for a hard mass in the lower rectum (Fig. 29-5). The feces may be out of reach higher in the colon. The digital exam often causes the urge to have a BM. Drugs, suppositories, or enemas may be ordered to remove the impaction.

Sometimes *digital removal of an impaction* is done. A lubricated, gloved finger is inserted into the rectum and hooked around a piece of feces. Then the finger and feces are removed. The stool is dropped into the bedpan. The process is repeated as needed.

See *Focus on Long-Term Care and Home Care: Fecal Impaction.*

See *Delegation Guidelines: Fecal Impaction.*

See *Promoting Safety and Comfort: Fecal Impaction.*

See procedure: *Checking For and Removing a Fecal Impaction.*

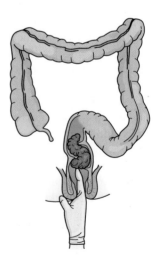

FIGURE 29-5 A gloved index finger is used to check for and remove a fecal impaction.

FOCUS ON LONG-TERM CARE AND HOME CARE

Fecal Impaction

Long-Term Care

The Centers for Medicare & Medicaid Services (CMS) monitors for problem areas in nursing centers. A serious problem, fecal impaction must be prevented. Tell the nurse if the resident is concerned about constipation. Follow center policy for recording BMs.

PROMOTING SAFETY AND COMFORT

Fecal Impaction

Safety

Checking for and removing impactions present dangers. The vagus nerve can be stimulated, which slows the heart rate. The heart rate can slow to unsafe levels in some persons. Rectal bleeding can also occur.

Comfort

The procedure is uncomfortable. It may embarrass the person.

DELEGATION GUIDELINES

Fecal Impaction

Checking for a fecal impaction is a nursing responsibility. If your state and agency allow the procedure to be delegated to you, make sure the conditions in *Delegation Guidelines: Bowel Needs* (p. 437) are met. If those conditions are met, you need this information from the nurse.

- What the doctor's order says
- If you should remove the impaction if you feel one
- When to take the person's pulse—before, during, and after the procedure (See *Promoting Safety and Comfort: Fecal Impaction*.)
- What pulse rates to report at once
- If the nurse needs to observe removed feces or possible BM
- What observations to report and record:
  - Pulse rates before, during, and after the procedure
  - Color, amount, consistency, and odor of removed feces
  - Signs of bleeding
  - Complaints of pain or discomfort
  - How the person tolerated the procedure
- When to report observations
- What patient or resident concerns to report at once

Checking For and Removing a Fecal Impaction

QUALITY OF LIFE

- Knock before entering the person's room.
- Address the person by name.
- Introduce yourself by name and title.

- Explain the procedure before starting and during the procedure.
- Protect the person's rights during the procedure.
- Handle the person gently during the procedure.

PRE-PROCEDURE

1 Follow *Delegation Guidelines:*
  a *Bowel Needs,* p. 437
  b *Fecal Impaction*
  See *Promoting Safety and Comfort:*
  a *Bowel Needs,* p. 437
  b *Fecal Impaction*
2 Practice hand hygiene.
3 Collect the following.
  - Bedpan and cover
  - Bath blanket
  - Toilet paper
  - Gloves

  - Lubricant
  - Waterproof under-pad
  - Basin of warm water
  - Soap or body wash
  - Washcloth
  - Bath towel
4 Practice hand hygiene.
5 Identify the person. Check the ID (identification) bracelet against the assignment sheet. Use 2 identifiers (Chapter 13). Also call the person by name.
6 Provide for privacy.
7 Raise the bed for body mechanics. Bed rails are up if used.

PROCEDURE

8 Lower the bed rail near you if up.
9 Cover the person with a bath blanket. Fan-fold top linens to the foot of the bed.
10 Position the person in Sims' position or in a left side-lying position (Chapter 18).
11 Check the person's pulse (Chapter 33). Note the rate and rhythm.
12 Practice hand hygiene. Put on the gloves.
13 Place the waterproof under-pad under the buttocks.

14 Expose the anal area.
15 Lubricate your gloved index finger.
16 Ask the person to take a deep breath through the mouth.
17 Insert the gloved finger during the deep breath.
18 Check for a fecal mass. Remove your finger and go to step 20 if:
  a You do not feel a fecal mass.
  b You feel a fecal mass but will not remove the impaction.

Continued

Checking For and Removing a Fecal Impaction—cont'd

PROCEDURE—cont'd

19 Remove the impaction.
   a Hook your index finger around a small piece of feces.
   b Remove your finger and the feces.
   c Drop the feces into the bedpan.
   d Clean your finger with toilet paper. Place the toilet paper in the bedpan.
   e Repeat steps 19, a-d until you no longer feel feces. Re-apply lubricant as needed.
   f *Check the person's pulse at intervals. Use your clean gloved hand. Note the rate and rhythm. Stop the procedure if the pulse rate has slowed or if the rhythm is irregular. Call for the nurse.*
20 Wipe the anal area with toilet paper.
21 Remove and discard the gloves. Practice hand hygiene. Put on clean gloves.
22 Check the person's pulse. Note the rate and rhythm.
23 Help the person onto the bedpan. Raise the head of the bed and raise the bed rail if used. Or assist the person to the bathroom or commode. The person wears a robe and slip-resistant footwear when up. The bed is in a low position safe and comfortable for the person.
24 Place the call light and toilet paper within reach. Remind the person not to flush the toilet.

25 Discard disposable items.
26 Remove and discard the gloves. Practice hand hygiene.
27 Leave the room if the person can be left alone.
28 Return when the person signals. Or check on the person every 5 minutes. Knock before entering.
29 Practice hand hygiene and put on gloves. Lower the bed rail if up.
30 Observe stools for amount, color, consistency, shape, and odor.
31 Provide perineal care as needed.
32 Remove the waterproof under-pad.
33 Empty, rinse, clean, and disinfect equipment. If the person had a BM, flush the toilet after the nurse observes it.
34 Return equipment to its proper place.
35 Remove and discard the gloves. Practice hand hygiene after removing and discarding the gloves.
36 Assist with hand hygiene. Wear gloves for this step. Practice hand hygiene after removing and discarding the gloves.
37 Cover the person. Remove the bath blanket.

POST-PROCEDURE

38 Provide for comfort. (See the inside of the back cover.)
39 Place the call light and other needed items within reach.
40 Lower the bed to a safe and comfortable level. Follow the care plan.
41 Raise or lower bed rails. Follow the care plan.
42 Unscreen the person.

43 Complete a safety check of the room. (See the inside of the back cover.)
44 Follow agency policy for used linens and used supplies.
45 Practice hand hygiene.
46 Report and record your observations.

Diarrhea

Diarrhea is the frequent passage of liquid stools. Feces move through the intestines rapidly. This reduces the time for fluid absorption. The need for a BM is urgent. Some people cannot get to a bathroom in time. Abdominal cramping, nausea, and vomiting may occur.

Causes of diarrhea include infections, some drugs, irritating foods, and microbes in food and water. Diet and drugs are ordered to reduce peristalsis. You need to:

- Assist with elimination needs promptly.
- Dispose of stools promptly. This prevents odors and the spread of microbes.
- Give good skin care. Liquid stools irritate the skin. So does frequent wiping with toilet paper. Skin breakdown and pressure injuries are risks.

Fluid lost through diarrhea must be replaced to prevent dehydration. *Dehydration is the excessive loss of water from tissues.* The person has pale or flushed skin, dry skin, and a coated tongue. Urine is dark and scant in amount *(oliguria).* Thirst, weakness, dizziness, and confusion also occur. Falling blood pressure and increased pulse and respirations are serious signs. Death can occur. The nursing process is used to meet fluid needs. The doctor may order IV (intravenous) fluids in severe cases (Chapter 32).

Microbes can cause diarrhea. Preventing their spread is important. Always follow Standard Precautions and the Bloodborne Pathogen Standard when in contact with stools.

See *Focus on Children and Older Persons: Diarrhea.*
See *Promoting Safety and Comfort: Diarrhea.*

FOCUS ON CHILDREN AND OLDER PERSONS

Diarrhea

Children
Infants and children have large amounts of body water. Dehydration is a risk. Death can be rapid. Report a liquid or watery stool at once. Ask the nurse to observe the stool. Note the number of wet diapers. Infants wet less when dehydrated.

Older Persons
Older persons are at risk for dehydration. The amount of body water decreases with aging. Many diseases affect body fluids. So do many drugs. Report signs of diarrhea at once. Ask the nurse to observe the stool. Death is a risk when dehydration is not recognized and treated.

PROMOTING SAFETY AND COMFORT

Diarrhea

Safety

The need for a BM is urgent when the person has diarrhea. Answer call lights promptly. Some people cannot get to a bathroom in time. Soiling results. Assist the person with hygiene needs and garment changes as needed. Do not judge the person. The person cannot control BMs.

Clostridioides difficile (Clostridium difficile [C. difficile]) is a microbe that causes diarrhea and intestinal infections. Commonly called *C. diff,* it can cause death. Persons at risk are older, are ill, or have prolonged use of antibiotics. Older persons in hospitals and nursing centers are at high risk. Signs and symptoms include:

- Watery diarrhea
- Fever
- Loss of appetite
- Nausea
- Abdominal pain or tenderness

The microbe is found in feces. A person becomes infected by touching items or surfaces contaminated with expelled feces and when touching his or her mouth or mucous membranes. *C. diff* can be found on bed linens, bed rails, toilets, bathroom fixtures, sinks, care supplies and equipment, walker handles, cart handles, bedside and over-bed tables, phones, TV remotes, personal electronics (computers, tablets, music players), and so on. You can spread the microbe if your contaminated hands or gloves:

- Touch a person
- Contaminate surfaces

Contact precautions are required (Chapter 17). Practice good hand-washing. Alcohol-based hand sanitizers are not as effective against *C. difficile* as soap and water. Care items and surfaces are disinfected with a bleach solution. Also follow Standard Precautions and the Bloodborne Pathogen Standard.

Fecal Incontinence

Fecal incontinence is the inability to control the passage of feces and flatus through the anus. Causes include:

- Intestinal diseases.
- Nervous system diseases and injuries.
- Fecal impaction or diarrhea.
- Some drugs.
- Chronic illness.
- Aging.
- Mental health disorders or dementia (Chapters 52 and 53). The person may not recognize needing to or having a BM.
- Unanswered call lights.
- Not getting to the bathroom in time. The person may have mobility problems or may walk slowly. The bathroom may be too far away or in use.
- Problems removing clothes.
- Not finding the bathroom in a new setting.

Fecal incontinence has emotional effects. Frustration, embarrassment, anger, and humiliation are common. The person may need:

- Bowel training
- Help with elimination after meals and every 2 to 3 hours
- Incontinence products to keep garments and linens clean
- Good skin care

See *Focus on Children and Older Persons: Fecal Incontinence.*

FOCUS ON **CHILDREN AND OLDER PERSONS**

Fecal Incontinence

Children

Infants and toddlers have fecal incontinence until toilet trained.

Older Persons

Persons with dementia may smear stools on themselves, furniture, and walls. Some are not aware of having BMs. Some resist care. Follow the care plan. The measures for urinary incontinence (Chapter 27) may be part of the care plan for fecal incontinence. Be patient. Ask for help from co-workers. Talk to the nurse if you have problems keeping the person clean.

Flatulence

Gas and air are normally in the stomach and intestines. They are expelled through the mouth (burping, belching, eructating) and anus. *Gas or air passed through the anus is called* **flatus**. *Flatulence is the excessive formation of gas or air in the stomach and intestines.* Causes include:

- Swallowing air while eating and drinking. This includes chewing gum, eating fast, drinking through a straw, and drinking carbonated beverages.
- Bacterial action in the intestines.
- Gas-forming foods—onions, beans, cabbage, cauliflower, radishes, and cucumbers.
- Constipation.
- Bowel and abdominal surgeries.
- Drugs that decrease peristalsis.

If flatus is not expelled, the intestines swell or enlarge *(distend)* from the pressure of gases. Abdominal cramping or pain, shortness of breath, and a swollen abdomen *(bloating)* occur. Exercise, walking, moving in bed, and the left side-lying position help to expel flatus. Enemas and drugs may be ordered to relieve flatulence.

BOWEL TRAINING

Bowel training has 2 goals.
- To gain control of BMs.
- To develop a regular pattern of elimination. Fecal impaction, constipation, and fecal incontinence are prevented.

Meals, especially breakfast, stimulate peristalsis and the urge for a BM. The person's usual time for a BM is noted on the care plan. So is toilet, commode, or bedpan use. The care plan includes a high-fiber diet, increased fluids, warm fluids, activity, and privacy. Follow the person's care plan for bowel training.

SUPPOSITORIES

A *suppository is a cone-shaped, solid drug that is inserted into a body opening. It melts at body temperature.* A rectal suppository is inserted into the rectum (Fig. 29-6).

A suppository may be ordered for constipation, fecal impaction, or bowel training. A BM occurs about 30 minutes later. If allowed by your state and agency, you may be asked to give rectal suppositories. Suppositories for other health problems must be given by the nurse.

See *Delegation Guidelines: Suppositories.*

See *Promoting Safety and Comfort: Bowel Needs,* p. 437.

DELEGATION GUIDELINES
Suppositories

Because they are drugs, inserting suppositories is a nursing responsibility. However, some states and agencies allow nursing assistants to insert certain suppositories. If inserting a rectal suppository is delegated to you, make sure that the conditions in *Delegation Guidelines: Bowel Needs* (p. 437) are met. If those conditions are met, you need this information from the nurse.
- How to position the person—Sims' or left side-lying position
- How to position the person after inserting the suppository and for how long—usually the Sims' or left side-lying position for 15 to 20 minutes
- What lubricant to use
- How soon to expect the urge for a BM
- What observations to report and record:
  - Bleeding or resistance when inserting the suppository
  - How long the person retained the suppository
  - Color, amount, consistency, shape, and odor of stools
  - Complaints of cramping, pain, or discomfort
  - Complaints of nausea or weakness
  - How the person tolerated the procedure
- How to record the procedure in the drug (medication) record
- When to report observations
- What patient or resident concerns to report at once

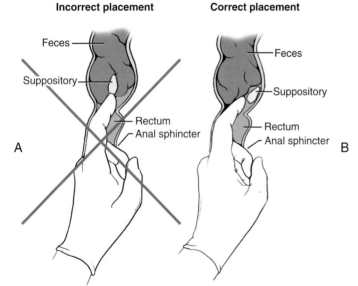

Incorrect placement — Feces, Suppository, Rectum, Anal sphincter

Correct placement — Feces, Suppository, Rectum, Anal sphincter

A   B

FIGURE 29-6 A, The rectal suppository is *not* inserted into feces. **B,** The suppository is inserted along the rectal wall. (Modified from Williams P: *deWit's fundamental concepts and skills for nursing,* ed 5, St Louis, 2018, Elsevier.)

ENEMAS

An *enema is the introduction of fluid into the rectum and lower colon.* Enemas are ordered to:
- Remove feces.
- Relieve constipation, fecal impaction, or flatulence.
- Clean the bowel of feces before certain surgeries and diagnostic procedures.

Safety and comfort measures for bowel needs are practiced when giving enemas (see Box 29-1). So are the rules in Box 29-2.

The enema ordered depends on the purpose—cleansing, constipation, fecal impaction, or flatulence. Consult with the nurse and use the agency's procedure manual to safely prepare and give enemas. You do not give enemas that contain drugs. Nurses give them.

See *Delegation Guidelines: Enemas.*

See *Promoting Safety and Comfort: Enemas.*

BOX 29-2 Giving Enemas

- Have the person void first. This increases comfort during the procedure.
- Give the enema ordered.
  - Cleansing enema (p. 446)—tap water enema, saline enema, or soapsuds enema (SSE)
  - Small-volume enema (p. 448)
  - Oil-retention enema (p. 450)
- Measure solution temperature with a water thermometer. See *Delegation Guidelines: Enemas*.
- Position the person as the nurse directs. The Sims' or left side-lying position is preferred.
- Ask the nurse and check the procedure manual for how far to insert the enema tubing. It is usually inserted 2 to 4 inches in adults.
- Lubricate the enema tip before inserting it.
- Stop tube insertion if you feel resistance, the person complains of pain, or bleeding occurs.

- Ask the nurse how high to raise the enema bag for a cleansing enema. For adults, it is usually held 12 inches above the anus.
- Give the amount of solution ordered. Give the solution slowly. Usually it takes 10 to 15 minutes to give 750 to 1000 mL.
- Hold the enema tube in place while giving the solution.
- Ask the nurse how long the person should try to retain the solution. The length of time depends on the amount and type of solution.
- Make sure the bathroom will be vacant when the person needs to have a BM. Make sure that another person will not use the bathroom. If the person uses the bedpan or commode, have the device ready.
- Ask the nurse to observe the enema results.

DELEGATION GUIDELINES

Enemas

Giving enemas is a nursing responsibility. If giving an enema to an adult is delegated to you, make sure the conditions in *Delegation Guidelines: Bowel Needs* (p. 437) are met. If those conditions are met, you need this information from the nurse.

- What enema to give—cleansing, small-volume, or oil-retention
- What lubricant to use
- When to give the enema
- What the solution temperature should be—usually 98.6°F to 100°F (Fahrenheit) (37.0°C to 37.8°C [centigrade]); sometimes warmer temperatures (105°F/40.5°C) are used for adults
- What position to use—Sims' or left side-lying position
- For a cleansing enema:
  - What size enema tube to use
  - The amount of solution ordered—usually 500 to 1000 mL for adults
  - What to add and how much—salt for a saline enema, castile soap for an SSE
  - How far to insert the enema tubing—usually 2 to 4 inches for adults
  - How high to hold the solution container—usually 12 inches above the anus
  - How fast to give the solution—750 to 1000 mL are usually given over 10 to 15 minutes
  - How many times to repeat the enema
- How long the person should try to retain the solution
- What observations to report and record:
  - The amount of solution given
  - Bleeding or resistance when inserting the tube
  - How long the person retained the enema solution
  - Color, amount, consistency, shape, and odor of stools
  - Complaints of cramping, pain, or discomfort
  - Complaints of nausea or weakness
  - How the person tolerated the procedure
- When to report observations
- What patient or resident concerns to report at once

PROMOTING SAFETY AND COMFORT

Enemas

Safety

Enemas are usually safe procedures. Many people give themselves enemas at home. However, enemas are dangerous for older persons and those with certain heart and kidney diseases.

Comfort

Before an enema procedure, have the bathroom ready for the person's use. Or have the commode or bedpan ready. Always keep a bedpan nearby in case the enema solution and stools are expelled. You promote mental comfort when the person knows the bathroom, commode, or bedpan is ready.

The person should retain the solution as long as possible. Provide for a comfortable Sims' or left side-lying position. When comfortable, it is easier to tolerate the procedure.

To prevent cramping:
- Use the correct water temperature. Cool water causes cramping.
- Give the solution slowly.

Cleansing Enemas

Cleansing enemas clean the bowel of feces and flatus. They relieve constipation and fecal impaction. They are given before certain surgeries and diagnostic procedures. Cleansing enemas take effect in 10 to 20 minutes.

A tap water, saline, or soapsuds enema is ordered. An *enemas until clear* order means that enemas are given until the return solution is clear and free of stools. Agency policy may allow repeating enemas 2 or 3 times. The nurse tells you what enema to give and how many times to repeat the enema.

- *Tap water enema*—obtained from a faucet. The colon may absorb some of the water into the bloodstream. This creates a fluid imbalance. *Only 1 tap water enema is given. Do not repeat the enema.* Repeated tap water enemas increase the risk of excessive fluid absorption.
- *Saline enema*—saline is a solution of salt and water. The solution is similar to body fluid. However, some of the salt solution may be absorbed, causing a fluid imbalance. The body retains water from the excess salt. For adults, 1 or 2 teaspoons of table salt are added to 500 to 1000 mL of tap water.
- *Soapsuds enema (SSE)*—for adults, 3 to 5 mL of castile soap is added to 500 to 1000 mL of tap water. Made of vegetable oil, castile soap is gentle and less irritating than stronger soaps. The SSE irritates the bowel's mucous lining. Repeated enemas can damage the bowel. So can using more than 3 to 5 mL of castile soap or stronger soaps.

See *Focus on Math: Cleansing Enemas.*
See *Focus on Children and Older Persons: Cleansing Enemas.*
See procedure: *Giving a Cleansing Enema to an Adult.*

FOCUS ON MATH

Cleansing Enemas

Cleansing enemas are given over 10 to 15 minutes. The nurse tells you the amount of solution to give and the amount of time to give it in. While giving the solution, monitor how fast the fluid flows. To calculate the amount to give per minute, divide the total amount (in milliliters [mL]) by the time (in minutes). Each minute as you give the enema, subtract this amount to check if the rate is too fast or too slow.

For example, you are to give a 750 mL saline enema over 15 minutes. Divide 750 mL by 15 minutes. The fluid in the bag should decrease by about 50 mL each minute.

$$750 \text{ mL} \div 15 \text{ minutes} = 50 \text{ mL/minute}$$

Note the start time. Check the amount at least each minute. After 1 minute, the solution should be at the 700 mL mark.

$$750 \text{ mL} - 50 \text{ mL} = 700 \text{ mL (after 1 minute)}$$

After 2 minutes, the solution should be about half-way between the 700 mL and 600 mL marks (650 mL).

$$700 \text{ mL} - 50 \text{ mL} = 650 \text{ mL (after 2 minutes)}$$

After 3 minutes, the solution should be at the 600 mL mark, and so on.

$$650 \text{ mL} - 50 \text{ mL} = 600 \text{ mL (after 3 minutes)}$$

If the solution is flowing too fast, clamp the tube and call for the nurse. The nurse may lower the bag to slow the flow. If the solution is flowing too slowly, call for the nurse. The nurse may adjust the tube or raise the bag to increase the flow.

FOCUS ON CHILDREN AND OLDER PERSONS

Cleansing Enemas

Children

Saline enemas are used for cleansing enemas in children. The nurse tells you the amount of solution to give. These are guidelines.

- Infants—120 to 240 mL
- Children 2 to 4 years—240 to 360 mL
- Children 4 to 10 years—360 to 480 mL
- Children 11 years and older—480 to 720 mL

How far to insert the tube depends on the child's age and needs. For example, no more than 1 inch for infants and no more than 4 inches for older children. The nurse tells you how far to insert the tube.

Infants cannot tell you they hurt. If cramping occurs, the child draws up the knees. The child's cry is higher-pitched than normal.

In children, cleansing enemas take effect in about 2 to 5 minutes.

Giving a Cleansing Enema to an Adult

QUALITY OF LIFE

- Knock before entering the person's room.
- Address the person by name.
- Introduce yourself by name and title.

- Explain the procedure before starting and during the procedure.
- Protect the person's rights during the procedure.
- Handle the person gently during the procedure.

PRE-PROCEDURE

1 Follow *Delegation Guidelines:*
  a *Bowel Needs*, p. 437
  b *Enemas*, p. 445
  See *Promoting Safety and Comfort:*
  a *Bowel Needs*, p. 437
  b *Enemas*, p. 445
2 Practice hand hygiene.
3 Collect the following before going to the person's room.
  - Disposable enema kit as directed by the nurse (enema bag, tube, clamp, and waterproof under-pad)
  - Water thermometer
  - Waterproof under-pad (if not in the enema kit)
  - Water-soluble lubricant
  - 3 to 5 mL (1 teaspoon) castile soap or 1 to 2 teaspoons of salt (if needed)
  - IV (intravenous) pole
  - Gloves

4 Arrange items in the person's room and bathroom.
5 Practice hand hygiene.
6 Identify the person. Check the ID bracelet against the assignment sheet. Use 2 identifiers (Chapter 13). Also call the person by name.
7 Put on gloves.
8 Collect the following.
  - Commode or bedpan and cover
  - Toilet paper
  - Bath blanket
  - Robe and slip-resistant footwear
  - Paper towels
9 Remove and discard the gloves. Practice hand hygiene. Put on clean gloves.
10 Provide for privacy.
11 Raise the bed for body mechanics. Bed rails are up if used.

PROCEDURE

12 Lower the bed rail near you if up.
13 Cover the person with a bath blanket. Fan-fold top linens to the foot of the bed.
14 Position the IV pole so the enema bag is 12 inches above the anus. Or it is at the height directed by the nurse.
15 Raise the bed rail if used.
16 Prepare the enema.
  a Close the clamp on the tube.
  b Adjust water flow until it is lukewarm.
  c Fill the enema bag for the amount ordered.
  d Measure water temperature with the water thermometer. The nurse tells you what water temperature to use.
  e Prepare the solution as directed by the nurse.
    1) *Tap water:* add nothing.
    2) *Saline enema:* add salt as directed.
    3) *SSE:* add castile soap as directed.
  f Stir the solution with the water thermometer. Scoop off any suds (SSE).
  g Seal the bag.
  h Hang the bag on the IV pole.

17 Lower the bed rail near you if up.
18 Position the person in Sims' position or in a left side-lying position.
19 Place a waterproof under-pad under the buttocks.
20 Expose the anal area.
21 Place the bedpan behind the person.
22 Position the enema tube in the bedpan. Remove the cap from the tubing.
23 Open the clamp. Let solution flow through the tube to remove air. Clamp the tube.
24 Lubricate the tube 2 to 4 inches from the tip.
25 Separate the buttocks to see the anus.
26 Ask the person to take a deep breath through the mouth.
27 Insert the tube gently 2 to 4 inches into the adult's rectum (Fig. 29-7). Do this when the person is exhaling. Stop if the person complains of pain, you feel resistance, or bleeding occurs.
28 Check the amount of solution in the bag.
29 Unclamp the tube. Give the solution slowly (Fig. 29-8).

Continued

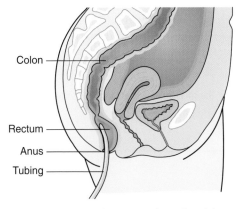

FIGURE 29-7 Enema tubing inserted into the adult rectum.

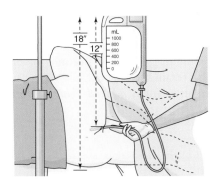

FIGURE 29-8 Giving an enema to an adult. The person is in Sims' position. The enema bag hangs from an IV pole. The bag is 12 inches above the anus and 18 inches above the mattress.

Giving a Cleansing Enema to an Adult—cont'd

PROCEDURE—cont'd

30 Ask the person to take slow, deep breaths. This helps the person relax.

31 Clamp the tube if the person needs to have a BM, has cramping, or starts to expel the solution. Also, clamp the tube if the person is sweating or complains of nausea or weakness. Unclamp when symptoms subside.

32 Give the amount of solution ordered. Stop if the person cannot tolerate the procedure.

33 Clamp the tube before it is empty. This prevents air from entering the bowel.

34 Hold toilet paper around the tube and against the anus. Remove the tube.

35 Discard toilet paper into the bedpan.

36 Wrap the tubing tip with paper towels. Place it inside the enema bag.

37 Encourage retention of the enema for the time ordered.

38 Assist the person to the bathroom or commode. The person wears a robe and slip-resistant footwear when up. The bed is at a low level that is safe and comfortable for the person. Or help the person onto the bedpan. Raise the head of the bed. Raise or lower bed rails according to the care plan.

39 Place the call light and toilet paper within reach. Remind the person not to flush the toilet.

40 Discard disposable items.

41 Remove and discard the gloves. Practice hand hygiene.

42 Leave the room if the person can be left alone.

43 Return when the person signals. Or check on the person every 5 minutes. Knock before entering the room or bathroom.

44 Practice hand hygiene and put on gloves. Lower the bed rail if up.

45 Observe enema results for amount, color, consistency, shape, and odor. Call the nurse to observe the results.

46 Provide perineal care as needed.

47 Remove the waterproof under-pad.

48 Empty, rinse, clean, disinfect, and dry equipment. Use clean, dry paper towels for drying. Flush the toilet after the nurse observes the results.

49 Return equipment to its proper place.

50 Remove and discard the gloves. Practice hand hygiene.

51 Assist with hand hygiene. Wear gloves for this step. Practice hand hygiene after removing and discarding the gloves.

52 Cover the person. Remove the bath blanket.

POST-PROCEDURE

53 Provide for comfort. (See the inside of the back cover.)

54 Place the call light and other needed items within reach.

55 Lower the bed to a safe and comfortable level. Follow the care plan.

56 Raise or lower bed rails. Follow the care plan.

57 Unscreen the person.

58 Complete a safety check of the room. (See the inside of the back cover.)

59 Follow agency policy for used linens and used supplies.

60 Practice hand hygiene.

61 Report and record your observations.

Small-Volume Enemas

Small-volume enemas irritate and distend the rectum to cause a BM. They are ordered for constipation or when the bowel does not need complete cleansing.

These enemas are ready to give. This solution is usually given at room temperature. To give the enema, the tip is inserted 2 inches into an adult's rectum (Fig. 29-9). Squeeze and roll up the plastic container from the bottom. Do not release pressure on the bottle. Otherwise, solution is drawn from the rectum back into the bottle.

Urge the person to retain the solution until he or she needs to have a BM. This usually takes 1 to 5 minutes or as long as 10 minutes. Staying in the Sims' or left side-lying position helps retain the enema.

See procedure: *Giving a Small-Volume Enema*.

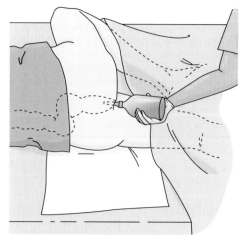

FIGURE 29-9 The small-volume enema tip is inserted 2 inches into the rectum.

Giving a Small-Volume Enema

QUALITY OF LIFE

- Knock before entering the person's room.
- Address the person by name.
- Introduce yourself by name and title.

- Explain the procedure before starting and during the procedure.
- Protect the person's rights during the procedure.
- Handle the person gently during the procedure.

PRE-PROCEDURE

1 Follow *Delegation Guidelines:*
  a *Bowel Needs*, p. 437
  b *Enemas*, p. 445
  See *Promoting Safety and Comfort:*
  a *Bowel Needs*, p. 437
  b *Enemas*, p. 445
2 Practice hand hygiene.
3 Collect the following before going to the person's room.
  - Small-volume enema
  - Waterproof under-pad
  - Gloves
4 Arrange items in the person's room.
5 Practice hand hygiene.

6 Identify the person. Check the ID bracelet against the assignment sheet. Use 2 identifiers (Chapter 13). Also call the person by name.
7 Put on gloves.
8 Collect the following.
  - Commode or bedpan and cover
  - Toilet paper
  - Robe and slip-resistant footwear
  - Bath blanket
9 Remove and discard the gloves. Practice hand hygiene. Put on clean gloves.
10 Provide for privacy.
11 Raise the bed for body mechanics. Bed rails are up if used.

PROCEDURE

12 Lower the bed rail near you if up.
13 Cover the person with a bath blanket. Fan-fold top linens to the foot of the bed.
14 Position the person in the Sims' or left side-lying position.
15 Place the waterproof under-pad under the buttocks.
16 Expose the anal area.
17 Position the bedpan by the person.
18 Remove the cap from the enema tip.
19 Separate the buttocks to see the anus.
20 Ask the person to take a deep breath through the mouth.
21 Insert the enema tip 2 inches into the adult's rectum (see Fig. 29-9). Do this as the person exhales. Insert the tip gently. Stop if the person complains of pain, you feel resistance, or bleeding occurs.
22 Squeeze and roll up the container gently. Release pressure on the bottle after you remove the tip from the rectum.
23 Put the container into the box, tip first. Discard the container and box.
24 Assist the person to the bathroom or commode when he or she has the urge to have a BM. The person wears a robe and slip-resistant footwear when up. The bed is at a low level that is safe and comfortable. Or help the person onto the bedpan and raise the head of the bed. Raise or lower bed rails according to the care plan.

25 Place the call light and toilet paper within reach. Remind the person not to flush the toilet.
26 Discard disposable items.
27 Remove and discard the gloves. Practice hand hygiene.
28 Leave the room if the person can be left alone.
29 Return when the person signals. Or check on the person every 5 minutes. Knock before entering the room or bathroom.
30 Practice hand hygiene. Put on gloves.
31 Lower the bed rail if up.
32 Observe enema results for amount, color, consistency, shape, and odor. Call the nurse to observe the results.
33 Provide perineal care as needed.
34 Remove the waterproof under-pad.
35 Empty, rinse, clean, disinfect, and dry equipment. Use clean, dry paper towels for drying. Flush the toilet after the nurse observes the results.
36 Return equipment to its proper place.
37 Remove and discard the gloves. Practice hand hygiene.
38 Assist with hand hygiene. Wear gloves for this step. Practice hand hygiene after removing and discarding the gloves.
39 Cover the person. Remove the bath blanket.

POST-PROCEDURE

40 Provide for comfort. (See the inside of the back cover.)
41 Place the call light and other needed items within reach.
42 Lower the bed to a safe and comfortable level. Follow the care plan.
43 Raise or lower bed rails. Follow the care plan.
44 Unscreen the person.

45 Complete a safety check of the room. (See the inside of the back cover.)
46 Follow agency policy for used linens and used supplies.
47 Practice hand hygiene.
48 Report and record your observations.

Oil-Retention Enemas

Oil-retention enemas relieve constipation and fecal impaction. The oil softens feces and lubricates the rectum so feces pass with ease. Depending on the type, the oil-retention enema may act quickly. For others, the oil is retained for 30 minutes to 1 to 3 hours. Most oil-retention enemas are ready-to-use. Follow the manufacturer's instructions.

See *Promoting Safety and Comfort: Oil-Retention Enemas.*
See procedure: *Giving an Oil-Retention Enema.*

PROMOTING SAFETY AND COMFORT

Oil-Retention Enemas

Safety

An oil-retention enema may be retained for at least 30 minutes. Leave the room after giving the enema. Check on the person often. Say when you will return. Remind the person to signal if help is needed. Report any problems at once.

Giving an Oil-Retention Enema

QUALITY OF LIFE

- Knock before entering the person's room.
- Address the person by name.
- Introduce yourself by name and title.
- Explain the procedure before starting and during the procedure.
- Protect the person's rights during the procedure.
- Handle the person gently during the procedure.

PRE-PROCEDURE

1 Follow *Delegation Guidelines:*
  a *Bowel Needs*, p. 437
  b *Enemas*, p. 445
  See *Promoting Safety and Comfort:*
  a *Bowel Needs*, p. 437
  b *Enemas*, p. 445
  c *Oil-Retention Enemas*
2 Practice hand hygiene.
3 Collect the following.
  - Oil-retention enema
  - Waterproof under-pads
  - Gloves
  - Bath blanket
4 Arrange items in the person's room.
5 Practice hand hygiene.
6 Identify the person. Check the ID bracelet against the assignment sheet. Use 2 identifiers (Chapter 13). Also call the person by name.
7 Provide for privacy.
8 Raise the bed for body mechanics. Bed rails are up if used.

PROCEDURE

9 Put on gloves.
10 Follow steps 12 through 23 in procedure: *Giving a Small-Volume Enema*, p. 449.
11 Cover the person. Leave him or her in the Sims' or left side-lying position.
12 Encourage retention of the enema until the urge to have a BM is felt.
13 Place more waterproof under-pads on the bed if needed.
14 Remove and discard the gloves. Practice hand hygiene.

POST-PROCEDURE

15 Provide for comfort. (See the inside of the back cover.)
16 Place the call light and other needed items within reach.
17 Lower the bed to a safe and comfortable level. Follow the care plan.
18 Raise or lower bed rails. Follow the care plan.
19 Unscreen the person.
20 Complete a safety check of the room. (See the inside of the back cover.)
21 Follow agency policy for used linens and used supplies.
22 Practice hand hygiene.
23 Report and record your observations.
24 Check the person often.

THE PERSON WITH AN OSTOMY

Sometimes part of the intestines is removed surgically. Cancer, bowel disease, and trauma (stab or bullet wounds) are common reasons. An ostomy is sometimes necessary. An *ostomy is a surgically created opening that connects an internal organ to the body's surface. The surgically created opening seen on the body's surface is called a* **stoma** (Fig. 29-10). An ostomy pouch is worn over the stoma to collect stools and flatus.

Colostomy

A *colostomy is a surgically created opening* (stomy) *between the colon* (colo) *and the body's surface.* Part of the colon is brought out onto the body's surface and a stoma is made. Feces and flatus pass through the stoma instead of the anus.

With a permanent colostomy, the diseased part of the colon is removed. A temporary colostomy gives the diseased or injured bowel time to heal. After healing, the bowel is surgically re-connected.

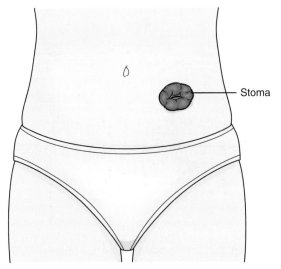

FIGURE 29-10 A stoma on the surface of the body.

The colostomy site depends on the site of disease or injury (Fig. 29-11). Stool consistency—liquid to formed—depends on the colostomy site. The more colon remaining to absorb water, the more solid and formed the stool. If the colostomy is near the end of the colon, stools are formed.

Stools irritate the skin. Skin care prevents skin breakdown around the stoma. The skin is washed and dried. A skin barrier applied around the stoma prevents stool contact with the skin. The skin barrier is part of the pouch or a separate device.

Ileostomy

An *ileostomy* *is a surgically created opening* (stomy) *between the ileum (small intestine* [ileo]) *and the body's surface.* Part of the ileum is brought out onto the body's surface and a stoma is made. The entire colon is removed (Fig. 29-12, p. 452).

Liquid stools drain constantly from an ileostomy. Water is not absorbed because the colon was removed. Feces in the small intestine contain digestive juices that are very irritating to the skin. The ostomy pouch must fit well. Stools must not touch the skin. Good skin care is required.

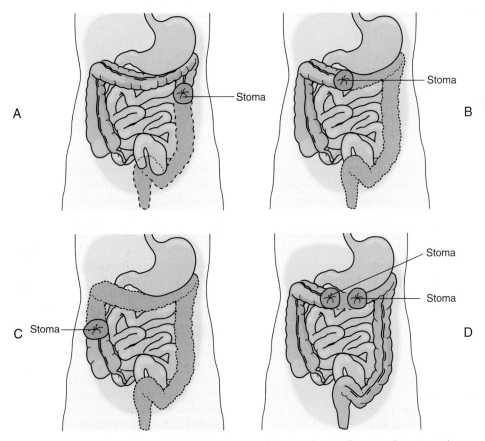

FIGURE 29-11 Colostomy sites. *Shading* shows the part of the bowel surgically removed. **A,** Sigmoid or descending colostomy. **B,** Transverse colostomy. **C,** Ascending colostomy. **D,** Double-barrel colostomy has 2 stomas. One allows for the excretion of feces. The other is for drugs to help the bowel heal. This type is usually temporary.

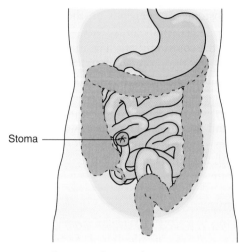

FIGURE 29-12 An ileostomy. The entire large intestine is removed. *Shading* shows the part of the bowel surgically removed.

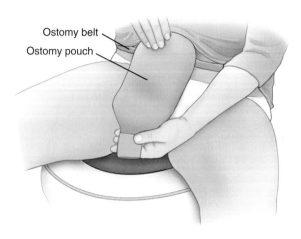

FIGURE 29-13 The ostomy pouch is secured to an ostomy belt. The pouch is emptied by directing it into the toilet and opening the outlet.

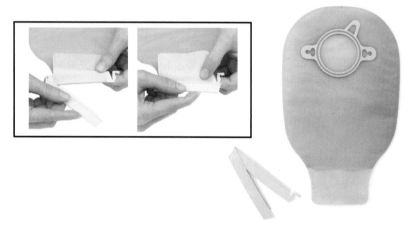

FIGURE 29-14 An ostomy pouch with a clamp. (Courtesy Hollister Incorporated, Libertyville, Ill.)

Ostomy Pouches

A plastic ostomy pouch with an adhesive back is applied to the skin. Some pouches are secured to ostomy belts (Fig. 29-13).

An outlet at the bottom of the pouch closes with a clip, clamp, or other closure (Fig. 29-14). The outlet is opened to empty the pouch of stools or to release flatus. The pouch bulges when stools are present. The pouch balloons or bulges when flatus is present.

The pouch is changed every 2 to 7 days and when it leaks. Frequent pouch changes can damage the skin.

Odors are prevented by:
- Using odor-free pouches.
- Performing good hygiene.
- Emptying the pouch.
- Avoiding gas-forming foods.
- Putting deodorants into the pouch.

The person wears normal clothes. Tight garments can prevent feces from entering the pouch. Also, bulging from stools and flatus can be seen with tight clothes.

Peristalsis decreases during sleep and increases after eating and drinking. After sleep, the stoma is less likely to expel feces. If the person showers or bathes with the pouch off, it is best done before breakfast. Showers and baths are delayed for 1 to 2 hours after a new pouch is applied. This gives adhesive time to seal to the skin.

See *Delegation Guidelines: Ostomy Pouches.*

DELEGATION GUIDELINES

Ostomy Pouches

Changing ostomy pouches is a nursing responsibility. If delegated to you, make sure the conditions in *Delegation Guidelines: Bowel Needs* (p. 437) are met. The nurse and care plan will provide needed information.

The nurse may ask you to remove an ostomy pouch before the person's shower or bath. The stoma may bleed slightly. You will not cause the person discomfort if you touch the stoma. The stoma does not have sensation.

Follow agency policy for pouch disposal. Pouches are not flushed down the toilet.

Emptying Ostomy Pouches. An ostomy pouch is emptied when it is about one-third ($\frac{1}{3}$) to one-half ($\frac{1}{2}$) full with stools or flatus. Depending on the person, ostomy type, and ostomy location, pouches are usually emptied 2 to 6 times a day. Because ileostomies constantly drain liquid feces, ileostomy pouches are emptied more often than colostomy pouches.

See *Focus on Children and Older Persons: Emptying Ostomy Pouches*.

See *Delegation Guidelines: Emptying Ostomy Pouches*.

See *Promoting Safety and Comfort: Emptying Ostomy Pouches*.

See procedure: *Assisting the Person to Empty an Ostomy Pouch*.

DELEGATION GUIDELINES
Emptying Ostomy Pouches

Assisting the person to empty an ostomy pouch may be a routine nursing task. If you are delegated the task, you need this information from the nurse and the care plan.
- If the person has a colostomy or ileostomy
- When to empty the pouch
- What special equipment and supplies to use
- What observations to report and record:
  - Color, amount, consistency, and odor of stools
  - Complaints of pain or discomfort
- When to report observations
- What patient or resident concerns to report at once

FOCUS ON **CHILDREN AND OLDER PERSONS**
Emptying Ostomy Pouches

Children
Children of all ages can have ostomies, even premature infants. If emptying a child's ostomy pouch is delegated to you, the nurse gives you needed information.

PROMOTING SAFETY AND COMFORT
Emptying Ostomy Pouches

Comfort
Empty ostomy pouches promptly when $\frac{1}{3}$ to $\frac{1}{2}$ full. Otherwise the pouch can leak stools or flatus. And an over-filled pouch can cause a bulge under clothing. Leaking and bulging can be embarrassing.

Never cut or puncture a pouch to release flatus. The pouch's odor barrier will no longer be intact. Also, stools can leak from the pouch.

Assisting the Person to Empty an Ostomy Pouch

QUALITY OF LIFE

- Knock before entering the person's room.
- Address the person by name.
- Introduce yourself by name and title.

- Explain the procedure before starting and during the procedure.
- Protect the person's rights during the procedure.
- Handle the person gently during the procedure.

PRE-PROCEDURE

1 Follow *Delegation Guidelines*:
  a *Bowel Needs*, p. 437
  b *Emptying Ostomy Pouches*
  See *Promoting Safety and Comfort*:
  a *Bowel Needs*, p. 437
  b *Emptying Ostomy Pouches*
2 Practice hand hygiene.
3 Put on gloves.
4 Arrange the following in the person's bathroom:
  • Toilet paper
  • Pre-moistened wipes
  • Plastic bag (for wipes)

5 Place a few sheets of toilet paper in the toilet bowl. This helps prevent splashing when the pouch is emptied.
6 Remove and discard the gloves. Practice hand hygiene.
7 Identify the person. Check the ID bracelet against the assignment sheet. Use 2 identifiers (Chapter 13). Also call the person by name.

Continued

Assisting the Person to Empty an Ostomy Pouch—cont'd

PROCEDURE

8 Put on gloves.
9 Assist the person to the bathroom. Close the bathroom door for privacy.
10 Help the person sit on the toilet and move garments out of the way. Make sure the person is comfortable.
11 Have the person spread his or her legs.
12 Position the pouch between the legs and over the toilet.
13 Hold the pouch outlet over the toilet. Open the clip or clamp and gently pinch the sides to open the outlet (see Fig. 29-13).
14 Allow the pouch to empty. If necessary, slide your thumb and index finger down the outside of the pouch to push out stools.
15 Clean the inside of the outlet with toilet paper or a pre-moistened wipe (Fig. 29-15). Make sure the inside is thoroughly clean. Discard toilet paper into the toilet. Discard the wipe into the plastic bag.

16 Clean the outside of the pouch outlet and the clip (clamp). Make sure the outside and the clip (clamp) are thoroughly clean. Use toilet paper or a pre-moistened wipe. Discard the toilet paper or wipe as in step 15.
17 Tie or seal the plastic bag (if used).
18 Close the pouch outlet with the clip (clamp). See Figure 29-14. Follow the manufacturer's instructions.
19 Observe the color, amount, consistency, and odor of stools. Flush the toilet.
20 Remove and discard the gloves. Practice hand hygiene.
21 Assist the person with hand hygiene. Wear gloves for this step.
22 Practice hand hygiene after removing and discarding gloves.
23 Help the person back to bed.

POST-PROCEDURE

24 Provide for comfort. (See the inside of the back cover.)
25 Place the call light and other needed items within reach.
26 Raise or lower the bed rails. Follow the care plan.
27 Complete a safety check of the room. (See the inside of the back cover.)

28 Follow agency policy for disposal of the plastic bag (if used). Wear gloves for this step.
29 Practice hand hygiene.
30 Report and record your observations.

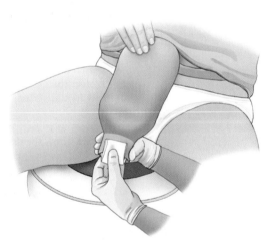

FIGURE 29-15 Cleaning the outlet of an ostomy pouch.

FOCUS ON **PRIDE**

The Person, Family, and Yourself

Personal and Professional Responsibility

You must know the legal limits of your role. Some states and agencies allow nursing assistants to insert some types of suppositories. For example, you may be allowed to insert suppositories in persons who use them for constipation. You cannot give a suppository for fever or vomiting. Know what you can and cannot do. Never perform a task beyond the legal limits of your role.

Rights and Respect

Bowel needs require privacy. Some persons are embarrassed to have a BM in a strange setting. To promote comfort and privacy:

- Ask others to leave the room.
- Close doors, privacy curtains, and window coverings.
- Turn on water or music to mask sounds.
- Cover the person.
- Allow enough time. Place the call light nearby and ask the person to call if help is needed.
- Knock before entering the room. Tell the person who you are. Ask if you can enter before opening the door completely.
- Use an agency-approved spray for odors.

Independence and Social Interaction

Some persons have had ostomies for a long time. They may have special routines or care measures. When you assist, ask what they prefer. To promote independence, allow personal choice and control as much as safely possible.

Delegation and Teamwork

The nurse may delegate a nursing responsibility to you. Giving an enema is an example. Never attempt a task that you are not comfortable doing. Make sure your state and agency allow you to perform the procedure. If those conditions are met, you can politely say: "I'm sorry, but I have not done that task before. I am not comfortable doing it on my own. Would you please show me how it is done?" Take pride in making the right choice to tell the nurse about your delegation concerns.

Ethics and Laws

All persons must be protected from abuse, mistreatment, and neglect. Examples include:

- Leaving a person sitting or lying in urine or stools
- Leaving a person on a toilet, commode, or bedpan for a long time
- Telling a person to void or have a BM in bed

Federal and state laws require the reporting and investigating of abuse, mistreatment, and neglect.

If found guilty, you will lose your job. The offense is noted on your registry. You cannot work in a nursing center or on a skilled care nursing unit in a hospital. Protect yourself from being accused. Check patients or residents often. Be careful and focused. Always treat the person with dignity.

FOCUS ON **PRIDE**: Application

You are asked to do an unfamiliar task. Do you seek help? Do you try to do it alone? Does asking for help bother you?

Guidance and assistance are part of the nurse's role in delegation. The nurse needs to know your comfort level with tasks. Never be ashamed to ask for guidance and assistance.

REVIEW QUESTIONS

Circle the BEST answer

1 Which is *true*?
   a A person must have a BM every day.
   b Stools are normally brown, soft, and formed.
   c Diarrhea occurs when feces move slowly through the bowel.
   d Constipation occurs when feces move quickly through the bowel.

2 Which should you ask the nurse to observe?
   a A black and tarry stool
   b The person's first BM of the day
   c Stool with an odor
   d Liquid stool from an ileostomy

3 The prolonged retention and buildup of feces in the rectum is called
   a Constipation
   b Fecal impaction
   c Diarrhea
   d Fecal incontinence

4 These measures promote normal BMs. Which is outside your role limits?
   a Provide oral fluids according to the care plan.
   b Assist with activity according to the care plan.
   c Give drugs to control diarrhea.
   d Provide privacy for bowel elimination.

5 A person has *C. difficile*. You should
   a Disinfect care items with soap and water
   b Use an alcohol-based hand sanitizer for hand hygiene
   c Wear a gown and gloves
   d Refuse to care for the person

6 Bowel training is aimed at
   a Bowel control and regular elimination
   b Ostomy control
   c Promoting toilet use
   d Preventing bleeding

Continued

REVIEW QUESTIONS—cont'd

7 Your state and agency allow you to insert rectal suppositories. You insert a suppository
  a Into the feces
  b Into the stoma
  c Along the rectal wall
  d With an enema tube

8 Which is used for a cleansing enema?
  a Mineral, olive, or cottonseed oil
  b A suppository
  c A 120-mL bottle of solution
  d Tap water, saline, or a soapsuds enema

9 Which is used for cleansing enemas in children?
  a Soapsuds
  b Saline
  c Oil
  d Tap water

10 When giving an enema
  a Use a cool solution
  b Give the solution slowly
  c Have the person void after giving the enema
  d Place the person in the supine position

11 In adults, the enema tube is inserted
  a 2 to 4 inches
  b 6 to 8 inches
  c 12 inches
  d Until you feel resistance

12 A small-volume enema is retained
  a For 2 minutes
  b At least 10 to 20 minutes
  c At least 30 minutes
  d Until the urge to have a BM is felt

13 Which statement about ostomies is *true*?
  a An ostomy has sensation.
  b A pouch is punctured to release flatus and odors.
  c The inside and the outside of the pouch outlet are cleaned when the pouch is emptied.
  d Changing ostomy pouches is a routine nursing task.

14 An ostomy pouch is usually emptied
  a Every 2 hours
  b When it is full
  c Every 2 to 7 days
  d When it is $\frac{1}{3}$ to $\frac{1}{2}$ full

Answers to Chapter 29 questions are on p. 886.

FOCUS ON PRACTICE

Problem Solving

You respond to a resident's call light. The resident needs to have a BM urgently. The bathroom is occupied by the roommate. What do you do?

Nutrition Needs

OBJECTIVES

- Define the key terms and key abbreviations in this chapter.
- Explain the purpose and use of the MyPlate symbol.
- Describe the functions and sources of nutrients.
- Explain how to read and use food labels.
- Describe the factors that affect eating and nutrition.
- Describe the special diets and between-meal snacks.
- Identify the signs, symptoms, and precautions for aspiration and regurgitation.

- Explain how to assist with measuring food intake.
- Explain how to assist with nutrition needs.
- Describe CMS requirements for serving food.
- Explain how to prevent foodborne illnesses.
- Perform the procedures described in this chapter.
- Explain how to promote PRIDE in the person, the family, and yourself.

KEY TERMS

anorexia The loss of appetite
aspiration Breathing fluid, food, vomitus, or an object into the lungs
calorie The fuel or energy value of food
cholesterol A soft, waxy substance found in the bloodstream and all body cells

dysphagia Difficulty *(dys)* swallowing *(phagia)*
nutrient A substance that is ingested, digested, absorbed, and used by the body
nutrition The processes involved in the ingestion, digestion, absorption, and use of food and fluids by the body

KEY ABBREVIATIONS

CMS	Centers for Medicare & Medicaid Services
F	Fahrenheit
FDA	Food and Drug Administration
GI	Gastro-intestinal
ID	Identification

mg	Milligram
NPO	*Nil per os;* nothing by mouth
oz	Ounce
USDA	United States Department of Agriculture

Food is a basic need. The person's diet affects physical and mental well-being and function. A poor diet and poor eating habits:

- Increase the risk for disease and infection.
- Cause chronic illnesses to become worse.
- Cause healing problems.
- Increase the risk for accidents and injuries.

Many factors affect dietary practices. They include culture, finances, and personal choice. (See *Caring About Culture: Meal Time Practices*, p. 458.) Dietary practices also include selecting, preparing, and serving food. The health team includes these factors in planning the person's nutrition needs.

NOTE: *Federal agencies often issue and revise nutrition-related guidelines. Dietary Guidelines for Americans (p. 459), MyPlate (p. 459), and food labels (p. 463) are examples. The Internet provides access to the most current information.*

See *Body Structure and Function Review: The Digestive System*, p. 458.

See *Focus on Long-Term Care and Home Care: Nutrition Needs*, p. 458.

See *Focus on Surveys: Nutrition Needs*, p. 459.

CARING ABOUT CULTURE

Meal Time Practices

Many cultural groups have their main meal at mid-day. They eat light meals in the evening. A main meal at lunch is common in *Austria, Brazil, Finland, Germany,* and *Greece.* In *Iran*, the most important meal is eaten at mid-day.

(NOTE: *Each person is unique. A person may not follow all of the beliefs and practices of his or her culture. Follow the care plan.*)

Modified from D'Avanzo CE: *Pocket guide to cultural health assessment,* ed 4, St Louis, 2008, Mosby.

FOCUS ON LONG-TERM CARE AND HOME CARE

Nutrition Needs

Long-Term Care

The Centers for Medicare & Medicaid Services (CMS) requires that the health team assess the resident's nutrition status. This includes:

* Drugs that affect taste or cause dry mouth, nausea, confusion, and so on
* Weight and height (Chapter 36)
* Appearance
* Food intake (p. 468)
* Fluid balance (Chapter 31)
* Factors affecting eating and nutrition (p. 464)

BODY STRUCTURE AND FUNCTION REVIEW

The Digestive System

The digestive system *(gastro-intestinal [GI] system)* breaks down food to be absorbed for use by the cells. This process is called *digestion.* The system also removes solid wastes from the body.

The digestive system involves the *GI tract* and the accessory organs of digestion (Fig. 30-1). The GI tract extends from the mouth to the anus.

Digestion begins in the *mouth (oral cavity).* The *teeth* cut, chop, and grind food into small pieces for swallowing. The *tongue* aids in chewing and swallowing. *Taste buds* on the tongue sense sweet, sour, bitter, and salty tastes. *Salivary glands* in the mouth secrete saliva. Saliva moistens food to ease swallowing and begin digestion. During swallowing, the tongue pushes food into the pharynx.

The *pharynx (throat)* is a muscular tube. Contraction of the pharynx pushes food into the esophagus. The *esophagus* is a muscular tube about 10 inches long. It extends from the pharynx to the stomach. Involuntary muscle contractions called *peristalsis* move food down the esophagus through the GI tract.

The *stomach* is a muscular, pouch-like sac. Strong stomach muscles stir and churn food to break it up into very small particles. The stomach secretes *gastric juices.* Gastric juices mix with food to form a semi-liquid substance called *chyme.* Through peristalsis, the chyme is pushed from the stomach into the small intestine.

The *small intestine* is about 20 feet long with 3 parts. The first part is the *duodenum.* There, more digestive juices are added to the chyme. One is called *bile.* Bile is a greenish liquid made in the *liver.* Bile is stored in the *gallbladder.* Juices from the *pancreas* and small intestine are added to the chyme. Digestive juices chemically break down food into nutrients for absorption.

Peristalsis moves the chyme through the other parts of the small intestine: *jejunum* and *ileum.* Tiny projections called *villi* line the small intestine. Villi absorb nutrients into the capillaries. Most nutrient absorption takes place in the jejunum and the ileum.

Some chyme is not digested. Undigested chyme passes from the small intestine into the *large intestine* (*large bowel* or *colon*). More fluid is absorbed. The solid waste that remains is eliminated through the *anus.* See Chapters 10 and 29.

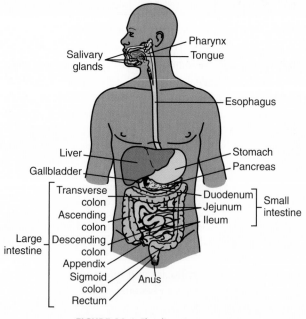

FIGURE 30-1 The digestive system.

BASIC NUTRITION

Nutrition is the processes involved in the ingestion, digestion, absorption, and use of food and fluids by the body. Foods and fluids contain nutrients. A *nutrient is a substance that is ingested, digested, absorbed, and used by the body.* Nutrients are grouped into fats, proteins, carbohydrates, vitamins, minerals, and water (p. 462).

Fats, proteins, and carbohydrates provide fuel for energy. A *calorie is the fuel or energy value of food.*

- 1 gram of fat—9 calories
- 1 gram of protein—4 calories
- 1 gram of carbohydrate—4 calories

A well-balanced diet and correct calorie intake are needed for growth, healing, and body function. A high-fat, high-calorie diet causes weight gain and obesity. A low-calorie diet promotes weight loss.

Dietary Guidelines

Dietary Guidelines for Americans are issued every 5 years by the federal government. The guidelines help people attain and maintain a healthy weight, prevent chronic diseases, and promote health. They focus on fewer calories, good food choices, and physical activity. For the most current guidelines, search the Internet for *Dietary Guidelines for Americans.*

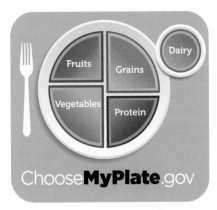

FIGURE 30-2 The MyPlate symbol. (Courtesy U.S. Department of Agriculture, Center for Nutrition and Policy Promotion.)

MyPlate

The MyPlate symbol (Fig. 30-2) encourages healthy eating from 5 food groups. Issued by the United States Department of Agriculture (USDA), MyPlate promotes wise food choices by:

- Balancing calories
  - Eating less
  - Avoiding over-sized portions
- Increasing certain foods
  - Making half of your plate fruits and vegetables
  - Making at least half of your grains whole grains
  - Drinking fat-free or low-fat (1%) milk
- Reducing certain foods
  - Choosing low-sodium foods
  - Drinking water instead of sugary drinks

See *Focus on Children and Older Persons: MyPlate.*

Physical Activity. The USDA recommends that adults do at least 1 of the following weekly.

- 2 hours and 30 minutes of moderate physical activity
- 1 hour and 15 minutes of vigorous physical activity

See Box 30-1 (p. 460) for examples of moderate and vigorous activities. Physical activity at least 3 days a week is best. Each activity should last at least 10 minutes. Adults also should do strengthening activities at least 2 days a week. Push-ups, sit-ups, and weight-lifting are examples.

See *Focus on Children and Older Persons: Physical Activity,* p. 460.

BOX 30-1	Physical Activities

Moderate Physical Activities
- Walking briskly (about 3½ miles per hour)
- Bicycling (less than 10 miles per hour)
- Gardening (raking, trimming bushes)
- Dancing
- Golf (walking and carrying clubs)
- Water aerobics
- Canoeing
- Tennis (doubles)

Vigorous Physical Activities
- Running and jogging (5 miles per hour)
- Walking very fast (4½ miles per hour)
- Bicycling (more than 10 miles per hour)
- Heavy yard work (chopping wood)
- Swimming (freestyle laps)
- Aerobics
- Basketball (competitive)
- Tennis (singles)

Modified from U.S. Department of Agriculture: Physical activity.

FOCUS ON CHILDREN AND OLDER PERSONS

Physical Activity

Children

For physical activity, the USDA recommends the following for children 6 to 17 years of age.
- 60 minutes or more each day of moderate to vigorous physical activity.
- Vigorous activity at least 3 days a week.
- Muscle and bone strengthening activities at least 3 days a week. Climbing and jumping are examples.

Older Persons

The USDA recommends that older persons follow the physical activity guidelines for adults. They should be as active as possible. Exercises that maintain or improve balance are helpful for persons at risk for falls.

Food Groups

The 5 food groups are:
- Grains group
- Vegetable group
- Fruit group
- Dairy group
- Protein foods group

The amount needed from each food group depends on age, biological sex, and physical activity. See Table 30-1 for sources, daily servings, serving sizes, and health benefits.

TABLE 30-1	Food Groups	
Food Sources	**Daily Servings and Serving Sizes**	**Health Benefits**
Grains		
• Grains are foods made from wheat, rice, oats, cornmeal, barley, or other cereal grains. Bread, pasta, oatmeal, breakfast cereals, tortillas, and grits are examples. • *Whole grains* have the entire grain kernel. Whole-wheat flour, bulgur (cracked wheat), oatmeal, whole cornmeal, and brown rice are examples. • *Refined grains* are processed to remove the grain kernel. White flour, white bread, and white rice are examples. They have less dietary fiber than whole grains.	**Daily Servings** • Women: 5 to 6 ounces (oz); at least 3 oz from whole grains • Men: 6 to 8 oz; at least 3 to 4 oz from whole grains **Serving Sizes** • 1 oz = 1 slice of bread • 1 oz = 1 cup breakfast cereal • 1 oz = ½ cup cooked rice, cereal, or pasta	• May reduce the risk of heart disease, obesity, and type 2 diabetes. • May prevent constipation. • May help with weight management. • May prevent certain birth defects. • Contain dietary fiber, several B vitamins (thiamin, riboflavin, niacin, folate [folic acid]), and minerals (iron, magnesium, and selenium).
Vegetables		
• Vegetables can be raw, cooked, fresh, frozen, canned, dried, or juiced. • *Dark green vegetables*—broccoli, collard greens, dark green leafy lettuce, kale, mustard greens, romaine lettuce, spinach, turnip greens, watercress. • *Red and orange vegetables*—acorn, butternut, and hubbard squashes; carrots; pumpkin; red peppers; sweet potatoes; tomatoes; tomato juice. • *Beans and peas*—black beans, black-eyed peas, garbanzo beans (chickpeas), kidney beans, pinto beans, soybeans, split peas. • *Starchy vegetables*—corn, green peas, potatoes. • *Other vegetables*—bean sprouts, cabbage, cauliflower, celery, cucumbers, green beans, green peppers, iceberg (head) lettuce, mushrooms, onions, summer squash, zucchini.	**Daily Servings** • Women: 2 to 2½ cups • Men: 2½ to 3 cups **Serving Sizes** • 1 cup = 1 cup raw or cooked vegetables or vegetable juice • 1 cup = 2 cups raw leafy greens	• May reduce the risk of stroke, high blood pressure, and heart disease. • May protect against certain cancers. • May help lower calorie intake. Most vegetables are low in fat and calories. • Contain no cholesterol (p. 462). • May prevent certain birth defects. • Contain potassium, dietary fiber, folate (folic acid), and vitamins A and C.

TABLE 30-1	Food Groups—cont'd	
Food Sources	**Daily Servings and Serving Sizes**	**Health Benefits**

Fruits

- Any fruit or 100% fruit juice counts as part of the fruit group.
- Fruits may be fresh, frozen, canned, or dried.
- Avoid fruits canned in syrup. Syrup contains added sugar. Choose fruits canned in 100% fruit juice or water.

Daily Servings
- Women: 1½ to 2 cups
- Men: 2 cups

Serving Sizes
- 1 cup = 1 cup fruit
- 1 cup = 1 cup fruit juice
- 1 cup = ½ cup dried fruit

- May reduce the risk of stroke, heart disease, and heart attack.
- May protect against certain cancers.
- May help prevent constipation.
- May prevent certain birth defects.
- May help lower fat and calorie intake. Most fruits are low in fat and calories.
- Contain no cholesterol.
- Are low in sodium (salt).
- Contain potassium, dietary fiber, vitamin C, and folate (folic acid).

Dairy

- All fluid milk products are part of the dairy group. So are many foods made from milk. Yogurt and cheese are examples.
- Low-fat or fat-free choices are best.
- Cream, cream cheese, and butter are not in this group.

Daily Servings
- Women: 3 cups
- Men: 3 cups

Serving Sizes
- 1 cup = 1 cup milk, yogurt, or soymilk
- 1 cup = 1½ oz natural cheese
- 1 cup = 2 oz processed cheese

- Help build bones and teeth and maintain bone mass. This may reduce the risk of osteoporosis.
- May reduce the risk of high blood pressure.
- Contains calcium, potassium, vitamin D, and protein.

Protein Foods

- All foods made from meat, poultry, seafood, eggs, processed soy products, nuts, and seeds are protein foods.
- Beans and peas are in this group and the vegetable group.
- For healthy choices, remember:
  - Choose lean or low-fat meat and poultry. Regular ground beef (75% to 80% lean) and chicken with skin are higher in fat.
  - Avoid fat for cooking. Fried chicken and eggs fried in butter are examples.
  - Seafood like salmon, trout, and herring may reduce heart disease risk.
  - Liver and other organ meats are high in cholesterol.
  - Egg yolks are high in cholesterol. Egg whites are cholesterol-free.
  - Processed meats (ham, sausage, hot dogs, luncheon and deli meats) have added sodium (salt).
  - Choose unsalted nuts and seeds to lower sodium intake.

Daily Servings
- Women: 5 to 5½ oz
- Men: 5½ to 6½ oz

Serving Sizes
- 1 oz = 1 oz lean meat, poultry, or fish
- 1 oz = 1 egg
- 1 oz = 1 tablespoon peanut butter
- 1 oz = ¼ cup cooked beans
- 1 oz = ½ oz nuts or seeds

- Contain protein, B vitamins (niacin, thiamin, riboflavin, and B6), vitamin E, iron, zinc, and magnesium.
- Many proteins are high in fat and cholesterol. Heart disease is a risk. However, this group provides nutrients needed for health and body maintenance.
- Seeds and certain nuts (peanuts, walnuts, almonds, pistachios) may reduce the risk of heart disease. High in calories, nuts should be eaten in small portions and in place of other protein foods.

Modified from U.S. Department of Agriculture: ChooseMyPlate.

Nutrients

No food or food group has every essential nutrient. A well-balanced diet ensures an adequate intake of essential nutrients.

- *Protein*—the most important nutrient, protein is needed for tissue growth and repair. Sources include meat, fish, poultry, eggs, milk and milk products, cereals, beans, peas, and nuts.
- *Carbohydrates*—provide energy and fiber for bowel elimination. Sources are fruits, vegetables, breads, cereals, and sugar.
  - *Dietary fiber (fiber)*—found in plant foods, fiber is not digested. It provides the bulky part of chyme for elimination.
  - *Sugars*—are broken down by the body into glucose. Glucose is used for energy.
- *Fats*—provide energy. They add flavor and help the body use certain vitamins. Unneeded dietary fat is stored as body fat *(adipose tissue)*. See "Fats and Oils."
- *Vitamins*—are needed for certain body functions. The body stores vitamins A, D, E, and K. Vitamins C and the B complex vitamins are not stored. They must be ingested daily. The lack of a certain vitamin results in illness. See Table 30-2.

- *Minerals*—are needed for bone and tooth formation, nerve and muscle function, fluid balance, and other body processes. Foods containing calcium help prevent musculo-skeletal changes. See Table 30-3.
- *Water*—is needed for all body processes (Chapter 31).

Fats and Oils

Some fats are healthy. Others are not. For example, fats from salmon, avocados, and olive oil are healthy fats. Unhealthy fats usually come from animal sources (meat and dairy foods) or are processed foods made from vegetable oils.

Solid fats are solid at room temperature. Butter, beef fat (tallow, suet), chicken fat, pork fat (lard), stick margarine, and shortening are examples. Desserts and baked goods, many cheeses, ice cream, and whole milk also contain fat.

Fats affect cholesterol levels. *Cholesterol is a soft, waxy substance found in the bloodstream and all body cells.* When certain cholesterol levels are high, the risk for heart disease increases. Eating less unhealthy fats can improve cholesterol and lower the risk for heart disease.

Oils are liquid fats. Oils come from plants and fish. Because they have nutrients (essential fats and vitamin E), the USDA includes oils in food patterns. However, *oils are not a food group.*

TABLE 30-2	Common Vitamins	
Vitamin	Major Functions	Sources
Vitamin A	Growth and development, immune function, reproduction, red blood cell formation, skin and bone formation, vision	Cantaloupe, carrots, dairy products, eggs, fortified cereals, green leafy vegetables, pumpkin, red peppers, sweet potatoes
Vitamin B1 (thiamin)	Changing food into energy, nervous system function	Beans and peas, enriched grain products (bread, cereal, pasta, rice), nuts, pork, sunflower seeds, whole grains
Vitamin B2 (riboflavin)	Changing food into energy, growth and development, red blood cell formation	Eggs, enriched grain products, meats, milk, mushrooms, poultry, seafood, spinach
Vitamin B3 (niacin)	Cholesterol production, changing food into energy, digestion, nervous system function	Beans, beef, enriched grain products, nuts, pork, poultry, seafood, whole grains
Vitamin B12	Changing food into energy, nervous system function, red blood cell formation	Dairy products, eggs, fortified cereals, meats, poultry, seafood
Folate (folic acid)	Prevention of birth defects, protein metabolism, red blood cell formation	Asparagus, avocado, beans and peas, enriched grain products, green leafy vegetables, orange juice
Vitamin C (ascorbic acid)	*Antioxidant* (substance that prevents cell damage), formation of substances that hold tissues together, immune function, wound healing	Broccoli, Brussels sprouts, cantaloupe, citrus fruits and juices, kiwi, peppers, strawberries, tomatoes and tomato juice
Vitamin D	Blood pressure control, bone growth, calcium balance, hormone production, immune and nervous system function	Eggs; fish; fish liver oil; fortified cereals, dairy products, margarine, orange juice, and soy drinks
Vitamin E	Antioxidant, formation of blood vessels, immune function	Fortified cereals and juices, green vegetables, nuts and seeds, peanuts and peanut butter, vegetable oils
Vitamin K	Blood clotting, strong bones	Green vegetables

Modified from U.S. Food and Drug Administration, Vitamins and Minerals Chart.

TABLE 30-3	Common Minerals	
Mineral	**Major Functions**	**Sources**
Calcium	Blood clotting, bone and teeth formation, blood vessel function, hormone secretion, muscle contraction, nervous system function	Almond, rice, coconut, and hemp milks; canned seafood with bones; dairy products; fortified cereals, juices, and soy drinks; green vegetables; tofu
Phosphorus	Acid-base balance, bone formation, energy production and storage, hormone function	Beans and peas; dairy products; meats; nuts and seeds; poultry; seafood; whole-grain, enriched, and fortified cereals and breads
Iron	Energy production, growth and development, immune function, red blood cell formation, reproduction, wound healing	Beans and peas; dark green vegetables; meats; poultry; prunes and prune juice; raisins; seafood; whole-grain, enriched, and fortified cereals and breads
Iodine	Growth and development, metabolism, reproduction, thyroid hormone function	Breads and cereals, dairy products, iodized salt, potatoes, seafood, seaweed, turkey
Sodium	Acid-base balance, blood pressure control, fluid balance, muscle and nerve function	Almost all foods, table salt (See p. 466.)
Potassium	Blood pressure control, carbohydrate metabolism, fluid balance, growth and development, heart function, muscle and nervous system function, protein formation	Bananas, beet greens, juices (carrot, pomegranate, prune, orange, tomato), milk, oranges, potatoes and sweet potatoes, prunes, spinach, tomatoes and tomato products, white beans, yogurt

Modified from U.S. Food and Drug Administration, Vitamins and Minerals Chart.

Adult women are allowed 5 to 6 teaspoons of oil daily. Adult men can have 6 to 7 teaspoons daily. Some foods are high in oil—nuts, olives, some fish, and avocados.

When making oil choices, remember:

- Oils are high in calories.
- The best oil choices come from fish, nuts, and vegetables (canola oil, corn oil, olive oil).
- Some foods are mainly oil. Mayonnaise, some salad dressings, and soft margarine (tub or squeeze) are examples.
- Oils from plant sources do not contain cholesterol.
- Enough oil is usually consumed daily from nuts, fish, cooking oil, and salad dressings.

Food Labels

Food labels are used to make informed food choices for a healthy diet (Fig. 30-3). Food labels contain information about:

- Serving size and the number of servings in each package. Nutrition information on the label is based on 1 serving.
- Calories. The number of calories in 1 serving. The number of servings eaten determines the number of calories eaten.
- Nutrients—total fat (saturated fat and *trans* fat are unhealthy fats), cholesterol, sodium, carbohydrate (dietary fiber, sugars, and added sugar), protein, vitamin D, calcium, iron, and potassium.

The *Percent Daily Value (%DV)* shows how much of a nutrient is in 1 serving of the food. The %DV helps you decide if a food is high or low in a nutrient. The value is based on a 2000-calorie daily diet. According to the Food and Drug Administration (FDA), a 5% DV is low. A DV of 20% or more is high.

Nutrition Facts	
8 servings per container	
Serving size	**2/3 cup (55g)**
Amount per serving	
Calories	**230**
	% Daily Value*
Total Fat 8g	**10%**
Saturated Fat 1g	**5%**
Trans Fat 0g	
Cholesterol 0mg	**0%**
Sodium 160mg	**7%**
Total Carbohydrate 37g	**13%**
Dietary Fiber 4g	**14%**
Total Sugars 12g	
Includes 10g Added Sugars	**20%**
Protein 3g	
Vitamin D 2mcg	10%
Calcium 260mg	20%
Iron 8mg	45%
Potassium 240mg	6%
* The % Daily Value (DV) tells you how much a nutrient in a serving of food contributes to a daily diet. 2,000 calories a day is used for general nutrition advice.	

FIGURE 30-3 Nutrition Facts Label. (From U.S. Food and Drug Administration, 2016.)

FACTORS AFFECTING EATING AND NUTRITION

Factors affecting eating and nutrition begin in childhood and continue throughout life. Follow the care plan to assist the person.

- *Culture.* Culture influences dietary practices, food choices, and food preparation. Frying, baking, smoking, or roasting food and eating raw food are some cultural practices. So is using sauces, herbs, and spices. See *Caring About Culture: Food Practices.*
- *Religion.* Selecting, preparing, and eating food often involve religion. For example, certain foods are not allowed. Or only certain foods or no foods are eaten during a *fast.* A person may follow all, some, or none of the dietary practices of his or her faith. Respect the person's religious practices.
- *Finances.* People with limited incomes often buy cheaper carbohydrate foods. Their diets often lack protein and certain vitamins and minerals.
- *Appetite.* Appetite relates to the desire for food. *Loss of appetite (anorexia)* can occur. Causes include illness, drugs, anxiety, pain, and depression. Unpleasant sights, thoughts, and smells are other causes.
- *Personal choice.* Food likes and dislikes are influenced by foods served in the home. Food choices depend on how food looks, how it is prepared, its smell, and ingredients. Usually food likes change with age and social experiences. Personal choice may involve a vegetarian diet. The focus is on plants for food—fruits, vegetables, dried beans and peas, grains, seeds, and nuts. Vegetarian eating patterns vary. For example:
  - Vegan diet—excludes all meat and animal products.
  - Lacto-vegetarian diet—includes dairy *(lacto)* products.
  - Lacto-ova vegetarian diet—includes dairy *(lacto)* products and eggs *(ova).*
- *Body reactions.* People should avoid foods that cause allergic reactions. Foods causing nausea, vomiting, diarrhea, indigestion, gas, or headaches are avoided.

- *Illness.* Appetite often decreases during illness and recovery from injuries. However, nutrition needs increase. The body must fight infection, heal tissue, and replace lost blood cells. Nutrients lost through vomiting and diarrhea need to be replaced.
- *Drugs.* Drugs can cause appetite loss, confusion, nausea, constipation, impaired taste, or changes in GI function. They can cause inflammation of the mouth, throat, esophagus, and stomach.
- *Chewing problems.* Mouth, teeth, and gum problems can affect chewing. Examples include oral pain, dry or sore mouth, gum disease (Chapter 23), dental problems, and dentures that fit poorly. Broken, decayed, or missing teeth also affect chewing (especially meats).
- *Swallowing problems.* Stroke; pain; confusion; dry mouth; and diseases of the mouth, throat, and esophagus can affect swallowing. See "The Dysphagia Diet" on p. 467.
- *Disability.* Disease or injury can affect the hands, wrists, and arms. Adaptive equipment (assistive devices) let the person eat independently (p. 469). The speech therapist and occupational therapist teach the person how to use them. Make sure each person has needed devices.
- *Impaired cognitive function.* Cognitive changes may affect the ability to use eating utensils. And they may affect eating, chewing, and swallowing.
- *Age.* Many GI changes occur with aging.

See *Focus on Children and Older Persons: Factors Affecting Eating and Nutrition.*

✿ CARING ABOUT CULTURE

Food Practices

Rice, corn, and beans are protein sources in *Mexico.* In the *Philippines,* rice is a main food. And fish, vegetables, and native fruits are preferred. A diet high in sugar and animal fat is common in *Poland.* In *China,* a meal of rice with meat, fish, and vegetables is common. High sodium content is from using soy sauce and dried and preserved foods.

(NOTE: Each person is unique. A person may not follow all of the beliefs and practices of his or her culture. Follow the care plan.)

Modified from D'Avanzo CE: Pocket guide to cultural health assessment, ed 4, St Louis, 2008, Mosby.

FOCUS ON **CHILDREN AND OLDER PERSONS**

Factors Affecting Eating and Nutrition

Older Persons

GI changes occur with aging.
- Taste and smell dull.
- Appetite decreases.
- Secretion of digestive juices decreases. Hard to digest, fried and fatty foods may cause indigestion.

Some people avoid the high-fiber foods needed for bowel elimination—apricots, celery, and fruits and vegetables with skins and seeds. High-fiber foods are hard to chew and can irritate the intestines.

Foods providing soft bulk are often ordered for chewing problems or constipation. Whole-grain cereals and cooked fruits and vegetables are examples.

Calorie needs are lower. Energy and activity levels are lower. Foods that contain calcium help prevent musculo-skeletal changes. Protein is needed for tissue growth and repair. Because of cost, diets may lack high-protein foods.

SPECIAL DIETS

Doctors may order special diets (Table 30-4).

* For a nutritional deficiency or a disease
* For weight gain or loss
* To remove or decrease certain substances in the diet

The health team considers the need for dietary changes, personal choices, religion, culture, and eating problems. They also consider food allergies and sensitivities. The nurse and dietitian teach the person and family about the diet.

Regular diet, *general diet*, and *house diet* mean no dietary limits or restrictions. Persons with diseases of the heart, kidneys, gallbladder, liver, stomach, or intestines often need special diets. High-protein diets are needed to heal wounds and pressure injuries. Adding bran to the diet provides fiber for bowel elimination. Allergies, excess weight, and other disorders also require special diets.

The sodium-controlled diet is often ordered (p. 466). So is a diabetes meal plan (p. 466). Persons with swallowing problems may need a dysphagia diet (p. 467). Surgery and some tests, procedures, and treatments require that nothing is eaten. The person has an *NPO order*. NPO stands for *nil per os*—nothing by mouth (Chapter 31).

TABLE 30-4	Special Diets	
Diet	**Use**	**Foods Allowed/Restricted**
Clear liquid—foods liquid at room temperature and clear or able to see through; non-irritating; non-gas forming; leave a small amount of residue	After surgery; for acute illness, infection, nausea, and vomiting; and to prepare for GI exams	Water, tea, and coffee *(without milk or cream)*; carbonated drinks; gelatin; fruit juices *without pulp* (apple, grape, cranberry); fat-free broth; hard candy, sugar, and Popsicles; *may need to avoid liquids with red coloring*
Full liquid—foods liquid at room temperature	Advance from clear-liquid diet after surgery; for stomach irritation, fever, nausea, and vomiting; for persons unable to chew, swallow, or digest solid foods	Foods on the clear-liquid diet; custard; eggnog; strained soups; strained fruit and vegetable juices; milk and milk-shakes; cooked cereals; plain ice cream and sherbet; plain pudding; yogurt
Mechanical soft—semi-solid foods that are easily digested	Advance from full-liquid diet; chewing problems, GI disorders, and infections	All liquids; eggs *(not fried)*; broiled, baked, or roasted meat, fish, or poultry that is chopped or shredded; mild cheeses (American, Swiss, cheddar, cream, cottage); strained fruit juices; refined bread *(no crust)* and crackers; cooked cereal; cooked or pureed vegetables; cooked or canned fruit *without skin or seeds*; plain pudding; plain cakes and soft cookies *without fruit or nuts*
Fiber- and residue-restricted—foods that leave a small amount of residue in the colon	Diseases of the colon and diarrhea	Coffee, tea, milk, carbonated drinks, strained fruit and vegetable juices; refined bread and crackers; creamed and refined cereal; rice; cottage and cream cheese; eggs *(not fried)*; plain puddings and cakes; gelatin; custard; sherbet and ice cream; canned or cooked fruit *without skin or seeds*; potatoes *(not fried)*; strained cooked vegetables; plain pasta; *no raw fruits or vegetables*
High-fiber—foods that increase residue and fiber in the colon to stimulate peristalsis	Constipation and GI disorders	All fruits and vegetables; whole-wheat bread; whole-grain cereals; fried foods; whole-grain rice; milk, cream, butter, and cheese; meats
Bland—foods that are non-irritating and low in roughage; foods served at moderate temperatures; no strong spices or condiments	Ulcers, gallbladder disorders, and some intestinal disorders; after abdominal surgery	Lean meats; white bread; creamed and refined cereals; cream or cottage cheese; gelatin; plain puddings, cakes, and cookies; eggs *(not fried)*; butter and cream; canned fruits and vegetables *without skin and seeds*; strained fruit juices; potatoes *(not fried)*; pastas and rice; strained or soft cooked carrots, peas, beets, spinach, squash, and asparagus tips; creamed soups from allowed vegetables; *no fried or spicy foods*
High-calorie—3000 to 4000 calories daily; includes 3 full meals and between-meal snacks	Weight gain and some thyroid problems	Dietary increases in all foods; large portions of regular diet with 3 between-meal snacks
Calorie-controlled—adequate nutrients while controlling calories to promote weight loss and reduce body fat	Weight loss	Foods low in fats and carbohydrates and lean meats; *avoid butter, cream, rice, gravies, salad oils, noodles, cakes, pastries, carbonated and alcoholic drinks, candy, potato chips, and similar foods*

Continued

TABLE 30-4	Special Diets—cont'd	
Diet	Use	Foods Allowed/Restricted
High-iron—foods high in iron	Anemia; after blood loss; for women during the reproductive years	Liver and other organ meats; lean meats; egg yolks; shellfish; dried fruits; dried beans; green leafy vegetables; lima beans; peanut butter; enriched breads and cereals
Fat-controlled (low cholesterol)—foods low in fat and prepared without adding fat	Heart, gallbladder, and liver diseases; disorders of fat digestion; diseases of the pancreas	Skim milk (fat-free) or buttermilk; cottage cheese *(no other cheeses allowed);* gelatin; sherbet; fruit; lean meat, poultry, and fish (baked, broiled, or roasted); fat-free broth; soups made with skim milk (fat-free); margarine; rice, pasta, breads, and cereals; vegetables; potatoes
High-protein—aids and promotes tissue healing	Burns, high fever, infection, and some liver diseases	Meat, milk, eggs, cheese, fish, poultry; breads and cereals; green leafy vegetables
Sodium-controlled—a certain amount of sodium is allowed	Heart disease, fluid retention, liver diseases, and some kidney diseases	Fruits and vegetables and unsalted butter are allowed; *adding salt at the table is not allowed; highly salted foods and foods high in sodium are not allowed; the use of salt during cooking may be restricted*
Gluten-free—foods without the gluten protein	Celiac disease	Beans; seeds; nuts; eggs; meats, fish, and poultry *(without breading, batter, or marinade);* fruits and vegetables; most dairy foods; gluten-free grains and starches (arrowroot, corn, cornmeal, hominy, flax, millet, rice, soy, and tapioca); gluten-free flours (rice, soy, corn, potato, bean); *no foods containing wheat, barley, triticale, or rye*
Diabetes meal plan—food and fluids are balanced with physical activity and drugs to manage blood glucose levels (Chapter 50)	Diabetes	Determined by nutrition and energy requirements and drugs to treat diabetes; *limit fried foods, foods high in fat and sodium, foods and drinks with added sugars;* sugar substitutes are allowed

The Sodium-Controlled Diet

According to the American Heart Association (AHA), the average amount of sodium in the daily diet is greater than 3400 mg (milligrams). Lowering sodium (commonly called salt) in the diet reduces the risk of high blood pressure, heart disease, and stroke. For most adults, the AHA recommends limiting sodium intake to no more than 2300 mg a day. The AHA says that no more than 1500 mg daily is a better goal.

With too much sodium, the body retains (holds) water. Tissues swell. There is excess fluid in the blood vessels. The heart works harder. With heart disease, the extra workload can cause serious problems or death.

Sodium control lowers the amount of sodium in the body. Less water is retained. Less water in the tissues and blood vessels reduces the heart's workload.

The doctor orders the amount of sodium allowed. Sodium-controlled diets involve:
- Omitting high-sodium foods (Box 30-2)
- Not adding salt to food at the table
- Limiting the amount of salt used in cooking
- Diet planning

Diabetes Meal Plan

Diabetes is a chronic illness in which the body cannot produce or use insulin properly (Chapter 50). The pancreas produces and secretes insulin. Insulin lets the body use sugar. Without enough insulin, sugar builds up in the bloodstream. It is not used by cells for energy. Treatment usually involves insulin or other drugs, diet, and exercise.

A meal plan for healthy eating is developed. It often involves:
- Food preferences (likes, eating habits, meal times, culture, and life-style). Food amounts and preparation methods may be restricted.
- Portion control. Healthy foods from each food group are eaten. The person's meal plan states the amounts allowed from each group.
- Carbohydrate counting (carb counting). The person keeps track of the amount of carbohydrates eaten each day.
- Eating meals and snacks at regular times. The person may need to eat at regular times to maintain a certain blood glucose (blood sugar) level.

Serve meals and snacks on time. Always check what was eaten. Report what the person did and did not eat. A between-meal snack makes up for what was not eaten (p. 474). The nurse tells you what to provide. The amount of insulin given depends on food intake and physical activity. Report changes in the person's eating habits.

BOX 30-2	High-Sodium Foods

Grains
- Baked goods—biscuits, muffins, cakes, cookies, pies, pastries, sweet rolls, donuts, and so on
- Breads and rolls
- Cereals—cold, instant hot
- Noodle mixes
- Pancakes
- Salted snack foods—pretzels, corn chips, popcorn, crackers, chips, and so on
- Stuffing mixes
- Waffles

Vegetables
- Canned vegetables
- Olives
- Pickles and other pickled vegetables
- Relish
- Sauerkraut
- Tomato sauce or paste
- Vegetable juices—tomato, V8, Bloody Mary mixes
- Vegetables with sauces, creams, or seasonings

Fruits
- None—fruits are not high in sodium

Dairy Group
- Buttermilk
- Cheese
- Commercial dips made with sour cream

Protein Foods
- Bacon and Canadian bacon
- Canned meats and fish—chicken, tuna, salmon, anchovies, sardines
- Caviar
- Chipped, dried, and corned beef and other meats
- Deli meats—turkey, ham, bologna, salami, pastrami, and so on

Protein Foods—cont'd
- Dried fish
- Ham
- Herring
- Hot dogs (frankfurters)
- Liverwurst
- Lox and smoked salmon
- Mackerel
- Pepperoni
- Salt pork
- Sausages
- Scrapple
- Shellfish—shrimp, crab, clams, oysters, scallops, lobster

Other
- Asian foods—Chinese, Japanese, East Indian, Thai, Vietnamese
- Baking soda and baking powder
- Catsup (ketchup)
- Cocoa mixes
- Commercially prepared dinners—frozen, canned, boxed, and so on
- Mayonnaise
- Mexican foods
- Mustard
- Pasta dishes—lasagna, manicotti, ravioli
- Peanut butter
- Pizzas
- Pot pies
- Salad dressings
- Salted nuts or seeds
- Sauces—soy, teriyaki, Worcestershire, steak, barbecue, pasta, chili, cocktail
- Seasoning salts—garlic, onion, celery, meat tenderizers, monosodium glutamate (MSG), and so on
- Soups—canned, packaged, instant, dried, bouillon

The Dysphagia Diet

Dysphagia means difficulty (dys) *swallowing* (phagia).
- A *slow swallow* means the person has difficulty getting enough food and fluids for good nutrition and fluid balance.
- An *unsafe swallow* means that food enters the airway (aspiration). *Aspiration is breathing fluid, food, vomitus, or an object into the lungs* (Chapter 32).

When feeding a person with dysphagia, you must:
- Know the signs and symptoms of dysphagia (Box 30-3, p. 468).
- Feed the person according to the care plan.
- Follow the person's ordered diet. Food and fluid thicknesses are changed to meet the person's needs (see Box 30-3).
- Follow aspiration precautions (see Box 30-3) and the care plan.
- Report changes in how the person eats.
- Report signs and symptoms of aspiration at once (see Box 30-3).

BOX 30-3	Dysphagia

Dysphagia Signs and Symptoms
- Avoids food that needs chewing.
- Avoids food with certain textures and temperatures.
- Tires during a meal.
- Has food spill out of the mouth while eating.
- "Pockets" or "squirrels" food in the cheeks. This means that food remains or is hidden in the mouth.
- Eats slowly, especially solid foods.
- Complains that food will not go down or that food is stuck.
- Coughs or chokes before, during, or after swallowing.
- Regurgitates food after eating (Chapter 32).
- Spits out food suddenly and almost violently.
- Has food come up through the nose.
- Has hoarseness—especially after eating.
- Makes gurgling sounds while talking or breathing after swallowing.
- Has a runny nose, sneezes, or has excessive drooling.
- Complains of frequent heartburn.
- Has a decreased appetite.

Dysphagia Diet
- The doctor, speech therapist, occupational therapist, dietitian, and nurse choose food and liquid thicknesses.
- Food thickness and texture are changed to ease swallowing.
  - *Mechanical soft*—foods have a moist, soft texture. Meats are chopped, blended, or ground. Vegetables are cooked well.
  - *Pureed*—foods have a smooth, uniform texture and hold their shape on a spoon. Foods are "pudding-like" and have no lumps.

Dysphagia Diet—cont'd
- Liquids are thickened as needed (Fig. 30-4).
  - *Nectar-thick liquid*—mildly thick. The liquid coats and drips off of a spoon. It can flow through a straw.
  - *Honey-thick liquid*—moderately thick. The liquid flows off of a spoon like honey. The person can drink it from a cup.
  - *Pudding-thick (spoon-thick) liquid*—extremely thick. The liquid stays on a spoon in a soft mound. It can be sipped or served with a spoon.

Aspiration Precautions
- Help the person with meals and snacks. Follow the care plan.
- Position the person upright as the nurse and care plan direct. The person remains upright for at least 1 hour after eating.
- Support the upper back, shoulders, and neck with a pillow.
- Follow the care plan for straw use. A straw may not be allowed.
- Check the person's mouth after eating for pocketing. Check inside the cheeks, under the tongue, and on the roof of the mouth. Remove any food.
- Provide mouth care after eating.
- Observe for signs and symptoms of aspiration. Report the following at once.
  - Choking
  - Coughing
  - Difficulty breathing during or after meals or snacks
  - Abnormal breathing or respiratory sounds
- Report and record your observations.

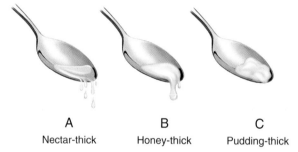

A
Nectar-thick

B
Honey-thick

C
Pudding-thick

FIGURE 30-4 A, Nectar-thick liquid. **B,** Honey-thick liquid. **C,** Pudding-thick (spoon-thick) liquid.

FOOD INTAKE

Food intake is measured in different ways. Follow agency policy for the method used.
- *Percentage of food eaten.* Food intake ranges from 0 to 100 percent (%). Some agencies record the percent of the whole meal tray. Others record the percent of each food item eaten. See Figure 30-5.
- *Calorie counts.* Note what the person ate and how much. For example, a chicken breast, rice, beans, fruit salad, and pudding were served. The person ate all the chicken, half the rice, and the fruit salad. The beans and pudding were not eaten. Note these on the flow sheet. A nurse or dietitian converts these portions into calories.

See *Focus on Math: Food Intake.*

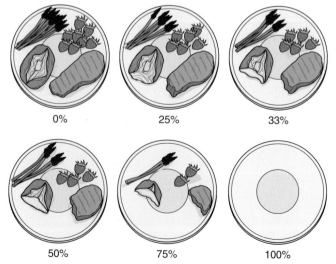

0%   25%   33%

50%   75%   100%

FIGURE 30-5 Percent of food eaten from the plate (0% means none was eaten; 100% means all was eaten).

FOCUS ON **MATH**

Food Intake

To measure food intake, you need to understand percents. Percents measure parts of a whole (Fig. 30-6). The "whole" is written as 100%.

To measure food intake, compare the food left to that served. Depending on agency policy and the food type, *estimate* or *calculate* food intake. *To estimate*, record the approximate amount of food eaten. See Figure 30-5. *To calculate:*

1 Subtract the amount left from the amount served. (This is the amount the person ate.)
2 Divide the number from step 1 by the amount served (the number of pieces making up the whole).
3 Multiply the number from step 2 by 100 for a percent. (*Percent* means out of 100.)

For example, 8 apple slices were served; 2 remain on the tray.

8 slices – 2 slices = 6 slices
The person ate 6 apple slices; 8 were served.
6 slices ÷ 8 slices = 0.75 of the slices served
0.75 × 100 = 75%
75% of the apple slices were eaten.

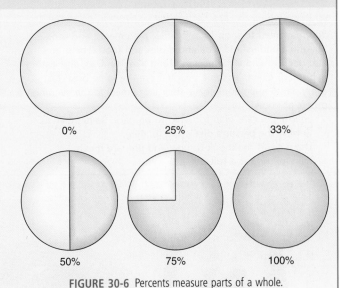

FIGURE 30-6 Percents measure parts of a whole.

MEETING NUTRITION NEEDS

A team approach is needed to meet a person's nutrition needs. The person, nursing team, doctor, dietitian, speech therapist, and occupational therapist are involved. So is the family if necessary. The person's likes, dislikes, and life-long habits are part of the care plan.

NOTE: *Tasks in this chapter may require more than 1 pair of gloves. Change gloves as needed. Use careful judgment. Remember to practice hand hygiene after removing gloves.*

See *Focus on Communication: Meeting Nutrition Needs.*

See *Focus on Long-Term Care and Home Care: Meeting Nutrition Needs.*

FOCUS ON **COMMUNICATION**

Meeting Nutrition Needs

The person may not eat everything served. You need to ask why and tell the nurse. You can say:
- "Please tell me why you didn't eat everything."
- "Was there something wrong with your food?"
- "Did your food taste okay?"
- "Was there something you didn't like?"
- "Was your food too hot or too cold?"
- "Would you like something else?"
- "Weren't you hungry?"

FOCUS ON **LONG-TERM CARE AND HOME CARE**

Meeting Nutrition Needs

Long-Term Care

The CMS has requirements for food served in nursing centers.
- Each person's nutrition needs are met.
- The person's religious and cultural needs and preferences are met.
- The person's diet is well balanced. It is nourishing and tastes good. Food is well seasoned. It is not too salty or too sweet.
- Food is appetizing. It has an appealing aroma and is attractive.
- Hot food is served hot. Cold food is served cold.
- Food is served promptly. If not, hot food cools and cold food warms.
- Food is prepared to meet each person's needs. Some people need food cut, ground, or chopped. Others have special diets (p. 465).
- Other foods are offered if the food served is refused. The substituted food must have a similar nutritional value to the first foods served.
- Each person receives at least 3 meals a day. A bedtime snack is offered.
- The center provides needed adaptive equipment (assistive devices) and utensils (Fig. 30-7, p. 470). They promote independence. Make sure the person has needed equipment.

Continued

FOCUS ON LONG-TERM CARE AND HOME CARE—cont'd

Meeting Nutrition Needs

Home Care

You may need to shop for groceries, plan meals, and cook. You must understand a balanced diet and food labels. You also need to know the person's food likes, dislikes, and eating habits. For example, some people have the same breakfast every day. Some people have their large meal in the evening, others at noon.

Follow the care plan for what to prepare. Remember to:
- Review the person's diet order (p. 465).
- Use a good cookbook to plan and prepare meals.
- Plan menus for a full week.

- Check recipe ingredients. Include needed items on your shopping list.
- Try to save money. Check newspapers, mailers, and the Internet for sales and coupons.
- Give all receipts to the person or family member.
- Store food properly. Refrigerate dairy products and most fresh fruits and vegetables right away. Do the same for meat, fish, or poultry that you will use that day. Freeze the rest and any frozen foods. Dried, packaged, canned, and bottled foods keep well in cabinets.
- See p. 476 for preventing "Foodborne Illness."

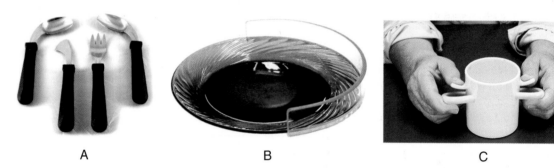

A   B   C

FIGURE 30-7 Adaptive equipment (assistive devices) for eating. **A,** Eating utensils have tapered and angled handles. The knife cuts with slicing and rocking motions. **B,** The plate guard helps keep food on the plate. **C,** The thumb grips on the cup help prevent spilling. (Images courtesy Elderstore, Alpharetta, Ga.)

Preparing for Meals

Preparing patients and residents for meals promotes comfort. To promote comfort:
- Assist with elimination needs.
- Provide oral hygiene. Make sure dentures are in place.
- Make sure eyeglasses and hearing aids are in place.
- Make sure incontinent persons are clean and dry.
- Position the person in a comfortable position.
- Reduce or remove unpleasant odors, sights, and sounds. See Chapter 21.
- Follow the care plan for pain-relief measures. See Chapter 35.
- Assist the person with hand hygiene.
  See *Delegation Guidelines: Preparing for Meals.*
  See *Promoting Safety and Comfort: Preparing for Meals.*
  See procedure: *Preparing the Person for a Meal.*

DELEGATION GUIDELINES

Preparing for Meals

Preparing for meals is a routine nursing task. You need this information from the nurse and the care plan.
- How much help the person needs
- Where the person will eat—room or dining room
- What the person uses for elimination—toilet, commode, bedpan, urinal, or specimen pan
- What type of oral hygiene to give
- If the person wears dentures
- If the person wears eyeglasses or hearing aids
- How to position the person—in bed, a chair, or wheelchair
- If the person needs help to the dining room
- If the person uses a wheelchair, walker, or cane
- When to report observations
- What patient or resident concerns to report at once

PROMOTING SAFETY AND COMFORT

Preparing for Meals

Safety

Before meals, the person needs to eliminate and have oral hygiene. Follow Standard Precautions and the Bloodborne Pathogen Standard. Also follow them to clean equipment and the room.

Preparing the Person for a Meal

QUALITY OF LIFE

- Knock before entering the person's room.
- Address the person by name.
- Introduce yourself by name and title.

- Explain the procedure before starting and during the procedure.
- Protect the person's rights during the procedure.
- Handle the person gently during the procedure.

PRE-PROCEDURE

1 Follow *Delegation Guidelines: Preparing for Meals.* See *Promoting Safety and Comfort: Preparing for Meals.*
2 Practice hand hygiene.
3 Collect the following.
   - Equipment for oral hygiene (Chapter 23)
   - Bedpan and cover (optional), urinal, commode, or specimen pan

   - Toilet paper
   - Wash basin
   - Soap
   - Washcloth and towel or hand wipes
   - Gloves
4 Provide for privacy.

PROCEDURE

5 Make sure eyeglasses and hearing aids are in place.
6 Assist with oral hygiene. Make sure dentures are in place. Wear gloves and practice hand hygiene after removing and discarding them.
7 Assist with elimination. Make sure the person is clean and dry if incontinent. Wear gloves and practice hand hygiene after removing and discarding them.
8 Assist with hand hygiene. Wear gloves and practice hand hygiene after removing and discarding them.
9 *For the person who will eat in bed:*
   a Raise the head of the bed to a comfortable position—Fowler's (45 to 60 degrees) or high-Fowler's (60 to 90 degrees). (NOTE: Some state competency tests require at least 45 degrees, others require 75 to 90 degrees.)
   b Remove items from the over-bed table. Clean the table.
   c Adjust the over-bed table in front of the person.

10 *For the person who will sit in a chair:*
   a Position the person in a chair or wheelchair.
   b Remove items from the over-bed table. Clean the table.
   c Adjust the over-bed table in front of the person.
11 *For the person who eats in the dining room,* assist the person to the dining room.

POST-PROCEDURE

12 Provide for comfort. (See the inside of the back cover.)
13 Place the call light and other needed items within reach.
14 Empty, clean, rinse, disinfect, and dry equipment. Use clean, dry paper towels for drying. Return equipment to its proper place. Wear gloves and practice hand hygiene after removing and discarding them.

15 Straighten the room. Eliminate unpleasant noise, odors, or equipment.
16 Unscreen the person.
17 Complete a safety check of the room. (See the inside of the back cover.)
18 Practice hand hygiene.

Serving Meals

Food is served in covered containers to keep foods at the correct temperature. Hot food is kept hot. Cold food is kept cold. Uncover food just before the person eats. Uncovered food changes temperature quickly.

Prepare persons for meals before food is served. If they are ready to eat, you can serve meals promptly. Food is kept at the correct temperature.

Some agencies have "room service" meal programs. A full menu (breakfast, lunch, dinner) is in the person's room. When ready to eat, the person calls the dietary department to place an order. Food is served a short while later. This program allows the person to eat when hungry. For a fee, visitors can order food to dine with the person.

Serve meals in the assigned order. In nursing centers, residents seated at tables are served at the same time.

If food is not served within 15 minutes, re-check food temperatures. Follow agency policy. If not at the correct temperature, get fresh food. Temperature guides and food thermometers are in dining rooms and in nursing unit kitchens. Some agencies allow re-heating in microwave ovens.

See *Focus on Long-Term Care and Home Care: Serving Meals,* p. 472.

See *Teamwork and Time Management: Serving Meals,* p. 472.

See *Delegation Guidelines: Serving Meals,* p. 472.

See *Promoting Safety and Comfort: Serving Meals,* p. 472.

See procedure: *Serving Meal Trays,* p. 473.

FOCUS ON LONG-TERM CARE AND HOME CARE

Serving Meals

Long-Term Care

The needs of nursing center residents vary. The following dining programs are common in nursing centers.

- *Social dining.* A table seats 4 to 6 residents (Fig. 30-8). Food is served as in a restaurant. Residents are oriented and can feed themselves.
- *Family dining.* Food is served in bowls and on platters. Residents serve and feed themselves as at home.
- *Low-stimulation dining.* Distractions are prevented. The health team decides where each person should sit.
- *Restaurant-style menus.* Food is selected from a menu to allow more food choices. The person is served as in a restaurant.
- *Open dining.* A buffet is open for several hours. Residents can eat any time while the buffet is open.

TEAMWORK AND TIME MANAGEMENT

Serving Meals

Meal trays are served in the order set by the health team. You will serve trays to your patients and residents and to those assigned to other nursing assistants. Your co-workers do the same. The goal is to serve trays promptly. This keeps food at the desired temperature.

DELEGATION GUIDELINES

Serving Meals

Serving meal trays is a routine nursing task. You need this information from the nurse and the care plan.

- The person's food allergies (if any)
- What adaptive equipment (assistive devices) are needed
- If the person needs help opening cartons, cutting food, buttering bread, and so on
- If the person's food intake (p. 468) and fluid intake (Chapter 31) are measured
- If calorie counts are done (p. 468)
- When to report observations
- What patient or resident concerns to report at once

PROMOTING SAFETY AND COMFORT

Serving Meals

Safety

Always check food temperature after re-heating. Food that is too hot can cause burns.

After eating, check the person's mouth for food (pocketing). Remove any food. Follow these safety measures.

- Use sponge swabs (Chapter 23) as needed. Wear gloves. Practice hand hygiene after removing and discarding them.
- Have the person tip the chin downward (toward the chest) to prevent aspiration.
- Call for the nurse if you cannot remove food easily.

Comfort

Check the person's position when serving a meal. The position may have changed after the person was prepared to eat. Provide other comfort measures as needed. See the inside of the back cover.

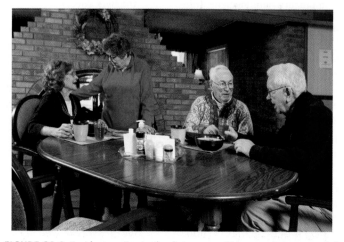

FIGURE 30-8 Residents eating in the dining room. Volunteers help as needed.

Serving Meal Trays

QUALITY OF LIFE

- Knock before entering the person's room.
- Address the person by name.
- Introduce yourself by name and title.
- Explain the procedure before starting and during the procedure.
- Protect the person's rights during the procedure.
- Handle the person gently during the procedure.

PRE-PROCEDURE

1 Follow *Delegation Guidelines: Serving Meals.* See *Promoting Safety and Comfort: Serving Meals.*
2 Practice hand hygiene.
3 Prepare the person for the meal if not already done. See procedure: *Preparing the Person for a Meal,* p. 471.

PROCEDURE

4 Check items on the tray with the dietary card. Make sure the tray is complete and has adaptive equipment (assistive devices).
5 Identify the person. Check the ID (identification) bracelet against the dietary card. Use 2 identifiers (Chapter 13). Also call the person by name.
6 Place the tray within the person's reach. Adjust the over-bed table as needed.
7 Remove food covers. Open cartons, cut food into bite-sized pieces, butter bread, and so on as needed (Fig. 30-9). Season food as the person prefers and the care plan allows.
8 Place the napkin, clothes protector, adaptive equipment (assistive devices), and eating utensils within reach. Help the person apply the clothes protector if needed.
9 Place the call light within reach.
10 Do the following when the person is done eating.
  a Measure and record fluid intake if ordered (Chapter 31).
  b Note the amount and type of foods eaten (p. 468).
  c Check for and remove any food in the mouth (pocketing). See *Promoting Safety and Comfort: Serving Meals.*
  d Remove the tray.
  e Clean spills. Change used linens and soiled clothing.
  f Help the person return to bed if needed.
  g Assist with oral hygiene and hand hygiene. Wear gloves. Practice hand hygiene after removing and discarding the gloves.

POST-PROCEDURE

11 Provide for comfort. (See the inside of the back cover.)
12 Place the call light and other needed items within reach.
13 Raise or lower bed rails. Follow the care plan.
14 Complete a safety check of the room. (See the inside of the back cover.)
15 Follow agency policy for used linens.
16 Practice hand hygiene.
17 Report and record your observations.

Feeding the Person

Weakness, paralysis, casts, confusion, and other limits can make self-feeding impossible. These persons are fed.

Serve food and fluids in the order the person prefers. Offer fluids during the meal. Fluids help the person chew and swallow.

Use teaspoons to feed the person. They are safer than forks. The teaspoon should be only one-third (⅓) full. This portion is chewed and swallowed easily. Some people need smaller portions. Follow the care plan.

Persons who need to be fed are often angry, humiliated, and embarrassed. Some are depressed, resentful, or refuse to eat. Let them do what they can. Some can handle "finger foods" (bread, cookies, crackers). If strong enough, let them hold milk or juice cups (never hot drinks). Follow ordered activity limits. Provide support. Encourage them to try, even if food is spilled.

Visually impaired persons often recognize foods from their aromas. Describe what is on the tray and what you are offering. For persons who feed themselves, describe foods and fluids and their place on the tray. Use the numbers on a clock for the location of foods (Fig. 30-10).

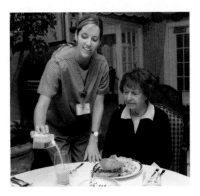

FIGURE 30-9 Cartons and containers are opened for the person.

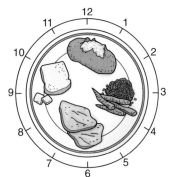

FIGURE 30-10 The numbers on a clock are used to help a visually impaired person locate food.

Many people pray before eating. Allow time and privacy for prayer. This shows respect and caring.

Meals provide social contact with others. Talk with the person. Also allow time to chew and swallow. Sit facing the person. Sitting is more relaxing. It shows that you have time. You can also see how well the person is eating and watch for swallowing problems.

See *Focus on Children and Older Persons: Feeding the Person.*

See *Focus on Surveys: Feeding the Person.*

See *Delegation Guidelines: Feeding the Person.*

See *Promoting Safety and Comfort: Feeding the Person.*

See procedure: *Feeding the Person.*

FOCUS ON CHILDREN AND OLDER PERSONS

Feeding the Person

Older Persons

Persons with dementia may become distracted during meals. Some do not sit long enough to eat. Others forget how to use eating utensils. Some persons resist efforts to help them eat. A confused person may throw or spit food.

These measures may be helpful for persons with dementia. Follow the person's care plan.

- Keep meal times and the setting consistent.
- Provide a calm, quiet setting. Limit noise and distractions. This helps the person focus.
- Limit the number of food choices.
- Offer several small meals during the day instead of larger ones.
- Use straws or cups with lids. These make drinking easier.
- Provide finger foods if the person has problems with utensils. A bowl may be easier to use than a plate.
- Provide healthy snacks. Keep snacks where the person can see them.

Be patient. Tell the nurse if you feel upset or impatient. The person has the right to be treated with dignity and respect.

FOCUS ON SURVEYS

Feeding the Person

Surveyors focus on nutrition needs. They observe if staff:

- Provide help with eating.
- Encourage the person to eat.
- Help the person use adaptive equipment (assistive devices).
- Feed the person if necessary.

Between-Meal Snacks

Many special diets involve between-meal snacks. Snacks provide extra nutrients. Common snacks are crackers, milk, juice, a milk-shake, cake, wafers, a sandwich, gelatin, and custard.

Snacks are served upon arrival on the nursing unit. Provide needed utensils, a straw, and a napkin. Follow the same considerations and procedures for serving meals and feeding the person.

DELEGATION GUIDELINES

Feeding the Person

Feeding patients and residents is a routine nursing task. Before feeding a person, you need this information from the nurse and the care plan.

- The person's food allergies (if any)
- Why the person needs help
- How much help the person needs
- How to position the person
- If the person can manage finger foods
- The person's activity limits
- The person's dietary restrictions
- Feeding portion size—$\frac{1}{3}$ teaspoonful or less
- Needed safety measures if the person has dysphagia
- If the person can use a straw
- What observations to report and record:
  - The amount and kind of food eaten
  - Complaints of nausea or dysphagia
  - Signs and symptoms of dysphagia
  - Signs and symptoms of aspiration
- When to report observations
- What patient or resident concerns to report at once

PROMOTING SAFETY AND COMFORT

Feeding the Person

Safety

Check food temperature. Very hot foods and fluids can burn the person.

Prevent aspiration. Check the person's mouth before offering more food or fluids. The mouth must be empty between bites and swallows.

The person must be alert enough to eat. Health problems, drug side effects, and fatigue can affect level of consciousness. *Do not try to feed a person who is drowsy.* Tell the nurse right away.

Comfort

The person will eat better if not rushed. Sit to show that you have time. Standing communicates being in a hurry.

Wipe the person's hands, face, and mouth as needed during the meal. Use the napkin or a wet washcloth. Then dry the person with a towel.

Feeding the Person

QUALITY OF LIFE

- Knock before entering the person's room.
- Address the person by name.
- Introduce yourself by name and title.

- Explain the procedure before starting and during the procedure.
- Protect the person's rights during the procedure.
- Handle the person gently during the procedure.

PRE-PROCEDURE

1 Follow *Delegation Guidelines: Feeding the Person.* See *Promoting Safety and Comfort:*
   - *Serving Meals,* p. 472
   - *Feeding the Person*
2 Practice hand hygiene.

3 Position the person in a comfortable position for eating—sitting in a chair or in Fowler's (45 to 60 degrees) or high-Fowler's (60 to 90 degrees). (NOTE: Some state competency tests require at least 45 degrees, others require 75 to 90 degrees.)
4 Get the tray. Place the tray on the over-bed table or dining table where the person can reach it.

PROCEDURE

5 Check items on the tray with the dietary card. Make sure the tray is complete.
6 Identify the person. Check the ID bracelet against the dietary card. Use 2 identifiers (Chapter 13). Also call the person by name.
7 Drape a napkin across the person's chest and underneath the chin. Or apply a clothes protector or towel.
8 Clean the person's hands. (NOTE: Some state competency tests require soap and water, others allow hand sanitizer or a hand wipe.)
9 Tell the person what foods and fluids are on the tray.
10 Prepare food for eating. Cut food into bite-sized pieces. Season food as the person prefers and as the care plan allows.
11 Place the chair where you can sit comfortably. Sit facing the person at eye level.
12 Serve foods in the order the person prefers. Identify foods as you serve them. Alternate between solid and liquid foods. Use a spoon for safety (Fig. 30-11). Allow enough time to chew and swallow. Do not rush the person. Also offer water, coffee, tea, or other fluids on the tray.

13 Check the person's mouth before offering more food or fluids. Make sure the mouth is empty between bites and swallows. Ask if the person is ready for the next bite or drink.
14 Use straws (if allowed) for liquids if the person cannot drink out of a glass or cup. Have 1 straw for each liquid. Provide short straws for weak persons. Follow the care plan for using straws.
15 Wipe the person's hands, face, and mouth as needed during the meal. Use the napkin or a hand wipe.
16 Follow the care plan if the person has dysphagia. (Some persons with dysphagia do not use straws.) Give thickened liquid with a spoon.
17 Talk with the person in a pleasant manner.
18 Encourage him or her to eat as much as possible.
19 Wipe the person's mouth with a napkin or a hand wipe. Discard the napkin or hand wipe.
20 Note how much and which foods were eaten (p. 468).
21 Measure and record fluid intake if ordered (Chapter 31).
22 Remove the tray.
23 Take the person to his or her room (if in a dining area).
24 Assist with oral hygiene and hand hygiene. Provide for privacy. Wear gloves. Practice hand hygiene after removing and discarding gloves.

POST-PROCEDURE

25 Provide for comfort. (See the inside of the back cover.)
26 Place the call light and other needed items within reach.
27 Raise or lower bed rails. Follow the care plan.
28 Complete a safety check of the room. (See the inside of the back cover.)

29 Return the food tray to the food cart.
30 Practice hand hygiene.
31 Report and record your observations.

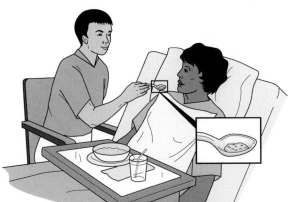

FIGURE 30-11 A spoon is used to feed the person. The spoon is one-third ($\frac{1}{3}$) full.

FOODBORNE ILLNESS

A foodborne illness (food poisoning) is caused by pathogens in food and fluids. Report the signs and symptoms listed in Box 30-4 to the nurse at once.

Food is not sterile. Therefore pathogens are present in food. Cooked and ready-to-eat foods can become contaminated from other food. For example, meat juices can spill or splash onto other food. Food handlers with poor hygiene can contaminate the food.

Pathogens grow rapidly between 40°F and 140°F (Fahrenheit). This range is called the "danger zone" by the USDA. You must keep food out of the "danger zone." To do so, keep cold food cold and hot food hot.

To keep food safe, the USDA recommends these 4 safety tips.

- *Clean*. Wash hands, utensils, and counter tops often.
- *Separate*. Avoid cross-contamination. Do not let raw meat, poultry, or their juices touch other foods that will not be cooked.
- *Cook*. Cook food to a safe internal temperature (Fig. 30-12). Use a food thermometer to check the internal temperature. When re-heating cooked food, re-heat to 165°F.
- *Chill*. Refrigerate or freeze food within 2 hours. If the air is 90°F or above, chill food within 1 hour.

See *Focus on Long-Term Care and Home Care: Foodborne Illness.*

BOX 30-4	Foodborne Illness—Signs and Symptoms

- Abdominal cramps or pain
- Backache
- Breathing problems
- Chills
- Diarrhea (may be bloody)
- Eyelids: droopy
- Fever
- Headache
- Muscle pain
- Nausea
- Speaking problems
- Swallowing problems
- Vision: double
- Vomiting

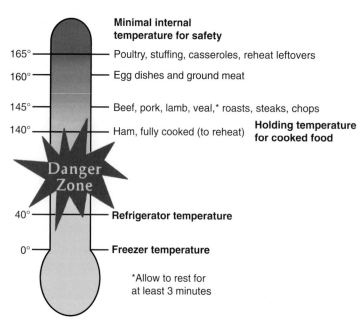

FIGURE 30-12 Food temperature guide. (Modified from U.S. Department of Agriculture: "Danger Zone" [40 °F–140 °F].)

FOCUS ON LONG-TERM CARE AND HOME CARE

Foodborne Illness

Home Care

You need to protect the patient and family from foodborne illnesses. Follow the clean, separate, cook, and chill safety tips.

Clean

- Practice hand-washing with soap and water (Chapter 16):
  - Before, during, and after preparing food
  - After handling raw meat, poultry, seafood, or their juices; or uncooked eggs
  - Before eating
  - After elimination
  - After changing a diaper or helping a child who has used the toilet
  - After touching an animal, animal feed, or animal waste
  - After touching garbage
  - Before and after caring for an ill person
  - Before and after treating a cut or wound
  - After blowing your nose, coughing, or sneezing
- Wash surfaces and utensils after each use.
  - Use hot, soapy water to wash cutting boards, dishes, utensils, and countertops. Do so especially if they held raw meat, poultry, seafood, or eggs.
  - Wash dish cloths often in the hot cycle of a washing machine.
- Wash fruits and vegetables.
  - First cut away damaged or bruised areas. Then rinse under running water.
  - Scrub firm produce (melons, cucumbers) with a clean produce brush.
  - Dry produce with a paper towel or clean cloth towel.
  - Do not wash bagged produce marked "pre-washed."
- Do not wash meat, poultry, or eggs.

Separate: Do Not Cross Contaminate

- Use separate cutting boards and plates for produce, meat, poultry, seafood, and eggs.
  - Use 1 cutting board for fresh produce or other foods that will not be cooked. Use another for raw meat, poultry, or seafood.
  - Replace cutting boards when worn.
  - Use separate plates and utensils for cooked and raw foods.
  - Wash thoroughly all plates, utensils, and cutting boards that have touched raw meat, poultry, seafood, or eggs. Do so before re-use with hot, soapy water.
- Keep certain types of food separate.
  - Shopping cart:
    - Separate raw meat, poultry, seafood, and eggs from other foods.
    - Place raw meat, poultry, and seafood in plastic bags while shopping if available.
    - Place raw meat, poultry, and seafood in separate bags when checking out. They should each be in separate bags from other foods.

Separate: Do Not Cross Contaminate—cont'd

  - At home:
    - Place raw meat, poultry, and seafood in containers or plastic bags that can be sealed.
    - Freeze raw meat, poultry, and seafood if not to be used within a few days.
  - Refrigerator:
    - Keep eggs in their original carton.
    - Store eggs in the main section of the refrigerator. Do not store them in the door.

Cook to the Right Temperature

- Use a food thermometer to make sure food is safe. Food is safely cooked when the internal temperature is high enough to kill pathogens.
- Use a food thermometer.
- Place the food thermometer in the thickest part of the food. The thermometer should not touch bone, fat, or gristle.
- Use a cooking chart to make sure food has reached a safe temperature.
- Keep food hot (140°F or above) after cooking.
  - Serve food right after cooking.
  - Keep food out of the danger zone (see Fig. 30-12) if not serving it right after cooking. Use a heat source—chafing dish, warming tray, slow cooker.
- Microwave food thoroughly (165°F or above).
  - Follow package directions for cooking to make sure food is thoroughly cooked.
  - Check the package directions for when to stir food during the cooking time. Stir food in the middle of the cooking time if no package instructions. For example, if you want to heat food for 4 minutes, stir after 2 minutes.
  - Follow package directions after cooking. For example, "Let stand for 2 minutes after cooking." Letting food sit for a few minutes allows colder areas to absorb heat from hotter areas.

Chill: Refrigerate and Freeze Food Properly

- Remember that microbes causing food poisoning multiply the fastest between 40°F and 140°F.
- Check that the refrigerator is set to 40°F or below and the freezer to 0°F. Use an appliance thermometer.
- Do not leave foods that will spoil out of the refrigerator for more than 2 hours.
- Refrigerate food within 1 hour if it was exposed to temperatures above 90°F.
- Place left-overs in shallow containers. Refrigerate promptly for quick cooling.
- Never thaw or marinate foods on the counter. Thaw or marinate meat, poultry, and seafood in the refrigerator.
- Check a food storage chart for when to throw out food.

Modified from U.S. Department of Health and Human Services: 4 steps to food safety, date reviewed April 12, 2019.

FOCUS ON **PRIDE**

The Person, Family, and Yourself

Personal and Professional Responsibility

You can help make meal time pleasant. Smile and greet each person as you serve food. Ask if help is needed. Talk with the person as you prepare food. When feeding, focus on the person. Meal time should be as pleasant as possible.

Rights and Respect

People often comment about food likes and dislikes. A person may say that the food is cold, bland, or tastes bad. People have the right to express what they prefer. Do not get angry or upset. The person should not feel as if he or she is complaining or being picky. Learning the person's likes and dislikes can improve nutrition. It also shows interest and concern for the person.

Independence and Social Interaction

Meals provide a time for social contact. A friendly, social setting is important. Some nursing centers have areas for residents to dine with guests. Families and friends may bring food from home. This helps meet love and belonging needs. Tell the nurse when the person receives food. The food must not interfere with the person's diet.

Delegation and Teamwork

Meals are a busy time. Teamwork is important. Staff work together to help residents to the dining area and serve food promptly. Staff must make sure everyone is served and nutrition needs are met. Have a helpful attitude.

Ethics and Laws

Each person is different. A person may have a food allergy or special diet. You must know what each person can and cannot have. You must protect the person from harm. Know each person's needs. If unsure, ask the nurse.

FOCUS ON **PRIDE**: *Application*

How do sights, sounds, smells, and personal preferences affect meal time? How can you help make it pleasant?

REVIEW QUESTIONS

Circle the BEST answer.

1 Nutrition is
  a Fats, proteins, carbohydrates, vitamins, and minerals
  b The processes involved in ingestion, digestion, absorption, and use of food and fluids by the body
  c The amount of food eaten
  d The balance between calories taken in and used by the body

2 Which is healthy?
  a Eating large portions
  b Eating from all 5 food groups
  c Increasing the amount of high-sodium foods
  d Eating more refined grains

3 What is the amount of grains needed daily for an adult woman?
  a 1 oz
  b 2 to 2½ oz
  c 3 oz
  d 5 to 6 oz

4 Which would meet an adult male's daily dairy needs?
  a 1 slice of bread, 1 cup of cheese, and ½ oz of nuts
  b 2 cups of milk and 1 cup of cooked rice
  c 1 cup of milk, 1 cup of yogurt, and 1½ oz of cheese
  d 2 tablespoons of peanut butter and 1 egg

5 Which food group contains the *most* cholesterol?
  a Grains
  b Vegetables
  c Fruit
  d Protein foods

6 These statements are about oils. Which is *true*?
  a The best oil choices come from fish, nuts, and vegetable oils.
  b Oils are low in calories.
  c Oils from plant sources contain cholesterol.
  d Oils are a food group.

7 Protein is needed for
  a Tissue growth and repair
  b Energy and the fiber for bowel elimination
  c Body heat and to protect organs from injury
  d Improving the taste of food

8 Which foods provide the *most* protein?
  a Butter and cream
  b Tomatoes and potatoes
  c Meats and fish
  d Corn and lettuce

9 Which is allowed on a gluten-free diet?
  a Breaded fish
  b Baked sweet potato
  c Whole-wheat bread
  d Flour tortillas

10 The sodium-controlled diet involves
  a Omitting high-sodium foods
  b Adding salt to food at the table
  c Using 3000 mg of salt in cooking
  d A sodium-intake flow sheet

REVIEW QUESTIONS—cont'd

11 Diabetes meal planning involves
   a Changing the thickness of foods
   b Eating larger food portions
   c Controlling sodium
   d Eating at regular times

12 Nursing centers must
   a Serve 2 meals a day
   b Serve food promptly
   c Serve food at room temperature to avoid burns
   d Serve food under-seasoned to lower sodium intake

13 A resident eats half of the food on the meal tray. Food intake for this meal is
   a 25%
   b 33%
   c 50%
   d 75%

14 Persons with dysphagia
   a Are fed in the semi-Fowler's position
   b Have a regular diet
   c Are fed according to the care plan
   d Eat alone in their rooms

15 A person coughs and drools while eating. You should
   a Give the person a drink
   b Puree the person's food
   c Give mouth care and continue feeding
   d Tell the nurse

16 Which is a sign of a swallowing problem?
   a Edema
   b Sore throat
   c Coughing while eating
   d Increased appetite

17 When feeding a person
   a Ask in what order the person likes foods served
   b Use a fork
   c Stand facing the person
   d Talk with your co-workers

18 You are re-heating cooked food. The food temperature should be
   a 40°F
   b 90°F
   c 140°F
   d 165°F

19 Which can cause foodborne illness?
   a Washing fruits before serving them
   b Keeping cooked foods at or above 140°F until served
   c Storing eggs in the main section of the refrigerator
   d Using 1 cutting board for raw meat and vegetables

20 You should
   a Wash poultry before cooking it
   b Thaw ground beef on a counter top
   c Refrigerate left-over food within 4 hours
   d Wash kitchen surfaces with hot, soapy water

Answers to Chapter 30 questions are on p. 886.

FOCUS ON **PRACTICE**

Problem Solving

After receiving a breakfast tray, a resident says: "I didn't ask for eggs this morning." You check the dietary card and notice the tray is for another person. What will you do? Why is this a problem?

Fluid Needs

OBJECTIVES

- Define the key terms and key abbreviations in this chapter.
- Describe fluid requirements.
- Identify the causes and signs and symptoms of dehydration.
- Explain how to assist with special fluid orders.
- Explain the purpose of intake and output records.
- Identify what to count as fluid intake and output.

- Explain how to assist with fluid needs.
- Explain how to provide drinking water.
- Perform the procedures described in this chapter.
- Explain how to promote PRIDE in the person, the family, and yourself.

KEY TERMS

dehydration A decrease in the amount of water in body tissues
edema The swelling of body tissues with water
electrolytes Minerals dissolved in water
graduate A measuring container for fluid

hydration Having an adequate amount of water in body tissues
intake The amount of fluid taken in; input
output The amount of fluid lost

KEY ABBREVIATIONS

ID	Identification	mL	Milliliter
I&O	Intake and output	NPO	*Nil per os;* nothing by mouth
IV	Intravenous	oz	Ounce

Water is needed to live. Death can result from too much or too little water. You will help meet fluid needs. Measuring intake and output and providing drinking water are examples.

FLUID BALANCE

Water is ingested through fluids and foods. Water is lost through urine, feces (stools), and vomit. It is also lost through the skin (perspiration) and the lungs (expiration).

Hydration means having an adequate amount of water in body tissues. To stay hydrated, fluid intake must roughly equal output.

- *Intake* (input) *is the amount of fluid taken in.*
- *Output is the amount of fluid lost.*

Edema occurs when fluid intake exceeds fluid output. *Edema is the swelling of body tissues with water.* It is common in people with heart and kidney diseases. Edema often occurs in the legs, ankles, and feet (Fig. 31-1). Liver disorders can cause swelling in the abdomen (Chapter 50). *Pulmonary edema* is a severe form of edema affecting the lungs (Chapter 49).

Dehydration occurs when output exceeds intake. *Dehydration is a decrease in the amount of water in body tissues.* Common causes and signs and symptoms of dehydration are listed in Box 31-1.

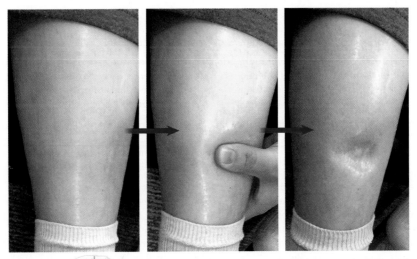

FIGURE 31-1 Eder~~~~~ ~~~~~~~~~ leg. The nurse applies pressure to the body part to check for edema. (Courtesy Kellie Wh~~~~)

BOX 31-1	**Dehydration**

Common Causes
- Bleeding
- Coma
- Dementia
- Diarrhea
- Drug therapy
- Fever
- Fluid intake: poor
- Fluid restriction
- Fluids: refusing
- Function problems: difficulty drinking, reaching fluids, communicating fluid needs
- Sweating: excess *(diaphoresis)*
- Urine production: increased
- Vomiting

Sig~~ ~~~ ~~~~~~~~

FOCUS ON **CHILDREN AND OLDER PERSONS**

Normal Fluid Requirements

Children
Infants and young children have more body water than adults do. Excess fluid losses cannot be tolerated. They quickly cause death in an infant or child.

Older Persons
The amount of body water decreases with age. So does the thirst sensation. Older persons need water but may not feel thirsty. Offer water often.

Older persons are at risk for diseases affecting fluid balance. Examples include heart disease, kidney disease, cancer, and diabetes. Some drugs cause the body to lose fluids. Others cause the body to retain water. Dehydration and edema are risks. Some persons have special fluid orders.

Electrolytes. *Electrolytes are minerals dissolved in water.* Sodium, potassium, calcium, and magnesium are some electrolytes. Electrolytes are needed for:
- Fluid balance
- Acid-base (pH) balance (Chapter 10)
- Movement of nutrients into the cells and wastes out of the cells
- Nerve, muscle, heart, and brain function

An *electrolyte imbalance* occurs when an electrolyte level is too low or too high. Dehydration and having too much body water are causes. Heart, kidney, and liver disorders can affect electrolyte levels. So can certain drugs and intravenous (IV) therapy (Chapter 32). Normal fluid and electrolyte levels are needed for body function.

SPECIAL FLUID ORDERS
The person may need a special fluid order to meet fluid needs. Intake and output (I&O) records are kept. Common fluid orders are listed in Table 31-1, p. 482. The order will be part of the person's care plan.

Normal Fluid Require~~~~~~~~
An adult needs 1500 mL (~~~~~~~~ ~~~ ~~~~~ ~y to survive. About 2000 to 250~~ ~~~~~ ~~ ~~~~~~~ ~ormal fluid balance. Water requ~~~~~~~~~ ~~~ ~~ ~ith hot weather, exercise, pregnan~~~ ~~~~~~~~ ~~~, fever, illness, and excess fluid loss~~~

See *Focus on Children an~ ~~~~~~ ~~~~~~~~ Normal Fluid Requirements.*

TABLE 31-1	Common Fluid Orders		
Fluid Order	Description	Some Uses	Care Measures
Encourage fluids	The person drinks an increased amount of fluid.	Dehydration, urinary tract infections, kidney stones	• Follow the care plan for the amount. • Keep a variety of fluids within the person's reach. • Offer fluids often and help the person drink if not able to do so alone.
Restrict fluids	Fluids are limited to a certain amount.	Edema, kidney failure, heart failure	• Follow the care plan for the amount allowed. • Offer fluids in small amounts and in small containers. • Remove the water mug or keep it out of sight. • Provide frequent oral hygiene to keep the mouth moist.
Nothing by mouth (NPO)	The person cannot eat or drink anything. NPO stands for *nil per os*—nothing *(nil)* by *(per)* mouth *(os)*.	Before and after surgery, before some laboratory tests and diagnostic procedures, to treat certain illnesses	• Post an NPO sign above the bed. • Remove the water mug from the room. • Provide frequent oral hygiene. The person must not swallow any fluid. • Follow the nurse's directions for how long the person will be NPO. The person is NPO for 6 to 12 hours before surgery and for some tests and procedures.
Thickened liquids	Water and all fluids are thickened by the dietary department.	Difficulty swallowing	• Serve thickened liquids as directed by the nurse and the care plan. Thickened commercial fluids are used. Or the dietary department thickens fluids. • Follow agency policy for how to record intake for thickened liquids. • See "The Dysphagia Diet" in Chapter 30.

INTAKE AND OUTPUT

You will measure and record intake and output (I&O).
- *Intake.* All oral fluids are measured and recorded—water, milk, coffee, tea, juices, soups, and soft drinks. So are foods that melt at room temperature—ice cream, sherbet, custard, gelatin, and Popsicles. The nurse measures and records IV fluids and tube feedings (Chapter 32).
- *Output.* Urine, vomitus, diarrhea, and wound drainage amounts are measured and recorded.

I&O records are used to plan and evaluate treatment. They also are kept for special fluid orders.

Measuring Intake and Output

Intake and output are measured in milliliters (mL). See Box 31-2 for amounts to know.

You must know the serving sizes of bowls, dishes, cups, pitchers, mugs, glasses, and other containers. This information may be on the I&O record (Fig. 31-2). Or the serving size is on the container.

A measuring container for fluid is called a **graduate**. Separate graduates are used for intake (left-over fluids) and for output—urine, vomitus, and drainage from suction. Like a measuring cup, the graduate is marked in ounces (oz) and milliliters (mL). For an accurate measurement, place the device on a flat surface and read it at eye level (Fig. 31-3).

BOX 31-2	I&O Measures
1 cubic centimeter (cc) = 1 mL	
1 teaspoon = 5 mL	
1 tablespoon = 15 mL	
1 oz = 30 mL	
1 cup = 240 mL	
1 pint = about 500 mL	
1 quart = about 1000 mL	
1 liter (L) = 1000 mL	

When intake or output is measured, the amount is recorded in the correct column on the I&O record (see Fig. 31-2). Amounts are totaled at the end of the shift and 24-hour day. The totals are recorded in the person's chart. They also are shared during the end-of-shift report.

The purpose of measuring I&O and how to help are explained to the person. Some persons measure and record their intake. Family members may help. The urinal, commode, bedpan, or specimen pan (Chapter 38) is used to void. Remind the person not to void in the toilet. Also remind the person to put toilet paper into the wastebasket.

See *Focus on Math: Measuring Intake and Output*, p. 484.
See *Delegation Guidelines: Measuring Intake and Output*.
See *Promoting Safety and Comfort: Measuring Intake and Output*, p. 484.
See procedure: *Measuring Intake and Output*, p. 485.

FLUID INTAKE AND OUTPUT FLOW SHEET
DATE *Oct 12*

RECORD TOTALS IN PATIENT'S MEDICAL RECORD			DIET/FLUID ORDERS *Regular*
Water glass	240 mL	Gelatin	120 mL
Juice glass	120 mL	Ice cream	90 mL
Milk carton	240 mL	Broth/strained soup	180 mL
Coffee cup	240 mL	Styrofoam cup	180 mL
Soft drink can	360 mL	Water mug	1000 mL
Tea glass	180 mL	Ice chips	½ amount of mL in cup

	INTAKE						OUTPUT		
	TIME	ORAL	TYPE & AMOUNT	TIME	IV	ENTERAL	TIME	SOURCE	AMOUNT
2300-0700		FLUIDS					*2330*	*Void*	*225 mL*
							0545	*Void*	*325 mL*
	0645	MUG/OTHER	*Water 200 mL*						
					8-HOUR SUB-TOTAL	*200 mL*	**8-HOUR SUB-TOTAL**		*550 mL*
0700-1500	*0830*	BREAKFAST	*Coffee 240 mL* *Milk 160 mL*				*0750*	*Void*	*200 mL*
							0930	*Void*	*225 mL*
							1145	*Void*	*250 mL*
							1330	*Void*	*200 mL*
	1015	SNACK	*Juice 120 mL*						
	1230	LUNCH	*Soft drink 240 mL* *Ice cream 90 mL* *Soup 90 mL*						
		SNACK							
	1450	MUG/OTHER	*Water 300 mL*						
					8-HOUR SUB-TOTAL	*1240 mL*	**8-HOUR SUB-TOTAL**		*875 mL*
1500-2300	1740	DINNER	Tea 180 mL Soft drink 100 mL				1505	Void	275 mL
							1655	Void	150 mL
							2010	Void	150 mL
							2115	Vomitus	100 mL
	1930	SNACK	Gelatin 120 mL						
	2230	MUG/OTHER	Water 325 mL						
					8-HOUR SUB-TOTAL	725 mL	**8-HOUR SUB-TOTAL**		675 mL
					24-HOUR TOTAL	2165 mL	**24-HOUR TOTAL**		2100 mL

FIGURE 31-2 A sample intake and output (I&O) record.

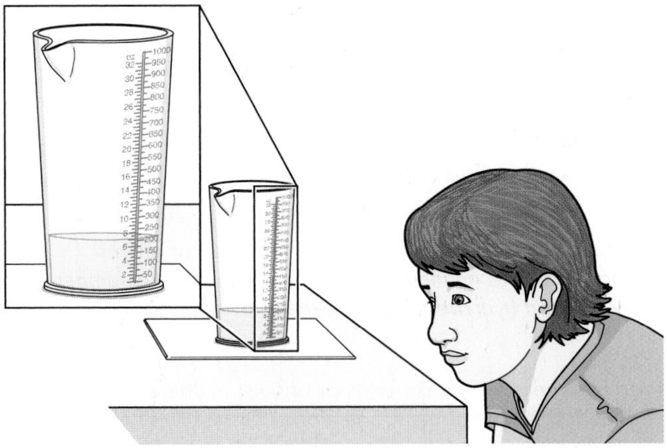

FIGURE 31-3 A graduate is on a flat surface. The amount is read at eye level.

DELEGATION GUIDELINES

Measuring Intake and Output

Measuring I&O is a routine nursing task. You need this information from the nurse and the care plan.

- If the person has a special fluid order (p. 481)
- When to report measurements—hourly or end-of-shift
- What the person uses for voiding—urinal, bedpan, commode, or specimen pan (Chapters 27 and 38)
- If the person has a catheter (Chapter 28)
- What patient or resident concerns to report at once

FOCUS ON MATH

Measuring Intake and Output

To measure I&O, you must accurately read measurements. You may have to do some math.

Measuring Intake

To measure intake, subtract the amount left in each liquid served from the full serving amount. For total intake, add the intake amounts from each liquid together.

Intake is measured in mL (milliliters). Some containers show the serving amount in oz (ounces). You need to convert (change) the serving amount from oz to mL. One oz equals 30 mL (1 oz = 30 mL). To convert, multiply the number of oz by 30. For example:

A coffee cup holds 8 oz. Multiply 8 oz by 30 (the number of mL in each oz). The full serving amount is 240 mL.

$$8 \text{ oz} \times 30 \text{ mL/oz} = 240 \text{ mL}$$
(mL/oz is read as "milliliters per ounce")

You measure 90 mL left in the cup. Subtract 90 mL (amount left) from 240 mL (serving amount). The person drank 150 mL.

$$240 \text{ mL (full serving)} - 90 \text{ mL (amount left)} = 150 \text{ mL intake}$$

Measuring Output

Measuring containers are marked in oz and mL. Urinals and specimen pans used to measure output may not have all lines labeled. To calculate unlabeled measurements (Fig. 31-4):

1 Choose the labeled line above the fluid level and the labeled line below it.

400 mL and 300 mL

2 Subtract these 2 numbers. The result is called the *difference*.

400 mL − 300 mL = 100 mL

3 Count the number of spaces between the 2 labeled lines in step 1.

4 spaces

4 Divide the difference in step 2 by the number of spaces.

100 mL ÷ 4 spaces = 25 mL
Each line increases by 25 mL.

Totaling Intake and Output

Intake and output amounts are each totaled at the end of the shift and 24-hour day. See Figure 31-2. Add the amounts for intake and the amounts for output. For example:

- Total shift intake amount: *During your shift a person drank 220 mL at breakfast, 390 mL at lunch, 90 mL as a snack, and 400 mL of water. The total intake for your shift is 1100 mL.*

$$220 \text{ mL} + 390 \text{ mL} + 90 \text{ mL} + 400 \text{ mL} = 1100 \text{ mL}$$

- Total shift output amount: *A person voided 3 times during your shift—200 mL, 250 mL, and 100 mL. The total output for your shift is 550 mL.*

$$200 \text{ mL} + 250 \text{ mL} + 100 \text{ mL} = 550 \text{ mL}$$

- Total 24-hour intake amount: *A person had 125 mL during the first shift, 1100 mL during the second shift, and 600 mL during the third shift. The total 24-hour day amount is 1825 mL.*

$$125 \text{ mL} + 1100 \text{ mL} + 600 \text{ mL} = 1825 \text{ mL}$$

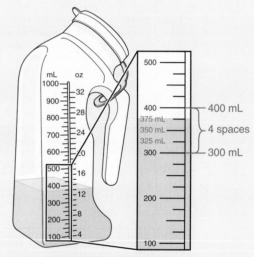

400 mL − 300 mL = 100 mL
100 mL ÷ 4 = 25 mL
Each line increases by 25 mL.

FIGURE 31-4 Calculating unlabeled measurements. Divide the difference between 2 labeled lines by the number of spaces between the 2 lines. Each line on this urinal increases by 25 mL. The measurements between 300 mL and 400 mL are 325 mL, 350 mL, and 375 mL.

PROMOTING SAFETY AND COMFORT

Measuring Intake and Output

Safety

Urine, vomitus, diarrhea, and wound drainage may contain microbes and blood. Microbes can grow in urinals, commodes, bedpans, specimen pans, kidney basins, and drainage systems. Follow Standard Precautions and the Bloodborne Pathogen Standard. Thoroughly clean the item with a disinfectant after it is used.

Remember to use separate graduates for intake and output.

NOTE: *A task may require more than 1 pair of gloves. Change gloves as needed. Use careful judgment. Remember to practice hand hygiene after removing gloves.*

Comfort

Promptly measure the contents of urinals, bedpans, commodes, specimen pans, and kidney basins. This helps prevent or reduce odors. Odors can disturb the person.

Measuring Intake and Output

QUALITY OF LIFE

- Knock before entering the person's room.
- Address the person by name.
- Introduce yourself by name and title.

- Explain the procedure before starting and during the procedure.
- Protect the person's rights during the procedure.
- Handle the person gently during the procedure.

PRE-PROCEDURE

1 Follow *Delegation Guidelines: Measuring Intake and Output*, p. 483. See *Promoting Safety and Comfort: Measuring Intake and Output.*
2 Practice hand hygiene.

3 Collect the following.
   - I&O record
   - 2 graduates:
     - A graduate for intake
     - A graduate for output
   - Gloves
   - Paper towels

PROCEDURE

4 Put on gloves.
5 Measure intake.
   a Pour liquid remaining in the container into the graduate used to measure intake. Avoid spills and splashes on the outside of the graduate.
   b Place the graduate on a flat surface. Measure the amount at eye level (see Fig. 31-3).
   c Check the serving amount on the I&O record. Or check the serving size of each container.
   d Subtract the remaining amount from the full serving amount. Note the amount. (For example, a cup holds 240 mL. The amount in the graduate is 50 mL. 240 mL – 50 mL = 190 mL.)
   e Pour fluid in the graduate back into the container.
   f Repeat steps 5, a-e for each liquid.
   g Add the amounts from each liquid together.
   h Record the time and amount on the I&O record.

6 Measure output.
   a Pour the fluid into the graduate used to measure output. Avoid spills and splashes on the outside of the graduate.
   b Place the device on a paper towel on a flat surface. Measure the amount at eye level.
   c Dispose of fluid in the toilet. Avoid splashes.
7 Clean, rinse, disinfect, and dry the graduates. Dispose of rinse in the toilet and flush. Use clean, dry paper towels for drying. Return the graduates to their proper place.
8 Clean, rinse, disinfect, and dry the voiding receptacle or other container. Dispose of rinse in the toilet and flush. Use clean, dry paper towels for drying. Return the item to its proper place.
9 Remove and discard the gloves. Practice hand hygiene.
10 Record the output amount on the person's I&O record.

POST-PROCEDURE

11 Provide for comfort. (See the inside of the back cover.)
12 Place the call light and other needed items within reach.

13 Complete a safety check of the room. (See the inside of the back cover.)
14 Report and record your observations.

PROVIDING DRINKING WATER

You provide fresh drinking water each shift and when the water mug is empty (Fig. 31-5).

Some agencies do not use the procedure on the next page. Instead, each mug is filled as needed. You take the mug to an ice and water dispenser. Fill the mug with ice first. Then add water. Follow the agency's procedure for providing fresh drinking water.

See *Focus on Communication: Providing Drinking Water*, p. 486.

See *Delegation Guidelines: Providing Drinking Water*, p. 486.

See *Promoting Safety and Comfort: Providing Drinking Water*, p. 486.

See procedure: *Providing Drinking Water*, p. 486.

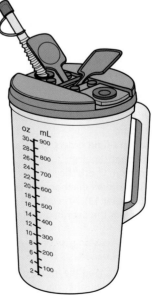

FIGURE 31-5 Water mug with straw. The mug is marked in milliliters (mL) and ounces (oz).

FOCUS ON COMMUNICATION
Providing Drinking Water

People vary about ice in their water. Ask what the person prefers. You can say:

- "Do you want ice in your water?"
- "How much ice do you want in your water?"
- "Do you like more ice or more water?"

Also ask where to place the mug. Be sure the person can reach it.

DELEGATION GUIDELINES
Providing Drinking Water

Providing drinking water is a routine nursing task. You need this information from the nurse and the care plan.

- The person's fluid orders
- If the person can have ice
- If the person uses a straw

PROMOTING SAFETY AND COMFORT
Providing Drinking Water

Safety

Water mugs can spread microbes. To prevent the spread of microbes:

- Label the mug with the person's name and room and bed number.
- Do not touch the rim or inside of the mug or lid.
- Do not let the ice scoop touch the mug, lid, or straw.
- Place the ice scoop in the scoop holder or on a towel for the scoop. Do not place it in the ice container or dispenser.
- Keep the ice chest closed when not in use.
- Make sure the mug is clean. Also check for cracks and chips. Provide a new mug as needed.

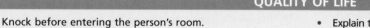

Providing Drinking Water

QUALITY OF LIFE

- Knock before entering the person's room.
- Address the person by name.
- Introduce yourself by name and title.

- Explain the procedure before starting and during the procedure.
- Protect the person's rights during the procedure.
- Handle the person gently during the procedure.

PRE-PROCEDURE

1. Follow *Delegation Guidelines: Providing Drinking Water*. See *Promoting Safety and Comfort: Providing Drinking Water*.
2. Obtain a list of special fluid orders from the nurse. Or use your assignment sheet.
3. Practice hand hygiene.
4. Collect the following.
   - Cart
   - Ice chest filled with ice
   - Cover for the ice chest

   - Scoop
   - Paper towels
   - Water mugs
   - Water pitcher filled with cold water (optional depending on agency procedure)
   - Towel for the scoop
5. Cover the cart with paper towels. Arrange equipment on top of the paper towels.

PROCEDURE

6. Take the cart to the person's room door. Do not take the cart into the room.
7. Check the person's fluid orders. Use the list from the nurse or your assignment sheet.
8. Identify the person. Check the identification (ID) bracelet against the fluid orders sheet or your assignment sheet. Use 2 identifiers (Chapter 13). Also call the person by name.
9. Take the mug from the over-bed table. Empty it into the bathroom sink.

10. Determine if a new mug is needed.
11. Use the scoop to fill the mug with ice (Fig. 31-6). Do not let the scoop touch the mug, lid, or straw.
12. Place the ice scoop on the towel.
13. Fill the mug with water. Get water from the room sink or bathroom sink or the water pitcher on the cart.
14. Place the mug on the over-bed table.
15. Make sure the mug is within the person's reach.

POST-PROCEDURE

16. Provide for comfort. (See the inside of the back cover.)
17. Place the call light and other needed items within reach.
18. Complete a safety check of the room. (See the inside of the back cover.)

19. Practice hand hygiene.
20. Repeats steps 6 through 19 for each person.

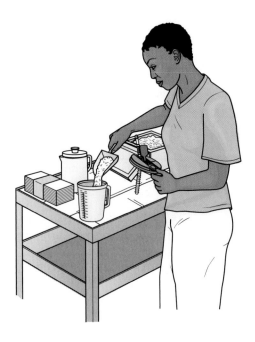

FIGURE 31-6 Providing drinking water.

FOCUS ON **PRIDE**

The Person, Family, and Yourself

Personal and Professional Responsibility

An *attentive* person is careful, alert, and thorough. These qualities are important when assisting with fluid needs. Follow each person's fluid order. Measure and record I&O correctly. Watch for signs and symptoms of dehydration. Report problems at once.

Rights and Respect

Patients and residents may complain about orders and treatments. For example, a resident does not like thickened liquids. Or a patient has an order to encourage fluids. The person is tired of being reminded to drink. Do not ignore complaints. They communicate needs. Listen and show respect.

Independence and Social Interaction

Personal choice promotes independence. Ask about the person's preferences. Drink choice, straw use, the amount of ice in drinks, and cream or sugar in coffee are examples.

Delegation and Teamwork

Some skills require math. Measuring I&O is an example. Math is hard for some persons. You may need extra practice. Tell your instructor. On the job, ask the nurse if you have a question. Do not be embarrassed to ask for help.

Ethics and Laws

Watch closely for changes in hydration. The case below is a real example of how poor hydration resulted in harm.

Mr. Phillip Caruso was admitted to a nursing center on January 22 after about 5 weeks of hospital care. On January 23, the doctor found him to be in stable condition. He showed signs of adequate hydration and responded to the doctor's commands.

The nursing center "did not keep a chart of Phillip's intake or output of fluids." According to the nurses, Mr. Caruso received:

- *3 meals a day.*
- *3 snacks [a day] with juice or milk.*
- *Drugs 4 times a day. He was given 4 oz of water with the drugs.*
- *Offers of something to drink every 2 hours during the night.*

Seven days later (January 29), Mr. Caruso was taken to the hospital. The emergency room doctor diagnosed severe dehydration. He was weak, confused, had tremors, and had dry skin with poor turgor. In the hospital, Mr. Caruso was treated with IV fluids and a catheter and for a urinary tract infection caused by the catheter.

Mr. Caruso returned to the nursing center on February 19. He died on May 14.

His family sued and charged the nursing center with negligence, abuse, and neglect for failing to give Mr. Caruso enough water. They claimed that the dehydration led to declines in his physical and mental condition.

The jury found in favor of the family. The jury awarded the family $195,000 and attorney fees. The nursing home appealed the case. Because of a legal technicality, a judge ordered a new trial.

(I. Caruso v Pine Manor Nursing Center, Ill., 1989.)

You can do your part to promote good fluid intake. Follow the person's care plan. Carefully record intake and output as ordered. Tell the nurse if you notice a change in the person's intake.

FOCUS ON **PRIDE**: *Application*

A patient with an order to restrict fluids complains of thirst. How can you meet the person's needs?

REVIEW QUESTIONS

Circle the BEST answer.

1 A person with diarrhea has scant, dark yellow urine. This is a sign of
   a Normal hydration
   b Edema
   c Infection
   d Dehydration

2 A person has edema. Which should you question?
   a Restrict fluids.
   b Encourage fluids.
   c Provide frequent oral hygiene.
   d Monitor I&O.

3 A person is NPO. You should
   a Provide a variety of fluids
   b Remove the water mug from the room
   c Offer fluids in small amounts and in small containers
   d Remove oral hygiene equipment from the room

4 Which are counted as fluid intake?
   a Broths and ice cream
   b Sauces and melted cheese
   c Thick stews and mashed potatoes
   d Butter and syrup

5 A person drank all of an 8 oz carton of milk. How many mL of fluid would you chart on the I&O record?
   a 8 mL
   b 60 mL
   c 120 mL
   d 240 mL

6 A person was served 240 mL of coffee and 120 mL of juice. You measure 50 mL of coffee and 60 mL of juice left. What do you chart for intake on the I&O record?
   a 110 mL
   b 250 mL
   c 370 mL
   d 480 mL

7 When measuring intake and output
   a Convert measurements to ounces
   b Use the same graduate for intake and output
   c Place the graduate on a flat surface and read it at eye level
   d Gloves are not needed

8 During your shift a patient vomited twice—125 mL and 75 mL. The patient had diarrhea once—50 mL. You empty 500 mL from the urine drainage bag. What is the total shift output amount?
   a 200 mL
   b 250 mL
   c 500 mL
   d 750 mL

9 Before providing fresh drinking water, you need to know the person's
   a Intake
   b Fluid orders
   c Diet
   d Preferred beverages

10 Which prevents contamination when passing drinking water?
   a Labeling the mug with the person's name
   b Keeping the ice chest open when not in use
   c Leaving the ice scoop in the ice container
   d Touching the mug with the ice scoop

Answers to Chapter 31 questions are on p. 886.

FOCUS ON **PRACTICE**

Problem Solving

A resident with an order for thickened liquids was served coffee without thickener. What will you do? What is the purpose of thickened liquid?

Nutritional Support and IV Therapy

OBJECTIVES

- Define the key terms and key abbreviations in this chapter.
- Identify the reasons for nutritional support and IV therapy.
- Explain how tube feedings are given.
- Describe scheduled and continuous feedings.
- Explain how to prevent aspiration.
- Describe the comfort measures for the person with a feeding tube.
- Describe parenteral nutrition.
- Describe the IV therapy sites.

- Identify the equipment used in IV therapy.
- Describe how to assist with the IV flow rate.
- Identify the safety measures for IV therapy.
- Identify the observations to report during nutritional support or IV therapy.
- Explain how to assist with nutritional support and IV therapy.
- Explain how to promote PRIDE in the person, the family, and yourself.

KEY TERMS

aspiration Breathing fluid, food, vomitus, or an object into the lungs

enteral nutrition Giving nutrients into the gastro-intestinal (GI) tract *(enteral)* through a feeding tube

flow rate The number of drops per minute *(gtt/min)* or milliliters per hour *(mL/hr)*

gastrostomy tube A feeding tube inserted through a surgically created opening *(stomy)* in the stomach *(gastro);* stomach tube

gavage The process of giving a tube feeding

intravenous (IV) therapy Giving fluids through a needle or catheter inserted into a vein; IV and IV infusion

jejunostomy tube A feeding tube inserted into a surgically created opening *(stomy)* in the *jejunum* of the small intestine

naso-enteral tube A feeding tube inserted through the nose *(naso)* into the small bowel *(enteral)*

naso-gastric (NG) tube A feeding tube inserted through the nose *(naso)* into the stomach *(gastro)*

parenteral nutrition Giving nutrients through a catheter inserted into a vein; *para* means *beyond; enteral* relates to the *bowel*

percutaneous endoscopic gastrostomy (PEG) tube A feeding tube inserted into the stomach *(gastro)* through a small incision *(stomy)* made through *(per)* the skin *(cutaneous);* a lighted instrument *(scope)* is used to see inside a body cavity or organ *(endo)*

regurgitation The backward flow of stomach contents into the mouth

KEY ABBREVIATIONS

GI	Gastro-intestinal	NG	Naso-gastric
gtt	Drops	NPO	Nothing by mouth
gtt/min	Drops per minute	oz	Ounce
IV	Intravenous	PEG	Percutaneous endoscopic gastrostomy
mL	Milliliter	TPN	Total parenteral nutrition
mL/hr	Milliliters per hour		

Many persons cannot eat or drink because of illness, surgery, or injury. They may have chewing, swallowing, or other eating problems. Some persons refuse to eat or drink. Others cannot eat enough to meet their nutritional needs. Nutritional support or intravenous (IV) therapy may be ordered to meet food and fluid needs.

See *Delegation Guidelines: Nutritional Support and IV Therapy.*

DELEGATION GUIDELINES

Nutritional Support and IV Therapy

Tasks involving nutritional support and IV therapy are nursing responsibilities. Your state and agency may allow you to assist with some of the care measures in this chapter. Before doing so, make sure that:

- Your state allows you to perform the task.
- The task is in your job description.
- You have had the necessary education and training.
- You know how to use the agency's equipment and supplies.
- You review the agency's procedure.
- You review the task with the nurse.
- A nurse is available to guide and assist you as needed.
- An RN (registered nurse) has identified and labeled all tubes, catheters, and needles.

  NOTE: A task may require more than 1 pair of gloves. Change gloves as needed. Use careful judgment. Remember to practice hand hygiene after removing gloves.

ENTERAL NUTRITION

Some persons cannot or will not ingest, chew, or swallow food. Or food cannot pass from the mouth into the esophagus and into the stomach or small intestine. Poor nutrition results. Common causes are:

- Cancer, especially cancers of the head, neck, and esophagus
- Trauma to the face, mouth, head, or neck
- Coma (Chapter 13)
- *Dysphagia* (difficulty swallowing)
- Dementia (Chapter 53)
- Eating disorders (Chapter 52)
- Nervous system disorders (Chapter 48)
- Prolonged vomiting
- Major trauma or surgery
- Acquired immunodeficiency syndrome (AIDS) (Chapter 47)
- Illnesses and disorders affecting eating and nutrition

Enteral nutrition is giving nutrients into the gastro-intestinal (GI) tract (enteral) through a feeding tube. Gavage is the process of giving a tube feeding. Tube feedings replace or supplement (add to) normal nutrition.

Types of Feeding Tubes

These feeding tubes are common.

- *Naso-gastric (NG) tube. A feeding tube is inserted through the nose* (naso) *into the stomach* (gastro) (Fig. 32-1). A doctor or an RN inserts the tube.
- *Naso-enteral tube. A feeding tube is inserted through the nose* (naso) *into the small bowel* (enteral) (Fig. 32-2). A doctor or RN inserts the tube.
- *Gastrostomy tube. A feeding tube is inserted through a surgically created opening* (stomy) *in the stomach* (gastro). It is also called a stomach tube. See Figure 32-3. A doctor inserts the tube.
- *Jejunostomy tube. A feeding tube is inserted into a surgically created opening* (stomy) *in the* jejunum *of the small intestine* (Fig. 32-4).
- *Percutaneous endoscopic gastrostomy (PEG) tube. A feeding tube is inserted into the stomach* (gastro) *through a small incision* (stomy) *made through* (per) *the skin* (cutaneous). *A lighted instrument* (scope) *is used to see inside a body cavity or organ* (endo). See Figure 32-5. A doctor inserts the tube.

NG and naso-enteral tubes are used for short-term nutritional support—usually less than 6 weeks. Gastrostomy, jejunostomy, and PEG tubes are used for long-term nutritional support—usually more than 6 weeks.

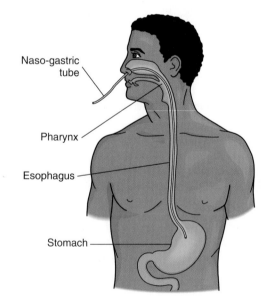

FIGURE 32-1 A naso-gastric (NG) tube is inserted through the nose and esophagus and into the stomach.

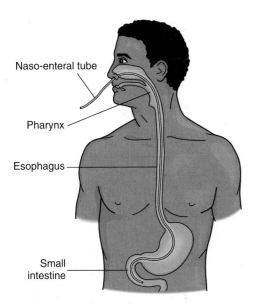

FIGURE 32-2 A naso-enteral tube is inserted through the nose and into the small intestine.

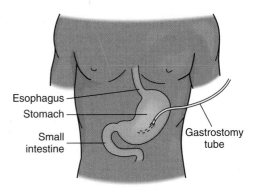

FIGURE 32-3 A gastrostomy tube.

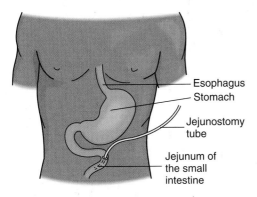

FIGURE 32-4 A jejunostomy tube.

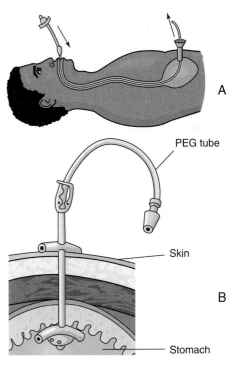

FIGURE 32-5 A, A percutaneous endoscopic gastrostomy (PEG) tube is inserted. **B,** PEG tube in place.

Formulas

The doctor orders the type of formula, the amount to give, and when to give tube feedings. Most formulas contain proteins, carbohydrates, fats, vitamins, and minerals. Commercial formulas are common.

See *Teamwork and Time Management: Formulas.*
See *Promoting Safety and Comfort: Formulas.*

TEAMWORK AND TIME MANAGEMENT

Formulas

The nurse and manufacturer's instructions tell you how long formula can hang. Check the time that the feeding started. Remind the nurse when the time limit is near. For example, a feeding started at 0800. It can hang for 8 hours (until 1600). At 1530 or 1545, tell the nurse how much time is left. Also report the amount of formula left.

PROMOTING SAFETY AND COMFORT

Formulas

Safety

Like food, microbes can grow in formula and cause illness if not stored properly. Un-opened formula is stored at room temperature. Open, un-used formula is stored in the refrigerator. The formula must be covered and labeled with the date and time. The formula is discarded after 24 hours.

Comfort

Cold fluids can cause cramping. Formula is given at room temperature. Refrigerated formula is warmed to room temperature. Follow the manufacturer's instructions for warming cold formula. The nurse may have you set the formula out at room temperature for 30 minutes before the feeding. Do not use a microwave or stove to warm formula.

Feeding Methods

Tube feedings can be given in 3 ways.

- *Syringe feeding* (Fig. 32-6, *A*)—formula is poured into a syringe. The syringe attaches to the feeding tube. The height of the syringe controls how fast the formula flows.
- *Gravity feeding* (Fig. 32-6, *B*)—formula is in a feeding bag. Tubing connects the bag to the feeding tube. The bag hangs on a pole. A clamp on the tubing and the height of the bag control how fast the formula flows.
- *Pump feeding* (Fig. 32-6, *C*)—a feeding pump is used. Formula is pumped from the bag, through connecting tubing, and into the feeding tube. Formula drips into the feeding tube at a certain rate.

After a syringe or gravity feeding, the nurse removes the syringe or connecting tubing. The nurse clamps and covers the end of the feeding tube with a cap or gauze. Clamping prevents air from entering the tube and fluid from leaking out. Covering the end also prevents leaking.

Feeding Times

Tube feedings are given at certain times. Or they are given over a 24-hour period.

Scheduled feedings (intermittent feedings) are given at certain times. (*Intermittent* means *to start, stop, and then start again.*) Between 3 and 8 feedings are given each day. Usually 8 to 12 ounces (oz) (240 to 360 milliliters [mL])

are given over about 30 minutes or less for an adult. The frequency, amount, and time are like a normal eating pattern.

Continuous feedings are usually given over 24 hours. A feeding pump is used (see Fig. 32-6, *C*). The person receives a certain amount each hour. A pump alarm sounds if something is wrong. When you hear an alarm, tell the nurse.

Observations

Diarrhea, constipation, delayed stomach emptying, and aspiration are risks. *Aspiration is breathing fluid, food, vomitus, or an object into the lungs.* Report the following at once.

- Nausea
- Discomfort during the feeding
- Vomiting
- Distended (enlarged and swollen) abdomen
- Coughing
- Complaints of indigestion or heartburn
- Redness, swelling, drainage, odor, or pain at the ostomy site
- Fever
- Signs and symptoms of respiratory distress (Chapter 43)
- Increased pulse rate
- Complaints of flatulence (Chapter 29)
- Diarrhea (Chapter 29)

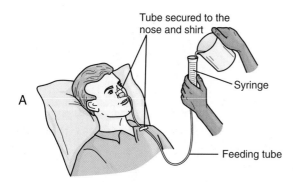

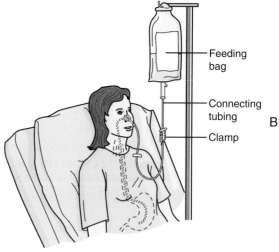

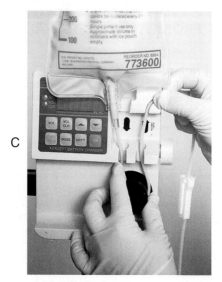

FIGURE 32-6 Tube feeding methods. **A,** Syringe feeding. A tube feeding is given with a syringe. **B,** Gravity feeding. Formula drips from a feeding bag into the feeding tube. **C,** Pump feeding. A pump is used. (**C,** from Potter PA, Perry AG, Stockert PA, Hall AM: *Fundamentals of nursing*, ed 9, St Louis, 2017, Mosby.)

Regurgitation and Aspiration

Aspiration is a major risk from tube feedings. It can cause pneumonia and death. Aspiration can occur:

- *During insertion.* NG tubes and naso-enteral tubes are passed through the nose into the esophagus and then into the stomach or small intestine. The tube can slip into the airway. An x-ray is taken to check tube placement.
- *From tube movement out of place.* Coughing, sneezing, vomiting, suctioning, and poor positioning are common causes. A tube can move from the stomach or intestines into the esophagus and then into the airway. The RN checks tube placement before every scheduled tube feeding. With continuous feedings, the RN checks tube placement every 4 hours. The RN attaches a syringe to the tube. GI secretions are withdrawn through the syringe. Then the pH of the secretions is measured (Chapter 38). *You never check feeding tube placement.*
- *From regurgitation. Regurgitation is the backward flow of stomach contents into the mouth.* Delayed stomach emptying and over-feeding are common causes.

Preventing Regurgitation and Aspiration. To help prevent regurgitation and aspiration:

- Position the person in Fowler's or semi-Fowler's position before the feeding. Follow the care plan and the nurse's directions.
- Maintain Fowler's or semi-Fowler's position after the feeding. This allows formula to move through the GI tract. The position is required for 1 to 2 hours after the feeding or at all times. Follow the care plan and the nurse's directions.
- Avoid the left side-lying position. It prevents the stomach from emptying into the small intestine.

During digestion, food slowly passes from the stomach into the small intestine. The stomach handles larger amounts of food than the small intestine. With intestinal tubes, feedings are given at a slow rate. The risk of regurgitation is less with intestinal tubes than with NG or gastrostomy tubes.

Persons with NG or gastrostomy tubes are at high risk for regurgitation. Before a feeding, the nurse checks that the stomach is emptying normally. The nurse aspirates (pulls into a syringe) stomach contents and measures the amount. This is called *residual. Residual* means *what remains.* Depending on the amount, the nurse decides to give or delay the feeding. The intent is to prevent aspiration from regurgitation caused by over-feeding.

See *Focus on Children and Older Persons: Preventing Regurgitation and Aspiration.*

FOCUS ON CHILDREN AND OLDER PERSONS

Preventing Regurgitation and Aspiration

Older Persons
Digestion slows with aging. Stomach emptying also slows. Older persons are at risk for regurgitation and aspiration. Less formula and longer feeding times prevent over-feeding.

Comfort Measures

Persons with feeding tubes usually are not allowed to eat or drink. They are NPO—nothing by mouth (Chapter 31). Dry mouth, dry lips, and sore throat cause discomfort. Sometimes hard candy or gum is allowed. These measures are common every 2 hours while the person is awake.

- Oral hygiene
- Lubricant for the lips
- Mouth rinses

Feeding tubes can irritate and cause pressure on the nose. They can change the shape of the nostrils or cause pressure injuries. These measures are common.

- Clean the nose and nostrils every 4 to 8 hours.
- Secure the tube to the nose (Fig. 32-7). Use tape or a tube holder. Tube holders have foam cushions that prevent pressure on the nose. Re-taping is not needed. Re-taping irritates the nose.
- Secure the tube to the person's garment at the shoulder area (see Fig. 32-6). This prevents the tube from pulling or dangling. Both can cause pressure on the nose. Do 1 of the following according to agency policy.
  - Loop a rubber band around the tube. Then pin the rubber band to the garment with a safety pin.
  - Tape the tube to the garment.

Assisting With Tube Feedings

The nurse may ask you to assist with tube feedings. With more training, some states and agencies allow nursing assistants to give tube feedings and remove NG tubes. *Remember, you never insert feeding tubes, check their placement, or check residual stomach contents. They are the RN's responsibility.*

See *Delegation Guidelines: Assisting With Tube Feedings,* p. 494.

See *Promoting Safety and Comfort: Assisting With Tube Feedings,* p. 494.

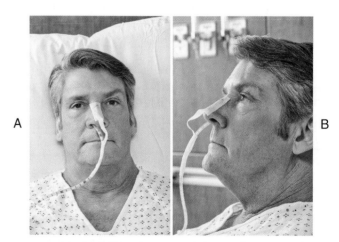

FIGURE 32-7 The feeding tube is secured to the nose. (From Perry AG, Potter PA, Ostendorf WR: *Nursing interventions & clinical skills,* ed 7, St Louis, 2020, Elsevier.)

Giving tube feedings and removing NG tubes are nursing responsibilities. If delegated to you, make sure that the conditions in *Delegation Guidelines: Nutritional Support and IV Therapy* (p. 490) are met.

If those conditions are met, you need this information from the nurse and the care plan.

- That the RN has checked tube placement and residual stomach contents
- The type of tube—NG, naso-enteral, gastrostomy, jejunostomy, or PEG
- What feeding method to use—syringe, gravity, or pump feeding
- What size syringe to use—usually 30 or 60 mL for an adult
- How to position the person for the feeding—Fowler's or semi-Fowler's
- How to position the person after the feeding—Fowler's or semi-Fowler's
- What formula to use
- How much formula to give
- How high to raise the syringe or hang the feeding bag (usually 18 to 24 inches above the stomach or intestines)
- The amount of flushing solution to use—usually 30 to 60 mL (1 to 2 oz) of water for an adult
- When to flush the feeding tube
- How fast to give the feeding if using a syringe—usually over 30 minutes or less
- The flow rate (in drops per minute) if a feeding bag is used (p. 498)
- The flow rate (in milliliters per hour) if a feeding pump is used (p. 498)
- If ice is kept around the bag for a continuous feeding
- If you are to remove an NG tube, when to remove the tube
- What observations to report and record
- When to report observations
- What patient or resident concerns to report at once

PARENTERAL NUTRITION

Parenteral nutrition is giving nutrients through a catheter inserted into a vein (Fig. 32-8). (Para *means* beyond. Enteral *relates to the* bowel.) A nutrient solution is given directly into the bloodstream. Nutrients do not enter the GI tract. Parenteral nutrition is often called *total parenteral nutrition (TPN)* or *hyperalimentation*. (*Hyper* means *high* or *excessive. Alimentation* means *nourishment.*)

The solution contains water, proteins, carbohydrates, vitamins, and minerals. It drips through a catheter inserted into a large vein. TPN is used when the person cannot receive oral or enteral feedings. Or it is used when oral or enteral feedings are not enough to meet nutrition needs.

Common reasons for TPN include:

- Disease, injury, or surgery to the GI tract
- Severe trauma, infection, or burns
- NPO for more than 5 to 7 days
- GI side effects from cancer treatments (Chapter 47)
- Prolonged coma
- Prolonged *anorexia* (loss of appetite)

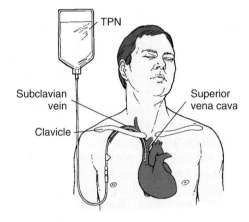

FIGURE 32-8 Parenteral nutrition. (From *Mosby's dictionary of medicine, nursing, and health professions,* ed 10, St Louis, 2017, Elsevier.)

Safety

Besides a feeding tube, the person may have an IV, a breathing tube (Chapter 44), and drainage tubes (Chapter 39). You must know the purpose of each tube. Have the nurse label each tube and its purpose. *Formula must enter only the feeding tube.* Otherwise, the person can die.

Before giving a tube feeding:

- Turn on the light. Do so even if the person is sleeping.
- Check and inspect the feeding tube and label with the nurse.
- Make sure an RN checks for tube placement.
- Make sure every tube, catheter, and needle is labeled.

- Trace the feeding tube back to the insertion site. Start at the end of the feeding tube. Trace the tube backward. For example, if the person has an NG tube, you will end at the nose. If the person has a gastrostomy tube, you will end at the abdomen. If you do not end at the correct place, do not give the tube feeding. Call for the nurse.

Nasal secretions may contain blood or microbes. So can drainage at an ostomy site. Wear gloves. Follow Standard Precautions and the Bloodborne Pathogen Standard.

Remind visitors to call for a nurse if any tube becomes disconnected. They could connect the wrong tubes together.

Observations

TPN risks include infection, fluid imbalances, and blood sugar imbalances. Report the following to the nurse at once.

- Fever, chills, and other signs and symptoms of infection (Chapter 16)
- Signs and symptoms of sugar imbalances (see "Diabetes" in Chapter 50)
- Chest pain
- Difficulty breathing or shortness of breath
- Cough
- Nausea and vomiting
- Diarrhea
- Thirst
- Rapid heart rate or an irregular heartbeat
- Weakness or fatigue
- Sweating
- *Pallor* (pale skin)
- Trembling
- Confusion or behavior changes

Assisting With TPN

The nurse is responsible for all aspects of TPN. To assist, carefully observe the person. Also assist with basic needs and activities of daily living. The person may be NPO. Provide frequent oral hygiene, lubricant to the lips, and mouth rinses as the nurse and care plan direct. Also follow other aspects of the person's care plan.

Many aspects of IV therapy apply to TPN.

IV THERAPY

Intravenous (IV) therapy (IV, IV infusion) is giving fluids through a needle or catheter inserted into a vein (Fig. 32-9). Fluid flows directly into the bloodstream. IV therapy is ordered to:

- Provide fluids when they cannot be taken by mouth.
- Replace minerals and vitamins lost from illness or injury.
- Provide sugar for energy.
- Give drugs and blood.

RNs are responsible for IV therapy. They start and maintain the infusion as ordered. RNs also give IV drugs and administer blood. State laws vary about your role and that of LPNs/LVNs in IV therapy.

IV Sites

Peripheral and central venous sites are used. *Peripheral* means *around (peri) a boundary (pheral).* The boundary is the center of the body near the heart. *Peripheral IV sites* are away from the center of the body. For adults, the back of the hand and inner forearm are useful sites (Fig. 32-10).

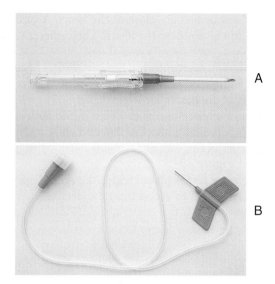

FIGURE 32-9 A, Intravenous catheter. **B,** Butterfly needle.

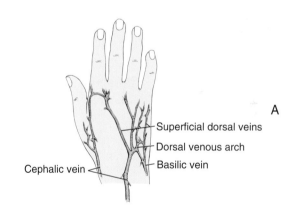
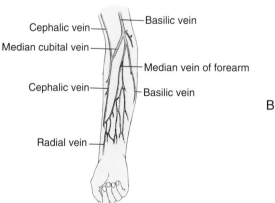

FIGURE 32-10 Peripheral IV sites. **A,** Back of the hand. **B,** Inner forearm. (From Potter PA, Perry AG, Stockert PA, Hall AM: *Fundamentals of nursing,* ed 8, St Louis, 2013, Mosby.)

Central venous sites are close to the heart. A catheter is threaded into a vein near the heart. The catheter is called a *central venous catheter* or a *central line.*

- A *peripherally inserted central catheter (PICC)* begins in a large peripheral vein in the upper arm. The catheter tip ends at the heart. See Figure 32-11, *A.*
- A *tunneled catheter* begins in a vein in the neck or chest. It is passed under the skin and ends at the heart. Part of the catheter remains outside the skin for use. See Figure 32-11, *B.*
- An *implanted port* is placed under the skin. A special needle is needed to access (use) the device. See Figure 32-11, *C.*

Central venous sites are used:
- For parenteral nutrition
- To give large amounts of fluid
- For long-term IV therapy
- To give drugs that irritate peripheral veins.
  See *Focus on Long-Term Care and Home Care: IV Sites.*
  See *Focus on Children and Older Persons: IV Sites.*

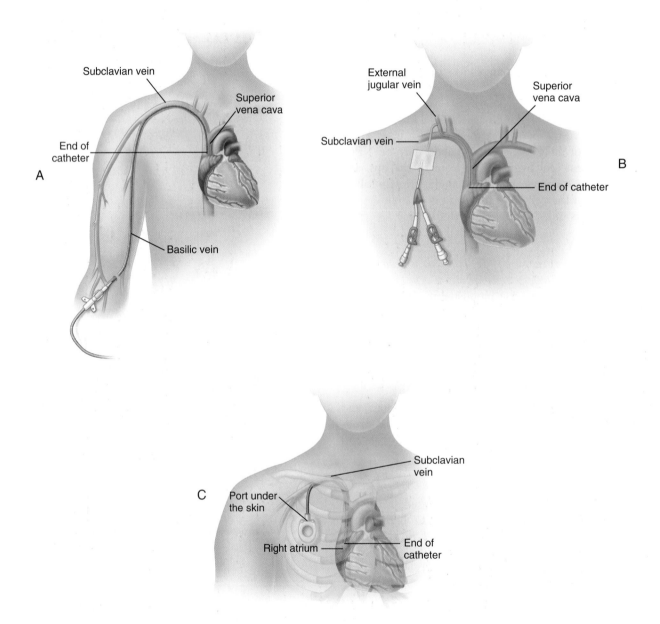

FIGURE 32-11 Central venous catheters. **A,** Peripherally inserted central catheter (PICC). **B,** Tunneled catheter. **C,** Implanted port. The device is under the skin. (Modified from Ignatavicious DD, Workman ML, Rebar C: *Medical-surgical nursing: patient-centered collaborative care,* ed 9, St Louis, 2018, Elsevier.)

IV Equipment

The basic equipment used in IV therapy is shown in Figure 32-13.

- The solution container is a plastic bag—*IV bag.*
- A *catheter* or *needle* is inserted into a vein (see Fig. 32-9).
- The *IV tube* or *infusion tubing* connects the IV bag to the catheter or needle.
- Fluid drips from the bag into the *drip chamber.*
- The *clamp* is used to regulate the flow rate.
- The IV bag hangs from an IV pole (IV standard) or ceiling hook.

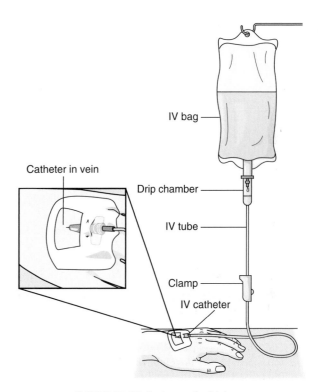

FIGURE 32-13 Equipment for IV therapy.

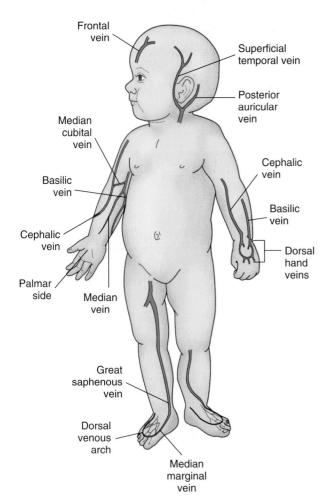

FIGURE 32-12 IV sites in children. (Modified from Hockenberry MJ, Wilson D: *Wong's nursing care of infants and children,* ed 10, St Louis, 2015, Mosby.)

Flow Rate

The doctor orders the amount of fluid to give *(infuse)* and the amount of time to give it in. With this information, the RN figures the flow rate. The *flow rate is the number of drops per minute (gtt/min) or milliliters per hour (mL/hr).* The abbreviation *gtt* means *drops.* The Latin word *guttae* means *drops.*

An electronic pump is often used (Fig. 32-14). The flow rate is displayed in mL/hr. An alarm sounds if something is wrong. Tell the nurse at once if you hear an alarm. If a pump is not used, the RN sets the clamp for the flow rate. *Never adjust any controls on IV pumps or change the position of the clamp.*

See *Focus on Math: Flow Rate.*

See *Teamwork and Time Management: Flow Rate.*

See *Promoting Safety and Comfort: Flow Rate.*

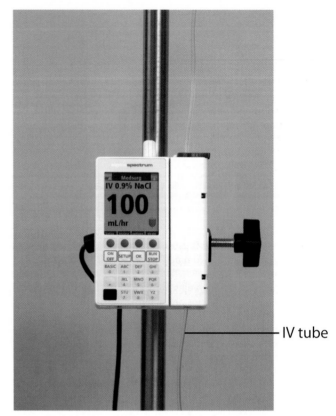

— IV tube

FIGURE 32-14 Electronic IV pump. (Modified from Williams PA: *Fundamental concepts and skills for nursing,* ed 5, St Louis, 2018, Elsevier.)

FOCUS ON MATH

Flow Rate

Counting Drops per Minute

You can check the flow rate when a pump is not used.

The nurse tells you the number of drops per minute (gtt/min). Use a watch. Count the number of drops that fall in the drip chamber in 1 minute (60 seconds). See Figure 32-15. Tell the nurse at once if:

- No fluid is dripping.
- The rate is too fast or too slow.
- The bag is empty or close to being empty.

For example: The nurse tells you the number of drops per minute is 25 gtt/min. You count 31 gtt/min.

> *31 gtt/min (rate counted) is greater than 25 gtt/min (correct rate).*
> *The rate is too fast. You tell the nurse.*

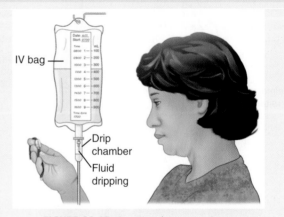

IV bag

Drip chamber

Fluid dripping

FIGURE 32-15 Counting drops per minute.

FOCUS ON **MATH**—cont'd

Flow Rate

Time Tape

A *time tape* tracks fluid given over a period of time (Fig. 32-16). The nurse marks the tape with times. If the rate is correct, the fluid level is at the nurse's mark on the tape at the correct time. To check the rate, compare the fluid level with the time on the tape.

- If the fluid is above the time line, the flow is too slow. Not enough fluid has been given.
- If the fluid is below the time line, the flow is too fast. Too much fluid has been given.

Tell the nurse at once if too little or too much fluid has been given.

For example, the doctor orders 1000 mL of fluid over 10 hours. The nurse calculates the flow rate and marks the time tape (see Fig. 32-16). The nurse starts the infusion at 0700 (7:00 AM). The nurse checks the fluid level for the first hour. You are asked to check the fluid level at 0900 (9:00 AM). At 0900, the fluid level is as shown in Figure 32-16. The fluid level is below the 0900 line. The flow is too fast. You tell the nurse.

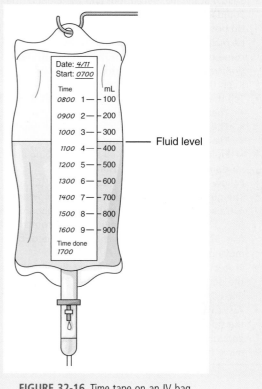

FIGURE 32-16 Time tape on an IV bag.

TEAMWORK AND TIME MANAGEMENT

Flow Rate

Patients and residents cared for by you and other staff may have IVs. When near the person or walking past the person's room, make sure the IV is dripping. Also check the amount of fluid in the bag. Report any problems to a nurse at once.

PROMOTING SAFETY AND COMFORT

Flow Rate

Safety

The person can suffer serious harm if the flow rate is too fast or too slow. The flow rate can change from:

- Position changes
- Kinked tubes
- Lying on the tube

Never change the position of the clamp or adjust any controls on infusion pumps. Tell the nurse at once about a problem with the flow rate.

Assisting With IV Therapy

You help meet the safety, hygiene, and activity needs of persons with IVs. Follow the safety measures in Box 32-1, p. 500. Report any sign or symptom listed in Box 32-1 at once.

Your state and agency may allow you to change dressings at peripheral IV sites. They also may let you discontinue (remove) a peripheral IV.

You never start or maintain IV therapy. Nor do you regulate the flow rate or change IV bags. You never give blood or IV drugs.

See *Focus on Communication: Assisting With IV Therapy*, p. 501.

See *Delegation Guidelines: Assisting With IV Therapy*, p. 501.

BOX 32-1	IV Therapy

Safety Measures

- Follow Standard Precautions and the Bloodborne Pathogen Standard.
- Do not move the needle or catheter. Correct position must be maintained. If the needle or catheter is moved, it may come out of the vein. Then fluid flows into tissues *(infiltration)*. Or the flow stops.
- Keep the IV site clean and dry.
- Tell the nurse if an IV pump alarm sounds. This may mean:
  - There is air in the tubing.
  - The infusion is done.
  - The pump's battery is low.
  - Fluid flow is blocked. Kinks in the tubing and closed clamps are common reasons.
- Follow the safety measures for restraints (Chapter 15). The nurse may splint (hold in position) or restrain the extremity to prevent movement. An armboard may be used (Fig. 32-17). Or the nurse may apply a protective device (Fig. 32-18). This helps prevent the needle or catheter from moving.
- Protect the IV bag, tubing, and needle or catheter when the person walks. Portable IV poles (IV standards) are used (Fig. 32-19).
- Assist with turning and re-positioning. Move the IV bag to the side of the bed where the person is lying. Allow enough slack in the tubing. The needle or catheter can move from pressure on the tube.

Signs and Symptoms of Complications

- Report the following at once.
  - Local—at the IV site
    - Bleeding
    - Blood backing up into the IV tube
    - Puffiness or swelling
    - Pale or reddened skin
    - Complaints of pain at or above the IV site
    - Hot or cold skin near the site
  - Systemic—involving the whole body
    - *Fever* (elevated body temperature)
    - Itching
    - Changes in blood pressure: increase or decrease
    - Pulse rate greater than 100 beats per minute
    - Irregular pulse
    - *Cyanosis* (bluish color)
    - Confusion or changes in mental function
    - Loss of consciousness
    - Difficulty breathing or shortness of breath
    - Decreasing or no urine output
    - Chest pain
    - Nausea

Armboard

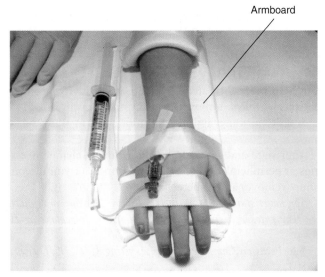

FIGURE 32-17 An armboard prevents movement at an IV site. (Modified from Roberts JR, Custalow CB, Thomsen TW: *Roberts and Hedges' clinical procedures in emergency medicine and acute care*, ed 7, Philadelphia, 2019, Elsevier.)

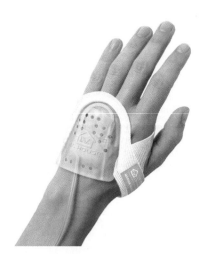

FIGURE 32-18 I.V. House Protective Device. (Courtesy I.V. House, St Louis, Mo.)

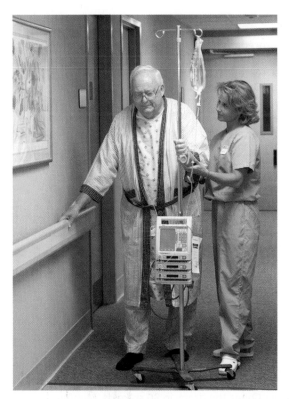

FIGURE 32-19 A person walking with an IV using a portable IV pole.

FOCUS ON COMMUNICATION

Assisting With IV Therapy

Arm position is important during IV therapy. You may need to remind the person:
- To position the arm a certain way
- About position limits

  For example, IV tubing is kinked from a bent arm. The fluid flow stops. You can say: "Please keep your arm straight. The fluid will not flow through your IV when your arm is bent."

DELEGATION GUIDELINES

Assisting With IV Therapy

Tasks involving IV therapy are nursing responsibilities. If changing a peripheral IV dressing or discontinuing (removing) a peripheral IV is delegated to you, make sure that the conditions in *Delegation Guidelines: Nutritional Support and IV Therapy* (p. 490) are met. If those conditions are met, you need this information from the nurse and the care plan.
- When to change the IV dressing
- If the person has an IV needle or catheter
- When to discontinue the IV
- If the person has 2 or more IVs, which IV to discontinue
- What supplies to use
- What observations to report and record (see Box 32-1)
- When to report observations
- What patient or resident concerns to report at once

FOCUS ON PRIDE

The Person, Family, and Yourself

Personal and Professional Responsibility

An IV in the arm can limit hand and arm movement. You may need to assist with hygiene, grooming, food and fluid, or activity needs. Assist only to the extent possible. The person should do as much as safely possible.

Rights and Respect

Persons needing nutritional support or IV therapy may be very ill. Sometimes decisions are made to stop therapy and allow the person to die. The person or family makes the decision after talking to the doctor. See Chapter 59. Respect the person and family and their decision.

Independence and Social Interaction

Emotional and social changes can occur when a feeding tube is needed. The person may miss the taste of food and social contact during meals. Feelings of sadness, loss, dependence, and loneliness can occur. You can:
- Listen.
- Provide emotional support.
- Encourage social contact.
- Tell the nurse about any concerns.

Delegation and Teamwork

Before any task, you must know how to protect IVs. For example:
- A person with an IV needs a shower. The nurse may have you apply a plastic bag, plastic wrap, or glove. Follow the nurse's instructions.
- A person receiving IV therapy needs to move from the bed to the chair. You must plan the move to avoid pulling on the IV site.

Ethics and Laws

When you hear an IV pump alarm, tell the nurse. Do so even if not assigned to the person. You do not adjust controls on IV pumps. Know the limits of your role. Performing tasks outside the limits of your role can harm the person. Legal action can be taken.

FOCUS ON PRIDE: Application

Consider the emotional impact of 1 treatment in this chapter. Describe how the person might feel. How can you provide mental comfort?

REVIEW QUESTIONS

Circle the BEST answer.

1 Enteral nutrition
   a Requires an NG tube
   b Is given into a central venous site
   c Is given into the GI tract
   d Requires an IV

2 The process of giving a tube feeding is called
   a Gavage
   b Parenteral nutrition
   c Aspiration
   d Regurgitation

3 For a tube feeding, the person is positioned in
   a Fowler's or semi-Fowler's position
   b The left side-lying position
   c The right side-lying position
   d The supine position

4 Formula for a tube feeding is given
   a At body temperature
   b At room temperature
   c Hot
   d Cold

5 Continuous feedings are given with a
   a Syringe
   b Feeding bag
   c PEG tube
   d Feeding pump

6 The nurse checks feeding tube placement to prevent
   a Aspiration
   b Bleeding
   c Over-feeding
   d Cramping

7 Which position prevents regurgitation after a tube feeding?
   a Fowler's or semi-Fowler's position
   b The supine position
   c The left or right side-lying position
   d The prone position

8 The risk of regurgitation is greatest with
   a Naso-enteral tubes
   b Total parenteral nutrition
   c NG and gastrostomy tubes
   d A jejunostomy tube

9 A person with a feeding tube is NPO. Which measure should you question?
   a Provide oral hygiene
   b Provide mouth rinses
   c Give clear liquids
   d Apply lubricant to the lips

10 A person has an NG tube. To prevent nasal irritation
   a Clean the tube every 4 to 8 hours
   b Replace the tape on the nose every 4 hours
   c Remove the tube every 4 hours
   d Secure the tube to the person's gown

11 A nurse asks you to give a tube feeding. The procedure is not in your job description. What should you do?
   a Give the tube feeding.
   b Do not accept the task.
   c Ask another nursing assistant to perform the task.
   d Ask another nurse what you should do.

12 A person is receiving TPN. The person complains of chest pain and difficulty breathing. What should you do?
   a Put the person in Fowler's position.
   b Call for the nurse.
   c Stop the TPN.
   d Provide oral hygiene.

13 A person is receiving TPN. You know that TPN
   a Involves a nutrient solution
   b Is given through a feeding tube
   c Can cause pressure injuries on the nose
   d Requires that the person be NPO

14 Which is a peripheral IV site?
   a A PICC
   b An implanted port
   c A central line
   d An IV on the back of the hand

15 What is the *correct* way to check an IV flow rate?
   a Count the drops in 30 seconds. Multiply the number by 2.
   b Count the drops for 1 minute.
   c Check if the fluid is dripping.
   d Measure the amount of fluid.

16 The IV flow rate is
   a The number of gtt/hr
   b The amount of fluid given in 1 minute
   c The number of gtt/min or mL/hr
   d The amount of fluid in the IV bag

17 You note that the IV bag is almost empty. You should
   a Clamp the IV tubing
   b Tell the nurse
   c Remove the IV
   d Adjust the flow rate

18 You see bleeding from an IV site. You should
   a Tell the nurse
   b Move the needle or catheter
   c Remove the IV
   d Clamp the IV tubing

Answers to Chapter 32 questions are on p. 886.

FOCUS ON **PRACTICE**

Problem Solving

You enter the room to check on a patient receiving a continuous tube feeding. The head of the bed is flat and the person says: "My mouth is dry." The feeding pump alarm begins to sound. What do you do first? What do you do next? What can you do within your role limits? What does the nurse need to do?

Vital Signs

OBJECTIVES

- Define the key terms and key abbreviations in this chapter.
- Explain why vital signs are measured.
- List the factors affecting vital signs.
- Identify the normal ranges for each temperature site.
- Explain when to use each temperature site.
- Explain how to use thermometers.
- Identify the pulse sites.
- Describe a normal pulse and normal respirations.
- Describe the practices for measuring blood pressure.
- Perform the procedures described in this chapter.
- Know the normal vital signs for the different age-groups.
- Explain how to promote PRIDE in the person, the family, and yourself.

KEY TERMS

afebrile Without *(a)* a fever *(febrile)*

apical-radial pulse Taking the apical and radial pulses at the same time

blood pressure (BP) The amount of force exerted against the walls of an artery by the blood

body temperature The amount of heat in the body that is a balance between the amount of heat produced and the amount lost by the body

bradycardia A slow *(brady)* heart rate *(cardia)*; less than 60 beats per minute

diastole The period of heart muscle relaxation; the heart is at rest

diastolic pressure The pressure in the arteries when the heart is at rest

febrile With a fever

fever Elevated body temperature

hypertension High blood pressure

hypotension Low blood pressure

pulse The beat of the heart felt at an artery as a wave of blood passes through the artery

pulse deficit The difference between the apical and radial pulse rates

pulse rate The number of heartbeats or pulses in 1 minute

respiration Breathing air into *(inhalation)* and out of *(exhalation)* the lungs

sphygmomanometer A cuff and measuring device used to measure blood pressure *(sphygmo* means *pulse; manometer* is *a device for measuring pressure)*

stethoscope An instrument used to listen to the sounds produced by the heart, lungs, and other body organs

systole The period of heart muscle contraction; the heart is pumping blood

systolic pressure The pressure in the arteries when the heart contracts

tachycardia A rapid *(tachy)* heart rate *(cardia)*; more than 100 beats per minute

thermometer A device used to measure *(meter)* temperature *(thermo)*

vital signs Temperature, pulse, respirations, and blood pressure; pulse oximetry and pain are included in some agencies

KEY ABBREVIATIONS

BP	Blood pressure	IV	Intravenous
C	Centigrade	mm	Millimeter
F	Fahrenheit	mm Hg	Millimeters of mercury
Hg	Mercury	TPR	Temperature, pulse, and respirations
ID	Identification		

Vital signs reflect the function of 3 body processes—regulation of body temperature, breathing, and heart function. The *vital signs of body function* are:

- *Temperature*
- *Pulse*
- *Respirations*
- *Blood pressure*
- *Pulse oximetry (in some agencies)*
- *Pain (in some agencies)*

Vital signs are often called TPR (temperature, pulse, and respirations) and BP (blood pressure). See "Pulse Oximetry" (p. 529 and Chapter 43) and "Pain" (p. 529 and Chapter 35).

NOTE: *A task may require more than 1 pair of gloves. Change gloves as needed. Use careful judgment. Remember to practice hand hygiene after removing gloves.*

MEASURING AND REPORTING VITAL SIGNS

A person's vital signs vary within certain limits. Box 33-1 lists factors that affect vital signs.

Vital signs detect even minor changes in normal body function. They tell about treatment response. They often signal life-threatening events. Part of the assessment step in the nursing process, vital signs are measured:

- During physical exams
- When the person is admitted to a health care agency
- When the person's condition requires
- Before and after surgery, complex procedures, and diagnostic tests
- After some care measures, such as ambulation (walking)
- After a fall or other injury
- When drugs affect the respiratory or circulatory system
- When the person complains of pain, dizziness, light-headedness, feeling faint, shortness of breath, a rapid heart rate, or not feeling well
- As stated on the care plan (usually daily, twice a day, or weekly in nursing centers)

You must accurately measure, record, and report vital signs. If unsure of your measurements, ask the nurse for help. Unless otherwise ordered, take vital signs with the person at rest—lying or sitting. Report the following at once.

- A vital sign that is changed from a prior measurement. The nurse tells you what change is important.
- An abnormal vital sign (a vital sign above or below the normal range).

See "Reporting and Recording" on p. 529.

See *Focus on Communication: Measuring and Reporting Vital Signs.*

See *Focus on Children and Older Persons: Measuring and Reporting Vital Signs.*

BOX 33-1	Factors Affecting Vital Signs

- Activity
- Age
- Anger
- Anxiety
- Drugs
- Eating
- Exercise
- Fear
- Biological sex (male or female)
- Illness
- Noise
- Pain
- Sleep
- Smoking
- Stress
- Weather
- Weight

FOCUS ON COMMUNICATION

Measuring and Reporting Vital Signs

Some persons like to know their vital signs. If agency policy allows, tell the person the measurements. With the person's consent, you can tell family members if they ask. This information is private and confidential. Roommates and visitors must not hear what you say. For greater privacy, write the measurements for the person.

A measurement may be abnormal. Or you are not able to feel a pulse or hear a blood pressure. Do not alarm the person. You can say:

- "I have a question about your blood pressure. I'll ask the nurse to take it."
- "Your pulse is a little slow (or fast). I'll have the nurse check it."
- "Your temperature is higher than normal. I'll use another thermometer and have the nurse check you."

FOCUS ON CHILDREN AND OLDER PERSONS

Measuring and Reporting Vital Signs

Children

How you measure vital signs varies with the child's age. Equipment also varies. Agency policy and the nurse direct what you do.

In young children, pulse and respirations are measured before procedures that may be frightening or uncomfortable. Such procedures may increase the pulse and respiratory rates. Measuring temperature and blood pressure are examples. The nurse tells you the order for vital signs. The nurse may have you measure temperature and blood pressure after pulse and respirations. If the child is crying, include that when reporting and recording measurements.

Older Persons

When measuring vital signs, the person with dementia may move, hit at you, or grab equipment. This is not safe for the person or you. Two staff members may be needed. One tries to calm and distract the person. The other measures the vital signs.

Try the procedure when the person is calmer. Or take the respirations and pulse at one time. Then take the temperature and blood pressure later.

Approach the person calmly. Use a soothing voice. Explain what you will do. Do not rush. Follow the care plan for the best way to calm and distract the person. If you cannot measure vital signs, tell the nurse at once.

BODY TEMPERATURE

Body temperature is the amount of heat in the body. It is a balance between the amount of heat produced and the amount lost by the body. Heat is produced as cells use food for energy. It is lost through the skin, breathing, urine, and feces (stools). Body temperature is fairly stable. It is lower in the morning and higher in the afternoon and evening. Body temperature is affected by the factors listed in Box 33-1, pregnancy, and the menstrual cycle.

You use thermometers to measure temperature. *A thermometer is a device used to measure* (meter) *temperature* (thermo). Thermometers have Fahrenheit (F) or centi-grade (C) scales. Use the degrees symbol (°) to record temperatures.

Temperature Sites

Temperature sites are listed in Box 33-2. Each site has a normal range (Table 33-1). Always report temperatures above or below the normal range.

BOX 33-2	Temperature Sites

Oral Site
Oral temperatures are *not* taken if the person:
- Is under 4 or 5 years of age.
- Is unconscious.
- Has had surgery or an injury to the face, neck, nose, or mouth.
- Is receiving oxygen.
- Breathes through the mouth.
- Has a naso-gastric tube.
- Is restless, confused, or disoriented.
- Is paralyzed on 1 side of the body.
- Has a sore mouth.
- Has a convulsive (seizure) disorder.

Rectal Site
The rectal site is used for infants and children under 3 years old. Rectal temperatures are taken when the oral site cannot be used. Rectal temperatures are *not* taken if the person:
- Has diarrhea.
- Has a rectal disorder or injury.
- Has heart disease.
- Had rectal surgery.
- Is confused or agitated.

Tympanic Membrane Site (Ear)
The site has fewer microbes than the mouth or rectum. The risk of spreading infection is reduced. The route is comfortable and non-invasive. Too much earwax can cause an incorrect measurement. This site is *not* used if the person has:
- An ear disorder
- Ear drainage

Temporal Artery Site (Forehead)
Body temperature is measured at the temporal artery in the forehead. The site is non-invasive.

Axillary Site (Underarm)
The axillary site is less reliable than the other sites. It is used when the other sites cannot be used. Do *not* use this site right after bathing.

Fever means an elevated body temperature. These terms are used to describe the person.
- *Febrile*—*with a fever.* (The Latin word *febris* means *fever.*)
- *Afebrile*—*without a fever.* (The prefix *a* means *without.*)
  See *Focus on Communication: Temperature Sites.*

See *Focus on Children and Older Persons: Temperature Sites.*

See *Promoting Safety and Comfort: Temperature Sites,* p. 506.

TABLE 33-1	Normal Body Temperatures	
Site	Baseline	Normal Range
Oral	98.6°F (37.0°C)	97.6°F to 99.6°F (36.5°C to 37.5°C)
Rectal	99.6°F (37.5°C)	98.6°F to 100.6°F (37.0°C to 38.1°C)
Axillary	97.6°F (36.5°C)	96.6°F to 98.6°F (35.9°C to 37.0°C)
Tympanic membrane	98.6°F (37.0°C)	98.6°F (37.0°C)
Temporal artery	99.6°F (37.5°C)	99.6°F (37.5°C)

FOCUS ON COMMUNICATION

Temperature Sites

Taking a rectal temperature can be embarrassing and uncomfortable. Be professional. Explain what you will do and why you must use the rectal site. For example:

> *I need to take a rectal temperature because you have a sore mouth. This electronic thermometer stays in place until it beeps. It takes a few seconds. Please tell me if you feel pain.*

A glass thermometer (p. 506) remains in the rectum for at least 2 minutes. To promote comfort, talk the person through the procedure. You can say: "I'm almost done. There's about 1 minute left. Are you doing okay?"

FOCUS ON CHILDREN AND OLDER PERSONS

Temperature Sites

Children
The oral site is not used for infants and children younger than 4 to 5 years. Use other routes as directed by the nurse and the care plan. See Box 33-2.

Older Persons
Older persons have lower body temperatures than younger persons. An oral temperature of 98.6°F may signal fever in an older person.

Tympanic membrane and temporal artery sites are used for persons who are confused and resist care. Oral and rectal sites are unsafe. The person may move, resist care, or bite down on the thermometer. This can injure the mouth, teeth, or rectum.

PROMOTING SAFETY AND COMFORT

Temperature Sites

Safety

Rectal temperatures are dangerous for persons with heart disease. The thermometer can stimulate the vagus nerve and slow the heart rate to dangerous levels.

Thermometer Types

There are different types of thermometers. See Figure 33-1 and Table 33-2. Electronic thermometers display the temperature on the front of the device. Follow the manufacturer's instructions and agency procedures to use, clean, and store thermometers.

See *Teamwork and Time Management: Thermometer Types.*

See *Focus on Long-Term Care and Home Care: Thermometer Types.*

See *Promoting Safety and Comfort: Thermometer Types.*

TEAMWORK AND TIME MANAGEMENT

Thermometer Types

The standard electronic, tympanic membrane, and temporal artery thermometers are shared with co-workers. Many types are kept in a battery charger when not in use. Tell your co-workers what thermometer you have. Work quickly but carefully. Return the device to the charging unit in a timely manner.

FOCUS ON LONG-TERM CARE AND HOME CARE

Thermometer Types

Home Care

Your home care agency may supply a digital thermometer. However, patients in home settings may have mercury-glass thermometers. If so, tell the nurse. Mercury is a hazardous substance (Chapter 13). The nurse can suggest that the person buy a digital thermometer or a glass thermometer with a mercury-free substance.

You may care for children in home settings. Do not use a mercury-glass thermometer to measure a child's temperature.

PROMOTING SAFETY AND COMFORT

Thermometer Types

Safety

Mercury-glass thermometers are not common today. Safer chemicals have replaced mercury. However, do not assume that a glass thermometer has a mercury-free mixture. If a thermometer breaks, tell the nurse at once. Do not touch the substance. Do not let the person do so. Follow agency procedures for handling hazardous materials. See Chapter 13.

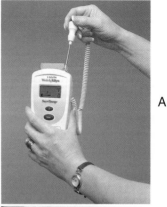
A

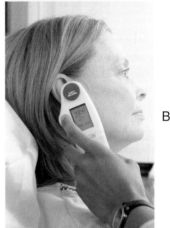
B

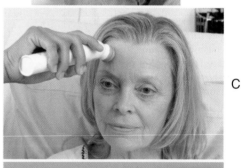
C

D

E

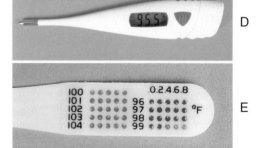

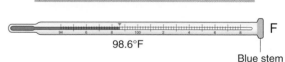
F
98.6°F
Blue stem

FIGURE 33-1 Thermometer types. **A,** Standard electronic thermometer. **B,** Tympanic membrane thermometer. **C,** Temporal artery thermometer. **D,** Digital thermometer. **E,** Disposable oral thermometer. **F,** Glass thermometer with a blue stem (for oral or axillary temperatures).

TABLE 33-2	Thermometer Types	
Thermometer Type	**Description**	**Guidelines for Use**
Standard electronic thermometer (see Fig. 33-1, *A*)	• Battery operated. • The *probe* is inserted at the measurement site. **Measurement sites:** • Oral • Rectal • Axillary	• Oral and axillary probes are *blue*. • Rectal probes are *red*. • Probe covers are disposable sheaths used to prevent the spread of infection. • Apply a new cover for each use. Discard after use. • Measures temperature in 4 to 15 seconds.
Tympanic membrane thermometer (see Fig. 33-1, *B*)	• Battery operated. **Measurement site:** • Tympanic membrane (ear)	• Do not use if there is ear drainage. • Probe covers are used. Discard after use. • Gently insert the covered probe into the ear. • Measures temperature in 1 to 3 seconds.
Temporal artery thermometer (see Fig. 33-1, *C*)	• Battery operated. **Measurement site:** • Temporal artery (forehead)	• Probe covers prevent the spread of infection. Discard after use. • Use the exposed side of the head. Do not use the side covered by hair, a dressing, a hat, or other covering. Do not use the side that was on a pillow. • Measures temperature in 3 to 4 seconds.
Digital thermometer (see Fig. 33-1, *D*)	• Small and battery operated. **Measurement sites:** • Oral • Rectal • Axillary	• Probe covers prevent the spread of infection. Discard after use. • Temperature is measured in 6 to 60 seconds.
Disposable oral thermometer (see Fig. 33-1, *E*)	• Measures temperature using small chemical dots that change color when heated. **Measurement site:** • Oral	• Each dot changes color at a certain temperature. • Temperature is measured in 45 to 60 seconds. • Disposable. Discard after use.

Glass thermometer (see Fig. 33-1, *F*)	• A hollow glass tube filled with a substance that expands and rises in the tube when heated. When cooled, the substance moves back down the tube.
	
	Measurement sites:
	• Oral
	• Rectal
	• Axillary
		• The *stem* part is held. The *tip* is inserted at the measurement site.
		  • Oral and axillary thermometers have a *blue* stem. They may have long and slender, stubby, or pear-shaped tips.
		  • Rectal thermometers have a *red* stem and a stubby tip.
		• Problems with use include:
		  • Long measurement times—oral 2 to 3 minutes, rectal 2 minutes, axillary 5 to 10 minutes.
		  • They break easily and can injure the measurement site.
		  • Mercury thermometers are hazardous. See *Promoting Safety and Comfort: Thermometer Types.*

Taking Temperatures

The nurse and care plan tell you:
• When to take the person's temperature
• What site to use
• What thermometer to use

There are many types of electronic thermometers. Follow the manufacturer's instructions. The procedure that follows is used as a guide.

See *Delegation Guidelines: Taking Temperatures*, p. 508.
See *Promoting Safety and Comfort: Taking Temperatures*, p. 508.
See procedure: *Taking a Temperature With an Electronic Thermometer*, p. 508.
See procedure: *Taking a Temperature With a Glass Thermometer*, p. 510.

Text continued on p. 512.

DELEGATION GUIDELINES

Taking Temperatures

Taking a temperature is a routine nursing task. Before doing so, you need this information from the nurse and the care plan.

- What site to use for each person—oral, rectal, axillary, tympanic membrane, or temporal artery
- What thermometer to use for each person
- How long to leave a glass thermometer in place
- When to take temperatures
- Which persons are at risk for a fever
- What observations to report and record
- When to report observations
- What patient or resident concerns to report at once:
  - A temperature changed from a past measurement
  - A temperature above or below the normal range for the site used

PROMOTING SAFETY AND COMFORT

Taking Temperatures

Safety

The mouth, rectum, axilla, and ear have many microbes and may contain blood. Probe covers are used or each person has his or her own thermometer. This prevents the spread of microbes and infection. Follow Standard Precautions and the Bloodborne Pathogen Standard when taking temperatures.

With rectal temperatures, your gloved hands may have contact with feces (stools). If so, remove gloves and practice hand hygiene. Then note the temperature on your note pad or assignment sheet. Put on clean gloves to complete the procedure.

Comfort

Do not leave a thermometer in place longer than needed. This affects comfort. For example, an oral glass thermometer is left in place for 2 to 3 minutes. Do not leave it in place longer.

Taking a Temperature With an Electronic Thermometer

QUALITY OF LIFE

- Knock before entering the person's room.
- Address the person by name.
- Introduce yourself by name and title.

- Explain the procedure before starting and during the procedure.
- Protect the person's rights during the procedure.
- Handle the person gently during the procedure.

PRE-PROCEDURE

1 Follow *Delegation Guidelines: Taking Temperatures*. See *Promoting Safety and Comfort: Taking Temperatures*.
2 For an oral temperature, ask the person not to eat, drink, smoke, or chew gum for at least 15 to 20 minutes before the measurement or as required by agency policy.
3 Practice hand hygiene.
4 Collect the following.
- Thermometer—standard electronic, tympanic membrane, or temporal artery
- Probe for a standard electronic thermometer (blue—oral or axillary; red—rectal)

- Probe covers
- Toilet paper (rectal temperature)
- Water-soluble lubricant (rectal temperature)
- Gloves
- Towel (axillary temperature)
5 Plug the probe into the thermometer if using a standard electronic thermometer.
6 Practice hand hygiene.
7 Identify the person. Check the identification (ID) bracelet against the assignment sheet. Use 2 identifiers (Chapter 13). Also call the person by name.

PROCEDURE

8 Provide for privacy. Position the person for an oral, rectal, axillary, or tympanic membrane temperature. The Sims' position is used for a rectal temperature.
9 Put on gloves if contact with blood, body fluids, secretions, or excretions is likely.
10 Insert the probe into a probe cover.
11 *For an oral temperature:*
- a Have the person open the mouth and raise the tongue.
- b Place the covered probe at the base of the tongue and to 1 side (Fig. 33-2).
- c Have the person lower the tongue and close the mouth.
- d Start the thermometer. Hold the probe in place until you hear a tone or see a flashing or steady light.

12 *For a rectal temperature:*
- a Place some lubricant on toilet paper.
- b Lubricate the end of the covered probe.
- c Expose the anal area.
- d Raise the upper buttock (Fig. 33-3).
- e Insert the probe $\frac{1}{2}$ inch into the rectum.
- f Start the thermometer. Hold the probe in place until you hear a tone or see a flashing or steady light.

Taking a Temperature With an Electronic Thermometer—cont'd

PROCEDURE—cont'd

13 *For an axillary temperature:*
 a Help the person remove an arm from the gown. Do not expose the person.
 b Dry the axilla with the towel.
 c Place the covered probe in the center of the axilla (Fig. 33-4, p. 510).
 d Place the person's arm over the chest.
 e Start the thermometer. Hold the probe in place until you hear a tone or see a flashing or steady light.

14 *For a tympanic membrane temperature:*
 a Have the person turn his or her head so the ear is in front of you.
 b Pull up and back on the adult's ear to straighten the ear canal (Fig. 33-5, p. 510). For children younger than 4 years of age, the nurse may have you pull the ear down and back.
 c Insert the covered probe gently.
 d Start the thermometer. Hold the probe in place until you hear a tone or see a flashing or steady light.

15 *For a temporal artery temperature:*
 a Place the device in the center of the forehead.
 b Press the scan button.
 c Slide the device right or left across the temporal artery (p. 514) (see Fig. 33-1, *C*). Use the side of the head that is exposed. Keep the thermometer flat on the forehead and in contact with the skin.
 d Release the scan button when the thermometer reaches the hairline.

16 Remove the probe from the site. Read the temperature on the display.

17 Press the eject button to discard the cover.

18 Note the person's name, temperature, and temperature site on your note pad or assignment sheet.

19 Return the probe to the holder.

20 Help the person put the gown back on (axillary temperature). For a rectal temperature:
 a Wipe the anal area with toilet paper to remove lubricant.
 b Cover the person.
 c Dispose of used toilet paper.
 d Remove and discard the gloves. Practice hand hygiene.

POST-PROCEDURE

21 Provide for comfort. (See the inside of the back cover.)
22 Place the call light and other needed items within reach.
23 Unscreen the person.
24 Complete a safety check of the room. (See the inside of the back cover.)
25 Return the thermometer to the charging unit. Follow agency policy for disinfection.
26 Practice hand hygiene.
27 Report and record the temperature. Note the temperature site. Report an abnormal temperature at once.

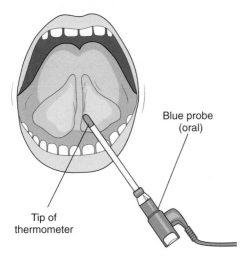

FIGURE 33-2 The thermometer is placed at the base of the tongue (under the tongue) and to 1 side.

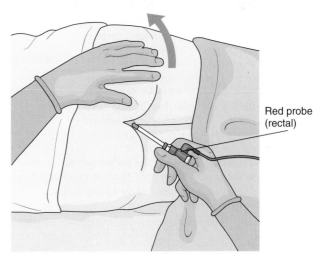

FIGURE 33-3 The rectal temperature is taken with the person in Sims' position. The buttock is raised to expose the anus.

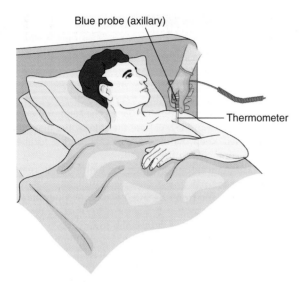

Blue probe (axillary)

Thermometer

FIGURE 33-4 The thermometer is in the center of the axilla and the person's arm is over the chest.

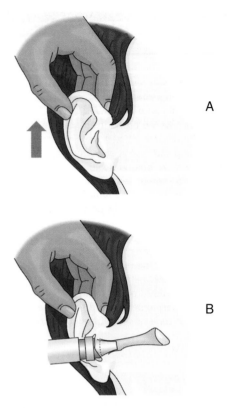

A

B

FIGURE 33-5 Tympanic membrane thermometer. **A,** The adult's ear is pulled up and back. **B,** The probe is inserted into the ear canal.

Taking a Temperature With a Glass Thermometer

QUALITY OF LIFE

- Knock before entering the person's room.
- Address the person by name.
- Introduce yourself by name and title.

- Explain the procedure before starting and during the procedure.
- Protect the person's rights during the procedure.
- Handle the person gently during the procedure.

PRE-PROCEDURE

1 Follow *Delegation Guidelines: Taking Temperatures,* p. 508. See *Promoting Safety and Comfort:*
   a *Thermometer Types,* p. 506
   b *Taking Temperatures,* p. 508
2 For an oral temperature, ask the person not to eat, drink, smoke, or chew gum for at least 15 to 20 minutes before the measurement or as required by agency policy.
3 Practice hand hygiene.

4 Collect the following.
   - Oral or rectal thermometer and holder
   - Tissues
   - Plastic covers if used
   - Gloves
   - Toilet paper (rectal temperature)
   - Water-soluble lubricant (rectal temperature)
   - Towel (axillary temperature)
5 Practice hand hygiene.
6 Identify the person. Check the ID bracelet against the assignment sheet. Use 2 identifiers (Chapter 13). Also call the person by name.
7 Provide for privacy.

Taking a Temperature With a Glass Thermometer—cont'd

PROCEDURE

8 Put on the gloves.

9 Rinse the thermometer under cold running water if it was soaking in a disinfectant. Do not use hot water. The substance can expand and break the thermometer. Dry it from the stem to the tip with tissues.

10 Check for breaks, cracks, or chips. Discard it following agency policy if it is broken, cracked, or chipped.

11 Shake down the thermometer below the lowest number. Hold the device by the stem. Stand away from walls, tables, and other hard surfaces. Flex and snap your wrist until the substance is below 94°F or 34°C (Fig. 33-6, p. 512).

12 Insert it into a plastic cover if used (Fig. 33-7, p. 512).

13 *For an oral temperature:*
   a Have the person moisten the lips.
   b Place the tip of the thermometer under the tongue and to 1 side (see Fig. 33-2).
   c Have the person lower the tongue and close the lips around the thermometer to hold it in place.
   d Ask the person not to talk or bite down on the thermometer.
   e Leave it in place for 2 to 3 minutes or as required by agency policy.

14 *For a rectal temperature:*
   a Position the person in the Sims' position.
   b Put a small amount of lubricant on toilet paper. Lubricant is used for easy insertion and to prevent injury.
   c Lubricate the tip of the thermometer.
   d Fold back top linens to expose the anal area.
   e Raise the upper buttock to expose the anus (see Fig. 33-3).
   f Insert the thermometer 1 inch into the rectum. Do not force the thermometer.
   g Hold the thermometer in place for 2 minutes or as required by agency policy. Continue to hold it while it is in the rectum.

15 *For an axillary temperature:*
   a Help the person remove an arm from the gown. Do not expose the person.
   b Dry the axilla with the towel.
   c Place the tip of the thermometer in the center of the axilla.
   d Have the person place the arm over the chest to hold the thermometer in place (see Fig. 33-4). Hold it and the arm in place if he or she cannot help.
   e Leave the thermometer in place for 5 to 10 minutes or as required by agency policy.

16 Remove the thermometer.

17 *After an oral or axillary temperature:*
   a Use a tissue to remove the plastic cover.
   b Wipe the thermometer with a tissue if no cover was used. Wipe from the stem to the tip.
   c Discard the tissue and cover (if used).
   d Read the thermometer (p. 512).
   e Help the person put the gown back on (axillary temperature).

18 *After a rectal temperature:*
   a Use toilet paper to remove the plastic cover.
   b Wipe the thermometer with toilet paper if no cover was used. Wipe from the stem to the tip.
   c Place used toilet paper on several thicknesses of clean toilet paper. Discard the cover (if used).
   d Read the thermometer (p. 512).
   e Place the thermometer on clean toilet paper.
   f Wipe the anal area with toilet paper to remove lubricant and any feces (stools). Set the used toilet paper on several thicknesses of clean toilet paper.
   g Cover the person.
   h Dispose of toilet paper in the toilet.
   i Remove and discard the gloves. Practice hand hygiene.

19 Note the person's name, temperature, and temperature site on your note pad or assignment sheet.

20 Shake down the thermometer.

21 Clean the thermometer following agency policy. (Wear gloves.) Agency policy may require that you:
   a Wipe the thermometer with tissues or toilet paper to remove mucus, feces (stools), or sweat. Wipe from the stem to the tip.
   b Rinse the thermometer under cold running water. Do not use hot water. Hot water causes the substance to expand and break the thermometer.

22 Store the thermometer in a holder or a container with a disinfectant solution. Follow agency policy.

23 Remove and discard the gloves. Practice hand hygiene.

POST-PROCEDURE

24 Provide for comfort. (See the inside of the back cover.)

25 Place the call light and other needed items within reach.

26 Unscreen the person.

27 Complete a safety check of the room. (See the inside of the back cover.)

28 Practice hand hygiene.

29 Report and record the temperature. Note the temperature site. Report an abnormal temperature at once.

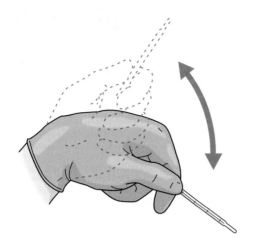

FIGURE 33-6 The wrist is snapped to shake down the thermometer. This moves the substance down in the tube.

Reading a Glass Thermometer. To read a glass thermometer:
- Hold it at the stem. Bring it to eye level (Fig. 33-8).
- Turn it until you can see the numbers and the long and short lines.
- Turn it back and forth slowly until you can see the silver or red line.
- Read from the tip toward the stem.
- Read the nearest degree (long line) to the left of the silver or red line.
- Read the nearest tenth of a degree (short line)—an even number on a Fahrenheit thermometer.
  See *Focus on Math: Reading a Glass Thermometer.*

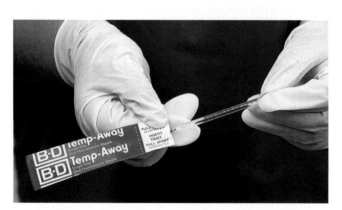

FIGURE 33-7 The thermometer is inserted into a plastic cover.

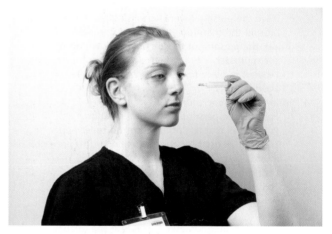

FIGURE 33-8 The thermometer is held at the stem. It is read at eye level.

FOCUS ON MATH

Reading a Glass Thermometer

To read a thermometer, you must understand whole numbers and decimals. Whole numbers are 0, 1, 2, 3, and so on. They are to the *left* of the decimal point. The numbers to the *right* of the decimal point (decimal place values) are part of a whole number. See Figure 33-9. Each whole number has 10 parts—the decimal place values. Decimal place values are read as "tenths"—1-tenth, 2-tenths, 3-tenths, and so on. Thermometers are read to 1 number past the decimal point (the "tenths" place).

To read a glass thermometer (Fig. 33-10):
1 Read the nearest long line to the left of the silver or red line.
  - Fahrenheit—each long line is 1 degree from 94°F to 108°F.
  - Centigrade—each long line is 1 degree from 34°C to 42°C.
2 Read the nearest tenth of a degree (short line).
  - Fahrenheit—each short line is 0.2 (2-tenths) of a degree (2-tenths, 4-tenths, 6-tenths, and 8-tenths).
  - Centigrade—each short line is 0.1 (1-tenth) of a degree (1-tenth, 2-tenths, 3-tenths, and so on to 9-tenths).

FOCUS ON MATH—cont'd

Reading a Glass Thermometer

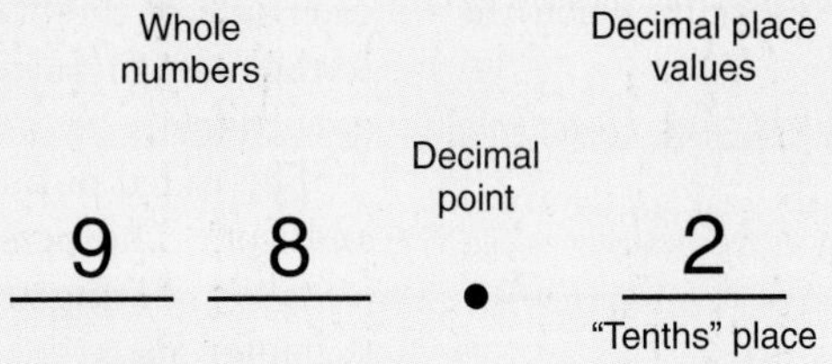
Whole numbers
Decimal place values
Decimal point
9
8
2
"Tenths" place

FIGURE 33-9 Values used to read thermometers.

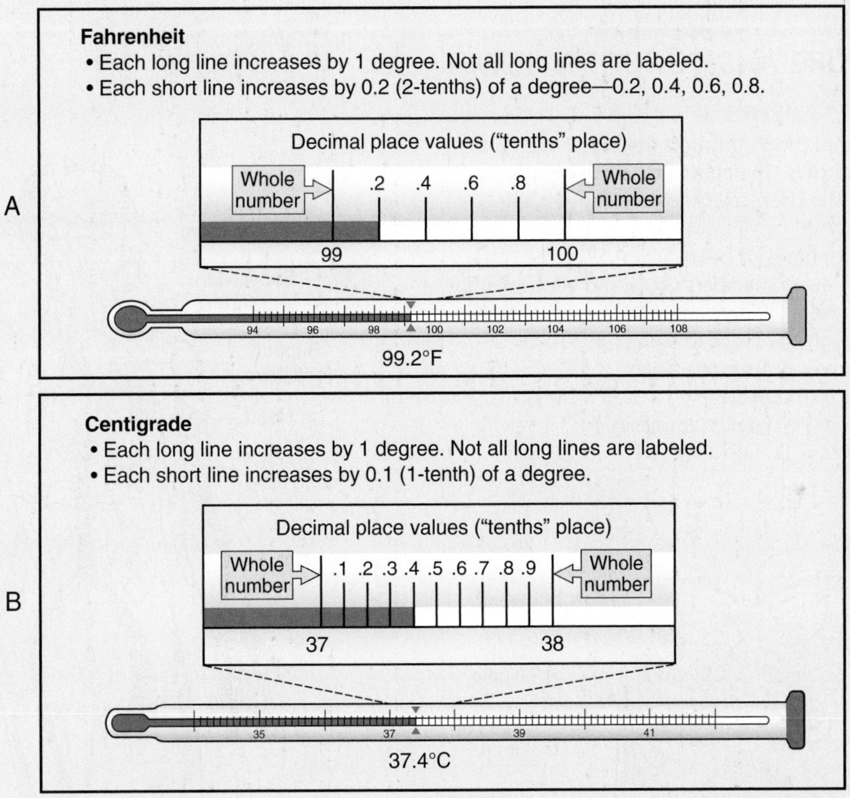
Fahrenheit
• Each long line increases by 1 degree. Not all long lines are labeled.
• Each short line increases by 0.2 (2-tenths) of a degree—0.2, 0.4, 0.6, 0.8.
Decimal place values ("tenths" place)
Whole number
.2 .4 .6 .8
Whole number
A
99
100
94
96
98
100
102
104
106
108
99.2°F
Centigrade
• Each long line increases by 1 degree. Not all long lines are labeled.
• Each short line increases by 0.1 (1-tenth) of a degree.
Decimal place values ("tenths" place)
Whole number
.1 .2 .3 .4 .5 .6 .7 .8 .9
Whole number
B
37
38
35
37
39
41
37.4°C

FIGURE 33-10 Reading thermometers. **A,** Fahrenheit thermometer. **B,** Centigrade thermometer.

PULSE

Arteries carry blood from the heart to all parts of the body. The *pulse* is the beat of the heart felt at an artery as a wave of blood passes through the artery. A pulse occurs when the heart beats.

See *Body Structure and Function Review: The Heart and Blood Vessels.*

Pulse Sites

The temporal, carotid, brachial, radial, femoral, popliteal, posterior tibial, and dorsalis pedis (pedal) pulses are on each side of the body (Fig. 33-13). The arteries are close to the body surface and lie over a bone. Therefore they are easy to feel.

The radial pulse is commonly used. It is easy to reach and find. The person is not exposed. The carotid pulse is taken during cardiopulmonary resuscitation (CPR) (Chapter 58).

The apical pulse is over the tip (apex) of the heart. This pulse is taken with a stethoscope. See "Using a Stethoscope."

See *Focus on Children and Older Persons: Pulse Sites.*

BODY STRUCTURE AND FUNCTION REVIEW

The Heart and Blood Vessels

The heart pumps blood through the blood vessels to the tissues and cells. The heart lies in the middle to lower part of the chest cavity toward the left side (Fig. 33-11).

There are 2 phases of heart action. *Diastole* is the resting phase. Heart chambers (*atria* and *ventricles*) fill with blood. *Systole* is the working phase. The heart contracts. Blood is pumped through the blood vessels (Fig. 33-12).

- *Arteries* carry blood away from the heart.
- *Veins* return blood to the heart.

See Chapter 10 for more detailed information.

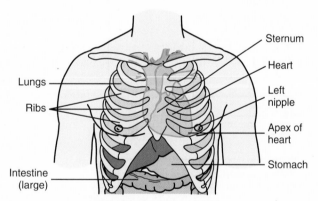

FIGURE 33-11 Location of the heart.

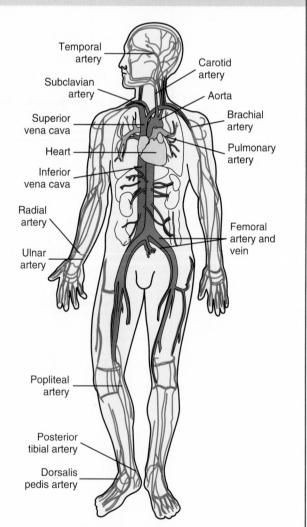

FIGURE 33-12 Blood vessels. Arteries are shown in *red.* Veins are *blue.*

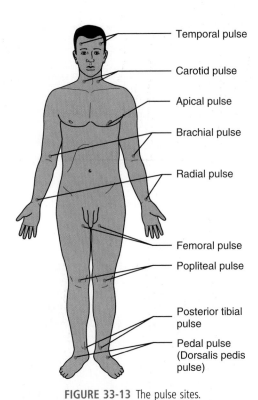

FIGURE 33-13 The pulse sites.

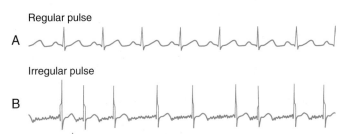

FIGURE 33-14 **A,** The electrocardiogram shows a regular pulse. The beats occur at regular intervals. (NOTE: Each tall spike is a beat.) **B,** These beats are at irregular intervals.

Pulse Rhythm and Force

The pulse *rhythm* should be in a regular pattern. The pause between beats is the same. An irregular pulse is when the beats are not evenly spaced or beats are skipped (Fig. 33-14).

Force relates to pulse strength. A forceful pulse is easy to feel. It is described as *strong, full,* or *bounding.* Hard-to-feel pulses are described as *weak, thready,* or *feeble.*

Electronic blood pressure equipment (p. 524) can also count pulses. The pulse rate and blood pressures are shown. Some show if the pulse is regular or irregular. However, you need to feel the pulse to determine its force.

Pulse oximetry equipment can also count pulses. See Chapter 43.

Using a Stethoscope

A *stethoscope is an instrument used to listen to the sounds produced by the heart, lungs, and other body organs.* You use it to hear apical pulses and for blood pressures. See Box 33-3 for how to use a stethoscope.

See *Focus on Communication: Using a Stethoscope,* p. 516.
See *Promoting Safety and Comfort: Using a Stethoscope,* p. 516.

FOCUS ON **CHILDREN AND OLDER PERSONS**

Pulse Sites

Children
The apical pulse is used for infants and children under 2 years. The nurse may ask you to use the radial site for children older than 2 years.

Pulse Rate

The *pulse rate is the number of heartbeats or pulses in 1 minute.* The rate varies for each age-group (Table 33-3). Pulse rate is affected by the factors in Box 33-1. Some drugs increase the pulse rate. Other drugs slow the pulse.

The adult pulse rate is between 60 and 100 beats per minute. A rate of less than 60 or more than 100 is abnormal. Report abnormal pulses at once.

- *Tachycardia is a rapid (tachy) heart rate (cardia). The heart rate is more than 100 beats per minute.*
- *Bradycardia is a slow (brady) heart rate (cardia). The heart rate is less than 60 beats per minute.*

TABLE 33-3	Pulse Ranges by Age
Age	Pulse Rate per Minute
Birth to 1 year	80-190
2 years	80-160
6 years	75-120
10 years	70-110
12 years and older	60-100

BOX 33-3	Using a Stethoscope

- Wipe the ear-pieces and chest-piece with antiseptic wipes before and after use. See Figure 33-15 (p. 516) for the parts of a stethoscope.
- Place the ear-piece tips in your ears. The bend of the tips points forward. Ear-pieces should fit snugly to block out noises. They should not cause ear pain or discomfort.
- Tap the diaphragm gently. You should hear the tapping. If not, turn the chest-piece at the tubing. Gently tap the diaphragm again. Proceed if you hear the tapping sound. Check with the nurse if you do not hear the tapping.
- Place the diaphragm over the pulse site. Hold it in place as in Figure 33-16 (p. 516).
- Prevent noise. Do not let anything touch the tubing. Ask the person to be silent. Make sure the room is quiet.

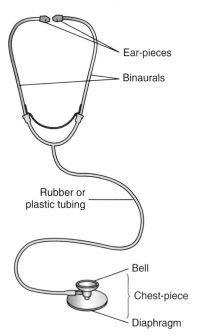

FIGURE 33-15 Parts of a stethoscope.

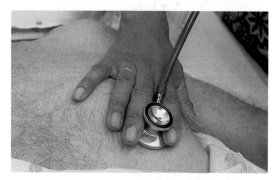

FIGURE 33-16 The stethoscope is held in place with the fingertips of the index and middle fingers.

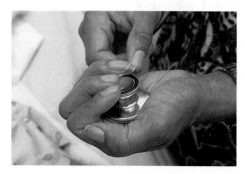

FIGURE 33-17 The diaphragm of the stethoscope is warmed in the palm of the hand.

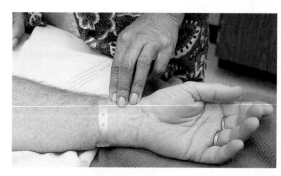

FIGURE 33-18 The 3 middle fingers are used to take the radial pulse.

FOCUS ON COMMUNICATION

Using a Stethoscope

Hearing through the stethoscope is hard when the person talks. Politely ask the person to be silent. Explain the procedure. Tell the person when and for how long to be silent. You can say:

I am going to check your pulse with a stethoscope. It is hard to hear your heart beat when you talk. Please do not talk when my stethoscope is on your chest. It will take about 1 minute.

The person may forget and begin talking. You can politely say: "This will only take 1 minute. Please stay quiet until I say that I'm done." Thank the person when you are done.

PROMOTING SAFETY AND COMFORT

Using a Stethoscope

Safety

Stethoscopes are in contact with many persons and staff. You must prevent infection. Wipe the ear-pieces and chest-piece with antiseptic wipes before and after use.

For Transmission-Based Precautions, dedicated equipment is kept in the room (Chapter 17). Equipment that must be shared is disinfected after use.

Comfort

Stethoscope diaphragms tend to be cold. Warm the diaphragm in your hand before putting it on the person (Fig. 33-17). Cold diaphragms can startle the person.

Taking Pulses

You will take radial, apical, and apical-radial pulses. You must count, report, and record accurately.

The radial pulse is used for routine vital signs. Place the first 2 or 3 fingertips against the radial artery. The radial artery is on the thumb side of the wrist (Fig. 33-18). Follow agency policy for how long to count. The following is common.

- Regular pulse—count the pulse for 30 seconds. Multiply by 2 for the number of pulses in 1 minute.
- Irregular pulse—count the pulse for 1 minute.

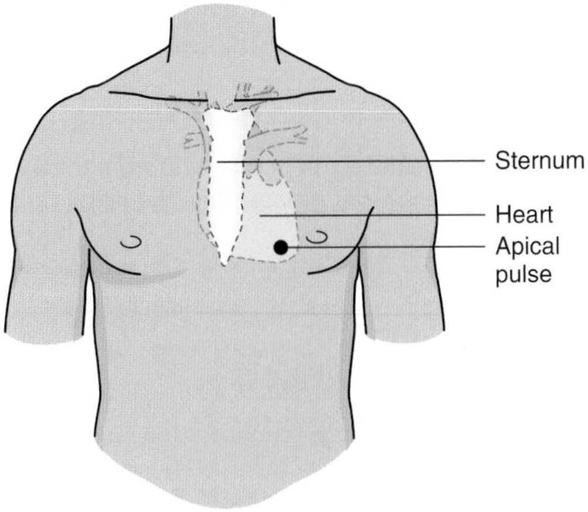

FIGURE 33-19 The apical pulse is located 2 to 3 inches to the left of the sternum (breastbone).

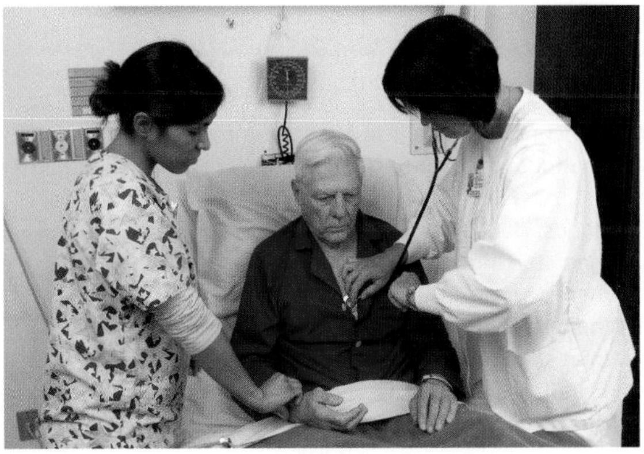

FIGURE 33-20 Taking an apical-radial pulse. One worker takes the apical pulse. The other takes the radial pulse.

The apical pulse is located 2 to 3 inches left of the sternum (Fig. 33-19). Use a stethoscope and count the pulse for 1 minute. The heartbeat normally sounds like a *lub-dub*. Count each *lub-dub* as 1 beat. Do not count the *lub* as 1 beat and the *dub* as another.

Apical pulses are taken on persons who:

- Have heart disease.
- Have irregular heart rhythms.
- Take drugs that affect the heart.

The apical and radial pulses should be the same. Sometimes heart contractions are not strong enough to create pulses in the radial artery. Then the radial rate is less than the apical rate. Heart disease is a common cause. To see if the apical and radial pulses are equal, 2 staff members are needed. One takes the radial pulse; the other takes the apical pulse (Fig. 33-20). *Taking the apical and radial pulses at the same time is called the* ***apical-radial pulse****.* The ***pulse deficit*** *is the difference between the apical and radial pulse rates.*

(NOTE: State competency tests require the use of a watch with a second [sweep] hand when taking pulses.)

See *Focus on Math: Taking Pulses*, p. 518.

See *Delegation Guidelines: Taking Pulses.*

See *Promoting Safety and Comfort: Taking Pulses.*

See procedure: *Taking a Radial Pulse*, p. 519.

See procedure: *Taking an Apical Pulse and an Apical-Radial Pulse*, p. 519.

Text continued on p. 520.

DELEGATION GUIDELINES

Taking Pulses

Taking a pulse is a routine nursing task. Before doing so, you need this information from the nurse and the care plan.

- What pulse to take for each person—radial, apical, or apical-radial
- When to take the pulse
- What other vital signs to measure
- How long to count the pulse—30 seconds or 1 minute
- If the nurse has concerns about certain patients or residents
- What observations to report and record:
  - The pulse site
  - The pulse rate—report a pulse rate less than 60 *(bradycardia)* or more than 100 *(tachycardia)* beats per minute at once
  - Pulse deficit for an apical-radial pulse
  - If the pulse is regular or irregular
  - Pulse force—strong (full, bounding) or weak (thready, feeble)
- When to report the pulse rate
- What patient or resident concerns to report at once

PROMOTING SAFETY AND COMFORT

Taking Pulses

Safety

Use your first 2 or 3 fingertips to take a pulse. Do not use your thumb. You could mistake the pulse in your thumb for the person's pulse. Reporting and recording the wrong pulse rate can harm the person.

FOCUS ON MATH

Taking Pulses

To count a pulse, use a watch with a second (sweep) hand. Start counting when the second (sweep) hand is at the 12, 3, 6, or 9 position. When counting a pulse for 30 seconds, do 1 of the following. See Figure 33-21.

- When starting at 12, count until position 6.
- When starting at 3, count until position 9.
- When starting at 6, count until position 12.
- When starting at 9, count until position 3.

For a 60-second pulse, count until the second (sweep) hand is back at the start position—12, 3, 6, or 9.

Radial Pulses

Pulse rate is measured in beats per minute. When you measure a regular pulse for 30 seconds, multiply the number by 2. This gives the number of beats per minute (60 seconds). For example, you count 36 beats in 30 seconds. For the number of beats per minute, multiply 36 by 2.

$$36 \text{ beats} \times 2 = 72 \text{ beats}$$
The pulse is 72 beats per minute.

Apical-Radial Pulses

For the *pulse deficit,* subtract the radial rate from the apical rate. (The radial rate is never greater than the apical rate.) For example:

- *The apical rate is 84 beats per minute. The radial rate is 84 beats per minute.*

$$84 \text{ apical beats} - 84 \text{ radial beats} = 0$$
The pulse deficit is 0.

- *The apical rate is 90 beats per minute. The radial rate is 86 beats per minute.*

$$90 \text{ apical beats} - 86 \text{ radial beats} = 4$$
The pulse deficit is 4.

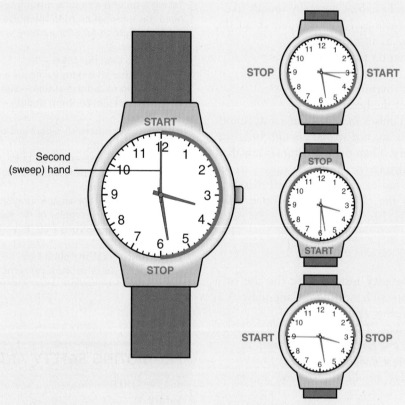

FIGURE 33-21 Using a watch with a second (sweep) hand to count for 30 seconds.

Taking a Radial Pulse

QUALITY OF LIFE

- Knock before entering the person's room.
- Address the person by name.
- Introduce yourself by name and title.

- Explain the procedure before starting and during the procedure.
- Protect the person's rights during the procedure.
- Handle the person gently during the procedure.

PRE-PROCEDURE

1 Follow *Delegation Guidelines: Taking Pulses,* p. 517. See *Promoting Safety and Comfort: Taking Pulses,* p. 517.
2 Practice hand hygiene.

3 Identify the person. Check the ID bracelet against the assignment sheet. Use 2 identifiers (Chapter 13). Also call the person by name.
4 Provide for privacy.

PROCEDURE

5 Have the person sit or lie down.
6 Locate the radial pulse on the thumb side of the person's wrist. Use your first 2 or 3 middle fingertips (see Fig. 33-18).
7 Note if the pulse is strong or weak and regular or irregular.
8 Count the pulse for 30 seconds. Multiply the number of beats by 2 for the number of pulses in 60 seconds (1 minute). This is the pulse rate. For example:
- You count 45 beats in 30 seconds.
- Multiply 45 beats by 2.
- 45 beats × 2 = 90 beats per minute.

9 Count the pulse for 1 minute if:
  a Directed by the nurse and the care plan.
  b Required by agency policy.
  c The pulse was irregular.
  d Required for your state competency test.
10 Note the following on your note pad or assignment sheet.
  a The person's name
  b Pulse site
  c Pulse rate
  d Pulse strength
  e If the pulse was regular or irregular

POST-PROCEDURE

11 Provide for comfort. (See the inside of the back cover.)
12 Place the call light and other needed items within reach.
13 Unscreen the person.
14 Complete a safety check of the room. (See the inside of the back cover.)

15 Practice hand hygiene.
16 Report and record the pulse rate and your observations. Report an abnormal pulse at once.

Taking an Apical Pulse and an Apical-Radial Pulse

QUALITY OF LIFE

- Knock before entering the person's room.
- Address the person by name.
- Introduce yourself by name and title.

- Explain the procedure before starting and during the procedure.
- Protect the person's rights during the procedure.
- Handle the person gently during the procedure.

PRE-PROCEDURE

1 Follow *Delegation Guidelines: Taking Pulses,* p. 517. See *Promoting Safety and Comfort:*
  a *Using a Stethoscope,* p. 516
  b *Taking Pulses,* p. 517
2 Ask a co-worker to help you (for an apical-radial pulse).
3 Practice hand hygiene.

4 Collect a stethoscope and antiseptic wipes.
5 Practice hand hygiene.
6 Identify the person. Check the ID bracelet against the assignment sheet. Use 2 identifiers (Chapter 13). Also call the person by name.
7 Provide for privacy.

Continued

Taking an Apical Pulse and an Apical-Radial Pulse—cont'd

PROCEDURE

8 Clean the stethoscope ear-pieces and chest-piece with the wipes.
9 *For an apical pulse:*
  a Have the person sit or lie down.
  b Expose the upper part of the left chest. Expose a woman's breasts only to the extent necessary.
  c Warm the diaphragm in your palm.
  d Place the stethoscope ear-pieces in your ears. The bend of the tips points forward.
  e Find the apical pulse. Place the diaphragm 2 to 3 inches to the left of the breastbone (see Fig. 33-19).
  f Count the pulse for 1 minute. (Count each lub-dub as 1 beat.) Note if it was regular or irregular.
10 *For an apical-radial pulse:*
  a Perform steps 9, a-d.
  b Find the apical pulse. See step 9, e. Your co-worker finds the radial pulse (see Fig. 33-20).
  c Give the signal to begin counting.
  d Count the apical pulse for 1 minute. Your co-worker counts the radial pulse for 1 minute.
  e Give the signal to stop counting. Ask your co-worker for the radial pulse rate.

11 Cover the person. Remove the stethoscope ear-pieces.
12 *For an apical-radial pulse,* subtract the radial pulse from the apical pulse for the pulse deficit. For example:
- You counted 72 apical beats per minute.
- Your co-worker counted 66 radial beats per minute.
- Subtract 66 (radial pulse) from 72 (apical pulse).
- 72 apical beats – 66 radial beats = 6. The pulse deficit is 6.
13 Note the person's name, pulse site(s), pulse rate(s), and pulse deficit on your note pad or assignment sheet. Note if the pulse was regular or irregular.

POST-PROCEDURE

14 Provide for comfort. (See the inside of the back cover.)
15 Place the call light and other needed items within reach.
16 Unscreen the person.
17 Complete a safety check of the room. (See the inside of the back cover.)
18 Clean the stethoscope ear-pieces and chest-piece with the wipes.

19 Return the stethoscope to its proper place. Follow agency policy for disinfection.
20 Practice hand hygiene.
21 Report and record your observations. Note if the pulse was regular or irregular. Record the pulse rate with *Ap* for apical. For an apical-radial pulse, record the apical and radial pulse rates and the pulse deficit. Report an abnormal pulse at once.

Checking Pedal Pulses. The pedal (dorsalis pedis) pulse is used to check blood flow in the foot. The dorsalis pedis artery is over a foot bone (Fig. 33-22). Often a nurse will mark the skin with an X where the pulse is found. This is so that all staff use the same site.

When a pedal pulse cannot be felt, a *Doppler* is used (Fig. 33-23). A Doppler uses ultrasound (sound waves) to find a pulse. The device is named after Christian J. Doppler. He developed the ultrasound method. When held over the pulse site, the Doppler makes a "whooshing" sound for each pulse.

Your role may include using a Doppler. If so, make sure that you:
- Have received the necessary training.
- Follow the nurse's directions.
- Follow the manufacturer's instructions.

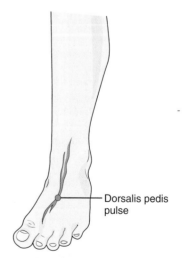

Dorsalis pedis pulse

FIGURE 33-22 The pedal pulse.

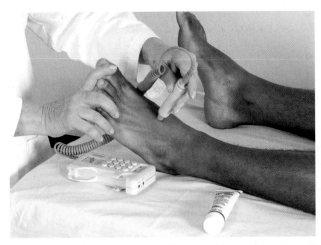

FIGURE 33-23 A Doppler is used to check a pedal pulse. (From Jarvis C: *Physical examination and health assessment*, ed 7, St Louis, 2016, Elsevier.)

RESPIRATIONS

Respiration means breathing air into (inhalation) *and out of* (exhalation) *the lungs.* Each respiration involves:

- 1 inhalation—the chest rises. Air enters the lungs.
- 1 exhalation—the chest falls. Air leaves the lungs.

The healthy adult has 12 to 20 respirations per minute. See Box 33-1 for the factors affecting vital signs. Heart and respiratory diseases often increase the respiratory rate.

Respirations are normally quiet, effortless, and regular. Both sides of the chest rise and fall equally. See Chapter 43 for abnormal respiratory patterns.

See *Body Structure and Function Review: The Respiratory System.*

Counting Respirations

Count respirations when the person is at rest. Position the person so you can see the chest rise and fall. To some extent, a person can control the rate and depth of breathing. People tend to change their breathing patterns when they know their respirations are being counted. Therefore do not tell the person that you are counting them.

Count respirations right after taking a pulse. Keep your fingers or stethoscope over the pulse site. The person assumes you are taking the pulse. To count respirations, watch the chest rise and fall. Count chest rises for 30 seconds. Multiply the number by 2 for the number of respirations in 1 minute. If you note an abnormal pattern, count respirations for 1 minute.

(NOTE: State competency tests require the use of a watch with a second [sweep] hand when counting respirations.)

See *Focus on Math: Counting Respirations*, p. 522.

See *Focus on Children and Older Persons: Counting Respirations*, p. 522.

See *Delegation Guidelines: Counting Respirations*, p. 522.

See procedure: *Counting Respirations*, p. 522.

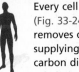

BODY STRUCTURE AND FUNCTION REVIEW

The Respiratory System

Every cell needs oxygen. The respiratory system (Fig. 33-24) brings oxygen into the lungs and removes carbon dioxide. *Respiration* is the process of supplying the cells with oxygen and removing carbon dioxide from them. Respiration involves *inhalation* (breathing in) and *exhalation* (breathing out). The terms *inspiration* (breathing in) and *expiration* (breathing out) are also used.

Air enters the body through the mouth and nose. Air passes through the *pharynx* (throat), *larynx* (voice box), and *trachea*. The trachea divides at its lower end into the *right bronchus* and *left bronchus*. Each bronchus enters a *lung*. The bronchi divide many times into smaller branches called *bronchioles*. The bronchioles further divide and end in tiny 1-celled air sacs called *alveoli*. They are supplied by capillaries.

Oxygen and carbon dioxide are exchanged between the alveoli and capillaries. Blood in the capillaries picks up oxygen from the alveoli. Then the blood returns to the heart and is pumped to the rest of the body. Alveoli pick up carbon dioxide from the capillaries for exhalation.

The lungs are separated from the abdominal cavity by a muscle called the *diaphragm*. A bony framework made up of the ribs, sternum, and vertebrae protects the lungs.

See Chapter 10 for more detailed information.

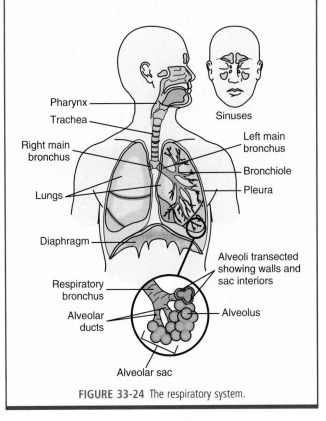

FIGURE 33-24 The respiratory system.

FOCUS ON MATH

Counting Respirations

Respirations are measured in breaths per minute. When you count regular respirations for 30 seconds, multiply the number by 2. This gives the number of respirations per minute (60 seconds). For example, you count 8 breaths in 30 seconds. For the number of breaths per minute, multiply 8 by 2.

$$8\ breaths \times 2 = 16\ breaths$$
The respiratory rate is 16 breaths per minute.

Like when taking pulses, you use a watch with a second (sweep) hand to count respirations. See *Focus on Math: Taking Pulses* for how to use a second (sweep) hand.

FOCUS ON CHILDREN AND OLDER PERSONS

Counting Respirations

Children
Infants and children have higher respiratory rates than adults. Count an infant's respirations for 1 minute.

Age	Respirations per Minute
Newborn	35
1 year	30
2 years	25
4 years	23
6 years	21
8 years	20
10-12 years	19
14 years	18
16 years	17
18 years	16–18

Modified from Hockenberry MJ, Wilson D, Rodgers CC: Wong's essentials of pediatric nursing, ed 10, St Louis, 2017, Elsevier.

DELEGATION GUIDELINES

Counting Respirations

Counting respirations is a routine nursing task. Before doing so, you need this information from the nurse and the care plan.

- How long to count respirations for each person—30 seconds or 1 minute
- When to count respirations
- If the nurse has concerns about certain patients or residents
- What other vital signs to measure

- What observations to report and record:
  - The respiratory rate
  - Equality and depth of respirations
  - If the respirations were regular or irregular
  - If the person has pain or difficulty breathing
  - Any respiratory noises
  - An abnormal respiratory pattern (Chapter 43)
- When to report observations
- What patient or resident concerns to report at once

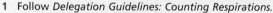

Counting Respirations

PROCEDURE

1. Follow *Delegation Guidelines: Counting Respirations.*
2. Keep your fingers or stethoscope over the pulse site.
3. Do not tell the person you are counting respirations.
4. Count chest rises. Each rise and fall of the chest is 1 respiration.
5. Note the following.
   - If respirations are regular
   - If both sides of the chest rise equally
   - The depth of respirations
   - If the person has any pain or difficulty breathing
   - An abnormal respiratory pattern

6. Count respirations for 30 seconds. Multiply the number by 2 for the number of respirations in 60 seconds (1 minute). This is the respiratory rate. For example:
   - You count 9 breaths in 30 seconds.
   - Multiply 9 breaths by 2.
   - 9 breaths × 2 = 18 breaths per minute.
7. Count respirations for 1 minute if:
   a Directed by the nurse and the care plan.
   b Required by agency policy.
   c They are abnormal or irregular.
   d Required for your state competency test.
8. Note the person's name, respiratory rate, and other observations on your note pad or assignment sheet.

POST-PROCEDURE

9. Provide for comfort. (See the inside of the back cover.)
10. Place the call light and other needed items within reach.
11. Unscreen the person.
12. Complete a safety check of the room. (See the inside of the back cover.)

13. Practice hand hygiene.
14. Report and record the respiratory rate and your observations. Report abnormal respirations at once.

BLOOD PRESSURE

Blood pressure (BP) is the amount of force exerted against the walls of an artery by the blood. BP is controlled by:
- The force of heart contractions
- The amount of blood pumped with each heartbeat
- How easily the blood flows through the blood vessels

Systole is the period of heart muscle contraction. The heart is pumping blood. **Diastole** *is the period of heart muscle relaxation. The heart is at rest.*

You measure systolic and diastolic pressures. The *systolic pressure is the pressure in the arteries when the heart contracts.* It is the higher pressure. The *diastolic pressure is the pressure in the arteries when the heart is at rest.* It is the lower pressure.

BP is measured in millimeters (mm) of mercury (Hg). The systolic pressure is recorded over the diastolic pressure. For example, a systolic pressure of 120 mm Hg (millimeters of mercury) and a diastolic pressure of 80 mm Hg are written as 120/80 mm Hg. This is read as "120 over 80 millimeters of mercury."

Normal and Abnormal Blood Pressures

BP can change from minute to minute. Factors affecting BP are listed in Box 33-4.

BP has normal ranges.
- *Systolic pressure*—90 mm Hg or higher but lower than 120 mm Hg
- *Diastolic pressure*—60 mm Hg or higher but lower than 80 mm Hg

Treatment is indicated for *hypertension (high blood pressure)* and *hypotension (low blood pressure).* Blood pressure is high when:
- The systolic pressure is 140 mm Hg or higher.
- The diastolic pressure is 90 mm Hg or higher.

When heart disease risk factors are present, a systolic pressure of 130 mm Hg or higher or a diastolic pressure of 80 mm Hg or higher may be considered hypertension. See Chapter 49.

Some people normally have low blood pressures. However, hypotension can signal a life-threatening problem. Blood pressure is low when:
- The systolic pressure is below 90 mm Hg.
- The diastolic pressure is below 60 mm Hg.

Report a systolic measurement at or above 120 mm Hg or below 90 mm Hg. Report a diastolic measurement at or above 80 mm Hg or below 60 mm Hg.

See *Focus on Communication: Normal and Abnormal Blood Pressures,* p. 524.

See *Focus on Children and Older Persons: Normal and Abnormal Blood Pressures,* p. 524.

BOX 33-4	Factors Affecting Blood Pressure

- *Age.* BP increases with age. It is lowest in infants and children. It is highest in adults.
- *Biological sex (male or female).* Women usually have lower blood pressures than men do. Blood pressures rise in women after menopause.
- *Family history.* High blood pressure tends to run in families.
- *Blood volume.* This is the amount of blood in the circulatory system. Severe bleeding lowers the blood volume. Therefore BP lowers. Giving IV (intravenous) fluids rapidly increases the blood volume. The BP rises.
- *Stress.* Stress includes anxiety, fear, and emotions. BP increases as the body responds to stress.
- *Pain.* Pain can increase BP. However, severe pain can cause shock. BP is seriously low in the state of shock (Chapter 58).
- *Exercise.* BP increases. BP is usually measured at rest.
- *Weight.* BP is higher in over-weight persons. It lowers with weight loss.
- *Race.* Black persons generally have higher blood pressures than others. They tend to get high blood pressure earlier in life.

- *Diet.* A high-sodium diet increases the amount of water in the body. The extra fluid volume increases BP.
- *Drugs.* Drugs can be given to raise or lower BP. Other drugs have the side effects of high or low BP. (A *side effect* is an undesirable reaction to a drug or therapy.)
- *Position.* BP is higher when lying down. It is lower in the standing position. Sudden changes in position can cause a drop in BP (postural hypotension). When the person stands BP may drop suddenly. Dizziness and fainting can occur.
- *Smoking.* BP increases. Nicotine in cigarettes causes blood vessels to narrow. The heart works harder to pump blood through narrowed vessels.
- *Alcohol.* Excessive alcohol intake can raise BP.
- *Certain health problems.* Some kidney diseases cause high blood pressure. High cholesterol, sleep apnea (Chapter 49), and diabetes (Chapter 50) are linked to high blood pressure.

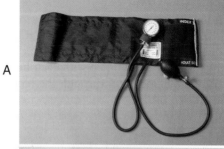

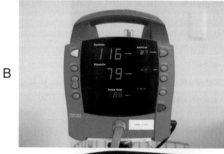

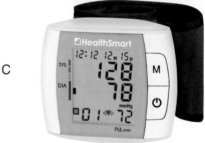

FIGURE 33-25 Blood pressure equipment. **A,** Aneroid manometer and cuff. **B,** Electronic manometer. **C,** Wrist manometer (monitor). (**C,** Courtesy Briggs Medical Service Company, Des Moines, Iowa.)

Blood Pressure Equipment

A *sphygmomanometer has a cuff and a measuring device for measuring blood pressure.* Sphygmo *means* pulse. *A device for measuring pressure is called a* manometer. These types are common.

- The *aneroid type* is a manual device with a round dial and a needle that points to the numbers (Fig. 33-25, *A*). (*Manual* relates to *being operated by hand.*)
- The *electronic type* shows the systolic and diastolic pressures and the pulse rate (Fig. 33-25, *B*).
- A *wrist manometer* (Fig. 33-25, *C*) measures blood pressure at the wrist. Some also show the pulse rate. Also called *wrist monitors*, this type is less reliable and is sensitive to body position. However, the device may be used for persons with bariatric needs. When measuring BP, the arm and wrist must be at heart level. Follow the manufacturer's instructions for use.

For the aneroid and electronic types, you wrap the blood pressure cuff around the upper arm. Tubing connects the cuff to the manometer. When inflated, the cuff causes pressure over the brachial artery. BP is measured as the cuff deflates.

- *Aneroid type.* A tube connects the cuff to a small, hand-held bulb. See Figure 33-26. Hold the bulb with the air-release valve up. To inflate the cuff (fill it with air), turn the air-release valve clockwise (to the right) to close the valve. Squeeze the bulb. To deflate the cuff (let air out), turn the valve counter-clockwise (to the left). Using a stethoscope, listen over the brachial artery as the cuff slowly deflates. Blood flowing through the arteries produces sounds.
  - The first sound heard is the systolic pressure.
  - The last sound heard is the diastolic pressure.
- *Electronic type.* No stethoscope is needed. A button is pressed to inflate the cuff. The cuff deflates automatically. The BP is displayed. Follow the manufacturer's instructions.

See *Focus on Children and Older Persons: Blood Pressure Equipment.*

See *Promoting Safety and Comfort: Blood Pressure Equipment.*

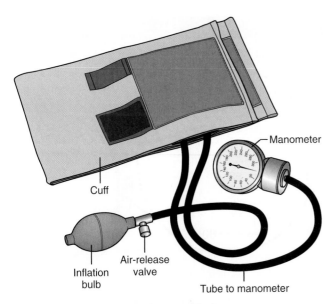

FIGURE 33-26 Parts of an aneroid sphygmomanometer.

FOCUS ON **CHILDREN AND OLDER PERSONS**

Blood Pressure Equipment

Children
Pediatric blood pressure cuffs are used for children. Infant and child sizes are available. The nurse tells you what size to use.

PROMOTING SAFETY AND COMFORT

Blood Pressure Equipment

Safety
Manometers with mercury are being phased out of health care. Some agencies may still use them. Handle mercury manometers carefully. If one breaks, call for the nurse at once. Do not touch the mercury. Do not let the person touch it. The agency follows special procedures for handling hazardous substances. See Chapter 13.

Comfort
Inflate the cuff only to the extent necessary. (See procedure: *Measuring Blood Pressure With an Aneroid Manometer*, p. 526.) The inflated cuff causes discomfort. The higher the inflation, the greater the discomfort.

Measuring Blood Pressure

You measure blood pressure in the brachial artery. Correct cuff size, cuff placement, and arm position are needed for an accurate measurement. Box 33-5 lists the guidelines for measuring blood pressure.

See *Focus on Math: Measuring Blood Pressure*, p. 526.

See *Delegation Guidelines: Measuring Blood Pressure*, p. 526.

See procedure: *Measuring Blood Pressure With an Aneroid Manometer*, p. 526.

See procedure: *Measuring Blood Pressure With an Electronic Manometer*, p. 528.

Text continued on p. 529.

BOX 33-5	Measuring Blood Pressure—Guidelines

- Do not take BP on an arm:
  - With an IV infusion
  - With an arm cast
  - With a dialysis access site
  - On the side of breast surgery
  - That is injured
- Ask the nurse if unsure of which arm to use.
- Let the person rest for 10 to 20 minutes before measuring BP.
- Measure BP with the person sitting or lying. Sometimes BP is measured in the standing position.
- Position the arm at the level of the heart. Support the arm with the palm up.
- Apply the cuff to the bare upper arm. Clothing can affect the measurement.
- Make sure the cuff is snug. A loose cuff causes a wrong reading.
- Use a larger cuff if the person has a large arm. Use a small cuff for a very small arm. Ask the nurse what size to use. Also check the care plan.
- Ask the person to be still during the measurement. Electronic BP manometers measure BP using sensors. Movement can affect accuracy.
- Ask the nurse for help if you have trouble measuring a BP. Frequent measurements at the same site can block blood flow and cause injury.

Aneroid Type

- Make sure the room is quiet. Talking, TV, music, and sounds from the hallway can affect hearing through a stethoscope.
- Have the manometer where you can clearly see it.
- Place the diaphragm of the stethoscope firmly over the brachial artery. The entire diaphragm has contact with the skin.
- Measure the systolic and diastolic pressures.
  - Expect the first sound at the point where you last felt the radial or brachial pulse (see procedure: *Measuring Blood Pressure With an Aneroid Manometer*, p. 526). The first sound is the systolic pressure.
  - The point where the sound disappears (the last sound heard) is the diastolic pressure.
- Take the BP again if you are not sure of accuracy. Wait 30 to 60 seconds to repeat the measurement. Do not repeat the measurement multiple times using the same arm. Ask the nurse to take the BP if you are unsure of the measurement.
- Tell the nurse at once if you cannot hear the blood pressure.

FOCUS ON MATH

Measuring Blood Pressure

$+-$ Aneroid manometers have long and short lines
$\times\div$ (Fig. 33-27).

- Long lines mark 10 mm Hg values.
- Short lines mark 2 mm Hg values.

Read the manometer as the cuff deflates. The needle is dropping.

- If the needle is at a long line, note this value. Long line values end in 0. For example: 70, 80, 90, 100, 110, 120, and so on.
- If the needle is between 2 long lines:
  - Note the value of the long line below the needle.
  - Note the short line. Count up from the long line below by even numbers. Short line values end with 2, 4, 6, or 8. See Figure 33-27.

For example, the needle is at the 3rd short line between 90 and 100. Count up by even numbers from 90. Line 1 is 92. Line 2 is 94. Line 3 is 96. The value is 96.

If needed, round up to the nearest 2 mm Hg. When you *round up* you choose the higher value. For example, the needle is between 82 and 80. Report and record the value as 82 mm Hg.

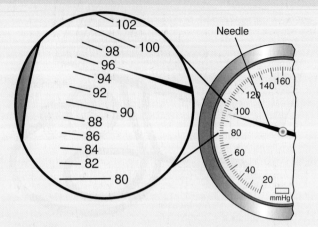

FIGURE 33-27 Reading the aneroid manometer. Long lines mark 10 mm Hg values. Short lines mark 2 mm Hg values.

DELEGATION GUIDELINES

Measuring Blood Pressure

Measuring BP is a routine nursing task. You need this information from the nurse and the care plan.

- When to measure BP
- What sphygmomanometer to use (p. 524)
- What arm to use
- The person's normal blood pressure range
- If the nurse has concerns about certain patients or residents

- If the person needs to be lying down, sitting, or standing
- What size cuff to use—regular, child-sized, extra-large, bariatric
- What observations to report and record
- When to report the BP measurement
- What patient or resident concerns to report at once

Measuring Blood Pressure With an Aneroid Manometer

QUALITY OF LIFE

- Knock before entering the person's room.
- Address the person by name.
- Introduce yourself by name and title.

- Explain the procedure before starting and during the procedure.
- Protect the person's rights during the procedure.
- Handle the person gently during the procedure.

PRE-PROCEDURE

1 Follow *Delegation Guidelines: Measuring Blood Pressure.*
  See *Promoting Safety and Comfort:*
  a *Using a Stethoscope,* p. 516
  b *Blood Pressure Equipment,* p. 525
2 Practice hand hygiene.
3 Collect the following.
  - Aneroid manometer
  - Stethoscope
  - Antiseptic wipes

4 Practice hand hygiene.
5 Identify the person. Check the ID bracelet against the assignment sheet. Use 2 identifiers (Chapter 13). Also call the person by name.
6 Provide for privacy.

Measuring Blood Pressure With an Aneroid Manometer—cont'd

PROCEDURE

7 Have the person sit or lie down.
8 Position the person's arm level with the heart. The palm is up.
9 Wipe the stethoscope ear-pieces and chest-piece with the wipes. Warm the diaphragm in your palm. Discard the wipes.
10 Stand no more than 3 feet away from the manometer.
11 Expose the upper arm.
12 Squeeze the cuff to expel (remove) any air. Close the valve on the bulb.
13 Find the brachial artery at the inner aspect of the elbow. (The brachial artery is on the little finger side of the arm.) Use your fingertips.
14 Locate the arrow on the cuff (Fig. 33-28, *A*). Align the arrow with the brachial artery (Fig. 33-28, *B*). Wrap the cuff around the upper arm at least 1 inch above the elbow. It is even and snug.
15 Place the stethoscope ear-pieces in your ears. Place the stethoscope's diaphragm over the brachial artery (Fig. 33-28, *C*). Do not place it under the cuff. (NOTE: For Methods 1 and 2, place the stethoscope after finding the radial pulse.)
16 Find the radial pulse. This step is for Methods 1 and 2.
17 *Method 1:*
  a Inflate the cuff until you cannot feel the pulse. Note this point.
  b Inflate the cuff 30 mm Hg beyond where you last felt the pulse.

18 *Method 2:*
  a Inflate the cuff until you cannot feel the pulse. Note this point.
  b Inflate the cuff 30 mm Hg beyond where you last felt the pulse.
  c Deflate the cuff slowly. Note the point when you feel the pulse.
  d Wait 30 seconds.
  e Inflate the cuff again, 30 mm Hg beyond where you felt the pulse return.
19 *Method 3:*
  a Inflate the cuff 160 mm Hg to 180 mm Hg.
  b Deflate the cuff if you hear a blood pressure sound. Re-inflate the cuff to 200 mm Hg.
20 Deflate the cuff at an even rate of 2 to 4 millimeters per second. Turn the valve counter-clockwise to deflate the cuff.
21 Note the point where you hear the first sound (Fig. 33-29, *A*, p. 528). This is the systolic reading. It is near the point where the pulse disappeared (Method 1) or returned (Method 2).
22 Continue to deflate the cuff completely. Note the point where the sound disappears (the last sound heard). This is the diastolic reading (Fig. 33-29, *B*, p. 528).
23 Deflate the cuff completely. Remove the cuff. Remove the stethoscope ear-pieces.
24 Note the person's name and BP on your note pad or assignment sheet. The BP in Figure 33-29 is written as 130/84 mm Hg.
25 Return the cuff to the case or wall holder.

POST-PROCEDURE

26 Provide for comfort. (See the inside of the back cover.)
27 Place the call light and other needed items within reach.
28 Unscreen the person.
29 Complete a safety check of the room. (See the inside of the back cover.)
30 Clean the stethoscope ear-pieces and chest-piece with the wipes. Discard the wipes.

31 Return the equipment to its proper place. Follow agency policy for disinfection.
32 Practice hand hygiene.
33 Report and record the BP. Note which arm was used. Report an abnormal BP at once.

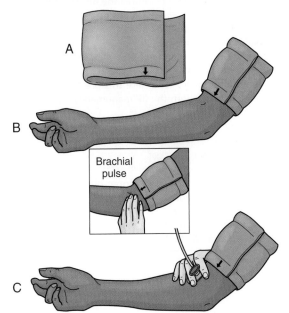

FIGURE 33-28 Measuring blood pressure. **A,** The arrow is used for correct cuff alignment. **B,** The cuff is placed so the arrow is aligned with the brachial artery. **C,** The diaphragm of the stethoscope is over the brachial artery.

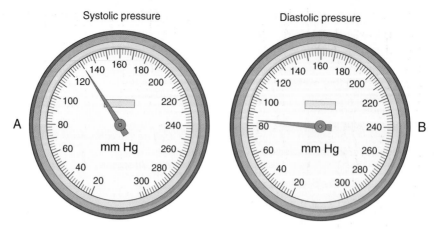

FIGURE 33-29 Manometer readings. **A,** This aneroid manometer is at 130 mm Hg for a systolic pressure. **B,** This aneroid manometer is at 84 mm Hg for a diastolic pressure. (NOTE: Both pressures are above the normal range.)

Measuring Blood Pressure With an Electronic Manometer

QUALITY OF LIFE

- Knock before entering the person's room.
- Address the person by name.
- Introduce yourself by name and title.

- Explain the procedure before starting and during the procedure.
- Protect the person's rights during the procedure.
- Handle the person gently during the procedure.

PRE-PROCEDURE

1 Follow *Delegation Guidelines: Measuring Blood Pressure,* p. 526.
2 Practice hand hygiene.
3 Collect the following:
   - Electronic BP manometer
   - BP cuff for use with the device (in the correct size for the person)

4 Practice hand hygiene.
5 Identify the person. Check the ID bracelet against the assignment sheet. Use 2 identifiers (Chapter 13). Also call the person by name.
6 Provide for privacy.

PROCEDURE

7 Have the person sit or lie down.
8 Position the arm level with the heart.
9 Expose the upper arm. The palm is up.
10 Squeeze the cuff to expel (remove) any air.
11 Turn on the electronic BP manometer.
12 Connect the cuff to the manometer's connection tubing.
13 Find the brachial artery at the inner aspect of the elbow. (The brachial artery is on the little finger side of the arm.) Use your fingertips.
14 Locate the arrow on the cuff. Align the arrow with the brachial artery. Wrap the cuff around the upper arm at least 1 inch above the elbow. It is even and snug.

15 Press the start button on the device. Leave the cuff in place while the device measures the BP. Ask the person to be still.
16 Remove the cuff after the BP is measured. The BP is displayed on the device.
17 Note the person's name and BP on your note pad or assignment sheet.
18 Follow agency policy for where to store the cuff (in the person's room or with the BP manometer).

POST-PROCEDURE

19 Provide for comfort. (See the inside of the back cover.)
20 Place the call light and other needed items within reach.
21 Unscreen the person.
22 Complete a safety check of the room. (See the inside of the back cover.)

23 Return the equipment to its proper place. Follow agency policy for disinfection.
24 Practice hand hygiene.
25 Report and record the BP. Note which arm was used. Report an abnormal BP at once.

PULSE OXIMETRY

Pulse oximetry measures the oxygen level in the blood. This is often measured with TPR and BP. It may be a vital sign in some agencies. See "Pulse Oximetry" in Chapter 43.

PAIN

Pain is a warning sign from the body. It signals tissue damage. Therefore many agencies consider it to be a vital sign. See "Pain" in Chapter 35.

REPORTING AND RECORDING

You must report and record accurately. You also must know what to report at once. Report:

- A change in any vital sign from a prior measurement. Follow the nurse's guidelines for what change the nurse considers important.
- A vital sign above or below the normal range. Normal ranges for an adult are:
  - Oral temperature—98.6°F (37.0°C). See Table 33-1 for normal temperatures at other sites.
  - Pulse—60 to 100 beats per minute.
  - Respirations—12 to 20 breaths per minute.
  - Blood pressure—90/60 mm Hg or higher but lower than 120/80 mm Hg.

Vital signs are recorded in the person's medical record. If measured often, a flow sheet or graphic sheet may be used (Fig. 33-30). Past and current measurements can be compared easily.

DAILY SUMMARY AND GRAPHIC

DATE	6/12					
HOUR	2400	0400	0800	1200	1600	2000
BP	118/72	124/76	122/78			
BP SITE	R arm	R arm	L arm			
TEMPERATURE						
TEMP ROUTE	Oral	Oral	Oral			
PULSE	76	74	78			
RESPIRATION	16	16	18			
PULSE OXIMETRY	97%	98%	97%			

Temperature scale: 104 / 40, 102.2 / 39, 100.4 / 38, 98.6 / 37, 96.6 / 36

FIGURE 33-30 Charting sample on a graphic sheet.

FOCUS ON **PRIDE**

The Person, Family, and Yourself

Personal and Professional Responsibility
Learning to measure vital signs takes practice. Do not be upset if you struggle at first. Plan when and what you will practice. Use class time wisely. Tell your instructor if you need more practice. Never be ashamed to ask for more practice time. Practice builds confidence.

Rights and Respect
The nurse may ask you to re-take a measurement. Or the nurse may re-check the measurement. Do not be offended. Show respect. Avoid negative thoughts or statements about the nurse or yourself. It does not mean the nurse does not trust you or that you have done something wrong. The nurse checks the measurements for safe care.

Independence and Social Interaction
Personal choice promotes independence. The person may prefer a certain arm for pulses and blood pressures. If safe to do so, use the arm the person prefers. Unless directed otherwise, let the person choose to sit or lie when vital signs are measured.

Delegation and Teamwork
You may care for persons needing Transmission-Based Precautions (Chapter 17). You must prevent the spread of infection from equipment. Some agencies have isolation carts or kits with equipment for vital signs. The equipment is left in the person's room. Do not use your own stethoscope or bring other equipment into the room or home. If equipment must be brought in, disinfect it after use. Special disinfectants may be needed. Follow agency policy to protect others from infection.

Ethics and Laws
Measurements must be accurate. Tell the nurse if you are unsure of any measurement. For example, you cannot feel a pulse or hear a blood pressure. Never make up a measurement. Reporting or recording false measurements is wrong. The person can be harmed. Take pride in doing the right thing by honest reporting and recording.

FOCUS ON **PRIDE**: Application

Plan to practice vital signs at school and at home. Practice on classmates, family, and friends. Who will you practice with? What will you practice most at school? What can you practice at home?

REVIEW QUESTIONS

Circle the BEST answer.

1 Which should you report at once?
  a An oral temperature of 98.4°F
  b A rectal temperature of 101.6°F
  c An axillary temperature of 97.6°F
  d An oral temperature of 99.0°F

2 A rectal temperature is taken when the person
  a Is unconscious
  b Has heart disease
  c Is confused
  d Has diarrhea

3 Which site is used to take an infant's temperature?
  a Oral site
  b Rectal site
  c Axillary site
  d Tympanic membrane site

4 To use an electronic thermometer
  a Shake down the thermometer before each use
  b Leave the thermometer in place for 2 minutes
  c Cover the probe with a probe cover
  d Use the blue probe for a rectal temperature

5 Which is usually used to take an adult's pulse?
  a The radial pulse
  b The apical pulse
  c The carotid pulse
  d The brachial pulse

6 For an adult, which pulse do you report at once?
  a A regular pulse at 64 beats per minute
  b A strong pulse at 78 beats per minute
  c A regular pulse at 90 beats per minute
  d An irregular pulse at 124 beats per minute

7 You count a regular pulse for 30 seconds. Which is *true*?
  a Divide the number of beats by 2 for the pulse rate.
  b If you count 44 beats, record a pulse rate of 44.
  c If you count 44 beats, record a pulse rate of 88.
  d Ask the nurse to check a regular pulse.

8 Which statement about the apical-radial pulse is *true*?
  a The radial pulse can be greater than the apical pulse.
  b The apical pulse can be greater than the radial pulse.
  c The apical and radial pulses are always equal.
  d The pulse deficit is always 0.

9 Which statement about measuring respirations is *true*?
  a Count the rise and fall of the chest as 2 respirations.
  b Count an abnormal pattern for 30 seconds.
  c A rate of 14 is abnormal for an adult.
  d Respirations are normally quiet.

10 Respirations are usually counted
  a After taking the temperature
  b Before taking the pulse
  c After taking the pulse
  d After taking the blood pressure

11 Which adult blood pressure is normal?
  a 80/54 mm Hg
  b 140/90 mm Hg
  c 112/78 mm Hg
  d 130/82 mm Hg

12 When measuring BP
  a Apply the cuff to the bare upper arm
  b Use the arm with an IV infusion
  c Make sure the cuff is loose
  d Place the stethoscope under the cuff

13 The systolic blood pressure is the point
  a Where the pulse is no longer felt
  b 30 mm Hg above where the pulse was felt
  c Where the first sound is heard
  d Where the last sound is heard

14 When taking a BP, you hear the last sound at the 1st short line above 70. You record the
  a Systolic pressure as 70
  b Diastolic pressure as 71
  c Systolic pressure as 72
  d Diastolic pressure as 72

15 You are not sure you heard a BP correctly. You should
  a Record what you think you heard
  b Measure the BP again after 60 seconds
  c Repeat the BP using the bell part of the stethoscope
  d Ask another nursing assistant to take the BP

Answers to Chapter 33 questions are on p. 886.

FOCUS ON PRACTICE

Problem Solving

A person's pulse is 110. The respiratory rate is 24. The oral temperature is 100.8°F. You think you heard the BP at 86/52. You are unsure of the measurement. What will you do? Are any of the vital signs abnormal? What must you do?

Exercise and Activity

OBJECTIVES

- Define the key terms and key abbreviations in this chapter.
- Describe bed rest.
- Explain how to prevent the complications from bed rest.
- Describe the devices that support and maintain body alignment.
- Explain the purpose of a trapeze.
- Describe range-of-motion exercises.
- Describe 4 walking aids.
- Perform the procedures described in this chapter.
- Explain how to promote PRIDE in the person, the family, and yourself.

KEY TERMS

abduction Moving a body part away from the mid-line of the body

adduction Moving a body part toward the mid-line of the body

ambulation The act of walking

atrophy The decrease in size or wasting away of tissue

bed rest Restricting a person to bed and limiting activity for health reasons

contracture Decreased motion and stiffness of a joint caused by shortening (contracting) of a muscle

deconditioning The loss of muscle strength from inactivity

dorsiflexion Bending the toes and foot up at the ankle

extension Straightening a body part

external rotation Turning the joint outward

flexion Bending a body part

footdrop The foot falls down at the ankle; permanent plantar flexion

hyperextension Excessive straightening of a body part

internal rotation Turning the joint inward

opposition Touching an opposite finger with the thumb

orthostatic hypotension See "postural hypotension"

orthotic A device used to support a muscle, promote a certain motion, or correct a deformity; *ortho* means *to straighten*

plantar flexion The foot *(plantar)* is bent *(flexion)*; bending the foot down at the ankle

postural hypotension Abnormally low *(hypo)* blood pressure when the person suddenly stands up *(postural)*; orthostatic hypotension

pronation Turning the joint downward

range of motion (ROM) The movement of a joint to the extent possible without causing pain

rotation Turning the joint

supination Turning the joint upward

syncope A brief loss of consciousness; fainting

KEY ABBREVIATIONS

ADL	Activities of daily living	PROM	Passive range of motion
ID	Identification	ROM	Range of motion

Exercise and activity are important for every body system. Physical and mental well-being are affected.

You assist the nurse and health team in promoting exercise and activity in all persons to the extent possible. The care plan and your assignment sheet include the person's activity level and needed exercises. The goal may be to:

- Improve independence for the home setting.
- Attain the highest level of function possible.
- Prevent loss of function.

See *Focus on Children and Older Persons: Exercise and Activity.*

FOCUS ON **CHILDREN AND OLDER PERSONS**

Exercise and Activity

Older Persons

Deconditioning is the loss of muscle strength from inactivity. When not active, older persons can become deconditioned quickly.

Persons with dementia may resist exercise and activity. Not understanding what is happening, they may fear harm. Some may become agitated and combative or cry out for help. Do not force the person to exercise or take part in activities. Stay calm and ask the nurse for help. Follow the care plan.

BED REST

Bed rest means restricting a person to bed and limiting activity for health reasons. Bed rest is ordered for a health problem or because of a change in the person's condition. Common reasons are to:

- Reduce oxygen needs.
- Reduce pain.
- Reduce swelling.
- Promote healing.
  These types of bed rest are common.
- *Strict or complete bed rest.* Everything is done for the person. All activities of daily living (ADL) are done in bed.
- *Bed rest.* The person performs some ADL. Self-feeding, oral hygiene, bathing, shaving, and hair care are often allowed.
- *Bed rest with commode privileges.* The commode is used at the bedside for elimination.
- *Bed rest with bathroom privileges (bed rest with BRP).* The bathroom is used for elimination.

Bed rest definitions vary among agencies. Follow the person's care plan and your assignment sheet for the activities allowed. Always ask the nurse what bed rest means for each person. Ask the nurse if you have questions about a person's activity limits.

Complications From Bed Rest

Bed rest and lack of exercise and activity can cause serious complications. Every system is affected. Pressure injuries, constipation, and fecal impaction can result. Urinary tract infections and renal calculi (kidney stones) can occur. So can blood clots (thrombi) and pneumonia (inflammation and infection of the lung).

The musculo-skeletal system is affected too. For normal movement, you help prevent the following.

- A *contracture is decreased motion and stiffness of a joint caused by shortening (contracting) of a muscle.* The contracted muscle is fixed into position, is deformed, and cannot stretch (Fig. 34-1). Common sites are the fingers, wrists, elbows, toes, ankles, knees, and hips. They can also occur in the neck and spine. The site is deformed and stiff.
- *Atrophy is the decrease in size or the wasting away of tissue.* Tissues shrink in size. *Muscle atrophy is a decrease in size or a wasting away of muscle* (Fig. 34-2).

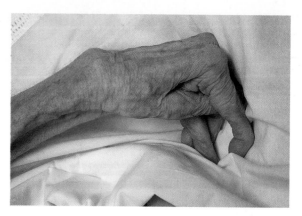

FIGURE 34-1 A contracture.

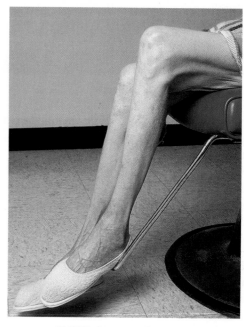

FIGURE 34-2 Muscle atrophy.

Postural hypotension is abnormally low (hypo) blood pressure when the person suddenly stands up (postural). When moving from a lying to sitting or standing position, the blood pressure drops. The person is dizzy, weak, and has spots before the eyes. Syncope can occur. *Syncope (fainting) is a brief loss of consciousness.* (The Greek word *synkoptein* means *to cut short.*) *Postural hypotension also is called* **orthostatic hypotension.** (*Ortho* and *static* mean *standing.* *Orthostatic* relates to *an upright posture.*)

Good nursing care prevents complications from bed rest. Good alignment, range-of-motion exercises (p. 535), and frequent position changes are important measures. These are part of the care plan.

See *Focus on Communication: Complications From Bed Rest.*

See *Promoting Safety and Comfort: Complications From Bed Rest.*

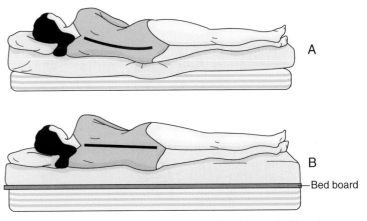

FIGURE 34-3 Bed boards. **A,** Mattress sagging without a bed board. **B,** A bed board is under the mattress. No sagging occurs.

FOCUS ON COMMUNICATION

Complications From Bed Rest

Postural hypotension can occur when moving from lying to sitting or standing. To check for postural hypotension, ask these questions.

- "Do you feel weak?"
- "Do you feel dizzy?"
- "Do you see spots before your eyes?"
- "Do you feel like fainting?"

PROMOTING SAFETY AND COMFORT

Complications From Bed Rest

Safety

Slowly changing positions is key to preventing postural hypotension. The person slowly progresses in stages from:

- Supine to Fowler's position
- Fowler's position to sitting on the side of the bed
- Sitting on the side of the bed to standing
- Standing to walking or sitting in a chair

While the person is supine, measure vital signs—blood pressure, pulse, respirations, and pulse oximetry (Chapter 43). For each stage:

- Ask about weakness, dizziness, or spots before the eyes. Return the person to the previous position if any occur. For example, the person complains of being dizzy while sitting on the side of the bed. Help the person return to the Fowler's position.
- Measure vital signs.

Report and record the person's vital signs, symptoms, and complaints. Call for the nurse at once if you have concerns about the person's condition.

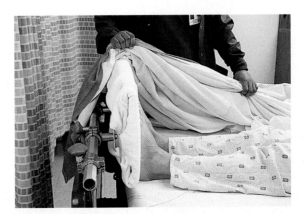

FIGURE 34-4 A foot-board. Feet are flush with the board to keep them in normal alignment.

Positioning Devices

Body alignment and positioning were discussed in Chapter 18. Supportive devices are often used to support and maintain a certain position.

- *Bed boards*—are placed under the mattress to prevent it from sagging (Fig. 34-3). The bed boards are covered with canvas or other material. Many are hinged at the middle for use with hospital beds. A hinged bed board allows the head of the bed to be raised. Bed boards may be used in home settings by persons with back problems.
- *Foot-board*—prevents plantar flexion that can lead to footdrop. In *plantar flexion, the foot* (plantar) *is bent* (flexion). *Footdrop is when the foot falls down at the ankle (permanent plantar flexion).* The foot-board is placed so the soles of the feet are flush against it (Fig. 34-4). Foot-boards also serve as bed cradles by keeping top linens off the feet and toes.

- *Trochanter roll*—prevents the hips and legs from turning outward (external rotation) (Fig. 34-5, p. 534). A bath blanket or bath towel is folded to the desired length and rolled up tightly. The flat end is placed under the person from the hip to the knee. The roll is tucked alongside the body.
- *Hip abduction wedge*—keeps the hips abducted (apart) (Fig. 34-6, p. 534). The wedge is placed between the person's legs. The device is common after hip replacement surgery.
- *Hand roll or hand grip*—prevents contractures of the thumb, fingers, and wrist (Fig. 34-7, p. 534). Foam rubber sponges, rubber balls, and finger cushions (Fig. 34-8, p. 534) also are used.
- *Splints*—keep the elbows, wrists, thumbs, fingers, ankles, or knees in normal position. They are usually secured in place with Velcro (Fig. 34-9, p. 534).
- *Bed cradle*—keeps the weight of top linens off the feet and toes (Fig. 34-10, p. 534). Heavy top linens can cause footdrop and pressure injuries.

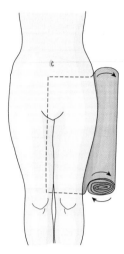

FIGURE 34-5 A trochanter roll is made from a bath blanket. It extends from the hip to the knee.

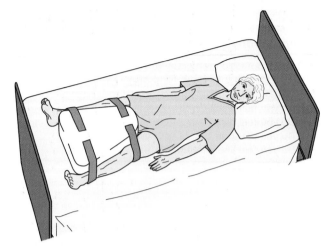

FIGURE 34-6 Hip abduction wedge.

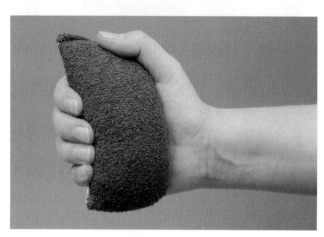

FIGURE 34-7 Hand grip.

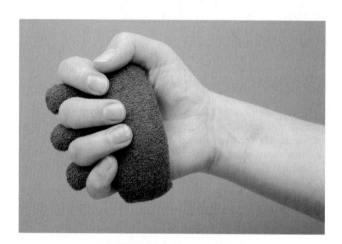

FIGURE 34-8 Finger cushion.

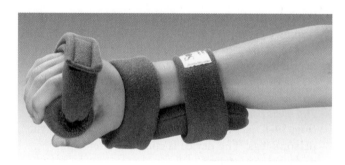

FIGURE 34-9 A splint. (Courtesy Ongoing Care Solutions, Inc., Pinellas Park, Fla.)

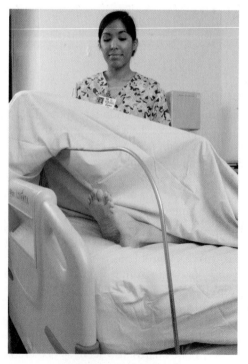

FIGURE 34-10 A bed cradle.

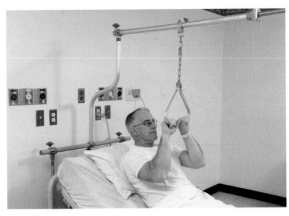

FIGURE 34-11 A trapeze is used to strengthen arm muscles.

Exercise

Exercise helps prevent contractures, muscle atrophy, and other complications from bed rest. Some exercise occurs with ADL. Other exercises are needed for muscles and joints. (See "Range-of-Motion Exercises" and "Ambulation," p. 539.)

A *trapeze* is used for exercises to strengthen arm muscles. The trapeze hangs from an over-bed frame (Fig. 34-11). The person grasps the bar with both hands to lift the trunk off the bed. The trapeze is also used to move up and turn in bed.

RANGE-OF-MOTION EXERCISES

*The movement of a joint to the extent possible without causing pain is the **range of motion (ROM)** of the joint.* Range-of-motion exercises involve moving the joints through their complete range of motion (Box 34-1). They are usually done at least 2 times a day.

* *Active* ROM exercises—are done by the person.
* *Passive* ROM (PROM) exercises—you move the joints through their range of motion.
* *Active-assistive* ROM exercises—the person does the exercises with some help.

Bathing, hair care, eating, reaching, dressing and undressing, and walking all involve joint movements. Persons on bed rest need more frequent ROM exercises. So do those who cannot walk, turn, or transfer themselves because of illness or injury.

See *Focus on Surveys: Range-of-Motion Exercises.*

See *Focus on Children and Older Persons: Range-of-Motion Exercises.*

See *Delegation Guidelines: Range-of-Motion Exercises*, p. 536.

See *Promoting Safety and Comfort: Range-of-Motion Exercises*, p. 536.

See procedure: *Performing Range-of-Motion Exercises*, p. 536.

Text continued on p. 539.

FOCUS ON **SURVEYS**

Range-of-Motion Exercises

The person's care plan must focus on his or her ROM. The goal may be 1 of the following.

* Increase range of motion.
* Prevent loss of or further decreases in range of motion. Surveyors may observe you performing ROM activities.

BOX 34-1   Range-of-Motion Exercises

Joint Movements

* *Abduction*—moving a body part away from the mid-line of the body
* *Adduction*—moving a body part toward the mid-line of the body
* *Opposition*—touching an opposite finger with the thumb
* *Flexion*—bending a body part
* *Extension*—straightening a body part
* *Hyperextension*—excessive straightening of a body part
* *Dorsiflexion*—bending the toes and foot up at the ankle
* *Plantar flexion*—bending the foot down at the ankle
* *Rotation*—turning the joint
* *Internal rotation*—turning the joint inward
* *External rotation*—turning the joint outward
* *Pronation*—turning the joint downward
* *Supination*—turning the joint upward

Safety Measures

* Cover the person with a bath blanket for warmth and privacy.
* Exercise only the joints the nurse tells you to exercise.
* Use good body mechanics.
* Expose only the body part being exercised.
* Support the part being exercised at all times.
* Move the joint slowly, smoothly, and gently.
* Do not force a joint beyond its present range of motion or to the point of pain. As each joint is exercised ask if the person:
  * Feels that the joint cannot move any farther.
  * Feels pain or discomfort in the joint.
  * Needs to stop or rest.
* Ask the person about pain or discomfort. Observe for signs of pain (Chapter 35). Restlessness and grimacing are examples.
* Stop if you meet resistance or suspect pain. Tell the nurse.

FOCUS ON **CHILDREN AND OLDER PERSONS**

Range-of-Motion Exercises

Children

Most play activities promote active ROM exercise. For example:

* Kicking a Mylar balloon or foam ball.
* Touching a Mylar balloon that is held or hung in different places. For example, hang a Mylar balloon from the trapeze.
* Playing basketball with bean-bags, wadded paper, or foam balls. Use a hoop or wastebasket as the target.
* Playing "pat-a-cake" or "Simon Says" (clap, kick, jump, and other motions).
* Having the child act like a bird, butterfly, spider, monkey, horse, or other animal.
* Playing video or computer games for finger and hand movements.
* Playing with finger paints, clay, or play dough.
* Having tricycle or wheelchair races.
* Playing "hide and seek." Hide a toy in the bed or room.
  Check with the nurse and care plan for the child's activity limits. Make sure the nurse approves of the play activity.

Modified from Hockenberry MJ and others: Wong's nursing care of infants and children, ed 10, St Louis, 2015, Mosby.

DELEGATION GUIDELINES
Range-of-Motion Exercises

Performing range-of-motion exercises may be a routine nursing task in your agency. (See *Promoting Safety and Comfort: Range-of-Motion Exercises.*) When delegated ROM exercises, you need this information from the nurse and the care plan.

- If ROM exercises are active, passive, or active-assistive
- Which joints to exercise
- What ROM exercises to do—abduction, adduction, flexion, extension, and so on (see Box 34-1)
- When to do the exercises
- How many times to repeat each exercise
- What observations to report and record:
  - The time the exercises were performed
  - The joints exercised and the exercises performed
  - The number of times the exercises were performed on each joint
  - Complaints of pain or signs of stiffness or spasm; specify the joint or body part involved
  - The degree to which the person took part in the exercises
  - When to report observations
- What patient or resident concerns to report at once

PROMOTING SAFETY AND COMFORT
Range-of-Motion Exercises

Safety
ROM exercises can cause injury if not done correctly. Muscle strain, joint injury, and pain are possible. Practice the measures in Box 34-1. Remind the person to tell you about any pain during the procedure.

ROM exercises to the neck can cause serious injury if not done correctly. Some agencies give nursing assistants special training before doing such exercises. Other agencies do not let nursing assistants do them. Know your agency's policy. Perform ROM exercises to the neck only if allowed by your agency, if you received needed training, and if they are delegated to you. In some agencies, only physical therapists do neck exercises.

Comfort
To promote physical comfort during ROM exercises, see Box 34-1. Provide privacy to promote mental comfort.

Performing Range-of-Motion Exercises

QUALITY OF LIFE

- Knock before entering the person's room.
- Address the person by name.
- Introduce yourself by name and title.
- Explain the procedure before starting and during the procedure.
- Protect the person's rights during the procedure.
- Handle the person gently during the procedure.

PRE-PROCEDURE

1. Follow *Delegation Guidelines: Range-of-Motion Exercises.* See *Promoting Safety and Comfort: Range-of-Motion Exercises.*
2. Practice hand hygiene.
3. Identify the person. Check the ID (identification) bracelet against the assignment sheet. Use 2 identifiers (Chapter 13). Also call the person by name.
4. Obtain a bath blanket.
5. Provide for privacy.
6. Raise the bed for body mechanics. Bed rails are up if used.

PROCEDURE

7. Lower the bed rail near you if up.
8. Position the person supine.
9. Cover the person with the bath blanket. Fan-fold top linens to the foot of the bed.
10. Exercise the neck *if allowed by your agency and if the nurse instructs you to do so* (Fig. 34-12, p. 538).
    a. Place your hands over the ears to support the head. Support the jaw with your fingers.
    b. Flexion—bring the head forward. The chin touches the chest.
    c. Extension—straighten the head.
    d. Hyperextension—bring the head backward until the chin points up.
    e. Rotation—turn the head from side to side.
    f. Lateral flexion—move the head to the right and to the left.
    g. Repeat flexion, extension, hyperextension, rotation, and lateral flexion 5 times—or the number of times stated on the care plan.
11. Exercise the shoulder (Fig. 34-13, p. 538).
    a. Support the wrist with 1 hand. Support the elbow with the other hand.
    b. Flexion—raise the arm straight up in front and over the head.
    c. Extension—bring the arm down to the side.
    d. Hyperextension—move the arm behind the body. (Do this if the person is in a straight-backed chair or is standing.)
    e. Abduction—move the straight arm away from the side of the body.
    f. Adduction—move the straight arm to the side of the body.
    g. Internal rotation—bend the elbow. Place it at the same level as the shoulder. Move the forearm and hand so the fingers point down.
    h. External rotation—move the forearm and hand so the fingers point up.
    i. Repeat flexion, extension, hyperextension, abduction, adduction, and internal and external rotation 5 times—or the number of times stated on the care plan.

Performing Range-of-Motion Exercises—cont'd

PROCEDURE—cont'd

12 Exercise the elbow (Fig. 34-14, p. 538).
 a Support the wrist with 1 hand. Support the elbow with your other hand.
 b Flexion—bend the arm so the same-side shoulder is touched.
 c Extension—straighten the arm.
 d Repeat flexion and extension 5 times—or the number of times stated on the care plan.
13 Exercise the forearm (Fig. 34-15, p. 538).
 a Continue to support the wrist and elbow.
 b Pronation—turn the hand so the palm is down.
 c Supination—turn the hand so the palm is up.
 d Repeat pronation and supination 5 times—or the number of times stated on the care plan.
14 Exercise the wrist (Fig. 34-16, p. 538).
 a Support the wrist with both of your hands.
 b Flexion—bend the hand down.
 c Extension—straighten the hand.
 d Hyperextension—bend the hand back.
 e Radial flexion (deviation)—turn the hand toward the thumb.
 f Ulnar flexion (deviation)—turn the hand toward the little finger.
 g Repeat flexion, extension, hyperextension, radial flexion (deviation), and ulnar flexion (deviation) 5 times—or the number of times stated on the care plan.
15 Exercise the thumb (Fig. 34-17, p. 538).
 a Support the person's hand with 1 hand. Support the thumb with your other hand.
 b Abduction—move the thumb out from the inner part of the index finger.
 c Adduction—move the thumb back next to the index finger.
 d Opposition—touch each fingertip with the thumb.
 e Flexion—bend the thumb into the hand.
 f Extension—move the thumb out to the side of the fingers.
 g Repeat abduction, adduction, opposition, flexion, and extension 5 times—or the number of times stated on the care plan.
16 Exercise the fingers (Fig. 34-18, p. 538).
 a Abduction—spread the fingers and thumb apart.
 b Adduction—bring the fingers and thumb together.
 c Flexion—make a fist.
 d Extension—straighten the fingers so the fingers, hand, and arm are straight.
 e Repeat abduction, adduction, flexion, and extension 5 times—or the number of times stated on the care plan.

17 Exercise the hip (Fig. 34-19, p. 539).
 a Support the leg. Place 1 hand under the knee. Place your other hand under the ankle.
 b Flexion—raise the leg.
 c Extension—straighten the leg.
 d Hyperextension—move the leg behind the body. (Do this if the person is standing.)
 e Abduction—move the leg away from the body.
 f Adduction—move the leg toward the other leg.
 g Internal rotation—turn the leg inward.
 h External rotation—turn the leg outward.
 i Repeat flexion, extension, hyperextension, abduction, adduction, and internal and external rotation 5 times—or the number of times stated on the care plan.
18 Exercise the knee (Fig. 34-20, p. 539).
 a Support the knee. Place 1 hand under the knee. Place your other hand under the ankle.
 b Flexion—bend the knee.
 c Extension—straighten the knee.
 d Repeat flexion and extension 5 times—or the number of times stated on the care plan.
19 Exercise the ankle (Fig. 34-21, p. 539).
 a Support the foot and ankle. Place 1 hand under the foot. Place your other hand under the ankle.
 b Dorsiflexion—pull the foot upward. Push down on the heel at the same time.
 c Plantar flexion—turn the foot down. Or point the toes.
 d Repeat dorsiflexion and plantar flexion 5 times—or the number of times stated on the care plan.
20 Exercise the foot (Fig. 34-22, p. 539).
 a Continue to support the foot and ankle.
 b Pronation—turn the outside of the foot up and the inside down.
 c Supination—turn the inside of the foot up and the outside down.
 d Repeat pronation and supination 5 times—or the number of times stated on the care plan.
21 Exercise the toes (Fig. 34-23, p. 539).
 a Flexion—curl the toes.
 b Extension—straighten the toes.
 c Abduction—spread the toes.
 d Adduction—put the toes together.
 e Repeat flexion, extension, abduction, and adduction 5 times—or the number of times stated on the care plan.
22 Cover the leg. Raise the bed rail if used.
23 Go to the other side. Lower the bed rail near you if up.
24 Repeat steps 11 through 21. Cover the leg when done.

POST-PROCEDURE

25 Provide for comfort. (See the inside of the back cover.)
26 Cover the person with the top linens. Remove the bath blanket.
27 Place the call light and other needed items within reach.
28 Lower the bed to a safe and comfortable level. Follow the care plan.
29 Raise or lower bed rails. Follow the care plan.
30 Fold and return the bath blanket to its proper place. Or follow agency policy for used linens.
31 Unscreen the person.
32 Complete a safety check of the room. (See the inside of the back cover.)
33 Practice hand hygiene.
34 Report and record your observations.

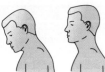

Flexion Extension Hyperextension Rotation Lateral flexion

FIGURE 34-12 Range-of-motion exercises for the neck.

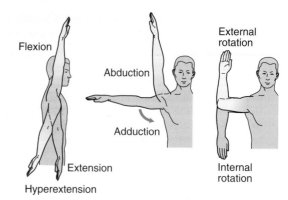

Flexion

Abduction

External rotation

Adduction

Extension

Hyperextension

Internal rotation

FIGURE 34-13 Range-of-motion exercises for the shoulder.

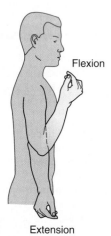

Flexion

Extension

FIGURE 34-14 Range-of-motion exercises for the elbow.

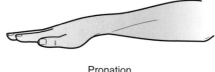

Pronation

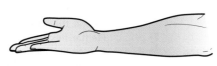

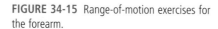

Supination

FIGURE 34-15 Range-of-motion exercises for the forearm.

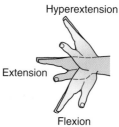

Hyperextension

Ulnar flexion (deviation)

Extension

Flexion

Radial flexion (deviation)

FIGURE 34-16 Range-of-motion exercises for the wrist.

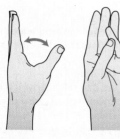
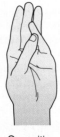
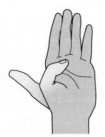

Abduction Adduction

Opposition to little finger

Flexion Extension

FIGURE 34-17 Range-of-motion exercises for the thumb.

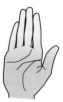

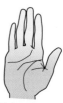

Abduction

Adduction

Flexion

Extension

FIGURE 34-18 Range-of-motion exercises for the fingers.

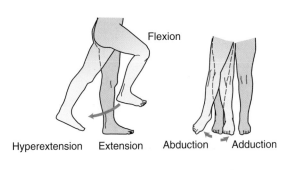

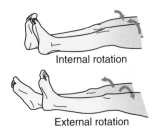

FIGURE 34-19 Range-of-motion exercises for the hip.

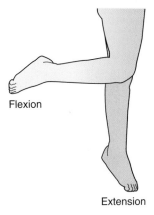

FIGURE 34-20 Range-of-motion exercises for the knee.

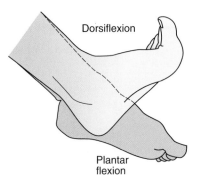

FIGURE 34-21 Range-of-motion exercises for the ankle.

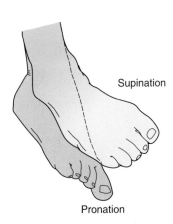

FIGURE 34-22 Range-of-motion exercises for the foot.

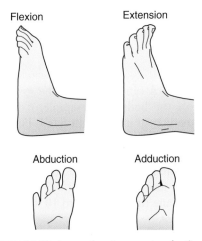

FIGURE 34-23 Range-of-motion exercises for the toes.

AMBULATION

Ambulation is the act of walking. Some people need help walking. They may be weak or unsteady from bed rest, illness, surgery, or injury. Walkers and canes are common for safety. Sometimes crutches (p. 543) and orthotic devices are needed (p. 545).

The walking aid ordered depends on the person's condition, size, support needed, and type of disability. A physical therapist (PT) teaches the person how to use the device.

Canes

Canes are used for weakness on 1 side of the body. They help provide balance and support. Single-tip and 4-point (quad) canes are common (Fig. 34-24). A 4-point cane gives more support than a single-tip cane but is harder to move.

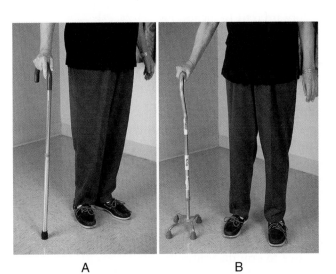

A   B

FIGURE 34-24 **A,** Single-tip cane. **B,** Four-point cane.

A   B   C

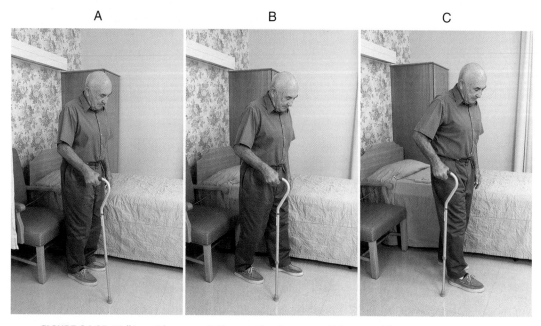

FIGURE 34-25 Walking with a cane. **A,** The cane (on the strong side) is moved forward about 6 to 10 inches. **B,** The leg opposite the cane (weak leg) is brought forward even with the cane. **C,** The leg on the cane side (strong side) is moved ahead of the cane and the weak leg.

Using a Cane. A cane is held on the *strong side* (unaffected side) of the body. For example, if the left leg is weak, the cane is held in the right hand. For proper cane position, the cane is held to the side and in front of the *strong foot.*

- Side—the cane tip is about 6 to 10 inches to the side of the strong foot.
- Front—the cane tip is about 6 to 10 inches in front of the strong foot.

The grip is level with the hip on the strong side. The person walks as follows.

- *Step 1:* The cane (on the strong side) is moved forward 6 to 10 inches (Fig. 34-25, *A*).
- *Step 2:* The weak leg (opposite the cane) is moved forward even with the cane (Fig. 34-25, *B*).
- *Step 3:* The strong leg is moved forward and ahead of the cane and the weak leg (Fig. 34-25, *C*).

Walkers

A walker gives more support than a cane. Wheeled walkers have wheels on the front legs and rubber tips on the back legs (Fig. 34-26). Rubber tips on the back legs prevent the walker from moving while the person is standing. To walk, the person pushes the walker about 6 to 8 inches in front of the feet.

Baskets, pouches, and trays attach to the walker for needed items. This allows more independence. The hands are free to grip the walker.

See *Promoting Safety and Comfort: Walkers.*

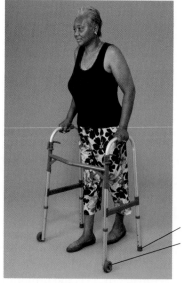

Rubber tip
Wheel on the outside of the walker

FIGURE 34-26 Wheeled walker.

PROMOTING SAFETY AND COMFORT
Walkers

Safety
Wheels are usually on the outside of the walker (see Fig. 34-26). With wheels on the outside, the walker is too wide for some doorways. Moving the wheels to the inside of the walker reduces the width. The person can go through narrower doorways.

Walker tennis balls are common. Placed on the rear legs, they allow the walker to slide easier on carpets and other surfaces (Fig. 34-27).

Walkers vary in design. Some have a braking action when weight is applied to the back legs. Some walkers have seats. The person sits to rest. Never push the walker when the person is seated.

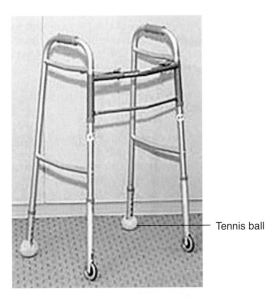

Tennis ball

FIGURE 34-27 Walker tennis balls on the rear legs of a walker. (From Fairchild SL, Kuchler R, Washington RD: *Pierson and Fairchild's principles & techniques of patient care*, ed 6, St Louis, 2018, Elsevier.)

Assisting With Ambulation

To walk, contractures and muscle atrophy must be prevented. Proper positioning and exercises are needed.

After bed rest, activity increases slowly and in steps. First the person sits on the side of the bed (dangles). Sitting in a chair may follow. Next the person walks a few steps. Distance increases as the person gains strength.

Follow the care plan when helping a person walk. Use a gait (transfer) belt (Chapter 14). The person uses wall hand rails or a cane or walker. Always check for postural hypotension (p. 532).

See *Focus on Communication: Assisting With Ambulation.*
See *Delegation Guidelines: Assisting With Ambulation.*
See *Promoting Safety and Comfort: Assisting With Ambulation.*
See procedure: *Assisting With Ambulation*, p. 542.

FOCUS ON COMMUNICATION
Assisting With Ambulation

Before ambulating, explain the activity. This promotes comfort and reduces fear. Explain:
- How far to walk
- What adaptive (assistive) devices are used
- That you will use a gait belt
- How you will assist
- What the person is to report to you
- How you will help if the person begins to fall
For example, you can say:

I am going to help you walk from your bed to the doorway and back. This belt helps support you while you walk. I will be at your side holding the belt at all times. Tell me right away if you feel unsteady, dizzy, weak, or faint. Also tell me if you feel any pain or discomfort. If you begin to fall, I will use the belt to pull you close to me and gently lower you to the floor. Do you have any questions?

DELEGATION GUIDELINES
Assisting With Ambulation

Assisting with ambulation is a routine nursing task. Before assisting with ambulation, you need this information from the nurse and the care plan.
- How much help the person needs
- If the person uses a cane, walker, crutches (p. 543), or an orthotic device (p. 545)
- Areas of weakness—right arm or leg, left arm or leg
- How far to walk the person
- What observations to report and record:
  - How well the person tolerated the activity
  - Shuffling, sliding, limping, or walking on tip-toes
  - Complaints of pain or discomfort
  - Complaints of postural hypotension—weakness, dizziness, spots before the eyes, feeling faint
  - The distance walked
- When to report observations
- What patient or resident concerns to report at once

PROMOTING SAFETY AND COMFORT
Assisting With Ambulation

Safety
Practice the safety measures to prevent falls (Chapter 14). Use a gait belt to help the person stand and during ambulation.

If a walker is used, remind the person not to pull on the walker to stand. The walker can tip. The person pushes on the mattress or the chair's armrests to stand (Chapter 20).

Remind the person to walk normally. Encourage the person to stand erect (upright) with the head up and the back straight. Discourage shuffling, sliding, and walking on tip-toes.

Comfort
The fear of falling affects mental comfort. Explain the purpose of the gait belt. Also explain how you will help the person if he or she starts to fall (Chapter 14).

Assisting With Ambulation

QUALITY OF LIFE

- Knock before entering the person's room.
- Address the person by name.
- Introduce yourself by name and title.

- Explain the procedure before starting and during the procedure.
- Protect the person's rights during the procedure.
- Handle the person gently during the procedure.

PRE-PROCEDURE

1 Follow *Delegation Guidelines: Assisting With Ambulation*, p. 541. See *Promoting Safety and Comfort: Assisting With Ambulation*, p. 541.
2 Practice hand hygiene.
3 Collect the following.
   - Slip-resistant shoes or footwear
   - Paper or towel to protect bottom linens
   - Gait (transfer) belt
   - Walker or cane (if needed)

4 Identify the person. Check the ID bracelet against the assignment sheet. Use 2 identifiers (Chapter 13). Also call the person by name.
5 Provide for privacy.

PROCEDURE

6 Lower the bed to a safe and comfortable level. Follow the care plan. Lock (brake) the bed wheels. Lower the bed rail if up.
7 Fan-fold top linens to the foot of the bed.
8 Place the paper or towel under the person's feet to protect bottom linens. Put the shoes on and fasten.
9 Help the person sit on the side of the bed. (See procedure: *Sitting on the Side of the Bed [Dangling]* in Chapter 19.)
10 Make sure the person's feet are flat on the floor.
11 Make sure that the person is properly dressed.
12 Apply the gait belt at the waist over clothing. (See procedure: *Using a Transfer/Gait Belt* in Chapter 14.)
13 Position the walker (if used) in front of the person. Or have the person hold the cane (if used) on the strong side.
14 Help the person stand. (See procedure: *Transferring the Person to a Chair or Wheelchair* in Chapter 20.) Grasp the gait belt at each side.
15 Stand at the weak side while the person gains balance. Hold the belt at the side and back.
16 Encourage the person to stand erect with the head up and the back straight.
17 *Positioning a walker or cane:*
   a Walker—the walker is 6 to 8 inches in front of the person.
   b Cane—the cane is held on the strong side.
      1) The cane tip is 6 to 10 inches to the side of the strong foot.
      2) The cane tip is 6 to 10 inches in front of the strong foot.

18 Help the person walk. Walk to the side and slightly behind the person on the person's weak side. Provide support with the gait belt (Fig. 34-28). Have the person use the hand rail on his or her strong side (unless using a walker or cane).
19 *For a walker or cane:*
   a Walker—with both hands, the person pushes the walker 6 to 8 inches in front of the feet.
   b Cane:
      1) The cane (on the strong side) is moved forward 6 to 10 inches (see Fig. 34-25, *A*).
      2) The weak leg (opposite the cane) is moved forward even with the cane (see Fig. 34-25, *B*).
      3) The strong leg is moved forward and ahead of the cane and the weak leg (see Fig. 34-25, *C*).
20 Encourage the person to walk normally. The heel strikes the floor first. Discourage shuffling, sliding, or walking on tip-toes.
21 Walk the ordered distance if the person tolerates the activity. Do not rush the person.
22 Help the person return to bed. Remove the gait belt. (See procedure: *Transferring the Person From a Chair or Wheelchair to Bed* in Chapter 20.)
23 Lower the head of the bed. Help the person to the center of the bed.
24 Remove the shoes. Remove the paper or towel over the bottom sheet. Discard the paper or follow agency policy for used linens.

POST-PROCEDURE

25 Provide for comfort. (See the inside of the back cover.)
26 Place the call light and other needed items within reach.
27 Raise or lower bed rails. Follow the care plan.
28 Return the shoes to their proper place.
29 Unscreen the person.

30 Complete a safety check of the room. (See the inside of the back cover.)
31 Practice hand hygiene.
32 Report and record your observations (Fig. 34-29).

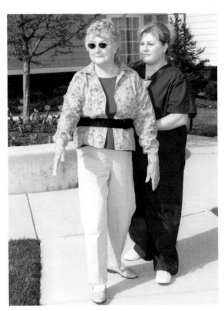

FIGURE 34-28 Assisting with ambulation. The nursing assistant walks at the person's side and slightly behind her. A gait belt is used for safety.

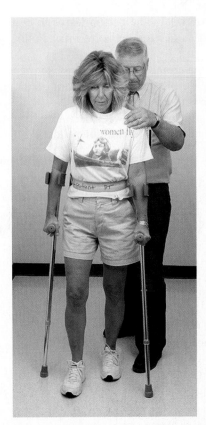

FIGURE 34-30 Forearm crutches. (From Fairchild SL, Kuchler R, Washington RD: *Pierson and Fairchild's principles & techniques of patient care,* ed 6, St Louis, 2018, Elsevier.)

DATE: 06/16	TIME: 1415
ACTIVITY AND POSITIONING	
☒ Ambulate	☐ Chair
☐ Self	☒ Bed
☒ Assist of 1	☒ Right side
☐ Assist of 2	☐ Left side
☐ Mechanical lift	☐ Back

Ambulated 25 feet in the hallway with assist of 1 and use of a gait belt. Reminded not to shuffle the feet. Showed no signs of distress or discomfort. Denied feeling dizzy, light-headed, or weak. No c/o pain. Assisted to bed after ambulating. Positioned on right side with a pillow behind the back, under the head, and between the legs. Denied any other needs.

SAFETY	
☒ Gait belt	☒ Belongings in reach
☒ Slip-resistant shoes	☒ Bed rails raised
☒ Call light in reach	☐ Bed rails lowered
☒ Bed in low position	

FIGURE 34-29 Charting sample.

Other Walking Aids

Injury, surgery, and deformity are some reasons for crutches or orthotic devices. The need may be temporary or permanent.

Crutches. Crutches are used when the person cannot use 1 leg or when 1 or both legs need to gain strength. Some persons with permanent leg weakness can use crutches. Forearm crutches are shown in Figure 34-30. Underarm crutches extend from the underarm to the ground (Fig. 34-31).

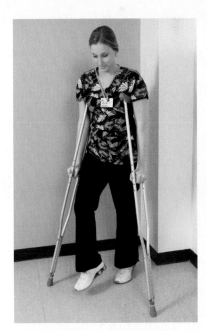

FIGURE 34-31 Underarm crutches.

Using Crutches. The person learns to crutch walk, use stairs, and sit and stand. Falls are a risk. Follow these safety measures.

- Check the crutch tips. They must not be worn down, torn, or wet. Replace worn or torn crutch tips. Dry wet tips with paper towels.
- Check crutches for flaws. Check wooden crutches for cracks and metal crutches for bends.
- Tighten all bolts.
- Have the person wear street shoes—flat with slip-resistant soles.
- Make sure clothes fit well. Loose clothes may get caught between the crutches and underarms. Loose clothes and long skirts can hang forward and block the person's view of the feet and crutch tips.
- Practice safety measures to prevent falls (Chapter 14).
- Keep crutches within the person's reach. Put them by the person's chair or against a wall.
- Know which crutch gait the person uses.
  - 4-point gait (Fig. 34-32)
  - 3-point gait (Fig. 34-33)
  - 2-point gait (Fig. 34-34)
  - Swing-to gait (Fig. 34-35)
  - Swing-through gait (Fig. 34-36)

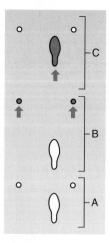

FIGURE 34-33 The 3-point gait. One leg is used. Both crutches are moved forward. Then the good foot is moved forward.

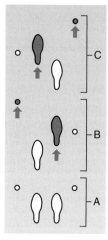

FIGURE 34-34 The 2-point gait. The person bears some weight on each foot. The left crutch and right foot are moved forward at the same time. Then the right crutch and left foot are moved forward.

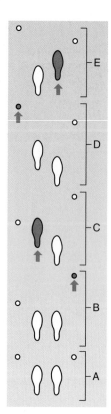

FIGURE 34-32 The 4-point gait. Both legs are used. The right crutch is moved forward and then the left foot. Then the left crutch is moved forward followed by the right foot.

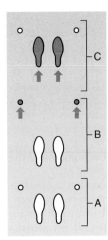

FIGURE 34-35 Swing-to gait. The person bears some weight on each leg. Both crutches are moved forward. Then the person lifts both legs and *swings to* the crutches.

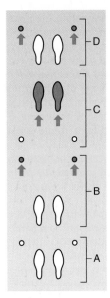

FIGURE 34-36 Swing-through gait. The person bears some weight on each leg. Both crutches are moved forward. Then the person lifts both legs and *swings through* the crutches.

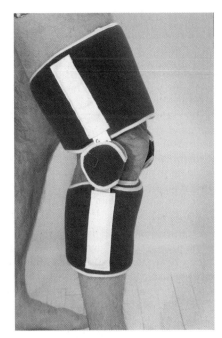

FIGURE 34-37 Knee brace. (Courtesy AliMed, Inc., Dedham, Mass.)

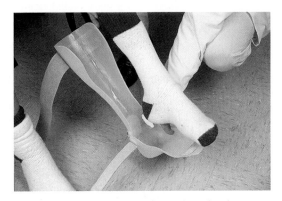

FIGURE 34-38 Ankle-foot orthosis (AFO).

Orthotic Devices. An *orthotic is a device used to support a muscle, promote a certain motion, or correct a deformity.* (Ortho *means* to straighten.) Paralysis and muscle weakness are common reasons for orthotic devices.

- *Braces.* Braces support weak body parts. They also prevent or correct deformities or prevent joint movement. A brace is applied over the ankle, knee, or back (Fig. 34-37).
- An ankle-foot orthosis (AFO) is worn with a shoe (Fig. 34-38). The AFO is secured with a Velcro strap. Used for footdrop, this type of brace is common after a stroke.

Keep skin and bony points under orthotics clean and dry. This prevents skin breakdown. Report redness or signs of skin breakdown at once. Also report complaints of pain or discomfort. The care plan tells you when to apply and remove a brace or AFO.

FOCUS ON **PRIDE**

The Person, Family, and Yourself

P ersonal and Professional Responsibility

Exercise and activity promote normal function of all body systems. Good conditioning has long-term effects. To promote activity, exercise, and well-being, you can:

- Encourage the person to be as active as possible.
- Resist the urge to do things that the person can safely do alone or with some help.
- Focus on the person's abilities.
- Give praise when the person is doing well, making progress, or gave a good effort.

R ights and Respect

Garments must provide privacy during exercise and activity. When ambulating, the person's gown must not be open in the back. During ROM exercises, cover the person with a bath blanket. Expose only the body part being exercised. Protect the right to privacy. Privacy promotes dignity and mental comfort.

I ndependence and Social Interaction

Nursing center activity programs promote physical, mental, and social well-being. Joints and muscles are exercised. Circulation is stimulated. Social interaction is mentally stimulating.

Bingo, movies, dances, exercise groups, shopping and museum trips, concerts, and guest speakers are common. Residents may tell you about favorite pastimes. Listen to interests. Suggest options that they may like. Allow personal choice to promote independence.

D elegation and Teamwork

To meet goals, all staff must follow the person's care plan. Progress slows or stops when only some staff follow the plan. For example, a person is to walk to and from the dining room at meal times. To save time, some staff push the person to the dining room in a wheelchair. Deconditioning results. Each staff member must do his or her part for the person's well-being.

E thics and Laws

Persons with contractures must be moved slowly and carefully. Otherwise pain and injury can occur. This case shows the result of a disregard for safe care.

A licensed nursing assistant (LNA) cared for a person with Alzheimer's disease. The resident was severely contracted. Her ability to communicate was poor. And she could not make decisions. The LNA admitted to:

- *Being observed pulling the resident's arms away from her body and allowing them to snap back*
- *Being observed pulling the resident's legs upward from the bed and allowing them to fall back down*
- *Failing to remove a bowel movement while cleaning the resident*

The Board found that the LNA abused and improperly cared for the resident. The unprofessional conduct violated the Administrative Rules of the Board of Nursing because of:

- *Abusing or improperly caring for a patient*
- *Performing unsafe or unacceptable patient care*
- *Failing to conform to acceptable standards of practice*
- *Engaging in conduct likely to harm the public*
  The LNA's license was suspended indefinitely.
  (State of Vermont Board of Nursing, 2000.)

Suspend indefinitely means that the LNA:

- Had to give her license to the Board.
- Could ask the Board to re-instate her license but had to prove that she:
  - Posed no danger to the public or practice of nursing.
  - Would safely and competently perform an LNA's duties.
  - Meets requirements for license renewal and re-instatement.

You can lose your ability to work as a nursing assistant for handling persons in ways that cause harm. Work carefully. Move patients and residents in a way that shows you care for their comfort, safety, and well-being.

FOCUS ON **PRIDE**: *Application*

How can you encourage independence and self-worth in persons needing help with exercise and activity?

REVIEW QUESTIONS

*Circle **T** if the statement is TRUE or **F** if it is FALSE.*

1 T F You must know the person's activity level.

2 T F A hip abduction wedge keeps the legs together.

3 T F A person is dizzy when walking. Help the person to sit.

4 T F A walker and a cane give the same support.

5 T F When using a cane, the feet move first.

6 T F When using a wheeled walker, the walker is pushed 6 to 8 inches in front of the person's feet.

7 T F An orthotic is used to support a muscle or promote a certain motion.

8 T F A person has a brace. Bony areas need protection from skin breakdown.

Circle the BEST answer.

9 The purpose of bed rest is to
   a Prevent postural hypotension
   b Reduce pain and promote healing
   c Prevent pressure injuries, constipation, and blood clots
   d Cause contractures and muscle atrophy

10 Which helps prevent plantar flexion?
   a An abduction wedge
   b A foot-board
   c A trochanter roll
   d Hand rolls

11 Which prevents the hip from turning outward?
   a A cane
   b A foot-board
   c A trochanter roll
   d A leg brace

12 A contracture is
   a The loss of muscle strength from inactivity
   b A decrease in the size of a muscle
   c A blood clot in the muscle
   d Decreased motion and stiffness of a joint

13 A trapeze is used to
   a Prevent footdrop
   b Prevent contractures
   c Strengthen arm muscles
   d Strengthen leg muscles

14 Active ROM exercises are performed by
   a The person
   b The physical therapist
   c You
   d The person with the help of another

15 When performing ROM exercises, which may cause injury?
   a Supporting the part being exercised
   b Moving the joint slowly, smoothly, and gently
   c Forcing the joint through its full range of motion
   d Exercising only the joints indicated by the nurse

16 Flexion involves
   a Bending the body part
   b Straightening the body part
   c Moving the body part toward the body
   d Moving the body part away from the body

17 Turning the joint downward is called
   a Dorsiflexion
   b Rotation
   c Supination
   d Pronation

18 When assisting with ambulation
   a Use a gait belt if the person is weak or unsteady
   b The person can shuffle or slide when walking after bed rest
   c Encourage the person to walk quickly
   d Walk on the person's strong side

19 A cane is held
   a At waist level
   b On the strong side
   c On the weak side
   d On either side

20 A person uses crutches. Which is a safety problem?
   a Crutch tips are wet.
   b The person wears slip-resistant shoes.
   c Crutches are within the person's reach.
   d Crutch bolts are tight.

Answers to Chapter 34 questions are on p. 886.

FOCUS ON **PRACTICE**

Problem Solving

You are assisting a resident to ambulate in the hallway with a walker and gait belt. The resident says: "I feel dizzy." No chair is nearby. A wheelchair is at the nurses' station at the end of the hallway. What will you do? How might you use planning and teamwork to avoid this in the future?

Comfort, Rest, and Sleep

OBJECTIVES

- Define the key terms and key abbreviations in this chapter.
- Explain why comfort, rest, and sleep are important.
- List the Centers for Medicare & Medicaid Services (CMS) room requirements for comfort, rest, and sleep.
- Explain why pain is personal.
- Describe 5 types of pain and the factors affecting pain.
- List the signs and symptoms of pain.
- List the nursing measures for comfort and pain relief.
- Explain the purposes of a back massage.
- Explain why meeting basic needs promotes rest.

- Identify when rest is needed.
- Describe the factors affecting sleep.
- Know the sleep requirements for each age-group.
- Explain how circadian rhythm affects sleep.
- Describe the common sleep disorders.
- List the nursing measures that promote rest and sleep.
- Perform the procedure described in this chapter.
- Explain how to promote PRIDE in the person, the family, and yourself.

KEY TERMS

acute pain Pain that is sharp or severe; may be felt suddenly from injury, disease, trauma, or surgery

chronic pain Pain that continues for a long time (longer than 12 weeks, occurs off and on, or is persistent [constant])

circadian rhythm Daily rhythm based on a 24-hour cycle that involves behavior, sleep, eating, and waking patterns; the day-night cycle or body rhythm

comfort A state of well-being; the person has no physical or emotional pain and is calm and at ease

discomfort See "pain"

distraction To focus the person's attention on something unrelated to pain

guided imagery Creating and focusing on a relaxing image

insomnia A chronic condition in which the person cannot sleep or stay asleep all night

pain To ache, hurt, or be sore; discomfort

phantom pain Pain that seems to come from a body part that is no longer there

radiating pain Pain felt at the site of tissue damage and that spreads to other areas

referred pain Pain from a body part that is felt in another body part

relaxation To be free from mental and physical stress

rest To be calm, at ease, and relaxed with no anxiety or stress

sleep A state of reduced consciousness, reduced voluntary muscle activity, and lowered metabolism

sleep deprivation The amount and quality of sleep are not adequate, causing reduced function and alertness

sleepwalking When the person leaves the bed and walks about while sleeping

KEY ABBREVIATIONS

CMS	Centers for Medicare & Medicaid Services	ID	Identification

Comfort, rest, and sleep are needed for well-being. The total person—the physical, emotional, social, and spiritual—is affected by comfort, rest, and sleep problems. Whatever the cause of such problems, quality of life is affected.

Rest and sleep restore energy and well-being. Pain, illness, and injury increase the need for rest and sleep. The body needs more energy for healing, repair, and daily functions.

See *Focus on Long-Term Care and Home Care: Comfort, Rest, and Sleep.*

FOCUS ON LONG-TERM CARE AND HOME CARE

Comfort, Rest, and Sleep

Long-Term Care

The Centers for Medicare & Medicaid Services (CMS) requires care that promotes well-being. Therefore nursing center rooms are designed and equipped for comfort.

- No more than 4 persons in a room
- A suspended curtain that goes around the bed for privacy
- A bed of proper height and size for the person
- A clean, comfortable mattress
- Linens (sheets, blankets, spreads) for the weather and climate
- A clean and orderly room
- An odor-free room
- A room temperature between 71°F and 81°F (Fahrenheit)
- A comfortable sound level
- Adequate ventilation and room humidity
- Adequate and comfortable lighting

COMFORT

Comfort is a state of well-being. The person has no physical or emotional pain. He or she is calm and at ease. Age, illness, and activity affect comfort. So do temperature, ventilation, noise, odors, and lighting. Such factors are controlled to meet the person's needs (Chapter 21). Pain is a major factor affecting comfort.

See *Focus on Communication: Comfort.*

FOCUS ON **COMMUNICATION**

Comfort

Do not assume the person is comfortable. For example, you can ask the following.

- "Are you comfortable?"
- "How can I help you be more comfortable?"
- "Are you warm enough?"
- "Do you need another blanket?"
- "Do you need another pillow?"
- "Should I adjust your pillow?"

Pain

Pain or discomfort means to ache, hurt, or be sore. Pain is subjective (Chapter 8). That is, you cannot see, hear, touch or feel, or smell another person's pain or discomfort. You must rely on what the person says.

Pain is personal. That is, pain differs for each person. What *hurts* to one person may *ache* to another. What one person calls *sore*, another may call *aching*. Many factors can affect pain (Box 35-1). If a person complains of pain or discomfort, the person has pain or discomfort. You must rely on what the person tells you. Believe the person. Report complaints of pain to the nurse for the nursing process.

Pain is a warning sign from the body. Often considered to be a vital sign (Chapter 33), it signals tissue damage. Pain often causes the person to seek health care. See Box 35-1 for the factors affecting pain.

See *Caring About Culture: Pain.*

BOX 35-1 Factors Affecting Pain

Past and current experiences. One's experiences and those of others help in learning about pain and what to expect. Pain severity, its cause, length of time, and pain relief affect the person's current response to pain.

Anxiety. Relates to feelings of fear, dread, worry, and concern. The person is uneasy, tense, and feels troubled or threatened. Pain can cause anxiety, which makes pain worse. Helping the person understand the cause of pain and what to expect helps to reduce anxiety and lessen pain.

Rest and sleep needs. Such needs increase with illness and injury. Pain seems worse when rest and sleep are affected.

Attention. Pain seems worse when it is the person's main focus. Pain seems worse when there are no distractions—TV, visitors, activity, and so on. Especially at night when unable to sleep, the person has time to think about pain.

Personal and family duties. Some people try to ignore or deny pain because of a job, school, or caring for children, a partner, or parents.

The meaning of pain. Pain can have different meanings. For example, pain can:

- Be a sign of weakness.
- Signal the need for tests and treatment.
- Bring pleasure, such as the pain of childbirth.
- Be useful. For example, the person does not have to work or can avoid certain people.
- Lead to doting and pampering. The person likes the attention.

Support from others. Dealing with pain is often easier when family and friends offer comfort and support. Touch, encouragement, or being available or nearby helps the person deal with pain. Facing pain alone is hard, especially for children and older persons.

Culture. Culture affects pain responses. In some cultures, the person in pain is stoic. To be *stoic* means *to show no reaction to joy, sorrow, pleasure, or pain.* Strong verbal and nonverbal pain reactions are seen in other cultures. See *Caring About Culture: Pain.*

Illness. Some diseases affect pain sensations. The person may not feel pain. Pain signals illness or injury. If pain is not felt, the person does not know to seek health care. Disease or injury may go undetected.

Age. See *Focus on Children and Older Persons: Pain,* p. 550.

CARING ABOUT CULTURE

Pain

Some people of *Mexico* and the *Philippines* may appear stoic in reaction to pain. In the *Philippines,* some people view pain as the will of God and believe that God will give strength to bear the pain.

In *Vietnam,* pain may be severe before some people request pain-relief measures. In *China,* showing emotion may be viewed as a weakness of character. If so, pain is often suppressed.

Non-English-speaking persons may have problems describing pain in English. The agency uses interpreters to communicate with the person.

(NOTE: Each person is unique. A person may not follow all of the beliefs and practices of his or her culture. Follow the care plan.)

Modified from D'Avanzo CE: Pocket guide to cultural health assessment, ed 4, St Louis, 2008, Mosby.

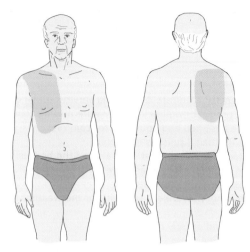

FIGURE 35-1 Gallbladder pain may radiate (spread) to the right upper abdomen, the back, and the right shoulder.

Signs and Symptoms. Promptly report any information you collect about pain. Write down what the person says. Use the person's exact words to report and record. The nurse needs the following information.

- *Location.* Where is the pain? Ask the person to point to the area of pain. Ask the person if the pain is anywhere else and to point to those areas.
- *Onset and duration.* When did the pain start? How long has it lasted?
- *Intensity.* Is the pain mild, moderate, or severe? Have the person rate the pain on a scale of 0 to 10, with 10 as the most severe (Fig. 35-2). Or use the *Wong-Baker FACES®* *Pain Rating Scale* (Fig. 35-3). Designed for children, the scale is useful for all age-groups. To use the scale, explain that each face shows how a person feels. Read the description for each face. Have the person choose the face best describing how he or she feels.
- *Description.* Have the person describe the pain. If necessary, offer some of the words listed in Box 35-2.
- *Factors causing pain.* These are called *precipitating factors.* To *precipitate* means *to cause.* Such factors include moving or turning in bed, coughing or deep breathing, and exercise. Ask what the person was doing before the pain started and when it started.
- *Factors affecting pain.* Ask what makes the pain better and what makes it worse.
- *Vital signs.* Measure pulse, respirations, and blood pressure (Chapter 33). Vital signs often increase with acute pain. They may be normal with chronic pain.
- *Other signs and symptoms.* Does the person have other symptoms—dizziness, nausea, vomiting, weakness, numbness or tingling, or others? Box 35-3 lists the signs and symptoms that often occur with pain.

See *Focus on Communication: Signs and Symptoms*, p. 552.
See *Focus on Surveys: Signs and Symptoms*, p. 552.

Types of Pain. Doctors use the type of pain for diagnosing. Nurses use the type for the nursing process.

- *Acute pain is sharp or severe. It may be felt suddenly from injury, disease, trauma, or surgery.* It may signal a new injury or a life-threatening event. There is tissue damage. Acute pain lasts a short time and lessens with healing.
- *Chronic pain continues for a long time (longer than 12 weeks, occurs off and on, or is persistent [constant]).* There is no longer tissue damage. Chronic pain remains long after healing. Arthritis is a common cause.
- *Radiating pain is felt at the site of tissue damage and spreads to other areas.* For example, low back pain can radiate to the buttocks and legs. Gallbladder disease can cause pain in the right upper abdomen, the back, and the right shoulder (Fig. 35-1).
- *Referred pain is pain from a body part that is felt in another body part.* For example, pain from a heart attack may only be felt in the shoulder or left arm. The person does not have chest pain.
- *Phantom pain seems to come from a body part that is no longer there.* For example, a person with an amputated leg may still sense leg pain.

PAIN: Ask patient to rate pain on scale of 0-10										
No pain										Worst pain imaginable
0	1	2	3	4	5	6	7	8	9	10

FIGURE 35-2 Pain rating scale. (From Williams P: *deWit's fundamental concepts and skills for nursing,* ed 5, St Louis, 2018, Elsevier.)

BOX 35-2	Words Used to Describe Pain

- Aching
- Burning
- Cramping
- Crushing
- Discomfort
- Dull
- Gnawing
- Heaviness
- Hurting
- Knife-like
- Numbness
- Piercing
- Pins and needles
- Pressure

- Radiating
- Ripping
- Sharp
- Shooting
- Soreness
- Spasms
- Squeezing
- Stabbing
- Tearing
- Tenderness
- Throbbing
- Tingling
- Vise-like

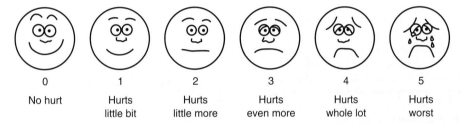

0	1	2	3	4	5
No hurt	Hurts little bit	Hurts little more	Hurts even more	Hurts whole lot	Hurts worst

FIGURE 35-3 Wong-Baker FACES® Pain Rating Scale. (From Hockenberry MJ and others: *Wong's nursing care of infants and children,* ed 10, St Louis, 2015, Mosby.)

BOX 35-3	Pain—Signs and Symptoms

Body Responses
- Appetite: changes in
- Dizziness
- Nausea
- Numbness
- Skin: pale *(pallor)*
- Sleep: difficulty with
- Sweating *(diaphoresis)*
- Tingling
- Vital signs (pulse, respirations, and blood pressure): increased
- Vomiting
- Weakness
- Weight loss

Behaviors
- Clenching the jaw
- Crying
- Frowning
- Gait: changes in; limping
- Gasping

Behaviors—cont'd
- Grimacing
- Groaning
- Grunting
- Holding the affected body part (splinting; guarding)
- Irritability
- Moaning
- Mood: changes in; depressed
- Pacing
- Positioning: maintaining 1 position; refusing to move; frequent position changes
- Pulling away when touched
- Quietness
- Resisting care
- Restlessness
- Rubbing a body part or area
- Screaming
- Speech: slow or rapid; loud or quiet
- Whimpering

FOCUS ON COMMUNICATION

Signs and Symptoms

A person may use words like "hurt" or "discomfort" instead of "pain." Children may use "owie" or "boo boo." Use words that the person uses.

Some persons have trouble rating pain intensity on a 0 to 10 scale. Instead, ask if the pain is mild, moderate, or severe.

FOCUS ON SURVEYS

Signs and Symptoms

Pain interferes with well-being—function, mobility, mood, sleep, and quality of life. The agency must:
- Recognize when a person has pain.
- Identify when pain might occur.
- Evaluate pain and its causes.
- Manage or prevent pain.

You may be the first to observe signs and symptoms of pain. You must recognize and report a change in the person's behavior and function. You follow the care plan for pain-relief measures. Therefore a surveyor may ask you about pain. Examples are:
- What are the signs and symptoms of pain?
- How do you ask a person to rate the intensity of pain?
- What factors can cause pain or make it worse?
- When and how do you report observations about pain?
- How do you assist the nurse with pain-relief measures?

BOX 35-4	Comfort and Pain-Relief Measures

- Position the person in good alignment. Use pillows for support.
- Keep bed linens clean, dry, tight, and wrinkle-free.
- Make sure the person is not lying on tubes.
- Assist with elimination needs.
- Adjust the room temperature to meet the person's needs.
- Provide blankets for warmth and to prevent chilling.
- Use correct moving and turning procedures.
- Wait 30 minutes after pain-relief drugs are given to give care or start activities.
- Give a back massage.
- Provide soft music to distract the person.
- Talk softly and gently.
- Use touch to provide comfort.
- Allow family and friends at the bedside as requested by the person.
- Avoid sudden or jarring movements of the bed or chair.
- Handle the person gently.
- Practice safety measures if the person takes strong pain-relief drugs or sedatives.
  - Keep the bed in a low position that is safe and comfortable for the person. Follow the care plan.
  - Raise bed rails as directed. Follow the care plan.
  - Check on the person every 10 to 15 minutes.
  - Provide help when the person needs to get up and when up and about.
- Apply warm or cold applications as directed by the nurse (Chapter 42).
- Provide a calm, quiet, darkened setting.

Nursing Measures

The nurse uses the nursing process to promote comfort and relieve pain. The care plan may include the measures in Box 35-4. See Figure 35-4.

Sometimes distraction, relaxation, and guided imagery are needed. If asked to assist, the nurse tells you what to do.

Distraction means to focus the person's attention on something unrelated to pain. Attention is moved away from the pain. Music, games, singing, praying, TV, and needle-work can distract attention (Fig. 35-5).

Relaxation means to be free from mental and physical stress. This state reduces pain and anxiety. The person is taught to breathe deeply and slowly and to contract and relax muscle groups. A comfortable position and a quiet room are important.

Guided imagery is creating and focusing on a relaxing image. The person is asked to create a pleasant scene. This is noted on the care plan so all staff use the same image. A calm, soft voice is used to help the person focus on the image. Soft music, a blanket for warmth, and a darkened room may help. The person is coached to focus on the image and to practice relaxation exercises.

Nurses give ordered pain-relief drugs. Such drugs can cause postural hypotension (Chapter 34), drowsiness, dizziness, and coordination problems. Protect the person from injury and falls. Follow the care plan for needed safety measures.

See *Focus on Children and Older Persons: Nursing Measures.*

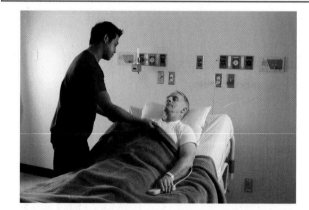

FIGURE 35-4 Measures are implemented to relieve pain. The person is in good alignment with pillows used for comfort. The room is darkened. Blankets provide warmth.

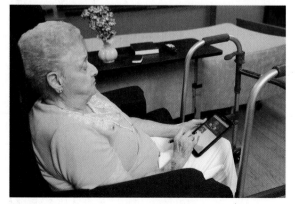

FIGURE 35-5 For distraction, this woman views family photos on an electronic device.

FOCUS ON CHILDREN AND OLDER PERSONS

Nursing Measures

Children

Pacifiers and favorite toys and blankets can comfort infants and young children. So can holding, rocking, touching, and talking or singing to them. Check with the nurse before you pick up and hold a child. Sometimes children are not held for treatment reasons.

The Back Massage. The back massage (back rub) can promote comfort and help relieve pain. It relaxes muscles and stimulates circulation. Good times for back massages are after re-positioning, after baths or showers, and with evening care. Back massages last 3 to 5 minutes. Observe the skin before the massage. Look for breaks in the skin, bruises, reddened areas, and other signs of skin breakdown.

Lotion reduces friction during the massage and softens the skin. Warm the lotion before applying it. Do 1 of the following.

- Rub some lotion between your hands.
- Place the bottle in the bath water.
- Hold the bottle under warm water.

Use firm strokes. Keep your hands in contact with the person's skin. After the massage, apply lotion to the elbows, knees, and heels. Those bony areas are at risk for skin breakdown.

See *Delegation Guidelines: The Back Massage.*
See *Promoting Safety and Comfort: The Back Massage.*
See procedure: *Giving a Back Massage.*

DELEGATION GUIDELINES

The Back Massage

Giving a back massage is a routine nursing task. Before giving a back massage, you need this information from the nurse and the care plan.

- If the person can have a back massage. See *Promoting Safety and Comfort: The Back Massage.*
- How to position the person.
- If the person has position limits. If yes, what are they?
- When to give a back massage.
- If the person needs back massages often for comfort and to relax.
- What observations to report and record:
  - Breaks in the skin
  - Bruising
  - Reddened areas
  - Signs of skin breakdown
- When to report observations.
- What patient or resident concerns to report at once.

PROMOTING SAFETY AND COMFORT

The Back Massage

Safety

Back massages can harm persons with certain heart diseases, back injuries and surgeries, skin diseases, and lung disorders. Check with the nurse and the care plan before giving back massages.

Do not massage reddened bony areas. Reddened areas signal skin breakdown and pressure injuries. Massage can cause more tissue damage.

Wear gloves if the person's skin is not intact. Do not massage areas of non-intact skin. Always follow Standard Precautions and the Bloodborne Pathogen Standard.

Comfort

The prone position is best for a massage. The side-lying position is often used. Older and disabled persons usually find the side-lying position more comfortable.

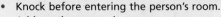

Giving a Back Massage

QUALITY OF LIFE

- Knock before entering the person's room.
- Address the person by name.
- Introduce yourself by name and title.

- Explain the procedure before starting and during the procedure.
- Protect the person's rights during the procedure.
- Handle the person gently during the procedure.

PRE-PROCEDURE

1 Follow *Delegation Guidelines: The Back Massage.* See *Promoting Safety and Comfort: The Back Massage.*
2 Practice hand hygiene.
3 Identify the person. Check the ID (identification) bracelet against the assignment sheet. Use 2 identifiers (Chapter 13). Also call the person by name.

4 Collect the following.
  - Bath blanket
  - Bath towel
  - Lotion
5 Provide for privacy.
6 Raise the bed for body mechanics. Bed rails are up if used.

Continued

Giving a Back Massage—cont'd

PROCEDURE

7 Lower the bed rail near you if up.
8 Position the person in the prone or side-lying position. The back is toward you.
9 Cover the person with a bath blanket. Expose the back, shoulders, and upper arms.
10 Lay the towel on the bed along the back. Do this if the person is in a side-lying position.
11 Warm the lotion.
12 Explain that the lotion may feel cool and wet.
13 Apply lotion to the lower back area.
14 Stroke up from the lower back to the shoulders. Then stroke down over the upper arms. Stroke up the upper arms, across the shoulders, and down the back (Fig. 35-6). Use firm strokes. Keep your hands in contact with the person's skin.
15 Repeat step 14 for at least 3 minutes.

16 Knead the back (Fig. 35-7).
   a Grasp the skin between your thumb and fingers.
   b Knead half of the back. Start at the lower back and move up to the shoulder. Then knead down from the shoulder to the lower back.
   c Repeat on the other half of the back.
17 Apply lotion to bony areas. Use circular motions with the tips of your index and middle fingers. *(Do not massage reddened bony areas.)*
18 Use fast movements to stimulate. Use slow movements to relax the person.
19 Stroke with long, firm movements to end the massage. Tell the person when you are finishing.
20 Straighten and secure clothing or sleepwear.
21 Cover the person. Remove the towel and bath blanket.

POST-PROCEDURE

22 Provide for comfort. (See the inside of the back cover.)
23 Place the call light and other needed items within reach.
24 Lower the bed to a safe and comfortable level. Follow the care plan.
25 Raise or lower bed rails. Follow the care plan.
26 Return lotion to its proper place.

27 Unscreen the person.
28 Complete a safety check of the room. (See the inside of the back cover.)
29 Follow agency policy for used linens.
30 Practice hand hygiene.
31 Report and record your observations.

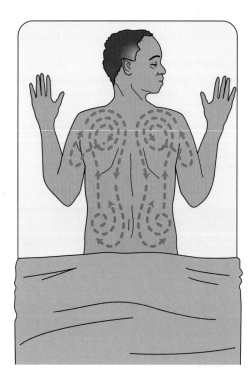

FIGURE 35-6 The person is in the prone position for a back massage. Stroke upward from the lower back to the shoulders, down over the upper arms, back up the upper arms, across the shoulders, and down to the lower back.

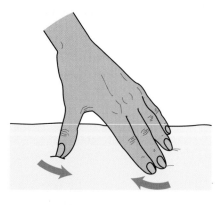
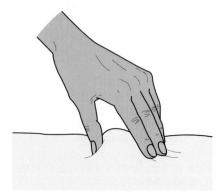

FIGURE 35-7 Knead by picking up tissue between the thumb and fingers.

REST

Rest means to be calm, at ease, and relaxed with no anxiety or stress. Rest may involve no activity. Or the person does calming and relaxing things. Reading, music, TV, needlework, and prayer are examples. Some people garden, bake, golf, walk, or do woodworking.

To promote rest, meet basic needs.

- *Physical needs.* Thirst, hunger, and elimination needs can affect rest. So can pain or discomfort. A comfortable position and good alignment are important. So is a quiet setting with clean, dry, and wrinkle-free linens. Some people rest easier in a clean, neat, and uncluttered room.
- *Safety and security needs.*
  - The person must feel safe from falling and injury. Keep the call light within reach.
  - Understanding the reason for care helps the person feel safe. So does knowing how care is given. Always explain procedures before doing them.
  - Many people have rituals or routines before resting. Going to the bathroom, brushing teeth, and washing the face and hands are examples. Some people pray. Some have a snack, lock doors, or make sure loved ones are safe at home. The person may want a certain blanket or afghan. Follow routines and rituals whenever possible.
- *Love and belonging needs.* Visits or calls from family and friends may relax the person. The person knows that others care. Reading cards and letters may be relaxing and restful (Fig. 35-8).
- *Self-esteem needs.* Patient gowns embarrass some people. Others fear exposure. Many persons rest better in their own sleepwear. Hygiene and grooming are important. This includes hair care and being clean and odor-free.

A 15- or 20-minute rest refreshes some people. Others need more time. Health care routines usually allow for afternoon rest.

Ill or injured persons need to rest often. Some rest before or after a procedure. For example, a bath tires a person. So does getting dressed. The person needs to rest before you make the bed. Some people like to rest after meals. Do not push the person beyond his or her limits. Allow rest when needed.

Distraction, relaxation, and guided imagery also promote rest. So does a back massage. Plan and organize care for uninterrupted rest.

The doctor may order bed rest for a person. See Chapter 34.

SLEEP

Sleep is a state of reduced consciousness, reduced voluntary muscle activity, and lowered metabolism. With reduced consciousness, the person can respond to loud noises or gentle shaking. There are no voluntary arm or leg movements during sleep. *Metabolism* is the burning of food to produce energy for the body. Less energy is needed during sleep. Thus metabolism is reduced during sleep. People wake up from sleep.

Sleep is a basic need. The mind and body rest. The body saves energy. Body functions slow. Vital signs are lower than when awake. Tissue healing and repair occur. Sleep lowers stress, tension, and anxiety. It refreshes and renews the person. The person regains energy and mental alertness. The person thinks and functions better after sleep.

Many factors affect the amount and quality of sleep. See Box 35-5, p. 556.

Circadian Rhythm

Sleep is part of circadian rhythm. *(Circa means about. Dies means day.) Circadian rhythm is a daily rhythm based on a 24-hour cycle that involves behavior, sleep, eating, and waking patterns.* Called the *day-night cycle* or *body rhythm,* circadian rhythm affects functioning. Some people function, think, and react better in the morning. They are more alert and active. Others do better in the evening.

Circadian rhythm includes a sleep-wake cycle. The person's *biological clock* signals when to sleep and when to wake up. For example, you sleep and wake up at certain times. You may awaken before the alarm clock goes off. That is part of your biological clock. Health care often interferes with a person's circadian rhythm and the sleep-wake cycle. Sleep problems easily occur.

Many people work evening and night shifts. Their bodies must adjust to changes in the sleep-wake cycle.

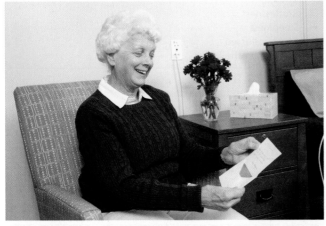

FIGURE 35-8 The resident reads cards and letters from family and friends.

BOX 35-5	Factors Affecting Sleep

Illness. Sleep needs increase. Various signs and symptoms (pain, nausea, frequent voiding, and so on), treatments and therapies, care devices, and uncomfortable positions can interfere with sleep. Sleep problems are common with Alzheimer's disease and other dementias (Chapter 53).

Nutrition. Sleep needs increase with weight gain and decrease with weight loss. Drinks and foods with caffeine (coffee, tea, colas, chocolate) prevent sleep. The protein *tryptophan* tends to help sleep. It is found in protein sources—milk, cheese, red meat, fish, poultry, and peanuts.

Exercise. Exercise helps people sleep well.

Sleep setting. The bed, pillows, noises, temperature, lighting, and a sleeping partner are part of the person's sleep setting. Any change in the usual setting can interfere with sleep.

Drugs and other substances. Sleeping pills promote sleep. Drugs for anxiety, depression, and pain may cause sleep. Some drugs cause nightmares and frequent voiding. Alcohol causes drowsiness and sleep. However, after drinking alcohol the person may awaken and have difficulty falling back asleep. A stimulant, caffeine prevents sleep. Caffeine is found in some drugs and some drinks and foods. See "Nutrition" above.

Life-style changes. Life-style relates to a person's daily routines and way of living. The person has usual sleep and wake times. Work, school, play, social events, and travel are some factors affecting the person's sleep-wake times.

Emotional problems. Fear, worry, depression, and anxiety affect sleep. Causes include problems with health, money, work, family, and relationships.

Age. Sleep needs vary for each age-group. The amount needed decreases with age (Table 35-1). Older persons have less energy than younger persons. They may nap during the day.

TABLE 35-1	Sleep Guidelines	
Age-Group	Age Range	Hours Each Day
Newborn	0 to 3 months	14 to 17 hours
Infant	4 to 12 months	12 to 16 hours
Toddler	1 to 2 years	11 to 14 hours
Pre-school	3 to 5 years	10 to 13 hours
School age	6 to 12 years	9 to 12 hours
Teenage	13 to 18 years	8 to 10 hours
Adult	18 to 60 years	7 or more hours
	61 to 64 years	7 to 9 hours
	65 years and older	7 to 8 hours

Modified from Centers for Disease Control and Prevention: How much sleep do I need?, Atlanta, Ga., updated March 2, 2017.

Sleep Disorders

Sleep disorders involve repeated sleep problems. The amount and quality of sleep are affected. See Box 35-5 for the factors affecting sleep and Box 35-6 for the signs and symptoms of sleep disorders.

- *Insomnia is a chronic condition in which the person cannot sleep or stay asleep all night.*
- *Sleep deprivation is when the amount and quality of sleep are not adequate, causing reduced function and alertness.* Sleep is interrupted. Factors that affect sleep can lead to sleep deprivation (see Box 35-5).
- *Sleepwalking is when the person leaves the bed and walks about while sleeping.* The person is not aware of sleepwalking and has no memory of the event. The event lasts 3 to 4 minutes or longer. You need to:
  - Protect the person from injury. Falls are a risk. Care tubings (intravenous, catheters, feeding) can cause injury if pulled out of the body when the person gets out of bed.
  - Awaken sleepwalkers gently. They startle easily.
  - Guide sleepwalkers back to bed.

See *Teamwork and Time Management: Sleep Disorders.*

BOX 35-6	Sleep Disorders—Signs and Symptoms

- Agitation
- Attention: decreased
- Coordination: problems with
- Disorientation
- Eyes: red, puffy, dark circles under the eyes
- Fatigue
- Hallucinations (Chapters 52 and 53)
- Irritability
- Memory: reduced word memory; problems finding the right word
- Mood: moodiness; mood swings
- Pulse: irregular
- Reasoning and judgment: decreased
- Responses to questions, conversations, or situations: slowed
- Restlessness
- Sleepiness
- Speech: slurred
- Tremors: in the hands

TEAMWORK AND TIME MANAGEMENT
Sleep Disorders

You may find a person sleepwalking. Help him or her back to bed even if not assigned to the person's care. Provide for comfort. Then tell the nurse what happened and what you did.

Promoting Sleep

The nurse assesses the person's sleep patterns. Report any of the signs and symptoms listed in Box 35-6 and your observations about how the person slept. Measures are planned to promote sleep (Box 35-7). Follow the care plan.

Bedtime rituals and routines are important. They are allowed if safe. The person may have a bedtime snack or perform hygiene in a certain order. Some watch TV in bed. Others read religious writings, pray, or say a rosary before sleep.

The person is involved in care planning. The person chooses when to nap or go to bed. The person chooses the measures that promote comfort, rest, and sleep. Follow the care plan and the person's wishes.

See *Focus on Long-Term Care and Home Care: Promoting Sleep*.

BOX 35-7	Promoting Sleep

- Plan care for uninterrupted rest.
- Encourage the person to avoid business or family matters before bedtime.
- Allow a flexible bedtime. Bedtime is when the person is tired, not a certain time.
- Provide a comfortable room temperature.
- Let the person take a warm bath or shower.
- Provide a bedtime snack.
- Avoid caffeine (coffee, tea, colas, chocolate).
- Avoid alcoholic beverages.
- Have the person void before going to bed.
- Make sure incontinent persons are clean and dry. Change a baby's diaper.
- Follow bedtime rituals and routines.
- Have the person wear loose-fitting sleepwear.
- Provide for extra warmth (blankets, socks) as needed.
- Make sure linens are clean, dry, and wrinkle-free.
- Position the person in good alignment and in a comfortable position.
- Support body parts as ordered.
- Give a back massage.
- Provide measures to relieve pain.
- Let the person read, listen to music, or watch TV. Read to children. You can read to an adult if he or she prefers.
- Assist with relaxation exercises as ordered.
- Sit and talk with the person.
- Reduce noise.
- Darken the room—close window coverings and the privacy curtain. Shut off or dim lights.
- Dim lights in hallways and the nursing unit.

FOCUS ON LONG-TERM CARE AND HOME CARE

Promoting Sleep

Long-Term Care

Some persons like to check on other residents before going to bed. Some have the duty of turning off lights at bedtime. These actions promote the person's dignity and mental comfort.

FOCUS ON **PRIDE**

The Person, Family, and Yourself

Personal and Professional Responsibility

Unmanaged pain decreases quality of life. You have an important role in assisting with pain relief. You talk with patients and residents and listen to their needs.

Report signs and symptoms of pain. Report what the person said and what you observed. The nurse uses this information to assess, plan, and evaluate pain relief.

Rights and Respect

Your care can either promote comfort and relaxation or cause stress, discomfort, and worry. For example:

- Are you prompt to meet needs?
- Do you ask about the person's preferences?
- Do you communicate in a respectful way?
- Do you allow time for rest?
- Do you leave the person's room clean, neat, and safe?

Take pride in providing care in a way that protects the right to quality of life.

Independence and Social Interaction

A person's emotional, spiritual, and social needs affect comfort. Time spent with friends and family can be comforting. For some, religious ceremonies or rituals promote peace and healing. Allow time and privacy for those needs. Small gestures show that you care. You can:

- Ask: "How are you feeling today?"
- Give the person time to pray before meals or at bedtime if this is something he or she values.
- Ask about the person's friends and family while giving care.

Delegation and Teamwork

The health team coordinates care and therapies with pain-relief measures and rest periods. It is common to wait 30 minutes after a pain-relief drug is given to perform procedures and provide care. The nurse tells you how long to wait. The person is allowed to rest after tiring activities, procedures, and therapies. Planning and communication are needed for effective teamwork and quality care.

Ethics and Laws

You may question what the person tells you about his or her pain. For example, a person rates headache pain as 9 on the 0 to 10 pain rating scale while working a crossword puzzle and listening to music. When you have a severe headache, you need to rest in a dark, quiet room. You doubt that the person's pain is really a 9 on the scale. You decide not to tell the nurse.

The person's pain really was severe. The crossword puzzle and music were distractions from the pain. Because you did not report the pain, the person did not receive pain-relief measures.

Ignoring a person's pain is wrong. Reporting a different pain rating is wrong. Avoid making judgments about the person's pain. Accurate reporting is needed for proper pain management.

FOCUS ON **PRIDE**: *Application*

Family and visitors often provide comfort. How will you welcome the person's visitors? How will you show you value them and their time with the person?

REVIEW QUESTIONS

Circle T if the statement is TRUE or F if it is FALSE.

1 T F   Pain is a warning from the body.

2 T F   Pain differs for each person.

3 T F   Pain can be seen.

4 T F   Changes in usual behavior may signal pain.

5 T F   A person's culture may affect reactions to pain.

6 T F   A back massage relaxes muscles and stimulates circulation.

7 T F   After lunch, a person asks for a back massage. You must wait until evening to give the massage.

8 T F   Persons with dementia usually sleep well at night.

9 T F   Tissue healing and repair occur during sleep.

10 T F   Voluntary muscle activity increases during sleep.

11 T F   Sleep refreshes and renews the person.

12 T F   Sleep increases stress, tension, and anxiety.

13 T F   Sleep deprivation can affect functioning.

14 T F   Older persons may nap during the day.

Circle the BEST answer.

15 A person has complained of knee pain on and off for several years. This type of pain is
a Acute pain
b Chronic pain
c Radiating pain
d Referred pain

16 A person is restless and complains of pain. You should
a Rate the intensity based on the person's behavior
b Give a pain-relief drug and tell the nurse
c Tell the nurse only if you think the person has pain
d Report the person's exact words

17 A person received a pain-relief drug. When should you give scheduled care?
a When you have time
b Right after the drug is given
c 30 minutes after the drug is given
d The next day

18 A drug was given for pain relief. To promote safety
a Keep the bed in the raised position
b Quickly change positions to avoid dizziness
c Check on the person every hour
d Provide help if the person needs to get up

19 Which measure promotes comfort and pain relief?
a Providing a blanket
b Speaking loudly
c Keeping the lights on in the room
d Asking about comfort every 5 minutes

20 When giving a back massage
a Massage for 15 to 20 minutes
b Warm the lotion before applying it
c Massage reddened areas
d Position the person in Fowler's position

21 A person tires easily. You are giving morning care. When should the person rest?
a After you complete morning care
b After the bath and before hair care
c After you make the bed
d When the person needs to

22 A healthy 70-year-old person needs about
a 11 to 12 hours of sleep per day
b 9 to 10 hours of sleep per day
c 7 to 8 hours of sleep per day
d 5 to 6 hours of sleep per day

23 Which prevents sleep?
a Cheese
b Chocolate
c Milk
d Beef

24 Which measure before bedtime promotes sleep?
a Having the person urinate
b Having the person walk
c Providing hot tea
d Leaving the hallway light on

Answers to Chapter 35 questions are on p. 886.

FOCUS ON PRACTICE

Problem Solving

Prioritize the following comfort needs. Which would you do first, second, third, and last?
- Provide a blanket.
- Report chest pain that began suddenly.
- Help a person who received a pain-relief drug 1 hour ago to the bathroom.
- Provide a back massage before bedtime.

Admissions, Transfers, and Discharges

OBJECTIVES

- Define the key terms and key abbreviations in this chapter.
- Describe your role in admissions, transfers, discharges, and moving the person to a new room.
- Explain how to help the person and family feel safe in the health care setting.
- Identify the rules for measuring weight and height.

- Explain why a person is moved to a new room within the agency.
- Perform the procedures described in this chapter.
- Explain how to promote PRIDE in the person, the family, and yourself.

KEY TERMS

admission Official entry of a person into a health care setting
discharge Official departure of a person from a health care setting

transfer Moving the person to another health care setting; moving the person to a new room within the agency

KEY ABBREVIATIONS

CMS	Centers for Medicare & Medicaid Services	in	Inch; inches
ft	Foot; feet	lb	Pound; pounds
ID	Identification		

*A*dmission *is the official entry of a person into a health care setting.* It causes anxiety and fear in patients, residents, and families. Worries and fears about serious health problems, treatments, surgeries, and pain are common.

The setting is new and strange. Patients, residents, and families may have concerns and fears about:
- Where to go, what to do, and what to expect
- Never returning home
- Who gives care, how care is given, and if the correct care is given
- Finding the bathroom
- Getting meals
- How to get help
- Being abused
- Strange sights and sounds
- Being apart from family and friends
- Making new friends
- Leaving homes and possessions behind

Moving to another room may cause similar concerns. So may transfer to another hospital or nursing center. Discharge to a home setting is usually a happy time. However, the person may need home care.

Transfer and discharge are defined as follows.
- *Transfer is moving the person to another health care setting.* In some agencies it also means *moving the person to a new room within the agency.*
- *Discharge is the official departure of a person from a health care setting.*

Admission, transfer, and discharge are critical events. So is moving to a new room. The new room may be on another nursing unit. These events involve:
- Privacy and confidentiality
- Understanding and communicating with the person
- Communicating with the health team
- Respect for the person and the person's property
- Being kind, courteous, and respectful
- Reporting and recording

See *Focus on Long-Term Care and Home Care: Admissions, Transfers, and Discharges*, p. 560.

See *Teamwork and Time Management: Admissions, Transfers, and Discharges*, p. 560.

See *Delegation Guidelines: Admissions, Transfers, and Discharges*, p. 560.

See *Promoting Safety and Comfort: Admissions, Transfers, and Discharges*, p. 560.

ADMISSIONS

The admission process usually starts in the admitting office. It may start in a hospital emergency room (ER). Admitting staff or a nurse obtains identifying information for the admission record—full name, age, birth date, and so on.

The person is given an identification (ID) number and ID bracelet (Chapter 13). The person or legal representative signs admitting papers and a general consent for treatment.

The nursing unit is told when to expect a new patient or resident. The person's room and bed number are given. In some agencies, the person can walk to the room if able. Most persons require transport by wheelchair or stretcher.

See *Focus on Long-Term Care and Home Care: Admissions.*

PREPARING THE ROOM

You prepare the room for the person's arrival. Figure 36-1 shows a room ready for a new resident.

See procedure: *Preparing the Person's Room.*

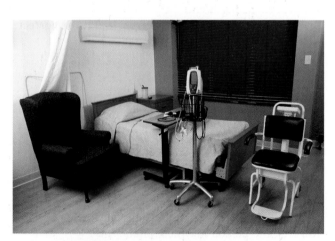

FIGURE 36-1 The room is ready for a new resident.

FOCUS ON LONG-TERM CARE AND HOME CARE

Admissions

Long-Term Care

In nursing centers, admission procedures are often started 2 or 3 days before the person enters the center. Needed information is obtained from the person or family member.

Some residents arrive by ambulance or wheelchair van. The attendants take them to their assigned rooms. Some arrive by car. The nurses or nursing assistants take them to their rooms. Often a family member is present.

A nurse or social worker explains the resident's rights to the person and family. They also receive written matter explaining them.

The person's photo is taken. The person may receive an ID bracelet. Photos or ID bracelets are used to identify the person (Chapter 13).

Persons with dementia and their families may need extra help during the admission process. Often confusion increases in a new setting. Fear, agitation, and wanting to leave are common. The family also is fearful. Many feel guilty about the need for nursing center care. You assist in helping the person and family feel safe and welcome.

Admission is often an emotional time for the person and family. They do not part until ready to do so. Remember, the center is now the person's home.

Preparing the Person's Room

PROCEDURE

1 Follow *Delegation Guidelines: Admissions, Transfers, and Discharges.*
2 Practice hand hygiene.
3 Collect the following.
  - Admission kit—wash basin, soap, toothpaste, toothbrush, water mug, and so on
  - Bedpan and urinal (for a man)
  - Nursing assistant admission checklist (Fig. 36-2, p. 562)
  - Thermometer
  - Stethoscope and blood pressure equipment
  - Pulse oximeter (Chapter 43)
  - Patient gown or sleepwear (if needed)
  - Towels and washcloths
  - IV (intravenous) pole (if needed)
  - Other items requested by the nurse
4 Place the following on the over-bed table.
  - Thermometer
  - Stethoscope and blood pressure equipment
  - Pulse oximeter (Chapter 43)
  - Nursing assistant admission checklist

5 Place the water mug on the bedside stand or over-bed table.
6 Place the following in the bedside stand.
  - Admission kit
  - Bedpan and urinal
  - Patient gown or sleepwear
  - Towels and washcloths
7 *If the person arrives by stretcher:*
  a Make a surgical bed (Chapter 22).
  b Raise the bed for a transfer from a stretcher.
8 *If the person is ambulatory or arrives by wheelchair:*
  a Leave the bed closed.
  b Lower the bed to a safe and comfortable level as directed by the nurse.
9 Attach the call light to the bed linens.
10 Place the IV pole (if needed) next to the head of the bed.
11 Practice hand hygiene.

Admitting the Person

A nurse usually greets and escorts the person and family to the room. You might do so if the person has no discomfort or distress.

Admission is your first chance to make a good impression. You must:
- Greet the person by name and title. Use the admission record to find out the person's name.
- Introduce yourself by name and title to the person, family, and friends.
- Make roommate introductions.
- Act in a professional manner.
- Treat the person with dignity and respect.

See *Focus on Long-Term Care and Home Care: Admitting the Person.*

FOCUS ON LONG-TERM CARE AND HOME CARE

Admitting the Person

Long-Term Care

Help the person feel safe and secure. Do not rush admission procedures. Rather, treat the person and family as guests in your home. Offer a beverage. Visit with them. Tell them nice things about the center.

Introduce residents in nearby rooms. Knowing other residents provides comfort and support. Residents understand, better than anyone else, what a nursing center is like.

The center is the person's home. Make the room as home-like as possible. You may help with unpacking and putting clothes away. The person may have pictures or photos to hang or display. Show care and compassion. Help the person feel safe, comfortable, and secure.

ADMISSION CHECKLIST

Preferred name _Sam_   **ID** _278-64593_

Measurements

Weight _195_ **lb**
- [ ] Standing scale
- [x] Chair scale
- [ ] Wheelchair scale
- [ ] Wheelchair weight _____ lb

Height _5_ **ft** _10_ **in**

Pain

Location _Low back_

Intensity _3_

Description _Aching_

Vital signs

Temperature _98.2_ °F
- [x] Oral
- [ ] Axillary
- [ ] Rectal
- [ ] Tympanic membrane

Pulse _78_

Respirations _20_

Blood pressure _122/84_ mm Hg

- [x] Right arm
- [x] Lying
- [ ] Left arm
- [ ] Sitting

Pulse oximetry _98_ %

Care Measures

Assist with garments
- [x] Dressed
- [ ] Patient gown
- [ ] Sleepwear

Items within reach
- [x] Filled water mug
- [x] Call light
- [x] TV and light controls
- [x] Needed/requested items

Assist to
- [x] Bed
- [ ] Chair
- [ ] Other _____

Belongings
- [x] Label personal property and care items.
- [x] Provide and label denture cup.
- [x] Complete the clothing and personal belongings lists.
- [x] Place clothes and personal items in closet, drawers, and bedside stand.

Orient Person and Family to Setting

Room
- [x] Call light
- [x] Bed, TV, and light controls
- [x] Items in the bedside stand
- [x] Over-bed table
- [x] Electrical outlets for charging electronic devices
- [x] Phone and phone calls
- [x] Bathroom and bathroom call light

Agency
- [x] Names of nurses, nursing assistants, and other staff
- [x] Visiting hours and policies
- [x] Internet access
- [x] Nurses' station
- [x] Lounge
- [x] Chapel or quiet area
- [x] Dining room
- [x] Meal and snack times

Safety and Comfort

- [x] Bed at a safe and comfortable level
- [x] Bed rails raised
- [ ] Bed rails lowered
- [x] Safety check of room

- [x] Ask about comfort needs
- [x] Comfort measures: _Provided a blanket, raised head of bed to level of comfort, reported pain to nurse_

Nursing assistant _C. Collins, CNA_   Checklist given to _J. Miller, RN_   Date _11/24_ Time _1415_

FIGURE 36-2 A sample nursing assistant admission checklist.

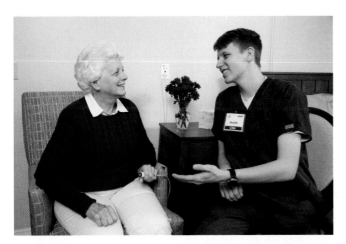

FIGURE 36-3 The nursing assistant introduces himself to the person.

🔶 **The Admission Procedure.** During the admission procedure the nurse may ask you to:
- Measure the person's weight and height.
- Measure vital signs and pulse oximetry.
- Obtain a urine specimen.
- Complete a clothing and personal belongings list.
- Orient the person to the room, the nursing unit, and the agency.
  See procedure: *Admitting the Person.*

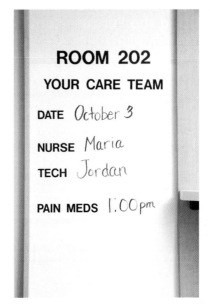

ROOM 202

YOUR CARE TEAM

DATE *October 3*

NURSE *Maria*

TECH *Jordan*

PAIN MEDS *1:00pm*

FIGURE 36-4 The names of nursing team members are posted on a marker board.

Admitting the Person

QUALITY OF LIFE

- Knock before entering the person's room.
- Address the person by name.
- Introduce yourself by name and title.

- Explain the procedure before starting and during the procedure.
- Protect the person's rights during the procedure.
- Handle the person gently during the procedure.

PRE-PROCEDURE

1 Follow *Delegation Guidelines: Admissions, Transfers, and Discharges,* p. 560. See *Promoting Safety and Comfort: Admissions, Transfers, and Discharges,* p. 560.

2 Practice hand hygiene.
3 Prepare the room. See procedure: *Preparing the Person's Room,* p. 561.

PROCEDURE

4 Identify the person. Use 2 identifiers (Chapter 13). Check the information in the admission record and on the ID bracelet.
5 Greet the person by name. Ask what name he or she prefers.
6 Introduce yourself to the person and others present (Fig. 36-3). Give your name and title. Explain that you assist the nurses in giving care.
7 Introduce the roommate.
8 Provide for privacy. Ask family or friends to leave the room unless the person prefers that someone stay. Tell them how much time you need and direct them to the waiting area.
9 Let the person stay dressed if his or her condition permits. Or help with changing into a patient gown or sleepwear.
10 Provide for comfort. The person is in bed or in a chair as directed by the nurse.
11 Assist the nurse with assessment.
  a Measure vital signs and pulse oximetry.
  b Measure weight and height (p. 564).
  c Collect information on the nursing assistant admission checklist.

12 Orient the person and family to the area.
  a Give names of the nurses and nursing assistants (Fig. 36-4).
  b Explain the purpose of items in the bedside stand.
  c Explain how to use the over-bed table.
  d Show how to use the call light.
  e Show the person the bathroom. Explain how to use the call light in the bathroom.
  f Show how to use bed, TV, and light controls.
  g Explain how to use the agency's phone. Place the phone within reach.
  h Explain how to connect to the Internet.
  i Show the electrical outlets for charging electronic devices.
  j Explain where to find the nurses' station, lounge, chapel, dining room, and other areas.
  k Identify staff—housekeeping, dietary, physical therapy, and others. Also identify students who are in the agency.
  l Explain when meals and snacks are served.
  m Explain visiting hours and policies.

Continued

Admitting the Person—cont'd

PROCEDURE—cont'd

13 Fill the water mug if oral fluids are allowed.
14 Place the call light within reach.
15 Place other controls and needed items within reach.
16 Provide a denture cup if needed. Label it with the person's name and room and bed number.
17 Label the person's property and personal care items with his or her name (if not done by the family). Follow agency policy for labeling items.

18 Complete a clothing and personal belongings list (Chapter 13). Follow agency policy for labeling clothing.
19 Help the person put away clothes and personal items. Use the closet, drawers, and bedside stand. (The family may help with this step.)

POST-PROCEDURE

20 Provide for comfort. (See the inside of the back cover.)
21 Lower the bed to a safe and comfortable level. Follow the nurse's directions.
22 Raise or lower bed rails as directed by the nurse.

23 Complete a safety check of the room. (See the inside of the back cover.)
24 Practice hand hygiene.
25 Report and record your observations.

Weight and Height

Weight and height are measured on admission. Then the person is weighed daily, weekly, or monthly. This is done to measure weight gain or loss.

Standing, chair, wheelchair, bed, and lift scales are used (Fig. 36-5). A standing scale is used for persons able to stand and walk. Chair, wheelchair, bed, and lift scales are used for persons who cannot stand. To measure weight and height, follow these guidelines.

- Follow the manufacturer's instructions for the scale used.
- Practice safety measures to prevent falls. See Chapters 13 and 14.
- Have the person wear a patient gown or sleepwear only. Clothes add weight. Footwear adds to the weight and height measurements.
- Protect the person from chilling and drafts. See Chapter 21.
- Have the person void before being weighed. A full bladder adds weight.
- Provide a dry incontinence product if needed. A wet product adds weight.
- Weigh the person at the same time of day. Before breakfast is the best time. Food and fluids add weight.
- Use the same scale for daily, weekly, and monthly weights. Scales weigh differently.
- Balance the scale at zero (0) before weighing the person. For balance scales, move the weights to zero. A digital scale should read at zero.

See *Focus on Math: Weight and Height.*

See *Teamwork and Time Management: Weight and Height,* p. 566.

See *Delegation Guidelines: Weight and Height,* p. 566.

See procedure: *Measuring Weight and Height With a Standing Scale,* p. 567.

See procedure: *Measuring Height—The Person Is in Bed,* p. 568.

Text continued on p. 569.

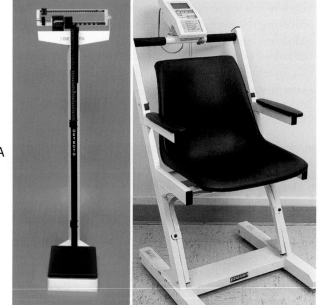

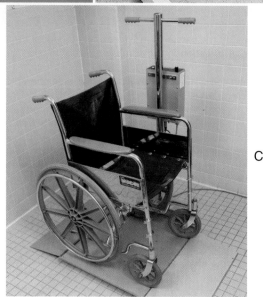

FIGURE 36-5 Types of scales. **A,** Standing scale. **B,** Chair scale. **C,** Wheelchair scale.

FOCUS ON **MATH**

Weight and Height

Weight—Reading the Scale

Standing scales (balance scales) have 2 bars with measurements (Fig. 36-6).

* The lower bar is divided into 50 pound (lb) values.
* The upper bar has long and short lines.
  * Long lines are 1 lb values.
  * Short lines are ¼, ½, and ¾ lb values.

The lower and upper bar values are added for the weight. *For example, the lower bar is at 100 lb and the upper bar is at 34 lb. The person's weight is 134 lb.*

100 lb + 34 lb = 134 lb

Weight—Measurements

Weight can be measured in pounds (lb) or kilograms (kg). There are 2.2 pounds in 1 kilogram (2.2 lb = 1 kg).

* To convert (change) kilograms to pounds, multiply the number of kilograms by 2.2. *For example: 100 kg is the same as 220 lb (100 kg × 2.2 = 220 lb).*
* To convert pounds to kilograms, divide the number of pounds by 2.2. *For example: 32 lb is the same as 14.5 kg (32 lb ÷ 2.2 = 14.5 kg).*

Know what measurement is used in your agency. Follow agency policy for reporting and recording.

Weight—Wheelchair Scales

To use a wheelchair scale:

1 Weigh the person's wheelchair while the person is in bed or in a chair. Note the wheelchair's weight.
2 Weigh the person in the wheelchair.
3 Subtract the weight in step 1 from the weight in step 2. This is the person's weight.

For example, the person's wheelchair weighs 35 lb. The weight of the person and the wheelchair is 200 lb.

200 lb (weight of the person and wheelchair) − 35 lb (wheelchair's weight) = 165 lb

The person weighs 165 lb.

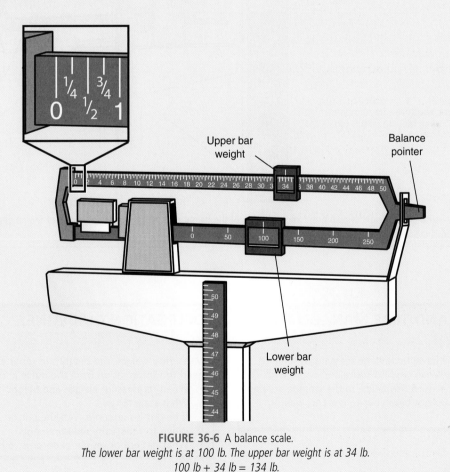

FIGURE 36-6 A balance scale.
The lower bar weight is at 100 lb. The upper bar weight is at 34 lb.
100 lb + 34 lb = 134 lb.
The weight is 134 lb.

Continued

FOCUS ON MATH—cont'd

Weight and Height

Height—Reading the Height Rod

The height rod has 2 sections—upper and lower. Raise or lower the upper section to adjust to the person's height. If the person is taller than the lower section, read the height at the movable part of the height rod.

The rod is marked with 1 inch (in) and $\frac{1}{4}$ inch values ($\frac{1}{4}$, $\frac{1}{2}$, $\frac{3}{4}$). Read height to the nearest $\frac{1}{4}$ inch. The numbers on the lower section increase moving up the rod. The numbers on the upper section increase moving down the rod.

See Figure 36-7.

Height—Measurements

For height, some agencies use feet and inches. Others only use inches. Know what measurements are used in your agency.

There are 12 inches (in) in 1 foot (ft) (1 ft = 12 in). To convert inches into feet and inches, divide the number of inches by 12. Use long division. If it does not divide evenly by 12, the number left over is the number of inches.

For example: Convert 64 inches into feet and inches.

$$\begin{array}{r} 5 \text{ Number of feet} \\ 12 \text{ Inches per foot} \overline{)\ 64\ \text{ Inches}} \\ -60 \\ \hline 4 \text{ Number of inches} \end{array}$$

64 inches = 5 ft 4 in

Upper section—the numbers increase moving *down* the rod.

Read height here.

Lower section—the numbers increase moving *up* the rod.

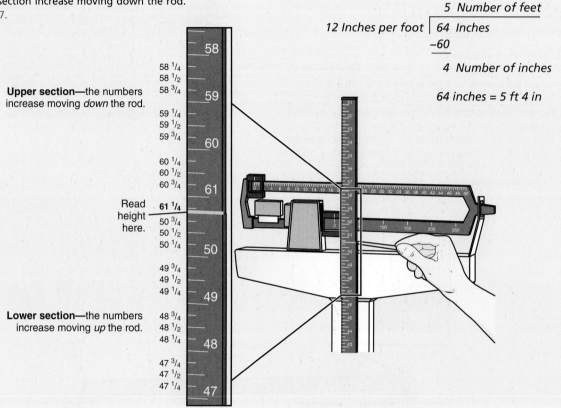

FIGURE 36-7 Height is read at the movable part of the height rod. (NOTE: The movable part of the height rod is marked with a yellow line.) This height rod measures 61$\frac{1}{4}$ inches (5 feet 1$\frac{1}{4}$ inches).

TEAMWORK AND TIME MANAGEMENT

Weight and Height

Nursing units usually have just 1 standing scale. In some agencies, chair, wheelchair, and lift scales are shared with other nursing units. Return the device to the storage area as quickly as possible. Do not have your co-workers wait or look for the scale.

DELEGATION GUIDELINES

Weight and Height

Measuring weight and height are routine nursing tasks. You need this information from the nurse and the care plan.
- When to measure weight and height
- What scale to use
- If height is measured with the person in bed
- When to report the measurements
- What patient or resident concerns to report at once

Measuring Weight and Height With a Standing Scale

QUALITY OF LIFE

- Knock before entering the person's room.
- Address the person by name.
- Introduce yourself by name and title.

- Explain the procedure before starting and during the procedure.
- Protect the person's rights during the procedure.
- Handle the person gently during the procedure.

PRE-PROCEDURE

1 Follow *Delegation Guidelines: Weight and Height.*
2 Ask the person to void.
3 Practice hand hygiene.
4 Bring the standing scale and paper towels to the person's room.
5 Practice hand hygiene.

6 Identify the person. Check the ID bracelet against the assignment sheet. Use 2 identifiers (Chapter 13). Also call the person by name.
7 Provide for privacy.

PROCEDURE

8 Place the paper towels on the scale platform.
9 Raise the height rod.
10 Move the weights to zero (0). The pointer is in the middle.
11 Have the person remove the robe and footwear. Assist as needed. (NOTE: For some state competency tests, shoes are worn.)
12 Help the person stand in the center of the scale. Arms are at the sides. The person does not hold on to anyone or any thing. See Figure 36-8.
13 Move the lower and upper weights until the balance pointer is in the middle (see Fig. 36-6).
14 Note the weight on your note pad or assignment sheet.

15 Ask the person to stand very straight.
16 Lower the height rod until it rests on the person's head (Fig. 36-9).
17 Read the height at the movable part of the height rod. Record the height in inches (or in feet and inches) to the nearest ¼ inch. See Figure 36-7.
18 Note the height on your note pad or assignment sheet.
19 Raise the height rod. Help the person step off of the scale.
20 Help the person put on a robe and slip-resistant footwear if he or she will be up. Or help the person back to bed.
21 Lower the height rod. Adjust the weights to zero (0) if this is your agency's policy.

POST-PROCEDURE

22 Provide for comfort. (See the inside of the back cover.)
23 Place the call light and other needed items within reach.
24 Raise or lower bed rails. Follow the care plan.
25 Unscreen the person.
26 Complete a safety check of the room. (See the inside of the back cover.)

27 Discard the paper towels.
28 Return the scale to its proper place.
29 Practice hand hygiene.
30 Report and record the measurements.

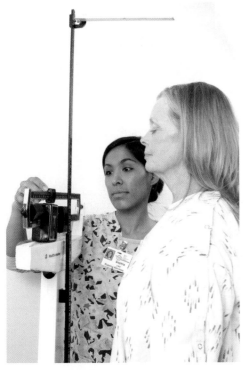

FIGURE 36-8 The person is weighed.

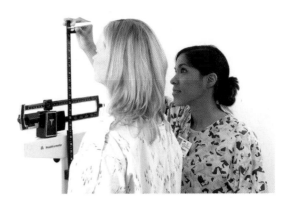

FIGURE 36-9 The height rod rests on the person's head.

Measuring Height—The Person Is in Bed

QUALITY OF LIFE

- Knock before entering the person's room.
- Address the person by name.
- Introduce yourself by name and title.

- Explain the procedure before starting and during the procedure.
- Protect the person's rights during the procedure.
- Handle the person gently during the procedure.

PRE-PROCEDURE

1 Follow *Delegation Guidelines: Weight and Height*, p. 566.
2 Practice hand hygiene.
3 Ask a co-worker to help you.
4 Collect a measuring tape and ruler.
5 Practice hand hygiene.

6 Identify the person. Check the ID bracelet against the assignment sheet. Use 2 identifiers (Chapter 13). Also call the person by name.
7 Provide for privacy.
8 Raise the bed for body mechanics. Bed rails are up if used.

PROCEDURE

9 Lower the bed rails (if up).
10 Position the person supine if the position is allowed.
11 Have your co-worker place and hold the beginning of the tape measure at the person's heel.
12 Pull the other end of the tape measure along the person's body. Pull it until it extends a few inches past the head.

13 Place the ruler flat across the top of the person's head and across the tape measure (Fig. 36-10). Make sure the ruler is level.
14 Read the height measurement. This is the point where the lower edge of the ruler touches the tape measure.
15 Note the height measurement on your note pad or assignment sheet.

POST-PROCEDURE

16 Provide for comfort. (See the inside of the back cover.)
17 Place the call light and other needed items within reach.
18 Lower the bed to a safe and comfortable level. Follow the care plan.
19 Raise or lower bed rails. Follow the care plan.

20 Complete a safety check of the room. (See the inside of the back cover.)
21 Return equipment to its proper place.
22 Practice hand hygiene.
23 Report and record the height.

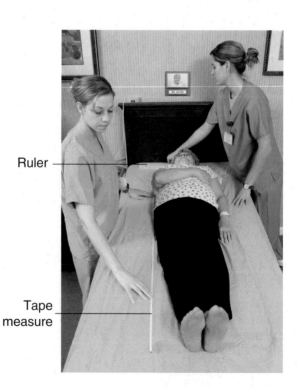

FIGURE 36-10 Height is measured in bed. The tape measure extends from the heel to the top of the head. The ruler is flat across the top of the person's head.

Ruler

Tape measure

MOVING THE PERSON TO A NEW ROOM

Sometimes a person is moved to a new room. Reasons include:

- A change in condition.
- The person requests a room change.
- Roommates do not get along.
- Care needs change.

The doctor, nurse, or social worker explains the reasons for the move to the person and family. You assist with the move or perform the entire procedure. The person is transported by wheelchair, stretcher, or the bed.

Support and reassure the person. If the new room is on another nursing unit, the person does not know the staff. Use good communication skills.

- Avoid pat answers. "It will be okay" is an example.
- Use touch to provide comfort.
- Introduce the person to the staff and roommate.
- Wish the person well as you leave him or her.
  See procedure: *Moving the Person to a New Room.*

Moving the Person to a New Room

QUALITY OF LIFE

- Knock before entering the person's room.
- Address the person by name.
- Introduce yourself by name and title.

- Explain the procedure before starting and during the procedure.
- Protect the person's rights during the procedure.
- Handle the person gently during the procedure.

PRE-PROCEDURE

1 Follow *Delegation Guidelines: Admissions, Transfers, and Discharges*, p. 560. See *Promoting Safety and Comfort: Admissions, Transfers, and Discharges*, p. 560.
2 Ask a co-worker to help you.
3 Practice hand hygiene.
4 Collect the following.
   - Wheelchair or stretcher
   - Utility cart
   - Bath blanket

5 Practice hand hygiene.
6 Identify the person. Check the ID bracelet against the assignment sheet. Use 2 identifiers (Chapter 13). Call the person by name.
7 Provide for privacy.

PROCEDURE

8 Place the person's belongings and care equipment on the cart.
9 Transfer the person to a wheelchair or stretcher (Chapter 20). Cover him or her with the bath blanket.
10 Transport the person to the new room. Your co-worker brings the cart.
11 Help transfer the person to the bed or chair. Help position the person (Chapters 18, 19, and 20).

12 Help arrange the person's belongings and equipment.
13 Report the following to the receiving nurse.
   - How the person tolerated the transfer
   - Observations made during the transfer
   - That a nurse from the previous unit will communicate with him or her.

POST-PROCEDURE

14 Return the wheelchair or stretcher and the cart to the storage area.
15 Practice hand hygiene.
16 Report and record the following.
   - The time of the transfer
   - Who helped you with the transfer
   - Where the person was taken
   - How the person was transferred (bed, wheelchair, or stretcher)
   - How the person tolerated the transfer
   - Who received the person
   - Other observations

17 Strip the bed and clean the unit. Practice hand hygiene and wear gloves for this step. (The housekeeping staff may do this step.)
18 Remove and discard the gloves. Practice hand hygiene.
19 Follow agency policy for used linens.
20 Make a closed bed.
21 Practice hand hygiene.

TRANSFERS AND DISCHARGES

Transfers and discharges are usually planned in advance. The person goes home or to another agency. If being discharged to home, the health team teaches the person and family about diet, exercise, drugs, procedures, and treatments. Home care, equipment, and therapies are arranged as needed. A doctor's appointment is given.

The nurse tells you when to start the transfer or discharge procedure and when the person is ready to leave. Usually a wheelchair is used. If leaving by ambulance, a stretcher is used.

Use good communication skills during a transfer or discharge. Wish the person and family well as they leave the agency.

A person may want to leave the agency without the doctor's permission. Tell the nurse at once. The nurse or social worker handles the matter.

See procedure: *Transferring or Discharging the Person*.

Transferring or Discharging the Person

QUALITY OF LIFE

- Knock before entering the person's room.
- Address the person by name.
- Introduce yourself by name and title.
- Explain the procedure before starting and during the procedure.
- Protect the person's rights during the procedure.
- Handle the person gently during the procedure.

PRE-PROCEDURE

1 Follow *Delegation Guidelines: Admissions, Transfers, and Discharges*, p. 560. See *Promoting Safety and Comfort: Admissions, Transfers, and Discharges*, p. 560.
2 Ask a co-worker to help you.
3 Practice hand hygiene.
4 Identify the person. Check the ID bracelet against the assignment sheet. Use 2 identifiers (Chapter 13). Also call the person by name.
5 Provide for privacy.

PROCEDURE

6 Help the person dress as needed.
7 Help the person pack. Check the bathroom and all drawers and closets. Make sure all items are collected.
8 Check off the clothing list and personal belongings list. Give the lists to the nurse.
9 Tell the nurse that the person is ready for the final visit. The nurse:
  a Gives prescriptions written by the doctor.
  b Provides discharge instructions.
  c Returns valuables from the safe.
  d Has the person sign the clothing and personal belongings lists.
10 *For the person leaving by wheelchair:*
  a Get a wheelchair and a utility cart for the person's items. Ask a co-worker to help you.
  b Help the person into the wheelchair.
  c Take the person to the exit area.
  d Lock (brake) the wheelchair wheels.
  e Help the person into the vehicle (Fig. 36-11).
  f Help put the person's items into the vehicle.
11 *For the person leaving by ambulance:*
  a Raise the bed rails.
  b Place the call light within reach.
  c Wait for the ambulance attendants.
  d Raise the bed for a transfer to the stretcher when the ambulance attendants arrive.

POST-PROCEDURE

12 Return the wheelchair and cart to the storage area.
13 Practice hand hygiene.
14 Report and record the following.
- The time of the discharge
- Who helped you with the procedure
- How the person was transported
- Who was with the person
- The person's destination
- Other observations
15 Strip the bed and clean the unit. Practice hand hygiene and wear gloves for this step. (The housekeeping staff may do this step.)
16 Remove and discard the gloves. Practice hand hygiene.
17 Follow agency policy for used linens.
18 Make a closed bed.
19 Practice hand hygiene.

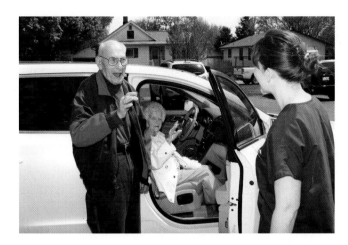

FIGURE 36-11 The resident in the car is being discharged.

FOCUS ON **PRIDE**

The Person, Family, and Yourself

P ersonal and Professional Responsibility

Admission to a hospital or nursing center is often hard for the person and family. Transfers and discharges also can cause fear and worry. To help the person adjust:

- Be courteous, caring, efficient, and competent.
- Be sensitive to fears and concerns.
- Handle the person's belongings carefully and with respect. Protect them from loss or damage.
- Focus on the person and family. Do not rush. Do not discuss other work you need to do.
- Treat the person and family like you want your loved ones treated.

R ights and Respect

Know your agency's rules for visitors. Do not assume that all units or agencies have the same rules. For example, psychiatric, intensive care, and pediatric units often have special rules. Give the person and visitors correct information. If you do not know, ask the nurse.

The person has the right to decide who can visit. Tell the nurse about the person's requests.

I ndependence and Social Interaction

A new setting brings social challenges. In a nursing center, the first hours and days can be lonely. The person can feel isolated and depressed.

You can help with these social challenges. Visit new residents and introduce them to other residents. Encourage them to take part in activities. Observe for and report social isolation or roommate troubles. Make sure your interactions are pleasant.

D elegation and Teamwork

The family often wants to be present during admissions, transfers, and discharges. They may have questions or need to answer questions. If the person consents, the family may be present.

Sometimes privacy is needed. For example, the nurse may need to ask about personal or embarrassing topics. Or the person needs to get dressed. The nurse may have you manage and assist the family when privacy is needed. The family is important. To show care and concern:

- Take them to the waiting area.
- Offer coffee or water while they wait.
- Show where they can get food and drinks.
- Tell them where they can make phone calls.
- Ask if there is anything they need.

E thics and Laws

Before discharge, the person receives discharge instructions. Common information includes drugs to continue or stop, new prescriptions, activity, diet, appointments, and special care instructions. The nurse explains the information, provides teaching, and answers questions. The information is given orally and in writing.

You may be tempted to give the person the information. Discharge teaching is beyond the scope of your role. You may provide wrong information. The person can be harmed.

If a person asks you about discharge instructions, say: "The nurse will give you information and answer your questions before you leave." Take pride in following the limits of your role.

FOCUS ON **PRIDE**: *Application*

Admissions, transfers, and discharges take time. You may be busy and have other tasks to do. How will you make the person feel that he or she is the most important at the time?

REVIEW QUESTIONS

Circle T if the statement is TRUE or F if it is FALSE.

1 T F You are admitting a new resident. You must introduce yourself by name and title.

2 T F A person arrives at the center by ambulance. You transport the person to his or her room.

3 T F The person is greeted by name and title during the admission process.

4 T F A person complains of pain. Report the complaint after completing your checklist.

5 T F The person will arrive by stretcher. You make an occupied bed.

6 T F You help orient the person to the new setting.

7 T F Clothing and personal belongings lists are made during the admission process.

8 T F Starting with admission, the person's rights are protected.

9 T F Persons with dementia adjust well to new settings.

10 T F A person objects to a transfer. An ombudsman can protect the person's rights.

Circle the BEST answer.

11 When the person arrives in the room, you
   a Record the person's identifying information
   b Measure vital signs
   c Explain the person's rights
   d Review the doctor's orders

12 You are going to measure weight with a standing scale. Which should you correct before weighing the person?
   a The person is wearing footwear.
   b The scale is balanced at zero (0).
   c There is a paper towel on the scale platform.
   d The person is in the center of the scale with arms at the sides.

13 When measuring height with a standing scale
   a Balance the height rod at zero (0)
   b Be sure footwear is worn
   c Read the height at the movable part of the height rod
   d Record height to the nearest inch

14 What is 68 inches in feet and inches?
   a 4 ft 0 in
   b 5 ft 6 in
   c 5 ft 8 in
   d 6 ft 8 in

15 Before transferring a person to another nursing unit, you
   a Gather the person's belongings
   b Explain the reason for the move
   c Tell the staff on the new unit to come get the person
   d Reassure the person by saying: "You'll be fine."

16 When discharging a person, you can
   a Teach the person about diet and drugs
   b Arrange for home care
   c Let the person leave when he or she is ready
   d Help the person into the vehicle

Answers to Chapter 36 questions are on p. 887.

FOCUS ON PRACTICE

Problem Solving

A person is waiting for a new room on another nursing unit. The room is not yet ready. Ready to move, the person is becoming anxious. How can you provide comfort and ease anxiety? How can you make the move efficient when the room is ready?

Assisting With the Physical Examination

- Define the key terms in this chapter.
- Explain what to do before, during, and after an examination (exam).
- Identify the equipment used for an exam.
- Describe how to prepare and drape a person for an exam.
- Explain the rules for assisting with an exam.
- Perform the procedure described in this chapter.
- Explain how to promote PRIDE in the person, the family, and yourself.

KEY TERMS

dorsal recumbent position The supine position with the legs together *(dorsal* means *the back of something; recumbent* means *to lie down);* horizontal recumbent position
genupectoral position See "knee-chest position" *(genu* means *knee; pectoral* refers to the *chest)*
horizontal recumbent position See "dorsal recumbent position"
knee-chest position The person kneels and rests the body on the knees and chest; the head is turned to 1 side, the arms are above the head or flexed at the elbows, the back is straight, and the body is flexed about 90 degrees at the hips; genupectoral position
laryngeal mirror An instrument used to examine the mouth, teeth, and throat

lithotomy position The woman lies on her back with the hips at the edge of the exam table, her knees are flexed, her hips are externally rotated, and her feet are in stirrups
nasal speculum An instrument *(speculum* means *mirror)* used to examine the inside of the nose *(nasal)*
ophthalmoscope A lighted instrument *(scope)* used to examine the internal eye *(ophthalmo)* structures
otoscope A lighted instrument *(scope)* used to examine the external ear *(oto)* and the eardrum (tympanic membrane)
percussion hammer An instrument used to tap body parts to test reflexes *(percussion* means *to strike hard);* reflex hammer
tuning fork An instrument vibrated to test hearing
vaginal speculum An instrument *(speculum)* used to open the vagina *(vaginal)* to examine it and the cervix

Doctors and advanced practice registered nurses (APRNs) perform physical exams. Exams are done to:
- Promote health.
- Determine fitness for work.
- Diagnose disease.

YOUR ROLE

Your role depends on agency policies and on what the examiner prefers. You may be asked to:
- Collect linens, equipment, and supplies.
- Prepare the exam room or the person's room.
- Cover the exam table with a clean drawsheet or paper.
- Provide for lighting.
- Transport the person to and from the exam room.
- Prepare the person for the exam (p. 574).
- Hand equipment and supplies to the examiner.
- Label specimen containers.
- Discard used supplies and clean equipment.
- Help the person dress or to a comfortable position after the exam.
- Follow agency policy for used linens.

EQUIPMENT

The instruments in Figure 37-1 (p. 574) are used in the exam.
- *Laryngeal mirror—used to examine the mouth, teeth, and throat.*
- *Nasal speculum—used to examine the inside of the nose.* Speculum *means* mirror; nasal *means* nose.
- *Ophthalmoscope—a lighted instrument* (scope) *used to examine the internal eye* (ophthalmo) *structures.*
- *Otoscope—a lighted instrument* (scope) *used to examine the external ear* (oto) *and the eardrum (tympanic membrane).* Some otoscopes can be changed into an ophthalmoscope.
- *Percussion hammer (reflex hammer)—used to tap body parts to test reflexes.* Percussion *means* to strike hard.
- *Tuning fork—vibrated to test hearing.*
- *Vaginal speculum—used to open the vagina* (vaginal) *to examine it and the cervix.* Speculum *means* mirror.

Some agencies prepare exam trays. If not, collect the items listed in the procedure: *Preparing the Person for an Examination,* p. 575. Arrange them on a tray or table.

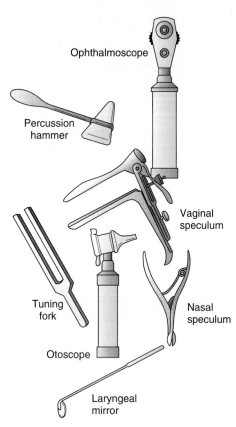

Ophthalmoscope

Percussion hammer

Vaginal speculum

Tuning fork

Nasal speculum

Otoscope

Laryngeal mirror

FIGURE 37-1 Physical exam instruments.

PREPARING THE PERSON

The physical exam can cause concerns. People may worry about findings. Some are confused or have fears about the procedure. Discomfort, embarrassment, exposure, and not knowing the procedure cause anxiety. Respect the person's feelings and concerns.

The nurse explains the exam's purpose and what to expect. Then the nurse obtains the person's consent. To assist the nurse:

- Provide for privacy.
  - Screen the person and close the room door.
  - Help the person put on a patient gown. Usually all clothes are removed. The gown reduces the naked feeling and fear of exposure.
- Have the person void to empty the bladder. This lets the examiner feel the abdominal organs. A full bladder can change the normal position and shape of organs. It also causes discomfort, especially when feeling the abdominal organs.
- Obtain a urine specimen if needed. Explain how to collect the specimen (Chapter 38). Label the container.
- Measure and record vital signs, weight, height, and pulse oximetry.
- Drape the person. Use a paper drape, bath blanket, sheet, or drawsheet.
- Position the person for the exam.
  See *Focus on Communication: Preparing the Person*.
  See *Focus on Children and Older Persons: Preparing the Person*.
  See *Delegation Guidelines: Preparing the Person*.
  See *Promoting Safety and Comfort: Preparing the Person*.
  See procedure: *Preparing the Person for an Examination*.

FOCUS ON COMMUNICATION

Preparing the Person

When preparing a person for an exam, do not assume the person knows what to do. Tell the person what clothing to remove, how to put on the gown (opening to the front or to the back), and where to sit. For example:

Please remove your clothes and put on this gown. The gown opens in the back. Under-garments can stay on. You can put your clothes on this chair. Here is a blanket to cover yourself. Please have a seat on the exam table after you change. Do you have any questions?

FOCUS ON CHILDREN AND OLDER PERSONS

Preparing the Person

Children
Babies wear diapers for an exam. Toddlers, pre-school children, and school-age children can wear underpants. Diapers or underpants are removed or lowered as needed during the exam.

Older Persons
Nursing center residents have an exam at least once a year. The person has the right to personal choice. The doctor or nurse explains the reason for the exam. The person is told who will do the exam and when and how it will be done.

The exam requires the person's consent. The person may want a different examiner. Or the person may want a family member present for the exam and when the results are explained.

DELEGATION GUIDELINES

Preparing the Person

In some agencies, preparing persons for exams is a routine nursing task. In others it is a nursing responsibility that may be delegated to you. To prepare a person for an exam, you need this information from the nurse and the care plan.

- When to prepare the person.
- What room to prepare—an exam room or the person's room.
- How to position the person.
- The equipment and supplies needed.
- If a urine specimen is needed. If yes, should you collect a random urine specimen or a midstream specimen (Chapter 38)?
- What patient or resident concerns to report at once.

PROMOTING SAFETY AND COMFORT

Preparing the Person

Safety
Protect the person from falls and injuries. Do not leave the person unattended.

Comfort
Warmth is important during an exam. Protect the person from chilling and drafts. Have an extra bath blanket nearby.

The physical exam often involves exposing and touching private areas—breasts, perineum, rectum. Sexual abuse has occurred in health care settings. The person may feel threatened or is actually being abused. He or she needs to call for help. Keep the call light within the person's reach at all times. And always act in a professional manner.

Preparing the Person for an Examination

QUALITY OF LIFE

- Knock before entering the person's room.
- Address the person by name.
- Introduce yourself by name and title.

- Explain the procedure before starting and during the procedure.
- Protect the person's rights during the procedure.
- Handle the person gently during the procedure.

PRE-PROCEDURE

1 Follow *Delegation Guidelines: Preparing the Person*. See *Promoting Safety and Comfort: Preparing the Person*.
2 Practice hand hygiene.
3 Collect the following.
   - Exam form
   - Flashlight
   - Blood pressure equipment
   - Stethoscope
   - Thermometer
   - Pulse oximeter (Chapter 43)
   - Scale
   - Tongue depressors (blades)
   - Laryngeal mirror
   - Ophthalmoscope
   - Otoscope
   - Nasal speculum
   - Percussion (reflex) hammer
   - Tuning fork
   - Vaginal speculum (for a female)
   - Tape measure
   - Gloves
   - Water-soluble lubricant
   - Cotton-tipped applicators

   - Specimen containers and labels
   - Disposable bag
   - Kidney basin
   - Towel
   - Bath blanket
   - Tissues
   - Drape (sheet, bath blanket, drawsheet, or paper drape)
   - Paper towels
   - Cotton balls
   - Waterproof under-pad
   - Eye chart (Snellen chart)
   - Slides
   - Patient gown
   - Alcohol wipes
   - Wastebasket
   - Container for soiled instruments
   - Marking pencils or pens
4 Practice hand hygiene.
5 Identify the person. Check the ID (identification) bracelet against the assignment sheet. Use 2 identifiers (Chapter 13). Also call the person by name.
6 Provide for privacy.

PROCEDURE

7 Have the person put on the gown. Tell him or her what clothes to remove and where to place them. Assist as needed.
8 Ask the person to void. Collect a urine specimen if needed. Provide for privacy.
9 Transport the person to the exam room. (Omit this step for an exam in the person's room.)
10 Measure weight and height (Chapter 36). Record the measurements on the exam form.
11 Help the person onto the exam table. Provide a step stool if necessary. (Omit this step for an exam in the person's room.)

12 Raise the far bed rail (if used). Raise the bed to a safe and comfortable working height. (Omit this step if an exam table is used.)
13 Measure vital signs and pulse oximetry. Record them on the exam form.
14 Position the person as directed.
15 Drape the person (p. 576).
16 Place a waterproof under-pad under the buttocks.
17 Raise the bed rail near you (if used).
18 Provide for adequate lighting.
19 Put the call light on for the examiner. Do not leave the person alone.

POSITIONING AND DRAPING

Some exam positions are uncomfortable and embarrassing. Before helping the person assume and maintain the position, explain:

* Why the position is needed
* How to assume the position
* How you will drape the person for warmth and privacy
* How long to expect to stay in the position

Exam Positions

The examiner may request 1 of the following exam positions.

* *Dorsal recumbent position (horizontal recumbent position)—the person is supine with the legs together.* (Dorsal *means* the back of something; recumbent *means* to lie down.) The position is used to examine the abdomen, chest, and breasts. To examine the perineal area, the knees are flexed and hips externally rotated. Drape the person as in Figure 37-2, *A.*
* *Lithotomy position—the woman lies on her back. Hips are at the edge of the exam table. Knees are flexed and hips externally rotated. Feet are in stirrups.* (See Fig. 37-2, *B.*) The position is used to examine the vagina and cervix. See draping for perineal care in Chapter 24. Some agencies provide socks for the feet and calves.
* *Knee-chest position—the person kneels and rests the body on the knees and chest. The head is turned to 1 side. The arms are above the head or flexed at the elbows. The back is straight. The body is flexed about 90 degrees at the hips.* (See Fig. 37-2, *C.*) The position is also called the *genupectoral position.* (Genu *means* knee. Pectoral *refers to the* chest.) The position is used to examine the rectum. Apply the drape in a diamond shape to cover the back, buttocks, and thighs.
* The *Sims' position*—is sometimes used to examine the rectum or vagina (Chapter 18). (See Fig. 37-2, *D.*) Apply the drape in a diamond shape. The examiner folds back the near corner to expose the rectum or vagina.

See *Focus on Children and Older Persons: Positioning and Draping.*

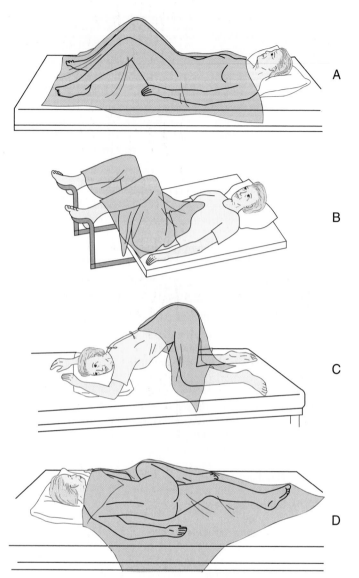

FIGURE 37-2 Positioning and draping for the physical exam. **A,** Dorsal recumbent position. **B,** Lithotomy position. **C,** Knee-chest position. **D,** Sims' position.

FOCUS ON CHILDREN AND OLDER PERSONS

Positioning and Draping

Older Persons
The knee-chest position is rarely used for older persons. The side-lying position is used to examine the rectum.

ASSISTING WITH THE EXAM

You may be asked to prepare, position, and drape the person. If assisting with the exam, follow the rules in Box 37-1.

See *Focus on Communication: Assisting With the Exam.*

See *Focus on Children and Older Persons: Assisting With the Exam.*

After the Exam

After the exam, the person dresses or returns to bed. First, the vagina or rectum is wiped or cleaned if lubricant was used to examine those structures. Assist and provide hand hygiene as needed. You also need to:

- Discard disposable items.
- Replace supplies on the exam tray.
- Clean re-usable items. This includes the otoscope and ophthalmoscope tips and stethoscope. Return items to the tray or storage area. Send a re-usable speculum to the supply department. It needs to be sterilized.
- Cover the exam table with a clean drawsheet or paper.
- Label specimens. Take them to the correct area with a requisition slip. See Chapter 38.
- Clean and straighten the person's unit or exam room.
- Follow agency policy for used linens.

See *Teamwork and Time Management: After the Exam.*

BOX 37-1 | **Assisting With the Physical Exam**

- Practice hand hygiene before and after the exam.
- Provide for privacy.
  - Close doors and window coverings.
  - Screen and drape the person.
- Position the person as directed by the examiner.
- Place instruments and equipment near the examiner.
- Stay in the room for the legal protection of the person and the examiner if:
  - The examiner's gender differs from the person's gender. A male is present for a male's exam. A female is present for a female's exam.
  - The person requests.
  - The examiner requests. The person's consent is needed.
- Protect the person from falling.
- Reassure the person throughout the exam.
- Anticipate the examiner's need for equipment and supplies.
- Expose only the body part being examined
- Place paper or paper towels on the floor if the person will stand.
- Follow Standard Precautions and the Bloodborne Pathogen Standard.
- Keep the call light within the person's reach.

FOCUS ON COMMUNICATION

Assisting With the Exam

Each examiner has a routine. To better assist, ask the examiner to explain the routine to you. Also ask what equipment and supplies are needed. For example:

- "I want to help in the best way I can. Please tell me how you will start the exam and how you will proceed."
- "Please ask for equipment and supplies as you need them. That way I can hand you the correct item."

FOCUS ON CHILDREN AND OLDER PERSONS

Assisting With the Exam

Children

A parent is present when children are examined. The parent may need to hold and keep a child still during some parts of the exam. Being kept still may frighten an infant. A child may fear harm or separation from the parent. A calm, comforting manner helps the child and parent. The parent may have fears too.

The equipment is the same as for adult exams. Toys are used to assess development. Vaginal speculums are not used.

Older Persons

Persons with dementia may resist the examiner's efforts. The person may be agitated and aggressive from confusion and fear. Do not restrain or force the person to have the exam. The exam is tried another time. Sometimes a family member can calm the person. Drugs may be ordered to help the person relax. The person's rights are always respected.

TEAMWORK AND TIME MANAGEMENT

After the Exam

Make sure the exam room is clean with supplies and equipment ready for the next exam. Otherwise you delay the person, the examiner, and the staff member assisting.

You may find an exam room that is not clean. Or exam equipment and supplies are not ready. Call for the nurse to see the problem before you proceed. The nurse can find out who last used the room or tray. The nurse can talk to the staff members involved.

FOCUS ON PRIDE

The Person, Family, and Yourself

P ersonal and Professional Responsibility

The person needs to feel safe and secure during the exam. The person should feel comfortable with the examiner and the assistant. Be professional and courteous. Provide care in a way that promotes dignity, self-esteem, and well-being.

R ights and Respect

The person has the right to privacy. Protect the person from exposure. Only the examiner and the assistant should see the person's body. The person must consent for others to be present. This includes family. Keep the person properly draped and screened. Expose only the body part being examined.

I ndependence and Social Interaction

Fears about the exam are common.
- Who will perform the exam? How will it be done?
- Why is the exam needed?
- Will an illness or cancer be found?
- Will surgery be needed? Will more drugs be needed? Will I die?
  To ease the person's fears:
- Greet the person. Introduce yourself by name and title.
- Talk with the person. Be pleasant.
- Tell the person good things about the examiner or agency. For example: "Your doctor is very kind and thorough." Your interactions affect the person's mental comfort.
Caring, kindness, and a positive attitude ease worries.

D elegation and Teamwork

Good teamwork involves being helpful, prepared, and knowledgeable. Know where to find the supplies and equipment used for exams. When you need an item, you can get it quickly.

Plan ahead. Test equipment before each use. For example, check that the ophthalmoscope and otoscope lights work. If not, correct the issue.

E thics and Laws

You must keep the person's information confidential. Talking about an exam with family, friends, or staff not involved in the person's care violates the *Health Insurance Portability and Accountability Act of 1996* (HIPAA). HIPAA protects the privacy and security of the person's health information (Chapter 5). Failure to follow HIPAA rules can result in fines, penalties, and criminal action.

FOCUS ON PRIDE: Application

Explain the importance of your role before, during, and after the physical exam. How do you prevent delays and promote comfort?

REVIEW QUESTIONS

Circle the BEST answer.

1 The otoscope is used to examine
  a Internal eye structures
  b The external ear and the eardrum
  c Reflexes
  d The vagina

2 When preparing for an exam, you
  a Explain the purpose of the exam
  b Leave to tell the nurse the person is ready
  c Position and drape the person
  d Obtain consent for the exam

3 Which part of an exam can you do?
  a Test reflexes.
  b Inspect the mouth, teeth, and throat.
  c Measure weight, height, and vital signs.
  d Observe the perineum and rectum.

4 A person is supine. The hips are flexed and externally rotated. The feet are supported in stirrups. The person is in the
  a Dorsal recumbent position
  b Knee-chest position
  c Sims' position
  d Lithotomy position

5 You will assist with a female resident's exam. Which is *true*?
  a Hand hygiene is practiced before and after the exam.
  b A male nursing team member stays in the room.
  c You may restrain her for the exam if needed.
  d A family member is not allowed in the room.

Answers to Chapter 37 questions are on p. 887.

FOCUS ON PRACTICE

Problem Solving

During an exam, you must leave the room several times for supplies. What problems does this cause? How could this have been prevented?

Collecting and Testing Specimens

OBJECTIVES

- Define the key terms and key abbreviations in this chapter.
- Explain why specimens are collected.
- Explain the rules for collecting specimens.
- Describe the different types of urine specimens.
- Describe 5 urine tests.
- Explain how to use reagent strips.
- Describe how to collect a stool specimen.

- Describe how to collect a sputum specimen.
- Describe the equipment used for blood glucose testing.
- Identify the skin puncture sites.
- Perform the procedures described in this chapter.
- Explain how to promote PRIDE in the person, the family, and yourself.

KEY TERMS

acetone See "ketone"
glucometer A device for measuring *(meter)* blood glucose *(gluco)*; glucose meter
glucosuria Sugar *(glucose)* in the urine *(uria)*
hematoma A swelling *(oma)* that contains blood *(hemat)*
hematuria Blood *(hemat)* in the urine *(uria)*
hemoptysis Bloody *(hemo)* sputum *(ptysis means to spit)*

ketone A substance appearing in urine from the rapid breakdown of fat for energy; acetone, ketone body
ketone body See "ketone"
melena A black, tarry stool
sputum Mucus from the respiratory system when expectorated (expelled) through the mouth

KEY ABBREVIATIONS

BM	Bowel movement	mL	Milliliter
ID	Identification	oz	Ounce
I&O	Intake and output	U/A	Urinalysis

Specimens *(samples)* are collected and tested to prevent, detect, and treat disease. Some specimens are tested at the bedside. Most are tested in the laboratory. All laboratory specimens require requisition slips with identifying information and the test ordered. The specimen container is labeled following agency policy. To collect specimens, follow the rules in Box 38-1.

See *Teamwork and Time Management: Collecting and Testing Specimens*, p. 580.

See *Promoting Safety and Comfort: Collecting and Testing Specimens*, p. 580.

BOX 38-1	Collecting Specimens

- Follow the rules for medical asepsis.
- Follow Standard Precautions and the Bloodborne Pathogen Standard.
- Use a clean container for each specimen.
- Use the correct container.
- Do not touch the inside of the container or the inside of the lid.
- Identify the person. Check the ID (identification) bracelet against the laboratory requisition slip or assignment sheet. Compare all information. Ask the person to state his or her first and last name and birthdate.
- Label the container in the person's presence. Provide clear, accurate information.
- Collect the specimen at the correct time.
- Ask a female if she is having a menstrual period. Tell the nurse. Menstruating may cause blood to be in the urine specimen.

- Ask the person not to have a bowel movement (BM) when collecting a urine specimen. Urine specimens must not contain stools.
- Ask the person to void before collecting a stool specimen. Stool specimens must not contain urine.
- Have the person put toilet paper in the toilet or in a disposable bag. Discard following agency policy. Urine and stool specimens must not contain tissue.
- Secure the lid on the specimen container tightly.
- Place the specimen container in a plastic bag with a *BIOHAZARD* label. Do not let the container touch the outside of the bag. Seal the bag.
- Take the specimen and requisition slip to the laboratory or storage area.

TEAMWORK AND TIME MANAGEMENT
Collecting and Testing Specimens

Nursing centers have storage areas for specimens. Specimens are picked up at a certain time and transported to a laboratory. Have specimens collected and in the storage area by the pick-up time. If not collected in time, results are delayed. A new specimen may be needed. The delay can harm the person. Using more supplies and equipment costs more money.

PROMOTING SAFETY AND COMFORT
Collecting and Testing Specimens

Safety

Correct identification is important when collecting and testing specimens. To identify the person, check the ID bracelet against all information on the requisition slip. Agency policy may require asking the person to identify himself or herself by both of the following.
- Stating or spelling his or her first and last name
- Stating his or her birthdate

Blood, body fluids, secretions, and excretions may contain microbes and blood. This includes urine, stool, and sputum specimens. Follow Standard Precautions and the Bloodborne Pathogen Standard when collecting, testing, and handling specimens.

> NOTE: A task may require more than 1 pair of gloves. Change gloves as needed. Use careful judgment. Remember to practice hand hygiene after removing gloves.

DELEGATION GUIDELINES
Urine Specimens

Collecting urine specimens is a routine nursing task. You need this information from the nurse and the care plan.
- Voiding device—bedpan, urinal, commode, or toilet with specimen pan
- The type of specimen needed
- What time to collect the specimen
- What special measures are needed
- If you need to test the specimen (p. 587)
- If measuring intake and output (I&O) is ordered (Chapter 31)
- What observations to report and record:
  - Problems obtaining the specimen
  - Color, clarity, and odor of urine
  - Blood in the urine
  - Particles in the urine
  - Complaints of pain, burning, urgency, difficulty voiding, or other problems
  - The time the specimen was collected
- When to report observations
- What patient or resident concerns to report at once

PROMOTING SAFETY AND COMFORT
Urine Specimens

Comfort

Clear specimen containers show urine. This may embarrass some people, including children. They do not like clear specimen containers that show urine. Cloudy containers are common.

URINE SPECIMENS

Urine specimens are collected for urine tests. Follow the rules in Box 38-1.

See *Delegation Guidelines: Urine Specimens.*
See *Promoting Safety and Comfort: Urine Specimens.*

The Random Urine Specimen

The random urine specimen is used for a routine urinalysis (U/A). No special measures are needed. It is collected any time in a 24-hour period. Many people collect the specimen themselves. Weak and very ill persons need help.

See procedure: *Collecting a Random Urine Specimen.*

Collecting a Random Urine Specimen

QUALITY OF LIFE

- Knock before entering the person's room.
- Address the person by name.
- Introduce yourself by name and title.

- Explain the procedure before starting and during the procedure.
- Protect the person's rights during the procedure.
- Handle the person gently during the procedure.

PRE-PROCEDURE

1 Follow *Delegation Guidelines: Urine Specimens*. See *Promoting Safety and Comfort*:
   a *Collecting and Testing Specimens*
   b *Urine Specimens*
2 Practice hand hygiene.
3 Collect the following before going to the person's room.
   - Laboratory requisition slip
   - Specimen container and lid
   - Voiding device (clean, un-used)—bedpan and cover (optional), urinal, or specimen pan (Fig. 38-1)
   - Specimen label
   - Disposable bag (if needed)
   - Plastic bag
   - *BIOHAZARD* label (if needed)
   - Gloves

4 Arrange your work area.
5 Practice hand hygiene.
6 Identify the person. Check the ID bracelet against the requisition slip. Compare all information. Also call the person by name. Ask the person to state his or her first and last name and birthdate.
7 Label the container in the person's presence.
8 Put on gloves
9 Collect a commode (if needed) and a graduate to measure output.
10 Provide for privacy.

PROCEDURE

11 Place the specimen pan on the toilet or commode container (see Fig. 38-1).
12 Ask the person to urinate into the voiding device. Have the person put toilet paper in the toilet. Or provide a disposable bag and follow agency policy for disposal. Toilet paper is not put in the bedpan or specimen pan.
13 Take the voiding device or commode container to the bathroom.
14 Pour about 120 mL (milliliters) (4 oz [ounces]) into the specimen container.
15 Place the lid on the specimen container tightly. Put the container in the plastic bag. Do not let the container touch the outside of the bag. Apply a *BIOHAZARD* label.

16 Measure urine if I&O are ordered. Include the specimen amount.
17 Empty, rinse, clean, disinfect, and dry equipment. Use clean, dry paper towels for drying. Return equipment to its proper place.
18 Remove and discard the gloves. Practice hand hygiene. Put on clean gloves.
19 Assist with hand hygiene.
20 Remove and discard the gloves. Practice hand hygiene.

POST-PROCEDURE

21 Provide for comfort. (See the inside of the back cover.)
22 Place the call light and other needed items within reach.
23 Raise or lower bed rails. Follow the care plan.
24 Unscreen the person.
25 Complete a safety check of the room. (See the inside of the back cover.)

26 Practice hand hygiene.
27 Take the specimen and requisition slip to the laboratory or storage area. Wear gloves if that is agency policy.
28 Remove and discard the gloves. Practice hand hygiene.
29 Report and record your observations.

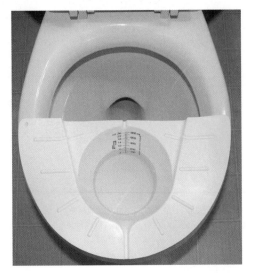

FIGURE 38-1 The specimen pan is at the front of the toilet on the toilet rim for a urine specimen. (NOTE: The toilet seat is lowered over the specimen pan for voiding.)

The Midstream Specimen

The midstream specimen is also called a *clean-voided specimen* or *clean-catch specimen*. The perineal area is cleaned first to reduce the number of microbes in the urethral area. The person starts to void into a device. Then the person stops the urine stream and a sterile specimen container is positioned. The person voids into the container until the specimen is obtained.

Stopping and starting the urine stream is hard for many people. You may need to position and hold the specimen container after the person starts to void (Fig. 38-2).

See *Focus on Communication: The Midstream Specimen.*

See *Promoting Safety and Comfort: The Midstream Specimen.*

See procedure: *Collecting a Midstream Specimen.*

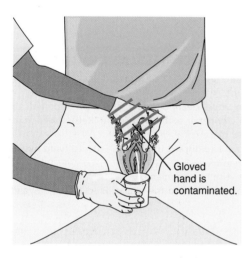

FIGURE 38-2 The labia are separated to collect a midstream specimen.

Gloved hand is contaminated.

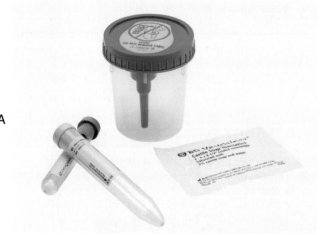

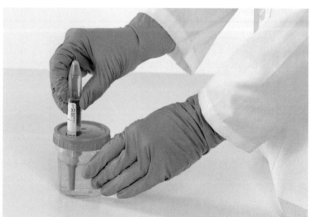

FIGURE 38-3 **A,** A urine specimen kit. This kit contains towelettes, a collection cup with a transfer device, and tubes with labels. **B,** Urine is transferred from the collection cup to a tube. (Courtesy Becton, Dickinson and Company, Franklin Lakes, N.J.)

Collecting a Midstream Specimen

QUALITY OF LIFE

- Knock before entering the person's room.
- Address the person by name.
- Introduce yourself by name and title.

- Explain the procedure before starting and during the procedure.
- Protect the person's rights during the procedure.
- Handle the person gently during the procedure.

PRE-PROCEDURE

1 Follow *Delegation Guidelines: Urine Specimens,* p. 580. See *Promoting Safety and Comfort:*
   a *Collecting and Testing Specimens,* p. 580
   b *Urine Specimens,* p. 580
   c *The Midstream Specimen*
2 Practice hand hygiene.
3 Collect the following before going to the person's room.
   - Laboratory requisition slip
   - Midstream specimen kit—specimen container, label, towelettes, sterile gloves
   - Plastic bag
   - Sterile gloves (if not part of the specimen kit and required by agency policy)
   - Disposable gloves
   - *BIOHAZARD* label (if needed)

4 Arrange your work area.
5 Practice hand hygiene.
6 Identify the person. Check the ID bracelet against the requisition slip. Compare all information. Also call the person by name. Ask the person to state his or her first and last name and birthdate.
7 Put on gloves.
8 Collect the following.
   - Voiding device—bedpan and cover (optional), urinal, commode, or specimen pan if needed
   - Supplies for perineal care (Chapter 24)
   - Graduate to measure output
   - Paper towels
9 Provide for privacy.

PROCEDURE

10 Provide perineal care (Chapter 24). (Wear gloves for this step. Practice hand hygiene after removing and discarding them.)
11 Open the specimen kit.
12 Put on the gloves. Apply sterile gloves if required by agency policy.
13 Open the packet of towelettes.
14 Open the specimen container. Do not touch the inside of the container or lid. The inside is sterile. Set the lid down with the inside up.
15 *For a female*—clean the perineal area with towelettes.
    a Spread the labia with your thumb and index finger. Use your non-dominant hand. (This hand is now contaminated. It must not touch anything sterile.)
    b Clean down the urethral area from front to back (top to bottom). Use a clean towelette for each stroke.
    c Keep the labia separated to collect the specimen (steps 17 through 20).
16 *For a male*—clean the penis with towelettes.
    a Hold the penis with your non-dominant hand. (This hand is now contaminated. It must not touch anything sterile.)
    b Clean the penis starting at the meatus. (Retract the foreskin if the male is uncircumcised.) Clean in a circular motion. Start at the center and work outward.
    c Hold the penis (and keep the foreskin retracted in the uncircumcised male) until the specimen is collected (steps 17 through 20).

17 Have the person void into a device.
18 Pass the specimen container into the urine stream. Keep the labia separated (see Fig. 38-2).
19 Collect about 30 to 60 mL (1 to 2 oz) of urine.
20 Remove the specimen container before the person stops voiding. Release the foreskin of the uncircumcised male.
21 Release the labia or penis. Let the person finish voiding into the device.
22 Put the lid on the specimen container. Touch only the outside of the container and lid. Wipe the outside of the container. Set the container on a paper towel.
23 Provide toilet paper when the person is done voiding.
24 Take the voiding device to the bathroom.
25 Measure urine if I&O are ordered. Include the specimen amount.
26 Empty, rinse, clean, disinfect, and dry equipment. Use clean, dry paper towels for drying. Return equipment to its proper place.
27 Remove and discard the gloves. Practice hand hygiene. Put on clean gloves.
28 Label the specimen container in the person's presence. Place the container in the plastic bag. The container must not touch the outside of the bag. Apply a *BIOHAZARD* label.
29 Assist with hand hygiene.
30 Remove and discard the gloves. Practice hand hygiene.

POST-PROCEDURE

31 Provide for comfort. (See the inside of the back cover.)
32 Place the call light and other needed items within reach.
33 Raise or lower the bed rails. Follow the care plan.
34 Unscreen the person.
35 Complete a safety check of the room. (See the inside of the back cover.)

36 Practice hand hygiene.
37 Take the specimen and requisition slip to the laboratory or storage area. Wear gloves if that is agency policy.
38 Remove and discard the gloves. Practice hand hygiene.
39 Report and record your observations.

The 24-Hour Urine Specimen

All urine voided during 24 hours is collected for a 24-hour urine specimen. To prevent microbe growth, the urine is chilled on ice or refrigerated. A preservative may be added to the collection container.

The person voids to start the test with an empty bladder. Discard this voiding. Save *all voidings* for the next 24 hours. The person and staff must clearly understand the procedure and the test period. This test is re-started if:

- A voiding was not saved.
- Toilet paper was discarded into the specimen.
- The specimen contains stools.

See *Promoting Safety and Comfort: The 24-Hour Urine Specimen*.

See procedure: *Collecting a 24-Hour Urine Specimen*.

PROMOTING SAFETY AND COMFORT

The 24-Hour Urine Specimen

Safety

The urine container or preservative may contain an acid. Pour urine into the container carefully and avoid splashes and splatters. Do not get the preservative or urine on your skin or in your eyes. If you do, flush your skin or eyes with a large amount of water. Tell the nurse what happened and check the safety data sheet (SDS) (Chapter 13). Also complete an incident report.

Keep the specimen chilled to prevent the growth of microbes. If not refrigerated, place the urine container in a bucket with ice. Add ice to the bucket as needed.

Assist the person with hand hygiene after every voiding. This prevents the spread of microbes that may be in the urine.

Collecting a 24-Hour Urine Specimen

QUALITY OF LIFE

- Knock before entering the person's room.
- Address the person by name.
- Introduce yourself by name and title.

- Explain the procedure before starting and during the procedure.
- Protect the person's rights during the procedure.
- Handle the person gently during the procedure.

PRE-PROCEDURE

1 Follow *Delegation Guidelines: Urine Specimens*, p. 580. See *Promoting Safety and Comfort*:
  a *Collecting and Testing Specimens*, p. 580
  b *Urine Specimens*, p. 580
  c *The 24-Hour Urine Specimen*
2 Practice hand hygiene.
3 Collect the following before going to the person's room.
  - Laboratory requisition slip
  - Urine container for a 24-hour collection
  - Voiding device (clean, un-used)—bedpan and cover (optional), urinal, or specimen pan
  - Specimen label
  - Preservative if needed
  - Bucket with ice if needed
  - Two 24-HOUR URINE labels
  - Funnel
  - Disposable bag
  - *BIOHAZARD* label
  - Gloves

4 Arrange your work area.
5 Place one 24-HOUR URINE label in the bathroom. Place the other near the bed.
6 Practice hand hygiene.
7 Identify the person. Check the ID bracelet against the requisition slip. Compare all information. Also call the person by name. Ask the person to state his or her first and last name and birthdate.
8 Label the urine container in the person's presence. Apply the *BIOHAZARD* label. Place the labeled container in the bathroom.
9 Put on gloves.
10 Collect a commode (if needed) and a graduate to measure output.
11 Provide for privacy.

Collecting a 24-Hour Urine Specimen—cont'd

PROCEDURE

12 Ask the person to void. Provide a voiding device. The specimen pan is on the front of the toilet or commode container (if used).

13 Measure and discard the urine. Note the time. This starts the 24-hour period.

14 Mark the time on the urine container.

15 Empty, rinse, clean, disinfect, and dry equipment. Use clean, dry paper towels for drying. Return equipment to its proper place.

16 Remove and discard the gloves. Practice hand hygiene. Put on clean gloves.

17 Assist with hand hygiene.

18 Remove and discard the gloves. Practice hand hygiene.

19 Mark the time the test began and the time it ends on the room and bathroom labels.

20 Remind the person to:
- Use the voiding device during the next 24 hours.
- Not have a BM when voiding.
- Put toilet paper in the toilet. Or provide a disposable bag. Follow agency policy for disposal.
- Put on the call light after voiding.

21 Return to the room when the person signals for you. Knock before entering the room.

22 Do the following after every voiding.
a Practice hand hygiene. Put on clean gloves.
b Measure urine if I&O are ordered.
c Use the funnel to pour urine into the urine container. Do not spill any urine. Tell the nurse if you spill or discard the urine. The test has to be re-started.
d Empty, rinse, clean, disinfect, and dry equipment. Use clean, dry paper towels for drying. Return equipment to its proper place.
e Remove and discard the gloves. Practice hand hygiene. Put on clean gloves.
f Assist with hand hygiene.
g Remove and discard the gloves. Practice hand hygiene.
h Follow "Post-Procedure" steps except for steps 28 and 33.

23 Ask the person to void at the end of the 24-hour period. Follow steps 22, a–g.

POST-PROCEDURE

24 Provide for comfort. (See the inside of the back cover.)

25 Place the call light and other needed items within reach.

26 Raise or lower bed rails. Follow the care plan.

27 Put on gloves.

28 Remove the labels from the room and bathroom.

29 Clean, rinse, dry, and return equipment to its proper place. Use clean, dry paper towels for drying. Discard disposable items.

30 Remove and discard the gloves. Practice hand hygiene.

31 Unscreen the person.

32 Complete a safety check of the room. (See the inside of the back cover.)

33 Take the specimen (labeled urine container) and requisition slip to the laboratory or storage area. Wear gloves if that is agency policy.

34 Remove and discard the gloves. Practice hand hygiene.

35 Report and record your observations.

Collecting a Urine Specimen From an Infant or Child

Sometimes urine specimens are needed from infants and children who are not toilet-trained. A collection bag ("wee bag") is applied over the urethra (Fig. 38-4). A parent or another staff member assists if the child is upset.

Voiding on request is hard for toilet-trained toddlers and young children. Potty chairs and specimen pans are useful. Remember to use terms the child understands. "Pee pee," "wee wee," "potty," and "tinkle" are examples. Or ask the parent what term the child uses and understands.

The nurse may have you give the child water or other fluids when a urine specimen is needed. Usually the child can void about 30 minutes after drinking fluids.

See procedure: *Collecting a Urine Specimen From an Infant or Child,* p. 586.

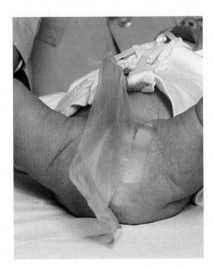

FIGURE 38-4 A urine collection bag applied to a baby girl's perineum.

Collecting a Urine Specimen From an Infant or Child

QUALITY OF LIFE

- Knock before entering the child's room.
- Address the child by name.
- Introduce yourself by name and title.

- Explain the procedure to the child and parents before starting and during the procedure.
- Protect the child's rights during the procedure.
- Handle the child gently during the procedure.

PRE-PROCEDURE

1. Follow *Delegation Guidelines: Urine Specimens*, p. 580. See *Promoting Safety and Comfort:*
   a *Collecting and Testing Specimens*, p. 580
   b *Urine Specimens*, p. 580
2. Practice hand hygiene.
3. Collect the following before going to the child's room.
   - Laboratory requisition slip
   - Collection bag ("wee bag")
   - *BIOHAZARD* label (if needed)
   - Specimen container
   - Plastic bag
   - Scissors

- Wash basin
- Bath towel
- 2 diapers
- Gloves

4. Arrange your work area.
5. Practice hand hygiene.
6. Identify the child. Check the ID bracelet against the requisition slip. Compare all information. Also call the child by name. Ask the parent to state the child's first and last name and the child's birthdate.
7. Provide for privacy.

PROCEDURE

8. Practice hand hygiene. Put on gloves.
9. Position the child on his or her back.
10. Remove and set aside the diaper.
11. Clean the perineal area with cotton balls. Use a new cotton ball for each stroke. Rinse and dry the area.
12. Remove and discard the gloves. Practice hand hygiene.
13. Put on clean gloves.
14. Flex the child's knees. Spread the legs.
15. Remove the adhesive backing from the collection bag.
16. Apply the bag to the perineum (see Fig. 38-4).
17. Cut a slit in the bottom of a new diaper.
18. Diaper the child.
19. Pull the collection bag through the slit in the diaper.
20. Remove and discard the gloves. Practice hand hygiene.
21. Raise the head of the crib if allowed. This helps urine collect in the bottom of the bag.
22. Check for crib safety. Medical crib rails are raised and locked before leaving the bedside.
23. Unscreen the child.
24. Dispose of the removed diaper. Follow agency policy. (Wear gloves for this step.)

25. Practice hand hygiene.
26. Check the child often. Check the bag for urine. (Provide for privacy and wear gloves for this step.)
27. Do the following if the child has voided.
    a Provide for privacy.
    b Practice hand hygiene. Put on clean gloves.
    c Remove the diaper.
    d Remove the collection bag gently.
    e Press the adhesive surfaces of the bag together. Make sure the seal is tight and there are no leaks. Or transfer the urine to the specimen container using the drainage tab.
    f Clean the perineal area. Rinse and dry well.
    g Diaper the child.
    h Remove and discard the gloves. Practice hand hygiene.
28. Put on clean gloves.
29. Label the collection bag or specimen container in the child's presence. Then place it in the plastic bag. Apply the *BIOHAZARD* label (if needed).

POST-PROCEDURE

30. Provide for comfort. (See the inside of the back cover.)
31. Check for crib safety. Medical crib rails are raised and locked before leaving the bedside.
32. Make sure the call light and other needed items are within reach for the child or parent.
33. Unscreen the child.
34. Clean, rinse, dry, and return equipment to its proper place. Use clean, dry paper towels for drying. Discard disposable items. (Wear gloves for this step.)

35. Complete a safety check of the room. (See the inside of the back cover.)
36. Remove and discard the gloves. Practice hand hygiene.
37. Take the specimen and requisition slip to the laboratory or storage area. Wear gloves if that is agency policy.
38. Remove and discard the gloves. Practice hand hygiene.
39. Report and record your observations.

Urinary Catheter Specimens

A straight catheter (Chapter 28) may be needed to collect a specimen. A nurse inserts the catheter into the bladder and removes it after collecting the specimen. You may need to collect supplies or help position the person. Assist as the nurse directs.

A urine specimen can be collected from an indwelling catheter (Chapter 28). Urine in the drainage bag is not used. The port on the drainage tubing is used to collect the specimen. The nurse:

1 Clamps the drainage tubing so fresh urine can collect in the catheter.
2 Cleans the port.
3 Connects a syringe to the port (Fig. 38-5).
4 Aspirates (draws up) urine into the syringe.
5 Unclamps the drainage tubing.
   See *Delegation Guidelines: Urinary Catheter Specimens.*

DELEGATION GUIDELINES
Urinary Catheter Specimens

Inserting a catheter is a nursing responsibility. With proper training and supervision, some states and agencies let nursing assistants perform this sterile procedure. See Chapter 28.

In some agencies, collecting a specimen from an indwelling catheter is a nursing responsibility that may be delegated to you. Before collecting a urinary catheter specimen, make sure that:

* Your state and agency allow you to perform the procedure.
* The procedure is in your job description.
* You have the necessary training.
* You know how to use the agency's equipment.
* You review the procedure with the nurse.
* The nurse is available to answer questions and to guide and assist you as needed.

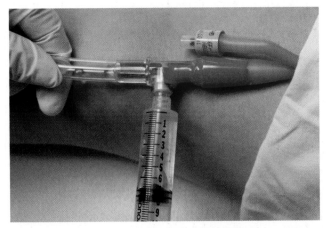

FIGURE 38-5 Collecting a specimen from a urinary catheter. A syringe is connected to the port on the drainage tubing. (From Perry AG, Potter PA, Ostendorf WR: *Nursing interventions & clinical skills,* ed 6, St Louis 2016, Elsevier.)

Testing Urine

The doctor orders the type and frequency of urine tests. Random urine specimens are needed. The nurse may have you do these simple tests.

* *Testing for pH*—Urine pH measures if urine is acidic or alkaline. Changes in normal pH (4.6 to 8.0) occur from illness, food, and drugs.
* *Testing for blood*—Injury and disease can cause hematuria. *Hematuria means blood* (hemat) *in the urine* (uria). Sometimes blood is seen in the urine. At other times it is unseen (*occult*).
* *Testing for glucose and ketones*—In diabetes, the pancreas does not secrete enough insulin (Chapter 50). The body needs insulin to use sugar for energy. If not used, sugar builds up in the blood. Some sugar appears in the urine. *Glucosuria means sugar* (glucose) *in the urine* (uria). Diabetes may cause ketones in the urine. *Ketones (ketone bodies, acetone) are substances appearing in urine from the rapid breakdown of fat for energy.* The body uses fat for energy if it cannot use sugar. Tests for glucose and ketones are usually done 4 times a day—30 minutes before meals and at bedtime. Test results are used for drug and diet decisions.
* *Testing for infection*—The presence of certain white blood cells can signal a urinary tract infection.
* *Testing for protein*—Protein in the urine can signal kidney and other diseases.
   See *Teamwork and Time Management: Testing Urine.*

TEAMWORK AND TIME MANAGEMENT
Testing Urine

Blood glucose testing is common for persons with diabetes (p. 595). Sometimes urine is tested for glucose and ketones. The nurse uses the test results to give the person diabetic drugs. The drugs are given at a certain time. The nurse needs the results before giving the drugs.

Using Reagent Strips. Reagent strips (test strips) have sections that change color when reacting with urine. To use a reagent (test) strip:

* Do not touch the test area on the strip.
* Dip the strip into urine.
* Compare the strip with the color chart on the bottle (Fig. 38-6, p. 588).
   See *Delegation Guidelines: Using Reagent Strips,* p. 588.
   See *Promoting Safety and Comfort: Using Reagent Strips,* p. 588.
   See procedure: *Testing Urine With Reagent Strips,* p. 588.

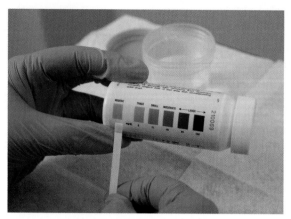

FIGURE 38-6 Reagent (test) strip for sugar and ketones.

PROMOTING SAFETY AND COMFORT

Using Reagent Strips

Safety

Accuracy is important. Promptly report results. Ordered drugs may depend on the results.

When using reagent (test) strips:
- Check the color of the strips. Do not use discolored strips.
- Check the expiration date on the bottle. Do not use the strips if the date has passed.
- Follow the manufacturer's instructions for an accurate result. Test results are used for diagnosis and treatment. A wrong result can cause serious harm.

DELEGATION GUIDELINES

Using Reagent Strips

Testing urine is a nursing responsibility that may be safely delegated to you. In some states and agencies testing urine with reagent strips is a routine nursing task. You need this information from the nurse and the care plan.
- What test is needed
- What equipment and reagent strips to use
- When to test urine
- Instructions for the test ordered
- If the nurse will observe test results
- What observations to report and record:
  - The time you collected and tested the specimen
  - Test results
  - Problems obtaining the specimen
  - Color, clarity, and odor of urine
  - Blood or particles in the urine
  - Complaints of pain, burning, urgency, difficulty voiding, or other problems
- When to report test results and observations
- What patient or resident concerns to report at once

Testing Urine With Reagent Strips

QUALITY OF LIFE

- Knock before entering the person's room.
- Address the person by name.
- Introduce yourself by name and title.

- Explain the procedure before starting and during the procedure.
- Protect the person's rights during the procedure.
- Handle the person gently during the procedure.

PRE-PROCEDURE

1 Follow *Delegation Guidelines: Using Reagent Strips*. See *Promoting Safety and Comfort*:
   a *Collecting and Testing Specimens*, p. 580
   b *Using Reagent Strips*
2 Practice hand hygiene.
3 Collect gloves and the reagent (test) strips ordered.
4 Practice hand hygiene.

5 Identify the person. Check the ID bracelet against the assignment sheet. Use 2 identifiers (Chapter 13). Also call the person by name. Ask the person to state his or her first and last name and birthdate.
6 Put on gloves.
7 Collect equipment for the urine specimen. (See procedure: *Collecting a Random Urine Specimen*, p. 581.)
8 Provide for privacy.

PROCEDURE

9 Collect the urine specimen. (See procedure: *Collecting a Random Urine Specimen*, p. 581.)
10 Remove a strip from the bottle. Put the cap tightly on the bottle at once.
11 Dip the strip test area into the urine.
12 Remove the strip after the correct amount of time. See the manufacturer's instructions.
13 Tap the strip gently against the urine container. This removes excess urine.

14 Wait the required amount of time. See the manufacturer's instructions.
15 Compare the strip with the color chart on the bottle (see Fig. 38-6). Read the results.
16 Discard disposable items and the specimen.
17 Empty, rinse, clean, disinfect, and dry equipment. Use clean, dry paper towels for drying. Return equipment to its proper place.
18 Remove and discard the gloves. Practice hand hygiene.

POST-PROCEDURE

19 Provide for comfort. (See the inside of the back cover.)
20 Place the call light and other needed items within reach.
21 Raise or lower bed rails. Follow the care plan.
22 Unscreen the person.

23 Complete a safety check of the room. (See the inside of the back cover.)
24 Practice hand hygiene.
25 Report and record the test results and other observations.

Straining Urine

A stone *(calculus)* can develop in a kidney, a ureter, or the bladder. Stones *(calculi)* vary in size (Chapter 51). They can be as small as grains of sand, pearl-sized, or larger. Some stones are removed by medical or surgical procedures. Others pass through urine. When stones are present, all urine is strained. Passed stones are sent to the laboratory.

The person drinks 8 to 12 glasses of water a day to help pass the stone. Expect the person to void in large amounts. See procedure: *Straining Urine*.

Straining Urine

QUALITY OF LIFE

- Knock before entering the person's room.
- Address the person by name.
- Introduce yourself by name and title.
- Explain the procedure before starting and during the procedure.
- Protect the person's rights during the procedure.
- Handle the person gently during the procedure.

PRE-PROCEDURE

1 Follow *Delegation Guidelines: Urine Specimens*, p. 580. See *Promoting Safety and Comfort*:
   a *Collecting and Testing Specimens*, p. 580
   b *Urine Specimens*, p. 580
2 Practice hand hygiene.
3 Collect the following before going to the person's room.
   - Laboratory requisition slip
   - Urine strainer
   - Specimen container
   - Specimen label
   - Voiding device (clean, un-used)—bedpan and cover (optional), urinal, or specimen pan
   - 2 STRAIN ALL URINE labels
   - Plastic bag
   - *BIOHAZARD* label (if needed)
   - Gloves

4 Arrange your work area.
5 Place 1 STRAIN ALL URINE label in the bathroom. Place the other near the bed.
6 Practice hand hygiene.
7 Identify the person. Check the ID bracelet against the requisition slip. Compare all information. Also call the person by name. Ask the person to state his or her first and last name and birthdate.
8 Label the specimen container in the person's presence.
9 Put on gloves.
10 Collect a commode (if needed) and a graduate to measure output.
11 Provide for privacy.

PROCEDURE

12 Have the person use the voiding device for urinating. The specimen pan is on the front of the toilet or commode container (if used). Ask the person to put on the call light after voiding.
13 Remove and discard the gloves. Practice hand hygiene.
14 Return to the room when the person signals for you. Knock before entering the room.
15 Practice hand hygiene. Put on clean gloves.
16 Place the strainer in the graduate.
17 Pour urine into the graduate. Urine passes through the strainer (Fig. 38-7, p. 590).
18 Place the strainer in the specimen container if any crystals, stones, or particles appear. Or transfer them to the specimen container as the nurse directs.

19 Place the specimen container in the plastic bag. Do not let the container touch the outside of the bag. Apply a *BIOHAZARD* label.
20 Measure urine if I&O are ordered.
21 Empty, rinse, clean, disinfect, and dry equipment. Use clean, dry paper towels for drying. Return equipment to its proper place.
22 Remove and discard the gloves. Practice hand hygiene. Put on clean gloves.
23 Assist with hand hygiene.
24 Remove and discard the gloves. Practice hand hygiene.

POST-PROCEDURE

25 Provide for comfort. (See the inside of the back cover.)
26 Place the call light and other needed items within reach.
27 Raise or lower bed rails. Follow the care plan.
28 Unscreen the person.
29 Complete a safety check of the room. (See the inside of the back cover.)

30 Practice hand hygiene.
31 Take the specimen container and requisition slip to the laboratory or storage area. Wear gloves if that is agency policy.
32 Remove and discard the gloves. Practice hand hygiene.
33 Report and record your observations.

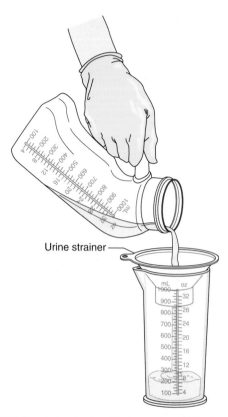

Urine strainer —

FIGURE 38-7 The strainer is placed in the graduate. Urine is poured through the strainer into the graduate.

STOOL SPECIMENS

Stools are studied for fat, microbes, worms, blood, and other abnormal contents. Ulcers, colon cancer, and hemorrhoids are common causes of bleeding. Often blood is seen if bleeding is low in the bowels. Stools are black and tarry from bleeding in the stomach or upper gastrointestinal tract. *Melena is a black, tarry stool.*

Bleeding may be in very small amounts. Then stools are tested for *occult blood. Occult* means *hidden* or *not seen.* The test screens for colon cancer and other digestive disorders. Occult blood test kits vary. Follow the manufacturer's instructions. The procedure that follows is an example of an occult blood test.

Urine must not contaminate the stool specimen. The person uses 1 device for voiding and another for a BM. Some tests require a warm stool. The specimen is taken at once to the laboratory or storage area. Follow the rules in Box 38-1.

See *Focus on Communication: Stool Specimens.*
See *Focus on Children and Older Persons: Stool Specimens.*
See *Delegation Guidelines: Stool Specimens.*
See *Promoting Safety and Comfort: Stool Specimens.*
See procedure: *Collecting and Testing a Stool Specimen.*

FOCUS ON COMMUNICATION
Stool Specimens

Before you begin, explain what the person needs to do and what you will do. Show the equipment and supplies and how to use them. For example:

> *I need to collect a specimen from a bowel movement. I'm going to place the specimen pan (show specimen pan) at the back of the toilet. Urinate into the toilet. Your bowel movement collects in the specimen pan. Please put toilet paper in the toilet, not in the specimen pan. After your bowel movement, put your call light on right away. I'll collect the specimen in this container (show the specimen container).*

Then ask if the person has questions. If you do not know the answer, tell the nurse. Make sure the person understands what to do. You can say: "Please tell me what you will do so I know that you understand."

FOCUS ON CHILDREN AND OLDER PERSONS
Stool Specimens

Children
If the child wears a diaper, you can obtain stool from the diaper. You may need to scrape the diaper.

DELEGATION GUIDELINES
Stool Specimens

Collecting a stool specimen is a routine nursing task. Testing a stool specimen is a nursing responsibility that may be safely delegated to you. Before collecting and testing a stool specimen, you need this information from the nurse.
- What time to collect and test the specimen
- What test is needed (if any)
- What equipment and special measures are needed
- Instructions for the test ordered
- If the nurse wants to observe the stool or test results
- What observations to report and record:
  - The time you collected and tested the specimen
  - Test results
  - Problems obtaining the specimen
  - Color, amount, consistency, and odor of stools
  - Complaints of pain or discomfort
- When to report observations
- What patient or resident concerns to report at once

PROMOTING SAFETY AND COMFORT
Stool Specimens

Safety
You must be accurate when testing stools. Follow the manufacturer's instructions for the test used. Promptly report the results to the nurse.

Comfort
Stools normally have an odor. A person may be embarrassed that you need a specimen. Complete the task quickly and carefully. Act in a professional manner.

Collecting and Testing a Stool Specimen

QUALITY OF LIFE

- Knock before entering the person's room.
- Address the person by name.
- Introduce yourself by name and title.

- Explain the procedure before starting and during the procedure.
- Protect the person's rights during the procedure.
- Handle the person gently during the procedure.

PRE-PROCEDURE

1 Follow *Delegation Guidelines: Stool Specimens.* See *Promoting Safety and Comfort:*
   a *Collecting and Testing Specimens,* p. 580
   b *Stool Specimens*
2 Practice hand hygiene.
3 Collect the following before going to the person's room.
   - Laboratory requisition slip
   - Occult blood test kit (if needed)
   - Device to collect the BM (clean, un-used)—bedpan and cover (optional) or specimen pan
   - Stool specimen container and lid (Fig. 38-8)
   - Specimen label
   - Tongue blades (if needed)
   - Disposable bag
   - Plastic bag
   - *BIOHAZARD* label (if needed)
   - Gloves

4 Arrange your work area.
5 Practice hand hygiene.
6 Identify the person. Check the ID bracelet against the requisition slip. Compare all information. Also call the person by name. Ask the person to state his or her first and last name and birthdate.
7 Label the specimen container in the person's presence.
8 Put on gloves.
9 Collect the following.
   - Device for voiding—bedpan and cover (optional), urinal, commode, or specimen pan
   - Toilet paper
10 Provide for privacy.

PROCEDURE

11 Have the person void. Provide the voiding device if not using the bathroom. Empty, rinse, clean, disinfect, and dry the device. Use clean, dry paper towels for drying. Return it to its proper place.
12 Put the specimen pan on the back of the toilet or commode (Fig. 38-9). Or provide the bedpan.
13 Ask the person not to put toilet paper into the bedpan, commode, or specimen pan. Have the person put toilet paper in the toilet. Or provide a disposable bag and follow agency policy for disposal.
14 Place the call light and toilet paper within reach. Raise or lower bed rails. Follow the care plan.
15 Remove and discard the gloves. Practice hand hygiene. Leave the room if the person can be left alone.
16 Return when the person signals. Or check on the person every 5 minutes. Knock before entering.
17 Practice hand hygiene. Put on clean gloves.
18 Lower the bed rail near you if up. Remove the bedpan (if used). Or assist the person off the toilet or commode (if used). Provide perineal care if needed.

19 Note the color, amount, consistency, and odor of stools.
20 Collect the specimen.
   a Use the spoon attached to the lid to pick up several spoonfuls of stool. Or use a tongue blade to take about 2 tablespoons of stool to the specimen container (Fig. 38-10, p. 592). Take the sample from:
      1) The middle of a formed stool
      2) Areas of pus, mucus, or blood and watery areas
      3) The middle and both ends of a hard stool
   b Put the lid on the specimen container tightly.
   c Place the container in the plastic bag. Do not let the container touch the outside of the bag. Apply a *BIOHAZARD* label according to agency policy.
   d Wrap the tongue blade in toilet paper. Discard it in the disposable bag.
21 Remove and discard the gloves. Practice hand hygiene. Put on clean gloves.

Continued

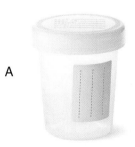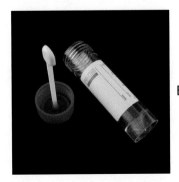

FIGURE 38-8 **A,** Stool specimen container. **B,** Stool specimen container with attached spoon. (**A,** © Fotofermer/Getty Images. **B,** From Healthlaw Medical Limited, Henso [Hangzhou] Co., Ltd. Hangzhou, China.)

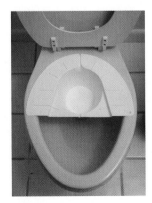

FIGURE 38-9 The specimen pan is placed at the back of the toilet for a stool specimen. (NOTE: The toilet seat is lowered over the specimen pan for the BM.)

Collecting and Testing a Stool Specimen—cont'd

PROCEDURE—cont'd

22 Test the specimen (if needed).
  a Open the test kit.
  b Use a tongue blade to obtain a small amount of stool.
  c Apply a thin smear of stool on *box A* on the test paper (Fig. 38-11, *A*).
  d Use another tongue blade to obtain stool from another part of the specimen.
  e Apply a thin smear of stool on *box B* on the test paper (Fig. 38-11, *B*).
  f Close the packet.
  g Turn the test packet to the other side. Open the flap. Apply developer (from the kit) to *boxes A* and *B*. Follow the manufacturer's instructions (Fig. 38-11, *C*).
  h Wait 10 to 60 seconds as required by the manufacturer.
  i Note the color changes on your assignment sheet (Fig. 38-11, *D*).
  j Dispose of the test packet.
  k Wrap the tongue blades with toilet paper. Discard them in the disposable bag.
23 Empty, rinse, clean, disinfect, and dry equipment. Use clean, dry paper towels for drying. Return equipment to its proper place.
24 Remove and discard the gloves. Practice hand hygiene. Put on clean gloves.
25 Assist with hand hygiene.
26 Remove and discard the gloves. Practice hand hygiene.

POST-PROCEDURE

27 Provide for comfort. (See the inside of the back cover.)
28 Place the call light and other needed items within reach.
29 Raise or lower bed rails. Follow the care plan.
30 Unscreen the person.
31 Complete a safety check of the room. (See the inside of the back cover.)
32 Deliver the specimen and requisition slip to the laboratory or storage area. Follow agency policy. Wear gloves if that is agency policy.
33 Remove and discard the gloves. Practice hand hygiene.
34 Report and record your observations and the test results.

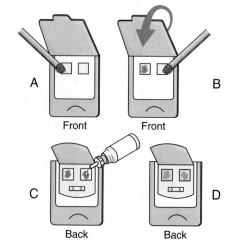

FIGURE 38-10 A tongue blade is used to transfer a small amount of stool from the bedpan to the specimen container.

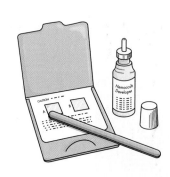

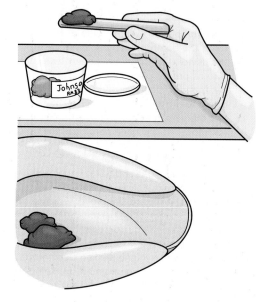

FIGURE 38-11 Testing for occult blood. **A,** Stool is smeared on *box A*. **B,** Stool is smeared on *box B* and then the flap is closed. **C,** Developer is applied to *boxes A* and *B* on the back side of the test packet. **D,** Color changes are noted.

SPUTUM SPECIMENS

Respiratory disorders cause the lungs, bronchi, and trachea to secrete mucus. *Mucus from the respiratory system is called* ***sputum*** *when expectorated (expelled) through the mouth.* Sputum is not saliva. Saliva ("spit") is a thin, clear liquid produced by the salivary glands in the mouth.

Sputum specimens are studied for blood, microbes, and abnormal cells. Sputum is coughed up from the bronchi and trachea. This is often painful and hard to do. Collecting a specimen is easier in the morning. Secretions collect in the trachea and bronchi during sleep. They are coughed up on awakening.

Follow the rules in Box 38-1. Also have the person rinse the mouth with water. Rinsing decreases saliva and removes food particles. Mouthwash is not used. It destroys some of the microbes in the mouth.

See *Focus on Children and Older Persons: Sputum Specimens.*

See *Delegation Guidelines: Sputum Specimens.*
See *Promoting Safety and Comfort: Sputum Specimens.*
See procedure: *Collecting a Sputum Specimen*, p. 594.

DELEGATION GUIDELINES
Sputum Specimens

Collecting a sputum specimen is a routine nursing task. You need this information from the nurse.

- When to collect the specimen
- The amount needed—usually 1 to 2 teaspoons
- If the person uses the bathroom
- If the person can hold the sputum container
- What observations to report and record:
  - The time the specimen was collected
  - The amount collected
  - How easily the person raised the sputum
  - Sputum color—clear, white, yellow, green, brown, or red
  - Sputum odor—none or foul odor
  - Sputum consistency—thick, watery, or frothy (with bubbles or foam)
  - *Hemoptysis*—*bloody* (hemo) *sputum* (ptysis *means* to spit)
  - If the person could not produce sputum
  - Any other observations
- When to report observations
- What patient or resident concerns to report at once

FOCUS ON **CHILDREN AND OLDER PERSONS**
Sputum Specimens

Children
Breathing treatments and suctioning (Chapter 44) are often needed to obtain sputum specimens in infants and small children. The RN (registered nurse) or respiratory therapist gives the breathing treatment. The nurse suctions the trachea for the specimen. The infant or child is likely to be upset during suctioning. You may need to hold the child still.

Older Persons
Older persons may lack the strength to cough up sputum. Coughing is easier after *postural drainage*. It drains secretions by gravity. Gravity causes fluids to flow down. The person is positioned so a lung part is higher than the airway (Fig. 38-12). The nurse or respiratory therapist does postural drainage. Assist as directed.

PROMOTING SAFETY AND COMFORT
Sputum Specimens

Safety
Transmission-Based Precautions are used if the person has or may have tuberculosis (TB) (Chapters 17 and 49). Wear a respirator to protect yourself (Chapter 17).

Comfort
The procedure can embarrass the person. Coughing and expectorating sounds can disturb others. Also, sputum is not pleasant to look at. Privacy is important. Cover the specimen container and place it in a bag. Some sputum specimen containers are cloudy to hide the contents.

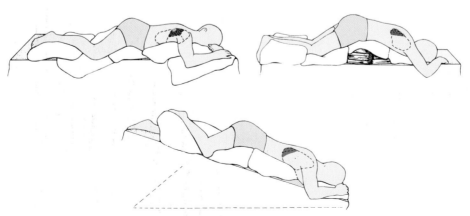

FIGURE 38-12 Some positions for postural drainage. (From Potter PA, Perry AG, Stockert PA, Hall AM: *Fundamentals of nursing*, ed 9, St Louis, 2017, Elsevier.)

Collecting a Sputum Specimen

QUALITY OF LIFE

- Knock before entering the person's room.
- Address the person by name.
- Introduce yourself by name and title.

- Explain the procedure before starting and during the procedure.
- Protect the person's rights during the procedure.
- Handle the person gently during the procedure.

PRE-PROCEDURE

1 Follow *Delegation Guidelines: Sputum Specimens*, p. 593.
   See *Promoting Safety and Comfort*:
   a *Collecting and Testing Specimens*, p. 580
   b *Sputum Specimens*, p. 593
2 Practice hand hygiene.
3 Collect the following before going to the person's room.
   - Laboratory requisition slip
   - Sputum specimen container and lid
   - Specimen label
   - Plastic bag
   - *BIOHAZARD* label (if needed)

4 Arrange your work area.
5 Practice hand hygiene.
6 Identify the person. Check the ID bracelet against the requisition slip. Compare all information. Also call the person by name. Ask the person to state his or her first and last name and birthdate.
7 Label the specimen container in the person's presence.
8 Collect gloves and tissues.
9 Provide for privacy. If able, the person uses the bathroom for the procedure.

PROCEDURE

10 Put on gloves.
11 Have the person rinse the mouth with clear water.
12 Have the person hold the container. Only the outside is touched.
13 Have the person cover the mouth and nose with tissues when coughing. Follow agency policy for used tissues.
14 Have the person take 2 or 3 breaths and cough up the sputum.
15 Have the person expectorate (spit) directly into the container (Fig. 38-13). Sputum must not touch the outside of the container.

16 Collect 1 to 2 teaspoons of sputum unless told to collect more.
17 Put the lid on the container.
18 Place the container in the plastic bag. Do not let the container touch the outside of the bag. Apply a *BIOHAZARD* label according to agency policy.
19 Remove and discard the gloves. Practice hand hygiene. Put on clean gloves.
20 Assist with hand hygiene.
21 Remove and discard the gloves. Practice hand hygiene.

POST-PROCEDURE

22 Provide for comfort. (See the inside of the back cover.)
23 Place the call light and other needed items within reach.
24 Raise or lower bed rails. Follow the care plan.
25 Unscreen the person.
26 Complete a safety check of the room. (See the inside of the back cover.)

27 Practice hand hygiene.
28 Deliver the specimen and the requisition slip to the laboratory or storage area. Follow agency policy. Wear gloves if that is agency policy.
29 Remove and discard the gloves. Practice hand hygiene.
30 Report and record your observations.

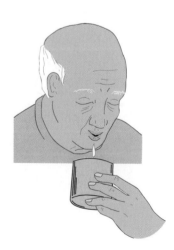

FIGURE 38-13 The person expectorates into the center of the specimen container.

⬛ BLOOD GLUCOSE TESTING

Blood glucose testing is used for persons with diabetes. The doctor uses the results to regulate drugs and diet.

A drop of capillary blood is collected through a skin puncture. A fingertip is the most common site for skin punctures.

Inspect the puncture site for trauma and skin breaks. Do not use swollen, bruised, cyanotic (bluish color), scarred, or calloused sites. Such areas have poor blood flow. A *callus* is a thick, hardened area on the skin. Calluses often form over frequently used areas, such as the tips of the thumbs and index fingers. Therefore thumbs and index fingers are not good skin puncture sites.

Use the side toward the tip of the middle or ring finger (Fig. 38-14). Do not use the center, fleshy part of the fingertip. The site has many nerve endings making punctures painful.

You use a sterile, disposable lancet to puncture the skin (Fig. 38-15). The person feels a brief, sharp pinch. A *lancet* is a short, pointed blade that punctures but does not cut the skin. The lancet is inside a protective cover. Do not touch the blade. Discard the blade into the sharps container after use.

A *glucometer (glucose meter) is a device for measuring* (meter) *blood glucose* (gluco). Reagent strips (test strips) are used. You apply a drop of blood to the reagent strip. The blood glucose level appears on the screen. How fast results are displayed depends on the type of glucometer. Some take 5 seconds.

You will learn to use your agency's device. Always follow the manufacturer's instructions. The procedure that follows is an example of how to measure blood glucose.

See *Teamwork and Time Management: Blood Glucose Testing.*

See *Delegation Guidelines: Blood Glucose Testing.*

See *Promoting Safety and Comfort: Blood Glucose Testing,* p. 596.

See procedure: *Measuring Blood Glucose,* p. 597.

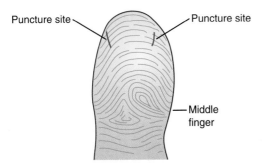

Puncture site — Puncture site

— Middle finger

FIGURE 38-14 Site for skin punctures.

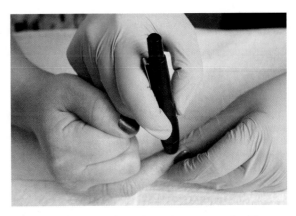

FIGURE 38-15 A lancet is used to puncture the skin.

TEAMWORK AND TIME MANAGEMENT
Blood Glucose Testing

Perform blood glucose testing at times directed by the nurse and the care plan. Drugs are given at a certain time. The nurse needs the blood glucose results before giving the drugs.

Glucometers are shared with other staff. Tell your co-workers when you have one. Work quickly but carefully. Return the device to the storage area in a timely manner.

DELEGATION GUIDELINES
Blood Glucose Testing

In some agencies, blood glucose testing is a nursing responsibility that may be delegated to you. If so, make sure that:
- Your state and agency allow you to perform the procedure.
- The procedure is in your job description.
- You have the necessary training.
- You know how to use the agency's equipment.
- You review the procedure with a nurse.
- The nurse is available to answer questions and to guide and assist you as needed.

If the above conditions are met, you need this information from the nurse and the care plan.
- What sites to avoid for a skin puncture
- When to collect and test the specimen—usually before meals and at bedtime
- If the person receives drugs that affect blood clotting (NOTE: If yes, it may take longer to stop bleeding. Apply pressure until bleeding stops.)
- What to report and record:
  - The time the specimen was collected
  - The blood glucose test result
  - The site used for the skin puncture
  - The amount of bleeding at the puncture site
  - Any signs of a *hematoma—a swelling* (oma) *that contains blood* (hemat)
  - How the person tolerated the procedure
  - Complaints of pain at the puncture site
  - Other observations or patient or resident complaints
- When to report observations and the test result
- What patient or resident concerns to report at once

PROMOTING SAFETY AND COMFORT
Blood Glucose Testing

Safety
Accurate results are important. Inaccurate results can harm the person. Follow the rules in Box 38-2.

You must know how to use the equipment. Use only the reagent strip specified by the manufacturer. Otherwise you will get inaccurate results.

Disinfect the glucometer before and after use. Follow the manufacturer's instructions for the disinfectant to use and how to use it.

Comfort
The third finger (ring finger) is used for children. The heel is used for skin punctures in infants who are not walking. See Figure 38-16.

Older persons often have poor circulation in their fingers. To increase blood flow, apply a warm washcloth or wash the hands in warm water.

BOX 38-2	Blood Glucose Testing

- Follow the manufacturer's instructions for the glucometer and disinfectant.
- Know how to use the equipment. Request any necessary training.
- Make sure the glucometer was tested for accuracy. Check the testing log.
- Enter a code or user-ID if required by the glucometer. This is provided by the agency. Do not share your user-ID with others.
- Make sure you have the correct reagent (test) strips for the glucometer you are using.
- Scan the bar code on the bottle of reagent strips if needed. Or compare the code on the bottle of reagent strips to the code on the glucometer (Fig. 38-17).
- Check the color of the reagent strips. Do not use discolored strips.
- Check the expiration date on the reagent strips. Do not use them if the date has passed.
- Report the result to the nurse at once.
- Record the result following agency policy.

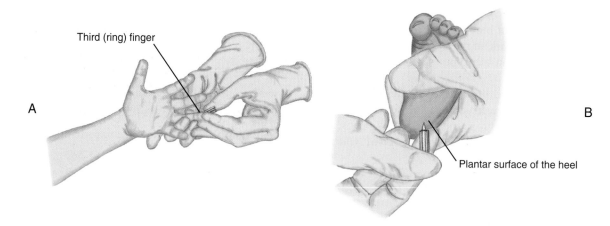

FIGURE 38-16 A, The third finger (ring finger) is used for skin punctures in children. **B,** Heel site is used for skin punctures in infants. (From James SR, Nelson KA, Ashwill JW: *Nursing care of children: principles and practice,* ed 4, Philadelphia, 2013, Saunders.)

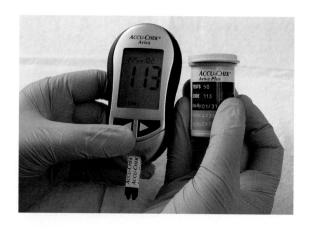

FIGURE 38-17 The code on the bottle of reagent (test) strips is compared to the code on the glucometer.

Measuring Blood Glucose

QUALITY OF LIFE

- Knock before entering the person's room.
- Address the person by name.
- Introduce yourself by name and title.

- Explain the procedure before starting and during the procedure.
- Protect the person's rights during the procedure.
- Handle the person gently during the procedure.

PRE-PROCEDURE

1 Follow *Delegation Guidelines: Blood Glucose Testing,* p. 595. See *Promoting Safety and Comfort:*
  a *Collecting and Testing Specimens,* p. 580
  b *Blood Glucose Testing*
2 Practice hand hygiene.
3 Collect the following.
  - Sterile lancet
  - Lancing device (if used)
  - Antiseptic wipes
  - Gloves
  - 2 × 2 gauze squares
  - Glucometer
  - Reagent (test) strips (Use the correct ones for the glucometer. Check the expiration date.)
  - Disinfectant

  - Paper towels
  - Warm washcloth
4 Read the manufacturer's instructions for the lancet and glucometer.
5 Disinfect the glucometer. Follow the manufacturer's instructions for the disinfectant.
6 Arrange your work area.
7 Identify the person. Check the ID bracelet against the assignment sheet. Use 2 identifiers (Chapter 13). Also call the person by name. Ask the person to state his or her first and last name and birthdate.
8 Provide for privacy.
9 Raise the bed for body mechanics. The far bed rail is up if used.

PROCEDURE

10 Help the person to a comfortable position.
11 Put on the gloves.
12 Prepare the supplies.
  a Open the antiseptic wipes.
  b Prepare the lancet. If using a lancing device, follow the manufacturer's instructions.
  c Turn on the glucometer.
  d Follow the prompts. You may need to enter a user-ID and the person's ID number. Scan the bar code on the bottle of test strips if needed. Or compare the code on the bottle of test strips to the code on the glucometer (see Fig. 38-17).
  e Remove a test strip from the bottle. Close the cap tightly.
  f Insert a test strip into the glucometer (Fig. 38-18, p. 598).
13 Perform a skin puncture to obtain a drop of blood.
  a Inspect the person's fingers. Select a puncture site.
  b Do the following to increase blood flow to the puncture site.
    1) Warm the finger. Rub it gently or apply a warm washcloth.
    2) Massage the hand and finger toward the puncture site.
    3) Lower the finger below the person's waist.
  c Hold the finger with your thumb and index finger. Use your non-dominant hand. Hold the finger until step 14, b.

  d Clean the site with an antiseptic wipe. *Do not touch the site after cleaning.*
  e Let the site dry.
  f Place the lancet or lancing device against the puncture site.
  g Push the button on the device to puncture the skin. (Follow the manufacturer's instructions.)
  h Apply gentle pressure below the puncture site.
  i Let a large drop of blood form.
14 Collect and test the specimen. Follow the manufacturer's instructions and agency procedures for the glucometer used.
  a Touch the test strip to the drop of blood (Fig. 38-19, p. 598). The glucometer will test the sample when enough blood is applied.
  b Apply pressure to the puncture site until bleeding stops. Use a gauze square. If able, let the person apply pressure to the site.
  c Read the result on the display (Fig. 38-20, p. 598). Note the result on your note pad or assignment sheet. Tell the person the result.
  d Turn off the glucometer.
15 Discard the lancet in the sharps container.
16 Discard the gauze square and test strip. Follow agency policy.
17 Remove and discard the gloves. Practice hand hygiene.

POST-PROCEDURE

18 Provide for comfort. (See the inside of the back cover.)
19 Place the call light and other needed items within reach.
20 Lower the bed to a safe and comfortable level. Follow the care plan.
21 Raise or lower bed rails. Follow the care plan.
22 Unscreen the person.
23 Discard used supplies.

24 Complete a safety check of the room. (See the inside of the back cover.)
25 Follow agency policy for used linens.
26 Disinfect the glucometer. Follow the manufacturer's instructions. (Wear gloves. Practice hand hygiene after removing and discarding the gloves.)
27 Return the glucometer to its proper place.
28 Report and record the test result tend your observations (Fig. 38-21, p. 598).

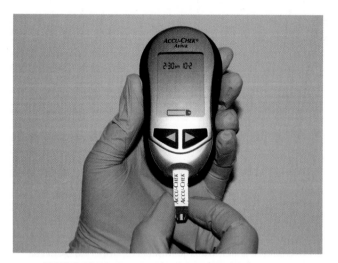

FIGURE 38-18 A reagent (test) strip is in the glucometer.

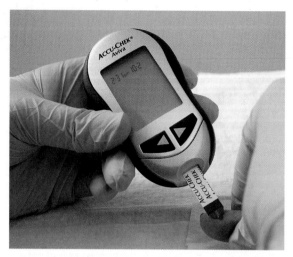

FIGURE 38-19 A drop of blood is applied to the reagent (test) strip.

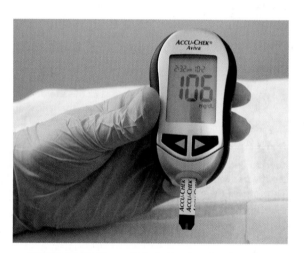

FIGURE 38-20 The result is displayed on the glucometer.

BLOOD GLUCOSE TESTING	
Puncture Site	**Observations**
Click to mark puncture site.	☒ Skin intact ☐ Bruising
	☐ Pain ☐ Cyanosis
	☐ Swelling ☐ Hematoma
	Bleeding amount
	☒ Small (stopped with brief pressure)
	☐ Moderate to large ☒ Pressure applied to site
Left hand Right hand	**Test Result and Reporting**
	Result: [106] mg/dL
	☒ Nurse notified of result and observations
	Nurse notified: [P. Young, RN]

FIGURE 38-21 Charting sample.

FOCUS ON **PRIDE**

The Person, Family, and Yourself

P ersonal and Professional Responsibility

You must collect specimens on the right person. Otherwise, one or both persons could be harmed. Before collecting a specimen, carefully identify the person.

In some agencies, collection information is written on the specimen container. Collection date and time and the collector's name or initials are examples. Follow agency policy to properly collect and label specimens.

R ights and Respect

Specimen collection can be embarrassing. To respect the right to privacy:

- Politely ask visitors to leave the room.
- Close doors, privacy curtains, and window coverings.
- Leave the room if it is safe to do so. If you cannot leave, tell the person why.

I ndependence and Social Interaction

Some persons can collect their own specimens. Doing so promotes independence and reduces embarrassment.

Explain the procedure and show the person the container. Tell the person where you are placing the container. When ready to collect the specimen, the person knows where to find the container.

D elegation and Teamwork

Before taking a specimen to the laboratory, tell the nurse and your co-workers. Ask if other staff need specimens delivered. Doing so saves staff time. This also prevents having too many staff members off the unit at the same time. Return from the laboratory promptly.

E thics and Laws

If you did not collect a specimen correctly, do not send it to the laboratory. Tell the nurse. Then collect the specimen at the next opportunity. Test results must be accurate for correct diagnosis and treatment. Take pride in honestly reporting mistakes.

FOCUS ON **PRIDE**: *Application*

What mistakes could occur in specimen collection? What can you do to prevent such mistakes? Explain why failing to report a mistake can be harmful.

REVIEW QUESTIONS

Circle the BEST answer.

1 Which specimen was collected *correctly?*
   a A stool specimen that contains urine
   b A urine specimen that contains toilet paper
   c A sputum specimen with a label and requisition slip
   d A urine specimen with a loose lid in a biohazard bag

2 A random urine specimen is collected
   a After sleep
   b Before meals
   c After meals
   d Any time

3 Perineal care is given before collecting a
   a Random specimen
   b Midstream specimen
   c 24-hour specimen
   d Stool specimen

4 A 24-hour urine specimen involves
   a Collecting all urine voided during a 24-hour period
   b Collecting a random specimen every hour for 24 hours
   c Testing urine for ketones every day
   d Measuring output every 24 hours

5 To collect a midstream specimen on a female
   a Spread the labia to expose the urethral area
   b Clean the urethral area from back to front
   c Collect urine at the start of the urine stream
   d Collect about 10 mL of urine

6 Urine is tested for glucose
   a To measure the pH
   b To check for blood
   c To check for sugar
   d To check for ketones

7 You need to strain a person's urine. Straining is done to find
   a Blood
   b Stones
   c Ketones
   d Acetone

8 You note a black, tarry stool. This is called
   a Melena
   b Feces
   c Hemostat
   d Occult blood

9 A warm stool specimen is needed. After collecting the specimen
   a Put it in an oven
   b Put it in a paper bag
   c Cover it with a towel
   d Take it to the laboratory or storage area

10 The best time to collect a sputum specimen is
   a On awakening
   b After meals
   c At bedtime
   d After oral hygiene

Continued

REVIEW QUESTIONS—cont'd

11 A sputum specimen is needed. Have the person
 a Use mouthwash
 b Rinse the mouth with clear water
 c Brush the teeth
 d Remove dentures

12 Which is the *best* site for a skin puncture?
 a The thumb
 b The index finger
 c The ring finger
 d The little finger

13 Which is needed to measure blood glucose?
 a Glucometer
 b Sterile specimen container
 c Color-changing reagent strip
 d Sphygmomanometer

14 Before using reagent strips for blood glucose testing
 a Make sure they are discolored
 b Label each strip with the person's name
 c Check the size of the test area
 d Check the expiration date

15 Which statement about reporting a blood glucose result is *true?*
 a Only report an abnormal result.
 b Report the result to the nurse at once.
 c Report the result after the person's meal.
 d Report the result any time before the person's next meal.

Answers to Chapter 38 questions are on p. 887.

FOCUS ON PRACTICE

Problem Solving

A midstream urine specimen is ordered. You give the patient the specimen cup and pack of towelettes and ask: "Do you know what to do?" The patient says: "Yes, I've done this before." You tell the patient to leave the specimen in the bathroom and signal for you when done.

 You return and notice the towelettes are un-opened. What do you do? Should you send the specimen to the laboratory? How could this have been prevented?

The Person Having Surgery

OBJECTIVES

- Define the key terms and key abbreviations in this chapter.
- Describe the common fears and concerns of surgical patients.
- Describe pre-operative and post-operative care.

- List the signs and symptoms to report after surgery.
- Perform the procedures described in this chapter.
- Explain how to promote PRIDE in the person, the family, and yourself.

KEY TERMS

anesthesia The loss *(an)* of all sensation *(esthesia)*, especially pain, produced by a drug

antiseptic A chemical applied to the skin to prevent the growth and reproduction of microbes

elective surgery Surgery done by choice to improve life or well-being

embolus A blood clot *(thrombus)* that travels through the vascular system until it lodges in a blood vessel

emergency surgery Surgery done at once to save life or function

general anesthesia A treatment with certain drugs that produces a deep sleep and the absence of all sensation, especially pain

local anesthesia The loss of sensation, produced by a drug, in a small area

post-operative After *(post)* surgery; post-op

pre-operative Before *(pre)* surgery; pre-op

regional anesthesia The loss of sensation, produced by a drug, in a large area

sedation A state of quiet, calmness, or sleep produced by a drug

surgical site infection (SSI) An infection that occurs after surgery in the body part where the surgery took place

thrombus A blood clot

urgent surgery Surgery needed for health; it can be delayed for a few days

KEY ABBREVIATIONS

AE	Anti-embolism; anti-embolic		NPO	*Nil per os;* nothing by mouth
ASC	Ambulatory surgery center		OR	Operating room
CBC	Complete blood count		PACU	Post-anesthesia care unit
ECG	Electrocardiogram		post-op	Post-operative
EKG	Electrocardiogram		pre-op	Pre-operative
ID	Identification		SCD	Sequential compression device
IV	Intravenous		SSI	Surgical site infection
NG	Naso-gastric		TED	Thrombo-embolic disease

The many reasons for surgery include to:

- Remove, repair, or replace a diseased or injured body part.
- Remove a tumor.
- Make a diagnosis.
- Relieve symptoms.
- Restore or improve function or appearance.

Surgeries are done in hospitals or ambulatory surgery centers (ASCs). Hospital patients are admitted 1 or 2 days before surgery or on the morning of surgery. Some patients have surgery after receiving emergency room care. Called *in-patients*, surgical patients stay for 1 or more days after surgery. Most hospitals offer ASC services.

ASCs are designed and equipped for certain surgical, diagnostic, or preventive procedures. Eye surgeries, colonoscopies to diagnose colon disorders, and pain management for back disorders are examples. Called *out-patients*, ASC patients go home in less than 23 hours. However, some ASCs offer over-night stays.

Surgeries are described as:
- *Elective surgery—done by choice to improve life or well-being.* It is not life-saving. Joint replacement surgery and cosmetic (plastic) surgery are examples. The surgery is scheduled in advance.
- *Urgent surgery—needed for health. It can be delayed for a few days.* Sometimes cancer surgery and coronary artery bypass surgery are delayed for a few days.
- *Emergency surgery—done at once to save life or function.* The need is sudden and not expected. Vehicle crashes, stabbings, and bullet wounds often require emergency surgery.

The person is prepared for what happens before, during, and after surgery. *Pre-operative (pre-op) refers to before (pre) surgery. Post-operative (post-op) refers to after (post) surgery.* Some people recover in nursing centers or rehabilitation centers. Some need home care.

PSYCHOLOGICAL CARE

Surgery causes many fears and concerns (Box 39-1). Past experiences affect feelings. Some persons have had surgery before. Others have not. Patients are affected when family and friends talk about their own surgeries. Some people do not share fears and concerns. They may cry, be quiet or withdrawn, or talk about other things. Some pace. Others are very cheerful.

Mental preparation is important. Respect the person's fears and concerns. Show warmth, sensitivity, and caring.

BOX 39-1	**Surgery Fears and Concerns**

Fear of …
- Anesthesia and its effects (p. 607)
- Cancer
- Complications from surgery
- Disability
- Disfigurement and scarring
- Dying during or after surgery
- Exposure
- Not waking up after surgery
- Pain: during surgery, after surgery
- Prolonged recovery
- Separation from family and friends
- Surgery on the wrong body part
- Tubes, needles, and other care equipment
- Waking up during surgery
- What happens after surgery—more surgery, treatments, care, and so on

Concerns about …
- Caring for children and other family members
- Finances—monthly bills, loan payments, mortgages, hospital bills, doctor bills
- House, lawn, and garden
- Pets
- Plants

Your Role

You can assist in the person's psychological care before and after surgery.
- Listen. The person may talk about fears and concerns.
- Refer questions to the nurse.
- Explain the care you will give and its need.
- Follow communication rules (Chapters 7 and 8).
- Use verbal and nonverbal communication (Chapter 7).
- Provide care with skill and ease.
- Report signs of fear or anxiety (Chapter 52).
- Report a request to see a member of the clergy. See *Focus on Communication: Your Role.*

FOCUS ON COMMUNICATION

Your Role

After surgery, the doctor talks to the patient and family about the results. Eager to know, they may ask you about reports. Refer their questions to the nurse. Never tell any results or diagnoses. You can say:
- "The doctor will talk to you about the surgery and the results. I'll tell the nurse that you're asking."
- "I'll get the nurse to answer your questions."

PRE-OPERATIVE CARE

The pre-operative (pre-op) period may be many days or a few minutes. If time allows, the person is prepared mentally and physically for anesthesia and surgery. The goal is to prevent complications before, during, and after surgery.

The nurse also provides patient information. The nurse explains what to expect before, during, and after surgery.
- *Pre-op care—*includes tests and their purpose, skin preparation, personal care, and the purpose and effects of pre-op drugs.
- *Deep breathing, coughing, and incentive spirometry—*are practiced. Post-op, they are done every 1 to 2 hours when the person is awake. See Chapter 43.
- *Post-anesthesia care unit (PACU)—*commonly called the *recovery room,* this is where the person wakes up after surgery (Fig. 39-1). PACU care is explained.
- *Vital signs—*are taken often until they are stable.
- *Food and fluids—*post-op, the person is NPO (*nil per os;* nothing by mouth) and has an IV (intravenous). Food and fluids are allowed when the person's condition is stable.
- *Turning and re-positioning—*are done at least every 1 to 2 hours post-op.
- *Early ambulation—*is done as soon as possible post-op.
- *Pain—*relates to the type and amount of pain to expect and how pain-relief drugs are given.
- *Treatments and equipment—*may involve a urinary catheter, NG (naso-gastric) tube, oxygen, wound suction, a cast, or traction.
- *Position restrictions—*are common after some surgeries. For example, the hip is abducted after hip replacement surgery (Chapter 48).

See *Teamwork and Time Management: Pre-Operative Care.*
See *Focus on Children and Older Persons: Pre-Operative Care.*

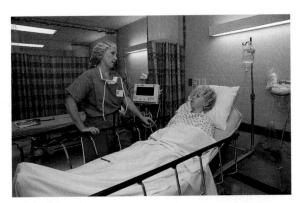

FIGURE 39-1 The post-anesthesia care unit (PACU).

TEAMWORK AND TIME MANAGEMENT

Pre-Operative Care

The nurse has a limited amount of time for pre-op care. You may be delegated several tasks. Tell the nurse when you complete each task. For example, you provide personal care (p. 604). Tell the nurse about your progress.

FOCUS ON **CHILDREN AND OLDER PERSONS**

Pre-Operative Care

Children

The child and parents are prepared for the surgery. Play is useful in helping the child understand what will happen. For example, a doll is used to show the surgery site. Operating room (OR) and PACU tours are given. The child and parents meet the OR and PACU nursing staff.

Special Tests

Pre-op, the doctor evaluates the person's health status. These tests are common.
- Chest x-ray.
- Complete blood count (CBC).
- Urinalysis (U/A).
- Electrocardiogram (ECG, EKG). See Figure 39-2.

Other tests depend on the person's condition and surgery. For expected blood loss, the person's blood is tested for blood type and compatible blood from a blood donor. This is called *type and crossmatch*.

The person is prepared for the tests as needed. Test results must be in the medical record before surgery.

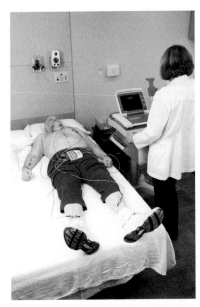

FIGURE 39-2 An electrocardiogram is taken.

Nutrition and Fluids

A light meal usually is allowed. Then the person is NPO for 6 to 8 hours before surgery. These measures reduce the risk of vomiting and aspiration during anesthesia and after surgery. An NPO sign is placed in the person's room. The water mug is removed.

Bowel Elimination

Bowel surgeries and procedures may require a *bowel prep*—cleansing the bowel of feces. Feces contain microbes. When the intestine is opened, feces can spill into the sterile abdominal cavity, causing a serious infection. The bowel prep helps prevent this contamination.

For the bowel prep, special fluids are ordered for the person to drink. Or enemas are ordered (Chapter 29).

Urinary Elimination

The person voids before the nurse gives pre-op drugs. If the person has a catheter, the drainage bag is emptied. The output is measured and recorded.

Catheters are commonly inserted in the OR. For pelvic and abdominal surgeries, the bladder must be empty. A full bladder is easily injured during surgery. Catheters also allow accurate output measurements during and after surgery.

Personal Care

Personal care before surgery may involve:

- *A complete bath, shower, or tub bath and shampoo.* A special soap or cleanser and shampoo are common. Their purpose is to reduce the number of microbes present. This lessens the risk of a wound infection. A patient gown and surgical cap are worn to the OR.
- *Make-up, nail polish, and non-natural nail removal.* The skin, lips, and nail beds are observed for color and circulation during and after surgery.
- *Hair care.* All hairpins, clips, combs, and other items are removed. So are wigs and hairpieces. A surgical cap keeps hair out of the face and operative site.
- *Oral hygiene.* Being NPO causes thirst and a dry mouth. The person must not swallow any water during oral hygiene.
- *Dentures.* Provide denture care and store dentures following agency policy. Some people do not like to be without their dentures. Let them wear dentures as long as possible. This promotes dignity and self-esteem.
- *Adaptive (assistive) devices and prostheses.* Eyeglasses, contact lenses, hearing aids, artificial eyes, and artificial limbs are removed. Hearing aids may be worn if the surgeon needs to talk to or instruct the patient during surgery. Follow agency policy for storage and safe-keeping.
- *Other.* Often elastic stockings (p. 610) are put on before transport to the OR. So are sequential compression devices (p. 613).

See *Promoting Safety and Comfort: Personal Care.*

PROMOTING SAFETY AND COMFORT

Personal Care

Safety

Check for loose teeth. Loose teeth are common in children. Adults may have loose teeth from periodontal disease (Chapter 23). Report loose teeth to the nurse. The nurse notes this in the medical record and alerts the OR staff. A loose tooth can fall out during anesthesia. The person can aspirate the tooth.

Jewelry

Jewelry is easily lost or broken in the OR and PACU. Transfers to and from the OR, PACU, and the person's room also present safety risks. And jewelry can cause pressure injuries (Chapter 41). Therefore all jewelry is removed and stored for safe-keeping. This includes body-piercing jewelry. Record jewelry removal and storage according to agency policy.

The person may want to wear a wedding ring or religious medal. Secure the item according to agency policy. Hand, arm, shoulder, and breast surgeries can cause swelling of the fingers on the affected side. Wedding rings are removed for such surgeries.

The Surgery Consent

The person's informed consent is needed for surgery. The patient and family are told about:

- The need for the surgery
- The surgery, risks, and possible complications
- Other treatment options
- The risks from not having surgery
- Who will do the surgery
- When the surgery will be done and how long it will take
- Expected length of recovery

Questions are answered. Misunderstandings are cleared up. A surgical consent is signed when the person understands the information. The doctor is responsible for securing the written consent. Often this is delegated to a nurse. *You do not obtain the person's written consent for surgery.*

The Pre-Operative Checklist

You may be delegated some tasks on the pre-operative checklist (Fig. 39-3). Promptly report when you complete each task and any observations. The checklist is completed before the nurse gives pre-op drugs.

Marking the Surgical Site. The surgeon marks the surgical site before the surgery. The patient is asked to confirm the site. Marking the site prevents surgery on the wrong part.

Site markings may be part of the pre-op checklist. The site is marked before pre-op drugs are given.

PRE-OPERATIVE CHECKLIST

Username: T. Murphy, RN   [Sign]

Date: March 7 📅   Time: 07 ▼ 00 ▼

Medical Record	Yes	No
Surgical consent signed	X	☐
NPO since Date: March 6 📅 Time: 22 ▼ 00 ▼	X	☐
Allergies verified Penicillin	X	☐
History and physical in medical record	X	☐
Advanced directives in medical record	X	☐

Test results in medical record:

X CBC		X U/A	
X Type and crossmatch		X EKG	
X Urine pregnancy for females		X Chest x-ray	

Complete Before Surgery	Yes	No
ID band is on	X	☐
Patient gown and surgical cap applied	X	☐
Surgical side/site marked and verified	X	☐
IV inserted	X	☐
AE stockings/SCD on	X	☐
Patient voided	X	☐
Urinary catheter inserted	X	☐

Personal Belongings	In Place	Removed	N/A
Make-up, nail polish, non-natural nails	☐	X	☐
Hairpins, clips, combs, wig, hairpiece	☐	☐	X
Dentures (full, partial)	☐	X	☐
Eyeglasses, contact lenses	☐	X	☐
Hearing aid(s)	☐	☐	X
Prostheses (eye, limb)	☐	☐	X
Jewelry	☐	X	☐

Measurements

Vitals Signs

Temperature   98.8   °F

Blood pressure   132/88   mm Hg

Pulse   68

Respirations   18

Pulse oximetry   98   %

Pain

Location   Right hip

Intensity   6

Weight and Height

Weight   165   lbs

Height   5   ft   4   in

FIGURE 39-3 A sample pre-operative checklist.

Skin Preparation

The incision is a portal of entry for microbes from the skin. A *surgical site infection (SSI) is an infection that occurs after surgery in the body part where the surgery took place. A skin prep* reduces the risk of SSI.

The area is cleaned with an antiseptic (Fig. 39-4). An **antiseptic** *is a chemical applied to the skin to prevent the growth and reproduction of microbes.* The incision and a large area around it are *prepped* (Fig. 39-5). The prep is done right before surgery.

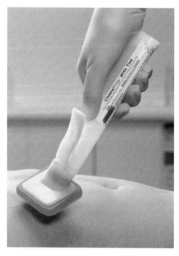

FIGURE 39-4 An antiseptic is applied to the skin to prevent infection. (Courtesy Becton, Dickinson and Company, Franklin Lakes, N.J.)

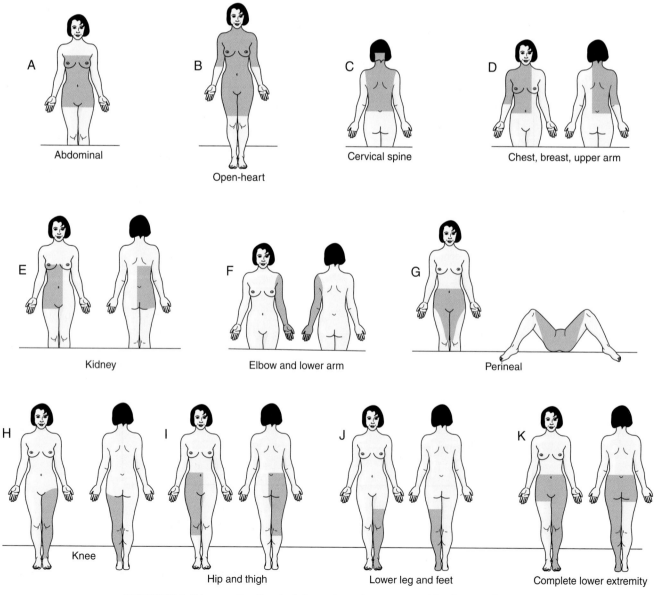

A Abdominal

B Open-heart

C Cervical spine

D Chest, breast, upper arm

E Kidney

F Elbow and lower arm

G Perineal

H Knee

I Hip and thigh

J Lower leg and feet

K Complete lower extremity

FIGURE 39-5 Skin prep sites. The *shaded area* shows the area prepped for the type of surgery.

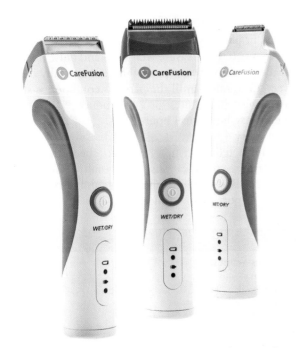

FIGURE 39-6 Surgical clippers. (Courtesy Becton, Dickinson and Company, Franklin Lakes, N.J.)

Hair Removal. Hair is not removed from the surgical site unless it will interfere with surgery. If the surgeon orders hair removal, it is done before the antiseptic is applied. Electric clippers are used for hair removal (Fig. 39-6). Or a hair removal cream may be used. Shaving with a razor can cause small cuts in the skin. This increases the risk for SSI.

Pre-Operative Drugs

Pre-operative drugs are given before transport to the OR. The drugs:
- Help the person relax and feel drowsy.
- Reduce respiratory secretions to prevent aspiration. A dry mouth also results.
- Prevent nausea and vomiting.

The person will feel sleepy and light-headed. The person is not allowed out of bed. To help prevent falls, accidents, and damaged equipment:
- Have the person void before the drugs are given. Then have the person use the bedpan or urinal to void.
- Raise the bed rails after the drugs are given.
- Move furniture to make room for the stretcher.
- Clear off the over-bed table and the bedside stand.

Transport to the Operating Room

OR staff transport the patient to the OR. First, identification checks are made. Then the patient is transported by bed or stretcher. Safety measures are practiced to prevent falls. Stretcher safety straps are secured. Side rails or bed rails are raised.

The family is shown where they can wait. Sometimes family members are allowed to go with the patient as far as the OR entrance.

See *Focus on Children and Older Persons: Transport to the Operating Room.*

SEDATION AND ANESTHESIA

Some procedures only require sedation. *Sedation is a state of quiet, calmness, or sleep produced by a drug.* Levels of sedation are minimal, moderate (conscious), and deep.

Produced by a drug, **anesthesia** *is the loss* (an) *of all sensation* (esthesia), *especially pain.*
- *General anesthesia is a treatment with certain drugs that produces a deep sleep and the absence of all sensation, especially pain.* Drugs are given IV or inhaled through a gas.
- *Regional anesthesia is the loss of sensation, produced by a drug, in a large area.* The person is awake. A drug is injected into a body part.
- *Local anesthesia is the loss of sensation, produced by a drug, in a small area.* A drug is injected at the site.

An *anesthesiologist* is a doctor specializing in giving sedation and anesthetics. An *anesthetist* is an RN (registered nurse) with advanced study in sedation and anesthetics.

POST-OPERATIVE CARE

After surgery the person is taken to the PACU to begin post-op (post-surgical) care. Recovery from sedation or anesthesia takes 1 to 2 hours. Vital signs are measured and observations are made often. The person is transported to his or her room when:
- Vital signs are stable.
- Respiratory function is good.
- The person can respond and call for help.

Preparing the Person's Room

The person's room must be ready for post-op care. After the person is taken to the OR, you can:
- Make a surgical bed. Lower the bed rails and raise the bed for a transfer from a stretcher. Take the bed to the OR department if this is agency policy.
- Place equipment and supplies in the room.
  - Thermometer
  - Stethoscope and blood pressure and pulse oximetry equipment
  - Kidney basin
  - Tissues
  - Waterproof under-pad
  - Vital signs flow sheet
  - I&O (intake and output) record
  - IV pole
  - Other items as directed by the nurse
- Move furniture out of the way for the stretcher or bed.

Return From the PACU

PACU staff transport the person and a unit nurse meets them in the person's room. Assist as needed for a stretcher-to-bed transfer. Also help position the person.

Vital signs and pulse oximetry are measured and observations made. They are compared with those from the PACU. The nurse checks the surgical site for bleeding. Catheter, IV, and other tube placements and functions are checked. Bed rails are raised. The call light and other needed items are placed within the person's reach. Necessary care and treatments are given. Then the family can join the person.

Measurements and Observations

Your role in post-op care depends on the person's condition. Often you will measure vital signs and pulse oximetry and make post-op observations. These are usually done:

- Every 15 minutes until the person's condition is stable
- Then every 30 minutes for 1 to 2 hours
- Then every hour for 4 hours
- Then every 4 hours

The nurse tells you how often to check the person. Many serious complications can result from surgery (Box 39-2). Be alert for the signs and symptoms in Box 39-2. Report them at once.

| BOX 39-2 | **Post-Op Complications and Observations** |

Complications

- Respiratory System
  - Pneumonia—inflammation and infection of lung tissue
  - Atelectasis—collapse of a portion of the lung
  - Pulmonary embolism—a blood clot from a vein that travels (embolus) in the bloodstream until it lodges in a lung
- Circulatory System
  - Hypovolemia—inadequate (hypo) amount (vol) of blood (emia)
  - Hemorrhage—the excessive loss (rrhage) of blood (hemo) in a short time
  - Hypovolemic shock—when organs and tissues do not get enough blood (shock) because of an inadequate (hypo) amount (vol) of blood (emia)
  - Thrombophlebitis—a blood clot (thrombo) causing inflammation (itis) of a vein (phleb)
  - Thrombus—a blood clot
  - Embolus—a blood clot that travels through the vascular system until it lodges in a blood vessel
- Urinary System
  - Urinary retention—urine collects (retention) in the bladder from being unable to void
  - Urinary tract infection—inflammation and infection of the urinary structures (bladder, ureters, urethra)
- Gastro-Intestinal System
  - Nausea
  - Vomiting
  - Constipation
  - Flatulence
  - Post-operative ileus—the absence of normal intestinal (ileus) function from the lack of peristalsis after surgery
- Integumentary System (Chapter 40)
  - Wound infection
  - Dehiscence—the separation of wound layers
  - Evisceration—the separation of the wound along with the protrusion of abdominal organs

Observations

- Abdominal: distention (swelling); pain; cramping
- Aching
- Anxiety
- Bleeding: from the incision, drainage tubes, suction tubes, or other sites
- Blood pressure: increase or decrease
- Chest pain
- Choking
- Condition: any change in

Observations—cont'd

- Confusion
- Cough: weak
- Discomfort in a leg
- Disorientation
- Drainage:
  - From wound (Chapter 40)
  - On or under dressings
  - On bed linens (including bottom linens and pillowcases)
  - Appearance from urinary catheter, NG tube, wound suction, and other tubes
- Hypoxia (Chapter 43)
- Intake and output
- IV flow rate
- Nausea
- Pain
- Pulse:
  - More than 100 beats per minute
  - Less than 60 beats per minute
  - Weak
  - Irregular
- Pulse oximetry measurement (Chapter 43)
- Respirations:
  - Shallow, slow breathing
  - Rapid
  - Gasping
  - Difficult (dyspnea)
  - Shortness of breath
  - Moist-sounding
  - Gurgling
- Restlessness
- Skin:
  - Moist or clammy
  - Pale (pallor)
  - Cyanosis (bluish color)
  - Cool
  - Warm or hot
- Sputum: clear, white, yellow, green, brown, or red; thick, watery, or frothy (with bubbles)
- Swelling in affected area
- Temperature: increase or decrease
- Thirst
- Urinary complaints: cannot void, burning, urgency, lower abdominal pain
- Urine: amount, character, and time of first voiding after surgery
- Vomiting

Positioning

The person is positioned for comfort and to prevent complications. There may be position restrictions after some surgeries. The person is usually positioned:

- To promote comfort
- For easy and comfortable breathing
- To prevent stress on the incision
- To prevent aspiration

When supine, the head of the bed is usually raised slightly. The person's head may be turned to the side.

The person is re-positioned at least every 1 to 2 hours. This prevents respiratory and circulatory complications. Turning may be painful. Provide support. Use smooth, gentle motions. Place pillows and positioning devices as the nurse directs (Chapters 18 and 34).

The nurse tells you when to re-position the person and the positions allowed. Usually you assist the nurse. The nurse may delegate these tasks when the person is stable and care is simple.

See *Focus on Children and Older Persons: Positioning.*

FOCUS ON **CHILDREN AND OLDER PERSONS**

Positioning

Older Persons
Many older persons have stiff and painful joints. Sore muscles, bones, and joints occur from the OR table. Turn and re-position older persons slowly and gently.

Preventing Respiratory and Circulatory Complications

Coughing and deep-breathing exercises help prevent respiratory complications, including post-operative pneumonia (see Box 39-2). So does incentive spirometry. See Chapter 43.

Circulation must be stimulated for blood flow in the legs. If blood flow is sluggish, blood clots may form. A *blood clot is called a thrombus.* Blood clots (thrombi) can form in the deep leg veins in the lower legs or thighs (Fig. 39-7, *A*). Many people do not have signs or symptoms. Report the following at once.

- Swollen area of a leg.
- Pain or tenderness in a leg. This may be only when standing or walking.
- Warmth in the part of the leg that is swollen or painful.
- Red or discolored skin.

A blood clot (thrombus) can break loose and travel through the bloodstream. It then becomes an embolus. An *embolus is a blood clot* (thrombus) *that travels through the vascular system until it lodges in a blood vessel* (Fig. 39-7, *B*). An embolus from a vein lodges in the lungs (pulmonary embolism) and can cause severe respiratory problems and death. Report chest pain or shortness of breath at once.

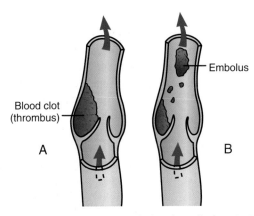

FIGURE 39-7 A, A blood clot is attached to the wall of a vein. The *arrows* show the direction of blood flow. **B,** Part of the thrombus breaks off and becomes an embolus. The embolus travels through the vascular system until it lodges in a distant vessel.

Circulation is stimulated and thrombi prevented by:

- Leg exercises
- Ambulation as soon as possible
- Elastic stockings (p. 610)
- Elastic bandages (p. 612)
- Sequential compression devices (p. 613)
- No prolonged standing or sitting

See *Focus on Children and Older Persons: Preventing Respiratory and Circulatory Complications.*

See *Promoting Safety and Comfort: Preventing Respiratory and Circulatory Complications.*

FOCUS ON **CHILDREN AND OLDER PERSONS**

Preventing Respiratory and Circulatory Complications

Older Persons
Older persons are at risk for respiratory complications. Respiratory muscles are weaker. The lungs are less elastic. The person has less strength for coughing. Coughing, deep breathing, and incentive spirometry are very important.

Older persons also are at risk for *thrombi* (blood clots) and *emboli* (more than 1 embolus). Blood is pumped through the body with less force. Circulation is already sluggish.

PROMOTING SAFETY AND COMFORT

Preventing Respiratory and Circulatory Complications

Comfort
For coughing exercises, "splinting" the incision promotes comfort. To *splint* means *to support or brace.* To splint the incision, the person holds a pillow or his or her hands over the incision. See Chapter 43.

Leg Exercises. Leg exercises promote venous blood flow and help prevent thrombi. The nurse tells you when to do the exercises. They are done at least every 1 or 2 hours while the person is awake. Assist if the person is weak.

These exercises are usually done 5 times.

- Make circles with the toes. This rotates the ankles.
- Dorsiflex and plantar flex the feet (Chapter 34).
- Flex and extend 1 knee and then the other (Fig. 39-8, *A*).
- Raise and lower the leg off the bed (Fig. 39-8, *B*). Repeat with the other leg.

After leg surgery, the surgeon may order other exercises and when to do them. Do not assist with leg exercises until the nurse tells you to.

Elastic Stockings. Elastic stockings put pressure on the veins. This promotes venous blood return to the heart. The stockings help prevent blood clots in leg veins.

Elastic stockings also are called AE stockings (AE means *anti-embolism* or *anti-embolic*). They also are called TED hose (TED means *thrombo-embolic disease*).

Persons at risk for thrombi include those who:

- Have heart and circulatory disorders.
- Are on bed rest.
- Have had surgery.
- Are older.
- Are pregnant.

Stockings come in thigh-high and knee-high lengths and various sizes. The nurse measures the person for the correct size.

The person may have 2 pairs of stockings. Wash 1 pair while the other pair is worn. Wash them by hand with a mild soap. Hang them to dry.

See *Delegation Guidelines: Elastic Stockings.*
See *Promoting Safety and Comfort: Elastic Stockings.*
See procedure: *Applying Elastic Stockings.*

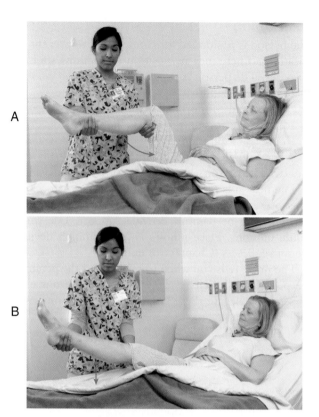

FIGURE 39-8 Leg exercises to stimulate circulation. **A,** The knee is flexed and then extended. **B,** The leg is raised and lowered.

DELEGATION GUIDELINES

Elastic Stockings

Applying elastic stockings is a routine nursing task. To apply elastic stockings, you need this information from the nurse and the care plan.

- What size to use—small, medium, large, extra-large, or bariatric
- What length to use—thigh-high or knee-high
- When to remove them and for how long—usually every 8 hours for 30 minutes
- What observations to report and record:
  - The size and length of stockings applied
  - When you applied the stockings
  - Skin color and temperature
  - Leg and foot swelling
  - Skin tears, wounds, or signs of skin breakdown
  - Complaints of pain, tingling, or numbness
  - When you removed the stockings and for how long
  - When you re-applied the stockings
  - When you washed the stockings
- When to report observations
- What patient or resident concerns to report at once

PROMOTING SAFETY AND COMFORT

Elastic Stockings

Safety
Apply the stocking so the toe opening is over the top of the toes or under the toes. Follow the manufacturer's instructions. Use the toe opening to check circulation, skin color, and skin temperature in the toes.

Stockings must not have twists, creases, or wrinkles. Twists can affect circulation. So can stockings that roll up, bunch up, or have the toe opening wrapped around the toes. Creases and wrinkles can cause skin breakdown.

Loose stockings do not exert pressure on the veins. Stockings that are too tight can affect circulation. Tell the nurse if the stockings are too loose or too tight.

Comfort
Apply stockings before the person gets out of bed. Otherwise the legs can swell from sitting or standing. Stockings are hard to put on swollen legs. The person is in bed while they are off. This prevents the legs from swelling.

Gently handle and move the person's foot and leg. Do not force the joints (toes, foot, ankle, knee, and hip) beyond their range of motion or to the point of pain.

Applying Elastic Stockings

QUALITY OF LIFE

- Knock before entering the person's room.
- Address the person by name.
- Introduce yourself by name and title.

- Explain the procedure before starting and during the procedure.
- Protect the person's rights during the procedure.
- Handle the person gently during the procedure.

PRE-PROCEDURE

1 Follow *Delegation Guidelines: Elastic Stockings*. See *Promoting Safety and Comfort: Elastic Stockings*.
2 Practice hand hygiene.
3 Obtain elastic stockings in the correct size and length. Note the location of the toe opening.

4 Identify the person. Check the ID (identification) bracelet against the assignment sheet. Use 2 identifiers (Chapter 13). Also call the person by name.
5 Provide for privacy.
6 Raise the bed for body mechanics. Bed rails are up if used.

PROCEDURE

7 Lower the bed rail.
8 Position the person supine.
9 Expose 1 leg. Fan-fold top linens to the foot of the bed or toward the other leg.
10 Gather or turn the stocking inside out down to the heel.
11 Slip the foot of the stocking over the toes, foot, and heel (Fig. 39-9, *A*). Properly position the heel pocket on the heel. The toe opening is over or under the toes. Follow the manufacturer's instructions.

12 Grasp the stocking top. Roll or pull the stocking up the leg. It turns right side out as it is rolled or pulled up.
13 Adjust the stocking as needed. Make sure the stocking does not cause pressure on the toes.
14 Remove twists, creases, or wrinkles. Make sure the stocking is even, snug, smooth, and wrinkle-free (Fig. 39-9, *B*).
15 Cover the leg. Repeat steps 9 through 14 for the other leg.
16 Cover the person.

POST-PROCEDURE

17 Provide for comfort. (See the inside of the back cover.)
18 Place the call light and other needed items within reach.
19 Lower the bed to a safe and comfortable level. Follow the care plan.
20 Raise or lower bed rails. Follow the care plan.

21 Unscreen the person.
22 Complete a safety check of the room. (See the inside of the back cover.)
23 Practice hand hygiene.
24 Report and record your observations.

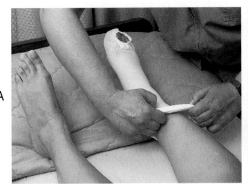
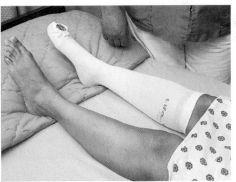

FIGURE 39-9 Applying elastic stockings. **A,** The stocking is slipped over the toes, foot, and heel. **B,** The stocking turns right side out as it is pulled up over the leg. The heel is positioned in the heel pocket of the stocking.

Elastic Bandages. Elastic bandages have the same purposes as elastic stockings. They also provide support and reduce swelling from injuries. Another use is to hold dressings in place. They are applied to arms and legs. To apply bandages:

- Use the correct size—length and width.
- Position the person in good alignment.
- Face the person during the procedure.
- Start at the lower (*distal*) part of the extremity. Work upward to the top (*proximal*) part.
- Expose the fingers or toes if possible. This allows circulation checks.
- Apply the bandage with firm, even pressure.
- Check the color and temperature of the extremity every hour.
- Re-apply a loose or wrinkled bandage.
- Replace a moist or soiled bandage.
  See *Focus on Communication: Elastic Bandages.*
  See *Delegation Guidelines: Elastic Bandages.*
  See *Promoting Safety and Comfort: Elastic Bandages.*
  See procedure: *Applying an Elastic Bandage.*

DELEGATION GUIDELINES
Elastic Bandages

Applying elastic bandages is a routine nursing task in some agencies. In others, it is a nursing responsibility that may be delegated to you. To apply elastic bandages, you need this information from the nurse and the care plan.

- Where to apply the bandage
- What width and length to use
- When to remove the bandage and for how long—usually every 8 hours for 30 minutes
- What observations to report and record:
  - The width and length applied
  - When you applied the bandage
  - Skin color and temperature
  - Swelling of the part
  - Skin tears, wounds, or signs of skin breakdown
  - Complaints of pain, itching, tingling, or numbness
  - A wet or soiled bandage
  - The amount and appearance of drainage
  - When you removed the bandage and for how long
  - When you re-applied the bandage
- When to report observations
- What patient or resident concerns to report at once

FOCUS ON COMMUNICATION
Elastic Bandages

Elastic bandages should promote comfort. To check for comfort, ask:

- "Does the bandage feel too tight?"
- "Do you feel pain, itching, or numbness?" If yes: "What do you feel?" "Where do you feel it?"

PROMOTING SAFETY AND COMFORT
Elastic Bandages

Safety
Elastic bandages must be firm and snug but not tight. A tight bandage can affect circulation.

Manufacturers supply bandages with loop and hook, clip, tape, or Velcro closures. Metal or plastic clips can injure the skin if they are loose, fall off, or cause pressure. Check the clips often for correct placement.

Comfort
A tight bandage can cause pain and discomfort. If the person complains of pain, tingling, or numbness, remove the bandage. Tell the nurse at once.

Applying an Elastic Bandage

QUALITY OF LIFE

- Knock before entering the person's room.
- Address the person by name.
- Introduce yourself by name and title.

- Explain the procedure before starting and during the procedure.
- Protect the person's rights during the procedure.
- Handle the person gently during the procedure.

PRE-PROCEDURE

1 Follow *Delegation Guidelines: Elastic Bandages.* See *Promoting Safety and Comfort: Elastic Bandages.*
2 Practice hand hygiene.
3 Collect an elastic bandage with closures as directed by the nurse.

4 Identify the person. Check the ID bracelet against the assignment sheet. Use 2 identifiers (Chapter 13). Also call the person by name.
5 Provide for privacy.
6 Raise the bed for body mechanics. Bed rails are up if used.

Applying an Elastic Bandage—cont'd

PROCEDURE

7   Lower the bed rail near you if up.
8   Help the person to a comfortable position in good alignment. Expose the part to bandage.
9   Make sure the area is clean and dry.
10 Hold the bandage with the roll up. The loose end is on the bottom (Fig. 39-10, *A*).
11 Apply the bandage to the lower (*distal*) and smallest part of the wrist, foot, ankle, or knee (Fig. 39-10, *B*).
12 Make 2 circular turns around the part.
13 Make over-lapping spiral turns in an upward (*proximal*) direction. Each turn over-laps ½ to ¾ of the previous turn (Fig. 39-10, *C*). Each over-lap is equal.

14 Apply the bandage smoothly with firm, even pressure. It is not tight.
15 End the bandage with 2 circular turns.
16 Secure the bandage with the manufacturer's closure. Clips are not under the body part.
17 Check the fingers or toes for coldness or *cyanosis* (bluish color). Ask about pain, itching, numbness, or tingling. Remove the bandage if any are noted. Report your observations.

POST-PROCEDURE

18 Provide for comfort. (See the inside of the back cover.)
19 Place the call light and other needed items within reach.
20 Lower the bed to a safe and comfortable level. Follow the care plan.
21 Raise or lower bed rails. Follow the care plan.

22 Unscreen the person.
23 Complete a safety check of the room. (See the inside of the back cover.)
24 Practice hand hygiene.
25 Report and record your observations.

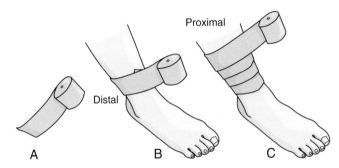

FIGURE 39-10 Applying an elastic bandage. **A,** The bandage roll is up. The loose end is at the bottom. **B,** The bandage is applied to the lower (*distal*) and smallest part with 2 circular turns. **C,** The bandage is applied with spiral turns in an upward (*proximal*) direction.

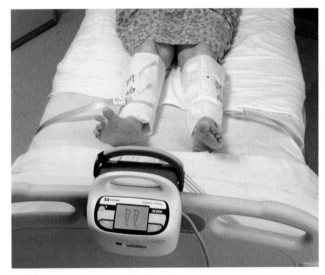

FIGURE 39-11 Sequential compression device. (From deWit SC, Stromberg HK, Dallred CV: *Medical-surgical nursing: concepts and practice*, ed 3, St Louis, 2017, Elsevier.)

Sequential Compression Devices. A sequential compression device (SCD) is a sleeve that straps around the leg (Fig. 39-11). Made of cloth or plastic, the SCD is secured in place with Velcro. Elastic stockings are often worn under SCDs.

A pump inflates the device with air. This promotes venous blood flow to the heart by causing pressure on the veins. Then the pump deflates the device.

SCDs are applied to both legs. After 1 side deflates, the other inflates. Applied pre-op, SCDs also are worn post-op.

Early Ambulation

Early ambulation prevents complications such as thrombi, pneumonia, atelectasis, constipation, and urinary tract infections. The person usually walks in the room or hallway the day of surgery. The person sits on the side of the bed first. Blood pressure and pulse are measured. If they are stable, the person is assisted out of bed.

The nurse tells you when the person can walk and how far to go. Distance increases as the person gains strength. Usually you assist the nurse the first time.

Wound Healing

The incision needs to heal. A dressing (bandage) may cover the incision for protection and to prevent infection. Your agency may let you do simple non-sterile dressing changes. See Chapter 40 for wound care.

Nutrition and Fluids

Post-op, the person has an IV. Continued IV therapy depends on the type of surgery and the person's condition. Anesthesia may cause nausea and vomiting. Diet progresses from NPO to clear liquids, to full liquids, to a regular diet. Frequent oral hygiene is important while NPO.

Some patients have NG tubes (Chapter 32). The NG tube may be attached to suction to keep the stomach empty. The person is NPO and has an IV.

Elimination

Anesthesia, surgery, and being NPO affect bowel and urinary elimination. Pain-relief drugs can cause constipation. Promote elimination as directed by the nurse and the care plan (Chapters 27 and 29). Fluid intake and a regular diet are needed for bowel elimination. Suppositories or enemas may be ordered for constipation.

Measure intake and output. The person must void within 6 to 8 hours after surgery. Report the time and amount of the first voiding. If the person does not void within 6 to 8 hours, a catheter may be needed. Some patients have a catheter after surgery. See Chapter 28.

Comfort and Rest

Pain is common after surgery. The degree of pain depends on:

- The extent of surgery.
- The incision site and size.
- If drainage tubes, casts, or other devices are present.
- Positioning during surgery. The position can cause muscle strains and discomfort.

Pain-relief drugs are ordered. The nurse uses the nursing process to promote comfort and rest. Many of the measures listed in Chapter 35 are part of the person's care plan.

Personal Hygiene

Personal hygiene is important for well-being. Wound drainage and skin prep solutions can irritate the skin and cause discomfort. NPO causes a dry mouth and breath odors. Moist, clammy skin from blood pressure changes or fever also cause discomfort.

Frequent oral hygiene, hair care, and a complete bed bath after surgery help refresh and renew the person. The gown and linens are changed when wet or soiled.

FOCUS ON **PRIDE**

The Person, Family, and Yourself

Personal and Professional Responsibility

What worries would you have about surgery—pain, loss of function, death, caring for your children and home, supporting your family? Imagine hours after being in an accident. You are told that your right leg was amputated.

Take time to listen to the person's fears and concerns. Avoid seeming rushed. Act professionally. Take pride in showing that you care.

Rights and Respect

The person has the right to accurate and complete information. You can answer questions about the care you give. If you do not know or are unsure of an answer, explain that you will ask the nurse.

Some questions are best answered by the nurse. For example: "How long will the surgery last?" or "What will be done for pain after surgery?" Even if you know the answer, say that you will ask the nurse to answer the question. Show good judgment. Only answer questions within the scope of your role.

Independence and Social Interaction

Some people prefer peace and quiet before and after surgery. Others want family and friends around. The support and conversation distracts from worries and pain. Each person is different. Ask what the person prefers. Tell the nurse. The nurse can talk with the family about the person's wishes and needs.

Delegation and Teamwork

You may be delegated parts of the person's post-op care. For example, you monitor vital signs. The patient and nurse rely on you. Complete post-op vital signs on time. Report abnormal values, sudden changes, and any concerns at once. Take pride in your role in post-op care. You can make a difference in the safety and quality of the person's care.

Ethics and Laws

When possible, the person signs the surgical consent. If unable, the person's spouse or nearest relative may be required to sign the consent. A parent or legal representative signs for a minor child. The legal representative signs for a person not mentally competent to sign.

FOCUS ON **PRIDE**: *Application*

Your attitude and conduct affect the person's surgical experience. You can either ease worries or increase stress. Explain how your behavior affects the person's outlook and comfort.

REVIEW QUESTIONS

Circle T *if the statement is TRUE or* F *if it is FALSE.*

1   T   F   Pins, clips, or combs keep the hair out of the face during surgery.

2   T   F   Nail polish is removed before surgery.

3   T   F   Make-up can be worn to the OR.

4   T   F   Sleepwear is worn to the OR.

5   T   F   Contact lenses are removed in the OR.

6   T   F   A surgical bed is made for the return from the PACU.

7   T   F   A decrease in blood pressure is reported at once.

8   T   F   The person walks for the first time 2 days after surgery.

9   T   F   Intake and output are measured after surgery.

10   T   F   The person should void within 6 to 8 hours after surgery.

Circle the BEST answer.

11 Which is true of elective surgery?
 a It is done at once.
 b The need is sudden and not expected.
 c It is scheduled at a later date.
 d General anesthesia is always used.

12 A person states: "I'm afraid of surgery." What should you do?
 a Call a member of the clergy.
 b Listen and use touch.
 c Change the subject.
 d Tell the family.

13 You assist with pre-op care by explaining
 a The reason for the surgery
 b The procedures you are doing
 c The risks and possible complications
 d What to expect during and after surgery

14 Before surgery, a person is
 a NPO
 b Allowed only water
 c Given breakfast
 d Given a tube feeding

15 A bowel prep is ordered to
 a Prevent bleeding
 b Relieve flatus
 c Prevent pain
 d Clean the intestines of feces

16 A skin prep is done to
 a Bathe the body completely
 b Sterilize the skin
 c Reduce the amount of microbes on the skin
 d Destroy non-pathogens and pathogens

17 After pre-op drugs are given, the patient
 a Must stay in bed
 b Can use the bathroom
 c Can use the commode to void
 d Can have sips of water

18 General anesthesia is
 a A specially educated nurse
 b A treatment causing deep sleep and absence of sensation
 c A treatment causing loss of sensation in a body part
 d A specially educated doctor

19 Coughing and deep breathing after surgery prevent
 a Bleeding
 b A pulmonary embolus
 c Respiratory complications
 d Pain and discomfort

20 Leg exercises
 a Stimulate circulation and prevent thrombi
 b Are done only for leg surgery
 c Are done every 4 hours
 d Are not needed if elastic stockings are worn

21 Post-op, a person's position is changed at least
 a Every 2 hours
 b Every 3 hours
 c Every 4 hours
 d Every shift

22 Elastic stockings
 a Hold dressings in place
 b Reduce swelling after injury
 c Prevent pressure injuries
 d Prevent blood clots

23 Elastic stockings are applied
 a When the person is standing
 b Before the person gets out of bed
 c After breakfast
 d For 30 minutes and then removed

24 The purpose of an elastic bandage is to
 a Prevent infection
 b Absorb drainage
 c Provide moisture for wound healing
 d Reduce swelling

25 When applying an elastic bandage
 a Position the part in good alignment
 b Cover the fingers or toes if possible
 c Apply it from the large to small part of the extremity
 d Apply it from the upper to lower part of the extremity

Answers to Chapter 39 questions are on p. 887.

FOCUS ON **PRACTICE**

Problem Solving

You are measuring a post-op patient's vital signs. The person is restless. The vital signs are similar to previous measurements. What do you do? Is there anything you need to report? If so, when?

Wound Care

OBJECTIVES

- Define the key terms and key abbreviations in this chapter.
- Describe skin tears, circulatory ulcers, and diabetic foot ulcers and the persons at risk.
- Explain how to help prevent skin tears, circulatory ulcers, and diabetic foot ulcers.
- Describe the process and complications of wound healing.
- Describe what to observe about wounds.
- Explain how to secure dressings.

- Explain the rules for applying dressings.
- Explain the purpose of binders and compression garments and how to apply them.
- Describe how to meet the basic needs of persons with wounds.
- Perform the procedure described in this chapter.
- Explain how to promote PRIDE in the person, the family, and yourself.

KEY TERMS

abrasion A partial-thickness wound caused by the scraping away or rubbing of the skin

arterial ulcer An open wound on the foot, ankle, or lower leg caused by poor arterial blood flow

chronic wound A wound that does not heal easily and within about 3 months

circulatory ulcer An open sore on the lower legs or feet caused by decreased blood flow through the arteries or veins; vascular ulcer

diabetic foot ulcer An open wound on the foot caused by complications from diabetes

excoriation Loss of the epidermis (top skin layer) caused by scratching or when skin rubs against skin, clothing, or other material

incision A cut produced surgically by a sharp instrument; it creates an opening into an organ or body space

laceration An open wound with torn tissues and jagged edges

penetrating wound An open wound that breaks the skin and enters a body area, organ, or cavity

puncture wound An open wound made by a sharp object

purulent drainage Thick green, yellow, or brown drainage

sanguineous drainage Bloody *(sanguis)* drainage

serosanguineous drainage Thin, watery drainage *(sero)* that is blood-tinged *(sanguineous)*

serous drainage Clear, watery fluid *(serum)*

skin tear A break or rip in the outer layers of the skin; the epidermis (top skin layer) separates from the underlying tissues

stasis ulcer See "venous ulcer"

ulcer A shallow or deep crater-like sore of the skin or mucous membrane

vascular ulcer See "circulatory ulcer"

venous ulcer An open sore on the lower legs or feet caused by poor venous blood flow; stasis ulcer

wound A break in the skin or mucous membrane

KEY ABBREVIATIONS

GI	Gastro-intestinal	ISTAP	International Skin Tear Advisory Panel
ID	Identification	PPE	Personal protective equipment

A *wound is a break in the skin or mucous membrane.* Wounds commonly result from:
- Surgery.
- *Trauma*—an accident or violent act that injures the skin, mucous membranes, bones, and organs. Falls, vehicle crashes, gunshots, stabbings, bites, burns, and frostbite are examples.
- Unrelieved pressure or friction (Chapter 41).
- Decreased blood flow through the arteries or veins.
- Nerve damage.

Wounds vary in depth. In a *partial-thickness wound*, the dermis and epidermis of the skin are broken. In a *full-thickness wound*, the dermis, epidermis, and subcutaneous tissues are penetrated. Muscle and bone may be involved.

Wounds are portals of entry for microbes. Infection is a major threat. Wound care includes preventing infection and further injury to the wound and nearby tissues. Blood loss and pain also are prevented.

The nurse uses the nursing process to keep the person's skin healthy. Some agencies have wound therapists or skin care teams to manage all skin problems. The team includes a nurse, physical therapist, and dietitian.

You may be involved in the care of the following wounds.

- *Abrasion*—*a partial-thickness wound caused by the scraping away or rubbing of the skin* (Fig. 40-1).
- *Excoriation*—*loss of the epidermis (top skin layer) caused by scratching or when skin rubs against skin, clothing, or other material* (Fig. 40-2).
- *Incision*—*a cut produced surgically by a sharp instrument. It creates an opening into an organ or body space* (Fig. 40-3).
- *Laceration*—*an open wound with torn tissues and jagged edges* (Fig. 40-4, p. 618).
- *Penetrating wound*—*an open wound that breaks the skin and enters a body area, organ, or cavity* (Fig. 40-5, p. 618).
- *Puncture wound*—*an open wound made by a sharp object* (knife, nail, metal, wood, glass). See Figure 40-6, p. 618.
- *Ulcer*—*a shallow or deep crater-like sore of the skin or mucous membrane* (p. 619).

See *Promoting Safety and Comfort: Wound Care.*

PROMOTING SAFETY AND COMFORT

Wound Care

Safety

Wounds are at high risk for infection.

- *Clean wound*—is not infected. Microbes have not entered the wound. Closed wounds are usually clean. So are intentional wounds (such as incisions) made into sterile body areas. The reproductive, urinary, respiratory, and gastro-intestinal (GI) systems are not entered.
- *Clean-contaminated wound*—occurs from the surgical entry of the reproductive, urinary, respiratory, or GI system. Some or all parts of these systems are not sterile and contain normal flora.
- *Contaminated wound*—has a high risk of infection. Unintentional wounds (such as trauma wounds from vehicle crashes) are usually contaminated. Contamination occurs from breaks in surgical asepsis, spillage of intestinal contents, and trauma. Tissues may show signs of inflammation.
- *Infected wound (dirty wound)*—contains large amounts of microbes and shows signs of infection. Examples include old wounds, surgical incisions made into infected areas, and trauma that ruptures the bowel.

Wound care may involve contact with blood, body fluids, secretions, or excretions. Follow Standard Precautions and the Bloodborne Pathogen Standard. Wear personal protective equipment (PPE) as needed. Gloves, gowns, masks, and eye protection are necessary when blood splashes and splatters are likely.

NOTE: A task may require more than 1 pair of gloves. Change gloves as needed. Use careful judgment. Remember to practice hand hygiene after removing gloves.

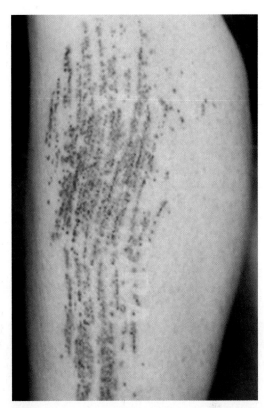

FIGURE 40-1 An abrasion. (From Lunn MM: *Essentials of medicolegal death investigation*, ed 1, San Diego, 2017, Academic Press.)

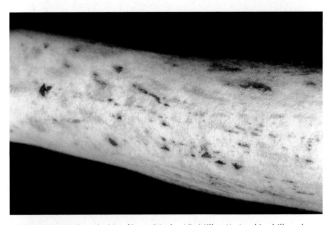

FIGURE 40-2 Excoriation. (From Marks JG, Miller JJ: *Lookingbill and Marks' principles of dermatology*, ed 6, London, 2019, Elsevier.)

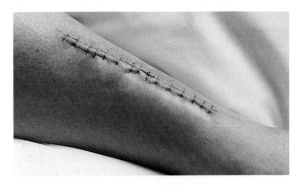

FIGURE 40-3 A surgical incision closed with staples. (From Perry AG, Potter PA, Ostendorf WR: *Nursing intervention and clinical skills*, ed 6, St Louis, 2016, Mosby.)

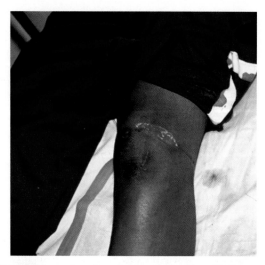

FIGURE 40-4 Laceration. (From Roberts JR, Custalow CB, Thomsen TW: *Roberts and Hedges' clinical procedures in emergency medicine and acute care*, ed 7, Philadelphia, 2019, Elsevier.)

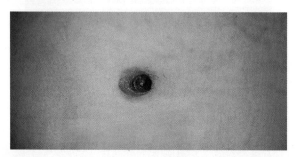

FIGURE 40-5 Penetrating wound. (From McCance KL, Huether SE: *Pathophysiology: the biologic basis for disease in adults and children*, ed 6, St Louis, 2010, Mosby.)

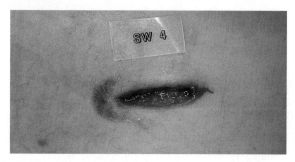

FIGURE 40-6 Puncture wound. (From McCance KL, Huether SE: *Pathophysiology: the biologic basis for disease in adults and children*, ed 6, St Louis, 2010, Mosby.)

SKIN TEARS

A *skin tear is a break or rip in the outer layers of the skin. The epidermis (top skin layer) separates from the underlying tissues* (Chapter 10). According to the International Skin Tear Advisory Panel (ISTAP), there are 3 types of skin tears.

- No skin loss (Fig. 40-7, *A*). The flap of skin can be placed back over the wound.
- Partial flap loss (Fig. 40-7, *B*). Part of the skin is lost. The remaining flap cannot be placed to cover the wound.
- Total flap loss (Fig. 40-7, *C*). The entire skin flap is lost. The wound is exposed.

The hands, arms, and lower legs are common sites for skin tears. Slight pressure can cause a skin tear.

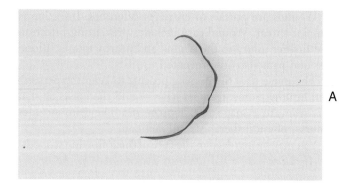

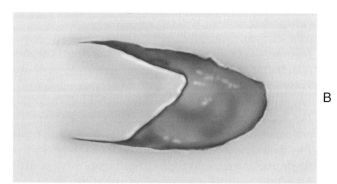

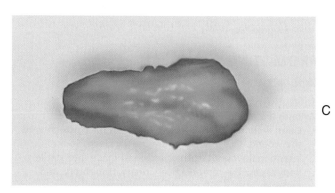

FIGURE 40-7 Skin tears. **A,** No skin loss. **B,** Partial flap loss. **C,** Total flap loss.

Causes

Skin tears are caused by:
- Friction, shearing (Chapter 19), pulling, or pressure on the skin.
- Falls or bumping a hand, arm, or leg on any hard surface. Beds, bed rails, chairs, wheelchair parts, walkers, and tables are dangers.
- Holding an arm or leg too tight.
- Removing tape or adhesives.
- Bathing, dressing, and other tasks.
- Pulling buttons and zippers across fragile skin.
- Jewelry—yours or the person's. Rings, watches, and bracelets are examples.
- Long or jagged fingernails (yours or the person's) and long or jagged toenails.

Skin tears are painful. Portals of entry for microbes, infection is a risk. Tell the nurse at once if you cause or find a skin tear. To prevent skin tears, follow the care plan and the measures in Box 40-1.

BOX 40-1	Preventing Skin Tears

- Follow the care plan and safety rules to:
  - Move, turn, position, or transfer the person.
    - Prevent shearing and friction.
    - Use an assist device to move and turn the person in bed.
    - Use pillows to support arms and legs.
  - Bathe the person.
  - Keep the skin moisturized and apply lotion.
  - Offer fluids.
- Keep your fingernails short and smoothly filed.
- Keep the person's fingernails short and smoothly filed. Report long, tough, or jagged toenails.
- Do not wear rings with large or raised stones. Do not wear bracelets.
- Check the person's rings and bracelets for broken, sharp, or jagged edges. If any are found, tell the nurse. The nurse will handle the matter.
- Be patient and calm when the person is confused, agitated, or resists care.
- Dress and undress the person carefully. Dress the person in soft clothes with long sleeves and long pants.
- Apply arm or leg protectors as ordered (Fig. 40-8).
- Provide a safe setting.
  - Remove clutter from the person's room and hallways.
  - Pad bed rails and wheelchair arms, footplates, and leg supports.
  - Provide good lighting so the person can see. The person must avoid bumping into furniture, walls, and equipment.
  - Provide a safe setting for wandering (Chapter 53).
- Remove tape carefully. To remove tape, hold the skin down and gently pull the tape ends toward the wound.
- Do not apply adhesive tape (p. 625).

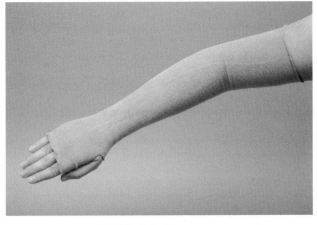

FIGURE 40-8 Skin protector.

Persons at Risk

Persons at risk for skin tears:

- Need help moving.
- Have poor nutrition.
- Have poor hydration.
- Have altered mental awareness.
- Have thin and fragile skin.

See *Focus on Children and Older Persons: Persons at Risk (Skin Tears)*.

FOCUS ON **CHILDREN AND OLDER PERSONS**

Persons at Risk (Skin Tears)

Older Persons

Persons who are confused may resist care. They often move quickly and without warning. Or they pull away during care. Some try to hit or kick. These sudden movements can cause skin tears.

Never force care on a person. Chapter 53 describes how to care for persons who are confused and resist care. Always follow the care plan.

Prevention and Treatment

Careful and safe care helps prevent skin tears and further injury. Follow the measures in Box 40-1. Also follow the care plan and the nurse's directions. They may include dressings (p. 625) and elastic bandages (Chapter 39) to protect the skin and promote healing.

CIRCULATORY ULCERS

Some diseases affect blood flow to and from the legs and feet, leading to circulatory ulcers. *Circulatory ulcers (vascular ulcers) are open sores on the lower legs or feet. They are caused by decreased blood flow through the arteries or veins.* Also called *leg and foot ulcers*, these wounds are painful and hard to heal. Infection and gangrene can develop. *Gangrene is a condition in which there is death of tissue.*

Circulatory ulcers include:

- *Venous ulcers (stasis ulcers) are open sores on the lower legs or feet caused by poor venous blood flow* (Fig. 40-9, p. 620). *Stasis* means *stopped or slowed fluid flow.* The heels and inner part of the ankles are common sites. Venous ulcers can occur from skin injury. Scratching and trauma are examples. Venous ulcers are painful. Infection is a risk. Healing is slow.
- *Arterial ulcers are open wounds on the foot, ankle, or lower leg caused by poor arterial blood flow.* They are found between the toes, on top of the toes, and on the outer side of the ankle (Fig. 40-10, p. 620).
- *Diabetic foot ulcers are open wounds on the foot caused by complications from diabetes.* Diabetes (Chapter 50) can affect the nerves and blood vessels. With nerve damage, the person can lose sensation in a foot or leg. The person may not feel pain, heat, or cold. When blood vessels are affected, blood flow decreases. Tissues and cells do not get needed oxygen and nutrients. Sores heal poorly. Infection and tissue death (gangrene) are risks. Sometimes the affected part must be amputated.

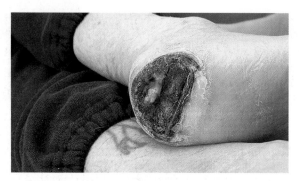

FIGURE 40-9 Venous ulcer.

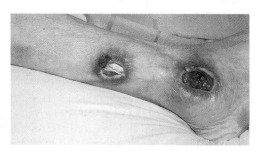

FIGURE 40-10 Arterial ulcer. (From Black JM, Hawks JH: *Medical-surgical nursing: clinical management for positive outcomes,* ed 8, St Louis, 2009, Saunders.)

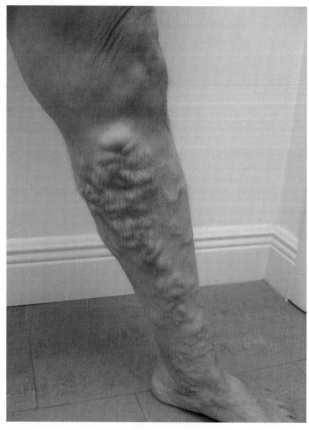

FIGURE 40-11 Varicose veins. Veins under the skin are dilated (wide) and bulging. (From Almeida JI: *Atlas of endovascular venous surgery,* ed 2, Philadelphia, 2019, Elsevier.)

Risk Factors

Risk factors for circulatory ulcers include:
- High blood pressure
- Diabetes
- Injury
- Narrowed arteries from aging
- Smoking
- History of blood clots (Chapter 39)
- Varicose veins (Fig. 40-11)
- Decreased mobility
- Obesity
- Surgery: leg, foot, bones, joints
- Advanced age
- *Phlebitis* (inflammation *[itis]* of a vein *[phleb]*)

Prevention and Treatment

Check the person's feet and legs daily. Report any sign of a problem at once. You must help prevent skin breakdown on the legs and feet. Follow the care plan to prevent and treat circulatory ulcers (Box 40-2). Diabetes foot care can prevent foot problems that cause diabetic foot ulcers (Box 40-3). The doctor orders drugs and treatments as needed.

Persons at risk need professional foot care. *You do not cut the toenails of persons with diseases affecting circulation.*

See *Focus on Long-Term Care and Home Care: Prevention and Treatment,* p. 622.

BOX 40-2 | **Preventing Circulatory Ulcers**

- Remind the person not to sit with the legs crossed.
- Re-position the person according to the care plan—at least every 2 hours.
- Do not use elastic or rubber band–type garters to hold socks or hose in place.
- Apply elastic stockings or elastic bandages as directed (Chapter 39).
- Do not dress the person in tight clothes.
- Provide good skin care daily and as needed. Keep the feet clean and dry. Clean and dry between the toes.
- Report toenails in need of trimming and filing.
- Do not scrub or rub the skin during bathing and drying.
- Keep linens clean, dry, and wrinkle-free.
- Avoid injury to the legs and feet.
- Make sure shoes fit well.
- Keep pressure off the heels and other bony areas. Use pillows or other devices as directed.
- Check the person's legs and feet. Report skin breaks or changes in skin color.
- Do not massage over pressure points (Chapter 41). *Never rub or massage reddened areas.*
- Use protective devices as directed.
- Follow the care plan for walking and exercises.

BOX 40-3 Diabetes Foot Care

Common Problems

- *Corns and calluses* (Fig. 40-12, *A*). These are thick layers of skin caused by too much rubbing or pressure on the same spot. They occur over bony areas.
- *Blisters* (Fig. 40-12, *B*). These form when shoes rub on the same spot. Ill-fitting shoes and wearing shoes without socks are causes.
- *Ingrown toenails* (Fig. 40-12, *C*). An edge of a toenail grows into the skin. This occurs when the skin is cut while trimming toenails or from tight shoes.
- *Bunions* (Fig. 40-12, *D*). A *bunion* is a bump on the outside edge of the big toe. The big toe slants toward the small toes. Heredity is a factor. Shoes that fit poorly (too tight or narrow), high heels, and pointy shoes are causes.
- *Plantar warts* (Fig. 40-12, *E*). *Plantar* means *sole*. Plantar warts occur on the soles (bottoms) of the feet. Caused by a virus, plantar warts are painful.
- *Hammer toes* (Fig. 40-12, *F*). One or more toes are flexed. Diabetic nerve damage can weaken foot muscles. Because of deformed toes, the person has problems walking. Shoes do not fit well. Sores can develop on the tops of the toes and on the bottoms of the feet.
- *Dry and cracked skin* (Fig. 40-12, *G*). Dry skin can occur from nerve damage or poor blood flow in the legs and feet. The dry skin can crack, causing portals of entry for microbes. Infection can occur.
- *Athlete's foot* (Fig. 40-12, *H*). This is a fungus causing itching, burning, redness, and cracked skin between the toes and on the soles of the feet. The cracks are portals of entry for microbes.
- *Fungal infection of the toenails* (Fig. 40-12, *I*). The toenails become thick and hard to cut. They may be yellow, brown, or black. A nail may fall off.

Care Measures

- Check the feet daily for:
  - Cuts
  - Sores
  - Blisters
  - Redness
  - Calluses
  - Infected toenails
  - Ingrown toenails
  - Drainage (p. 624)
  - Warm skin

Care Measures—cont'd

- Wash the feet daily in warm water with mild soap.
  - Test the water temperature with your elbow or use a water thermometer. Because burns are a risk, water temperature should be 90°F to 95°F (Fahrenheit).
  - Do not soak the feet in water. The skin could dry out.
  - Dry the feet well, especially between the toes.
- Apply talcum powder or cornstarch between the toes. This keeps the skin between the toes dry.
- Apply a thin layer of lotion, cream, or petroleum jelly on the tops and bottoms of the feet (not between the toes). Do so after washing and drying to keep the skin soft and smooth.
- Have the person wear closed-toed shoes and clean socks, stockings, or nylons. This prevents blisters and sores.
  - Socks, stockings, and nylons do not have holes or seams.
  - Lightly padded socks are best.
  - Tight socks or knee-high stockings are avoided.
  - Athletic and walking shoes are best.
  - Open-toed shoes, sandals, flip-flops, pointy shoes, and high-heels are not worn.
  - Vinyl and plastic shoes are not worn. They do not stretch and do not allow air movement inside the shoes.
- Check for sharp edges or objects in the shoes. Make sure the lining is smooth.
- Do not allow the person to walk barefoot. The person could step on something and hurt the foot.
- Provide socks at night for cold feet.
- Promote blood flow to the feet. Have the person:
  - Elevate the feet when sitting.
  - Wiggle the toes for 5 minutes 2 or 3 times a day.
  - Move the ankles up and down and in and out.
  - Avoid crossing the legs.
- Do not trim or cut toenails or cut corns or calluses or try to smooth them. Professional foot care is needed.

Modified from National Institute of Diabetes and Digestive and Kidney Diseases: Diabetes and foot problems, *January 2017.*

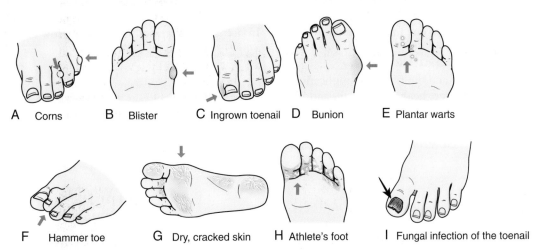

A Corns   B Blister   C Ingrown toenail   D Bunion   E Plantar warts

F Hammer toe   G Dry, cracked skin   H Athlete's foot   I Fungal infection of the toenail

FIGURE 40-12 Foot problems common with diabetes. (Redrawn from National Institute of Diabetes and Digestive and Kidney Diseases: *Prevent diabetes problems: keep your feet healthy,* Bethesda, Md, February 2014, U.S. Department of Health and Human Services.)

WOUND HEALING

The healing process has 3 phases.
- *Phase 1* (3 days). Bleeding stops. A scab forms, preventing microbes from entering the wound. An increased blood supply to the wound brings nutrients and healing substances. Signs and symptoms of inflammation appear—redness, swelling, heat or warmth, and pain. Loss of function may occur.
- *Phase 2* (days 3 to 21). Cells multiply to repair the wound. Some wounds do not heal in a timely manner. A *chronic wound* *does not heal easily and within about 3 months.*
- *Phase 3* (day 21 to 2 years). The scar gains strength. The red, raised scar becomes thin and pale.

Types of Wound Healing

Healing occurs in 3 ways (Fig. 40-13).
- *First (primary) intention.* The wound is closed. Sutures (stitches), staples, clips, special glue, or adhesive strips hold the wound edges together.
- *Second intention.* Contaminated and infected wounds are cleaned and dead tissue removed. Wound edges are not brought together. The wound gaps. Healing takes longer, leaving a larger scar. Infection is a great risk.
- *Third intention.* The wound is left open and closed later. It combines first and second intention. Infection and poor circulation are reasons for third intention.

Complications of Wound Healing

Many factors affect healing and the risk for complications. They include wound type, age, health, nutrition, and lifestyle. Age, smoking, circulatory disease, and diabetes affect circulation. Some drugs prolong bleeding.

Good nutrition is needed. Protein is needed for tissue growth and repair.

Hemorrhage and Shock. *Hemorrhage* is the excessive loss *(rrhage)* of blood *(hemo)* in a short time (Chapter 58). *Shock* results when tissues and organs do not get enough blood (Chapter 58). Both are life-threatening.
- *Internal hemorrhage. Internal* means *inside.* You cannot see bleeding inside tissues and body cavities. A hematoma may form. A *hematoma* is a swelling *(oma)* that contains blood *(hemat)*. The area is swollen and reddish blue in color. Shock, vomiting blood, coughing up blood, and loss of consciousness signal internal hemorrhage.
- *External hemorrhage. External* means *outside.* You can see bleeding outside the body. Common signs are bloody drainage and dressings soaked with blood. Gravity causes fluid to flow down. Check under the body part for pooling of blood.

See Chapter 58 for the signs and symptoms of hemorrhage and shock. Hemorrhage and shock are emergencies. Alert the nurse at once. Assist as requested.

Infection. Contamination can occur during or after injury or surgery. An infected wound appears inflamed (reddened) and has drainage. The wound is painful and tender. The person has a fever.

Immune system changes and antibiotics increase the risk of infection. Specific antibiotics kill specific pathogens. In doing so, other pathogens may grow and multiply.

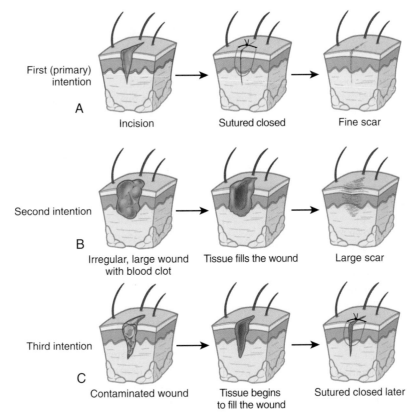

First (primary) intention

A

Incision → Sutured closed → Fine scar

Second intention

B

Irregular, large wound with blood clot → Tissue fills the wound → Large scar

Third intention

C

Contaminated wound → Tissue begins to fill the wound → Sutured closed later

FIGURE 40-13 Wound healing. **A,** First (primary) intention. **B,** Second intention. **C,** Third intention. (Modified from Lewis SL et al.: *Medical-surgical nursing: assessment and management of clinical problems,* ed 10, St Louis, 2017, Elsevier.)

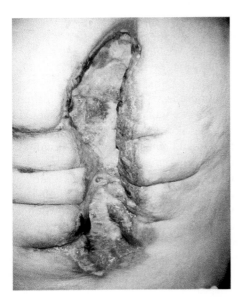

FIGURE 40-14 Wound dehiscence. (Courtesy KCI Licensing, Inc., San Antonio, Tex.)

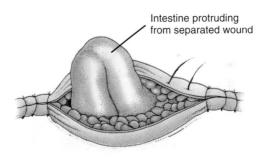

Intestine protruding from separated wound

FIGURE 40-15 Wound evisceration. (Modified from Ignatavicius DD, Workman ML: *Medical-surgical nursing: critical thinking for collaborative care,* ed 5, St Louis, 2006, Saunders.)

Dehiscence and Evisceration.

Dehiscence is the separation of wound layers (Fig. 40-14). *(Dehiscence* is from the Latin word meaning *to gap.)* It may involve the skin layer or underlying tissues. Abdominal wounds are commonly affected.

Evisceration is the separation of the wound along with the protrusion of abdominal organs (Fig. 40-15). *(E* means *out from. Viscera* relates to the *internal organs.)* Coughing, vomiting, and abdominal distention (swelling) place stress on the wound. The person often describes the sensation of the wound "popping open."

Dehiscence and evisceration are surgical emergencies. Tell the nurse at once. The nurse covers the wound with large sterile dressings saturated with saline. Help prepare the person for surgery as directed.

Wound Appearance

The wound and any drainage are observed for healing and complications. See Box 40-4 for observations to make when assisting with wound care. Report and record your observations according to agency policy.

See *Focus on Long-Term Care and Home Care: Wound Appearance.*

BOX 40-4   Wound Observations

- Wound site:
  - Surgery or trauma may involve multiple wounds.
- Wound size and depth are measured by the nurse in centimeters (cm). See Figure 40-16.
- Wound appearance:
  - Is the wound red and swollen?
  - Is the area around the wound warm to touch?
  - Are sutures, staples, or clips intact or broken?
  - Are wound edges closed or separated?
  - Did the wound break open?
- Drainage:
  - Is the drainage serous, sanguineous, serosanguineous, or purulent?
  - What is the amount of drainage?
- Odor:
  - Does the wound or drainage have an odor?
- Surrounding skin:
  - Is surrounding skin intact?
  - What is the color of surrounding skin?
  - Are surrounding tissues swollen?

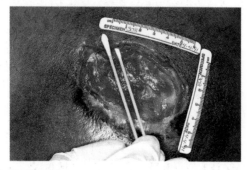

FIGURE 40-16 The size and depth of the wound are measured. (From Potter PA, Perry AG, Stockert PA, Hall AM: *Fundamentals of nursing*, ed 8, St Louis, 2013, Mosby.)

FOCUS ON LONG-TERM CARE AND HOME CARE

Wound Appearance

Home Care

The nurse may use electronic images to assess the wound. Before you take photos or videos, make sure the person has signed the required consents. (The nurse obtains the consents.)

Make sure the date and time stamp features on your electronic device are working. Check that the date and time are correct.

Electronic images do not replace accurate observations. See Box 40-4.

Wound Drainage

During injury and wound healing, fluid and cells escape from tissues. The amount and kind of drainage depends on wound size and site, bleeding, and infection. Wound drainage is observed and measured. See Figure 40-17.

- *Serous drainage—clear, watery fluid* (serum). *Serous* comes from the word *serum.* Serum is the clear, thin, fluid portion of blood. Serum does not contain blood cells or platelets. Fluid in a blister is serous.
- *Sanguineous drainage—bloody* (sanguis) *drainage.* The Latin word *sanguis* means *blood.* Hemorrhage is suspected when large amounts are present. Bright drainage means fresh bleeding. Older bleeding is darker.
- *Serosanguineous drainage—thin, watery drainage* (sero) *that is blood-tinged* (sanguineous).
- *Purulent drainage—thick green, yellow, or brown drainage.*

Drainage must leave the wound for healing. Trapped drainage causes swelling of underlying tissues. The wound may heal at the skin level but underlying tissues do not close. Infection and complications can occur.

When large amounts of drainage are expected, the doctor inserts a drain. A *Penrose drain* is a rubber tube that opens and drains onto a dressing (Fig. 40-18). An open drain, microbes can enter the drain and wound.

Closed drainage systems prevent microbes from entering the wound. A drain is attached to suction. The *Hemovac* (Fig. 40-19) and *Jackson-Pratt* (Fig. 40-20) systems are examples. Other systems depend on the wound type, size, and site.

You may assist the nurse in observing the wound drainage. For a closed drainage system, follow agency policy and the manufacturer's instructions.

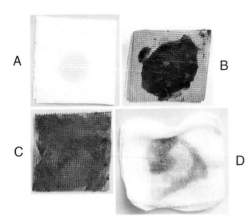

FIGURE 40-17 Wound drainage. **A,** Serous drainage. **B,** Sanguineous drainage. **C,** Serosanguineous drainage. **D,** Purulent drainage. (From Potter PA, Perry AG, Stockert PA, Hall AM: *Fundamentals of nursing*, ed 9, St Louis, 2017, Elsevier.)

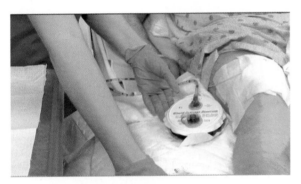

FIGURE 40-19 Hemovac. Drains are sutured to the wound and connected to a reservoir. (From Mosby's Nursing Video Skills 4.0, St. Louis, Basic Intermediate and Advanced Skills, St Louis, 2014, Mosby.)

DRESSINGS

Wound dressings have many functions. They:
- Protect wounds from injury and microbes.
- Absorb drainage.
- Remove dead tissue.
- Promote comfort.
- Cover unsightly wounds.
- Provide a moist environment for wound healing.
- Apply pressure (pressure dressings) to help control bleeding.

Dressing type and size depend on the type of wound, its size and site, and the amount of drainage (Fig. 40-21, p. 626). Infection is a factor. The dressing's function and the frequency of dressing changes are other factors.

Some dressings have special agents for wound healing. If you assist with a dressing change, the nurse explains its use to you.

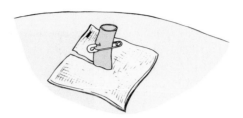

FIGURE 40-18 Penrose drain. (From Potter PA, Perry AG, Stockert PA, Hall AM: *Fundamentals of nursing*, ed 9, St Louis, 2017, Elsevier.)

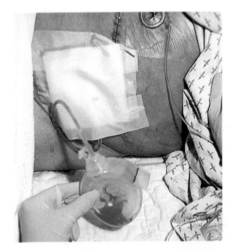

FIGURE 40-20 Jackson-Pratt drainage system. (From Potter PA, Perry AG, Stockert PA, Hall AM: *Fundamentals of nursing*, ed 9, St Louis, 2017, Elsevier.)

Securing Dressings

Dressings must be secured over wounds. Microbes can enter the wound and drainage can escape if the dressing is dislodged. Tape and Montgomery straps (p. 626) secure dressings. Binders (p. 629) hold dressings in place.

Tape. Adhesive, paper, plastic, cloth, and elastic tapes are common. Adhesive tape sticks well. However, adhesive problems include:
- It is hard to remove from the skin.
- It can irritate the skin.
- Skin tears or abrasions can occur when tape is removed.
- Adhesive tape allergies are common.

Paper, plastic, and cloth tapes usually do not cause allergic reactions. Elastic tape allows movement of the body part.

Tape comes in $\frac{1}{2}$, $\frac{3}{4}$, 1, 2, and 3 inch widths. Tape is applied to the top, middle, and bottom of the dressing. The tape must be wide enough and long enough to extend beyond each side of the dressing (Fig. 40-22, p. 626). *Do not apply tape to circle the entire body part. If swelling occurs, circulation to the part is impaired.*

See *Focus on Communication: Tape*, p. 626.

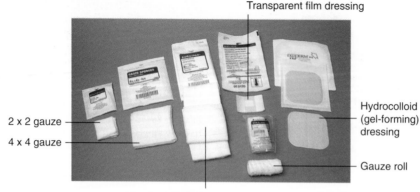

FIGURE 40-21 Types of dressings. (Modified from Williams P: *deWit's fundamental concepts and skills for nursing*, ed 5, St Louis, 2018, Elsevier.)

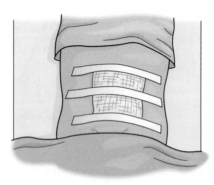

FIGURE 40-22 Tape is applied at the top, middle, and bottom of the dressing. The tape extends beyond both sides of the dressing.

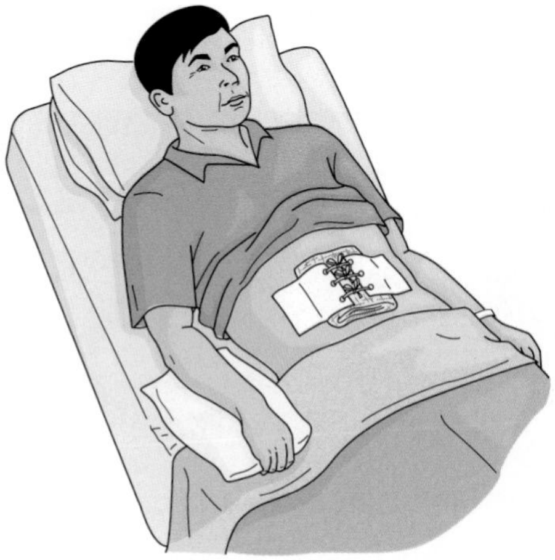

FIGURE 40-23 Montgomery straps.

FOCUS ON COMMUNICATION

Tape

Before applying tape, ask if the person has an allergy to tape. You can ask:

- "Do any types of tape irritate your skin?"
- "Do you have an allergy to tape?"

Montgomery Straps. Montgomery straps (Fig. 40-23) are used for large dressings and frequent dressing changes. A Montgomery strap has a tape strip and cloth tie. With the dressing in place, the tape strips are placed on both sides of the dressing. Then the straps are secured over the dressing.

The straps are undone for the dressing change. The tape strips stay in place. They are removed if soiled. Montgomery straps protect the skin from frequent tape application and removal.

Applying Dressings

A wound may not require a dressing and may be left "open to air." Or a transparent dressing covers the wound, which allows it to be seen for observations. Still other wounds require dressings that range from simple to complex.

See *Focus on Children and Older Persons: Applying Dressings.*

See *Teamwork and Time Management: Applying Dressings.*

See *Delegation Guidelines: Applying Dressings.*

See *Promoting Safety and Comfort: Applying Dressings.*

See procedure: *Applying a Dry, Non-Sterile Dressing,* p. 628.

FOCUS ON CHILDREN AND OLDER PERSONS

Applying Dressings

Children

Dressing changes may frighten children. Tape removal can be painful. Wound appearance can be frightening. A calm, cooperative child helps prevent contamination of the sterile field. A parent or caregiver holds the child so the wound can be reached easily. Holding or playing with a toy can comfort the child.

TEAMWORK AND TIME MANAGEMENT
Applying Dressings

Collect all needed items before you start. Have extra dressings, tape, and other supplies on hand. Leave un-used items in the room for the next dressing change. Wound contamination can occur if you need to leave the room during the procedure.

DELEGATION GUIDELINES
Applying Dressings

Applying dressings is a nursing responsibility that may be delegated to you in some agencies. When applying a dressing is delegated to you, make sure that:
- Your state allows you to perform the procedure.
- The procedure is in your job description.
- You have the necessary training.
- You know how to use the equipment.
- You review the procedure with the nurse.
- A nurse is available to answer questions and to guide and assist you as needed.
  If the above conditions are met, follow the rules in Box 40-5. You will need this information from the nurse.
- When to change the dressing
- When a pain-relief drug will take effect
- What to do if the dressing sticks to the wound
- How to clean the wound
- What dressings to use
- How to secure the dressing—tape or Montgomery straps
- What kind of tape to use—adhesive, paper, plastic, cloth, or elastic
- What size tape to use—½, ¾, 1, 2, or 3 inch width
- What observations to report and record:
  - Supplies used to dress the wound and secure the dressing
  - A red or swollen wound
  - An area around the wound that is warm to touch
  - If wound edges are closed or separated
  - A wound that has broken open
  - Drainage appearance—clear, bloody, or watery and blood-tinged; thick and green, yellow, or brown (p. 624)
  - The amount of drainage
  - Wound or drainage odor
  - Intactness and color of surrounding tissues
  - Possible dressing contamination—urine; feces; other body fluids, secretions, or excretions; dislodged dressing
  - Pain
  - Fever
- When to report observations
- What patient or resident concerns to report at once

BOX 40-5   Applying Dressings

- Let pain-relief drugs take effect, usually 30 minutes. The dressing change can cause discomfort. After giving the drug, the nurse tells you how long to wait.
- Meet fluid and elimination needs before you begin.
- Collect equipment and supplies before you begin.
- Do not bend or reach over your work area.
- Control your nonverbal communication. Wound odors, appearance, and drainage may be unpleasant. Do not communicate your thoughts or reactions to the person.
- Remove soiled dressings so the person cannot see the soiled side. The drainage and its color may upset the person.
- Do not force the person to look at the wound. A wound can affect body image and self-esteem. The nurse helps the person deal with the wound.
- Remove tape by gently pulling the tape ends toward the wound.
- Remove dressings gently. They may stick to the wound, drain, or surrounding skin. If the dressing sticks, the nurse may have you wet the dressing with a saline solution. A wet dressing is easier to remove.
- Touch only the outer edges of new dressings as you would for a sterile field (Chapter 16).
- Report and record your observations. See *Delegation Guidelines: Applying Dressings*.

PROMOTING SAFETY AND COMFORT
Applying Dressings

Safety
Tape removal can cause skin tears in persons with thin, fragile skin. Use extreme care to remove tape.

Do not apply tape to irritated, injured, or non-intact skin. Tape can further damage the skin.

Dressings containing blood are regulated waste. Follow the Bloodborne Pathogen Standard and agency policy to dispose of soiled dressings.

Comfort
Wounds and dressing changes can cause discomfort or pain. Allow time for a pain-relief drug to take effect before a dressing change. Gently apply and remove tape and dressings.

The person may not report discomfort from a dressing. You should ask:
- "Is the dressing comfortable?"
- "Does the tape cause pain or itching?"

Applying a Dry, Non-Sterile Dressing

QUALITY OF LIFE

- Knock before entering the person's room.
- Address the person by name.
- Introduce yourself by name and title.

- Explain the procedure before starting and during the procedure.
- Protect the person's rights during the procedure.
- Handle the person gently during the procedure.

PRE-PROCEDURE

1 Follow *Delegation Guidelines: Applying Dressings*, p. 627.
   See *Promoting Safety and Comfort:*
   a *Wound Care*, p. 617
   b *Applying Dressings*, p. 627
2 Practice hand hygiene.
3 Collect the following.
   - Gloves
   - PPE (personal protective equipment) as needed
   - Tape or Montgomery straps
   - Dressings as directed by the nurse
   - 4 × 4 gauze (see Fig. 40-21)
   - Saline solution as directed by the nurse
   - Cleaning solution as directed by the nurse

   - Adhesive remover
   - Dressing set with scissors and forceps
   - Plastic bag
   - Bath blanket
4 Practice hand hygiene.
5 Identify the person. Check the ID (identification) bracelet against the assignment sheet. Use 2 identifiers (Chapter 13). Also call the person by name.
6 Provide for privacy.
7 Arrange your work area. You should not have to reach over or turn your back on your work area.
8 Raise the bed for body mechanics. Bed rails are up if used.

PROCEDURE

9 Lower the bed rail near you if up.
10 Help the person to a comfortable position.
11 Cover the person with a bath blanket. Fan-fold top linens to the foot of the bed.
12 Expose the affected body part.
13 Make a cuff on the plastic bag. Place the bag within reach.
14 Practice hand hygiene.
15 Don needed PPE. Put on gloves.
16 Remove tape or undo Montgomery straps.
   a *Tape:* hold the skin down. Gently pull the tape toward the wound.
   b *Montgomery straps:* undo the straps. Fold the straps away from the wound.
17 Remove any adhesive from the skin. Pick up a gauze square with the forceps. Wet a 4 × 4 gauze dressing with adhesive remover. Clean away from the wound.
18 Remove dressings with a gloved hand or the forceps (Fig. 40-24). Start with the top dressing and remove each layer. Keep the soiled side away from the person's sight. Put dressings in the plastic bag. They must not touch the outside of the bag.

19 Remove the dressing over the wound very gently. It may stick to the wound or drain site. Moisten the dressing with saline if it sticks to the wound. Discard the dressing as in step 18.
20 Observe the wound, drain site, and wound drainage.
21 Remove the gloves and put them in the bag. Practice hand hygiene.
22 Open the new dressings.
23 Put on clean gloves.
24 Clean the wound with saline as directed by the nurse. See Figure 40-25.
25 Apply dressings as directed by the nurse (Fig. 40-26). See "Surgical Asepsis" in Chapter 16.
26 Secure the dressings. Use tape or Montgomery straps.
27 Remove the gloves. Put them in the bag.
28 Remove and discard PPE.
29 Practice hand hygiene.
30 Cover the person. Remove the bath blanket.

POST-PROCEDURE

31 Provide for comfort. (See the inside of the back cover.)
32 Place the call light and other needed items within reach.
33 Lower the bed to a safe and comfortable level. Follow the care plan.
34 Raise or lower bed rails. Follow the care plan.
35 Return equipment and supplies to their proper place. Leave extra dressings and tape in the room.
36 Discard used supplies in the bag. Tie the bag closed. Discard the bag following agency policy. (Wear gloves for this step.)

37 Clean your work area. Follow the Bloodborne Pathogen Standard.
38 Unscreen the person.
39 Complete a safety check of the room. (See the inside of the back cover.)
40 Remove and discard the gloves. Practice hand hygiene.
41 Report and record your observations.

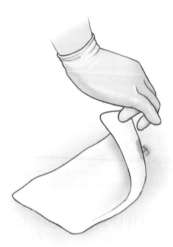

FIGURE 40-24 Removing a dressing. Keep the soiled side away from the person's sight.

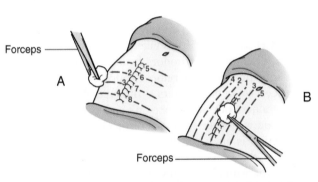

FIGURE 40-25 Cleaning a wound. **A,** Start at the wound and stroke out to the surrounding skin. Use new gauze for each stroke. **B,** Clean the wound from the top to the bottom. Start at the wound. Then clean the surrounding areas. Use new gauze for each stroke. (From Potter PA, Perry AG, Stockert PA, Hall AM: *Fundamentals of nursing,* ed 9, St Louis, 2017, Elsevier.)

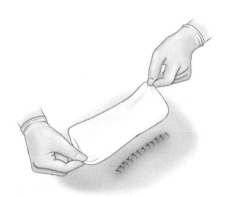

FIGURE 40-26 Applying a dressing. Wear clean gloves. Touch only the outer edges of the dressing. Do not touch the part that will contact the wound.

BINDERS AND COMPRESSION GARMENTS

Binders are wide bands of elastic fabric. They support wounds and hold dressings in place. They also prevent or reduce swelling, promote comfort, and prevent injury. These binders are common.

- *Abdominal binder*—provides abdominal support and holds dressings in place (Fig. 40-27). The top part is at the waist. The lower part is over the hips. Binders are secured in place with Velcro or with hook and loop closures.
- *Breast binder*—supports the breasts after surgery (Fig. 40-28). It is secured in place with Velcro or padded zippers.

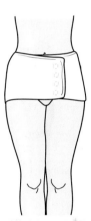

FIGURE 40-27 Abdominal binder. The top part is at the waist. The lower part is over the hips.

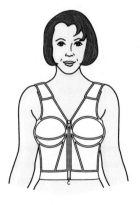

FIGURE 40-28 Breast binder.

Compression garments are made of a tight, stretchy fabric (Fig. 40-29). Commonly worn after plastic surgery, they help:

- Reduce swelling.
- Prevent fluid buildup at the surgical site.
- Hold the skin against the body.
- Achieve the desired shape.

Box 40-6 lists the rules for applying binders and compression garments.

See *Focus on Communication: Binders and Compression Garments.*

See *Promoting Safety and Comfort: Binders and Compression Garments.*

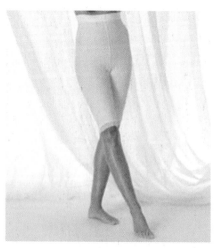

FIGURE 40-29 Compression garment. (Courtesy Rainey Compression Essentials, Atlanta, Ga.)

BOX 40-6   Binders and Compression Garments

- Follow the manufacturer's instructions.
- Position the person in good alignment.
- Apply the device for firm, even pressure over the area.
- Apply the device so it is snug. It must not interfere with breathing or circulation.
- Re-apply the device if it is out of position or causes discomfort.
- Change the device if moist or soiled. This prevents the growth of microbes.
- Tell the nurse at once if the person's breathing changes.
- Check the skin under and around the device. Tell the nurse at once if there is redness, irritation, or other signs of a skin problem.

FOCUS ON COMMUNICATION

Binders and Compression Garments

The person may not tell you about pain or discomfort. You need to ask:

- "Is the binder (or garment) too tight or too loose?"
- "Does the binder (or garment) cause pain?"
- "Do you feel pressure from the binder (or garment)?" If yes: "Where? Please show me."

PROMOTING SAFETY AND COMFORT

Binders and Compression Garments

Safety

Apply binders and compression garments properly. Doing so helps prevent discomfort, skin irritation, and circulatory and respiratory problems. Correct application is needed for safety and for the device to work properly.

Comfort

A binder or compression garment should promote comfort. Tell the nurse if the device causes pain or discomfort.

HEAT AND COLD APPLICATIONS

Heat and cold applications promote healing and comfort. They also reduce tissue swelling. See Chapter 42.

MEETING BASIC NEEDS

Wounds may be large or small, simple or complex. A wound can affect basic needs. However, it is only part of the person's care. Remember, the *person* has the wound.

Pain and discomfort may affect breathing and moving. Turning, re-positioning, and walking may be painful. Be gentle. Let pain-relief drugs take effect before giving care.

Pain, discomfort, and odors from wound drainage can affect appetite. Promptly remove soiled dressings from the room. Use room deodorizers as directed. Also keep drainage containers out of the person's sight. Tell the nurse if the person wants certain foods or drinks.

Infection is always a threat. Follow Standard Precautions and the Bloodborne Pathogen Standard. Carefully observe the wound for signs and symptoms of infection.

Delayed healing is a risk for persons who are older, obese, or have poor nutrition. Protein is needed for tissue growth and repair. Poor circulation and diabetes also affect healing, increasing the risk of infection.

Safety and security needs are affected. Scarring, disfigurement, delayed healing, and infection are common fears. So are fears about the wound "popping open." Medical bills are other concerns. The person may need care for a long time.

Victims of violence may fear future attacks and worry about finding and convicting the attacker and about family safety. Victims of intimate partner, child, and elder abuse often hide the source of their injuries.

Others might see wounds on the head, face, arms, or legs. Clothing is useful in hiding some wounds. Disfiguring wounds can affect sexual performance or feelings of sexual attraction. With amputation, the person has to adapt to perform daily activities and work. Eye injuries can cause vision changes. Abdominal trauma and surgery can affect eating and elimination.

Along with body image, love and belonging and self-esteem needs are affected. The person may be sad and tearful or angry and hostile. Adjustment may require rehabilitation and counseling. Be gentle and kind, give thoughtful care, and practice good communication.

FOCUS ON **PRIDE**

The Person, Family, and Yourself

Personal and Professional Responsibility

As a nursing assistant, you have responsibilities for wound care. For example, if you are careless during a transfer, you can cause a skin tear. If you rush during a bath, you may not notice a wound between skin folds. If you do not apply shoes properly, a foot ulcer can develop.

How you provide care affects the person's health, safety, and quality of life. Take pride in working safely and carefully.

Rights and Respect

A person may have questions about wound care such as why an incision has no dressing. Tell the person that you will ask the nurse to explain reasons for care. Wait until questions are answered before performing the care measure.

Independence and Social Interaction

Wounds, dressings, drainage and drainage devices, and wound odors may disturb patients, residents, and visitors. Visitors may feel uncomfortable. To promote comfort and interaction with family and friends:

* Keep the wound or dressing covered if able.
* Ask visitors to leave the room during dressing changes or when exposing the wound or dressing.
* Remove soiled dressings from the room promptly.
* Keep drainage containers out of sight if able. Some large containers can be covered with a towel if directed by the nurse.
* Use a room deodorizer for odors as directed.

Delegation and Teamwork

Wound care can be painful and tiring. To promote comfort and rest:

* Ask when pain-relief drugs will be given and take effect. Allow rest periods before and after care.
* Be prepared. Leaving to get supplies causes care and procedures to take longer than planned.
* Assist the nurse as instructed. You may need to position the person or raise a body part while the nurse changes a dressing. Teamwork reduces the amount of energy the person must use.

Ethics and Laws

Agency practices vary for charging supplies. Ethical practice involves honestly following agency rules. Not charging supplies correctly costs the nursing unit and agency money. Taking supplies home for your own use is unethical. This is stealing. Take pride in following agency rules and being an honest and reliable member of the nursing team.

FOCUS ON **PRIDE**: *Application*

Define *body image*. Is body image the same for all persons? Is it the same throughout a person's life? Explain. How might a wound affect body image?

REVIEW QUESTIONS

Circle the BEST answer.

1. A person has a laceration from a fall. The wound is
   a. At risk for infection
   b. An incision
   c. A chronic wound
   d. A clean wound

2. A person had rectal surgery. The person has a
   a. Clean wound
   b. Dirty wound
   c. Clean-contaminated wound
   d. Contaminated wound

3. Skin rubbing against skin can cause
   a. Excoriation
   b. An incision
   c. A laceration
   d. A penetrating wound

4. Which can cause skin tears?
   a. Trimmed and smooth nails
   b. Soft clothing
   c. Rings
   d. Padded wheelchair footplates

5. A person has a circulatory ulcer. Which measure should you question?
   a. Do not cut or trim toenails.
   b. Hold socks in place with elastic garters.
   c. Apply elastic stockings.
   d. Re-position the person every hour.

6. Diabetic foot ulcers are caused by
   a. Gangrene
   b. Amputation
   c. Infection
   d. Nerve and blood vessel damage

7. A person has diabetes. When providing foot care
   a. Dry well between the toes
   b. Apply lotion between the toes
   c. Trim the toenails
   d. Use hot water

8. A person with diabetes wears socks with shoes to prevent
   a. Corns
   b. Bunions
   c. Blisters
   d. Plantar warts

Continued

REVIEW QUESTIONS—cont'd

9 A wound is separating. This is called
   a Primary intention
   b Third intention
   c Dehiscence
   d Evisceration

10 Clear, watery drainage from a wound is called
   a Purulent drainage
   b Serous drainage
   c Sero-purulent drainage
   d Serosanguineous drainage

11 Dressings
   a Protect the wound from injury
   b Prevent drainage
   c Provide a dry environment for healing
   d Support the wound and reduce swelling

12 To secure a dressing, apply tape
   a Around the entire part
   b Along the sides of the dressing
   c To the top, middle, and bottom of the dressing
   d As the person prefers

13 A person has frequent dressing changes. The nurse will likely have the dressings secured with
   a A binder
   b Montgomery straps
   c Paper or cloth tape
   d An elastic bandage

14 How long should you wait for a pain-relief drug to take effect?
   a 5 minutes
   b 10 minutes
   c 15 minutes
   d 30 minutes

15 To remove tape
   a Pull it away from the wound
   b Pull it toward the wound
   c Use forceps
   d Use a saline solution

16 An abdominal binder is used to
   a Prevent blood clots
   b Prevent wound infection
   c Provide support and hold dressings in place
   d Decrease swelling and circulation

Answers to Chapter 40 questions are on p. 887.

FOCUS ON PRACTICE

Problem Solving

An older resident has thin, fragile skin. You notice a new skin tear on the person's arm. What do you do? How can you prevent skin tears?

Pressure Injuries

41

OBJECTIVES

- Define the key terms and key abbreviations in this chapter.
- Describe the causes and risk factors for pressure injuries.
- Identify the persons at risk for pressure injuries.
- Describe the stages of pressure injuries and the Kennedy terminal ulcer.

- Identify the sites for pressure injuries.
- Explain how to prevent pressure injuries.
- Identify the complications from pressure injuries.
- Explain how to promote PRIDE in the person, the family, and yourself.

KEY TERMS

avoidable pressure injury A pressure injury that develops from the improper use of the nursing process
bedfast Confined to bed
bony prominence An area where the bone sticks out or projects from the flat surface of the body; pressure point
chairfast Confined to a chair
colonized The presence of bacteria on the wound surface or in wound tissue; the person does not have signs and symptoms of an infection
epidermal stripping Removing the epidermis (outer skin layer) as tape is removed from the skin
eschar Thick, leathery dead tissue that may be loose or adhered to the skin; it is often black or brown
intact skin Normal skin and skin layers without damage or breaks

pressure injury Localized damage to the skin and underlying soft tissue; the injury is usually over a bony prominence or related to a medical or other device and results from pressure or pressure in combination with shear
pressure point See "bony prominence"
shear When layers of the skin rub against each other; when the skin remains in place and underlying tissues move and stretch, tearing underlying capillaries and blood vessels and causing tissue damage
skin breakdown Changes or damage to intact skin—normal skin and skin layers
slough Dead tissue that is shed from the skin; it is usually light colored, soft, and moist; may be stringy at times
unavoidable pressure injury A pressure injury that occurs despite efforts to prevent one through proper use of the nursing process

KEY ABBREVIATIONS

CMS   Centers for Medicare & Medicaid Services

NPIAP   National Pressure Injury Advisory Panel

The National Pressure Injury Advisory Panel (NPIAP) defines *pressure injury* (Fig. 41-1, p. 634) *as:*
- *Localized damage to the skin and underlying soft tissue.*
- *The injury is usually over a bony prominence or related to a medical or other device.*
- *The injury results from pressure or pressure in combination with shear.*

A **bony prominence (pressure point)** *is an area where the bone sticks out or projects from the flat surface of the body.* The back of the head, shoulder blades, elbows, hips, spine, sacrum, knees, ankles, heels, and toes are bony prominences (Fig. 41-2, p. 634).

Pressure injuries result from intense or prolonged pressure and shear. *Shear is when layers of the skin rub against each other. Or shear is when the skin remains in place and underlying tissues move and stretch, tearing underlying capillaries and blood vessels. Tissue damage occurs.*

Possibly painful, a pressure injury may involve intact skin or an open ulcer.
- *Intact skin is normal skin and skin layers without damage or breaks* (Fig. 41-3, p. 635).
- An ulcer is a shallow or deep crater-like sore of the skin or mucous membrane (see Fig. 41-1).

Some agencies and organizations use the term *pressure ulcer*. The term *bedsore* is commonly used by patients, residents, and families. Pressure injury, pressure ulcer, and bedsore essentially mean the same thing.

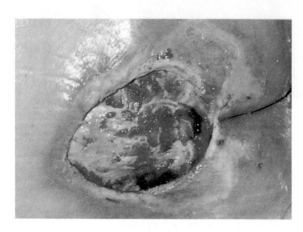

FIGURE 41-1 A pressure injury. (From Ostomy Wound Management, *Proceedings from the November National V.A.C.* ® 51[2A, supp]: 7S, Feb 2005, HMP Communications. Used with permission.)

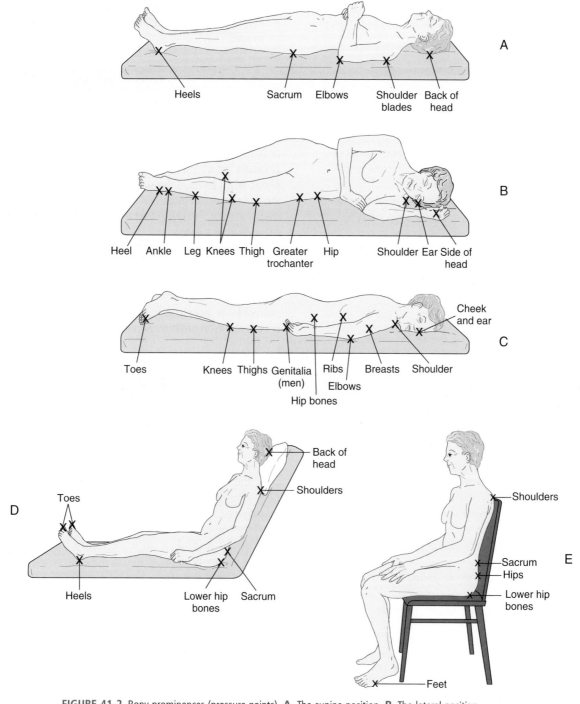

FIGURE 41-2 Bony prominences (pressure points). **A,** The supine position. **B,** The lateral position. **C,** The prone position. **D,** Fowler's position. **E,** Sitting position.

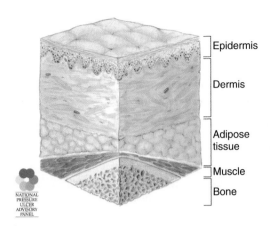

FIGURE 41-3 Intact skin. (Used with permission of the National Pressure Injury Advisory Panel.)

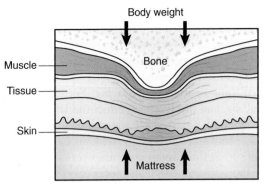

FIGURE 41-4 Tissue under pressure. The skin is squeezed between 2 hard surfaces—the bone and the mattress. (Redrawn from Agency for Healthcare Research and Quality: *Understanding your body: what are pressure ulcers?* Rockville, Md, November 2007, U.S. Department of Health and Human Services.)

RISK FACTORS

Pressure and shearing are the major causes of pressure injuries. They also cause skin breakdown that can lead to pressure injuries. *Skin breakdown involves changes or damage to intact skin.*

Unrelieved pressure squeezes tiny blood vessels. For example, pressure occurs when the skin over a bony area is squeezed between hard surfaces (Fig. 41-4). The bone is 1 hard surface. The other is usually the mattress or seat. Squeezing or pressure prevents blood flow to the skin and underlying tissues. Oxygen and nutrients cannot get to the cells. Skin and tissues die.

Shear occurs when the person slides down in the bed or chair. Blood vessels and tissues are damaged. Blood flow to the area is reduced.

See Box 41-1 for pressure injury risk factors. Agencies must identify persons at risk for pressure injuries. The health team assesses the person's physical and mental health. A person's risk may increase during an illness, from condition changes, because of injury or surgery, or from medical devices. The person's care plan must include measures to reduce or remove risk factors. See "Persons at Risk," p. 636.

See *Teamwork and Time Management: Risk Factors.*

BOX 41-1	Pressure Injury Risk Factors

- Aging and age-related skin changes
- Skin breakdown and non-intact skin
- Dry skin
- Fragile and weak capillaries
- General thinning of the skin
- Loss of the fatty layer under the skin
- Decreased sensation to touch, heat, and cold
- Decreased mobility
- Limited activity: for example, sitting in a chair or lying in bed most or all of the day
- Chronic diseases (diabetes, high blood pressure)
- Diseases that decrease circulation and oxygen to tissues; poor circulation to an area
- Fever
- Poor nutrition
- Poor hydration
- Incontinence: urinary, fecal
- Moisture in dark body areas: skin folds, under breasts, perineal area
- Pressure on bony parts (pressure points)
- Poor fingernail and toenail care
- Friction (rubbing of 1 surface against another) and shearing
- *Edema* (the swelling of body tissues with water)

TEAMWORK AND TIME MANAGEMENT

Risk Factors

You must help prevent pressure injuries. As you walk in hallways, look to see if a person has slid down in bed or in a chair. Do the same when people are in dining and lounge areas. Help re-position the person. Ask a co-worker to help you as needed. Report the re-positioning to the nurse.

PERSONS AT RISK

Persons at risk for pressure injuries are those who:

- Are *bedfast* (*confined to bed*) or *chairfast* (*confined to a chair*). Pressure occurs from lying or sitting in the same position too long.
- Need some or total help moving. For example, coma, paralysis, and hip fractures affect the ability to move.
- Are agitated, have muscle spasms, or have involuntary muscle movements. The movements cause rubbing (friction) against linens and other surfaces.
- Are incontinent. Urine and feces (stools) irritate the skin, leading to skin breakdown. They are also sources of moisture.
- Are exposed to moisture. Urine, feces (stools), wound drainage, sweat, and saliva are sources of moisture. Moisture irritates the skin. It also increases the risk of friction and shearing during re-positioning.
- Have poor nutrition or poor fluid balance. A balanced diet nourishes the skin. Fluid balance is needed for healthy skin.
- Have limited awareness. The person does not know to move or change positions. Some drugs and health problems can affect awareness.
- Have problems sensing pain or pressure. The person does not know to alert the staff to these symptoms of tissue damage.
- Have circulatory problems. Cells and tissues die when starved of oxygen and nutrients.
- Are obese, have weight loss, or are very thin. Loss of muscle and fat reduces padding between bones and surfaces.
- Have medical devices. A pressure injury can develop where a medical device causes pressure on the skin.
- Have an existing or healed pressure injury. See "Pressure Injury Stages."

See *Focus on Children and Older Persons: Persons at Risk.*

FOCUS ON CHILDREN AND OLDER PERSONS

Persons at Risk

Children

Ill infants and children and those with mobility problems are at risk for pressure injuries. The back of the head is a common site. Incontinence (urinary and fecal) is also a risk factor.

Pressure, friction, shearing, poor nutrition, infection, medical devices, and epidermal stripping are causes. *Epidermal stripping is removing the epidermis (outer skin layer) as tape is removed from the skin.* Newborns are at risk because of their fragile skin.

Older Persons

Older persons have thin, fragile skin that is easily injured. Some have chronic diseases affecting mobility, nutrition, circulation, and awareness.

The Centers for Medicare & Medicaid Services (CMS) requires that nursing centers identify persons at risk for pressure injuries. A person can develop a pressure injury within 2 to 6 hours after the onset of pressure.

PRESSURE INJURY STAGES

Pressure injuries range from reddened intact skin to tissue loss with bone exposure. See Box 41-2 for pressure injury stages.

See *Focus on Communication: Pressure Injury Stages.*

See *Focus on Long-Term Care and Home Care: Pressure Injury Stages.*

Text continued on p. 640.

BOX 41-2   Pressure Injury Stages

Stage 1 pressure injury: non-blanchable erythema of intact skin. To *blanch* means *to become white.* When pressure is applied to the skin, blood is pressed away. This causes the skin to become white or pale. When pressure is relieved, the skin returns to its normal color. *Erythema* means *red or redness. Non-blanchable erythema* means *that the reddened skin does not become white or pale when pressure is applied and removed* (Fig. 41-5). With Stage 1 pressure injury, intact skin has a reddened area that is non-blanchable. See Figure 41-6.

Stage 2 pressure injury: partial-thickness skin loss with exposed dermis. The wound is pink or red and moist. It may involve a broken or intact blister. Fat and deeper tissues are not visible. See Figure 41-7, p. 638.

Stage 3 pressure injury: full-thickness skin loss. The skin is gone. Fat can be seen in the ulcer. Slough and/or eschar may be present. See Figure 41-8, p. 638.
- *Slough is dead tissue that is shed from the skin. It is usually light colored, soft, and moist. It may be stringy at times* (Fig. 41-9, p. 638).
- *Eschar is thick, leathery dead tissue that may be loose or adhered to the skin. It is often black or brown* (Fig. 41-10, p. 638).

Stage 4 pressure injury: full-thickness skin and tissue loss. The skin is gone. Muscle, tendon, ligament, cartilage, or bone is exposed. Slough and/or eschar may be seen. See Figure 41-11, p. 639.

Unstageable pressure injury: obscured full-thickness skin and tissue loss. *Obscure* means *not plain or clear.* There is skin and tissue loss. The extent of tissue damage cannot be seen because of slough or eschar. When slough or eschar is removed, the injury can be seen. See Figure 41-12, p. 639.

Deep tissue pressure injury: persistent non-blanchable deep red, maroon, or purple discoloration. Intact or non-intact skin is deep red, maroon, or purple and remains non-blanchable. The wound is dark or is a blood-filled blister. See Figure 41-13, p. 640.

Modified from European Pressure Ulcer Advisory Panel, National Pressure Injury Advisory Panel, and Pan Pacific Pressure Injury Alliance: Prevention and treatment of pressure ulcers/injuries: quick reference guide, Emily Haesler (Ed.), 2019, EPUAP/NPIAP/PPPIA.

Pressure Injury Stages

Report areas of redness, skin color changes, blisters, or skin or tissue loss. Describe what you see as best as you can. Tell the nurse the site. The nurse needs to assess the area. For example, you can say:

- "I saw a reddened area on Mr. Drake's left heel. It was about the size of a quarter. The skin looked intact. Please look at it."
- "I noticed a red area with a blister on Ms. Walsh's left buttock. I didn't see any drainage. Please look at it. I'll help you turn her."

Pressure Injury Stages

Home Care

Home care patients can develop pressure injuries. Check the person's skin during every visit. Report and record your observations.

Remind family members to check the person's skin. They need to call the nurse if pressure injury signs are noted.

Blanchable vs Non-Blanchable

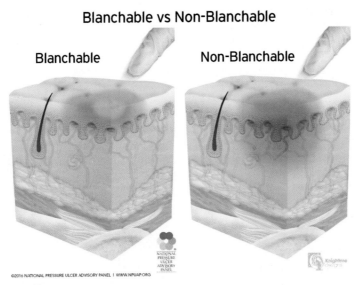

FIGURE 41-5 Blanchable and non-blanchable skin. (Used with permission of the National Pressure Injury Advisory Panel, January 2017.)

Stage 1 Pressure Injury – Darkly Pigmented   Stage 1 Pressure Injury – Lightly Pigmented

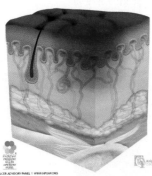 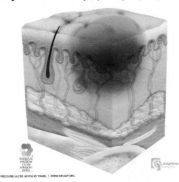 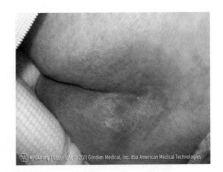

FIGURE 41-6 Stage 1 pressure injury. NOTE: *Pigment gives color to the skin. Intact skin with a localized area of non-blanchable erythema, which may appear differently in darkly pigmented skin. Presence of blanchable erythema or changes in sensation, temperature, or firmness may precede visual changes. Color changes do not include purple or maroon discoloration; these may indicate deep tissue pressure injury.* (Illustrations, photo, and definition used with permission and as required by the National Pressure Injury Advisory Panel, January 2017.)

Stage 2 Pressure Injury

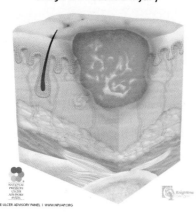

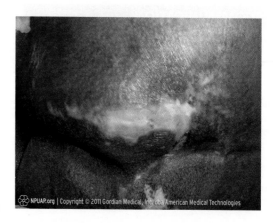

FIGURE 41-7 Stage 2 pressure injury. *Partial-thickness loss of skin with exposed dermis. The wound bed is viable, pink or red, moist, and may also present as an intact or ruptured serum-filled blister. Adipose (fat) is not visible and deeper tissues are not visible. Granulation tissue, slough and eschar are not present. These injuries commonly result from adverse microclimate and shear in the skin over the pelvis and shear in the heel. This stage should not be used to describe moisture associated skin damage (MASD) including incontinence associated dermatitis (IAD), intertriginous dermatitis (ITD), medical adhesive related skin injury (MARSI), or traumatic wounds (skin tears, burns, abrasions). (Illustration, photo, and definition used with permission and as required by the National Pressure Injury Advisory Panel, January 2017.)*

Stage 3 Pressure Injury

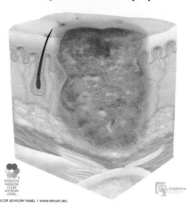

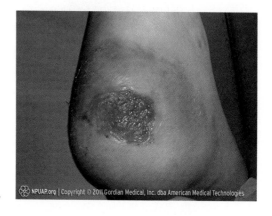

FIGURE 41-8 Stage 3 pressure injury. *Full-thickness loss of skin, in which adipose (fat) is visible in the ulcer and granulation tissue and epibole (rolled wound edges) are often present. Slough and/or eschar may be visible. The depth of tissue damage varies by anatomical location; areas of significant adiposity can develop deep wounds. Undermining and tunneling may occur. Fascia, muscle, tendon, ligament, cartilage and/or bone are not exposed. If slough or eschar obscures the extent of tissue loss this is an Unstageable Pressure Injury. (Illustration, photo, and definition used with permission and as required by the National Pressure Injury Advisory Panel, January 2017.)*

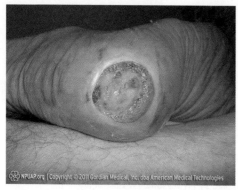

FIGURE 41-9 Slough. (Used with permission of the National Pressure Injury Advisory Panel, January 2017.)

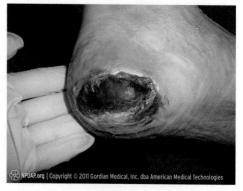

FIGURE 41-10 Eschar. (Used with permission of the National Pressure Injury Advisory Panel, January 2017.)

Stage 4 Pressure Injury

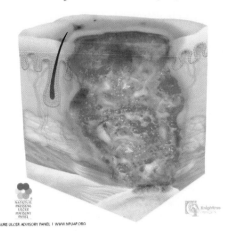

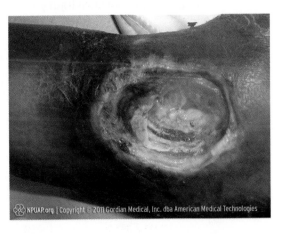

FIGURE 41-11 Stage 4 pressure injury. *Full-thickness skin and tissue loss with exposed or directly palpable fascia, muscle, tendon, ligament, cartilage or bone in the ulcer. Slough and/or eschar may be visible. Epibole (rolled edges), undermining and/or tunneling often occur. Depth varies by anatomical location. If slough or eschar obscures the extent of tissue loss this is an Unstageable Pressure Injury. (Illustration, photo, and definition used with permission and as required by the National Pressure Injury Advisory Panel, January 2017.)*

Unstageable Pressure Injury – Dark Eschar   Unstageable Pressure Injury – Slough and Eschar

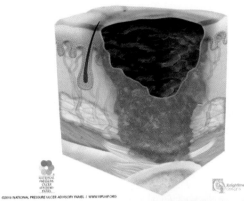

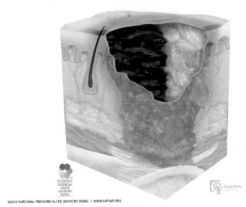

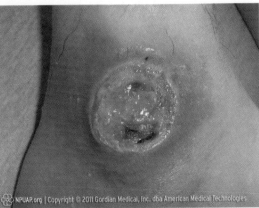

FIGURE 41-12 Unstageable pressure injury. *Full-thickness skin and tissue loss in which the extent of tissue damage within the ulcer cannot be confirmed because it is obscured by slough or eschar. If slough or eschar is removed, a Stage 3 or Stage 4 pressure injury will be revealed. Stable eschar (i.e. dry, adherent, intact without erythema or fluctuance) on the heel or ischemic limb should not be softened or removed. (Illustrations, photo, and definition used with permission and as required by the National Pressure Injury Advisory Panel, January 2017.)*

Deep Tissue Pressure Injury

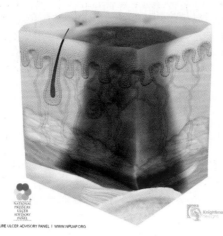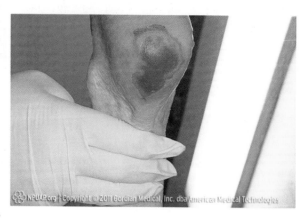

FIGURE 41-13 Deep tissue pressure injury (DTPI). *Intact or non-intact skin with localized area of persistent non-blanchable deep red, maroon, purple discoloration or epidermal separation revealing a dark wound bed or blood filled blister. Pain and temperature change often precede skin color changes. Discoloration may appear differently in darkly pigmented skin. This injury results from intense and/or prolonged pressure and shear forces at the bone-muscle interface. The wound may evolve rapidly to reveal the actual extent of tissue injury, or may resolve without tissue loss. If necrotic tissue, subcutaneous tissue, granulation tissue, fascia, muscle or other underlying structures are visible, this indicates a full thickness pressure injury (Unstageable, Stage 3 or Stage 4). Do not use DTPI to describe vascular, traumatic, neuropathic, or dermatologic conditions. (Illustration, photo, and definition used with permission and as required by the National Pressure Injury Advisory Panel, January 2017.)*

Kennedy Terminal Ulcer

Persons receiving end-of-life care (Chapter 59) are at risk for pressure injuries. Described by Karen Kennedy-Evans, the *Kennedy terminal ulcer* occurs over a bony prominence 2 to 3 days before death. The sacrum is the most common site. The cause is thought to be *skin failure*—the skin (along with other body organs) shuts down 10 to 14 days before death.

The onset is sudden. Shaped like a pear, butterfly, or horseshoe, the ulcer can be red, yellow, purple, or black (Fig. 41-14). At first it may look like a small black spot or a dried bowel movement. Within a few hours it can increase to the size of a quarter or larger. Usually Stage 2 with a blister at first, it rapidly progresses to Stage 3 or 4.

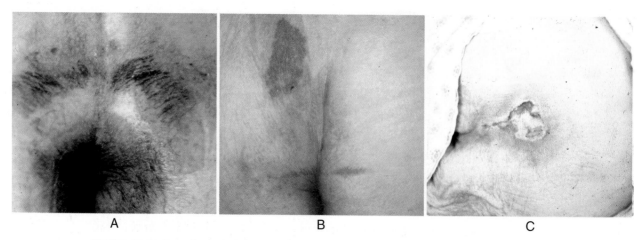

A   B   C

FIGURE 41-14 Kennedy terminal ulcer. **A** and **B,** First 4 to 8 hours. **C,** After 8 hours. (From Kennedy KL: *Understanding the Kennedy terminal ulcer*, Tucson, 2014.)

SITES

Pressure injuries usually occur over bony prominences (pressure points). These areas bear the body's weight in certain positions (see Fig. 41-2). Pressure from body weight can reduce the blood supply to the skin. The sacrum and heels are common sites for pressure injuries.

Medical device–related pressure injuries can develop at sites where devices are used for diagnostic or treatment purposes. For example, eyeglasses can cause pressure and friction on the ears. Oxygen tubing (Chapter 43) can cause pressure on the nose, face, and ears. Pressure can occur on an ear from the mattress when in a side-lying position. Tubes, casts, braces, and other devices can cause pressure on the hands, arms, legs, and feet. Pressure can occur on the buttocks from bedpans.

Mucosal membrane pressure injuries are found in mucous membranes where a medical device is used. A urinary catheter can cause pressure and friction on the meatus. A feeding tube can cause pressure in the nose.

Pressure injuries can occur where skin has contact with skin. Common sites are between abdominal folds, the legs, the buttocks, the thighs, and under the breasts.

PREVENTION AND TREATMENT

Preventing pressure injuries is much easier than trying to heal them. Unfortunately, some pressure injuries cannot be prevented. Called *unavoidable pressure injuries, they occur despite efforts to prevent them through proper use of the nursing process.* The Kennedy terminal ulcer is an example. An *avoidable pressure injury develops from improper use of the nursing process.*

Health care agencies are required to have pressure injury prevention programs that involve:

- Identifying persons at risk. The health team assesses the person's risk factors and skin condition.
- Prevention measures for those at risk. Good nursing care, cleanliness, and skin care are essential. Managing moisture, good nutrition and fluid balance, and relieving pressure also are key measures. Box 41-3 lists common measures used to prevent skin damage and pressure injuries. Always follow the person's care plan.

Some agencies use symbols or colored stickers as pressure injury alerts. Placed on the person's door or medical record, the alerts remind the staff that the person is at risk.

See *Focus on Surveys: Prevention and Treatment.*

FOCUS ON SURVEYS

Prevention and Treatment

Because pressure injuries are very serious, they are a focus of surveys. During a survey you might be asked about:

- How you are involved in the person's care
- What measures the agency uses to prevent pressure injuries
- What skin changes you should report and when
- To whom you should report skin changes
- Your knowledge of measures in the person's care plan

BOX 41-3	**Preventing Pressure Injuries**

Moving and Positioning

- Follow the person's re-positioning schedule (Fig. 41-15, p. 642). Re-position bedfast persons at least every 1 to 2 hours. Re-position chairfast persons at least every hour. Some persons are re-positioned every 15 minutes.
- Remind persons sitting in recliners, chairs, or wheelchairs to shift positions at least every 15 minutes.
- Position the person according to the care plan. Use pillows for support as directed. The 30-degree lateral position is recommended (Fig. 41-16, p. 642).
- Do not position the person:
  - On a pressure injury
  - On a reddened area
  - On tubes or other medical devices
- Do not leave a person on a bedpan longer than needed.
- Do not let the person sit on donut-shaped cushions.
- Prevent shearing and friction during moving and transfer procedures. Do not drag the person. Use assist devices as directed. See Chapters 19 and 20.
- Use slow, gradual turns and movements when re-positioning persons who are critically ill.
- Prevent shearing. Do not raise the head of the bed more than 30 degrees. Follow the care plan for:
  - When to raise the head of the bed
  - How far to raise the head of the bed
  - How long (in minutes) to raise the head of the bed

Moving and Positioning—cont'd

- Use pillows, foam wedges, or other devices to prevent bony areas from contact with bony areas. The ankles, knees, hips, and sacrum are examples.
- Keep the heels and ankles off the bed. Use pillows or other devices as directed. Place the pillows or devices under the lower legs from mid-calf to the ankles.
- Use protective devices as directed (p. 643).
- Elevate the legs when the person is sitting in a recliner.
- Tilt the person's seat, if safely possible, when in a chair or wheelchair. Tilting prevents the person from sliding forward.
- Support the feet properly when the person is sitting upright in a chair or wheelchair. Use a footstool if the person's feet do not touch the floor when sitting in a chair. The body slides forward when the feet do not touch the floor. For the person in a wheelchair, position the feet on the footrests.

Skin Care

- Inspect the skin every time you give care. This includes during or after transfers, re-positioning, bathing, and elimination procedures. Report any concern at once.
- Follow the person's bathing schedule. Some persons do not need a bath or shower every day.
- Do not use hot water to bathe or clean the skin. Hot water can irritate the skin.
- Use a cleansing agent as directed. Soap can dry and irritate the skin.

Continued

BOX 41-3　Preventing Pressure Injuries—cont'd

Skin Care—cont'd

- Provide good skin care.
  - The skin is clean and dry after bathing.
  - The skin is free of moisture from a bath or shower and from urine, feces (stools), perspiration, wound drainage, and other secretions.
  - Skin under the breasts and in the groin area is clean and dry.
- Follow measures to prevent incontinence.
- Prevent skin exposure to moisture. Check persons who are incontinent of urine or feces (stools) often. Provide good skin care and change linens and garments at the time of soiling. Use incontinence products as directed.
- Apply an ointment or moisture barrier if the person is incontinent of urine or feces (stools). Follow the care plan.
- Check persons often who perspire heavily or have wound drainage. Change linens and garments as needed. Provide good skin care.
- Apply moisturizer to dry areas—hands, elbows, hips, ankles, heels, and so on. The nurse tells you what to use and what areas need attention.
- Give a back massage when re-positioning the person. Do not massage bony areas.
- Do not massage over pressure points. *Never rub or massage reddened areas.*
- Keep linens clean, dry, and wrinkle-free.
- Make sure the bed or chair is free of objects. Crumbs, pins, pencils, pens, and coins are examples.

Skin Care—cont'd

- Do not irritate the skin. Avoid scrubbing or vigorous rubbing when bathing or drying the person.
- Use pillows and blankets to prevent skin from being in contact with skin.
- Make sure clothes do not increase the risk for pressure injuries.
  - Avoid seams, buttons, or zippers that press against the skin.
  - Avoid tight clothes.
  - Keep clothes from bunching up or wrinkling.
- Make sure socks and shoes are in good repair. Socks should not have holes, wrinkles, or creases. Make sure there is nothing in the shoes before the person puts them on.
- Do not apply heat or cold (Chapter 42) directly on a pressure injury.
- See Chapter 40 for diabetes foot care.

Medical Devices

- Use the correct device. Follow the care plan for what size and shape to use.
- Apply and secure the device correctly. Follow the manufacturer's directions.
- Move or re-position the device according to the care plan.
- Check the skin under a medical device for edema and signs of skin breakdown or a pressure injury (see Box 41-2).
- Protect the skin under the device as directed by the nurse.
- Do not position the person on top of a medical device.
- Ask about the person's comfort. Tell the nurse if the device is causing discomfort or is too loose or too tight.

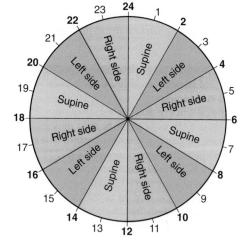

FIGURE 41-15 Turn clock. The clock shows the times to turn the person and to what position.

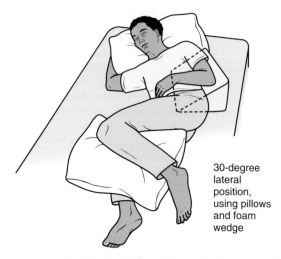

30-degree lateral position, using pillows and foam wedge

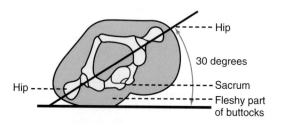

FIGURE 41-16 The 30-degree lateral position. Pillows are under the head, shoulder, and leg. This position inclines (lifts up) the hip to avoid pressure on the hip. The person does not lie on the hip as in the side-lying position.

Protective Devices

Wound care products, drugs, treatments, dressings, and equipment are ordered to promote healing. Support surfaces relieve or reduce pressure. Such surfaces include foam, air, alternating air, gel, or water mattresses.

Protective devices are often used to prevent and treat skin breakdown and pressure injuries. These devices are common.

- *Bed cradle.* A bed cradle is a metal frame placed on the bed and over the person (Chapter 34). Top linens are brought over the cradle to prevent pressure on the legs, feet, and toes. Tuck and miter linens under the mattress bottom and sides. This protects against drafts and chilling.
- *Elbow and heel protectors.* These devices are made of foam padding, pressure-relieving gel, sheepskin, and other cushioning materials. They fit the shape of elbows and heels (Fig. 41-17). Some are inside sleeves or mesh. Others are secured in place with straps. The devices promote comfort and reduce shear and friction.
- *Heel elevators.* These raise the heels and feet off the bed (Fig. 41-18). They prevent pressure. Some also prevent footdrop (Chapter 34).

- *Gel- or fluid-filled pads and cushions.* These devices have a pressure-relieving gel or fluid (Fig. 41-19). They are used for chairs and wheelchairs to prevent pressure. If the outer case is vinyl, the device may be placed in a fabric cover to protect the skin. Some covers are 2 colors (Fig. 41-20) to remind the staff to re-position the person.
- *Special beds.* Some beds have air flowing through the mattresses. An *alternating pressure mattress* (Fig. 41-21) has many tubes that fill and release air at certain times. This changes where pressure is placed on the body. Some beds rotate from side to side. Alignment stays the same. Pressure points change as the bed rotates. They are useful for persons with spinal cord injuries.
- *Other equipment.* Pillows, trochanter rolls, foot-boards, and other positioning devices are used (Chapter 34). They maintain good alignment.

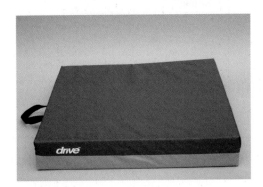

FIGURE 41-19 Gel cushion.

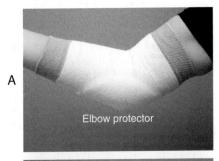

A

Elbow protector

B

Heel protector

FIGURE 41-17 Elbow and heel protectors.

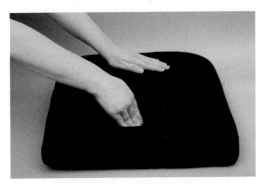

FIGURE 41-20 Two-color foam cushion.

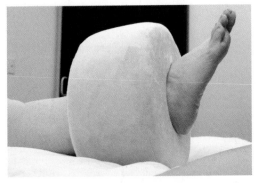

FIGURE 41-18 Heel elevator.

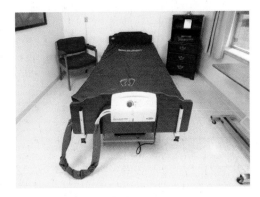

FIGURE 41-21 Alternating pressure mattress.

Dressings

A variety of dressings are available to treat pressure injuries. The dressing selected by the nursing team depends on the size, depth, and location of the pressure injury. Keeping the wound moist and the amount of drainage are other factors.

COMPLICATIONS

Infection is the most common complication. According to the CMS, all Stage 2, 3, and 4 pressure injuries are colonized with bacteria. *Colonized refers to the presence of bacteria on the wound surface or in wound tissue. The person does not have signs and symptoms of an infection.* A wound is *infected* when bacteria invade the tissues around or in the pressure injury. The person has signs and symptoms of infection (Chapter 16). Pain and delayed healing may signal an infection.

Osteomyelitis is a risk if the pressure injury is over a bony prominence. The risk is great if the wound is not healing. *Osteomyelitis* means inflammation *(itis)* of the bone *(osteo)* and bone marrow *(myel)*. Pain is severe. Treatment includes bed rest and antibiotics. Careful and gentle positioning is needed. Surgery may be done to remove dead bone and tissue.

Pressure injuries can cause pain. Pain management is important. Pain may affect movement and activity. Immobility is a risk factor for pressure injuries. And it may delay healing of an existing pressure injury.

REPORTING AND RECORDING

Report and record any signs of skin breakdown or pressure injury at once. See Figure 41-22. See "Wound Appearance" in Chapter 40.

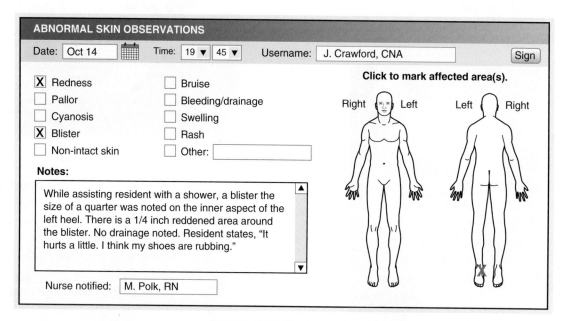

FIGURE 41-22 Charting sample.

FOCUS ON **PRIDE**

The Person, Family, and Yourself

P ersonal and Professional Responsibility

You have an important role in preventing and treating pressure injuries. Your attitude and quality of work affect the person. If you take your role seriously and believe you have a positive impact, the person benefits. If you are careless and lack concern for the person's well-being, harm can result.

You are an important part of the nursing team. Take pride in your role. Work to the best of your ability.

R ights and Respect

You have the right and responsibility to speak for patients and residents. This is called being an *advocate*. You may be the first to notice a pressure injury. Reporting your observations can prevent further harm and result in prompt actions to promote healing. Take pride in being a voice for your patients and residents.

I ndependence and Social Interaction

A pressure injury is a serious matter. Infection, pain, amputation, and longer hospital or nursing center stays are complications. Healing can take a long time. As time passes, family and friends may not visit as often. Or the person may feel like a burden to others. Loneliness and depression can occur.

Do not neglect mental and social needs. Be kind. Show compassion. Take time to listen. Give care in a way that improves quality of life.

D elegation and Teamwork

Always report and record the completion of delegated tasks. Be accurate and honest. Never report or record something you did not do. Also, do not report or record before completing a task.

For example, a nursing assistant did not report placing a resident on the bedpan at 2250 (10:50 PM). The next shift began at 2300 (11:00 PM). At 0700 (7:00 AM), the resident was still on the bedpan. A pressure injury had developed. At risk for pressure injuries, the resident was to be re-positioned every 2 hours. The chart showed re-positioning had been done every 2 hours from 2300 (11:00 PM) to 0700 (7:00 AM).

Poor communication, false recording, and negligence will cause harm. You must be thorough, honest, and careful when completing, reporting, and recording delegated tasks.

E thics and Laws

Agencies must have a plan to predict, prevent, and treat pressure injuries early. Assessments are done on admission and regularly. The agency must take action to address risks.

Know your agency's policies and procedures for identifying those at risk for pressure injuries. Follow the measures in Box 41-3 and the care plan to do your part to prevent pressure injuries.

FOCUS ON **PRIDE**: *Application*

Describe the physical, mental, and social effects a pressure injury can have. How can you help meet the person's needs?

REVIEW QUESTIONS

Circle T *if the statement is TRUE or* F *if it is FALSE.*

1 T F Skin breakdown can lead to a pressure injury.

2 T F Unrelieved pressure squeezes tiny blood vessels. Tissues do not receive needed oxygen and nutrients.

3 T F Persons who are bedfast or chairfast are at risk for pressure injuries.

4 T F Pressure injuries can develop on the ears.

5 T F Pressure injuries can develop where medical devices are on the skin.

6 T F You assess the person's risk for pressure injuries.

7 T F Pressure injuries can involve muscles, tendons, and bones.

8 T F All pressure injuries are avoidable.

9 T F To prevent pressure injuries, the head of the bed is raised higher than 30 degrees.

10 T F You should inspect the person's skin every time you provide care.

11 T F A person is at risk for pressure injuries. A bath is needed every day.

12 T F You are giving a back massage. You should massage bony areas.

13 T F You can use pillows and blankets to prevent skin from being in contact with skin.

Circle the BEST answer.

14 A pressure injury is
a An open wound
b A localized injury to the skin and underlying tissue
c A bony prominence
d Dead tissue

15 A person is in Fowler's position. This places pressure on
a The knees and ankles
b The ribs and breasts
c The cheek and ear
d The sacrum and heels

Continued

REVIEW QUESTIONS—cont'd

16 Pressure injuries are the result of
 a Moisture
 b Medical devices
 c Aging
 d Unrelieved pressure

17 Which contributes to the development of pressure injuries?
 a Shear
 b Slough
 c Eschar
 d Skin blanching

18 A pressure injury can develop within
 a 2 to 6 hours
 b 6 to 10 hours
 c 10 to 14 hours
 d 14 to 18 hours

19 Which is a risk factor for pressure injuries?
 a Balanced diet
 b Intact skin
 c Incontinence
 d Increased circulation

20 Which is the most common site for a Kennedy terminal ulcer?
 a Back of the head
 b Hip
 c Sacrum
 d Heel

21 In a light-skinned person, a Stage 1 pressure injury has
 a A blister
 b A reddened area
 c Drainage
 d Gangrene

22 A care plan includes the following. Which should you question?
 a Re-position the person every 2 hours.
 b Scrub the skin during bathing.
 c Apply lotion to dry areas.
 d Keep linens clean, dry, and wrinkle-free.

23 You should position the person
 a On an existing pressure injury
 b On a reddened area
 c On tubes or other medical devices
 d Using assist devices

24 What is the preferred position for preventing pressure injuries?
 a 30-degree lateral position
 b Semi-Fowler's position
 c Prone position
 d Supine position

25 Which keeps the heels and ankles off the bed?
 a Bed cradles
 b Pillows
 c Air flotation bed
 d Trochanter rolls

26 A person in a chair should shift his or her position every
 a 15 minutes
 b 30 minutes
 c Hour
 d 2 hours

27 A person is sitting in a chair. The feet do not touch the floor. What should you do?
 a Have the person slide forward until the feet touch the floor.
 b Let the feet dangle.
 c Stack pillows under the person's feet.
 d Position the feet on a footstool.

28 Which helps treat pressure injuries?
 a Donut-shaped cushions
 b Weight loss
 c Gel or fluid-filled pads and cushions
 d Cleansing with soap and hot water

29 To prevent skin breakdown from moisture
 a Avoid using lotion on dry areas
 b Check incontinent persons every 4 hours
 c Dry under the breasts and in the groin area well
 d Change linens once daily for persons who perspire heavily

30 You see a reddened area on the person's skin. What should you do?
 a Rub the area.
 b Apply a moisturizer.
 c Apply a moisture barrier.
 d Tell the nurse.

31 You assist the nurse with pressure injuries by
 a Assessing pressure injury risk factors
 b Diagnosing pressure injury stages
 c Performing pressure injury prevention measures
 d Deciding how to treat pressure injuries

32 A pressure injury is colonized. This means that
 a The wound is infected
 b Bacteria are present
 c The person has osteomyelitis
 d The person has a gauze dressing

Answers to Chapter 41 questions are on p. 887.

FOCUS ON **PRACTICE**

Problem Solving

A resident at risk for pressure injuries complains when awakened for care. You and a co-worker enter the room for re-positioning. The person is asleep. What will you do? What is the risk of waiting to re-position? How can you provide safe, quality care that avoids causing frustration?

Heat and Cold Applications

OBJECTIVES

- Define the key terms and key abbreviations in this chapter.
- Explain the purpose, effects, and complications of heat and cold applications.
- Identify the persons at risk for complications from heat and cold applications.
- Describe moist and dry heat applications.
- Describe moist and dry cold applications.
- Describe the rules for applying heat and cold.
- Explain how cooling and warming blankets are used.
- Perform the procedure described in this chapter.
- Explain how to promote PRIDE in the person, the family, and yourself.

KEY TERMS

compress A soft pad applied over a body area
constrict To narrow
cyanosis Bluish (cyano) color

dilate To expand or open wider
pack Wrapping a body part with a wet or dry application

KEY ABBREVIATIONS

C   Centigrade
F   Fahrenheit

ID   Identification

Heat and cold applications are applied to the skin. They are used to:
- Promote healing.
- Promote comfort.
- Reduce tissue swelling.

Heat and cold have opposite effects on body functions. Heat increases circulation—tissues receive more oxygen and nutrients. Cold decreases circulation—tissues receive less oxygen and nutrients. Severe injuries and changes in body function can occur. The risks are great.

See *Focus on Children and Older Persons: Heat and Cold Applications.*

See *Delegation Guidelines: Heat and Cold Applications.*

FOCUS ON CHILDREN AND OLDER PERSONS

Heat and Cold Applications

Children
Infants and young children have fragile skin. At risk for burns, they need careful attention. Always respond when a child cries. Crying can communicate pain.

DELEGATION GUIDELINES

Heat and Cold Applications

Applying heat and cold applications is a nursing responsibility that may be delegated to you in some agencies. Before applying heat or cold make sure that:
- Your state allows you to perform the procedure.
- The procedure is in your job description.
- You have the necessary training.
- You know how to use the equipment.
- You review the procedure with a nurse.
- A nurse is available to answer questions and to guide and assist you as needed.

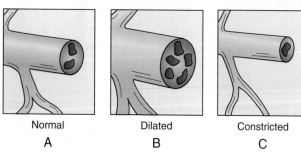

Normal
A

Dilated
B

Constricted
C

FIGURE 42-1 A, A blood vessel under normal conditions. **B,** Dilated blood vessel. **C,** Constricted blood vessel.

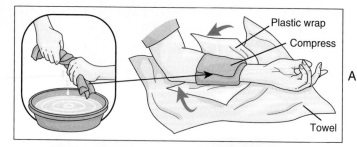

Plastic wrap
Compress
A
Towel

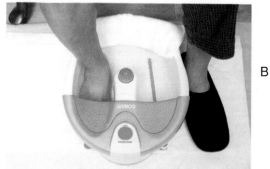

B

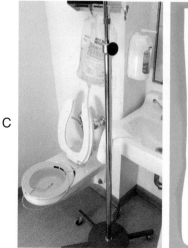

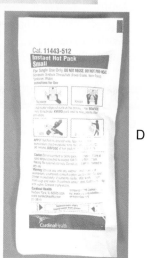

C

D

FIGURE 42-2 Moist heat applications. **A,** Compress. **B,** Hot soak. **C,** Disposable sitz bath. **D,** Hot pack. (NOTE: Compresses can be hot or cold. And some hot packs can also be used as cold packs.)

HEAT APPLICATIONS

Heat applications can be applied to almost any body part. They are used for musculo-skeletal injuries or problems (sprains, arthritis). Heat:

- Relieves pain.
- Relaxes muscles.
- Promotes healing.
- Reduces tissue swelling.
- Decreases joint stiffness.

When heat is applied to the skin, blood vessels in the area dilate. *Dilate means to expand or open wider* (Fig. 42-1). Blood flow increases. Excess fluid is removed from the area faster. The skin is red and warm.

Complications

High temperatures can cause burns. Report pain, excess redness, and blisters at once. Also observe for pale skin. When heat is applied too long, blood vessels *constrict (narrow)* (see Fig. 42-1). Blood flow decreases. Tissues receive less oxygen. Tissue damage occurs and the skin is pale.

Older and fair-skinned persons have fragile skin that is easily burned. Persons with problems sensing heat and pain also are at risk. Nervous system damage, altered awareness, and circulatory disorders affect sensation. So do confusion and some drugs.

Metal implants pose risks. Metal conducts heat. Deep tissues can be burned. Pacemakers (cardiac devices) and some joint replacements are made of metal. Do not apply heat to an implant area.

Heat is not applied to a pregnant woman's abdomen. The heat can affect fetal growth.

Moist and Dry Heat Applications

With a *moist heat application,* water has contact with the skin. Water conducts heat. Moist heat has greater and faster effects than dry heat. Heat penetrates deeper with a moist application. To prevent injury, moist heat applications have lower (cooler) temperatures than dry heat applications. Moist heat applications (Fig. 42-2) include:

- *Hot compress.* A *compress is a soft pad applied over a body area.* It is usually made of cloth. Sometimes an aquathermia pad is applied over the compress to maintain the temperature of the compress.

- *Hot soak.* A body part is in water. This is usually used for smaller parts—a hand, lower arm, foot, or lower leg. A tub is used for larger areas.
- *Sitz bath.* The perineal and rectal areas are immersed in warm or hot water. (*Sitz* means *seat* in German.) Sitz baths are common for hemorrhoids, after rectal or female pelvic surgeries, and after childbirth. They are used to:
  - Clean perineal and anal wounds
  - Promote healing
  - Relieve pain and soreness
  - Increase circulation
  - Stimulate voiding
- *Hot pack.* A *pack involves wrapping a body part with a wet or dry application.* There are single-use (disposable) and re-usable packs. Some are used for heat or cold. Follow the manufacturer's instructions to activate the heat or cold. To clean re-usable packs, follow agency policy and the manufacturer's instructions.

With *dry heat applications*, water does not have contact with the skin. A dry heat application stays at the desired temperature longer. Dry heat does not penetrate as deep as moist heat. Because water is not used, dry heat needs higher (hotter) temperatures for the desired effect. Burns remain a risk.

Some *hot packs* and warming therapy pads are dry heat applications. The *aquathermia pad* (Aqua-K, K-Pad) is a common therapy pad (Fig. 42-3). Tubes inside the pad are filled with distilled water. (Distilled water is water that has been purified with contaminants removed.) Heated water flows to the pad through a hose. Another hose returns water to the electric heating unit. Reheated water flows back into the pad.

See *Focus on Long-Term Care and Home Care: Moist and Dry Heat Applications.*

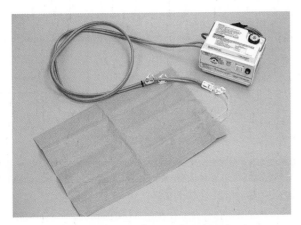

FIGURE 42-3 The aquathermia pad.

COLD APPLICATIONS

Cold applications are often used to treat sprains and fractures. Cold applications:

- Reduce pain.
- Prevent swelling.
- Decrease circulation and bleeding.
- Cool the body when fever is present.

Cold has the opposite effect of heat. When cold is applied to the skin, blood vessels constrict (see Fig. 42-1). Blood flow decreases.

Cold is useful right after an injury. Decreased blood flow reduces bleeding. Less fluid collects in the tissues. Cold numbs the skin. This helps reduce or relieve pain in the part.

Complications

Complications include pain, burns, blisters, and poor circulation. Burns and blisters occur from intense cold. They also occur from dry cold in direct contact with the skin.

When cold is applied for a long time, blood vessels dilate. Blood flow increases. Prolonged application of cold has the same effect as heat applications.

Older and fair-skinned persons have fragile skin. They are at great risk for complications. So are persons with sensory impairments.

Moist and Dry Cold Applications

Moist cold applications penetrate deeper than dry ones. Therefore moist cold applications are warmer than dry cold applications.

The cold compress is a moist cold application (see Fig. 42-2, *A*). Filled with crushed ice, dry cold applications include ice bags, ice collars, and ice gloves (Fig. 42-4).

Cold packs can be moist or dry applications (see Fig. 42-2, *D*). Commercial cold packs are single-use (disposable) or re-usable. To activate the cold, you strike, knead, or squeeze the pack. Keep re-usable cold packs in the freezer. Clean them after use. Discard single-use cold packs after use.

See *Focus on Long-Term Care and Home Care: Moist and Dry Cold Applications*, p. 650.

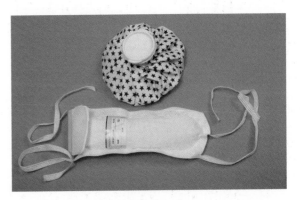

FIGURE 42-4 Ice bags.

Applying Heat and Cold

Protect the person from injury during heat and cold applications. Follow the rules in Box 42-1. See Table 42-1 for heat and cold temperature ranges.

See *Focus on Communication: Applying Heat and Cold.*

See *Teamwork and Time Management: Applying Heat and Cold.*

See *Delegation Guidelines: Applying Heat and Cold.*

See *Promoting Safety and Comfort: Applying Heat and Cold.*

See procedure: *Applying Heat and Cold Applications.*

BOX 42-1	Applying Heat and Cold

- Know how to use the equipment. Follow the manufacturer's instructions for commercial devices.
- Measure the temperature of moist applications. Follow agency policy or use a water thermometer.
- Follow agency policies for safe temperature ranges. See Table 42-1.
- Do not apply *very hot* (above 106°F or 41.1°C) applications. Tissue damage can occur. A nurse applies *very hot* applications.
- Ask the nurse what temperature to use.
  - Heat—cooler temperatures for persons at risk.
  - Cold—warmer temperatures for persons at risk.
- Have the nurse show you the application site.
- Cover dry heat or cold applications before applying them. Use a flannel cover, towel, or other cover as directed.
- Provide for privacy. Properly screen and drape the person. Expose only the body part involved.
- Maintain comfort and body alignment during the procedure.
- Observe the skin every 5 minutes during the procedure. See *Delegation Guidelines: Applying Heat and Cold.*
- Do not let the person change the temperature of the application.
- Know how long to leave the application in place. Heat and cold are applied no longer than 15 to 20 minutes.
- Follow the rules for electrical safety when using electrical appliances for heat. See Chapter 13.
- Place the call light within the person's reach.
- Complete a safety check before leaving the room. (See the inside of the back cover.)

TABLE 42-1	Heat and Cold Temperature Ranges	
Temperature	**Fahrenheit (F) Range**	**Centigrade (C) Range**
Hot	99°F to 106°F	37°C to 41°C
Warm	93°F to 98°F	34°C to 37°C
Tepid	80°F to 92°F	26°C to 34°C
Cool	65°F to 79°F	18°C to 26°C
Cold	50°F to 64°F	10°C to 18°C

Modified from Perry AG, Potter PA, Ostendorf WR: *Nursing interventions & clinical skills*, ed 6, St Louis, 2016, Mosby.

FOCUS ON COMMUNICATION

Applying Heat and Cold

The person may not report pain or discomfort. The person may not know what symptoms to report. For heat and cold applications, you need to ask:

- "Does the application feel too hot or too cold?"
- "Do you feel any pain, numbness, or burning?"
- "Do you feel weak, faint, or drowsy?" If yes: "Tell me how you feel."

TEAMWORK AND TIME MANAGEMENT

Applying Heat and Cold

After applying heat or cold, check the person and the application every 5 minutes. Plan your work so you can stay in or near the person's room. For example:

- Make the bed and straighten the person's unit.
- Provide care to the person's roommate if assigned to him or her.
- Help the person complete the daily or weekly menu.
- Read cards and letters to the person, with his or her consent.
- Address envelopes and other correspondence for the person.
- Take time to visit with the person.

DELEGATION GUIDELINES
Applying Heat and Cold

To apply heat or cold, you need this information from the nurse and the care plan.

- What application to apply
- How to cover the application
- What temperature to use (see Table 42-1)
- The application site
- How long to leave the application in place
- What observations to report and record:
  - Complaints of pain or discomfort, numbness, or burning
  - Excess redness
  - Blisters
  - Pale, white, or gray skin
  - *Cyanosis—bluish* (cyano) *color*
  - Shivering
  - Rapid pulse, weakness, faintness, and drowsiness (sitz bath)
  - Time, site, and length of application
- When to report observations
- What patient or resident concerns to report at once

PROMOTING SAFETY AND COMFORT
Applying Heat and Cold

Safety
Keep the call light within reach and check the person every 5 minutes. Also follow these safety measures.

- *Sitz bath.* Blood flow increases to the perineum and rectum. Therefore less blood flows to other areas. Observe for signs of weakness, fainting, or fatigue. Also protect the person from injury, chills, and burns.
- *Commercial hot and cold packs.* Read warning labels and follow the manufacturer's instructions.
- *Aquathermia pad:*
  - Follow electrical safety measures (Chapter 13).
  - Check the device for damage or flaws.
  - Follow the manufacturer's instructions.
  - Place the heating unit on an even, uncluttered surface. This prevents it from being knocked over or knocked off the surface.
  - Check the hoses for kinks or bubbles. Water must flow freely.
  - Place the pad in a flannel cover. The flannel absorbs perspiration at the application site. (Some agencies use towels or pillowcases.)
  - Secure the pad in place with ties, tape, or rolled gauze. Do not use pins. They can puncture the pad and cause leaks.
  - Do not place the pad under a body part. Heat cannot escape. Burns can result if heat cannot escape.
  - Give the temperature setting key to the nurse. This prevents anyone from changing the temperature. The temperature is usually set at 105°F (40.5°C) with a key.

Some persons have medicated patches or ointments applied to the skin. Do not apply heat over such areas.

Comfort
Cold applications can cause chills and shivering. Provide for warmth. Use bath blankets or other blankets as needed.

Applying Heat and Cold Applications

QUALITY OF LIFE

- Knock before entering the person's room.
- Address the person by name.
- Introduce yourself by name and title.

- Explain the procedure before starting and during the procedure.
- Protect the person's rights during the procedure.
- Handle the person gently during the procedure.

PRE-PROCEDURE

1 Follow *Delegation Guidelines:*
  a *Heat and Cold Applications,* p. 647
  b *Applying Heat and Cold*
  See *Promoting Safety and Comfort: Applying Heat and Cold.*
2 Practice hand hygiene.
3 Collect equipment.
- *For a hot compress:*
  - Basin
  - Water thermometer
  - Small towel, washcloth, or gauze squares
  - Plastic wrap or aquathermia pad
  - Ties, tape, or rolled gauze
  - Bath towel
  - Waterproof under-pad

- *For a hot soak:*
  - Water basin or arm or foot bath
  - Water thermometer
  - Waterproof under-pad
  - Bath blanket
  - Towel
- *For a sitz bath:*
  - Disposable sitz bath
  - Water thermometer
  - 2 bath blankets, bath towels, and a clean gown
- *For an aquathermia pad:*
  - Aquathermia pad and heating unit
  - Distilled water
  - Flannel cover or other cover as directed
  - Ties, tape, or rolled gauze

Continued

Applying Heat and Cold Applications—cont'd

PRE-PROCEDURE—cont'd

- • *For a hot or cold pack:*
  - • Commercial pack
  - • Pack cover
  - • Ties, tape, or rolled gauze (if needed)
  - • Waterproof under-pad
- • *For an ice bag, ice collar, or ice glove:*
  - • Ice bag, collar, or glove
  - • Crushed ice
  - • Flannel cover or other cover as directed
  - • Paper towels

- • *For a cold compress:*
  - • Large basin with ice
  - • Small basin with cold water
  - • Gauze squares, washcloths, or small towels
  - • Waterproof under-pad

4 Identify the person. Check the ID (identification) bracelet against the assignment sheet. Use 2 identifiers (Chapter 13). Also call the person by name.

PROCEDURE

5 Provide for privacy.
6 Position the person for the procedure.
7 Place the waterproof under-pad (if needed) under the body part.
8 *For a hot compress* (see Fig. 42-2, *A*):
  a Fill the basin ½ to ⅔ (one-half to two-thirds) full with hot water as directed. Measure water temperature.
  b Place the compress in the water and wring out.
  c Apply the compress over the area. Note the time.
  d Cover the compress as directed. Do 1 of the following.
     1) Apply plastic wrap and then a bath towel. Secure the towel in place with ties, tape, or rolled gauze.
     2) Apply an aquathermia pad.
9 *For a hot soak* (see Fig. 42-2, *B*):
  a Fill the container ½ (one-half) full with hot water. Measure water temperature.
  b Place the part into the water. Pad the edge of the container with a towel. Note the time.
  c Cover the person with a bath blanket for warmth.
10 *For a sitz bath* (see Fig. 42-2, *C*):
  a Place the sitz bath on the toilet seat.
  b Fill the sitz bath ⅔ (two-thirds) full with water. Measure water temperature.
  c Secure the gown above the waist.
  d Help the person sit on the sitz bath. Note the time.
  e Provide for warmth. Place a bath blanket around the shoulders. Place the other over the legs.
  f Stay with the person if he or she is weak or unsteady.
11 *For an aquathermia pad* (see Fig. 42-3):
  a Fill the heating unit to the fill line with distilled water.
  b Remove the bubbles. Place the pad and tubing below the heating unit. Tilt the heating unit from side to side.
  c Set the temperature as the nurse directs (usually 105°F [40.5°C]). Remove the key.
  d Place the pad in the cover.
  e Set the heating unit on the bedside stand. Keep the pad and connecting hoses level with the unit.
  f Plug in the unit. Let water warm to the desired temperature.
  g Apply the pad to the part. Note the time.
  h Secure the pad in place with ties, tape, or rolled gauze.

12 *For a hot or cold pack* (see Fig. 42-2, *D*):
  a Squeeze, knead, or strike the pack as directed by the manufacturer.
  b Place the pack in the cover.
  c Apply the pack. Note the time.
  d Secure the pack in place with ties, tape, or rolled gauze. Some packs are secured with Velcro straps.
13 *For an ice bag, collar, or glove* (see Fig. 42-4):
  a Fill the device with water. Put in the stopper. Turn the device upside down to check for leaks.
  b Empty the device.
  c Fill the device ½ to ⅔ (one-half to two-thirds) full with crushed ice or ice chips.
  d Remove excess air. Bend, twist, or squeeze the device. Or press it against a firm surface.
  e Place the cap or stopper on securely.
  f Dry the device with paper towels.
  g Place the device in the cover.
  h Apply the device. Note the time.
  i Secure the device with ties, tape, or rolled gauze.
14 *For a cold compress* (see Fig. 42-2, *A*):
  a Place the small basin with cold water into the large basin with ice.
  b Place the compresses into the cold water.
  c Wring out a compress.
  d Apply the compress to the part. Note the time.
15 Place the call light and other needed items within reach. Unscreen the person if appropriate.
16 Raise or lower bed rails. Follow the care plan.
17 Do the following every 5 minutes.
  a Check the person for signs and symptoms of complications (see *Delegation Guidelines: Applying Heat and Cold*, p. 651). Remove the application if any occur. Tell the nurse at once.
  b Check the application for cooling (hot application) or warming (cold application).
18 Remove the application after 15 to 20 minutes.

POST-PROCEDURE

19 Provide for comfort. (See the inside of the back cover.)
20 Place the call light and other needed items within reach.
21 Raise or lower bed rails. Follow the care plan.
22 Unscreen the person.
23 Clean, rinse, dry (with clean, dry paper towels), and return re-usable items to their proper place. Follow agency policy for used linens. Wear gloves.

24 Complete a safety check of the room. (See the inside of the back cover.)
25 Remove and discard the gloves. Practice hand hygiene.
26 Report and record your observations.

COOLING AND WARMING BLANKETS

Cooling and warming blankets are used to cool or warm the body. Cooling is used for fever and heat-related illnesses. Warming is used for *hypothermia*—a very low *(hypo)* body temperature *(thermia)*. See Chapter 58 for cold- and heat-related illnesses.

Treatment may involve a cooling or warming blanket made of rubber or plastic. Warm or cool fluid flows through tubes in the blanket. Vital signs are measured often.

See *Focus on Children and Older Persons: Cooling and Warming Blankets.*

FOCUS ON CHILDREN AND OLDER PERSONS
Cooling and Warming Blankets

Children
Rapid temperature changes can occur in infants and children. Observe them closely. Measure temperature and other vital signs as the nurse directs. Report the following at once.
- The temperature measurement and other vital signs measurements
- Changes in vital signs
- Changes in the child's condition

FOCUS ON PRIDE
The Person, Family, and Yourself

Personal and Professional Responsibility
You are responsible for the tasks you perform. Never perform a task that is not in your job description or you are not comfortable doing. The person may be harmed. Do not be afraid, embarrassed, or ashamed to ask the nurse about your concerns. Take pride in acting responsibly.

Rights and Respect
Respect the right to privacy. Be sure the person is properly screened and covered. This will vary by application site, method, and personal preference. For example:
- A sitz bath is ordered. Ensure that the person is covered and no one enters the bathroom during the procedure.
- A resident receiving a hot soak to a foot wants the privacy curtain to remain pulled.
- A patient has an ice bag on 1 hand. So roommates can talk, the patient would like to be unscreened during the application.

Independence and Social Interaction
Patients and residents can plan if they know what will happen. For example, a person wants to make a phone call before a hot compress. Or a person wants a hot soak done before visitors arrive. You promote independence when you involve the person in planning.

Delegation and Teamwork
Safety and comfort measures require time and planning. Heat and cold are usually applied for 15 to 20 minutes. The procedure involves:
- Meeting elimination needs before the procedure
- Positioning the person for comfort
- Placing needed items within reach—call light, water mug, reading material, electronic devices, phone, remotes, other requested items
- Checking the person often
- Reporting and recording task completion and your observations

Ethics and Laws
Complications from heat and cold can be severe. Safety is a priority. Harm and legal action can result if you:
- Apply a heat or cold application without an order.
- Use the equipment without training.
- Apply an application that is too hot or too cold.
- Do not cover an application as directed.
- Neglect to check the person often.
- Leave the application on longer than directed.
- Fail to report complications to the nurse.
  Follow the rules in Box 42-1. Take pride in protecting the person from injury.

FOCUS ON PRIDE: *Application*

Providing comfort is an important part of every task. What special considerations are needed for heat and cold applications? How will you know if you have met the person's comfort needs?

REVIEW QUESTIONS

Circle the BEST answer.

1 Heat applications
   a Decrease blood flow
   b Constrict vessels before dilating them
   c Tighten muscles
   d Relieve pain

2 The *greatest* threat from heat applications is
   a Infection
   b Burns
   c Chilling
   d Skin tears

3 Who has the *greatest* risk for complications from heat applications?
   a An adult with dark skin
   b An older person with nerve damage
   c An adult with a wound
   d A pregnant woman

4 Which statement about moist and dry heat applications is *true?*
   a With moist applications, water has contact with the skin.
   b Moist heat has fewer effects than dry heat.
   c Dry heat penetrates deeper than moist heat.
   d Lower temperatures are required for dry heat applications.

5 A hot application is usually
   a 80°F to 92°F
   b 93°F to 98°F
   c 99°F to 106°F
   d Above 106°F

6 A nurse asks you to apply a hot pack. Which should you question?
   a Check that the pack's temperature is at least 110°F (43.3°C).
   b Place the pack in a cover.
   c Secure the pack in place with ties.
   d Check the person for complications every 5 minutes.

7 Which statement about sitz baths is *true?*
   a Sitz baths last 25 to 30 minutes.
   b Weakness and fainting can occur.
   c The lower body is immersed in warm water.
   d Sitz baths decrease circulation to the perineum and rectum.

8 When using an aquathermia pad
   a Do not cover the pad
   b Place the pad under the person
   c Check for kinks in the hoses
   d Secure the pad in place with pins

9 Cold applications
   a Prevent swelling and decrease circulation
   b Dilate blood vessels
   c Prevent the spread of microbes
   d Increase bleeding

10 Which signals a complication of a cold application?
    a Cool skin
    b Cyanosis
    c Decreased swelling
    d Fever

11 For a cold application
    a Use cooler temperatures for persons at risk
    b Observe the skin every 10 minutes
    c Place the application on a bluish skin area
    d Provide for warmth and privacy

12 Before applying an ice bag
    a Place the bag in the freezer
    b Measure the temperature of the bag
    c Place the bag in a cover
    d Provide perineal care

13 Moist cold compresses are left in place no longer than
    a 20 minutes
    b 30 minutes
    c 45 minutes
    d 60 minutes

14 A cooling blanket is used for
    a Hypothermia
    b Heat-related illnesses
    c Cyanosis
    d Shivering

Answers to Chapter 42 questions are on p. 887.

FOCUS ON **PRACTICE**

Problem Solving

You are to remove a hot pack. The person says: "My knee feels much better with that on. Can you leave it on longer?" What do you do? Is it safe or are there risks to leaving the application in place? Explain.

Oxygen Needs

OBJECTIVES

- Define the key terms and key abbreviations in this chapter.
- Describe the factors affecting oxygen needs.
- List the signs and symptoms of altered respiratory function.
- Describe pulse oximetry.
- Explain the measures to meet oxygen needs.

- Explain how to safely assist with oxygen therapy.
- Describe the devices used to give oxygen.
- Perform the procedures described in this chapter.
- Explain how to promote PRIDE in the person, the family, and yourself.

KEY TERMS

allergy A sensitivity to a substance that causes the body to react with signs and symptoms

apnea The lack or absence *(a)* of breathing *(pnea)*

atelectasis The collapse of a portion of a lung

Biot's respirations Rapid and deep respirations followed by 10 to 30 seconds of apnea

bradypnea Slow *(brady)* breathing *(pnea)*; respirations are fewer than 12 per minute

Cheyne-Stokes respirations Respirations gradually increase in rate and depth and then become shallow and slow; breathing may stop *(apnea)* for 10 to 20 seconds

cyanosis Bluish color *(cyano)* to the skin, lips, mucous membranes, and nail beds

dyspnea Difficult, labored, or painful *(dys)* breathing *(pnea)*

hemoptysis Bloody *(hemo)* sputum *(ptysis means to spit)*

hyperventilation Breathing *(ventilation)* is rapid *(hyper)* and deeper than normal

hypoventilation Breathing *(ventilation)* is slow *(hypo)*, shallow, and sometimes irregular

hypoxemia A reduced amount *(hypo)* of oxygen *(ox)* in the blood *(emia)*

hypoxia Cells do not have enough *(hypo)* oxygen *(oxia)*

Kussmaul respirations Very deep and rapid respirations

orthopnea Breathing *(pnea)* deeply and comfortably only when sitting *(ortho)*

orthopneic position Sitting up *(ortho)* and leaning over a table to breathe *(pneic)*

oxygen concentration The amount (percent [%]) of hemoglobin containing oxygen

pollutant A harmful chemical or substance in the air or water

pulse oximetry Measures *(metry)* the oxygen *(oxi)* concentration in arterial blood

respiratory arrest When breathing stops

respiratory depression Slow, weak respirations at a rate of fewer than 12 per minute

sputum Mucus from the respiratory system when expectorated (expelled) through the mouth

tachypnea Rapid *(tachy)* breathing *(pnea)*; respirations are more than 20 per minute

KEY ABBREVIATIONS

CO_2	Carbon dioxide	O_2	Oxygen
ID	Identification	RBC	Red blood cell
L/min	Liters per minute	SpO_2	Saturation of peripheral oxygen (oxygen concentration)

Oxygen (O_2) is a gas. It has no taste, odor, or color. It is a basic need required for life. The person dies within minutes if breathing stops. Brain and other organ damage can occur without enough oxygen. Illness, surgery, and injuries affect the amount of oxygen in the body.

You assist with oxygen needs. You must give safe and effective care.

NOTE: *A task may require more than 1 pair of gloves. Change gloves as needed. Use careful judgment. Remember to practice hand hygiene after removing gloves.*

See *Body Structure and Function Review: The Respiratory System*, p. 656.

BODY STRUCTURE AND FUNCTION REVIEW
The Respiratory System

Every body cell needs oxygen. The respiratory system (Fig. 43-1) brings oxygen (O_2) into the lungs and removes carbon dioxide (CO_2). *Respiration* is the process of supplying the cells with O_2 and removing CO_2 from them. Respiration involves breathing in *(inhalation, inspiration)* and breathing out *(exhalation, expiration)*.

Air enters the body through the *nose*. Then the air passes into the *pharynx* (throat)—a tube-shaped passage-way for air and food. Air passes from the pharynx into the *larynx* (voice box). Then air passes from the larynx into the *trachea* (windpipe).

The trachea divides at its lower end into the *right bronchus* and *left bronchus*. Each bronchus enters a *lung*. Upon entering the lungs, each bronchus divides many times into smaller branches *(bronchioles)*. The bronchioles subdivide, ending up in tiny 1-celled air sacs *(alveoli)*.

O_2 and CO_2 are exchanged between the alveoli and capillaries. Blood in the capillaries picks up O_2 from the alveoli. That blood is returned to the left side of the heart and pumped to the rest of the body. Alveoli pick up CO_2 from the capillaries for exhalation.

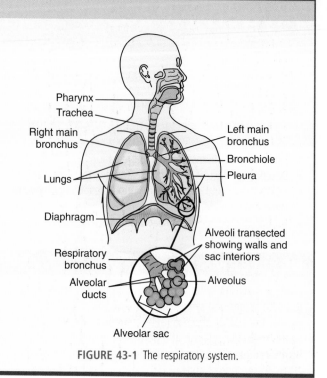

FIGURE 43-1 The respiratory system.

FACTORS AFFECTING OXYGEN NEEDS

Any disease, injury, or surgery involving the respiratory or circulatory system affects the intake and use of O_2. Altered function of any system (for example, the nervous, musculo-skeletal, or urinary system) can also affect oxygen needs. Body systems depend on each other. Respiratory complications may result. Oxygen needs are affected by:

- *The circulatory system.* Narrowed vessels affect blood flow. Capillaries and cells must exchange O_2 and CO_2.
- *Red blood cell count.* Red blood cells (RBCs) contain hemoglobin. Hemoglobin picks up O_2 in the lungs and carries it to the cells. The bone marrow must produce enough RBCs. Blood loss also reduces the number of RBCs.
- *The nervous system.* Nervous system diseases and injuries can affect respiratory muscles. O_2 and CO_2 blood levels also affect brain function. When O_2 is lacking, respirations increase to bring in more oxygen. When CO_2 increases, respirations increase to rid the body of CO_2.
- *Aging.* Respiratory muscles weaken. Lung tissue is less elastic. Strength for coughing decreases. *Pneumonia* (inflammation and infection of the lungs) can develop.
- *Exercise.* O_2 needs increase with exercise. Respiratory rate and depth increase to bring in O_2. Persons with heart and respiratory diseases may have enough oxygen at rest. However, even slight activity can increase O_2 needs. Activity may be limited.
- *Fever.* O_2 needs increase. Respiratory rate and depth increase.

- *Pain.* O_2 needs increase, causing respirations to increase. Chest and abdominal injuries and surgeries often involve respiratory muscles. It hurts to breathe.
- *Drugs.* Some drugs depress the respiratory center in the brain. *Respiratory depression means slow, weak respirations at a rate of fewer than 12 per minute. Respiratory arrest is when breathing stops.* Narcotics (morphine, fentanyl, Demerol, and others) can have these effects. (*Narcotic* comes from the Greek word *narkoun.* It means *stupor* or *to be numb.*) Substance abusers are at risk for respiratory depression and respiratory arrest.
- *Smoking.* Smoking is a major risk factor for lung cancer, chronic bronchitis, emphysema, and coronary artery disease (Chapter 49).
- *Allergies.* An *allergy is a sensitivity to a substance that causes the body to react with signs and symptoms.* Runny nose, wheezing, and congestion are common. Mucous membranes in the upper airway swell. Severe swelling can close the airway. Shock and death are risks. Pollens, dust, foods, drugs, insect bites, powders, flowers, perfumes, sprays, animals, and cigarette smoke often cause allergies.
- *Pollutants.* A *pollutant is a harmful chemical or substance in the air or water.* Examples are dust, fumes, toxins, asbestos, coal dust, and sawdust. They damage the lungs.
- *Nutrition.* The body needs iron and vitamins (vitamin B_{12}, vitamin C, and folate) to produce RBCs.
- *Alcohol.* Alcohol depresses the brain. Excessive amounts reduce the cough reflex and increase the risk of aspiration. Obstructed airway and pneumonia are risks from aspiration.

ALTERED RESPIRATORY FUNCTION

Respiratory function involves 3 processes. Respiratory function is altered if even 1 process is affected.

- Air moves into and out of the lungs.
- O_2 and CO_2 are exchanged between the alveoli and capillaries.
- The blood carries O_2 to the cells and removes CO_2 from them.

Hypoxemia and hypoxia are risks and can threaten life. *Hypoxemia is a reduced amount* (hypo) *of oxygen* (ox) *in the blood* (emia). It can lead to hypoxia. *Hypoxia means that cells do not have enough* (hypo) *oxygen* (oxia). Cells cannot function properly. The brain is very sensitive to inadequate O_2. Restlessness, dizziness, and disorientation are early signs. Report the signs and symptoms of altered respiratory function in Box 43-1 at once.

BOX 43-1 | **Altered Respiratory Function**

- Restlessness
- Dizziness
- Disorientation and confusion
- Behavior and personality changes
- Concentrating and following directions: problems with
- Anxiety and apprehension
- Fatigue
- Agitation
- Pulse rate: increased
- Respirations:
  - Increased rate and depth
  - Noisy, wheezing, wet-sounding, *stridor* (a loud, high-pitched sound from airway blockage)
  - Dyspnea or other abnormal breathing pattern
- Sitting position—upright, leaning forward, hunched over a table
- *Cyanosis—bluish color* (cyano) *to the skin, lips, mucous membranes, and nail beds*
- Shortness of breath or complaints of being "winded" or "short-winded"
- Cough (note type, frequency, and time of day)
  - Dry and hacking
  - Harsh and barking
  - Productive (produces sputum) or non-productive
- *Sputum—mucus from the respiratory system when expectorated (expelled) through the mouth*
  - Color—clear, white, yellow, green, brown, or red
  - Odor—none or foul odor
  - Consistency—thick, watery, or frothy (with bubbles or foam)
  - *Hemoptysis—bloody* (hemo) *sputum* (ptysis *means to spit*); note if the sputum is bright red, dark red, blood-tinged, or streaked with blood
- Chest pain (note location)
  - Constant or comes and goes
  - Person's description—stabbing, knife-like, aching
  - What makes it worse—movement, coughing, yawning, sneezing, sighing, deep breathing, position
- Vital signs: changes in

Abnormal Breathing Patterns

Adults normally breathe 12 to 20 times per minute. Infants and children have faster rates. Normal respirations are quiet, effortless, and regular. Both sides of the chest rise and fall equally. Abnormal breathing patterns (Fig. 43-2, p. 658) and some causes include:

- *Tachypnea—rapid* (tachy) *breathing* (pnea). *Respirations are more than 20 per minute.* Fever, exercise, pain, pregnancy, and airway obstruction are among the causes.
- *Bradypnea—slow* (brady) *breathing* (pnea). *Respirations are fewer than 12 per minute.* Drug over-dose and nervous system disorders are causes.
- *Apnea—the lack or absence* (a) *of breathing* (pnea). It occurs in cardiac arrest and respiratory arrest. Sleep apnea is another type of apnea (Chapter 49).
- *Hypoventilation—breathing* (ventilation) *is slow* (hypo), *shallow, and sometimes irregular.* Lung disorders affecting the alveoli are causes. Pneumonia is an example. Other causes include obesity, airway obstruction, and drug side effects. Nervous system and musculo-skeletal disorders affecting the respiratory muscles also are causes.
- *Hyperventilation—breathing* (ventilation) *is rapid* (hyper) *and deeper than normal.* Causes include asthma, emphysema, infection, fever, nervous system disorders, hypoxia, anxiety, pain, and some drugs.
- *Dyspnea—difficult, labored, or painful* (dys) *breathing* (pnea). Heart disease and anxiety are causes.
- *Cheyne-Stokes respirations—respirations gradually increase in rate and depth and then become shallow and slow. Breathing may stop* (apnea) *for 10 to 20 seconds.* Drug over-dose, heart failure, renal failure, and brain disorders are causes. Cheyne-Stokes are common when death is near.
- *Orthopnea—breathing* (pnea) *deeply and comfortably only when sitting* (ortho). Causes are emphysema, asthma, pneumonia, angina, and other heart and respiratory disorders.
- *Biot's respirations—rapid and deep respirations followed by 10 to 30 seconds of apnea.* They occur with nervous system disorders.
- *Kussmaul respirations—very deep and rapid respirations.* They signal diabetic coma.

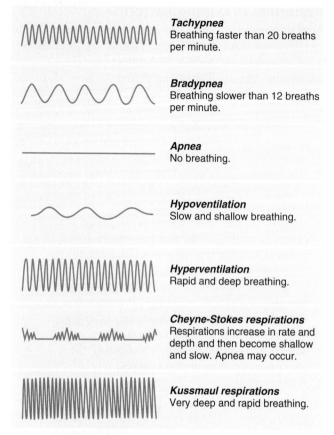

Tachypnea
Breathing faster than 20 breaths per minute.

Bradypnea
Breathing slower than 12 breaths per minute.

Apnea
No breathing.

Hypoventilation
Slow and shallow breathing.

Hyperventilation
Rapid and deep breathing.

Cheyne-Stokes respirations
Respirations increase in rate and depth and then become shallow and slow. Apnea may occur.

Kussmaul respirations
Very deep and rapid breathing.

FIGURE 43-2 Some abnormal breathing patterns.

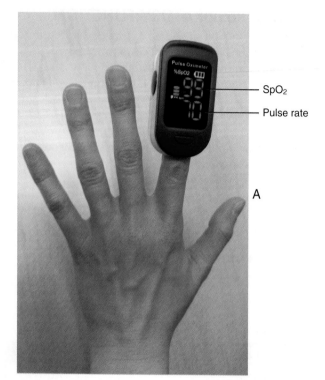

SpO₂

Pulse rate

A

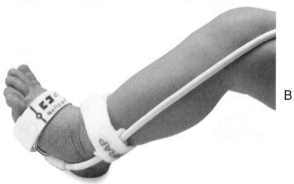

B

FIGURE 43-3 A, A pulse oximetry sensor is attached to a finger. The device displays the O₂ concentration and pulse. **B,** A pulse oximetry sensor for children. (**B,** From Covidien ©2015. All rights reserved. Used with permission of Covidien.)

PULSE OXIMETRY

Various tests may be ordered to detect lung changes. A chest x-ray and other complex tests are examples. You may be involved in pulse oximetry and collecting sputum specimens (Chapter 38). *Pulse oximetry measures (metry) the oxygen (oxi) concentration in arterial blood. Oxygen concentration is the amount (percent [%]) of hemoglobin containing O_2.* An agency may use 1 of these terms.

- *Pulse oximetry* or *pulse ox.*
- *O_2 saturation* or *O_2 sat.*
- *SpO_2* (saturation of peripheral oxygen). *Saturation* means *to be filled. Peripheral* relates to *the surface.* SpO_2 measures the amount of hemoglobin near the surface of the skin that is filled with oxygen.

The normal oxygen concentration range is between 95% and 100%. For example, if 97% of all hemoglobin (100%) carries O_2, tissues get enough oxygen. If only 90% contains O_2, tissues do not get enough oxygen. As low as 85% may be normal for persons with some chronic diseases.

A sensor attaches to a finger, toe, earlobe, nose, or forehead (Fig. 43-3). Light beams on 1 side of the sensor pass through tissues. A detector on the other side measures the amount of light passing through the tissues. With this information, the oximeter measures the O_2 concentration.

Good blood flow to the site is needed. Avoid swollen sites and sites with skin breaks. Bright light, nail polish, non-natural nails, and movements affect measurements. For a good sensor site:

- Place a towel over the sensor to block bright lights.
- Remove nail polish or use another site.
- Do not use finger sites with non-natural nails.
- Use the earlobe if there are shivering, seizure, or tremor movements.
- Do not measure blood pressure on the side of a finger site. Blood pressure cuffs affect blood flow.

Oxygen concentration is often measured with vital signs. The pulse rate may be shown on the pulse oximeter along with the oxygen concentration. Report and record measurements according to agency policy.

Oximeter alarms are set for continuous monitoring. An alarm sounds if:

- O_2 concentration is low.
- The pulse rate is too fast or slow.
- Other problems occur.

    See *Focus on Children and Older Persons: Pulse Oximetry*.
    See *Delegation Guidelines: Pulse Oximetry*.
    See *Promoting Safety and Comfort: Pulse Oximetry*.
    See procedure: *Using a Pulse Oximeter*.

FOCUS ON **CHILDREN AND OLDER PERSONS**

Pulse Oximetry

Children
Different sensors may be used for children (see Fig. 43-3, *B*). The sensor is attached to the sole of the foot, palm of the hand, toe, or earlobe. If the child moves a lot, the earlobe is a better site.

DELEGATION GUIDELINES

Pulse Oximetry

Pulse oximetry measurement is a routine nursing task. You need this information from the nurse and the care plan.

- What site to use
- How to use the equipment
- What sensor to use
- What tape to use (if needed)
- The person's normal SpO_2 range
- Alarm limits for SpO_2 and pulse rate (if set)
- When to do the measurement
- What pulse site to use: apical or radial
- How often to check the site for continuous monitoring (usually at least every 2 hours)

- What observations to report and record:
  - The date and time
  - The SpO_2 and display pulse rate (see Fig. 43-3, *A*)
  - Apical or radial pulse rate
  - What the person was doing at the time
  - Oxygen flow rate (p. 667) and the device used (p. 666)
  - Reason for the measurement: routine, continuous monitoring, or condition change
- When to report observations
- What patient or resident concerns to report at once:
  - An SpO_2 below the alarm limit (usually 95%)
  - A pulse rate above or below the alarm limit
  - The signs and symptoms listed in Box 43-1

PROMOTING SAFETY AND COMFORT

Pulse Oximetry

Safety
The person's condition can change quickly. Pulse oximetry does not lessen the need for good observation. Observe for signs and symptoms of altered respiratory function (see Box 43-1).

Comfort
A clip-on sensor feels like a clothespin. It should not hurt or cause discomfort. Ask the person to tell you at once if it causes pain, discomfort, or too much pressure. Change the sensor site as directed by the nurse.

Using a Pulse Oximeter

QUALITY OF LIFE

- Knock before entering the person's room.
- Address the person by name.
- Introduce yourself by name and title.

- Explain the procedure before starting and during the procedure.
- Protect the person's rights during the procedure.
- Handle the person gently during the procedure.

PRE-PROCEDURE

1 Follow *Delegation Guidelines: Pulse Oximetry*. See *Promoting Safety and Comfort: Pulse Oximetry*.
2 Practice hand hygiene.
3 Collect the following before going to the person's room.
   - Oximeter
   - Sensor (if not part of the device)
   - Tape (if needed)
   - Alcohol wipe

4 Arrange your work area.
5 Practice hand hygiene.
6 Identify the person. Check the identification (ID) bracelet against your assignment sheet. Use 2 identifiers (Chapter 13). Also call the person by name.
7 Provide for privacy.

Continued

Using a Pulse Oximeter—cont'd

PROCEDURE

8   Provide for comfort.
9   Select and clean the site with an alcohol wipe. If measuring blood pressure, use 1 arm for blood pressure and a site on the other arm for pulse oximetry.
10 Clip or tape the sensor to the site. If needed, connect the sensor to the oximeter.
11 Turn on the oximeter.
12 *For continuous monitoring:*
    a   Set the high and low alarm limits for SpO₂ and pulse rate.
    b   Turn on audio and visual alarms.

13 Check the apical or radial pulse with the pulse on the display. The pulse rates should be about the same. Note both pulses on your assignment sheet.
14 Read the SpO₂ on the display. Note the value on the flow sheet and your assignment sheet.
15 Leave the sensor in place for continuous monitoring. Otherwise, turn off the device and remove the sensor.

POST-PROCEDURE

16 Provide for comfort. (See the inside of the back cover.)
17 Place the call light and other needed items within reach.
18 Unscreen the person.
19 Complete a safety check of the room. (See the inside of the back cover.)

20 Return the device to its proper place (except for continuous monitoring). Follow agency policy for disinfection.
21 Practice hand hygiene.
22 Report and record the SpO₂, the pulse rates, and your other observations.

MEETING OXYGEN NEEDS

Air must move deep into the alveoli where O₂ and CO₂ (carbon dioxide) are exchanged. Disease, injury, and surgery can prevent air from reaching the alveoli. Pain, immobility, and some drugs interfere with deep breathing and coughing. Therefore secretions collect in the airway and lungs. Microbes can grow in the secretions. Infection is a threat.

Oxygen needs must be met. The following measures are common in care plans.

- Positioning
- Deep breathing and coughing
- Incentive spirometry (p. 663)
    See *Focus on Communication: Meeting Oxygen Needs.*

FIGURE 43-4 The person is in the orthopneic position. A pillow is on the over-bed table for comfort.

Frequent position changes are needed. Unless position limits were ordered, the person must not lie on 1 side for a long time. Secretions pool. The lungs cannot expand on that side. Position changes are needed at least every 2 hours. Follow the care plan.

If the person must lie flat for a procedure, raise the head of the bed as soon as possible. Raise it at once if the person has difficulty breathing and is allowed semi-Fowler's or Fowler's position. Call for the nurse at once.

Deep Breathing and Coughing

Deep breathing and coughing help meet oxygen needs. Deep breathing moves air into most parts of the lungs. Coughing removes mucus. Deep-breathing and coughing exercises are done after surgery or injury and during bed rest. They are painful after surgery or injury. Breaking an incision open while coughing is a fear.

Deep breathing and coughing are usually done every 1 to 2 hours while awake. They help prevent pneumonia and atelectasis. *Atelectasis is the collapse of a portion of a lung.* It occurs when mucus collects in the airway. Air cannot get to a part of the lung. The lung collapses. Surgery, bed rest, lung diseases, and paralysis are risk factors.

FOCUS ON **COMMUNICATION**

Meeting Oxygen Needs

The questions you ask the person assist with the nursing process. For example:
- "Do you need more pillows?"
- "Do you want the head of your bed raised more?"
- "How often are you coughing?"
- "Are you coughing anything up?"
- "Are you coughing up mucus? Please use a tissue to cough up mucus, then put on your call light. The nurse will observe the mucus."

Positioning

Breathing is usually easier in the semi-Fowler's and Fowler's positions. Persons with difficulty breathing often prefer the *orthopneic position—sitting up (ortho) and leaning over a table to breathe (pneic).* Place a pillow on the table to increase comfort (Fig. 43-4).

See *Focus on Communication: Deep Breathing and Coughing.*

See *Focus on Children and Older Persons: Deep Breathing and Coughing.*

See *Delegation Guidelines: Deep Breathing and Coughing.*

See *Promoting Safety and Comfort: Deep Breathing and Coughing.*

See procedure: *Assisting with Deep-Breathing and Coughing Exercises.*

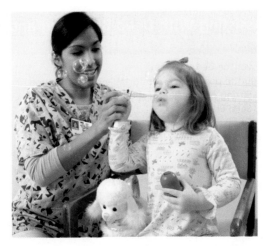

FIGURE 43-5 The child blows bubbles for a deep-breathing exercise.

FOCUS ON **COMMUNICATION**

Deep Breathing and Coughing

To encourage cough etiquette (Chapter 16), you can say:

Please cover your nose and mouth with tissues when coughing. I'll put these tissues where you can reach them. Here is a waste container for your used tissues. Where would you like it? Also, please wash your hands after coughing. Let me know if you need help.

FOCUS ON **CHILDREN AND OLDER PERSONS**

Deep Breathing and Coughing

Children
Party favors are useful for helping children deep breathe. They include paper blowouts, horns, whistles, pinwheels, and others. They are fun and colorful. Blowing bubbles also promotes deep breathing. Before blowing bubbles, the child takes a deep breath (Fig. 43-5).

DELEGATION GUIDELINES

Deep Breathing and Coughing

Assisting with deep-breathing and coughing exercises is a routine nursing task. To assist, you need this information from the nurse and the care plan.
- When to do them and how often
- How many deep breaths and coughs are needed
- What observations to report and record:
  - The number of deep breaths and coughs
  - How the person tolerated the procedure
- When to report observations
- What patient or resident concerns to report at once

PROMOTING SAFETY AND COMFORT

Deep Breathing and Coughing

Safety
Respiratory hygiene and cough etiquette are needed for a productive cough (Chapter 16). The person needs to:
- Cover the nose and mouth to cough or sneeze.
- Use tissues to contain respiratory secretions.
- Dispose of tissues in the nearest waste container after use.
- Wash the hands after coughing, sneezing, or contact with respiratory secretions.

While the person is covering the nose and mouth, you need to splint a chest or abdominal incision with your hands or a pillow. See step 8, b in procedure: *Assisting With Deep-Breathing and Coughing Exercises.* Wear gloves to splint the incision.

Assisting With Deep-Breathing and Coughing Exercises

QUALITY OF LIFE

- Knock before entering the person's room.
- Address the person by name.
- Introduce yourself by name and title.

- Explain the procedure before starting and during the procedure.
- Protect the person's rights during the procedure.
- Handle the person gently during the procedure.

PRE-PROCEDURE

1 Follow *Delegation Guidelines: Deep Breathing and Coughing.* See *Promoting Safety and Comfort: Deep Breathing and Coughing.*
2 Practice hand hygiene.

3 Identify the person. Check the ID bracelet against the assignment sheet. Use 2 identifiers (Chapter 13). Also call the person by name.
4 Provide for privacy.

Continued

Assisting With Deep-Breathing and Coughing Exercises—cont'd

PROCEDURE

5 Lower the bed rail if up.

6 Help the person to a comfortable sitting position.
   * Sitting on the side of the bed
   * Semi-Fowler's
   * Fowler's

7 *For deep breathing:*
   a Have the person place the hands over the rib cage (Fig. 43-6).
   b Have the person breathe as deeply as possible. Have the person inhale through the nose.
   c Ask the person to hold the breath for 2 to 3 seconds.
   d Ask the person to exhale slowly through pursed lips (Fig. 43-7). Have the person exhale until the ribs move as far down as possible.
   e Repeat this step 4 more times.

8 *For coughing:*
   a *If the person does not have a productive cough:* have the person place both hands over the chest or abdominal incision. One hand is on top of the other (Fig. 43-8, *A*). Or the person holds a pillow or folded towel over the chest or abdominal incision (Fig. 43-8, *B*).
   b *If the person has a productive cough:*
      1) Have the person practice cough etiquette.
      2) Splint the chest or abdominal incision with your hands or a pillow. Wear gloves.
   c Have the person take in a deep breath as in step 7.
   d Ask the person to cough strongly 2 times with the mouth open.

9 Assist with hand hygiene.

POST-PROCEDURE

10 Provide for comfort. (See the inside of the back cover.)

11 Place the call light and other needed items within reach.

12 Raise or lower bed rails. Follow the care plan.

13 Unscreen the person.

14 Complete a safety check of the room. (See the inside of the back cover.)

15 Practice hand hygiene.

16 Report and record your observations (Fig. 43-9).

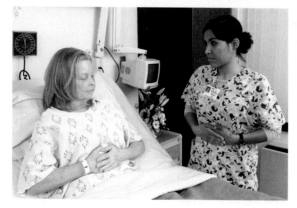

FIGURE 43-6 The hands are over the rib cage for deep breathing.

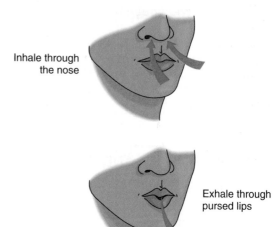

Inhale through the nose

Exhale through pursed lips

FIGURE 43-7 The person inhales through the nose and exhales through pursed lips during the deep-breathing exercise.

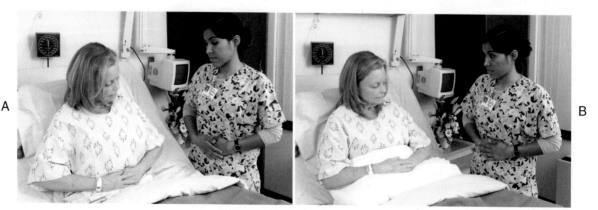

A   B

FIGURE 43-8 The incision is supported for the coughing exercise. **A,** The hands are over the incision. **B,** A pillow is held over the incision.

DATE: 04/19	TIME: 1530
OXYGEN NEEDS: CARE MEASURES	

☒ Deep breathe   ☐ Turn
  ⑤ Times   ☒ Back
☒ Cough   ☐ Right side
  ② Times   ☐ Left side
☐ Incentive spirometry   ☐ Suction
  ☐ Times
  Volume ☐ mL

Assisted patient with deep-breathing and coughing exercises. Incision splinted with a pillow. Patient states: "It is getting easier." Denied pain or discomfort. Over-bed table with water mug and tissues in reach. Call light in reach.

Nurse notified: K. Somers, RN

FIGURE 43-9 Charting sample.

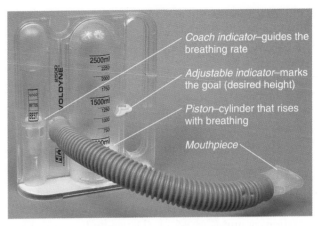

FIGURE 43-10 Parts of a spirometer.

Coach indicator–guides the breathing rate

Adjustable indicator–marks the goal (desired height)

Piston–cylinder that rises with breathing

Mouthpiece

Incentive Spirometry

Incentive means *to encourage.* A *spirometer* is a machine that measures *(meter)* the amount (volume) of air inhaled with an inspiration *(spiro)* (Fig. 43-10). Incentive spirometry also is called *sustained maximal inspiration (SMI). Sustained* means *constant. Maximal* means *the most* or *the greatest.* And *inspiration* relates to *breathing in.* The person inhales as deeply as possible and holds the breath for 3 to 5 seconds.

The goals are to improve lung function and prevent complications. Like yawning or sighing, breathing is long, slow, and deep. Air moves deep into the lungs. Secretions loosen. O_2 and CO_2 exchange occurs between the alveoli and capillaries.

The nurse teaches the person how to use the incentive spirometer. The device is used as follows. The person:

1 Sits on the side of the bed, in Fowler's position, or in a chair.
2 Places the spirometer upright.
3 Exhales normally.
4 Seals the lips around the mouthpiece.
5 Takes a slow, deep breath until the piston rises to the desired height. A marker on the spirometer shows the desired height.
6 Holds the breath for 3 to 5 seconds to keep the piston floating.
7 Removes the mouthpiece and exhales slowly.
8 Rests for a few seconds.
9 Repeats steps 3 through 8 at least 10 to 15 times. The doctor orders the number of breaths.
10 Coughs after at least 10 breaths.
11 Repeats steps 1 through 10 at least every 1 to 2 hours while awake.

See *Delegation Guidelines: Incentive Spirometry.*

DELEGATION GUIDELINES

Incentive Spirometry

Assisting with incentive spirometry is a routine nursing task. To assist, you need this information from the nurse and the care plan.
- How often the person needs incentive spirometry
- How many breaths the person needs to take
- The desired height of the floating piston
- How to clean the mouthpiece
- What observations to report and record:
  - How many breaths the person took
  - The height of the floating piston
  - If the person coughed after the procedure
  - How the person tolerated the procedure
- When to report observations
- What patient or resident concerns to report at once

ASSISTING WITH OXYGEN THERAPY

Oxygen therapy may be ordered when oxygen needs are affected (p. 656) and for altered respiratory function (see Box 43-1). Oxygen therapy is needed constantly or for symptom relief—chest pain or shortness of breath. Persons with respiratory diseases may have enough oxygen at rest. With mild exercise or activity, they become short of breath. Oxygen therapy helps relieve shortness of breath.

Oxygen is treated as a drug. The doctor orders when to give O_2, the amount, and the device to use. Harm can result from too much or not enough oxygen. *You do not give oxygen.* The nurse and respiratory therapist start and maintain oxygen therapy. You help provide safe care.

Oxygen Sources

Oxygen is supplied as follows.

- *Wall outlet.* O_2 is piped into each person's unit (Fig. 43-11).
- *Oxygen tank.* Portable oxygen tanks are used for emergencies, for transfers, and by persons who walk or use wheelchairs (Fig. 43-12). A gauge tells how much O_2 is left (Fig. 43-13).
- *Oxygen concentrator.* The machine removes oxygen from the air (Fig. 43-14). A power source is needed. An oxygen tank is needed for power failures and mobility.
- *Liquid oxygen system.* A portable unit is filled from a stationary unit (Fig. 43-15). Depending on unit size and the flow rate (p. 667), the portable unit has enough O_2 for about 8 to 20 hours of use. A dial shows the amount of O_2 in the unit.

See *Focus on Long-Term Care and Home Care: Oxygen Sources.*

See *Teamwork and Time Management: Oxygen Sources.*

See *Promoting Safety and Comfort: Oxygen Sources.*

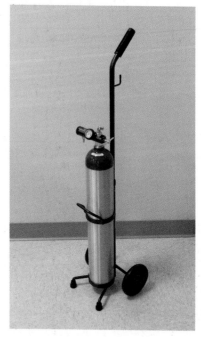

FIGURE 43-12 A portable oxygen tank.

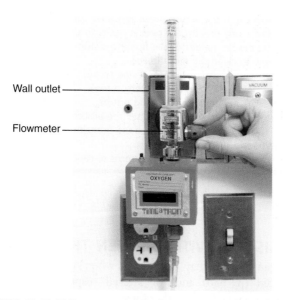

FIGURE 43-11 Wall oxygen outlet. The flowmeter is used to set the oxygen flow rate.

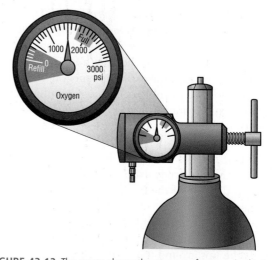

FIGURE 43-13 The gauge shows the amount of oxygen in the tank.

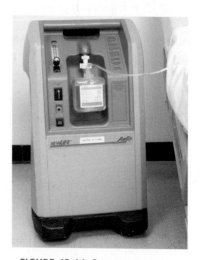

FIGURE 43-14 Oxygen concentrator.

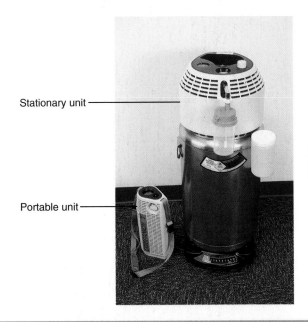

Stationary unit ——

Portable unit ——

FIGURE 43-15 A portable liquid oxygen unit and stationary unit. (From Perry AG, Potter PA, Ostendorf WR: *Clinical nursing skills & techniques*, ed 8, St Louis, 2014, Mosby.)

FOCUS ON LONG-TERM CARE AND HOME CARE

Oxygen Sources

Home Care

Oxygen tanks, oxygen concentrators, and liquid oxygen systems are used in home care. They are maintained by a medical supply company. Keep the company's name and phone number near the phone.

The patient and family must practice safety measures for using and storing oxygen. This includes measures to prevent fires. The nurse instructs them to:

- Practice fire prevention measures (Chapter 13) including:
  - Keeping a fire extinguisher in the room
  - Making sure smoke alarms are in working order
- Do not allow smoking in the room where oxygen is used.
  - Post NO SMOKING signs in the room and on the room door.
  - Remove smoking materials—cigarettes, cigars, pipes, electronic cigarettes, matches, lighters, and so on.
- Remove materials that can ignite, spark, or explode.
  - Personal products—nail polish remover, body oils, petroleum products (lotions and creams), or products containing alcohol
  - Alcoholic beverages
  - Oils and greases
  - Lithium batteries

- Practice electrical safety (Chapter 13) including:
  - Using 3-pronged plugs.
  - Turning off electrical items before unplugging them.
  - Using electrical items that are in good repair. Examples include TVs, radios, music players, computers and other electronic devices, toys, and so on.
  - Avoiding the use of electrical items that may spark. Such items include electric blankets, shavers, and heaters; hair dryers; wool and synthetic fabrics; and some toys.
- Store and use oxygen safely.
  - Keep oxygen sources and tubing at least 5 to 10 feet away from heat sources and open flames. Examples include:
    - Candles
    - Stoves, ovens, and cooktops
    - Heating ducts and pipes
    - Radiators
    - Space heaters—electrical and kerosene
    - Oil and kerosene lamps
  - Keep oxygen sources upright.
  - Keep oxygen sources in well-ventilated areas and away from the sun.
  - Do not drape or cover an oxygen source with clothing, blankets, or other materials.
  - Turn off oxygen when it is not in use.
  - Turn off oxygen if a fire occurs. Get the person and family out of the home. Call 911 to report a fire.

TEAMWORK AND TIME MANAGEMENT

Oxygen Sources

Oxygen tanks and liquid oxygen systems contain a certain amount of O_2. When the O_2 level is low, a new tank is needed or the liquid oxygen system is refilled. Check the O_2 level often. Report a low O_2 level at once.

PROMOTING SAFETY AND COMFORT

Oxygen Sources

Safety

Liquid oxygen is very cold. If touched, it can freeze the skin. Tampering with equipment is unsafe and could damage the equipment. Follow agency procedures and the manufacturer's instructions for liquid oxygen.

Many activities increase the need for O_2. These include moving in bed, transfer procedures, and walking. Do not remove the person's O_2. If needed, ask the nurse for longer tubing. Or ask the nurse to change to a portable oxygen tank.

Oxygen Devices

The nurse tells you what device was ordered for giving O_2. These devices are common.

- *Nasal cannula* (Fig. 43-16). The prongs are inserted into the nostrils. A band goes behind the ears and under the chin to keep the device in place. A cannula allows for eating and drinking. Tight prongs can irritate the nose. Pressure injuries on the ears and cheekbones are possible.
- *Simple face mask* (Fig. 43-17). It covers the nose and mouth. The mask has small holes in the sides. CO_2 escapes when exhaling.
- *Partial-rebreather mask* (Fig. 43-18). A bag is added to the simple face mask for exhaled air. When breathing in, the person inhales O_2 and some exhaled air. Some room air also is inhaled. The bag should not totally deflate when inhaling.
- *Non-rebreather mask* (Fig. 43-19). Exhaled air and room air cannot enter the bag. Exhaled air leaves through holes in the mask. When inhaling, only O_2 from the bag is inhaled. The bag must not totally collapse during inhalation.
- *Venturi mask* (Fig. 43-20). Precise amounts of O_2 are given. Color-coded adapters show the amount of O_2 given.

Talking and eating are hard to do with a mask. Listen carefully. Moisture can build up under the mask. Keep the face clean and dry to help prevent irritation from the mask. For eating, the nurse changes the oxygen mask to a cannula.

Pressure injuries can develop where medical devices cause pressure on the skin. Check the areas where oxygen devices contact the skin. Report any sign of a pressure injury at once. See Chapter 41.

See *Focus on Children and Older Persons: Oxygen Devices.*

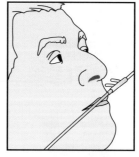
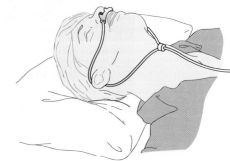

FIGURE 43-16 Nasal cannula. NOTE: The prong openings face downward.

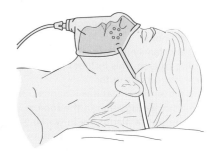

FIGURE 43-17 Simple face mask.

FOCUS ON CHILDREN AND OLDER PERSONS

Oxygen Devices

Children

Oxygen devices for children include cannulas, face masks, partial- and non-rebreather masks, and Venturi masks. Oxygen hoods are used for infants (Fig. 43-21).

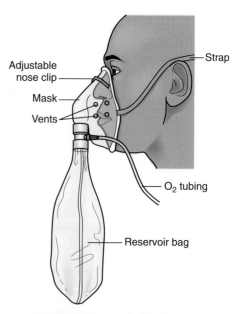

Adjustable nose clip
Strap
Mask
Vents
O_2 tubing
Reservoir bag

FIGURE 43-18 Partial-rebreather mask.

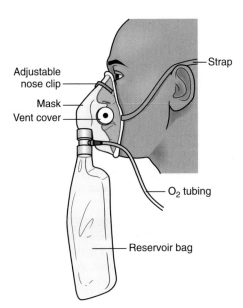

FIGURE 43-19 Non-rebreather mask.

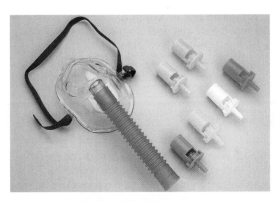

FIGURE 43-20 Venturi mask.

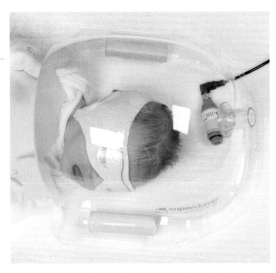

FIGURE 43-21 Oxygen hood. (From Maxtec, West Salt Lake City, Utah.)

Oxygen Flow Rates

The *flow rate* is the amount of oxygen given. It is measured in liters per minute (L/min). The ordered flow rate may be 1 to 15 liters of O_2 per minute. The nurse or respiratory therapist sets the flow rate with a flowmeter (see Fig. 43-11).

The nurse and care plan tell you the person's flow rate. Always check the flow rate. Tell the nurse at once if it is too high or too low. A nurse or respiratory therapist will adjust the flow rate. Some states and agencies let nursing assistants adjust O_2 flow rates. Know your agency's policy.

Oxygen Set-Up

Oxygen is a dry gas. If not humidified (made moist), O_2 dries the airway's mucous membranes. Distilled water is added to the humidifier (Fig. 43-22). (Distilled water is water that has been purified with contaminants removed.)

When added to the humidifier, distilled water creates water vapor. Oxygen picks up the water vapor as it flows into the system. Bubbling in the humidifier means water vapor is being produced. Low flow rates (1 to 2 L/min) by cannula are usually not humidified.

See *Teamwork and Time Management: Oxygen Set-Up.*
See *Delegation Guidelines: Oxygen Set-Up,* p. 668.
See *Promoting Safety and Comfort: Oxygen Set-Up,* p. 668.
See procedure: *Setting Up Oxygen,* p. 668.

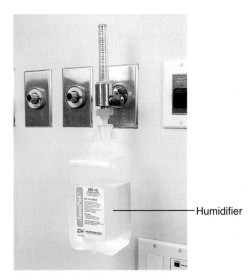

FIGURE 43-22 Oxygen set-up with a humidifier.

TEAMWORK AND TIME MANAGEMENT

Oxygen Set-Up

As you walk past the room of any person receiving humidified O_2, always check the humidifier. Check for and tell the nurse if:
- There is no bubbling.
- The water level is low.

DELEGATION GUIDELINES

Oxygen Set-Up

Setting up oxygen is a nursing responsibility that may be delegated to you in some agencies. If setting up O_2 is delegated to you, you need this information from the nurse.
- The person's name and room and bed numbers
- What oxygen device to use
- If you need a humidifier

PROMOTING SAFETY AND COMFORT

Oxygen Set-Up

Safety

You do not give oxygen. Tell the nurse when the O_2 system is set up. The nurse turns on the O_2, sets the flow rate, and applies the O_2 device. *You do not adjust the flow rate unless allowed by your state and agency.*

Practice medical asepsis. Do not let the connecting tubing hang on the floor.

You must give safe care. Follow the rules in Box 43-2. Also follow the rules for fire and the use of oxygen (Chapter 13).

BOX 43-2   Oxygen Safety

- Do not remove the oxygen device.
- Make sure the device is secure but not tight.
- Check for irritation from the device:
  - Behind the ears
  - Under the nose (cannula)
  - Around the face (mask)
  - On the cheekbones
- Keep the face clean and dry when a mask is used.
- Do not shut off the O_2 flow unless there is a fire. *Turn off the O_2 flow if there is a fire. Remove the oxygen device.*
- Do not adjust the flow rate unless allowed by your state and agency.
- Tell the nurse at once if the:
  - Flow rate is too high or too low
  - Humidifier is not bubbling

- Maintain an adequate water level in the humidifier.
- Secure tubing in place. Tape, clamp, or pin it to the person's garment following agency policy. Do not puncture the tubing.
- Make sure there are no kinks in the tubing.
- Make sure the person does not lie on any part of the tubing.
- Make sure the oxygen tank is secure in its holder.
- Report at once signs and symptoms of altered respiratory function or abnormal breathing patterns. See p. 657.
- Follow the care plan for oral hygiene.
- Make sure the oxygen device is clean and free of mucus.
- See "Fire and Oxygen" in Chapter 13.

Setting Up Oxygen

QUALITY OF LIFE

- Knock before entering the person's room.
- Address the person by name.
- Introduce yourself by name and title.

- Explain the procedure before starting and during the procedure.
- Protect the person's rights during the procedure.
- Handle the person gently during the procedure.

PRE-PROCEDURE

1 Follow *Delegation Guidelines: Oxygen Set-Up.* See *Promoting Safety and Comfort: Oxygen Set-Up.*
2 Practice hand hygiene.
3 Collect the following before going to the person's room.
   - Oxygen device with connecting tubing
   - Flowmeter
   - Humidifier (if ordered)
   - Distilled water (if using a humidifier)

4 Arrange your work area.
5 Practice hand hygiene.
6 Identify the person. Check the ID bracelet against the assignment sheet. Use 2 identifiers (Chapter 13). Also call the person by name.

PROCEDURE

7 Make sure the flowmeter is in the OFF position.
8 Attach the flowmeter to the wall outlet or to the tank.
9 Fill the humidifier with distilled water.
10 Attach the humidifier to the bottom of the flowmeter.
11 Attach the oxygen device and connecting tubing to the humidifier. *Do not set the flowmeter. Do not apply the O_2 device on the person.*

12 Place the cap securely on the distilled water. Store the water according to agency policy.
13 Discard the packaging from the O_2 device and connecting tubing.

POST-PROCEDURE

14 Provide for comfort. (See the inside of the back cover.)
15 Place the call light and other needed items within reach.
16 Complete a safety check of the room. (See the inside of the back cover.)

17 Practice hand hygiene.
18 Tell the nurse when you are done. The nurse will:
   - Turn on the O_2 and set the flow rate.
   - Apply the O_2 device on the person.

FOCUS ON **PRIDE**

The Person, Family, and Yourself

Personal and Professional Responsibility

You are responsible for reporting the person's complaints. A person may say: "I can't breathe" or "I'm not getting enough air." Do not dismiss the complaint. Tell the nurse at once. You cannot feel what the person does. Trust what the person tells you.

Rights and Respect

People have the right to a safe setting. Smoking is not allowed where oxygen is used and stored. NO SMOKING signs are common in rooms and hallways. You may need to remind the person or visitors not to smoke. Be polite and respectful. Show the person where smoking is allowed.

Independence and Social Interaction

Needing long-term oxygen therapy changes a person's life. Portable oxygen sources increase independence. Small oxygen tanks and portable liquid oxygen units are examples. Such devices allow freedom and promote quality of life.

Delegation and Teamwork

If asked to give oxygen or adjust a flow rate, politely refuse. Refusing to perform a task is your right and duty when the task is beyond the legal limits of your role. Do not ignore the request. Tell the nurse that you can assist. Gathering supplies is an example. Or ask if you can help with a different task.

Ethics and Laws

The following case shows how harm resulted from unsafe use of oxygen by a certified nursing assistant (CNA) who was not trained or qualified to handle oxygen.

A CNA took a group of residents outside to smoke. One resident, who used oxygen, was taken outside with her oxygen tank. Center policy stated that oxygen was to be used and handled only by nurses. The CNA tried to turn off the oxygen but she did not turn it off completely. The resident's cigarette set fire to the oxygen and caused severe facial burns.

Ethics and Laws—cont'd

The CNA lost her job. The state's board of nursing asked the CNA for a written response to complaints against her. The CNA did not respond.

The CNA's conduct provided grounds for disciplinary action. The CNA was charged with:

- *Committing an act that deceives, defrauds, or harms the public*
- *Conduct or practice that is or may be harmful to the health of a patient or the public*
- *Failing to follow policies and procedures designed to protect the patient or resident*
- *Violating the rights or dignity of a patient or resident*
- *Neglecting or abusing a resident physically, verbally, emotionally, or financially*
- *Accepting care tasks that the CNA lacks the education or competence to perform*
- *Failing to cooperate with the board during an investigation by:*
  - *Not providing a complete, written explanation of the matter*
  - *Not completing and returning a board-issued questionnaire within 30 days*

The CNA's certificate was revoked.
(Arizona State Board of Nursing, 2010.)

Performing tasks that you are not trained to do can cause harm. You can lose your job and your ability to work as a nursing assistant. Take pride in following the limits of your role and providing safe care.

FOCUS ON **PRIDE**: *Application*

What are the limits to your role when assisting with oxygen therapy? Why are such limits important? Explain the value of your role. How do you help the nurse and patient or resident?

REVIEW QUESTIONS

Circle the BEST answer.

1 Alcohol and narcotics affect oxygen needs because they
   a Depress the brain
   b Are pollutants
   c Cause allergies
   d Cause infection

2 Hypoxia is
   a Not enough oxygen in the blood
   b The amount of hemoglobin that contains oxygen
   c Not enough oxygen in the cells
   d The lack of carbon dioxide

3 An early sign of altered respiratory function is
   a Cyanosis
   b Increased pulse
   c Restlessness
   d Dyspnea

4 A person breathes deeply and comfortably only while sitting. This is called
   a Apnea
   b Orthopnea
   c Bradypnea
   d Kussmaul respirations

5 Tachypnea means that respirations are
   a Slow
   b Rapid
   c Absent
   d Difficult or painful

6 Which should you report to the nurse at once?
   a A respiratory rate of 18 per minute
   b An SpO_2 of 97%
   c Bubbling in a humidifier
   d Dyspnea

Continued

REVIEW QUESTIONS—cont'd

7 A person's SpO_2 is 98%. Which is *true*?
   a The pulse oximeter is wrong.
   b The pulse is 98 beats per minute.
   c The measurement is within normal range.
   d The person has hypoxia.

8 A person has non-natural nails. Which is another pulse oximetry sensor site?
   a The wrist
   b The chest
   c The upper arm
   d An earlobe

9 You are assisting with deep breathing and coughing. You need to explain the procedure again if the person
   a Inhales through pursed lips
   b Sits in a comfortable position
   c Inhales deeply through the nose
   d Holds a pillow over an incision

10 A person has a productive cough. You remind the person to
   a Use a face mask
   b Cover the nose and mouth when coughing
   c Cough and deep breathe twice daily
   d Inhale through the mouth

11 Liquid oxygen can freeze the skin.
   a True
   b False

12 Which is useful for deep breathing?
   a Pulse oximeter
   b Incentive spirometer
   c Simple face mask
   d Partial-rebreather mask

13 Which oxygen device allows for eating?
   a Simple face mask
   b Partial-rebreather mask
   c Venturi mask
   d Nasal cannula

14 Oxygen flow rate is measured in
   a mm Hg
   b mL/h
   c L/min
   d SpO_2

15 When assisting with oxygen therapy, you can
   a Turn the oxygen on and off
   b Start the oxygen
   c Decide what device to use
   d Keep connecting tubing secure and free of kinks

16 A person has humidified oxygen. The water level should move up with inspiration and down with expiration.
   a True
   b False

17 A person is receiving O_2. Which is *unsafe*?
   a Smoking materials are in the room.
   b Electrical items are turned off, then unplugged.
   c 3-pronged electrical items are used.
   d There is a fire extinguisher in the room.

18 A person is receiving O_2. Which should you question?
   a Provide oral hygiene.
   b Use a portable tank for walking.
   c Adjust the flow rate if it is too high or too low.
   d Secure tubing in place.

Answers to Chapter 43 questions are on p. 887.

FOCUS ON **PRACTICE**
Problem Solving

You are a student training in the clinical setting. A nursing assistant asks you to change a person's O_2 flow rate. Nursing assistants in your state are not allowed to adjust O_2 flow rates. How will you respond? What will you do if the nursing assistant adjusts the flow rate?

Respiratory Support and Therapies

OBJECTIVES

- Define the key terms and key abbreviations in this chapter.
- Explain how to assist in the care of persons with artificial airways.
- Describe the principles and safety measures for suctioning.

- Explain how to assist in the care of persons on mechanical ventilation.
- Explain how to assist in the care of persons with chest tubes.
- Explain how to promote PRIDE in the person, the family, and yourself.

KEY TERMS

hemothorax Blood *(hemo)* in the pleural space *(thorax)*

intubation Inserting an artificial airway

mechanical ventilation Using a machine to move air into and out of the lungs

patent Open and unblocked

pleural effusion The escape and collection of fluid *(effusion)* in the pleural space

pneumothorax Air *(pneumo)* in the pleural space *(thorax)*

suction The process of withdrawing or sucking up fluid (secretions)

tracheostomy A surgically created opening *(stomy)* in the neck into the trachea *(tracheo)*

KEY ABBREVIATIONS

CO_2	Carbon dioxide		O_2	Oxygen
ET	Endotracheal		RT	Respiratory therapist

Some persons have serious problems affecting the respiratory system. They need complex procedures and equipment. The nurse may ask you to assist in their care.

See *Body Structure and Function Review: The Respiratory System* (Chapter 43).

See *Promoting Safety and Comfort: Respiratory Support and Therapies.*

PROMOTING SAFETY AND COMFORT

Respiratory Support and Therapies

Safety
Respiratory secretions may contain microbes or blood. Follow Standard Precautions and the Bloodborne Pathogen Standard.

ARTIFICIAL AIRWAYS

Artificial airways keep the airway *patent (open and unblocked).* They are needed:

- When disease, injury, secretions, or aspiration obstructs the airway.
- For mechanical ventilation (p. 675)
- By some persons who are semi-conscious or unconscious
- During surgery and recovery from anesthesia
  Intubation means inserting an artificial airway
  (Fig. 44-1, p. 672). Airways are usually plastic and disposable.

- *Oro-pharyngeal airway*—inserted through the mouth and into the pharynx (see Fig. 44-1, *A*). A nurse or respiratory therapist (RT) inserts the airway.
- *Endotracheal (ET) tube*—inserted through the mouth or nose into the trachea (see Fig. 44-1, *B*). A lighted scope is used to guide insertion by a doctor, specially trained nurse, or RT. The cuff on the tube is inflated to seal the airway. The seal prevents air and fluid leaks around the cuff.
- *Tracheostomy tube*—inserted through a surgically created opening *(stomy)* into the trachea *(tracheo)* (see Fig. 44-1, *C*). Like ET tubes, cuffed tracheostomy tubes are common. Doctors perform tracheostomies.

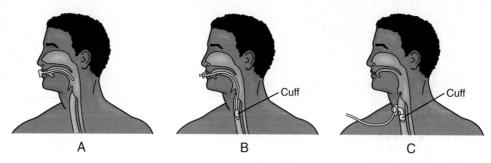

A B C

FIGURE 44-1 Artificial airways. **A,** Oro-pharyngeal airway. **B,** Endotracheal tube with cuff. **C,** Tracheostomy tube with cuff. (NOTE: Inflated cuffs keep endotracheal and tracheostomy tubes in place.)

Vital signs and pulse oximetry are measured often. Observe for signs and symptoms of altered respiratory function (Chapter 43). If an airway comes out or is dislodged, tell the nurse at once.

Gagging and choking feelings are common. Imagine something in your mouth, nose, or throat. Comfort and reassure the person. Remind the person that the airway helps breathing. Use touch to show you care.

Frequent oral hygiene is needed. Follow the care plan. See *Focus on Communication: Artificial Airways.*

Tracheostomies

A *tracheostomy is a surgically created opening* (stomy) *in the neck into the trachea* (tracheo). Tracheostomies are often temporary. When no longer needed, the stoma is allowed to heal or is closed surgically.

Tracheostomies are permanent when the larynx is surgically removed. Cancer, airway injuries, long-term coma, spinal cord injuries, and diseases causing weakness or paralysis of the respiratory muscles may require a permanent tracheostomy.

A tracheostomy tube has 3 parts (Fig. 44-2).

- The *obturator* has a round end. It is used to guide insertion of the outer cannula (tube). Then it is removed. The obturator is kept at the bedside in case the tracheostomy tube falls out and needs insertion.
- The *outer cannula* is secured in place with ties around the neck or a Velcro collar. The outer cannula is not removed. It keeps the tracheostomy patent. *Call for the nurse at once if the outer cannula comes out.*
- The *inner cannula* is inserted into the outer cannula and locked in place. It is removed for cleaning and mucus removal to keep the airway patent. Most tracheostomy tubes have inner cannulas.

The tube must not come out *(extubation)*. If not secure, it could come out with coughing or if pulled on. A loose tube moves up and down, damaging the trachea. The tube must remain patent. If able, the person coughs up secretions. Otherwise suctioning is needed. *Call for the nurse at once if you note signs and symptoms of altered respiratory function.*

FOCUS ON COMMUNICATION

Artificial Airways

An artificial airway affects the person's ability to speak. Some tracheostomy tubes allow speech. Paper and pencils, Magic Slates, and communication boards are ways to communicate. Hand signals, nodding the head, and hand squeezes are common for simple "yes" and "no" answers. Follow the care plan. Always keep the call light and other needed items within reach.

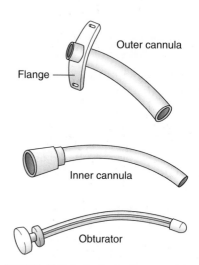

FIGURE 44-2 Parts of a tracheostomy tube.

Safety Measures. Nothing must enter the stoma. Water and inhaled substances are examples. Otherwise the person can aspirate. These safety measures are needed.

- Dressings do not have loose gauze or lint.
- The stoma or tube is covered when outdoors. The person wears a stoma cover or shield, scarf, or shirt or blouse that covers the neck. The cover allows air to pass through for inhalation but prevents dust, insects, and other small particles from entering the stoma.
- The stoma is not covered with plastic, leather, or similar materials. Air cannot pass through such materials. Therefore air cannot be inhaled through the stoma and the person cannot breathe.
- Tub baths are taken. For showers, a shower guard is worn. A hand-held nozzle is used to direct water away from the stoma.
- The person is assisted with shampooing. Water must not enter the stoma.
- The stoma is covered when shaving.
- Swimming is not allowed. Water will enter the tube or stoma.
- Medical-alert jewelry is worn. The person carries a medical-alert ID (identification) card.

Assisting With Tracheostomy Care.
Tracheostomy care (trach care) is a nursing responsibility. The nurse may ask you to assist. Trach care is done to prevent infection, promote healing, and promote comfort. It also is done as needed for excess secretions, soiled ties or collar, or soiled or moist dressings. The nurse tells you when trach care is needed and what supplies to collect. Assist as directed.

Trach care involves:

- Cleaning the inner cannula to remove mucus and keep the airway patent. A disposable inner cannula is discarded and new one is inserted. Re-usable cannulas are cleaned with a small bottle brush or a pipe cleaner and a cleaning agent.
- Cleaning the stoma to prevent infection and skin breakdown.
- Applying clean ties or a Velcro collar. Clean ties are applied before removing the used ones. Hold the outer cannula in place until the nurse secures the new ties or collar. The ties or collar must be secure but not tight. For an adult, a finger should slide under the ties or collar (Fig. 44-3, *A*).

See *Focus on Children and Older Persons: Assisting With Tracheostomy Care.*

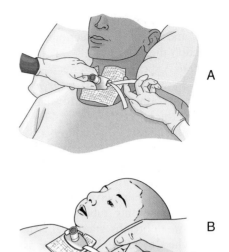

FIGURE 44-3 **A,** For an adult, a finger is inserted under the ties. **B,** For children, only a fingertip is inserted under the ties.

FOCUS ON **CHILDREN AND OLDER PERSONS**

Assisting With Tracheostomy Care

Children

Some children have congenital defects that are present at birth. (The Latin word *congenitus* means *to be born with.*) Tracheostomies are needed for some congenital defects affecting the neck and airway.

Some infections cause swelling of the airway structures. This obstructs air flow. So does foreign body aspiration. These problems may require emergency tracheostomies.

Tracheostomy ties must be secure but not tight. Only a fingertip should slide under the ties (Fig. 44-3, *B*). Ties are too loose if you can slide your whole finger under them.

Assist the nurse by holding the child still. Position the child's head as the nurse directs.

SUCTIONING

Secretions can collect in the airway. Retained secretions:

- Obstruct air flow into and out of the airway.
- Provide an environment for microbes.
- Interfere with oxygen (O_2) and carbon dioxide (CO_2) exchange.

Usually coughing removes secretions. Some persons cannot cough or the cough is too weak to remove secretions. They need suctioning.

Suction is the process of withdrawing or sucking up fluid (secretions). A tube connects to a suction source—wall outlet or suction machine—at 1 end and to a suction catheter at the other end. The catheter is inserted into the airway. Secretions are suctioned through the catheter.

The upper airway (nose, mouth, and pharynx) and lower airway (trachea and bronchi) are suctioned. These routes are used to suction the airway.

- *Oro-pharyngeal.* A suction catheter is passed through the mouth *(oro)* into the pharynx *(pharyngeal).* The Yankauer suction catheter is used to suction the mouth and for thick secretions (Fig. 44-4).
- *Naso-pharyngeal.* The suction catheter is passed through the nose *(naso)* into the pharynx *(pharyngeal).*
- *Lower airway.* The suction catheter is passed through an ET or tracheostomy tube (Fig. 44-5).

The person's lungs are hyperventilated before suctioning an ET or tracheostomy tube. *Hyperventilate* means to give extra *(hyper)* breaths *(ventilate).* An Ambu bag (Fig. 44-6) attached to an oxygen source is used. The oxygen delivery device is removed from the ET or tracheostomy tube and the Ambu bag is attached. To give a breath, the bag is squeezed with both hands. The nurse or RT gives 3 to 5 breaths.

Hyperventilating the lungs is the responsibility of a nurse or RT. Check if your state and agency allow you to use an Ambu bag attached to an oxygen source.

To assist the nurse with suctioning, follow the safety measures in Box 44-1.

See *Focus on Children and Older Persons: Suctioning.*

See *Delegation Guidelines: Suctioning.*

See *Promoting Safety and Comfort: Suctioning.*

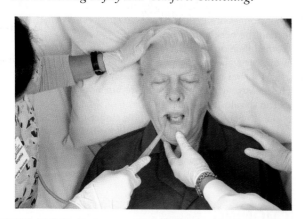

FIGURE 44-4 The Yankauer suction catheter is used to suction the mouth and for large amounts of thick secretions.

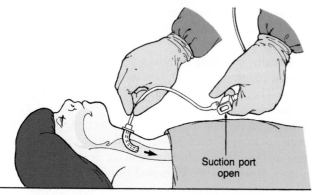

FIGURE 44-5 A tracheostomy tube is suctioned. (Modified from Hockenberry MJ, Wilson D, Rodgers CC: *Wong's essentials of pediatric nursing,* ed 10, St Louis, 2017, Elsevier.)

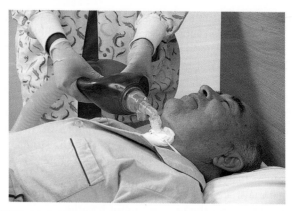

FIGURE 44-6 The Ambu bag is squeezed with 2 hands to hyperventilate the lungs.

BOX 44-1	Assisting With Suctioning

- Review the procedure with the nurse. Know what you are expected and allowed to do.
- Report coughing and the signs and symptoms of altered respiratory function (Chapter 43). Suctioning is done as needed, not on a schedule.
- Position the person as directed by the nurse—semi-Fowler's position with the head turned to 1 side or lateral position with the head turned to 1 side.
- Follow Standard Precautions and the Bloodborne Pathogen Standard. Secretions may contain blood and are potentially infectious.
- Follow sterile technique (Chapter 16) when assisting with naso-pharyngeal suctioning and the suctioning of ET and tracheostomy tubes. This helps prevent microbes from entering the airway.
- Collect the catheter type and size as directed by the nurse. If too large, it can injure the airway.
- Collect and keep suction catheter supplies and equipment at the bedside as directed by the nurse. They are ready when the person needs suctioning.
- Check the pulse, respirations, and pulse oximeter measurements before, during, and after the procedure. Also observe level of consciousness. Tell the nurse if any of these occur:
  - A change in pulse rate or pulse rate less than 60 beats per minute.
  - Irregular pulse rhythm.
  - An increase or decrease in blood pressure.
  - Altered respiratory function.
  - A decrease in oxygen saturation. Normal range is 95% to 100%. See Chapter 43.

DELEGATION GUIDELINES

Suctioning

Suctioning is a nursing responsibility or that of an RT. Some states and agencies allow nursing assistants to perform oro-pharyngeal suctioning. If delegated to you, make sure that:

- Your state allows you to perform the procedure.
- The procedure is in your job description.
- You have the necessary training.
- You know how to use the equipment.
- You review the procedure with a nurse.
- A nurse is available to answer questions and to guide and assist you as needed.

If the above conditions are met, you need the following information from the nurse and the care plan.

- What kind and size of suction catheter to use
- How to position the person—semi-Fowler's or lateral position
- What suction pressure to use
- What observations to report and record:
  - The amount, color, and consistency of secretions
  - Signs and symptoms of altered respiratory function (Chapter 43)
  - How the person tolerated the procedure
- When to report observations
- What patient or resident concerns to report at once (see Box 44-1)

PROMOTING SAFETY AND COMFORT

Suctioning

Safety

If not done correctly, suctioning can cause serious harm. The person does not get oxygen during suctioning. Suction is applied for only 5 to 10 seconds. Altered respiratory function and life-threatening problems can occur from the respiratory, cardiovascular, and nervous systems. Cardiac arrest is a risk. Infection and airway injuries are possible.

MECHANICAL VENTILATION

Mechanical ventilation is using a machine to move air into and out of the lungs (Fig. 44-7). An ET or tracheostomy tube is needed.

Problems that interfere with breathing or normal oxygen levels include:

- Weak muscle effort, obstructed airway, and damaged lung tissue
- Nervous system diseases and injuries affecting the respiratory center in the brain
- Nerve damage interfering with messages between the lungs and the brain
- Drug over-dose depressing the brain

Ventilator alarms sound when something is wrong. One alarm means the person is disconnected from the ventilator and can die from the lack of oxygen. The nurse shows you how to reconnect the ET or tracheostomy tube. When any alarm sounds, first check if the tube is attached to the ventilator. If not, re-attach it to the ventilator. Then tell the nurse at once about the alarm. Do not re-set alarms.

Persons needing mechanical ventilation are often very ill. Other problems and injuries are common. Some persons are confused, disoriented, or cannot think clearly. The machine, fear of dying, and needing the machine life-long are concerns. Some are relieved to get enough oxygen. Mechanical ventilation can be painful for those with chest injuries or chest surgery. Tubes and hoses restrict movement, causing more discomfort.

The nurse may have you assist with the person's care. See Box 44-2, p. 676.

See *Focus on Long-Term Care and Home Care: Mechanical Ventilation*, p. 676.

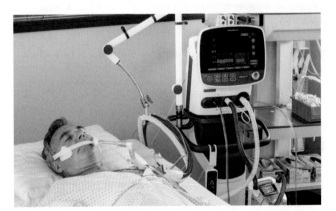

FIGURE 44-7 A mechanical ventilator. (© Hamilton Medical.)

BOX 44-2	Assisting With Mechanical Ventilation

- Keep the call light and other needed items within reach.
- Answer call lights promptly. The person depends on others for basic needs.
- Make sure hoses and connecting tubes have slack. They must not pull on the artificial airway.
- Explain who you are and what you are going to do. Do this each time you enter the room.
- Give the day, date, and time every time you give care.
- Report signs of altered respiratory function or discomfort at once.
- Do not change machine settings or re-set alarms.
- Follow the care plan for communication. The person cannot talk. Use agreed-upon hand or eye signals for "yes" and "no." Everyone must use the same signals. Some persons can use the communication aids described in Chapter 7. Ask questions with simple answers. It may be hard to write long responses.
- Watch what you say and do. This includes when you are near and away from the person and family. They are aware of your verbal and nonverbal communication. Do not say or do anything that could upset the person.
- Use touch to comfort and reassure the person. Also tell the person about the weather, pleasant news events, and gifts and cards.
- Meet basic needs. Follow the care plan.
- Tell the person when you are leaving the room and when you will return.
- Complete a safety check before leaving the room. (See the inside of the back cover.)

FOCUS ON **LONG-TERM CARE AND HOME CARE**

Mechanical Ventilation

Long-Term Care
Mechanical ventilation may be needed for a few hours. Or it may be needed for several days or longer. When possible, the person is weaned from the ventilator. That is, the person needs to breathe without the machine. The RT and nurse plan the weaning process. Weaning can take many weeks.

Home Care
Some ventilator-dependent persons receive home care. The nurse teaches you and the family how to care for the person. You must be able to reach the nurse by phone. Make sure delegated tasks are allowed by your state and agency.

CHEST TUBES

Air, blood, or fluid can collect in the pleural space (sac or cavity). This occurs when the chest is entered because of injury or surgery.

- *Pneumothorax is air* (pneumo) *in the pleural space* (thorax).
- *Hemothorax is blood* (hemo) *in the pleural space* (thorax).
- *Pleural effusion is the escape and collection of fluid* (effusion) *in the pleural space.*

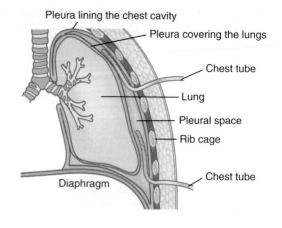

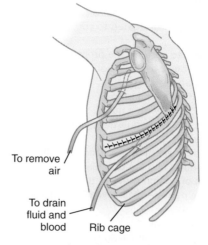

FIGURE 44-8 Chest tubes inserted into the pleural space. (Modified from Lewis SL, Bucher L, Heitkemper MM, Harding MM: *Medical-surgical nursing: assessment and management of clinical problems*, ed 10, St Louis, 2017, Elsevier.)

Pressure from air, blood, or fluid in the pleural space collapses the lung. Air cannot reach affected alveoli for O_2 and CO_2 exchange. Altered respiratory function results. Pressure on the heart affects the heart's ability to pump blood.

The doctor inserts chest tubes to remove the air, blood, or fluid (Fig. 44-8). The sterile procedure is done in surgery, the emergency room, or at the bedside. A nurse assists.

Chest tubes attach to a drainage system (Fig. 44-9). The system must be air-tight so air does not enter the pleural space. Water-seal drainage keeps the system air-tight. The bottles in Figure 44-10 show how the system works.

- A chest tube attaches to connecting tubing.
- Connecting tubing attaches to a tube in the drainage container.
- The tube in the drainage container extends under the water. The water prevents air from entering the chest tube and then the pleural space.

See Box 44-3 for care of the person with chest tubes.

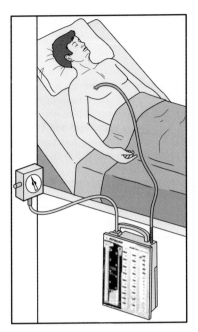

FIGURE 44-9 Chest tube attached to a disposable water-seal drainage system. (Redrawn from Atrium Medical, Maquet Getinge Group, Hudson, NH.)

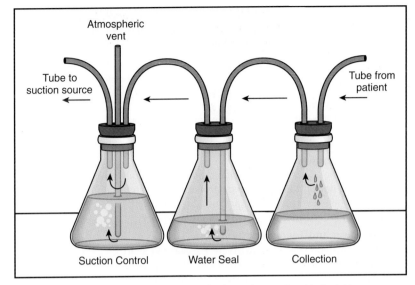

FIGURE 44-10 Water-seal drainage system. (Redrawn from Atrium Medical, Maquet Getinge Group, Hudson, NH.)

BOX 44-3	**Assisting With Chest Tubes**

- Keep the drainage system below the chest.
- Report the following at once.
  - Vital signs and pulse oximetry measurements. The nurse tells you when to take them.
  - Signs and symptoms of altered respiratory function. See Chapter 43.
  - Complaints of pain or difficulty breathing.
  - Changes in chest drainage. This includes increases in drainage or the appearance of bright red drainage.
  - If bubbling in the drainage system increases, decreases, or stops.
  - If any part of the drainage system is loose or disconnected.
- Keep connecting tubing coiled on the bed. Allow enough slack so the chest tubes are not dislodged when the person moves. If tubing hangs in loops, drainage collects in the loops.

- Prevent tubing kinks. Kinks obstruct the chest tube. Air, blood, or fluid collects in the pleural space.
- Record chest drainage according to agency policy.
- Turn and position the person as directed. Be careful and gentle to prevent the chest tubes from dislodging.
- Assist with deep-breathing and coughing exercises and incentive spirometry as directed. See Chapter 43.
- Keep sterile petrolatum gauze at the bedside as directed by the nurse. It is needed if a chest tube comes out.
- Call for help at once if a chest tube comes out. Cover the insertion site with sterile petrolatum gauze or other dressing according to agency policy. Stay with the person. Follow the nurse's directions.
- Complete a safety check before leaving the room. (See the inside of the back cover.)

FOCUS ON **PRIDE**

The Person, Family, and Yourself

Personal and Professional Responsibility

The person's airway must be clear for survival. Tell the nurse at once if you suspect a problem. Delay can cause harm or death.

Observing the person and reporting concerns are important parts of your role. Take pride in safely assisting with respiratory support and therapies.

Rights and Respect

Persons requiring respiratory support may be comatose or sedated. However, the person may hear and understand. Show dignity and respect when providing care.

- Tell the person when he or she will be moved or touched.
- Explain what the person will feel and where it will be felt.
- Talk to the person. Tell about pleasant things.
- Focus on the person. Do not ignore the person or talk with co-workers about personal matters.
- Use touch to show you care.

Continued

FOCUS ON **P R I D E—cont'd**

The Person, Family, and Yourself

Independence and Social Interaction

Mechanical ventilation brings fears and worries for the family. Quality time with the person can bring the family peace and ease stress. To provide social support, you can:

- Encourage the family to talk to the person. If the person cannot respond, explain that he or she may hear and understand.
- Allow private time.
- Promote the use of touch. Provide chairs so the family can sit by the person to hold a hand, stroke the hair, and so on.
- Allow family involvement in care measures. Brushing hair, applying lotion, and giving nail care are examples.

Delegation and Teamwork

Some team members have 1 focus of care. For example, an RT provides respiratory treatments and therapies. Develop a good working relationship with the RT. Politely offer to help as needed. The RT is a good source for respiratory issues. Ask questions and thank the RT for answering them.

Ethics and Laws

Many respiratory support measures and therapies in this chapter are outside the scope of your role. Serious problems can occur from the wrong care. Know your limits. Assist with care measures as directed. Remember your legal and ethical responsibilities. You have the right to refuse a function or task that is beyond your legal scope, preparation, skill level, and job description.

FOCUS ON **PRIDE**: *Application*

Imagine if a family member required mechanical ventilation. What concerns and fears would you have? Describe the quality of care you would expect. How would you like to be treated? How will you apply these qualities in your interactions with the person and family?

REVIEW QUESTIONS

Circle the BEST answer.

1 A person has a tracheostomy. Which is *true?*
   a The person must not cough.
   b The obturator is kept at the nurses' station.
   c The tube must remain patent.
   d The nurse removes the outer cannula for cleaning.

2 A person with a tracheostomy *cannot*
   a Shampoo
   b Shave
   c Shower with a hand-held nozzle
   d Swim

3 The nurse is changing tracheostomy ties. You must
   a Remove the inner cannula
   b Clean the stoma
   c Remove the dressing
   d Hold the outer cannula in place

4 You cannot slide a finger under the tracheostomy ties. This means that the ties
   a Are secure   c Need to be replaced
   b Are too tight   d Need to be removed

5 Which signals the need for suctioning?
   a A pulse rate of 90 beats per minute
   b Signs and symptoms of altered respiratory function
   c It has been 2 hours since the last suctioning
   d Being unable to speak

6 Suctioning the lower airway requires
   a Sterile technique
   b Mechanical ventilation
   c A Yankauer catheter
   d Chest tubes

7 Your role in suctioning involves
   a Selecting the type of suction catheter
   b Hyperventilating the lungs
   c Deciding when to suction the airway
   d Keeping needed supplies at the bedside

8 You note the following while assisting with suctioning. Which should you report at once?
   a A pulse rate of 82 beats per minute
   b A regular heart rhythm
   c Oxygen saturation of 92%
   d Thick secretions

9 A person has an ET tube with mechanical ventilation. Which is *true?*
   a The ET tube must stay attached to the ventilator.
   b You should remove slack from hoses and tubing.
   c The person cannot respond or sense touch.
   d You can re-set alarms on the ventilator.

10 A ventilator alarm sounds. What should you do?
   a Re-set the alarm.
   b Check if the airway is attached to the machine.
   c Do nothing.
   d Ask the person what is wrong.

11 A person has a pneumothorax. This is
   a Fluid in the pleural space
   b Blood in the pleural space
   c Air in the pleural space
   d Secretions in the pleural space

12 Assisting with chest tube care involves
   a Avoiding deep breathing and coughing
   b Making sure tubing is not kinked
   c Keeping the drainage system at chest level
   d Hanging tubing in loops

Answers to Chapter 44 questions are on p. 887.

FOCUS ON PRACTICE

Problem Solving

The nurse suctioned a patient's tracheostomy tube 2 hours ago. Now the person's breathing is noisy and wet-sounding. Coughing has a harsh sound. Is this normal? What do you do? How often is suctioning done?

Rehabilitation Needs

OBJECTIVES

- Define the key terms and key abbreviations in this chapter.
- Describe how rehabilitation involves the whole person.
- Identify the complications to prevent.
- Identify the common reactions to rehabilitation.

- Explain your role in rehabilitation.
- List the common rehabilitation programs and services.
- Explain how to promote PRIDE in the person, the family, and yourself.

KEY TERMS

activities of daily living (ADL) The activities usually done during a normal day in a person's life
disability Any lost, absent, or impaired physical or mental function
prosthesis An artificial replacement for a missing body part
rehabilitation The process of restoring the person to his or her highest possible level of physical, psychological, social, and economic function

restorative aide A nursing assistant with special training in restorative nursing and rehabilitation skills
restorative nursing care Care that helps persons regain health and strength for safe and independent living

KEY ABBREVIATIONS

ADL	Activities of daily living
CMS	Centers for Medicare & Medicaid Services

ROM Range-of-motion

Disease, injury, and surgery can affect body function. So can birth injuries and birth defects (Chapter 54). Often more than 1 function is lost.

A *disability is any lost, absent, or impaired physical or mental function.* Causes are acute or chronic (Box 45-1).
- An *acute problem* has a short course with complete recovery. A fracture (broken bone) is an example.
- A *chronic problem* has a long course. The problem is controlled—not cured—with treatment. Arthritis and paralysis are chronic health problems.

Disabilities can affect eating, bathing, dressing, walking, and work ability. These daily activities and others are hard or seem impossible. The degree of disability affects how much function is possible. The person may depend totally or in part on others for basic needs.

Rehabilitation is the process of restoring the person to his or her highest possible level of physical, psychological, social, and economic function. Physical, occupational, and speech-language therapists are among the health team members involved (Chapter 1). The goals of rehabilitation are to:
- Prevent or reduce the degree of disability.
- Improve abilities for the highest level of independence. Self-care or returning to work may be a goal. If improved function is not possible, the goal is to prevent further loss of function for the best possible quality of life.
- Help the person adjust to the disability.

Some persons return home after rehabilitation. The process may continue in home or community settings.

See *Focus on Long-Term Care and Home Care: Rehabilitation Needs*, p. 680.

BOX 45-1	Common Problems Requiring Rehabilitation

- Amputation
- Birth defects
- Brain tumor
- Burns
- Cancer
- Chronic obstructive pulmonary disease

- Fractures
- Head injury
- Intellectual and developmental disabilities (Chapter 54)
- Joint replacement surgery

- Myocardial infarction (heart attack)
- Spinal cord injury or tumor
- Stroke
- Substance abuse—drug, alcohol
- Wound healing

RESTORATIVE NURSING

Some patients and residents need more care after their rehabilitation program ends. *Restorative nursing care is care that helps persons regain health and strength for safe and independent living.* Restorative nursing measures promote:
* Healing
* Self-care
* Elimination
* Positioning
* Mobility
* Communication
* Cognitive function

Rehabilitation and restorative nursing may occur at the same time. For example, a person needs physical therapy for rehabilitation after joint replacement surgery. The person also needs restorative nursing care to help with walking and to promote healing of the surgical incision. Both rehabilitation and restorative nursing focus on the whole person.

Restorative Aides

Some agencies have restorative aides. A *restorative aide is a nursing assistant with special training in restorative nursing and rehabilitation skills.* These aides assist the nursing and health teams as needed. Required training varies among states. If no state requirements, the agency provides needed training.

THE WHOLE PERSON

Health problems and disabilities affect the whole person with physical, psychological, and social effects. Suppose an illness left you paralyzed from the waist down.
* Would you be angry, afraid, or depressed?
* How would you move about?
* How would you care for yourself and your family?
* How would you worship, shop, or visit friends?
* Could you work and support yourself?

Adjustments are physical, psychological, social, and economic. Abilities—what the person can do—are stressed. Complications may cause further disability.

See *Focus on Children and Older Persons: The Whole Person.*

Physical Aspects

Rehabilitation starts when the person first seeks health care. Complications are prevented from bed rest, a long illness, surgery, or injury. Bowel and bladder problems are prevented. So are contractures and pressure injuries. Good alignment, turning and re-positioning, range-of-motion (ROM) exercises, and supportive devices are needed (Chapters 18, 19, and 34). Good skin care also prevents pressure injuries (Chapters 24 and 41).

Elimination. Some persons need bladder training (Chapter 27). The method depends on the person's problems, abilities, and needs. Some need bowel training (Chapter 29). Bowel control and regular elimination are goals. Fecal impaction, constipation, and fecal incontinence are prevented.

Self-Care. Self-care is a major goal. *Activities of daily living (ADL) are the activities usually done during a normal day in a person's life.* ADL include bathing, oral hygiene, dressing, eating, elimination, and moving about. The health team evaluates the person's ADL abilities and the need for self-help devices.

Sometimes the hands, wrists, and arms are affected. Adaptive (assistive) devices are often changed, made, or bought for the person's needs.
* Eating devices include glass holders, plate guards, and silverware with curved handles or cuffs (Chapter 30). Some devices attach to splints (Fig. 45-1).
* Electric toothbrushes have back-and-forth brushing motions for oral hygiene.
* Adaptive (assistive) devices for hygiene promote independence.

Adaptive (assistive) devices are useful for cooking, dressing, writing, phone calls, and other tasks. Some are shown in Figure 45-2. Also see Chapters 24, 25, and 26.

See *Focus on Surveys: Self-Care.*

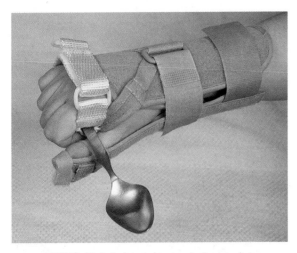

FIGURE 45-1 Eating device attached to a splint.

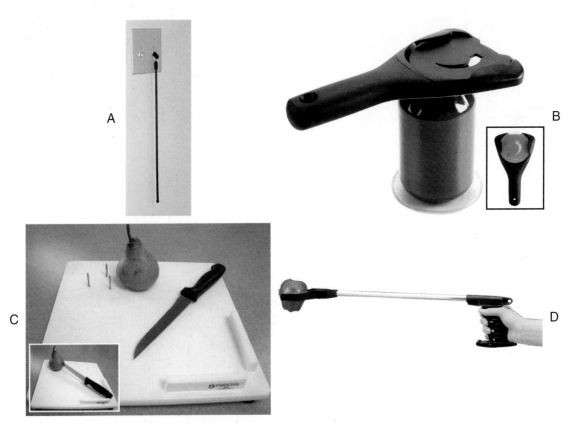

FIGURE 45-2 **A,** Light switch extender. **B,** Jar opener. **C,** Cutting board. **D,** Reacher. (A and C, Courtesy Parsons ADL, Inc. Tottenham, Ontario. B, Courtesy OXO International, Inc., New York, NY. D, Image provided by Performance Health.)

Mobility. The person may need to learn how to move in bed. Or the person may need crutches or a walker, cane, or brace (Chapter 34). Physical and occupational therapies are common for musculo-skeletal and nervous system problems (Fig. 45-3). Some people need wheelchairs. If possible, they learn wheelchair transfers. Such transfers include to and from the bed, toilet, bathtub, sofa, and chair and in and out of vehicles (Figs. 45-4, 45-5, and 45-6).

An amputation also affects mobility. A *prosthesis is an artificial replacement for a missing body part*. The person learns how to use the artificial arm or leg (Chapter 48). The goal is for the device to be like the missing body part in function and appearance.

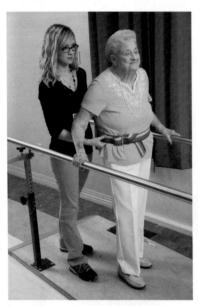

FIGURE 45-3 The person is assisted with walking in physical therapy.

Transfer board

FIGURE 45-4 The person uses a transfer board (sliding board) to transfer from wheelchair to bed.

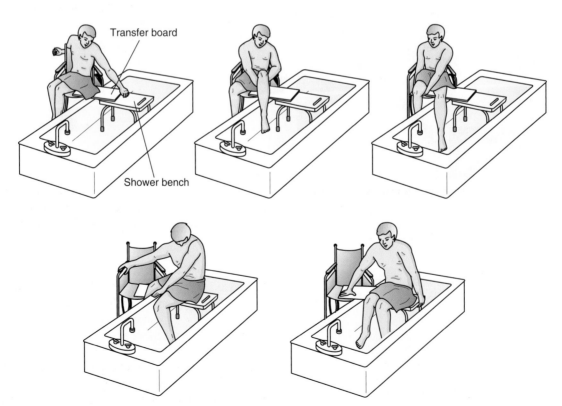

FIGURE 45-5 A wheelchair to tub transfer. A transfer board (sliding board) and shower bench are used.

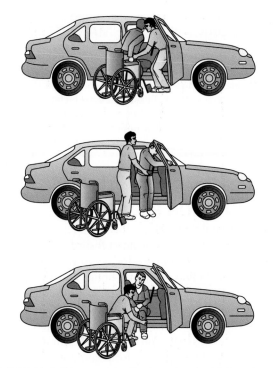

FIGURE 45-6 The person transfers from the wheelchair to the car.

Nutrition. Dysphagia may occur after a stroke. *Dysphagia* means difficulty *(dys)* swallowing *(phagia)*. The person may need a dysphagia diet (Chapter 30). If possible, the person learns exercises to improve swallowing. Persons who cannot swallow need enteral nutrition (Chapter 32).

Mechanical Ventilation. Some persons needing mechanical ventilation (Chapter 44) are weaned from the ventilator. That is, the person learns to breathe without the machine. The process may take many weeks. Other persons learn to live with life-long mechanical ventilation.

Communication

Aphasia (Chapter 46) may occur from a stroke. *Aphasia* is the total or partial loss *(a)* of the ability to use or understand language *(phasia)*. It results from damage to parts of the brain responsible for language and speech. Speech therapy and communication devices are helpful (Chapters 7 and 46).

See *Focus on Communication: Communication.*

FOCUS ON COMMUNICATION

Communication

Persons with speech disorders may need other communication methods. Pictures, reading, writing, facial expressions, and gestures are examples. All health team members and the family use the same method with the person. Changing methods can cause confusion and delay progress.

Psychological and Social Aspects

A disability can affect function and appearance. Self-esteem and relationships may suffer. Feelings of being unwhole, useless, unattractive, unclean, or undesirable are common. Some deny the disability, expecting therapy to correct the problem. Some persons are depressed, angry, and hostile.

A good attitude is important. So is being motivated and accepting limits. The focus is on abilities and strengths. Progress may be slow. Learning a new task is a reminder of the disability. Despair, frustration, fear, and other emotions may occur.

Remind persons of their progress. Give support, reassurance, and encouragement. Psychological and social needs are part of the care plan. Spiritual support helps some persons.

See *Focus on Communication: Psychological and Social Aspects.*

FOCUS ON COMMUNICATION

Psychological and Social Aspects

Emotional needs are great during rehabilitation. Good communication and support provide encouragement.
- Listen to the person.
- Show concern, not pity.
- Focus on what the person can do. Point out even slight progress.
- Be polite but firm. Do not let the person control you.
- Do not shout at or insult the person. Such behaviors are abuse and mistreatment.
- Do not argue with the person.
- Tell the nurse about problems. The person may need other support measures.

Economic Aspects

Some persons return to their jobs. Those who cannot do so are assessed for work skills, work history, interests, and talents. A job skill may be restored or a new one learned. The goal is gainful employment. Help is given finding a job.

THE REHABILITATION TEAM

Rehabilitation is a team effort. The person is the key team member. The person, family, doctor, and nursing and health teams set goals and plan care. The focus is to regain function and independence.

The team meets often to discuss the person's progress. The rehabilitation plan is changed as needed. The person and family attend the meetings when possible. Families provide support and encouragement. Often they help with home care.

Your Role

You help promote the person's independence. Preventing decline in function also is a goal. The many procedures, care measures, and rules in this book apply. Safety, communication, legal, and ethical aspects apply. So do the measures in Box 45-2.

See *Focus on Communication: Your Role.*

See *Teamwork and Time Management: Your Role.*

BOX 45-2	Assisting With Rehabilitation Needs

Physical Needs
- Follow the care plan and the nurse's instructions.
- Follow the person's daily routine.
- Provide for safety.
- Report early signs and symptoms of complications. They include pressure injuries, contractures, and bowel and bladder problems.
- Keep the person in good alignment.
- Turn and re-position the person as directed.
- Use safe transfer methods.
- Practice measures to prevent pressure injuries.
- Perform ROM exercises as instructed.
- Remember that muscles will atrophy if not used. And that contractures can develop.
- Know how to use and apply adaptive (assistive) devices.
- Provide and apply needed adaptive (assistive) devices.

Psychological and Social Needs
- Protect the person's rights. Privacy and personal choice are very important.
- Encourage performing ADL to the extent possible.
- Allow time to complete tasks. Do not rush the person.
- Give praise for even a little progress.
- Provide emotional support and reassurance.
- Try to understand and appreciate the person's situation, feelings, and concerns.
- Do not pity the person or give sympathy.
- Provide for spiritual needs.
- Practice the methods developed by the rehabilitation team. You will better assist the person.
- Practice the task that the person must do. This helps you guide and direct the person.
- Stress what the person can do. Focus on abilities and strengths, not on disabilities and weaknesses.
- Have a hopeful outlook.

REHABILITATION PROGRAMS

Common rehabilitation programs include:
- *Cardiac rehabilitation*—for heart disorders
- *Brain injury rehabilitation*—for nervous system disorders including traumatic brain injury
- *Spinal cord rehabilitation*—for spinal cord injuries
- *Stroke rehabilitation*—after a stroke
- *Respiratory rehabilitation*—for respiratory system disorders such as chronic obstructive pulmonary disease, after lung surgery, for respiratory complications from other health problems, and for mechanical ventilation
- *Orthopedic rehabilitation*—for fractures, joint replacement surgery, and other musculo-skeletal problems
- *Amputee rehabilitation*—for amputation of a limb
- *Hearing, speech, and vision rehabilitation*—for persons who are hard of hearing or deaf, have speech problems, are blind, or have severe vision problems
- *Drug and alcohol treatment*—for persons addicted to drugs or alcohol
- *Behavioral health treatment*—for those with mental health disorders
- *Rehabilitation for complex medical and surgical conditions*—wound care, diabetes, and burns are examples

After hospital care, the person may transfer to a nursing center or rehabilitation agency. Home care agencies, adult day-care centers, and assisted living residences (Chapter 57) may also provide rehabilitation services.

See *Focus on Children and Older Persons: Rehabilitation Programs.*

See *Focus on Long-Term Care and Home Care: Rehabilitation Programs.*

QUALITY OF LIFE

Successful rehabilitation improves quality of life. A hopeful and winning outlook is needed. The more the person can do alone, the better his or her quality of life. To promote quality of life:

- Protect the right to privacy.
- Encourage personal choice.
- Protect the right to be free from abuse and mistreatment.
- Learn to deal with your anger and frustration.
- Encourage activities.
- Provide a safe setting.
- Show patience, understanding, and sensitivity.

Continued

FOCUS ON **P R I D E—cont'd**

The Person, Family, and Yourself

Independence and Social Interaction

Quality of life improves the more the person can do for himself or herself. To promote independence:

- Stress the person's abilities and strengths.
- Let the person choose activities of interest.
- Remain patient. Do not rush the person.
- Resist the urge to do things for the person that he or she can do.
- Offer encouragement and support.
- Have the person use adaptive (assistive) devices as needed.
- Encourage personal choice. Personal choice allows control.

Delegation and Teamwork

Disability affects the whole person. Frustration is common. Many persons are angry and discouraged. Such feelings can be hard to control. Outbursts may occur.

You must learn to deal with your frustration. The person does not choose loss of function. If the process upsets you, think how the person must feel.

Delegation and Teamwork—cont'd

You must:

- Show patience, understanding, sensitivity, and respect.
- Be calm and act in a professional manner.
- Control your words and actions.

The nurse can suggest ways to help you control or express your feelings. You may need to assist with other persons for a while. Take pride in being a part of a strong, supportive team.

Ethics and Laws

The person may not want to practice rehabilitation procedures or methods. He or she may want you to give care instead. To make progress, the person needs to follow the rehabilitation plan. Do not let the person control you. Report any problems to the nurse.

FOCUS ON **PRIDE**: *Application*

Do you have a family member or friend with a disability? How does the disability affect the whole person? How does it affect your friendship or the family?

REVIEW QUESTIONS

Circle T if the statement is TRUE and F if it is FALSE.

1 T F You should give praise for even slight progress.

2 T F Only chronic health problems require rehabilitation.

3 T F A person is not allowed food until exercises are done. This is abuse and mistreatment.

4 T F Personal preferences are considered in the rehabilitation plan.

5 T F Rehabilitation for older persons is usually faster-paced than for younger persons.

6 T F You need to stress what the person can do.

7 T F Making changes in the home limits rehabilitation progress.

8 T F You should know how to use and apply adaptive (assistive) devices.

9 T F You need to convey hopefulness to the person.

Circle the BEST answer.

10 Rehabilitation and restorative nursing care focus on
- a What the person cannot do
- b Self-care
- c The whole person
- d Mobility and communication

11 Rehabilitation involves preventing
- a Angry feelings
- b Contractures and pressure injuries
- c The use of adaptive (assistive) devices
- d Nursing center care

12 A person has weakness on the right side. ADL are
- a Done by the person to the extent possible
- b Done by you
- c Delayed until the right side can be used
- d Supervised by a therapist

13 To provide emotional support during rehabilitation
- a Remind the person of his or her limits
- b Give sympathy and show pity
- c Talk about your feelings
- d Listen and give praise

14 During therapy, a person wants music played. You should
- a Explain that music is not allowed
- b Choose some music
- c Ask the person to choose some music
- d Ask a therapist to choose some music

15 A person's right side is weak. You move the call light to the left side. You promote quality of life by
- a Encouraging self-care
- b Allowing personal choice
- c Providing for safety
- d Taking part in activities

Answers to Chapter 45 questions are on p. 887.

FOCUS ON **PRACTICE**

Problem Solving

A person's care plan includes long-handled devices for dressing and bathing. During the bath, you provide a long-handled sponge. The person says: "I don't feel like using that today. Will you wash my feet for me?" What will you say and do? How will your response affect the person's progress?

Hearing, Speech, and Vision Problems

OBJECTIVES

- Define the key terms and key abbreviations in this chapter.
- Describe the common ear, speech, and eye disorders.
- Describe how to communicate with persons who have hearing loss.
- Explain the purpose of a hearing aid.
- Describe how to care for hearing aids.
- Explain how to communicate with persons who have speech disorders.

- Explain how to assist persons who are visually impaired or blind.
- Explain how to protect an ocular prosthesis from loss or damage.
- Perform the procedure described in this chapter.
- Explain how to promote PRIDE in the person, the family, and yourself.

KEY TERMS

aphasia The total or partial loss *(a)* of the ability to use or understand language *(phasia)*

blindness The absence of sight

braille A touch reading and writing system that uses raised dots for each letter of the alphabet; the first 10 letters also represent the numbers 0 through 9

Broca's aphasia See "expressive aphasia"

cerumen Earwax

deafness Hearing loss in which it is impossible for the person to understand speech through hearing alone

expressive aphasia Difficulty expressing or sending out thoughts through speech or writing; Broca's aphasia

global aphasia Difficulty expressing or sending out thoughts and difficulty understanding language; mixed aphasia

hearing loss Not being able to hear the range of sounds associated with normal hearing

low vision Vision loss that cannot be corrected with eyeglasses, contact lenses, drugs, or surgery; vision loss interferes with every-day activities

mixed aphasia See "global aphasia"

receptive aphasia Difficulty understanding language; Wernicke's aphasia

tinnitus A ringing, roaring, hissing, or buzzing sound in the ears or head

vertigo Dizziness

Wernicke's aphasia See "receptive aphasia"

KEY ABBREVIATIONS

ADA	Americans With Disabilities Act of 1990	**ASL**	American Sign Language
AMD	Age-related macular degeneration		

Hearing, speech, and vision are important for self-care, work, most activities, and safety and security needs. For example, you see dark clouds and hear tornado warning sirens. You know to seek shelter. With speech, you alert others.

Hearing, speech, and vision disorders occur in all age-groups. Common causes are birth defects, injuries, infections, diseases, and aging.

HEARING DISORDERS

The ear functions in hearing and balance. Hearing is needed for clear speech, responding to others, safety, and awareness of surroundings.

See *Body Structure and Function Review: The Ear*, p. 688.

BODY STRUCTURE AND FUNCTION REVIEW
The Ear

A sense organ, the ear (Fig. 46-1) functions in hearing and balance. It has 3 parts: the *external ear, middle ear,* and *inner ear.*

Sound waves are guided through the external ear (outer part) into the *auditory canal.* Glands in the auditory canal secrete a waxy substance called *cerumen.* The auditory canal extends about 1 inch into the *eardrum.* The eardrum *(tympanic membrane)* separates the external and middle ear.

The middle ear contains the *eustachian tube* and 3 small bones called *ossicles.* The eustachian tube connects the middle ear and the throat. Air enters the eustachian tube so there is equal pressure on both sides of the eardrum. The ossicles amplify sound received from the eardrum and transmit the sound to the inner ear. The 3 ossicles are:

- The *malleus*—looks like a hammer.
- The *incus*—looks like an anvil.
- The *stapes*—is shaped like a stirrup.

The inner ear consists of *semicircular canals* and the *cochlea.* The cochlea looks like a snail shell. It contains fluid that carries sound waves from the middle ear to the *acoustic nerve.* The acoustic nerve then carries messages to the brain.

The 3 semicircular canals are involved with balance. They sense the head's position and changes in position. They send messages to the brain.

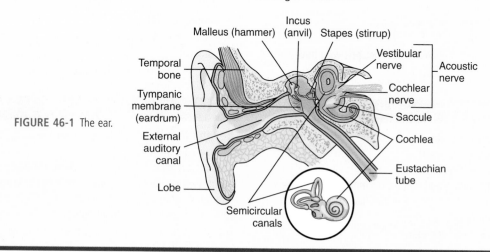

FIGURE 46-1 The ear.

Otitis Media

Otitis media is an infection *(itis)* of the middle *(media)* ear *(ot).* It often begins with sore throats, colds, the flu, allergies, or other respiratory infections that spread to the middle ear. Viruses and bacteria are causes.

Otitis media is acute or chronic. Chronic otitis media can damage the structures needed for hearing. Permanent hearing loss can occur.

Fluid builds up in the ear. Pain (earache), hearing loss, fever, and tinnitus occur. *Tinnitus is a ringing, roaring, hissing, or buzzing sound in the ears or head.* An untreated infection can spread to nearby structures in the head. The doctor orders antibiotics, pain-relief drugs, or drugs to relieve congestion.

See *Focus on Children and Older Persons: Otitis Media.*

FOCUS ON **CHILDREN AND OLDER PERSONS**
Otitis Media

Children

Otitis media is common in infants and children. Infants cannot tell you about an earache. The child may:

- Have ear pain or an earache
- Have a fever.
- Tug or pull at the ears.
- Roll the head back.
- Cry more than usual.
- Be fussy and irritable.
- Have fluid draining from the ear.
- Sleep poorly.
- Be dizzy or have problems with balance.
- Have trouble hearing.
- Not respond to quiet sounds.

Older Persons

Otitis media can occur in adults. They may have some of the same signs and symptoms as children. Persons with dementia may show behavior changes.

Meniere's Disease

Meniere's disease involves the inner ear. Usually 1 ear is affected. Symptoms are sudden. They include:

- *Vertigo—dizziness*
- Tinnitus
- Hearing loss
- Feeling of fullness or pressure in the ear

An attack usually involves vertigo, tinnitus, and hearing loss. Vertigo causes whirling and spinning sensations. The dizziness causes severe nausea and vomiting. An episode can last 20 minutes or 2 to 24 hours.

Drugs may be ordered to prevent dizziness, nausea, and fluid in the ear. A low-salt diet may decrease fluid in the inner ear. Smoking, caffeine, and alcohol are avoided. Safety is needed during vertigo.

- Have the person lie down on a firm surface.
- Prevent falls. Assist with walking and use bed rails according to the care plan.
- Have the person keep the head still and focus on an object that does not move. The person avoids turning the head. To talk to the person, stand directly in front of him or her.
- Avoid sudden movements. The person moves slowly.
- Prevent flashing lights (such as from TV) and bright lights.

Hearing Loss

Hearing loss is not being able to hear the range of sounds associated with normal hearing. Losses are mild to deafness. *Deafness is hearing loss in which it is impossible for the person to understand speech through hearing alone.*

Causes include damage to the outer, middle, or inner ear or to the acoustic nerve. See Box 46-1 for the risk factors and signs and symptoms of hearing loss.

Temporary hearing loss can occur from *earwax (cerumen).* Hearing improves after the earwax is removed.

See *Focus on Communication: Hearing Loss.*

See *Promoting Safety and Comfort: Hearing Loss.*

FOCUS ON COMMUNICATION

Hearing Loss

The National Association of the Deaf (NAD) uses the terms *deaf* and *hard of hearing* to describe persons with hearing loss. Do not use the terms *deaf and dumb, deaf-mute,* or *hearing-impaired.* Such terms offend persons who are hard of hearing.

PROMOTING SAFETY AND COMFORT

Hearing Loss

Safety
Do not try to remove earwax. This is done by a doctor or a nurse. Do not insert anything, including cotton swabs, into the ear.

BOX 46-1	**Hearing Loss**

Risk Factors

- Aging—ear structures change
- Loud noise—a short blast (explosion, gunshot), occupational exposure (farming, factory work), recreational exposure (loud music including with earbuds, snowmobile, motorcycle, airplane)
- Heredity—greater risk for ear damage or changes from aging
- Some drugs—antibiotics, chemotherapy
- Some illnesses—ear infection, stroke, tumor
- Trauma—head injury

Signs and Symptoms

- Problems:
  - Hearing on the phone
  - Hearing with background noise or in noisy areas
  - Following conversations when 2 or more people are speaking
  - Understanding women and children
- Straining to understand a conversation
- Hearing voices as mumbled or slurred
- Misunderstanding what others say
- Answering questions or responding inappropriately
- Asking others to repeat themselves
- Speaking too loudly
- Leaning forward to hear
- Turning and cupping the better ear toward the speaker
- Turning up the TV, radio, music, or other sound sources so loud that others complain

---

Effects on the Person. A person may deny hearing loss or not notice gradual hearing loss. Others may see changes in the person's behavior or attitude but not suspect hearing loss.

Psychological and social changes may occur. People may shun social events to avoid embarrassment because of giving wrong answers or responses. Or they try to control conversations. They may feel lonely, bored, and left out. Only parts of conversations are heard. They think others are talking about them or are talking softly on purpose. Straining and working hard to hear can cause fatigue, frustration, and irritability.

Hearing is needed for clear speech. Pronouncing words and voice volume depend on hearing yourself. Hearing loss may result in slurred speech or pronouncing words wrong. Some people have monotone speech or drop word endings. It may be hard to understand the person. Do not assume or pretend that you understand. Serious problems can result. See "Speech Disorders" on p. 693.

See *Focus on Children and Older Persons: Effects on the Person,* p. 690.

FOCUS ON CHILDREN AND OLDER PERSONS

Effects on the Person

Children

Hearing problems may be present at birth or develop as the child grows. Hearing is needed for speech and language development. Children learn to talk by imitating sounds and voices.

Medical attention is needed if a child does not hear well or speak clearly. See Box 46-2. Items checked "No" may signal hearing loss. Report concerns about a child's hearing to the nurse.

Communication. The measures in Box 46-3 promote hearing and communication. Some persons wear hearing aids (p. 692) or lip-read (speech-read). They watch facial expressions, gestures, and body language. American Sign Language (ASL) (Figs. 46-2 and 46-3, p. 692) uses signs made with the hands and other movements such as facial expressions, gestures, and postures. (Different sign languages are used in different countries. For example, British Sign Language is different from ASL.)

Some people have *hearing dogs*. The dog alerts the person to sounds. Phones, doorbells, smoke alarms, alarm clocks, babies' cries, sirens, and on-coming cars are examples.

BOX 46-2	Hearing Checklist for Children

Items marked "No" may signal hearing loss.

No	Yes	**Birth to 3 Months**
___	___	Reacts to loud sounds.
___	___	Calms down or smiles when spoken to.
___	___	Recognizes your voice and calms down if crying.
___	___	When feeding, starts or stops sucking in response to sound.
___	___	Coos and makes pleasure sounds.
___	___	Has a special way of crying for different needs.
___	___	Smiles when he or she sees you.

4 to 6 Months

No	Yes	
___	___	Follows sounds with his or her eyes.
___	___	Responds to changes in the tone of your voice.
___	___	Notices toys that make sounds.
___	___	Pays attention to music.
___	___	Babbles in a speech-like way and uses many different sounds, including sounds that begin with *p*, *b*, and *m*.
___	___	Laughs.
___	___	Babbles when excited or unhappy.
___	___	Makes gurgling sounds when alone or playing with you.

7 Months to 1 Year

No	Yes	
___	___	Enjoys playing peek-a-boo and pat-a-cake.
___	___	Turns and looks in the direction of sounds.
___	___	Listens when spoken to.
___	___	Understands words for common items such as "cup," "shoe," or "juice."
___	___	Responds to requests ("Come here.").
___	___	Babbles using long and short groups of sounds ("tata," "upup," "bibibi").
___	___	Babbles to get and keep attention.
___	___	Communicates using gestures such as waving or holding up arms.
___	___	Imitates different speech sounds.
___	___	Has 1 or 2 words ("Hi," "dog," "Dada," or "Mama") by first birthday.

1 to 2 Years

No	Yes	
___	___	Knows a few parts of the body and can point to them when asked.
___	___	Follows simple commands ("Roll the ball.") and understands simple questions ("Where's your shoe?").
___	___	Enjoys simple stories, songs, and rhymes.

1 to 2 Years—cont'd

No	Yes	
___	___	Points to pictures, when named, in books.
___	___	Acquires new words on a regular basis.
___	___	Uses some 1- or 2-word questions ("Where kitty?" or "Go bye-bye?").
___	___	Puts 2 words together ("More cookie.").
___	___	Uses many different consonant sounds at the beginning of words.

2 to 3 Years

No	Yes	
___	___	Has a word for almost everything.
___	___	Uses 2- or 3-word phrases to talk about and ask for things.
___	___	Uses *k*, *g*, *f*, *t*, *d*, and *n* sounds.
___	___	Speaks in a way that is understood by family members and friends.
___	___	Names objects to ask for them or to direct attention to them.

3 to 4 Years

No	Yes	
___	___	Hears you when you call from another room.
___	___	Hears the TV or radio at the same sound level as other family members.
___	___	Answers simple "Who?" "What?" "Where?" and "Why?" questions.
___	___	Talks about activities at day care, pre-school, or friends' homes.
___	___	Uses sentences with 4 or more words.
___	___	Speaks easily without repeating syllables or words.

4 to 5 Years

No	Yes	
___	___	Pays attention to a short story and answers simple questions about it.
___	___	Hears and understands most of what is said at home and in school.
___	___	Uses sentences that give many details.
___	___	Tells stories that stay on topic.
___	___	Communicates easily with other children and adults.
___	___	Says most sounds correctly except for a few (*l*, *s*, *r*, *v*, *z*, *ch*, *sh*, and *th*).
___	___	Uses rhyming words.
___	___	Names some letters and numbers.
___	___	Uses adult grammar.

Modified from National Institute on Deafness and Other Communication Disorders: Your baby's hearing and communicative development checklist, NIH Publication No. 10-4040, Bethesda, Md, updated March 6, 2017, National Institutes of Health.

BOX 46-3　Measures to Promote Hearing

The Setting

- Reduce or eliminate background noises. Turn off radios, music players, TVs, air conditioners, fans, and so on.
- Provide a quiet place to talk. Avoid areas with loud sound.
- Have the person sit where able to hear best.

The Person

- Make sure the person's hearing aid is turned on, working, and properly placed in or behind the ear (p. 692).
- Have the person wear needed eyeglasses or contact lenses. The person needs to see your face to lip-read (speech-read).

You

- Gain attention. Alert the person to your presence. Raise an arm or hand or lightly touch the person's hand, arm, or shoulder. Do not startle or approach the person from behind.
- Position yourself at the person's level. Sit if the person is sitting. Stand if the person is standing.
- Face the person when speaking. Do not turn or walk away while you are talking. Do not talk from the doorway or another room.
- Have light shine on your face. Shadows and glares affect the ability to see your face clearly.
- Maintain eye contact with the person.
- Speak clearly, distinctly, and at a normal rate. Do not talk too fast or too slow.
- Speak in a normal tone of voice. Do not shout or mumble.
- State the person's name before starting a conversation. This gains the person's attention and focus.

You—cont'd

- Adjust the pitch of your voice as needed. Ask if the person can hear you better.
  - If no hearing aid, lower the pitch. Higher-pitched voices are harder to hear than lower-pitched voices.
  - If a hearing aid is worn, raise the pitch slightly.
- Do not cover your mouth, smoke, eat, or chew gum while talking. Mouth movements are affected.
- Keep your hands away from your face.
- Stand or sit on the side of the better ear.
- State the topic of conversation first.
- Say when you are changing the subject. State the new topic.
- Use short sentences and simple words.
- Pause between sentences. Ensure understanding before speaking again.
- Use gestures and facial expressions as useful clues.
- Write out important names, words, numbers, addresses, appointments, and so on.
- Re-phrase if the person does not seem to understand. Do not repeat the same words again and again.
- Keep conversations and discussions short. This avoids tiring the person.
- Be alert to messages sent by your facial expressions, gestures, and body language.
- Be alert to the person's nonverbal communication. For example, watch for puzzled looks and expressions of anger, frustration, excitement, fatigue, and so on.

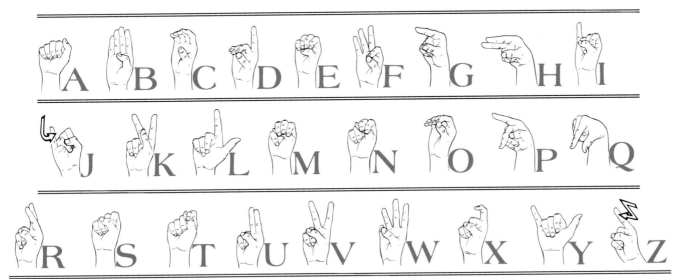

FIGURE 46-2 Manual alphabet. (Courtesy National Association of the Deaf, Silver Spring, Md.)

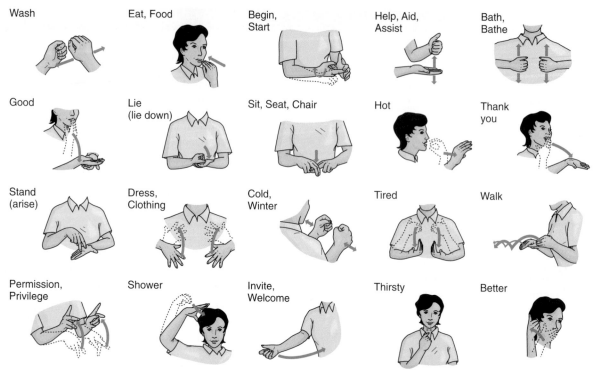

FIGURE 46-3 American Sign Language examples.

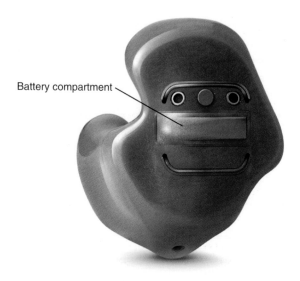

FIGURE 46-4 An in-the-ear hearing aid. (Courtesy Sivantos Group, Henri-Dunant-Street 100, 91058 Erlangen, Germany.)

Hearing Aids. *Hearing aids* fit behind or in the ear (Fig. 46-4). They make sounds louder. They do not correct, restore, or cure hearing problems. The person hears better because the device makes sounds louder. Background noise and speech are louder. The measures in Box 46-3 apply.

Hearing aids are costly. See Box 46-4 for hearing aid care measures.

BOX 46-4   Hearing Aids—Care Measures

- Hold and handle hearing aids gently. This includes when removing, inserting, or cleaning the device and when inserting batteries.
- Do the following if a hearing aid does not seem to work properly.
  - Check if the hearing aid is *on.* The device has an *on* and *off* switch.
  - Check the battery position.
  - Insert a new battery if needed. Use the correct battery size.
  - Clean the hearing aid. Follow the manufacturer's instructions.
- Hold the hearing aid over a soft cloth or soft surface to change the battery or to clean the device.
- Do not expose the hearing aid to heat or extreme cold.
- Have the person remove the hearing aid before using a hair dryer, hair spray, spray perfumes, shaving lotions, or powders.
- Protect the hearing aid from water. The person does not wear a hearing aid during a bath or shower.
- Clean the hearing aid according to the manufacturer's instructions.
- Check meal trays and bed linens for hearing aids. The person may have removed the hearing aid and set it aside.
- Remove and turn off the hearing aid at bedtime. This saves battery life. Remove the battery if the person prefers.
- Place the hearing aid in its storage case when not worn. Place the storage case in the top drawer of the bedside stand.

Other Hearing Devices. Other devices can help the person with hearing loss.

- *Phone amplifying devices.* Special phone receivers make sounds louder. Some phones work with hearing aids.
- Extension bells that make phones ring louder.
- *Telephone and relay services.* The *Americans With Disabilities Act (ADA) of 1990* requires that states provide telephone use for persons who are deaf or hard of hearing. The Telecommunications Relay Service (TRS) is shown in Figure 46-5. The hard of hearing person (caller) uses a tele-typewriter or other device to send a message to the person called. A relay assistant speaks the typed message to the person called. The message back to the hard of hearing person (caller) is typed by the relay assistant for the caller to read. The relay assistant must maintain the confidentiality of all conversations. Emergency 911 and other services are available to meet the person's needs.
- *Internet services and equipment.* The *Twenty-First Century Communications and Video Accessibility Act* requires that persons with disabilities be able to access and use Internet services and equipment.
- *TV and radio listening systems.* These are used with or without hearing aids. The person does not have to turn the volume up high.
- Smoke alarms with strobe lights.
- Doorbells that can be heard throughout the house.

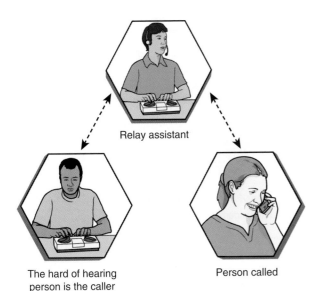

Relay assistant

The hard of hearing person is the caller

Person called

FIGURE 46-5 Telecommunications Relay Service (TRS). The person with a hearing disability types a message to the person called. The relay assistant communicates messages between the calling party and the party called.

SPEECH DISORDERS

Speech disorders affect oral communication. Hearing loss, developmental disabilities (Chapter 54), and brain injury are common causes. These problems are common.

- *Aphasia.* See "Aphasia" on p. 694.
- *Apraxia of speech.* *Apraxia* means not (*a*) to act, do, or perform (*praxia*). The person cannot use speech muscles to make words for understandable speech. The person understands and knows what to say. The motor speech area in the brain is damaged.
- *Dysarthria.* *Dysarthria* means difficult or poor (*dys*) speech (*arthria*). Nerve damage affects mouth and face muscles. Slurred, soft, slow, or hoarse speech can occur.

To communicate with the speech-impaired person, practice the measures in Box 46-5.

Some persons need speech rehabilitation. A speech-language pathologist helps the person:

- Use remaining abilities.
- Restore or improve language abilities to the extent possible.
- Learn communication methods.
- Strengthen speech muscles.

Improvement depends on many factors. They include the cause, amount, and area of brain or nerve damage; age; health; and willingness and ability to learn.

BOX 46-5	**Communicating With Speech-Impaired Persons**

The Person
- Have the person repeat or re-phrase statements as needed.
- Repeat what the person has said. Ask if you understood correctly.
- Have the person write down key words or the message.
- Have the person point, gesture, or draw key words.

You
- Follow the care plan for a consistent approach.
- Provide a calm, quiet setting. Turn off the TV, radio, music, and other distractions.
- Include the person in conversations.
- Listen and give the person your full attention.
- Use short, simple sentences.
- Repeat as needed.
- Write down key words as needed.
- Speak in a normal tone. Do not talk in a babyish or child-like way.
- Ask questions to which you know the answers. This helps you learn how the person speaks.
- Allow the person enough time to talk.
- Determine the topic being discussed. This helps you understand main points. Watch lip movements.
- Watch facial expressions, gestures, and body language. They give clues about what is being said.
- Do not correct the person's speech.

Aphasia

Aphasia is the total or partial loss (a) *of the ability to use or understand language* (phasia). Parts of the brain responsible for language are damaged. The person has problems reading, writing, and speaking. Stroke, head injury, brain infections, dementia, and brain tumors are common causes.

Expressive aphasia (Broca's aphasia) relates to difficulty expressing or sending out thoughts through speech or writing. The person knows what to say but has problems speaking, reading, and writing. The person may:

- Omit small words such as "is," "and," "of," and "the."
- Speak in 1-word or short sentences (less than 4 words). "Walk dog" can mean "I will take the dog for a walk" or "You take the dog for a walk."
- Put words in the wrong order. The person may say "room bath" for "bathroom."
- Think one thing but say another. The person may want food but ask for a book.
- Call people the wrong names.
- Make up words.
- Produce sounds and no words.
- Swear for no reason.

Receptive aphasia (Wernicke's aphasia) is difficulty understanding language. The person has trouble understanding what is said or written. Words do not make sense. What the person says has no meaning. The person may not be aware of mistakes.

Some people have both expressive and receptive aphasia. *Global aphasia (mixed aphasia) involves difficulty expressing or sending out thoughts and difficulty understanding language.* The person has problems speaking and understanding language.

Emotional needs are great. Frustration, depression, and anger are common. Communication is needed to function and relate to others. The person wants to communicate but cannot. Be patient and kind.

EYE DISORDERS

Vision problems range from mild loss to complete blindness. *Blindness is the absence of sight.* Vision loss is sudden or gradual. One or both eyes are affected.

See Box 46-6 for the signs and symptoms of vision problems.

See *Body Structure and Function Review: The Eye.*

BODY STRUCTURE AND FUNCTION REVIEW

The Eye

Receptors for vision are in the eyes (Fig. 46-6). Bones of the skull, eyelids and eyelashes, and tears protect the eyes from injury. The eye has 3 layers.

- The *sclera,* the white of the eye, is the outer layer. It is made of tough connective tissue.
- The *choroid* is the second layer. Blood vessels, the *ciliary muscle,* and the *iris* make up the choroid. The iris gives the eye its color. The opening in the middle of the iris is the *pupil.* Pupil size varies with the amount of light entering the eye. The pupil *constricts* (narrows) in bright light. It *dilates* (widens) in dim or dark places.
- The *retina* is the inner layer. It has receptors for vision and the nerve fibers of the *optic nerve.* The *macula* is near the center of the retina. The area contains cells that are sensitive to light, color, and the fine detail needed for central vision.

Light enters the eye through the *cornea*—the transparent part of the outer layer that lies over the eye. Light rays pass to the *lens,* which lies behind the pupil. The light is then reflected to the retina. Light is carried to the brain by the optic nerve.

The *aqueous chamber* separates the cornea from the lens. The chamber is filled with a fluid called *aqueous humor.* The fluid helps the cornea keep its shape and position. The *vitreous humor* is behind the lens. It is a gelatin-like substance that supports the retina and maintains the eye's shape.

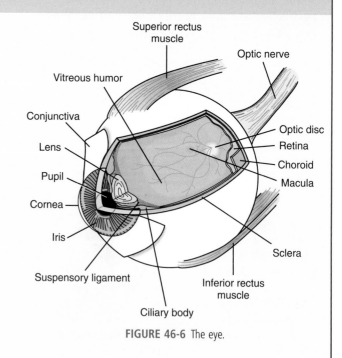

FIGURE 46-6 The eye.

| BOX 46-6 | Vision Problems—Signs and Symptoms |

The Person Complains Of:
- Hazy, blurred, cloudy, or double vision
- Pain or discomfort by or in the eye: sudden or recurring
- Flashes of light
- Halos, rainbows, or rings around lights
- Spots or "floaters"
- Sensitivity or pain to light or glares
- Headaches
- Pain or pressure on the forehead or behind the eyes
- Sudden change or loss of vision in 1 eye
- Burning, itching, or redness in 1 eye
- Drainage from an eye
- Tearing
- Seeing a curtain come down over the eye
- Problems seeing at night
- An eye injury
- A swollen eye

You Observe the Person:
- Squinting
- Bumping into things
- Shuffling, tripping, or being hesitant when walking
- Being overly cautious when going up or down stairs
- Having problems reaching for things:
  - Over-reaches
  - Does not reach far enough
  - Gropes for things
- Having changed how the person reads, watches TV, drives, or walks
- Complaining about not enough lighting to read or do things
- Holding reading matter near the face or at an angle
- Having trouble identifying faces or objects
- Wearing clothes that do not match
- Having trouble eating:
  - Cutting food
  - Getting food on a fork or spoon
  - Spilling or dropping food
  - Pouring liquids
- Having problems seeing at night

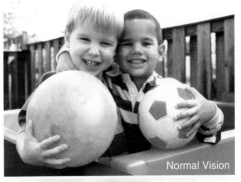

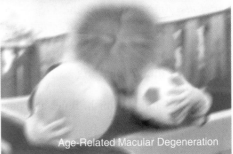

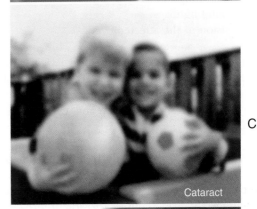

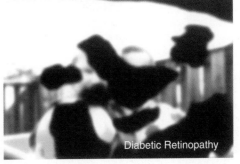

FIGURE 46-7 Vision loss with eye disorders. **A,** Normal vision. **B,** Vision loss from macular degeneration. **C,** Vision loss from a cataract. **D,** Vision loss from diabetic retinopathy. (A and C, Modified from National Eye Institute: *Facts about cataract,* Bethesda, Md, September 2015, National Institutes of Health. B, Modified from National Eye Institute: *Don't lose sight of age-related macular degeneration,* Bethesda, Md, NIH Publication No. 12-3462, revised 2012, National Institutes of Health. D, Modified from National Eye Institute: *Facts about diabetic eye disease,* Bethesda, Md, September 2015, National Institutes of Health.)

Age-Related Macular Degeneration

Age-related macular degeneration (AMD) blurs central vision. *Central vision* is what you see "straight-ahead." AMD causes a blind spot in the center of vision (Fig. 46-7, *A and B*). Central vision is needed to read, write, drive, cook, and see faces and for fine detail.

AMD damages the macula in the center of the retina. The retina receives light and sends messages to the brain through the optic nerve. Normal signals are not sent to the brain. Onset is gradual and painless.

Risk Factors. AMD risk increases after age 60. Besides age, risk factors include:
- Smoking.
- Race. Whites are at greater risk than any other group.
- Family history.

Treatment. For advanced AMD, no treatment can prevent vision loss. Laser surgery may stop or slow the disease progress. It may save what is left of central vision. The following can reduce the risk of AMD.

- Eating a healthy diet high in green, leafy vegetables and fish
- Not smoking
- Maintaining normal blood pressure and cholesterol levels
- Regular exercise

Cataracts

A cataract is clouding of the lens (Fig. 46-8). The normal lens is clear. *Cataract* comes from the Greek word for *waterfall*. Trying to see is like looking through a waterfall. Cataracts can occur in 1 or both eyes. Signs and symptoms include:

- Cloudy, blurry, or dimmed vision (see Fig. 46-7, *A and C*).
- Colors seem faded and brownish. Blues and purples are hard to see.
- Sensitivity to light and glares.
- Poor vision at night.
- Halos around lights.
- Double vision in the affected eye.

Risk Factors. Most cataracts are caused by aging. A family history, diabetes, smoking, excessive alcohol use, and prolonged exposure to sunlight are risk factors. So are high blood pressure, obesity, and eye injuries and surgeries.

Treatment. Surgery is the only treatment. The lens is removed and a plastic lens is implanted. Surgery is done when the cataract affects daily activities. Driving, reading, and watching TV are examples. Vision improves after surgery.

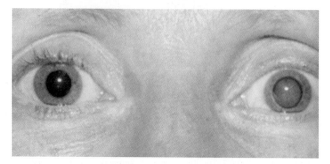

FIGURE 46-8 The right eye is normal. The left eye has a cataract. (From Swartz MH: *Textbook of physical diagnosis*, ed 7, Philadelphia, 2014, Saunders.)

Post-operative care includes:
- Have the person wear ordered eyeglasses or eye shield as directed. If ordered, the shield is worn for sleep, including naps.
- Follow measures for visually impaired or blind persons when an eye shield is worn. There may be vision loss in the other eye.
- Remind the person not to rub or press the affected eye.
- Do not bump the eye.
- Place the over-bed table and bedside stand on the un-operative side.
- Place the call light and needed items within reach.
- Report eye drainage or complaints of pain at once.
- Remind the person not to bend, stoop, cough, or lift things.

Diabetic Retinopathy

In diabetic retinopathy, blood vessels in the retina are damaged. A complication of diabetes, it is a leading cause of blindness among working adults. Usually both eyes are affected.

Vision blurs (see Fig. 46-7, *A and D*). The person may see spots "floating." Often there are no early warning signs.

Risk Factors. Everyone with diabetes (Chapter 50) is at risk. The risk increases the longer the person has diabetes. For example, a person with diabetes for 20 years is at greater risk than someone with diabetes for 10 years.

Treatment. The person needs to control diabetes, blood pressure, and cholesterol. Some drugs injected into the eye and laser surgery may help. In another procedure, blood is removed from the center of the eye.

Glaucoma

With glaucoma, fluid builds up in the eye causing pressure on the optic nerve. The optic nerve is damaged. Vision loss with eventual blindness occurs.

Glaucoma can affect 1 or both eyes. Onset is sudden or gradual. Peripheral vision (side vision) is lost. The person sees through a tunnel (Fig. 46-9), has blurred vision, and sees halos around lights. Severe eye pain, nausea, and vomiting occur with sudden onset.

Risk Factors. Glaucoma is a leading cause of vision loss in the United States. Persons at risk include:
- African Americans over 40 years of age
- Everyone over 60 years of age, especially Mexican Americans
- Those with a family history of the disease

Treatment. Glaucoma has no cure. Prior damage cannot be reversed. Drugs and surgery can control glaucoma and prevent further damage to the optic nerve.

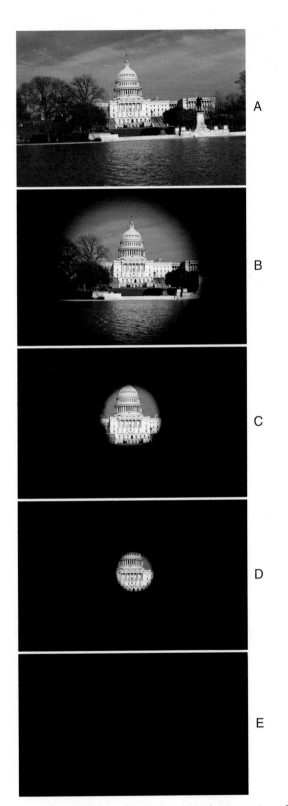

FIGURE 46-9 Vision loss from glaucoma. **A,** Normal vision. **B,** Loss of peripheral vision begins. **C, D,** and **E,** Vision loss continues, with eventual blindness.

Low Vision

Low vision is vision loss that cannot be corrected with eyeglasses, contact lenses, drugs, or surgery. The vision loss interferes with every-day activities. Reading, shopping, cooking, watching TV, writing, driving, and other every-day tasks are hard to do.

While wearing eyeglasses or contact lenses, the person has problems:

- Recognizing faces of family and friends
- Doing tasks that require close vision—reading, cooking, sewing, and so on
- Picking out and matching clothing colors
- Reading signs (traffic, stores)
- Doing things because lighting seems dimmer

Risk Factors. Low vision risk factors include:

- Eye diseases and their causes including glaucoma, cataracts, and AMD
- Diabetes
- Eye injuries
- Birth defects
- Aging
- Stroke

Treatment. The person learns to use visual and adaptive (assistive) devices. Examples include:

- Prescription reading glasses
- Large-print reading materials
- Hand-held and video magnifiers
- Telescopic aids for far vision
- Paper with bold lines and a black felt-tip marker for writing
- Audio tapes
- Electronic reading machines
- Computers with large print and speech systems
- Closed-circuit TV
- Phones, clocks, and watches with large numbers and that talk
- Lighting that can be adjusted
- Dark-colored light switches and electrical outlets against light-colored walls
- Motion lights that turn on when the person enters a room

Impaired Vision and Blindness

Some people are totally blind. Others sense some light but have no usable vision. Others have some usable vision but cannot read newsprint. The legally blind person sees at 20 feet what a person with normal vision sees at 200 feet. See Box 46-6 for the signs and symptoms of vision problems.

Loss of sight is serious. Adjustments can be hard and long. Special education and rehabilitation programs help the person adjust to the vision loss and learn to be independent. The goal is to be as active as possible and have quality of life. The person learns to use visual and adaptive (assistive) devices, braille, long canes, and guide dogs. Follow the practices in Box 46-7, p. 698.

See *Focus on Long-Term Care and Home Care: Impaired Vision and Blindness*, p. 699.

Text continued on p. 700.

BOX 46-7   Caring for Blind and Visually Impaired Persons

The Setting

- Report worn or loose carpeting and other flooring. Also report the use of throw rugs or plastic runners.
- Keep furniture, equipment, electrical cords, and other items out of areas where the person will walk.
- Report furniture that has wheels.
- Keep chairs pushed in under the table or desk.
- Keep room doors fully open or fully closed.
- Keep drawers and cabinet, cupboard, and closet doors fully closed.
- Report burnt-out light bulbs.
- Provide preferred lighting. Tell the person when the lights are on or off.
- Adjust window coverings to prevent glares. Sunny days and bright, snowy days cause glares.
- Keep the call light and TV, light, and other controls within reach.
- Turn on night-lights in the person's room and bathroom and in hallways.
- Practice safety measures to prevent falls (Chapter 14).
- Orient the person to the room. Describe the layout. Include the location and purpose of furniture and equipment.
- Let the person touch and find furniture and equipment.
- Do not re-arrange furniture and equipment.
- Use colors and contrast. Solid, bright colors (red, orange, yellow) are best. Avoid pastels, patterns, prints, designs, and stripes. White or yellow against black provides strong contrast. Place light-colored objects against dark backgrounds or dark-colored objects against light backgrounds. For example, use a white plate with a dark placemat or tablecloth.
- Provide the same meal-time setting. Arrange things in the same way for each meal.
    - Have the person sit in good light.
    - Arrange the place setting.
        - The knife and spoon are to the right of the plate.
        - The fork and napkin are to the left of the plate.
        - The glass or cup is to the right of the plate if the person is right-handed. It is to the left of the plate if left-handed.
    - Arrange main dishes, side dishes, seasonings, and condiments in a straight line or in a semi-circle just beyond the place setting.
    - Explain the location of food and beverages. Use the face of a clock (Chapter 30). Or guide the person's hand to each item on the tray or place setting.
    - Cut meat, open containers, butter bread, and perform other tasks as needed.
- Complete a safety check before leaving the room. (See the inside of the back cover.)

The Person

- Have the person wear comfortable shoes that fit correctly.
- Have the person use hand and stair railings and grab (safety) bars.
- Assist with walking as needed. Offer to guide and help the person. Respect the person's answer. If help is accepted:
    - Offer your arm. State which arm is offered. Tap the back of your hand against the person's hand.
    - Have the person hold on to your arm just above the elbow (Fig. 46-10). Do not grab the person's arm.
    - Walk at a normal pace. Walk 1 step ahead of the person. Stand next to the person at the top and bottom of stairs and when crossing streets.
    - Never push, pull, or guide the person in front of you.
    - Pause to change direction, step up, or step down.
    - Warn of stairs, elevators, escalators, doors, turns, furniture, and other obstructions. State if steps are up or down.
    - Have the person hold on to a railing, the wall, or a strong surface if you need to step away. Tell the person that you are leaving and what to hold on to.
- Guide the person to a seat by placing your guiding arm on the seat. The person moves a hand down your arm to the seat.
- Let the person do as much as possible. Do not do things that the person can do. Cutting and seasoning food, getting dressed, and putting on shoes are examples.
- Provide visual and adaptive (assistive) devices. Follow the care plan.

You

- Identify yourself when you enter the room. Give your name, title, and reason for being there. Do not touch the person until he or she is aware of your presence.
- Ask the person how much he or she can see. Do not assume the person is totally blind or has some vision.
- Identify others. Say where each person is and what the person is doing.
- Offer to help. Simply say: "May I help you?" Respect the person's answer.
- Leave the person's belongings where you found them. Do not move or re-arrange things. If you must move things, tell the person what you moved and where.

BOX 46-7	Caring for Blind and Visually Impaired Persons—cont'd

Communication

- Face the person when speaking. Speak slowly and clearly.
- Use a normal tone of voice. Do not shout or speak loudly.
- Address the person by name. This shows that you are directing a comment or question to him or her.
- Speak directly to the person. Do not talk just to others who are present.
- Feel free to use words such as "see," "look," "read," or "watch TV." You can use "blind" and "visually impaired." You also can use colors, sizes, shapes, patterns, designs, and so on.
- Describe people, places, and things thoroughly. Do not leave out a detail because you do not think it is important.
- Warn of dangers—calmly and clearly. You can say "wait" first. Then describe the danger. For example: "Wait, there is ice on the sidewalk."
- Greet the person by name when he or she enters a room. This alerts the person to your presence. Tell the person who you are. Also identify others in the room.
- Listen to the person. Give verbal cues that you are listening. Say: "yes," "okay," "I see," "tell me more," "I don't understand," and so on.

Communication—cont'd

- Answer questions. Provide specific and descriptive responses.
- Give step-by-step explanations as you give care. Say when the procedure is over.
- Give specific directions.
  - "Right behind you," "on your left," or "in front of you" are examples. Avoid phrases like "over here" or "over there."
  - Tell the distance. For example: "three steps in front of you" or "at the end of the hallway by the nurses' station."
  - Give landmarks if possible. Sounds and scents can serve as "landmarks." "By the kitchen" is an example.
- Tell the person when you are leaving the room or the area. If appropriate, state where you are going. For example: "I'm going to go into your bathroom now."
- Tell the person when you are ending a conversation. For example: "Thank you for sharing stories about your children."

FOCUS ON LONG-TERM CARE AND HOME CARE

Impaired Vision and Blindness

Home Care

The practices in Box 46-7 apply in the home for a safe setting. Outdoor walks and stairs must be free of toys, ice, and snow. Furniture, closets, drawers, shelves, and other items are arranged for the person's needs. Always replace items where you found them. Do not re-arrange the person's things.

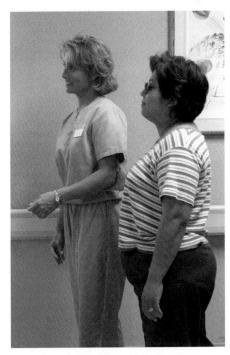

FIGURE 46-10 The blind person walks slightly behind the nursing assistant. She touches the nursing assistant's arm lightly.

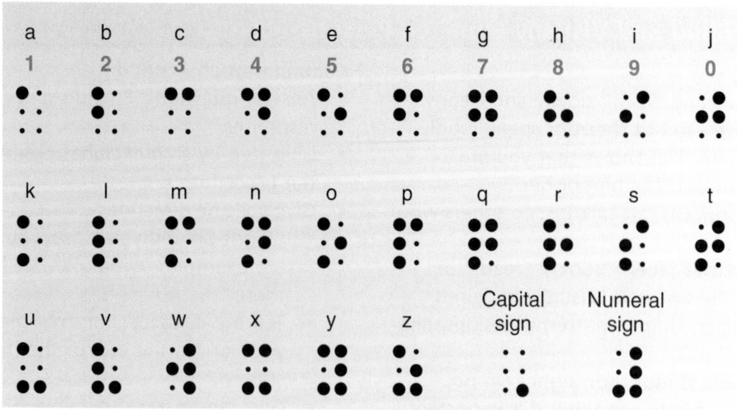

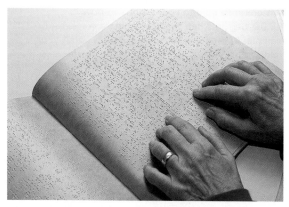

FIGURE 46-11 Braille.

FIGURE 46-12 Braille is read by moving the fingers left to right across the braille lines.

Braille. *Braille is a touch reading and writing system that uses raised dots for each letter of the alphabet* (Fig. 46-11). *The first 10 letters also represent the numbers 0 through 9.* Braille is read by moving the hands from left to right along each line of braille (Fig. 46-12).

Special devices allow computer access—keyboards, displays, and printers. A "braille display" lets the person read the information. Braille printers produce printouts in braille.

Mobility. Blind and visually impaired persons learn to move about using a long cane or a guide dog. Both are used world-wide.

- Long canes are white or silver-gray with red tips. Do not interfere with the arm holding the cane. The person stores the cane when not in use. If you store it, tell the person where.
- The guide dog sees for the person. The dog responds to the master's commands. Commands are disobeyed to avoid danger. For example, the guide dog disobeys a command to cross the street if a car is coming. Do not pet, feed, or distract a guide dog. Such actions can place the person in danger.

PROMOTING SAFETY AND COMFORT

Corrective Lenses

Safety

Dirty eyeglasses can cause many of the signs and symptoms in Box 46-6. The person may worry about an eye problem when you simply need to clean the eyeglasses.

Eyeglasses are costly. Protect them from loss or damage. When not worn, put them in their case. Place the case in the top drawer of the bedside stand.

Some agencies let nursing assistants remove and insert contact lenses. If allowed to insert and remove contacts, follow agency procedures.

DELEGATION GUIDELINES

Eyeglasses

Cleaning eyeglasses is a routine nursing task. Do not wait until the nurse tells you to clean them. Clean them daily and as needed.

To clean eyeglasses, find out if you need a special cleaning solution. Then follow the manufacturer's instructions.

Corrective Lenses

Eyeglasses and contact lenses correct many vision problems. Eyeglasses are worn for reading, for seeing at a distance, or for all activities. Contact lenses are usually worn while awake. Some contacts can be worn day and night for up to 30 days.

See *Promoting Safety and Comfort: Corrective Lenses.*

Eyeglasses. Lenses are hardened glass or plastic. Clean them daily and as needed. Wash glass lenses with warm water. Dry them with a lens cloth or cotton cloth. Plastic lenses scratch easily. Use special cleaning solutions and cloths.

See *Delegation Guidelines: Eyeglasses.*
See procedure: *Caring for Eyeglasses.*

Caring for Eyeglasses

QUALITY OF LIFE

- Knock before entering the person's room.
- Address the person by name.
- Introduce yourself by name and title.

- Explain the procedure before starting and during the procedure.
- Protect the person's rights during the procedure.
- Handle the person gently during the procedure.

PRE-PROCEDURE

1 Follow *Delegation Guidelines: Eyeglasses.* See *Promoting Safety and Comfort: Corrective Lenses.*
2 Practice hand hygiene.

3 Collect the following.
   - Eyeglass case
   - Cleaning solution or warm water
   - Disposable lens cloth or cotton cloth

PROCEDURE

4 Remove the eyeglasses.
   a Hold the frames in front of the ears (Fig. 46-13, *A*).
   b Lift the frames from the ears. Bring the eyeglasses down away from the face (Fig. 46-13, *B*).
5 Clean the lenses with a cleaning solution or warm water. Clean in a circular motion. Dry the lenses with the cloth.
6 *For the person not wearing eyeglasses:*
   a Open the eyeglass case.
   b Fold the glasses. Put them in the case. Do not touch the clean lenses.
   c Place the case in the top drawer of the bedside stand.

7 *For the person wearing eyeglasses:*
   a Hold the frames at each side. Place them over the ears.
   b Adjust the eyeglasses so the nose-piece rests on the nose.
   c Return the case to the top drawer of the bedside stand.

POST-PROCEDURE

8 Provide for comfort. (See the inside of the back cover.)
9 Place the call light and other needed items within reach.
10 Return the cleaning solution to its proper place.
11 Discard the disposable cloth.

12 Complete a safety check of the room. (See the inside of the back cover.)
13 Practice hand hygiene.
14 Report and record your observations.

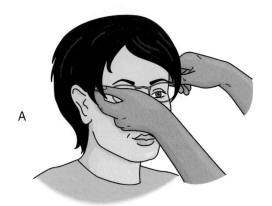
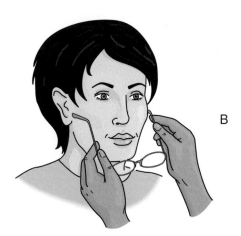

FIGURE 46-13 Removing eyeglasses. **A,** Hold the frames in front of the ears. **B,** Lift the frames from the ears. Bring the glasses down away from the face.

Contact Lenses. Contact lenses fit on the eye. There are hard and soft contacts. Disposable ones are discarded daily, weekly, or monthly. Contacts are cleaned, removed, and stored according to the manufacturer's instructions.

Report and record the following.

- Eye redness or irritation
- Eye drainage
- Complaints of eye pain, blurred or fuzzy vision, or uncomfortable lenses

Ocular Prostheses

Injury or disease may require removing an eyeball. The person is fitted with an ocular (eye) prosthesis. See Figure 46-14. This artificial eye does not provide vision. It matches the other eye in color and shape. The other eye may have normal, some, or no vision.

Worn all the time, even for sleep, the prosthesis usually needs little care. Usually cleaning is needed every 2 to 3 weeks. The prosthesis is briefly removed for cleaning and then re-inserted. To clean an ocular prosthesis:

1 Practice hand hygiene.
2 Collect a kidney basin, denture cup, or other container as directed by the nurse. Line the container with a soft cloth or 4 × 4 gauze. This prevents scratches and damage.
3 Have the person put the eye in the container.
4 Line the sink with a towel.
5 Wash the eye, using your fingertips, with mild soap and warm water. Baby shampoo is often recommended. Rinse well. Do not use a cloth to wash or dry the eye. (Wear gloves for this step.)
6 Line a container with a new soft cloth or 4 × 4 gauze.
7 Place the eye in the container. Remove gloves and practice hand hygiene.
8 Have the person insert the prosthesis.
See *Promoting Safety and Comfort: Ocular Prostheses.*

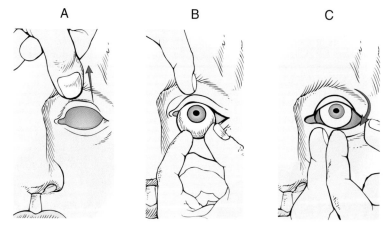

FIGURE 46-14 Inserting an ocular prosthesis. **A,** Lift the upper lid. **B,** Slide the prosthesis under the lid. **C,** Release the upper lid. (From Lewis SM, Heitkemper MM, Dirksen SR: *Medical-surgical nursing: assessment and management of clinical problems,* ed 5, St Louis, 2000, Mosby.)

PROMOTING SAFETY AND COMFORT

Ocular Prostheses

Safety

When an ocular prosthesis is removed, you must prevent chips, scratches, and other damage. It must not fall on the floor or other hard surface. Always hold the eye over a towel or other soft surface.

The prosthesis is the person's property. Protect it from loss or damage.

FOCUS ON **PRIDE**

The Person, Family, and Yourself

Personal and Professional Responsibility

Hearing aids, contact lenses, and eyeglasses are costly to repair or replace. Protect devices from loss or damage. If a device is lost or damaged, tell the nurse. Take pride in being responsible and honest.

Rights and Respect

Many persons with hearing, speech, and vision problems have overcome great challenges. They take pride in how they have adapted. They deserve to be treated with dignity and respect. Do not pity the person. Treat the person like an adult, not like a child. Focus on the person's abilities, not disabilities.

Always refer to the person first. Then state the disability if needed. For example, a nurse says: "Please take Mrs. Jones a warm blanket. She is blind, so remember to knock and introduce yourself before entering the room. She will place the blanket as she prefers."

Independence and Social Interaction

Adjusting to a hearing, speech, or vision problem is often long and hard. Take time to listen. Be patient, understanding, and sensitive to the person's needs and feelings. Allow the person to be in control to the extent possible. This helps promote independence to improve quality of life.

Delegation and Teamwork

Hearing loss requires changes in communication. Communication measures are part of the care plan. Using gestures, written notes, or an ASL interpreter are examples.

Follow the care plan. A consistent approach is needed. The health team communicates with the person in the same way. Take pride in being part of a caring health team.

Ethics and Laws

The *Americans With Disabilities Act (ADA) of 1990* protects the rights of persons with disabilities. It includes persons with limited hearing, speech, and vision. The ADA covers rights such as employment, access to services and places, and the use of communication devices.

To comply with the ADA, agencies often provide:
- Braille on signs for areas with public access. Lobbies restrooms, elevators, and cafeterias are examples.
- Communication devices for hearing or speech problems. For example, a device with a keyboard and small screen is connected to a phone line. The device is used instead of a phone.
- Sign language interpreters.
- Information in large print and braille.

Know your agency's resources for persons with disabilities. Offer to help. If not sure how to help, ask the nurse. Take pride in helping others.

FOCUS ON **PRIDE**: *Application*

Hearing, speech, and vision problems do not affect intelligence. Some behaviors insult the person. Treating the person like a child and talking to others but not the person are examples. What are other examples? Identify ways to show dignity and respect.

REVIEW QUESTIONS

Circle the BEST answer.

1 Care of the person with Meniere's disease includes
   a Wearing a hearing aid
   b Preventing falls from vertigo
   c Speech therapy
   d Treating infection

2 Which is a sign of hearing loss?
   a An adult tugs or pulls at the ears.
   b A 5-month-old babbles and makes gurgling sounds.
   c An adult asks others to repeat themselves.
   d A 10-month-old uses gestures to communicate.

3 When talking to a person with hearing loss
   a Shout
   b Change the subject if the person does not seem to understand
   c Avoid using gestures and facial expressions
   d Use short sentences and simple words

4 A hearing aid
   a Corrects a hearing problem
   b Makes sounds louder
   c Makes speech clearer
   d Lowers background noise

5 A hearing aid does not seem to be working. Your *first* action is to
   a See if it is turned on
   b Wash it with soap and water
   c Have it repaired
   d Remove the batteries

6 A person has aphasia. You know that
   a The person cannot hear
   b Mouth and face muscles are affected
   c The person has a language disorder
   d The person cannot speak

7 A person with receptive aphasia has trouble
   a Talking
   b Writing
   c Understanding messages
   d Using gestures

8 A person has a speech disorder. You should
   a Correct the person's speech
   b Discourage the writing of words
   c Leave the TV on while talking
   d Ask the person to repeat as needed

Continued

REVIEW QUESTIONS—cont'd

9 A person with a cataract
   a Has cloudy, blurry, or dim vision
   b Loses central vision
   c Has eye pain
   d Is blind

10 A person had cataract surgery. Which would you question?
   a Remind the person not to bend or cough.
   b Let the person rub the eye.
   c Place the over-bed table on the un-operative side.
   d Have the person wear an eye shield during naps.

11 A person has AMD. Which is *true?*
   a There is a blind spot in the center of the eye.
   b Lost vision can be restored with surgery.
   c Peripheral (side) vision is lost.
   d Vision is blurry with spots.

12 With low vision
   a There is no usable vision
   b Surgery can correct vision loss
   c Visual and adaptive devices are needed
   d Every-day activities are not affected

13 Who is at risk for low vision?
   a The person with diabetic retinopathy
   b The person with global aphasia
   c The person with Meniere's disease
   d The person who is blind

14 Braille involves
   a A long cane for walking
   b Raised dots arranged for letters of the alphabet
   c A guide dog
   d Corrective lenses

15 Which are dangers for blind or visually impaired persons?
   a Closed drawers
   b Doors that are fully open
   c Equipment in hallways
   d Night-lights

16 A person is blind. The meal-time setting should
   a Be the same for every meal
   b Provide variety for mental stimulation
   c Include plates, napkins, and placemats with designs
   d Be at the same time everyday

17 A person is visually impaired. You should
   a Move furniture to provide variety
   b Avoid words such as "see" and "look"
   c Assume that the person has no sight
   d Explain procedures step-by-step

18 A person is blind. To give directions you can say
   a "Over there"
   b "Right here"
   c "Across the room"
   d "On your left"

19 When eyeglasses are not worn they should be
   a Soaked in a cleansing solution
   b Taken to the nurses' station
   c Put in the eyeglass case
   d Placed on the over-bed table

20 To care for an ocular prosthesis
   a Dry the eye with a cloth
   b Wash the eye with mild soap and warm water
   c Scrub the eye with 4 × 4 gauze
   d Store the eye in an empty container

Answers to Chapter 46 questions are on p. 887.

FOCUS ON PRACTICE

Problem Solving

A resident asks for help completing the weekly menu. You are to read each option and mark the choices. Hard of hearing, the resident struggles to hear you. You repeat the meal options many times. What will you do? How can you promote hearing?

Cancer, Immune System, and Skin Disorders

- Define the key terms and key abbreviations in this chapter.
- Explain the differences between benign tumors and cancer.
- Identify cancer signs, symptoms, and risk factors.
- Explain the common cancer treatments.
- Describe the needs of persons with cancer.
- Describe the common immune system disorders.
- Describe the human immunodeficiency virus (HIV) and acquired immunodeficiency syndrome (AIDS).

- Explain how to assist in the care of persons with AIDS.
- Describe the cause, signs and symptoms, and treatment of shingles.
- Explain how to promote PRIDE in the person, the family, and yourself.

KEY TERMS

benign tumor A tumor that does not spread to other body parts
biopsy A procedure in which a piece of tissue is removed for testing
cancer See "malignant tumor"
malignant tumor A tumor that invades and destroys nearby tissues and can spread to other body parts; cancer

metastasis The spread of cancer to other body parts
mole A brown, tan, or black spot on the skin that is flat or raised and round or oval
stomatitis Inflammation *(itis)* of the mouth *(stomat)*
tumor A new growth of abnormal cells that is benign or malignant

KEY ABBREVIATIONS

AIDS	Acquired immunodeficiency syndrome		**STD**	Sexually transmitted disease
CDC	Centers for Disease Control and Prevention		**TB**	Tuberculosis
HIV	Human immunodeficiency virus			

Understanding cancer, immune system, and skin disorders gives meaning to the required care. Refer to Chapter 10 while you study this chapter.

CANCER

Cells reproduce for tissue growth and repair. Cells divide in an orderly way. Sometimes cell division and growth are out of control. A mass or clump of cells develops. This *new growth of abnormal cells is called a* **tumor**. *Tumors are benign or malignant* (Fig. 47-1, p. 706).

- *Benign tumors do not spread to other body parts* (see Fig. 47-1, *A*). They can grow to a large size but rarely threaten life. They usually do not grow back when removed.
- *Malignant tumors (cancer) invade and destroy nearby tissues. They can spread to other body parts* (see Fig. 47-1, *B*). They may be life-threatening. Sometimes they grow back after removal.

Metastasis is the spread of cancer to other body parts (Fig. 47-2, p. 706). If not treated and controlled, cancer cells break off the tumor and travel to other body parts. New tumors grow at those sites.

A biopsy is often needed to diagnose cancer. A *biopsy is a procedure in which a piece of tissue is removed for testing.* The tissue sample is removed with a needle, using a scope, or with surgery. Sometimes the entire tumor and tissue around the tumor are removed. The sample is examined for cancer.

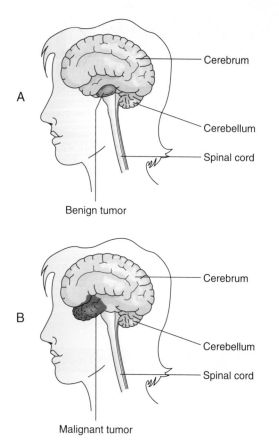

FIGURE 47-1 Tumors. **A,** A benign tumor grows within a local area. **B,** A malignant tumor invades other tissues.

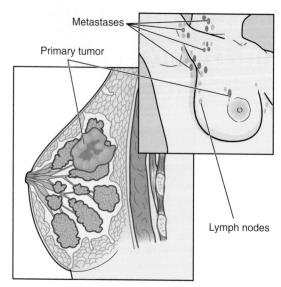

FIGURE 47-2 A tumor in the breast has metastasized to the lymph nodes.

Cancer Signs and Symptoms

Cancer can occur almost anywhere. See Box 47-1 for some signs and symptoms of cancer. Pain may be an early symptom in some cancers. Bone cancer is an example. However, pain often means the cancer has metastasized. If detected early, cancer can be treated and controlled.

See *Focus on Children and Older Persons: Cancer Signs and Symptoms.*

FOCUS ON CHILDREN AND OLDER PERSONS

Cancer Signs and Symptoms

Children

The most common childhood cancers are:

- Leukemia—a cancer of the blood and bone marrow. The bone marrow is a spongy substance found inside bones. Blood cells are made in the bone marrow. Leukemia is the most common form of childhood cancer.
- Brain and spinal cord tumors.
- Lymphomas—tumors of the lymph tissues.

Early signs and symptoms are often similar to common illnesses and injuries. Fever, fatigue, swollen glands, weight loss, bruising, and tender joints or bones are examples. Children should see a doctor when signs and symptoms are severe or do not go away.

BOX 47-1	**Cancer—Signs and Symptoms**

Brain Tumor
- Headache—morning headache, headache that goes away after vomiting
- Seizures
- Vision, hearing, and speech problems
- Loss of appetite
- Frequent nausea and vomiting
- Changes in personality, mood, ability to focus, or behavior
- Loss of balance and trouble walking
- Weakness
- Unusual sleepiness, change in activity level

Pancreatic Cancer
- *Jaundice*—yellowish skin and eyes
- Light colored stools
- Dark urine
- Pain in the upper or middle abdomen and back
- Weight loss
- Loss of appetite
- Fatigue

Uterine Cancer
- Unusual vaginal bleeding or discharge
- Vaginal bleeding after menopause
- *Dysuria*—painful or difficult urination
- Pain during sex
- Pelvic pain

Cervical Cancer
- Vaginal bleeding (including bleeding after sex)
- Unusual vaginal discharge
- Pelvic pain
- Pain during sex

Breast Cancer
- Lump or thickening in or near the breast or underarm
- Change in the size or shape of the breast
- Dimple or puckering in the breast skin, dimples that look like the skin of an orange
- Nipple turned inward into the breast
- Fluid (other than breast-milk) from the nipple, especially if bloody
- Scaly, red, or swollen skin on the breast, nipple, or areola (the dark area of skin around the nipple)

Bladder Cancer
- Blood in the urine (urine looks rusty or bright red)
- Urinary frequency
- Painful urination
- Low back pain

Colon Cancer
- Change in bowel habits
- Blood in the stool (bright red or very dark)
- Diarrhea, constipation, feeling that the bowel does not empty completely
- Stools that are narrower than usual
- Frequent gas pains, bloating, fullness, cramping
- Weight loss
- Fatigue
- Vomiting

Kidney Cancer
- Blood in the urine
- Lump in the abdomen
- Pain in the side that does not go away
- Loss of appetite
- Weight loss
- Signs of *anemia* (a decrease in red blood cells or hemoglobin; *an* means *lack of*, *emia* means *blood condition*)—shortness of breath, fatigue, rapid pulse, dizziness, pale skin

Leukemia
- Weakness
- Fatigue
- Fever or night sweats
- Easy bruising or bleeding
- Flat, pinpoint spots under the skin caused by bleeding
- Shortness of breath
- Weight loss, loss of appetite
- Pain in the bones or stomach
- Pain or feeling of fullness below the ribs
- Painless lumps in the neck, underarm, stomach, or groin
- Having many infections

Lung Cancer
- Chest discomfort or pain
- Cough that does not go away or worsens over time
- Trouble breathing, wheezing
- Blood in sputum
- Hoarseness
- Loss of appetite
- Weight loss
- Fatigue
- Dysphagia
- Swelling in the face, neck veins, or both

Lymphoma
- Swelling in the lymph nodes in the neck, underarm, groin, or stomach
- Fever
- Night sweats
- Fatigue
- Weight loss
- Skin rash or itchy skin
- Pain in the chest, abdomen, or bones

Mouth and Lip Cancer
- Sore on the lip or in the mouth that does not heal
- Lump or thickening on the lips, gums, or in the mouth
- A white or red patch on the gums, tongue, or lining of the mouth
- Lip or mouth bleeding, pain, or numbness
- Voice change
- Loose teeth or dentures that no longer fit well
- Trouble chewing, swallowing, or moving the tongue or jaw
- Jaw swelling
- Sore throat or feeling that something is caught in the throat

Continued

BOX 47-1	Cancer—Signs and Symptoms—cont'd

Melanoma

- Change in the size, shape, or color of a *mole (a brown, tan, or black spot on the skin that is flat or raised and round or oval)* (Fig. 47-3)
- Mole with irregular edges
- Mole with more than 1 color
- Uneven mole shape—1 half does not match the other half
- Mole that itches, oozes, bleeds, or has an ulcer (Chapter 40)
- New moles growing near an existing mole
- Skin color changes

Skin Cancer

- A sore that does not heal
- Skin that is raised, smooth, shiny, and pearly
- Skin that is firm and looks like a scar (may be white, yellow, or waxy)
- Raised and red or reddish-brown skin
- Scaling, bleeding, or crusty areas

Prostate Cancer

- Weak urine stream
- Urine stream that starts and stops
- Sudden urge to urinate
- Frequent urination, especially at night
- Trouble starting the urine flow
- Urinary retention
- Pain or burning with urination
- Blood in the urine or semen
- Pain in the back, hips, or pelvis
- Signs of anemia—shortness of breath, fatigue, rapid pulse, dizziness, pale skin

Thyroid Cancer

- A lump (nodule) in the neck
- Dyspnea
- Dysphagia, pain with swallowing
- Hoarseness

Modified from National Cancer Institute:

- Adult central nervous system tumors treatment (PDQ®)–patient version, *updated October 11, 2019.*
- Pancreatic cancer treatment (PDQ®)–patient version, *updated May 23, 2018.*
- Endometrial cancer treatment (PDQ®)–patient version, *updated June 12, 2019.*
- Cervical cancer treatment (PDQ®)–patient version, *updated November 8, 2019.*
- Breast cancer treatment (PDQ®)–patient version, *updated November 21, 2019.*
- Bladder cancer treatment (PDQ®)–patient version, *updated October 30, 2019.*
- Colon cancer treatment (PDQ®)–patient version, *updated May 15, 2019.*
- Renal cell cancer treatment (PDQ®)–patient version, *updated November 8, 2019.*
- Adult acute lymphoblastic leukemia treatment (PDQ®)–patient version, *updated July 23, 2019.*
- Non-small cell lung cancer treatment (PDQ®)–patient version, *updated October 16, 2019.*
- Adult non-Hodgkin lymphoma treatment (PDQ®)–patient version, *updated November 8, 2019.*
- Lip and oral cavity cancer treatment (adult) (PDQ®)–patient version, *updated September 5, 2019.*
- Melanoma treatment (PDQ®)–patient version, *updated November 8, 2019.*
- Skin cancer treatment (PDQ®)–patient version, *updated November 8, 2019.*
- Prostate cancer treatment (PDQ®)–patient version, *updated June 12, 2019.*
- Thyroid cancer treatment (adult) (PDQ®)–patient version, *updated May 16, 2019.*

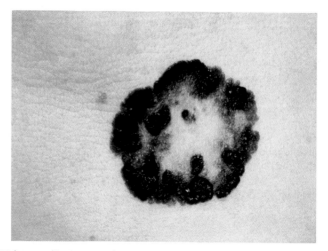

FIGURE 47-3 Melanoma. (From Centers for Disease Control and Prevention, Department of Health and Human Services/Carl Washington, M.D., Emory Univ. School of Medicine; Mona Saraiya, MD, MPH.)

Risk Factors

Cancer is the second leading cause of death in the United States. The National Cancer Institute describes these risk factors.

- *Age.* Advancing age is the most important risk factor. However, cancer can occur at any age.
- *Tobacco.* This includes using tobacco (smoking, snuff, and chewing tobacco) and being around tobacco (second-hand smoke). This risk can be avoided.
- *Radiation.* Sources are sun light, x-rays, and radon gas that forms in the soil and some rocks.
- *Infections.* Certain viruses and bacteria increase the risk of cancers—cervix, penis, vagina, anus, mouth, nose and throat, lung, liver, lymphoma, leukemia, Kaposi's sarcoma (associated with AIDS, p. 712), stomach.
- *Immuno-suppressive drugs.* Such drugs are often used for organ transplant patients to prevent rejection of the transplant. They lower the body's ability to stop cancer from forming.
- *Alcohol.* Alcohol is linked to the increased risk of cancers of the mouth, throat, esophagus, larynx, liver, and breast.
- *Hormones.* The female hormones estrogen and progesterone are known to increase the risk of breast and uterine cancers.
- *Diet and obesity.* A healthy diet, physical activity, and a healthy weight may reduce the risk of some cancers. Obesity is linked to post-menopausal breast cancer and cancers of the colon, rectum, uterus, esophagus, kidney, pancreas, and gallbladder.
- *Environment.* Air pollution, second-hand smoke, and asbestos are linked to lung cancer. Drinking water with large amounts of arsenic is linked to skin, bladder, and lung cancers.

Treatment

Treatment depends on the tumor type, its site and size, and if it has spread. The treatment goal may be to:

- Cure the cancer. Remove cancer from the body and kill cancer cells.
- Control the disease. Help the person live longer.
- Reduce symptoms from the cancer and its treatments.

Some cancers respond to 1 type of treatment. Others require 2 or more types. Cancer treatments also damage healthy cells and tissues. Side effects depend on the type and extent of the treatment.

Surgery. Surgery removes tumors. It is done to cure or control cancer or to relieve pain. See Chapter 39.

Radiation Therapy. Radiation therapy *(radiotherapy)* kills cancer cells. X-ray beams are aimed at the tumor. Sometimes radioactive material is implanted in or near the tumor. Radiation therapy:

- Destroys certain tumors.
- Shrinks a tumor before surgery.
- Destroys cancer cells that remain after surgery.
- Controls tumor growth to prevent or relieve pain.

Cancer cells and normal cells receive radiation. Healthy cells are damaged. Skin changes occur at the treatment site—dryness, itching, swelling, peeling, redness, blistering, hair loss. Special skin care measures are ordered. Dry mouth, sore throat, and *dysphagia* (difficulty swallowing) can result from radiation to the head and neck. Extra rest is needed for fatigue. Discomfort, nausea, vomiting, diarrhea, and loss of appetite *(anorexia)* are other side effects.

See *Promoting Safety and Comfort: Radiation Therapy.*

Chemotherapy. Chemotherapy involves drugs that kill cancer cells. It is used to:

- Cure the cancer.
- Shrink a tumor before surgery.
- Slow growth of the cancer.
- Prevent the cancer from spreading.
- Kill cells that break off the tumor to prevent metastasis.
- Relieve symptoms caused by the cancer.

PROMOTING SAFETY AND COMFORT

Radiation Therapy

Safety

Radiation implants (seeds, ribbons, capsules) are placed near the tumor. Therefore the person's body gives off radiation. Practice these safety measures.

- Tell the nurse if you are or may be pregnant or are younger than 18. The nurse needs to change your assignment.
- Follow agency policy for wearing a badge or device to measure radiation exposure.
- Talk to the person from the doorway if you do not need to enter the room. Radiation exposure decreases with distance.
- Don protective gloves and shoe coverings before entering the person's room.
- Work quickly.
- Follow the limits for time in the person's room and for the distance between you and the person.
- Leave trash, linens, and food trays in the room. These items will be removed by staff trained to do so.
- Remove and discard your gloves and shoe coverings before leaving the room.
- Wash your hands after leaving the room.

Comfort

The person has a private room to protect others from radiation exposure. A visitor may be limited to 30 minutes or less a day. Visitors may stand at the doorway rather than enter the room. Children under 18 years of age and pregnant women are not allowed to visit.

Therefore the person may feel sad, lonely, and depressed. Assure the person that care needs will be met. Treat the person with caring, kindness, and dignity.

Chemotherapy affects the whole body. Cancer cells and normal cells are affected. Side effects depend on the drug used.

- Fatigue.
- Hair loss (*alopecia*).
- Gastro-intestinal irritation. Poor appetite, nausea, vomiting, and diarrhea can occur. *Stomatitis, an inflammation* (itis) *of the mouth* (stomat), may occur.
- Decreased blood cell production. Bleeding and infection are risks. The person may be weak and tired.
- Changes in thinking and memory.
- Emotional changes.

The drug usually stays in the person's body for 3 to 7 days. It is excreted through body fluids—urine, feces, vomit, tears, saliva, semen, and vaginal secretions. Safety measures are listed in Box 47-2.

Hormone Therapy. Some cancers need hormones to grow. Hormone therapy involves drugs or surgery to remove hormone sources from the body. For example, to treat breast cancer, drugs are given to block hormones from the ovaries or the ovaries are removed. For prostate cancer, drugs are given to block hormones from the testicles or the testicles are removed.

Side effects include hot flashes, fatigue, nausea, and loss of sexual desire. Men may have weakened bones, diarrhea, and enlarged and tender breasts. Women may have vaginal dryness, menstrual changes (if pre-menopausal), and mood changes. Fertility is affected in men and women. Men may experience impotence (Chapter 55).

Immunotherapy. Immunotherapy helps the immune system fight the cancer. Side effects include flu-like symptoms—fever, chills, weakness, dizziness, nausea and vomiting, muscle or joint aches, fatigue, headache, dyspnea, and blood pressure changes. Pain, swelling, redness, itching, and rash may occur.

Other Therapies. Other therapies include:
- *Targeted therapy.* There are differences in how cancer cells grow, divide, and spread. Targeted drugs focus on these differences to treat cancer. Most healthy cells are not harmed. Targeted therapy may be used alone or with surgery, chemotherapy, or radiation.
- *Stem cell transplants.* A stem cell is a cell from which new cell types develop. The new cells have certain functions—blood cells, brain cells, bone cells, and so on. High doses of chemotherapy or radiation therapy can kill cancer cells and blood cells in the bone marrow. Fewer blood cells are produced. The person is given blood-forming stem cells. New blood cells develop from the stem cells.
- *Complementary and alternative medicine (CAM).* *Complementary medicine* is used with standard cancer treatments. *Alternative medicine* is used instead of standard cancer treatments. CAM includes massage therapy, herbal products, vitamins, special diets, spiritual healing, aromatherapy, and acupuncture. Aromatherapy involves the use of fragrant oils to improve symptoms. Acupuncture involves inserting small needles at certain points in the skin to control pain and other symptoms.

The Person's Needs

Persons with cancer have many needs. They include:
- Pain relief or control
- Rest and exercise
- Fluids and nutrition
- Preventing skin breakdown
- Preventing bowel problems—constipation from pain-relief drugs; diarrhea from some cancer treatments
- Dealing with treatment side effects
- Psychological and social needs
- Spiritual needs
- Sexual needs

BOX 47-2   Safety During Chemotherapy

General Safety
- Wear gloves for any contact with the person's body fluids, secretions, or excretions. Wash your hands after removing and discarding the gloves.
- Wash the hands or any body part or area that has contact with the person's body fluids, secretions, or excretions. Do so at once. Use soap and water. This applies to you, the person, and others.

Elimination and Vomiting
- Wear gloves to handle bedpans, urinals, or kidney basins.
- Empty and rinse bedpans, urinals, and kidney basins after use.
- Flush after the person uses the toilet or you empty a bedpan, urinal, or kidney basin. Put the lid down first to avoid splashing. Flush twice if young children or pets will have contact with the toilet.
- Wash bedpans, urinals, and kidney basins at least once a day with soap and water. Or provide the person with new items. Follow agency policy.

Elimination and Vomiting—cont'd
- Wear gloves when changing and handling diapers, incontinence products, waterproof under-pads, and ostomy pouches.
- Double-bag diapers, incontinence products, waterproof under-pads, and ostomy pouches. Follow agency policy.
- Place ostomy waste in a tied plastic bag or a zip-lock bag. Then place the bag in another plastic bag. Discard following agency policy.

Laundry
- Follow agency policy for soiled linens and clothing. In the home setting:
  - Wash soiled linens as soon as possible. Or place them in a plastic bag. Discard the plastic bag in the trash after washing the items.
  - Wash soiled items separately from other linens or garments.
  - Wash soiled items twice.

Modified from UPMC: Patient education: safe handling of chemotherapy waste material, Pittsburgh, Pa, 2019, UPMC.

Psychological and social needs are great. Anger, fear, and depression are common. Some surgeries are disfiguring. The person may feel unwhole, unattractive, or unclean. The person and family need support.

Spiritual needs are important. A spiritual leader may provide comfort. To many people, spiritual needs are just as important as physical needs.

Persons dying of cancer often receive hospice care (Chapters 1 and 59). Support is given to the person and family.

See *Focus on Communication: The Person's Needs.*

FOCUS ON **COMMUNICATION**

The Person's Needs

Knowing what to say to a person with cancer can be hard. Do not avoid the person. Talk as you would with any other person. Avoid comments like "I'm sure you will be fine" or "It will be okay."

Often the person needs to talk and have someone listen. Listen and use touch to show you care. Being there when needed is important. You may not have to say anything. Just listen.

IMMUNE SYSTEM DISORDERS

The immune system protects the body from microbes, cancer cells, and other harmful substances. It defends against threats inside and outside the body. Immune system disorders occur from problems with the immune response. The response may be inappropriate, too strong, or lacking.

See *Body Structure and Function Review: The Immune System.*

Autoimmune Disorders

Autoimmune disorders occur when the immune system attacks the body's own *(auto)* healthy cells, tissues, or organs. The body parts affected depend on the type of disorder (Fig. 47-4, p. 712). Common autoimmune disorders include:

- *Celiac disease.* The person cannot tolerate gluten—a substance in wheat, rye, barley, and some drugs. When gluten is ingested, the immune system causes damage to the small intestines. Signs and symptoms include abdominal bloating and pain, diarrhea or constipation, weight loss or gain, and fatigue.
- *Graves' disease.* The thyroid gland produces excess *(hyper)* amounts of the thyroid hormone. The person has irritability, problems sleeping, weight loss, sweating, muscle weakness, shaky hands, and bulging eyes (Fig. 47-5, p. 712).
- *Hashimoto's disease.* The thyroid gland does not produce enough thyroid hormone. The person has fatigue, weakness, weight gain, sensitivity to cold, muscle aches, stiff joints, facial swelling, and constipation.

BODY STRUCTURE AND FUNCTION REVIEW

The Immune System

The immune system protects the body from disease and infection. Abnormal body cells can grow into tumors. Sometimes the body produces substances that cause the body to attack itself. Microbes (bacteria, viruses, and other germs) can cause an infection.

The immune system gives the body *immunity*—protection against a disease or condition. The person will not get or be affected by the disease.

- *Specific immunity* is the body's reaction to a certain threat.
- *Non-specific immunity* is the body's reaction to anything it does not recognize as a normal body substance.

Special cells and substances function to produce immunity.

- *Antibodies*—normal body substances that recognize other substances. They are involved in destroying abnormal or unwanted substances.
- *Antigens*—substances that cause an immune response. Antibodies recognize and bind with unwanted antigens. This leads to the destruction of unwanted substances and the production of more antibodies.
- *Phagocytes*—white blood cells that digest and destroy microbes and other unwanted substances.
- *Lymphocytes*—white blood cells that produce antibodies. Lymphocyte production increases as the body responds to an infection.
  - *B lymphocytes (B cells)*—cause the production of antibodies that circulate in the plasma. The antibodies react to specific antigens.
  - *T lymphocytes (T cells)*—destroy invading cells. *Killer T cells* produce poisons near the invading cells. Some T cells attract other cells. The other cells destroy the invaders.

When the body senses an antigen from an unwanted substance, the immune system acts. Phagocyte and lymphocyte production increases. Phagocytes destroy the invaders through digestion. The lymphocytes produce antibodies that identify and destroy the unwanted substances.

- *Lupus.* This disease can damage the joints, skin, kidneys, heart, lungs, and other body parts. A rash across the nose and cheeks is common. See Figure 47-6, p. 712.
- *Multiple sclerosis* (Chapter 48).
- *Rheumatoid arthritis* (Chapter 48).
- *Type 1 diabetes* (Chapter 50).
- *Inflammatory bowel disease* (Chapter 50).

Most autoimmune disorders are chronic. Treatment depends on the disorder and the tissues and organs affected. Treatment is aimed at:

- Relieving symptoms
- Replacing needed hormones
- Suppressing the immune system

Body Parts That Can Be Affected by Autoimmune Diseases

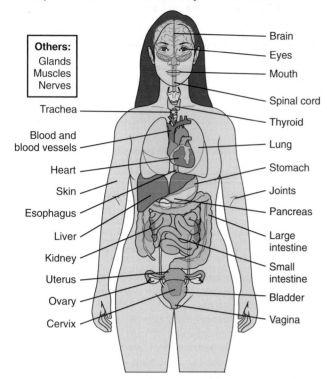

FIGURE 47-4 Body parts affected by autoimmune disorders. (Redrawn from Office on Women's Health, U.S. Department of Health and Human Services: *Autoimmune diseases,* updated April 1, 2019.)

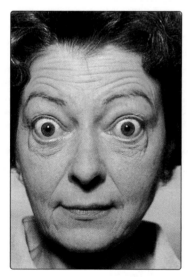

FIGURE 47-5 Bulging eyes occurs in Graves' disease. (From Gaw A, Murphy M, et al: *Clinical biochemistry: an illustrated colour text,* ed 5, Philadelphia, 2013, Elsevier.)

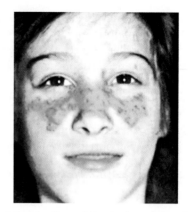

FIGURE 47-6 Called the "butterfly" rash, the rash from lupus is across the nose and cheeks. (From Kliegman RM, et al: *Nelson textbook of pediatrics,* ed 20, Philadelphia, 2016, Elsevier.)

HIV/AIDS

Acquired immunodeficiency syndrome (AIDS) is caused by the *human immunodeficiency virus (HIV).* HIV attacks the immune system. Therefore it destroys the body's ability to fight infections and disease.

HIV is spread through certain body fluids—blood, semen, vaginal fluids, rectal fluids, and breast-milk. HIV is *not spread* by air, water, saliva, tears, sweat, insects, casual contact (shaking hands, hugging, dancing, sharing dishes), closed mouth or social kissing, or toilet seats.

HIV is transmitted *mainly* by:
- Having sex with someone who has HIV.
  - Anal sex
  - Vaginal sex
  - Multiple sex partners
- Sharing needles, syringes, rinse water, or other equipment used to prepare injection drugs.

The Centers for Disease Control and Prevention (CDC) reports that HIV *may* be spread by:
- HIV-infected mothers to children during pregnancy, birth, or breast-feeding.
- Being stuck with an HIV-contaminated needle or other sharp object
- Receiving blood transfusions, blood products, or organ or tissue transplants contaminated with HIV
- Eating food pre-chewed by an HIV-infected person if the food mixes with blood
- Being bitten and skin broken by an HIV-infected person
- Oral sex
- Contact between broken skin, wounds, or mucous membranes and HIV-infected blood or blood-contaminated body fluids
- Deep, open-mouth kissing if blood is exchanged when the person with HIV has sores or bleeding gums

Box 47-3 lists the stages and signs and symptoms of HIV and AIDS. HIV can be transmitted to others during any stage. Some HIV-infected persons are symptom-free for more than 10 years. However, they carry HIV and can spread it to others.

Drugs are available to treat or reduce HIV symptoms. They also reduce complications and prolong life. AIDS has no vaccine and no cure at present. Without treatment, persons with AIDS live about 3 years.

You may care for persons who are HIV positive, are HIV carriers, or have AIDS (Box 47-4). You may have contact with the person's blood or body fluids. Protect yourself and others. Follow Standard Precautions and the Bloodborne Pathogen Standard. A person may have the HIV virus but no symptoms. In some persons, HIV or AIDS is not yet diagnosed.

See *Focus on Children and Older Persons: HIV/AIDS.*
See *Promoting Safety and Comfort: HIV/AIDS,* p. 714.

BOX 47-3 **AIDS—Stages and Signs and Symptoms**

Acute Infection
- May occur within 2 to 4 weeks after HIV infection.
- Flu-like symptoms often described as the "worst flu ever."
  - Fever
  - Chills
  - Rash
  - Night sweats
  - Muscle aches
  - Sore throat
  - Fatigue
  - Swollen lymph nodes
  - Mouth ulcers
- Symptoms may last a few days to several weeks.

Clinical Latency Stage (Chronic HIV Infection)
- *Latency* means *present and developing but not obvious or visible.*
- The HIV is living and developing without producing symptoms.
- The person has no HIV-related symptoms or only mild ones. HIV can still be spread to others even if there are no symptoms.
- This stage can last 10 years or longer. Some people progress to the next stage faster.

AIDS
- The immune system is badly damaged.
- The person is at risk for infections, illnesses, and cancers. They include pneumonia, tuberculosis (TB), Kaposi's sarcoma, nervous system disorders, mental health disorders, and dementia.
- Signs and symptoms:
  - Rapid weight loss
  - Recurring fever
  - Night sweats
  - Fatigue: extreme and unexplained
  - Swollen lymph glands: underarms, groin, neck
  - Diarrhea lasting more than a week
  - Sores: mouth, anus, genitals
  - Pneumonia
  - Red, brown, pink, or purple blotches: on or under the skin; inside the mouth, nose, or eyelids
  - Memory loss
  - Depression

BOX 47-4 **Caring for the Person With AIDS**

- Follow Standard Precautions and the Bloodborne Pathogen Standard.
- Provide daily hygiene. Avoid irritating soaps.
- Follow the care plan for oral hygiene. A toothbrush with soft bristles is best.
- Provide oral fluids as ordered.
- Measure and record intake and output.
- Measure weight daily.
- Encourage deep-breathing and coughing exercises as ordered.
- Prevent pressure injuries.
- Assist with range-of-motion exercises and ambulating as ordered.
- Encourage self-care. The person may use adaptive (assistive) devices (walker, commode, eating devices).
- Encourage the person to be as active as possible.
- Change linens and garments when damp or wet.
- Listen and provide emotional support.

FOCUS ON CHILDREN AND OLDER PERSONS

HIV/AIDS

Older Persons
According to the CDC, older persons are more likely to have late-stage HIV infection when diagnosed. Causes include:
- Not being tested for HIV
- Not thinking they are at risk for HIV
- Dismissing HIV symptoms as normal aging

Older persons have many of the same HIV risk factors as younger persons. When not concerned about pregnancy, women may be less likely to practice safe sex. Thinning and drying of vaginal tissue may also increase risk in older women. Older persons are also less likely to discuss sexual activity and drug use with their doctors.

More immune system damage occurs when HIV treatment is started later. The CDC reported that over 6640 people age 50 and older were newly diagnosed with HIV in 2017. The CDC estimated that at the end of 2016, about 327,000 people aged 55 and older had HIV.

PROMOTING SAFETY AND COMFORT

HIV/AIDS

Safety

The CDC recommends HIV testing at least once for everyone ages 13 to 64. Pregnant women and those planning to become pregnant should be tested as early as possible. A person with HIV will test positive (HIV-positive). If HIV is not present, the person tests negative (HIV-negative).

According to the CDC, testing should be done once a year if the person:

* Is a man who is sexually active with men (gay)
* Is a man who is sexually active with men and women (bi-sexual)
* Has had sex with an HIV-positive partner
* Has had more than 1 partner since his or her last HIV test
* Has shared needles or equipment used to prepare injection drugs
* Has exchanged sex or drugs for money
* Has another sexually transmitted disease (STD) (Chapter 51), hepatitis (Chapter 50), or TB (Chapter 49)
* Has had sex with anyone who has done anything listed above
* Does not know the sexual history of a sexual partner

HIV Prevention. The CDC recommends the following measures to prevent HIV.

* Choosing less risky sexual behaviors. Anal sex carries the highest risk. Oral sex is less risky than anal or vaginal sex.
* Using condoms consistently and correctly.
* Reducing the number of sexual partners. The greater the number of partners, the greater the risk of a partner with HIV.
* Taking pre-exposure prophylaxis (PrEP) drugs. (*Prophylaxis* means *prevention measures.*) Such drugs are indicated for:
  * HIV-negative persons who have an on-going sexual relationship with an HIV-positive partner.
  * Gay or bi-sexual men who have had anal sex without a condom.
  * Gay or bi-sexual men diagnosed with an STD in the past 6 months.
  * Bi-sexual men and heterosexual men or women who do not regularly use condoms during sex with partners of unknown HIV status or with partners who are at risk for HIV. Such partners include bi-sexual men and persons who inject drugs.
* Seeing a doctor within 3 days after possible exposure to HIV. The doctor may order post-exposure prophylaxis (PEP).
* Testing and treatment for other STDs.
* Encouraging HIV-positive partners to get and continue treatment.

SKIN DISORDERS

There are many types of skin disorders. Alopecia, hirsutism, dandruff, lice, and scabies are discussed in Chapter 25. Skin tears and pressure injuries are discussed in Chapters 40 and 41. Burns are discussed in Chapter 58.

See *Body Structure and Function Review: The Integumentary System.*

BODY STRUCTURE AND FUNCTION REVIEW

The Integumentary System

The *integumentary system,* or *skin,* is the largest system. It is the body's natural covering. There are 2 skin layers (Fig. 47-7).

* The *epidermis* is the outer layer. It has living cells and dead cells. Dead cells constantly flake off and are replaced by living cells. Living cells also die and flake off. Living cells of the epidermis contain *pigment.* Pigment gives skin its color. The epidermis has no blood vessels and few nerve endings.
* The *dermis* is the inner layer. It is made up of connective tissue. Blood vessels, nerves, sweat glands, oil glands, and hair roots are found in the dermis.

Sweat glands help regulate body temperature. Sweat is secreted through the skin's pores. The body is cooled as sweat evaporates. *Oil glands* secrete an oily substance into the space near the hair shaft. Oil travels to the skin surface. This helps keep the hair and skin soft and shiny.

The skin has many functions.

* Provides the body's protective covering.
* Prevents microbes and other substances from entering the body.
* Prevents excess amounts of water from leaving the body.
* Protects organs from injury.
* Contains sensory structures. Nerve endings in the skin sense both pleasant and unpleasant stimulation. They sense cold, pain, touch, and pressure to protect the body from injury.
* Helps regulate body temperature. Blood vessels dilate (widen) when the temperature outside the body is high. More blood is brought to the body surface for cooling during evaporation. When blood vessels constrict (narrow), the body retains heat. This is because less blood reaches the skin.
* Stores fat and water.

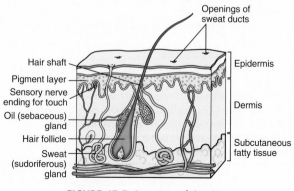

FIGURE 47-7 Structures of the skin.

Shingles

Shingles (herpes zoster) is caused by the same virus that causes chicken pox. The virus lies dormant in nerve tissue. *(Dormant* means *to be inactive.)* The virus can become active years later.

A rash or blisters can occur. At first there is burning or tingling pain, numbness, or itching. This occurs in an area on 1 side of the body or 1 side of the face. After 1 to 5 days, a rash with fluid-filled blisters appears (Fig. 47-8). Pain is often described as intense and burning. Itching is common. Fever, headache, chills, and nausea may occur.

Persons who have had chicken pox are at risk. So are persons with weakened immune systems from HIV infection, certain cancers, immuno-suppressive drugs, and stress. The risk of getting shingles increases with age.

Anti-viral drugs and pain-relief drugs are used. For many healthy people, the rash is gone in 2 to 4 weeks. Pain can last for months or years after the rash heals. Vaccines are available to prevent shingles. The CDC recommends that persons age 50 and older be vaccinated against shingles.

According to the CDC, shingles lesions are infectious until they crust over. The person needs to cover the rash, avoid touching or scratching the rash, and practice hand hygiene often.

Avoid contact with an infected person if you:
- Have never had chicken pox or the vaccine to prevent chicken pox.
- Are pregnant and have not had chicken pox or the vaccine to prevent chicken pox.
- Have a weakened immune system.

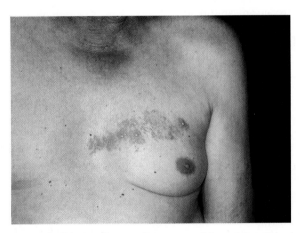

FIGURE 47-8 Shingles. (Courtesy Department of Dermatology, School of Medicine, University of Utah, Salt Lake City, Utah.)

FOCUS ON **PRIDE**

The Person, Family, and Yourself

Personal and Professional Responsibility
Oncology is the study of cancer. Oncology staff are experienced with the care and needs of persons with cancer. Staff need to be kind, caring, patient, and compassionate. Good communication skills are needed to provide quality care and to work well with the team.

Rights and Respect
People often form opinions about others. Opinions may be based on life-style, appearance, or even a disease. You cannot always control your opinions or feelings. However, they must not affect the care you give. Treat all persons with dignity and respect.

Independence and Social Interaction
The person and family have many reactions to illness—fear, anger, worry, guilt. Families respond in different ways. Family bonds are stronger when the family relies on each other during stress. A helpful and supportive family benefits the person's quality of life.

Delegation and Teamwork
Some disorders are life-threatening. AIDS and some malignant tumors are examples. Caring for dying persons is a challenge. You may have emotions and responses similar to the family. Share your feelings with the nursing team. Listen when others need to talk.

Ethics and Laws
Oncology staff often care for persons many times. Staff get to know the person's likes, dislikes, and preferences. Staff learn about the person's family, school or work, hobbies, and so on. Interest in the person adds to quality of care.

Maintaining professional boundaries can be hard when caring for persons you see often and get to know well. However, you must protect the person's privacy and rights. Watch your behavior closely to avoid crossing boundaries (Chapter 5). Tell the nurse if you suspect a person is crossing boundaries.

FOCUS ON **PRIDE**: *Application*
Many of the disorders in this chapter are life-changing. The disorder does not affect only the person. Choose 1 disorder in this chapter. Discuss the impact on the person and others.

REVIEW QUESTIONS

Circle **T** *if the statement is TRUE and* **F** *if it is FALSE.*

1 T F A benign tumor can cause metastasis.
2 T F Chemotherapy and radiation damage healthy cells and tissues.
3 T F A person has a radiation implant. You are exposed to radiation when near the person.
4 T F For chemotherapy, agency policy may require double-bagging incontinence products.
5 T F A person has an autoimmune disorder. The person's body has attacked its own cells, tissues, and organs.
6 T F Celiac disease causes the thyroid gland to produce excess thyroid hormone.
7 T F Autoimmune disorders are usually chronic.
8 T F A person infected with HIV does not have signs and symptoms. The person can spread the virus to others.
9 T F Persons who have had chicken pox are at risk for shingles.
10 T F With shingles, a painful rash covers the body.

Circle the BEST answer.

11 A person has cancer. You know that
   a The tumor will not threaten life
   b The tumor can spread to other body parts
   c The tumor is benign
   d The person's mouth is inflamed

12 Who has the greatest risk of cancer?
   a The person who smokes
   b The person who is physically active
   c The person who limits time in the sun
   d The person who is 43 years old

13 In persons with cancer, pain
   a Is usually an early sign of cancer
   b Often means that the cancer has spread
   c Is followed by a rash with blisters
   d Occurs with a fever

14 Care after cancer surgery will likely include
   a Pain-relief measures
   b Mouth care for stomatitis
   c Skin care for burns at the treatment site
   d Measures to prevent hair loss

15 Chemotherapy will likely cause
   a Burns
   b Skin breakdown
   c Nausea and vomiting
   d Weight gain

16 A cancer patient becomes sad while talking about treatment. You should
   a Change the subject
   b Call for the nurse
   c Tell the person: "You will be fine"
   d Listen

17 HIV is spread through
   a Body fluids
   b Coughing and sneezing
   c Using public phones and restrooms
   d Hugging or dancing with an infected person

18 Which poses the *lowest* risk for HIV transmission?
   a Sex with an infected person
   b Needle-sharing
   c Sharing dishes with an infected person
   d Being born to an infected mother

19 HIV can be prevented by
   a Taking immuno-suppressive drugs
   b Getting an HIV vaccine
   c Using complementary and alternative medicine
   d Avoiding risky sexual behaviors

20 A person has shingles. You know that
   a Healing occurs in 3 to 5 days
   b Itching and pain are common
   c Lesions are not infectious
   d Antibiotics are used for treatment

Answers to Chapter 47 questions are on p. 887.

FOCUS ON **PRACTICE**

Problem Solving

You work for a home health agency. Your only visit today is a patient with AIDS. You have a cough and fever. Do you go to work or call to say you cannot work? Explain the reason for your decision.

Nervous System and Musculo-Skeletal Disorders

OBJECTIVES

- Define the key terms and key abbreviations in this chapter.
- Describe the care required for stroke, Parkinson's disease, multiple sclerosis, and amyotrophic lateral sclerosis.
- Describe the care required for traumatic brain injury, spinal cord injury, and autonomic dysreflexia.
- Describe the care required for arthritis and osteoporosis.
- Explain how to assist in the care of persons after total joint replacement surgery.

- Explain how to assist in the care of persons in casts, in traction, and with hip fractures.
- Describe the effects of amputation.
- Explain how to promote PRIDE in the person, the family, and yourself.

KEY TERMS

amputation The removal of all or part of an extremity
arthritis Joint (*arthr*) inflammation (*itis*)
arthroplasty The surgical replacement (*plasty*) of a joint (*arthro*)
closed fracture The bone is broken but the skin is intact; simple fracture
comminuted fracture The bone is shattered or broken into 3 or more pieces
compound fracture See "open fracture"
fracture A broken bone
gangrene A condition in which there is death of tissue

hemiplegia Paralysis (*plegia*) on 1 side (*hemi*) of the body
open fracture The broken bone has pierced the skin; compound fracture
paralysis Loss of muscle function, sensation, or both
paraplegia Paralysis in the legs and lower trunk (*para* means *beyond*; *plegia* means *paralysis*)
quadriplegia Paralysis in the arms, legs, and trunk (*quad* means *4*; *plegia* means *paralysis*); tetraplegia
simple fracture See "closed fracture"
tetraplegia See "quadriplegia" (*tetra* means *4*; *plegia* means *paralysis*)

KEY ABBREVIATIONS

AD	Autonomic dysreflexia	MS	Multiple sclerosis
ADL	Activities of daily living	RA	Rheumatoid arthritis
ALS	Amyotrophic lateral sclerosis	ROM	Range-of-motion
CVA	Cerebrovascular accident	TBI	Traumatic brain injury
JA	Juvenile arthritis	TIA	Transient ischemic attack

Understanding nervous and musculo-skeletal disorders gives meaning to the required care. Refer to Chapter 10 while you study this chapter.

NERVOUS SYSTEM DISORDERS

Healthy nervous system function is needed to speak, understand, feel, see, hear, touch, think, control bowels and bladder, and move. Injuries and disease can result in short- or long-term health problems.

See *Body Structure and Function Review: The Nervous System*, p. 718.

BODY STRUCTURE AND FUNCTION REVIEW
The Nervous System

The nervous system controls, directs, and coordinates body functions. It consists of the brain and spinal cord (Fig. 48-1) and nerves throughout the body.

Nerves connect to the spinal cord. Nerves carry messages or impulses to and from the brain. A *stimulus* is anything that excites or causes a body part to function, become active, or respond. A stimulus causes a nerve impulse. A reflex results. A *reflex* is the body's response (function or movement) to a stimulus. Reflexes are involuntary, unconscious, and immediate. The person cannot control reflexes.

Some nerve fibers have a protective covering called a *myelin sheath.* Nerve fibers covered with myelin conduct impulses faster than those fibers without it.

The Central Nervous System

The *brain* and *spinal cord* make up the central nervous system. The brain is covered by the skull. The 3 main parts of the brain are the *cerebrum,* the *cerebellum,* and the *brainstem* (Fig. 48-2).

The cerebrum is the center of thought and intelligence. The cerebrum is divided into 2 halves called *right* and *left hemispheres.* The right hemisphere controls movement and activities on the body's left side. The left hemisphere controls the right side.

The outside of the cerebrum is called the *cerebral cortex.* It controls reasoning, memory, consciousness, speech, voluntary muscle movement, vision, hearing, sensation, and other activities.

The cerebellum regulates and coordinates body movements. It controls balance and the smooth movements of voluntary muscles.

The brainstem contains the *midbrain, pons,* and *medulla.* The midbrain and pons relay messages between the medulla and the cerebrum. The medulla controls heart rate, breathing, blood vessel size, swallowing, coughing, and vomiting. The brain connects to the spinal cord at the lower end of the medulla.

The spinal cord lies within the spinal column. It contains pathways that conduct messages to and from the brain. The brain and spinal cord are covered and protected by 3 layers of connective tissue called *meninges.*

Cerebrospinal fluid circulates around the brain and spinal cord. Cerebrospinal fluid cushions shocks that could easily injure brain and spinal cord structures.

The Peripheral Nervous System

The peripheral nervous system has 12 pairs of *cranial nerves* and 31 pairs of *spinal nerves.* The cranial nerves conduct impulses between the brain and the head, neck, chest, and abdomen. They conduct impulses for smell, vision, hearing, pain, touch, temperature, and pressure. They also conduct impulses for voluntary and involuntary muscles. Spinal nerves carry impulses from the skin, extremities, and internal structures not supplied by the cranial nerves.

Some peripheral nerves form the *autonomic nervous system.* This system controls involuntary muscles and certain body functions—heartbeat, blood pressure, intestinal contractions, and glandular secretions.

The autonomic nervous system is divided into the *sympathetic nervous system* and the *parasympathetic nervous system.* They balance each other. The sympathetic nervous system speeds up functions. The parasympathetic nervous system slows functions.

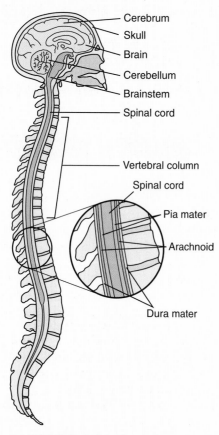

- Cerebrum
- Skull
- Brain
- Cerebellum
- Brainstem
- Spinal cord
- Vertebral column
- Spinal cord
- Pia mater
- Arachnoid
- Dura mater

FIGURE 48-1 Central nervous system.

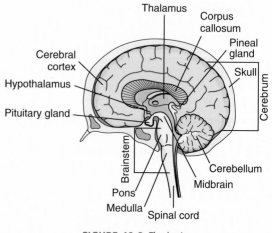

- Thalamus
- Corpus callosum
- Pineal gland
- Skull
- Cerebrum
- Cerebral cortex
- Hypothalamus
- Pituitary gland
- Brainstem
- Cerebellum
- Midbrain
- Pons
- Medulla
- Spinal cord

FIGURE 48-2 The brain.

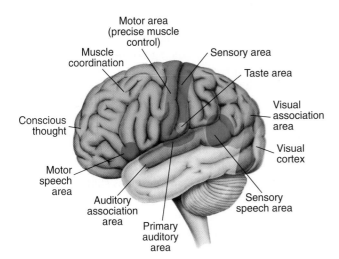

FIGURE 48-3 Functions lost from a stroke depend on the area of brain damage. (Modified from Patton KT, Thibodeau GA: *The human body in health & disease*, ed 7, St Louis, 2018, Elsevier.)

Stroke

Stroke (*brain attack* or *cerebrovascular accident [CVA]*) occurs when 1 of these happens.

- A blood vessel in the brain bursts and bleeds into the brain (cerebral hemorrhage).
- A blood clot blocks a blood vessel in the brain. Blood flow stops.

Brain cells in the affected area do not get enough oxygen and nutrients. Brain damage occurs. Functions controlled in the area of brain damage are lost (Fig. 48-3).

Stroke is a leading cause of disability and death in the United States. See Box 48-1 for warning signs. The person needs emergency care. Blood flow to the brain must be restored as soon as possible.

Warning signs may last a few minutes. This is called a *transient ischemic attack (TIA)*. (*Transient* means *temporary* or *short term. Ischemic* means *to hold back* [ischein] *blood* [hemic].) Blood supply to the brain is interrupted for a short time. A TIA may occur before a stroke. All stroke-like symptoms signal the need for emergency care.

Risk Factors. Risk factors include:
- High blood pressure
- Smoking or second-hand smoke
- Heart disease
- Diabetes
- High cholesterol
- TIAs
- Age 55 and older
- Being over-weight
- Lack of physical activity
- Family history of stroke, heart disease, or TIAs
- Drug or alcohol abuse (Chapter 52)
- Biological sex—men are at higher risk than women
- Race—African Americans have a higher risk than other races
- Hormones—use of birth control pills

BOX 48-1	Stroke—Warning Signs

- Sudden numbness or weakness of the face, arm, or leg, especially on 1 side of the body
- Sudden confusion, trouble speaking or understanding speech
- Sudden trouble seeing in 1 or both eyes
- Sudden trouble walking, dizziness, loss of balance or coordination
- Sudden, severe headache with no known cause

From National Institute of Neurological Disorders and Stroke: Know stroke, *Bethesda, Md, July 2013.*

Signs and Symptoms. Stroke can occur suddenly. The person may have warning signs (see Box 48-1). The person also may have nausea, vomiting, and memory loss. Unconsciousness, noisy breathing, high blood pressure, slow pulse, redness of the face, and seizures may occur. So can *hemiplegia—paralysis* (plegia) *on 1 side* (hemi) *of the body*. The person may lose bowel and bladder control and the ability to speak. (See "Aphasia" in Chapter 46.)

Effects on the Person. If the person survives, some brain damage is likely. The entire body may be affected. Functions lost depend on the area of brain damage (see Fig. 48-3). They include:
- Loss of face, hand, arm, leg, or body control
- Hemiplegia
- Changing emotions (crying easily or mood swings sometimes for no reason)
- Difficulty swallowing (*dysphagia*)
- Aphasia or slowed or slurred speech (Chapter 46)
- Changes in sight, touch, movement, and thought
- Impaired memory
- Urinary frequency, urgency, or incontinence
- Loss of bowel control or constipation
- Depression and frustration
- Behavior changes

The person may forget about or ignore the weaker side. This is called *neglect*. It is from the loss of vision or movement and feeling on that side. Sometimes thinking is affected. The person may not recognize or know how to use common items. Activities of daily living (ADL) and other tasks are hard to do. The person may forget what to do and how to do it. If the person does know, the body may not respond.

Rehabilitation starts at once. The goal is to regain the highest possible level of function (Box 48-2, p. 720).

See *Focus on Long-Term Care and Home Care: Effects on the Person (Stroke)*, p. 720.

BOX 48-2	Stroke Care Measures

- Position the person in the side-lying position to prevent aspiration.
- Keep the bed in semi-Fowler's position.
- Approach the person from the strong (unaffected) side. The person may have loss of vision on the affected side.
- Turn and re-position the person at least every 2 hours.
- Use assist devices to move, turn, re-position, and transfer the person.
- Encourage incentive spirometry and deep breathing and coughing.
- Prevent contractures. Assist with range-of-motion (ROM) exercises.
- Prevent pressure injuries.
- Meet food and fluid needs. A dysphagia diet is common (Chapter 30).
- Apply elastic stockings to prevent *thrombi* (blood clots) in the legs.
- Meet elimination needs. Follow the care plan for:
  - Catheter care or bladder training
  - Bowel training
- Practice safety precautions.
  - Keep the call light and other needed items within reach on the strong (unaffected) side.
  - Check the person often. Follow the care plan.
  - Use bed rails according to the care plan.
  - Prevent falls and other injuries.
- Encourage as much self-care as possible. This includes turning, positioning, and transferring. The person uses adaptive (assistive) devices and walking aids as needed.
- Do not rush the person. Movements are slower after a stroke.
- Follow established communication methods.
- Give support, encouragement, and praise.
- Complete a safety check before leaving the room. (See the inside of the back cover.)

FOCUS ON LONG-TERM CARE AND HOME CARE

Effects on the Person (Stroke)

Long-Term Care

Some persons return home after rehabilitation. For others, long-term care is often permanent. Many measures listed in Box 48-2 are part of the person's care.

Home Care

Many stroke survivors return home. Family assistance and home health care are often needed. Many measures in Box 48-2 continue. The health team recommends home changes to help the person function.

Parkinson's Disease

Parkinson's disease is a progressive disorder affecting movement. Persons over the age of 60 are at risk. Signs and symptoms are mild at first on 1 side of the body (Fig. 48-4). They worsen over time and may involve both sides of the body. Signs and symptoms include:

- *Tremors*—often start in the hand. Pill-rolling movements (rubbing the thumb and index finger) may occur. The person may have trembling in the hands, arms, legs, jaw, and face.
- *Slow movement*—the person develops short, shuffling steps. Simple tasks are hard to do.
- *Rigid, stiff muscles*—in the arms, legs, neck, and trunk.
- *Stooped posture and impaired balance*—it is hard to walk. Falls are a risk.
- *Mask-like expression*—the person cannot blink and smile. A fixed stare is common.
- *Speech changes*—soft, monotone, or slurred speech.

Other signs and symptoms develop over time. They include swallowing and chewing problems, constipation, sleep problems, depression, and emotional changes (fear, insecurity). Memory loss and slow thinking can occur.

With no cure, drugs are ordered to control the disease. Exercise and physical therapy help improve strength, posture, balance, and mobility. Therapy is needed for speech and swallowing problems. The person may need help with eating and self-care. Normal elimination is a goal. Safety measures are needed to prevent falls and injuries.

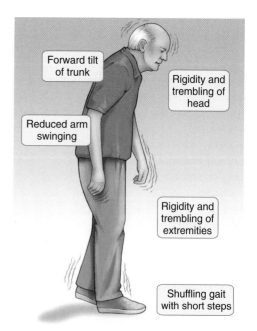

FIGURE 48-4 Signs of Parkinson's disease. (From Patton KT, Thibodeau GA: *The human body in health & disease*, ed 7, St Louis, 2018, Elsevier.)

Multiple Sclerosis

Multiple means *many*. *Sclerosis* means *hardening or scarring*. In multiple sclerosis (MS), the myelin (which covers nerve fibers) in the brain and spinal cord is destroyed. Nerve impulses between the body and the brain are not sent in a normal way. Functions are impaired or lost.

Symptoms can occur at any age but usually between the ages of 15 and 60. Women and whites are at greater risk than other groups. The risk increases if a family member has MS. Signs and symptoms vary widely depending on the nerves affected. They may include:

- Blurred or double vision; blindness in 1 eye
- Muscle weakness—usually on 1 side of the body at first
- Balance and coordination problems
- Tingling, prickling, or numb sensations
- Partial or complete paralysis
- Pain
- Speech problems
- Tremors
- Dizziness
- Concentration, attention, memory, and judgment problems
- Depression
- Bladder problems
- Problems with sexual function
- Hearing loss
- Fatigue

MS can present in many ways. For example:

- Symptoms appear for a while then seem to go away. The person is in *remission*. Later, symptoms flare up again *(relapse)*.
- More symptoms appear. The person's condition worsens.
- The person has remissions and relapses at first. Eventually symptoms become worse. More symptoms occur with each flare-up. The person's condition declines.

MS has no cure. Some drugs can slow the disease and help control symptoms. Persons with MS are kept as active and as independent as possible. The care plan reflects changing needs. Skin care, hygiene, and ROM exercises are important. So are turning, positioning, and deep breathing and coughing. Elimination needs are met. Injuries and complications from bed rest are prevented.

See *Focus on Long-Term Care and Home Care: Multiple Sclerosis.*

FOCUS ON LONG-TERM CARE AND HOME CARE

Multiple Sclerosis

Home Care

The person may need help with housekeeping to avoid fatigue. As mobility decreases, the person depends more on others. Occupational and physical therapists are often involved in the person's care.

Amyotrophic Lateral Sclerosis

Amyotrophic lateral sclerosis (ALS) attacks nerve cells in the brain and spinal cord that control voluntary muscles. Muscles in the arms and legs and those used for chewing and talking are voluntary. Commonly called Lou Gehrig's disease, it is rapidly progressive and fatal. (Lou Gehrig was a New York Yankees baseball player who died of the disease.)

ALS usually strikes persons between 40 and 75 years of age. Most die 3 to 5 years after onset.

Affected nerve cells in the brain and spinal cord stop sending messages to the voluntary muscles. The muscles weaken, waste away *(atrophy)*, and twitch. Over time, the brain cannot start voluntary movements or control them. The person cannot move the arms, legs, and body. Muscles for speaking, chewing and swallowing, and breathing also are affected. Eventually respiratory muscles fail. The person needs a ventilator to breathe (Chapter 44).

The disease usually does not affect the mind, intelligence, or memory. However, some persons develop dementia. Sight, smell, taste, hearing, and touch are not affected. Usually bowel and bladder functions remain intact.

ALS has no cure. Some drugs can slow the disease and improve symptoms. However, damage cannot be reversed. The person is kept active and independent to the extent possible. The care plan reflects changing needs. It may include:

- Physical, occupational, and speech-language therapies
- ROM exercises
- Mobility aides—braces, walker, wheelchair
- Comfort and pain-relief measures
- Communication methods
- Dysphagia diet or feeding tube
- Respiratory support—suctioning, mechanical ventilation
- Safety measures to prevent falls and injuries
- Psychological and social support
- Hospice care

Head Injuries

Head injuries result from trauma to the scalp, skull, or brain. Injuries range from a minor bump to a serious, life-threatening brain injury. Falls, vehicle accidents, violence (assaults, gunshots), and sports injuries are common causes.

Head injuries are open or closed. Bleeding may occur.

- Closed—the skull did not break but the brain is injured.
- Open (penetrating)—an object broke the skull and entered the brain.

Symptoms may develop at the time of the injury. Or they can take several hours or days to develop. Symptoms are from bleeding or swelling inside the skull.

Most head injuries need emergency care. See Chapter 58.

Traumatic Brain Injury. Traumatic brain injury (TBI) occurs from an injury to the brain—bump, blow, jolt, or an object entering the brain. Common causes include:

- *Falls.* Older persons and children are at risk for falling out of bed, slipping in the shower or bathtub, falling down steps, and falling from ladders.
- *Vehicle accidents.* Cars, motorcycles, and bikes are often involved. Persons who were walking or jogging have been injured.
- *Violence.* Gunshots, intimate partner violence (Chapter 5), and child abuse can result in TBI.
- *Sports.* Many sports increase the risk of TBI—football, soccer, boxing, baseball, hockey, lacrosse, skateboarding, and other high-impact sports.
- *Explosive blasts and combat injuries.* TBI can occur from penetrating injuries, blows to the head, and falls. Military personnel are at risk.

Brain tissue is bruised or torn. Bleeding is in the brain or in nearby tissues. Spinal cord injuries are likely.

Men, infants and children, young adults, and older persons are at risk for TBI. Death can occur at the time of injury or later. See Box 48-3 for the signs and symptoms of TBI.

If the person survives, some permanent damage is likely. Disabilities depend on the severity and site of injury. They include:

- Cognitive problems—thinking, memory, and reasoning.
- Sensory problems—sight, hearing, touch, taste, and smell.
- Communication problems—expressing or understanding language.
- Emotional problems—depression, anxiety, personality changes, aggressive behavior, acting out, socially inappropriate behavior.
- Changes in level of consciousness:
  - Coma—the person is unconscious, does not respond, is unaware, and cannot be aroused.
  - Vegetative state—the person is unconscious and unaware of surroundings. He or she may open the eyes, make sounds, or move. The person cannot speak or follow commands.
  - Brain death (Fig. 48-5). Despite complete loss of brain function, the heart continues to beat. Reflex activity, movement, and spontaneous respirations are absent.

Emergency care involves drugs and surgery to limit brain damage. Rehabilitation is required. Physical, occupational, speech-language, and mental health therapies depend on the person's needs. Nursing care depends on the person's needs and abilities.

See *Focus on Children and Older Persons: Traumatic Brain Injury.*

BOX 48-3 **Traumatic Brain Injury—Signs and Symptoms**

- Loss of consciousness: a few seconds to a few minutes or longer
- Being dazed, confused, or disoriented
- Headache: gets worse or does not go away
- Nausea or vomiting: repeated
- Fatigue or drowsiness
- Neck pain
- Problems sleeping; sleeping more than usual; cannot be awakened
- Dizziness; loss of balance
- Blurred vision
- Ringing in the ears
- Bad taste in the mouth
- Memory, thinking, attention, and concentration problems
- Convulsions or seizures
- Large eye pupil: 1 or both eyes
- Clear fluids draining from the nose or ears
- Weakness or numbness: fingers and toes; arms and legs
- Coordination: loss of
- Behavior: unusual—agitation, restlessness
- Speech: slurred

Modified from National Institutes of Neurological Disorders and Stroke: Traumatic brain injury information page, page modified March 27, 2019, National Institutes of Health.

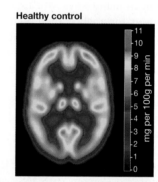

Healthy control

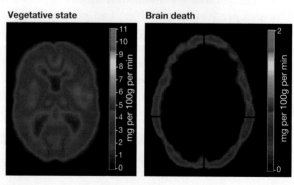

Vegetative state

Brain death

FIGURE 48-5 Altered consciousness. (Images courtesy *Nature Reviews Neuroscience,* McMillan Publishers Limited, 2014.)

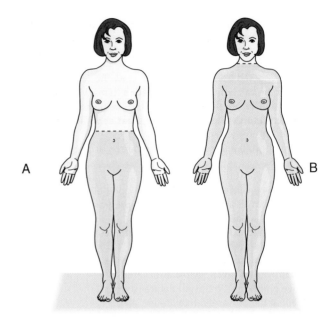

FIGURE 48-6 The *shaded areas* show the area of paralysis. **A,** Paraplegia. **B,** Quadriplegia (tetraplegia).

Spinal Cord Injury

A spinal cord injury usually results from a sudden, traumatic blow to the spine. The trauma fractures or dislocates vertebrae in the spine. Spinal cord tissue is torn or bruised. Spinal cord injuries can seriously damage the nervous system. *Paralysis (loss of muscle function, sensation, or both)* can result. Emergency care is needed.

Young adult men have the highest risk. Common causes are vehicle accidents, falls, violence (knife and gunshot wounds), sports injuries, alcohol use, cancer, and other diseases.

Problems depend on the amount of damage to the spinal cord and the level of injury. Damage to the spinal cord may be incomplete or complete.

- Incomplete—some sensory (feeling) and muscle (movement) function below the level of the injury remains.
- Complete—no sensory or muscle function below the level of the injury remains.

The higher the level of injury, the more functions lost (Fig. 48-6).

- Lumbar injuries—occur in the low back. Sensory and muscle function in the legs is lost. The person has paraplegia. *Paraplegia is paralysis in the legs and lower trunk.* (Para *means* beyond; plegia *means* paralysis.)
- Thoracic injuries—occur in the middle and upper back. Sensory and muscle function below the chest is lost. The person has paraplegia.
- Cervical injuries—occur at the neck. Sensory and muscle function of the arms, legs, and trunk is lost. *Paralysis in the arms, legs, and trunk is called* **quadriplegia** *or* **tetraplegia.** (Quad *and* tetra *mean* 4. Plegia *means* paralysis.)

The person with a spinal cord injury has 1 or more of these signs and symptoms.

- Severe back, neck, or head pain or pressure
- Loss of movement
- Loss of sensation—heat, cold, touch
- Bladder and bowel incontinence
- Problems with balance and walking
- Breathing problems
- Twisted or odd position of neck or back
- Spasms

Cervical traction with a special bed may be needed (p. 730). The spine is kept straight at all times. See Box 48-4 (p. 724) for care measures. Emotional needs are great. Reactions to paralysis and loss of function are often severe.

If the person lives, rehabilitation is needed. The person learns to function at the highest possible level with adaptive (assistive) and other devices. Some persons live independently at home or with home care. Others need long-term care or assisted-living settings.

BOX 48-4	Paralysis—Care Measures

- Practice safety measures to prevent falls. Use bed rails as directed.
- Keep the bed in a low position. Follow the care plan.
- Keep the call light and other needed items within reach. If unable to use the call light, check the person often.
- Prevent burns. Check bath water, heat applications, and food for proper temperature.
- Turn (logroll) and re-position the person at least every 2 hours.
- Prevent pressure injuries. Follow the care plan.
- Use supportive devices to maintain good alignment.
- Follow bowel and bladder training programs.
- Keep intake and output records.
- Maintain muscle function and prevent contractures. Assist with ROM exercises.
- Assist with food and fluid needs. Provide adaptive (assistive) devices as ordered.
- Give emotional and psychological support.
- Follow the person's rehabilitation plan.
- Complete a safety check of the room. (See the inside of the back cover.)

BOX 48-5	Autonomic Dysreflexia

- Monitor urinary output.
- Follow measures for catheter care. Do not let the drainage bag get too full.
- Prevent urinary tract infections.
- Promote bowel elimination. Prevent constipation and fecal impaction.
- Prevent skin injuries—skin tears, pressure injuries, cuts, bruises, burns, and so on.
- Check the feet for ingrown toenails, blisters, pressure injuries, and so on.
- Have the person wear loose and comfortable clothing.
- Remove wrinkles from clothing and linens.
- Re-position the person at least every 2 hours. Avoid prolonged pressure from the bed or chair.
- Report complaints of pain and menstrual cramps.

Autonomic Dysreflexia (AD). This syndrome occurs with spinal cord injuries above the mid-thoracic (middle back) level. The autonomic nervous system over-reacts to a stimulus (*reflexia*). A full bladder, constipation, fecal impaction, and skin disorders are examples. Causing the sudden onset of excessively high blood pressure, AD is life-threatening. Stroke, seizures, heart attack, and death are risks. Report any of the following at once.

- High blood pressure
- Headache: throbbing or pounding
- Pulse: slow or rapid; irregular
- Blurred vision
- Muscle spasms, especially the jaw
- Sweating
- Skin and face: flushing, reddening
- Cold, clammy skin
- "Goose bumps"
- Nasal congestion
- Nausea
- Anxiety
- Dizziness
- Fainting
- Bowel or bladder problems
- Restlessness

To treat AD, the head of the bed is raised or the person sits upright if allowed. Tight clothing is removed. And the cause is treated. See Box 48-5.

See *Promoting Safety and Comfort: Autonomic Dysreflexia*.

PROMOTING SAFETY AND COMFORT

Autonomic Dysreflexia

Safety
Constipation and fecal impaction can cause autonomic dysreflexia. So can checking for an impaction or giving enemas. Do not perform these procedures if the person is at risk for AD. The procedures are best done by a nurse.

MUSCULO-SKELETAL DISORDERS

Musculo-skeletal disorders affect movement. Injury and aging are common causes. Daily living, social activities, and quality of life are affected.

See *Body Structure and Function Review: The Musculo-Skeletal System*.

BODY STRUCTURE AND FUNCTION REVIEW

The Musculo-Skeletal System

Bones

Bones are hard, rigid structures.

- *Long bones* bear the body's weight. Leg bones are long bones.
- *Short bones* allow skill and ease in movement. Bones in the wrists, fingers, ankles, and toes are short bones.
- *Flat bones* protect the organs. They include the ribs, skull, pelvic bones, and shoulder blades.
- *Irregular bones* are the vertebrae in the spinal column. They allow various degrees of movement and flexibility.

Joints

A *joint* is the point at which 2 or more bones meet (Fig. 48-7). Joints allow movement (Chapter 34).

- *Ball-and-socket joint* allows movement in all directions. The rounded end of 1 bone fits into the hollow end of another bone. The hips and shoulders are ball-and-socket joints.
- *Hinge joint* allows movement in 1 direction. The elbow is a hinge joint.
- *Pivot joint* allows turning from side to side. A pivot joint connects the skull to the spine.

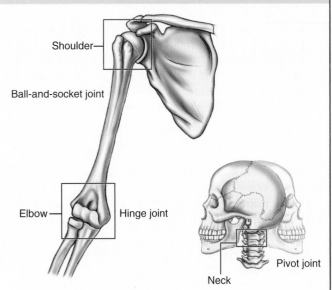

FIGURE 48-7 Types of joints. (Modified from Herlihy B: *The human body in health and illness,* ed 6, St Louis, 2018, Elsevier.)

Arthritis

Arthritis means joint (arthr) *inflammation* (itis). Affected joints have swelling, stiffness, and reduced range of motion. The joints are hard to move.

The 2 main types of arthritis are:

- *Osteoarthritis.* Cartilage at the ends of bones is damaged and wears away, allowing the bones to rub together. The hands, knees, hips, and spine are often affected (Fig. 48-8).
- *Rheumatoid arthritis (RA).* An autoimmune disorder (Chapter 47), RA attacks the lining of the joint causing inflammation and painful swelling. Many joints are affected at the same time. The wrists, hands, and knees are commonly affected. RA can also affect the neck, shoulders, elbows, hips, ankles, and feet. RA occurs on both sides of the body. For example, both the right and left wrists are affected. RA can cause fever and fatigue. RA can affect other tissues and organs. The lungs, heart, and eyes are examples.

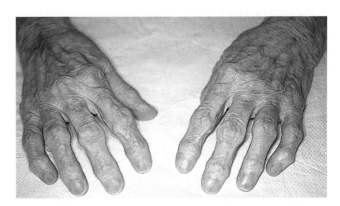

FIGURE 48-8 Bony growths called *Heberden nodes* occur in the finger joints. (From Swartz MH: *Textbook of physical diagnosis,* ed 7, Philadelphia, 2014, Saunders.)

Risk Factors. Arthritis risk factors include:

- *Aging.* The risk increases with age.
- *Being over-weight.* Stress is placed on the weight-bearing joints—hips and knees. Stress also is placed on the spine.
- *Biological sex.* Arthritis is more common in women.
- *Joint injury.* A previous joint injury or over-use of a joint may develop into osteoarthritis.
- *Family history.* Arthritis tends to run in families.

Treatment. Osteoarthritis and RA have no cure. Treatments are similar.

- *Pain control.* Drugs decrease swelling and inflammation and relieve pain.
- *Heat and cold.* Heat relieves pain, increases blood flow, and reduces stiffness. Heat applications, a warm bath or shower, and water therapy in a heated pool are helpful. Cold applied for 20 minutes is useful after joint use and for severe pain. Cold slows circulation to reduce swelling. Nerve endings are numbed, which dulls the pain. See Chapter 42.
- *Exercise.* Exercise helps joint flexibility. It helps with weight control and promotes fitness. The person is taught needed exercises. Walking, biking, swimming, and water aerobics have a low risk of joint stress or injury.
- *Rest and joint care.* Good body mechanics, posture, and regular rest protect the joints. Relaxation methods are helpful.
- *Adaptive (assistive) devices.* Canes and walkers provide support. Splints support weak joints and promote alignment. Devices for hands and wrists are useful.
- *Weight control.* Weight loss reduces stress on weight-bearing joints and prevents further joint injury.
- *Healthy life-style.* The focus is on fitness, exercise, rest, managing stress, and good nutrition.
- *Safety.* Falls are prevented. Help is given with ADL as needed. Elevated toilet seats are helpful when hips and knees are affected. So are chairs with higher seats and armrests.
- *Joint replacement surgery.* *Arthroplasty is the surgical replacement (plasty) of a joint (arthro).* The damaged joint is removed and replaced with an artificial joint *(prosthesis).* Hip and knee replacements are common (Fig. 48-9). See Box 48-6 for care measures. Ankle, foot, shoulder, elbow, and finger joints also can be replaced. The surgery is done to relieve pain, restore joint function, or correct a deformed joint.

See *Focus on Children and Older Persons: Arthritis.*

BOX 48-6	Care After Joint Replacement—Hip and Knee

- Incentive spirometry and deep-breathing and coughing exercises to prevent respiratory complications.
- Elastic stockings to prevent *thrombi* (blood clots) in the legs.
- Physical therapy and exercises to strengthen the hip or knee.
- Measures to protect the hip as shown in Figure 48-10.
- Food and fluids for tissue healing and to restore strength.
- Safety measures to prevent falls.
- Measures to prevent infection. Wound, urinary tract, and skin infections must be prevented.
- Measures to prevent pressure injuries.
- Assist devices for moving, turning, re-positioning, and transfers.
- Long-handled devices for reaching things.
- Assistance with walking and a walking aid—cane, walker, or crutches.

FOCUS ON CHILDREN AND OLDER PERSONS

Arthritis

Children

Arthritis in children is called juvenile arthritis (JA). The child has joint swelling, pain, and stiffness in the hands, knees, or feet that does not go away. Symptoms are worse after sleep. Other signs include:

- Limping in the morning or after a nap
- Clumsiness
- Fever
- Rash
- Swollen lymph nodes

Children of all ages and ethnic groups can be affected. JA is thought to be an autoimmune disorder.

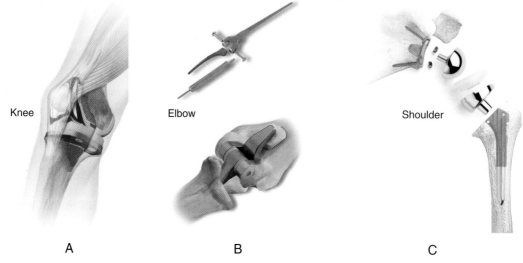

Knee   Elbow   Shoulder

A   B   C

FIGURE 48-9 A, Knee replacement prosthesis. **B,** Elbow replacement prosthesis. **C,** Shoulder replacement prosthesis. (Courtesy Zimmer, Inc., A Bristol-Meyers Squibb Company, Warsaw, Ind.)

Do

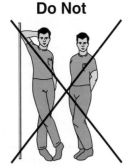

Do not cross your operated leg past the mid-line of the body or turn your kneecap in toward your body.

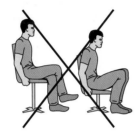

Do not sit in low chairs or cross your legs.

To sit: Use a high chair with arms or add pillows to elevate the seat.

Avoid flexing your hips past 90 degrees.

To bend: Keep the operative leg behind you or as instructed by your therapist.

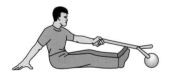

To reach: Use long-handled grabbers or as your therapist advises.

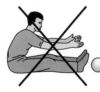

Use an elevated toilet.

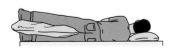

Sleep with a pillow between the legs.

FIGURE 48-10 Measures to protect the hip after hip replacement surgery. (Modified from Monahan FD and others: *Phipps' medical-surgical nursing: health and illness perspectives,* ed 8, St Louis, 2007, Mosby.)

Fractures

A fracture is a broken bone. Depending on the type of fracture, tissues around the fracture—muscles, blood vessels, nerves, and tendons—may be injured. Fractures are open or closed (Fig. 48-11, p. 728).

- *Open fracture (compound fracture)—the broken bone has pierced the skin.*
- *Closed fracture (simple fracture)—the bone is broken but the skin is intact.*

In a **comminuted fracture** the bone is shattered or broken into 3 or more pieces (Fig. 48-12, p. 728). (*Comminuted* comes from the Latin word *comminuere*, which means *to break into pieces*.) The fracture may be open or closed. Surrounding tissues may be injured.

Falls, accidents, sports injuries, bone tumors, and osteoporosis (p. 732) are some causes. Signs and symptoms of a fracture are:

- Severe pain
- Swelling and tenderness
- Problems moving the part
- Deformity (the part looks out of place)
- Bruising and skin color changes at the fracture site
- Bleeding (internal or external)
- Numbness and tingling

For healing, bone ends are brought into and held in normal position. This is called *reduction and fixation.*

- Reduction—the bone is moved back into place.
  - Closed reduction—the bone is not exposed.
  - Open reduction—the bone is surgically exposed and moved into alignment.
- Fixation—the bone is held (fixed) in place.
  - External fixation—Pins, screws, or wires are set into the bone outside the skin (Fig. 48-13, p. 728). The device is removed after healing or when the person is healthy enough for internal fixation of the fracture.
  - Internal fixation—Nails, rods, pins, screws, plates, or wires are surgically placed to keep the bone in place. The device is under the skin (Fig. 48-14, p. 728). After healing, the device is left in place or removed.

Casts, splints, and traction also are used. Healing can take 6 to 8 weeks or longer depending on age, type of fracture, and general health.

See *Focus on Children and Older Persons: Fractures,* p. 728.

Do Not

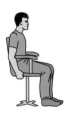

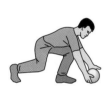

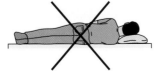

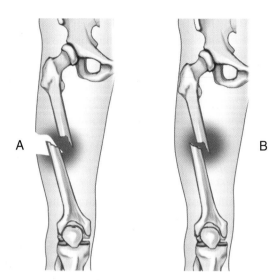

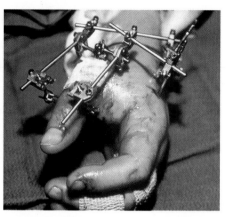

FIGURE 48-13 External fixators. (Courtesy Howmedica, Inc., Allendale, Pa.)

FIGURE 48-11 A, Open fracture. **B,** Closed fracture. (From Patton KT, Thibodeau GA: *The human body in health & disease,* ed 7, St Louis, 2018, Elsevier.)

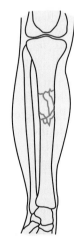

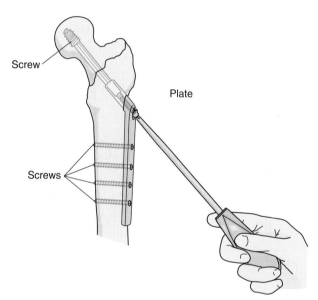

FIGURE 48-12 A comminuted fracture is broken into 3 or more pieces. (From Monahan FD and others: *Phipps' medical-surgical nursing: health and illness perspectives,* ed 8, St Louis, 2007, Mosby.)

FIGURE 48-14 Devices used for internal fixation of a fracture. (Modified from Monahan FD and others: *Phipps' medical-surgical nursing: health and illness perspectives,* ed 8, St Louis, 2007, Mosby.)

FOCUS ON **CHILDREN AND OLDER PERSONS**

Fractures

Children
Falls and accidents involving motor vehicles, bikes, skateboards, and roller blades are common causes of fractures in children. Fractures may signal child abuse in infants and children.

Casts. Casts are made to fit the affected body part using plaster or fiberglass (Fig. 48-15). Cotton padding is applied to protect the skin. Then wet plaster or fiberglass strips or rolls are wrapped around the part. Fiberglass casts dry quickly. A plaster cast dries in 24 to 48 hours. It is odorless, white, and shiny when dry. When wet, it is gray and cool and has a musty smell. The nurse may ask you to assist with care (Box 48-7).

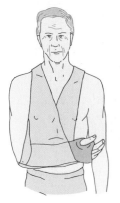
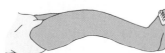
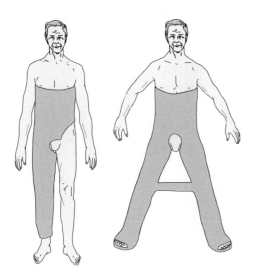

Short arm cast   Long leg cast

Single hip spica   Double hip spica

FIGURE 48-15 Examples of casts.

BOX 48-7   Cast Care

The Cast
- Do not cover the cast with blankets, plastic, or other material. A cast gives off heat as it dries. Covers prevent the escape of heat. Burns can occur if heat cannot escape.
- Promote drying of the cast. All cast surfaces need exposure to air. Follow the nurse's directions to:
  - Turn the person. The person is turned at least every 2 hours.
  - Use a fan to move air over the cast.
- Maintain the shape of the cast.
  - Do not place a wet cast on a hard surface. It flattens the cast.
  - Use pillows to support the entire length of the cast (Fig. 48-16, p. 730).
  - Support the wet cast with your palms to turn and position the person (Fig. 48-17, p. 730). Fingertips can dent the cast, causing pressure areas and skin breakdown.
  - Report rough cast edges. The nurse may cover the cast edges with tape.
  - Keep the cast dry. A wet cast loses its shape. For casts near the perineal area, the nurse may apply a waterproof material after the cast dries.
- Do not remove stockinette or padding around the cast edges.

Positioning
- Position the person as directed.
- Elevate a casted arm or leg on pillows to reduce swelling.
- Have enough help to turn and re-position the person. Plaster casts are heavy and awkward. Balance is lost easily.

Safety
- Follow the care plan for elimination needs. A fracture pan may be needed.
- Do not let the person insert things into the cast. Itching under the cast causes an intense desire to scratch. Scratching items can open the skin—pencils, coat hangers, knitting needles, back scratchers, and so on. Infection is a risk. Scratching items can wrinkle the cotton padding. Or they can be lost into the cast. Both can cause pressure and skin breakdown.
- Do not put powder on the skin under the cast.
- Do not let the person wear rings on the fingers or toes. The fingers or toes may swell or be swollen.
- Complete a safety check before leaving the room. (See the inside of the back cover.)

Reporting and Recording
- Report these signs and symptoms at once.
  - *Pain*—pressure injury, poor circulation, nerve damage
  - *Swelling and a tight cast*—reduced blood flow to the part
  - *Pale skin*—reduced blood flow to the part
  - *Cyanosis* (bluish skin color)—reduced blood flow to the part
  - *Odor*—infection
  - *Inability to move the fingers or toes*—pressure on a nerve
  - *Numbness*—pressure on a nerve, reduced blood flow to the part
  - *Temperature changes*—cool skin means poor circulation; hot skin means inflammation
  - *Drainage on or under the cast*—infection or bleeding
  - *Chills, fever, nausea, and vomiting*—infection

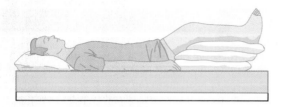

FIGURE 48-16 Pillows support the entire length of the wet cast.

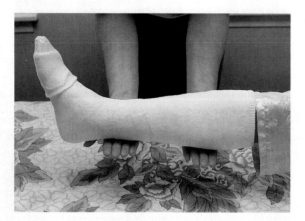

FIGURE 48-17 The cast is supported with the palms.

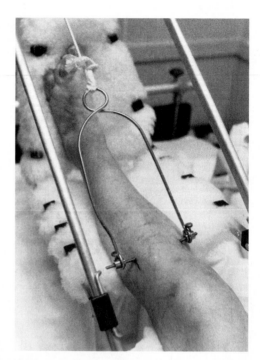

FIGURE 48-19 Skeletal traction is attached to the bone. (From Monahan FD and others: *Phipps' medical-surgical nursing: health and illness perspectives,* ed 8, St Louis, 2007, Mosby.)

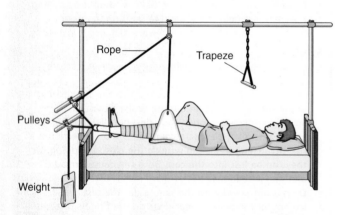

FIGURE 48-18 Traction set-up. Note the weight, pulleys, and rope. A trapeze is used to raise the upper body off the bed. (Modified from Monahan FD and others: *Phipps' medical-surgical nursing: health and illness perspectives,* ed 8, St Louis, 2007, Mosby.)

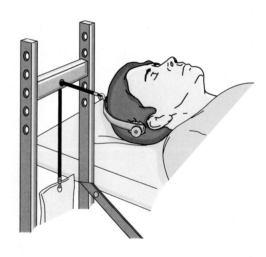

FIGURE 48-20 Tongs are inserted into the skull for cervical traction. (From Monahan FD and others: *Phipps' medical-surgical nursing: health and illness perspectives,* ed 8, St Louis, 2007, Mosby.)

Traction. With traction, a steady pull from 2 directions keeps the bone in place. Weights, ropes, and pulleys are used (Fig. 48-18). Traction is applied to the neck, arms, legs, or pelvis.

Skin traction is applied to the skin. Boots, wraps, tape, or splints are used. Weights are attached to the device (see Fig. 48-18). For *skeletal traction,* wires or pins are inserted through the bone (Fig. 48-19). For cervical traction, tongs are applied to the skull (Fig. 48-20). Weights are attached to the bone.

To assist with the person's care, see Box 48-8.

BOX 48-8	Traction Care

- Keep the person in good alignment.
- Do not remove the traction.
- Keep the weights off the floor. Weights must hang freely from the traction set-up (see Fig. 48-18).
- Do not add or remove weights.
- Check for frayed ropes. Report fraying at once.
- Perform ROM exercises for uninvolved joints as directed.
- Position the person as directed. Usually only the supine position is allowed. Slight turning may be allowed.
- Provide the fracture pan for elimination.
- Give skin care as directed.
- Put bottom linens on the bed from the top down. The person uses a trapeze to raise the body off the bed (see Fig. 48-18).
- Check pin, nail, wire, or tong sites for redness, drainage, and odors. Report observations at once.
- Observe for the signs and symptoms listed under cast care (see Box 48-7). Report them at once.
- Complete a safety check before leaving the room. (See the inside of the back cover.)

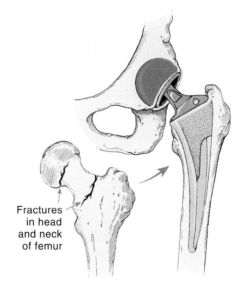

Fractures in head and neck of femur

FIGURE 48-21 Hip fracture repaired with a prosthesis. (Modified from Cooper K, Gosnell K: *Adult health nursing,* ed 8, St Louis, 2019, Elsevier.)

Hip Fractures. Common in older persons, hip fractures require surgical repair or a hip replacement (Fig. 48-21). Risk factors include:

- *Age.* Older persons are at risk.
- *Biological sex.* Hip fractures are more common in women.
- *Osteoporosis.* See p. 732.
- *Drugs.* Some drugs can weaken bones or have dizziness as a side effect.
- *Nutrition.* Calcium and vitamin D are needed for healthy bones.
- *Inactivity.* Weight-bearing exercise and activities are needed to strengthen bones.
- *Smoking and alcohol use.* These can cause bone loss.

Falls are the most common cause of hip fractures. However, fractures have occurred upon standing or twisting. Signs and symptoms include:

- Being unable to move after falling
- Severe hip or groin pain
- Shorter leg on the injured side
- Turning the leg outward on the injured side
- Not being able to stand on the injured side
- Swollen and bruised area around the hip

Post-operative problems present life-threatening risks. They include pneumonia, urinary tract infections, and *thrombi* (blood clots) in the leg veins or lungs. Pressure injuries, constipation, and confusion are other problems.

Adduction, internal rotation, external rotation, and severe hip flexion are avoided after surgery. Physical therapy is common after surgery. Some persons also need occupational therapy for self-care activities. Adaptive (assistive) devices are used for dressing and bathing. A walker is usually needed at first. See Box 48-9 for the care required for a hip fracture.

BOX 48-9	Hip Fracture Care

- Give good skin care. Skin breakdown can be rapid.
- Prevent pressure injuries.
- Prevent wound, skin, and urinary tract infections.
- Encourage incentive spirometry and deep-breathing and coughing exercises as directed.
- Turn and position the person as directed. Usually the person is not positioned on the operative side.
- Prevent external rotation of the hip. Use trochanter rolls, pillows, or sandbags.
- Keep the leg abducted at all times. Use pillows (Fig. 48-22, p. 732) or a hip abduction wedge (abductor splint). Do not exercise the affected leg.
- Provide a straight-back chair with armrests. The person needs a high, firm seat.
- Place the chair on the unaffected side.
- Use assist devices to move, turn, re-position, and transfer the person.
- Do not let the person stand on the operated leg unless allowed by the doctor.
- Elevate the leg following the care plan. With an internal fixation device, the leg is not elevated when the person sits in a chair. Elevating the leg puts strain on the device.
- Apply elastic stockings to prevent *thrombi* (blood clots) in the legs.
- Remind the person not to cross his or her legs.
- Assist with walking according to the care plan. The person may use a walker.
- Follow measures to protect the hip. See Box 48-6 and Figure 48-10.
- Practice safety measures to prevent falls.
- Complete a safety check before leaving the room. (See the inside of the back cover.)

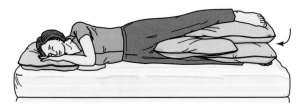

FIGURE 48-22 Pillows are used to keep the hip in abduction. (From Monahan FD and others: *Phipps' medical-surgical nursing: health and illness perspectives,* ed 8, St Louis, 2007, Mosby.)

Osteoporosis

With osteoporosis, the bone *(osteo)* becomes porous and brittle *(porosis)*. Bones are thin and weak. They are fragile and break easily. Spine, hip, and wrist fractures are common. Risk factors include:

* Aging.
* Biological sex. Women are at higher risk because of the loss of estrogen after menopause. White and Asian women are at risk.
* Being thin and small.
* A family history of osteoporosis.
* A diet low in calcium and vitamin D.
* Tobacco and alcohol use.
* Eating disorders (Chapter 52).
* Bed rest, immobility, and lack of exercise. Bones must bear weight for strength and to form properly.

A fracture is often the first sign of osteoporosis. Even slight activity can cause a fracture—turning in bed, getting up from a chair, coughing, lifting an object, bending forward, and so on. A fracture in the spine can cause:

* Sloped shoulders
* Curving in the back
* Loss of height
* Stooped or hunched posture (Fig. 48-23)
* Back pain

Prevention is important. Calcium and vitamin supplements may be ordered to prevent bone loss and build new bone. Estrogen is ordered for some women. Other preventive measures include:

* Exercising weight-bearing joints—walking, jogging, stair climbing, weight-lifting, dancing, and so on.
* Eating foods that contain calcium and vitamin D.
* No smoking.
* Limiting alcohol. For women, no more than 1 drink a day.
* Good posture and body mechanics.
* Safety measures to prevent falls.
* Safe moving, transfer, turning, and positioning procedures.

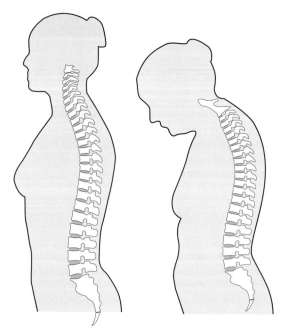

FIGURE 48-23 Osteoporosis in the spine. (Modified from Office of Women's Health: *Osteoporosis,* page updated May 20, 2019, U.S. Department of Health & Human Services.)

Loss of Limb

An *amputation* is the removal of all or part of an extremity. Severe injuries, tumors, severe infection, gangrene, and vascular disorders are common causes. Diabetes can cause vascular changes leading to amputation.

Gangrene is a condition in which there is death of tissue. Causes include poor blood flow from infection, injuries, and vascular disorders. Tissues do not get enough oxygen and nutrients. Tissues become black, cold, shriveled, and die (Fig. 48-24). Surgery is needed to remove dead tissue. Gangrene can spread throughout the body and cause death.

Much support is needed. The amputation affects the person's life—body image, appearance, daily activities, moving about, work, and so on. Fear, shock, anger, denial, and depression are common emotions.

A *prosthesis* is an artificial replacement for a missing body part (Fig. 48-25). For a proper fit, the stump is shaped into a cone (Fig. 48-26). Exercises are done to strengthen other limbs. Occupational and physical therapists help the person learn to use the prosthesis.

The person may feel that the limb is still there. Aching, tingling, and itching are common sensations. Or the person complains of pain in the amputated part *(phantom pain).* This is a normal reaction. It may occur for a short time or for many years.

Because of other health problems, many older persons cannot use a leg prosthesis. They need to use wheelchairs. After amputation, most older persons need long-term care or home care.

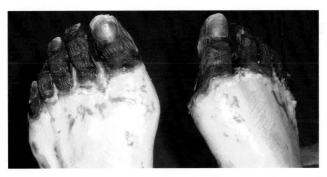

FIGURE 48-24 Gangrene. (From Centers for Disease Control and Prevention/Christina Nelson, MD, MPH, 2012.)

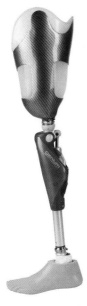

FIGURE 48-25 Above-the-knee prosthesis. (Courtesy Otto Bock Health Care, Minneapolis, Minn.)

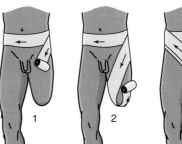
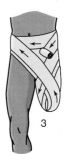
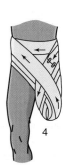

FIGURE 48-26 A mid-thigh amputation is bandaged to shape the stump. (From Monahan FD and others: *Phipps' medical-surgical nursing: health and illness perspectives,* ed 8, St Louis, 2007, Mosby.)

FOCUS ON **PRIDE**

The Person, Family, and Yourself

Personal and Professional Responsibility

Nervous system and musculo-skeletal system disorders affect the whole person. Social, psychological, physical, and spiritual needs must be met. Care must focus on the whole person.

Rights and Respect

With some disorders, function declines over time. The family watches the person struggle to move, perform ADL, or live. The person, family, and caregivers need support and encouragement. Treat them with dignity, respect, and kindness.

Independence and Social Interaction

The disorders in this chapter affect independence. The person may rely on family and caregivers for support and daily needs. The person may feel angry or depressed. To promote independence:

- Focus on the person's abilities, not disabilities.
- Praise the person's progress.
- Allow personal choice.
- Encourage the person to try.

Delegation and Teamwork

Teamwork promotes safe and efficient care. Value your team members. Thank them for helping. Offer to help others. Take pride in being a good team member.

Ethics and Laws

Accidents happen. Mistakes do not always mean negligence. To be found negligent, evidence must show that you did not act in a reasonable and careful manner. As a result, the person or the person's property was harmed.

Always work carefully. If an accident occurs, tell the nurse what happened. Take pride in being honest and accountable.

FOCUS ON **PRIDE**: *Application*

Many disorders in this chapter have no cure. Problems remain or worsen. Describe the impact on the person and family. How does this differ from disorders that heal?

REVIEW QUESTIONS

Circle the BEST answer.

1 A stroke also is called
   a A cerebrovascular accident
   b Aphasia
   c Hemiplegia
   d A transient ischemic attack

2 Warning signs of stroke occur
   a With exertion
   b Suddenly
   c Between the ages of 20 and 40
   d At rest

3 A person had a stroke. Which should you question?
   a Leave the bed in semi-Fowler's position.
   b Perform ROM exercises every 2 hours.
   c Turn and re-position the person every 2 hours.
   d Place needed items on the weak (affected) side.

4 Which statement about Parkinson's disease is *true?*
   a There is a cure.
   b Mental function is affected first.
   c Tremors, slow movements, and a shuffling gait occur.
   d Paralysis occurs but mental function is intact.

5 Which statement about multiple sclerosis is *true?*
   a There is a cure.
   b Only voluntary muscles are affected.
   c It is triggered by excessively high blood pressure.
   d Symptoms may disappear for a while.

6 Amyotrophic lateral sclerosis affects nerve cells that control
   a Involuntary muscles
   b Voluntary muscles
   c The brain
   d The lungs

7 A person has amyotrophic lateral sclerosis. Which can you perform?
   a Range-of-motion exercises
   b Tracheostomy suctioning
   c Feeding tube insertion
   d Fall risk assessment

8 Persons with head or spinal cord injuries require
   a Rehabilitation
   b Drugs to cure paralysis
   c A prosthesis
   d Chemotherapy

9 Which carries the *lowest* risk for traumatic brain injury?
   a Falling in the bathroom
   b Motorcycle accident
   c Transferring with a mechanical lift
   d Child abuse

10 A person has quadriplegia from a spinal cord injury. Which should you question?
   a Keep the bed in a low position.
   b Assist with active ROM exercises.
   c Follow the bowel training program.
   d Turn and re-position every hour.

11 Autonomic dysreflexia occurs
   a After spinal cord injuries
   b In Parkinson's disease
   c With Lou Gehrig's disease
   d Following stroke

12 Autonomic dysreflexia is usually triggered by
   a High blood sugar
   b High blood pressure
   c A full bladder
   d A virus

13 Arthritis affects the
   a Joints
   b Bones
   c Voluntary muscles
   d Involuntary muscles

14 A person has arthritis. Care includes
   a Keeping joints abducted
   b Applying traction to affected areas
   c Wearing a cast to prevent movement
   d Rest balanced with exercise

15 A person had hip replacement surgery. Which should you question?
   a Do not cross the legs.
   b Provide a chair with a low seat.
   c Keep a hip abduction wedge between the legs.
   d Provide a long-handled brush for bathing.

16 A cast needs to dry. Which should you question?
   a Turn the person so the cast dries evenly.
   b Cover the cast with blankets and plastic.
   c Elevate the cast on pillows.
   d Support the cast by the palms when lifting.

REVIEW QUESTIONS—cont'd

17 A person has an arm cast. Which is normal?
a Numbness and inability to move the fingers
b Chills and nausea
c Cool skin and cyanosis
d Pulse rate of 76 and a respiratory rate of 18

18 A person is in traction. Care includes
a Avoiding ROM exercises
b Keeping the weights on the floor
c Removing the weights if the person is uncomfortable
d Using a fracture pan for elimination

19 After hip surgery the operated leg is kept
a Abducted
b Adducted
c Externally rotated
d Flexed

20 A person with osteoporosis is at risk for
a Fractures
b An amputation
c Phantom pain
d Paralysis

21 After an amputation, the person
a Needs a wheelchair
b Has quadriplegia
c Is fitted with a prosthesis
d Needs arthroplasty

Answers to Chapter 48 questions are on p. 887.

FOCUS ON **PRACTICE**
Problem Solving

After a stroke a person has hemiplegia, aphasia, and dysphagia. How will you modify the care measures listed below? Apply learning from this and other chapters.
- Transferring from the bed to the wheelchair
- Dressing and undressing
- Assisting with food and fluids
- Explaining a procedure
- Performing a safety check of the room

OBJECTIVES

- Define the key terms and key abbreviations in this chapter.
- Describe congenital heart defects.
- Identify cardiovascular disorder risk factors and complications.
- Describe the care required for hypertension, coronary artery disease, angina, myocardial infarction, heart failure, and dysrhythmias.

- Describe the care required for chronic obstructive pulmonary disease, asthma, and sleep apnea.
- Explain the differences between a cold and influenza and the care required.
- Describe the care required for pneumonia and tuberculosis.
- Describe the care required for lymphedema and lymphoma.
- Explain how to promote PRIDE in the person, the family, and yourself.

KEY TERMS

apnea The lack or absence *(a)* of breathing *(pnea)*
arrhythmia See "dysrhythmia"
congenital To be born with
dysrhythmia An abnormal *(dys)* heart rhythm *(rhythmia)*; arrhythmia
hypertension High blood pressure

lymphedema A buildup of lymph in the tissues causing edema (swelling)
pneumonia Inflammation and infection of lung tissue
sleep apnea Pauses *(a)* in breathing *(pnea)* that occur during sleep

KEY ABBREVIATIONS

CAD	Coronary artery disease	MI	Myocardial infarction
CDC	Centers for Disease Control and Prevention	mm Hg	Millimeters of mercury
CHF	Congestive heart failure	O_2	Oxygen
CO_2	Carbon dioxide	RBC	Red blood cell
COPD	Chronic obstructive pulmonary disease	TB	Tuberculosis
ICD	Implanted cardioverter defibrillator	WBC	White blood cell
IV	Intravenous		

Cardiovascular and respiratory system disorders are leading causes of death in the United States. Many people have these disorders. Disorders also occur in the lymphatic system. Understanding these disorders gives meaning to the care you give.

CARDIOVASCULAR DISORDERS

The circulatory (cardiovascular) system delivers blood to the body's cells. Problems occur in the heart or blood vessels. See Chapter 40 for circulatory ulcers.

See *Body Structure and Function Review: The Circulatory System.*

See *Focus on Children and Older Persons: Cardiovascular Disorders*, p. 738.

BODY STRUCTURE AND FUNCTION REVIEW

The Circulatory System

The circulatory system is made up of the *blood, heart,* and *blood vessels.* The heart pumps blood through the blood vessels.

The Blood

The blood consists of blood cells and *plasma.* Plasma is mostly water. It carries blood cells to other body cells. Plasma also carries substances (nutrients, hormones, and chemicals) that cells need to function.

Red blood cells (RBCs) are called *erythrocytes. Hemoglobin* in the RBCs gives blood its red color. As RBCs circulate through the lungs, hemoglobin picks up oxygen (O_2). Hemoglobin carries O_2 to the cells. When blood is bright red, hemoglobin in the RBCs is filled with O_2. As blood circulates through the body, O_2 is given to the cells. Cells release carbon dioxide (CO_2) (a waste product). It is picked up by the hemoglobin. RBCs filled with CO_2 make the blood look dark red.

Blood also contains *white blood cells (WBCs)* and *platelets (thrombocytes).* WBCs are called *leukocytes.* They protect the body against infection. Platelets are needed for blood clotting.

The Heart

The heart is a muscle. It pumps blood through the blood vessels to the tissues and cells. The heart has 4 chambers (Fig. 49-1). Upper chambers receive blood and are called *atria.* The *right atrium* receives blood from body tissues. The *left atrium* receives blood from the lungs. Lower chambers are called *ventricles.* Ventricles pump blood. The *right ventricle* pumps blood to the lungs for O_2. The *left ventricle* pumps blood to all parts of the body.

Valves are between the atria and ventricles (see Fig. 49-1). The valves allow blood flow in 1 direction. They prevent blood from flowing back into the atria from the ventricles. The *tricuspid valve* is between the right atrium and the right ventricle. The *mitral valve (bicuspid valve)* is between the left atrium and the left ventricle.

Heart action has 2 phases.
- *Diastole*—the resting phase. Heart chambers fill with blood.
- *Systole*—the working phase. The heart contracts. Blood is pumped through the blood vessels when the heart contracts.

The heart has its own electrical system that stimulates the heart to contract. The electrical signal begins in the *sinoatrial (SA) node* (see Fig. 49-1). The SA node sets the pace of the heart. It stimulates the heart to beat at 60 to 100 beats per minute. The electrical signal spreads through the heart, causing the heart to contract.

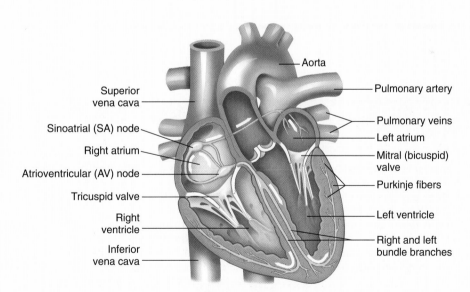

FIGURE 49-1 Structures of the heart. Chambers and major vessels that carry blood full of O_2 are shown in red. Chambers and major vessels that carry blood low in O_2 are shown in blue. Valves are white. The heart's electrical system is yellow. (Modified from Patton KT, Thibodeau GA: *The human body in health & disease,* ed 6, St Louis, 2014, Mosby.)

Continued

BODY STRUCTURE AND FUNCTION REVIEW—cont'd

The Circulatory System

The Blood Vessels

Blood flows to body tissues and cells through the blood vessels. There are 3 groups of blood vessels: arteries, capillaries, and veins (Fig. 49-2).

Arteries carry blood away from the heart. Arterial blood is rich in O_2. The *aorta* (see Fig. 49-2) is the largest artery. It receives blood directly from the left ventricle. The aorta branches into other arteries that carry blood to all parts of the body. These arteries branch into smaller parts within the tissues. The smallest branch of an artery is an *arteriole.*

Arterioles connect to *capillaries.* Capillaries are very tiny blood vessels. Nutrients, O_2, and other substances pass from capillaries into the cells. The capillaries pick up waste products (including CO_2) from the cells. Veins carry waste products back to the heart.

Veins return blood to the heart. They connect to the capillaries by *venules.* Venules are small veins. Venules branch together to form veins. The many veins also branch together as they near the heart to form 2 main veins—the *inferior vena cava* and the *superior vena cava* (see Fig. 49-2). Both empty into the right atrium. The inferior vena cava carries blood from the legs and trunk. The superior vena cava carries blood from the head and arms. Venous blood is dark red. It has little O_2 and a lot of CO_2.

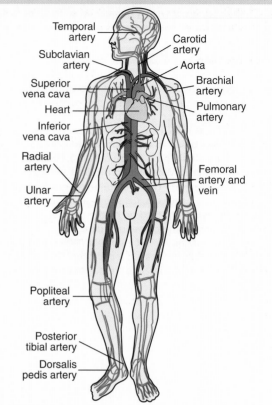

FIGURE 49-2 Arterial and venous systems. Arterial system is red. Venous system is blue.

FOCUS ON CHILDREN AND OLDER PERSONS

Cardiovascular Disorders

Children

Some babies have congenital heart defects. *Congenital means to be born with.* Defects occur during pregnancy as the baby's heart develops. The defect can involve the heart walls, heart valves, or the blood vessels near the heart. Blood flow is affected. The flow can slow down, go in the wrong direction or place, or be blocked.

Usually the cause is unknown. Risk factors include:

- Family history. A family history of defects may increase the risk.
- Environment. Smoking during pregnancy and second-hand smoke increase risk. So does taking certain drugs early in pregnancy. Drinking alcohol during pregnancy also increases the risk.
- Some medical conditions during pregnancy. Diabetes and a viral infection with rubella (German measles) are examples.

The common signs of congenital heart defects are:

- *Cyanosis* (bluish tint to the skin, lips, and fingernails)
- Fatigue
- Heart murmurs (heart sounds other than "lub-dub" during an apical pulse)
- Poor circulation
- Fast breathing

Heart defects are found during pregnancy or when the child is very young. Some are not diagnosed until the child is older. Treatment may involve:

- Drugs.
- Correcting the defect with a catheter. A catheter is inserted into a blood vessel and then into the heart.
- Surgery.
- A heart transplant.

With successful treatment, many children with heart defects grow into healthy adults. Some need life-long treatment.

Hypertension

With every heartbeat, blood is pumped into arteries. Blood pressure is the force of blood pressing against artery walls. Pressure is higher when the heart beats *(systole)*. Pressure is lower when the heart rests *(diastole)*.

Hypertension means high blood pressure. Blood pressure is high when:

- The systolic pressure is 140 mm Hg (millimeters of mercury) or higher.
- The diastolic pressure is 90 mm Hg or higher.

When risk factors are present (Box 49-1), a systolic pressure between 130 and 139 mm Hg or a diastolic pressure between 80 and 89 mm Hg may signal hypertension. Report abnormal blood pressures at once.

Hypertension often does not cause symptoms. Measuring blood pressure regularly is important. Over time, hypertension causes the heart to work harder, leading to other disorders. Heart attack (p. 741), heart failure (p. 741), stroke (Chapter 48), and kidney failure (Chapter 51) are examples.

Life-style changes can lower blood pressure. A diet low in fat and salt, a healthy weight, and regular exercise are needed. No smoking is allowed. Alcohol and caffeine are limited. Managing stress and sleeping well also lower blood pressure. Certain drugs lower blood pressure.

BOX 49-1	Cardiovascular Disorders— Risk Factors

Factors You *Cannot* Change

- Age—45 years or older for men; 55 years or older for women
- Biological sex—risk increases for women after menopause; having diabetes increases the risk more in women than in men
- Race—African Americans are at greater risk
- Family history—tends to run in families; early onset in a close family member increases the risk

Factors You *Can* Change

- Being over-weight
- Stress
- Smoking and tobacco use
- Poor diet—high in fat, salt, sugar, and cholesterol
- Excessive alcohol use
- Lack of exercise
- Not getting enough sleep
- High blood pressure
- Unhealthy blood cholesterol levels
- Diabetes

Modified from MedlinePlus: How to prevent heart disease, Bethesda, Md, updated November 6, 2019, U.S. National Library of Medicine.

Coronary Artery Disease

The *coronary arteries* supply the heart muscle with blood. In coronary artery disease (CAD) (coronary heart disease, heart disease), the coronary arteries become hardened and narrow. One or all are affected. The heart muscle gets less blood and O_2.

The most common cause is atherosclerosis (Fig. 49-3). Plaque—made up of cholesterol, fat, and other substances—collects on artery walls. The narrowed arteries block some or all blood flow. Blood clots can form along the plaque and block blood flow.

Major complications of CAD are angina, heart attack, heart failure, irregular heartbeats, and sudden death. The more risk factors present (see Box 49-1), the greater the chance of CAD and its complications.

Treatment goals are to:

- Relieve symptoms (see "Angina," p. 740)
- Slow or stop atherosclerosis
- Lower the risk of blood clots
- Widen or bypass clogged arteries
- Prevent complications

CAD requires life-style changes (see "Hypertension"). Drugs may be given to:

- Lower cholesterol
- Lower blood pressure
- Prevent blood clots
- Decrease the heart's workload and relieve symptoms
- Delay medical and surgical procedures that open or bypass diseased arteries (Fig. 49-4, p. 740)

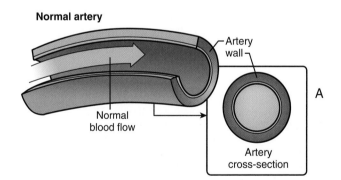

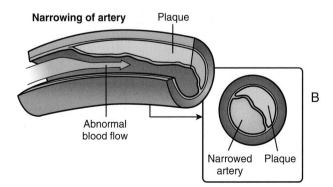

FIGURE 49-3 A, Normal artery. **B,** Plaque on the artery wall in atherosclerosis.

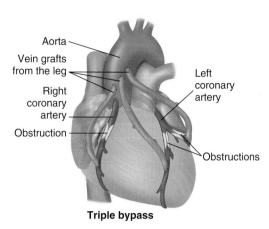

Triple bypass

FIGURE 49-4 Coronary artery bypass surgery. Arteries or veins from other parts of the body are used to bypass (go around) narrowed coronary arteries. (Modified from Patton KT, Thibodeau GA: *The human body in health & disease*, ed 7, St Louis, 2018, Elsevier.)

Cardiac Rehabilitation. CAD complications may require cardiac rehabilitation (cardiac rehab). The cardiac rehab team includes doctors (the person's doctor, a heart specialist, a heart surgeon), nurses, exercise specialists, physical and occupational therapists, dietitians, and mental health professionals.

Cardiac rehab programs include:

- Exercise. Exercise begins slowly. At first, the heart is monitored during exercise. Activity increases over time. Exercise outside of rehab is encouraged. Walking and yard work are examples.
- Healthy eating. The person learns how to make healthy food choices. Diet planning for health problems such as diabetes, obesity, hypertension, and high cholesterol is included.
- Education. The person learns ways to stay healthy. Quitting smoking and managing other health problems are examples.
- Support. The rehab team provides support for life-style changes. Some persons need help coping with anxiety and depression (Chapter 52).

Angina

Angina is chest pain from reduced blood flow to part of the heart muscle (*myocardium*). (*Angina* comes from the Latin word *angor* that means *strangling*.) It occurs when the heart needs more O_2. Normally blood flow to the heart increases when O_2 needs increase. Exertion, a heavy meal, stress, and excitement increase the heart's need for O_2. So does smoking and very hot or cold temperatures. In CAD, narrowed vessels prevent increased blood flow.

Chest pain is described as tightness, pressure, squeezing, or burning in the chest. Pain can occur in the shoulders, arms, neck, jaw, or back (Fig. 49-5). The person may also have nausea, fatigue, dyspnea, sweating, light-headedness, and weakness.

Rest often relieves symptoms in a few minutes. Persons with angina need to know:

- The usual pattern of their symptoms. This includes the causes, usual description and duration of the pain, and if rest or drugs relieve pain.
- What drugs to use and how to use them. *Nitroglycerin* dissolved under the tongue is common.
- How to control angina. Avoiding triggers like physical exertion, stress, and large meals are examples.
- The limits of physical activity. The person should stop activity before symptoms occur. For example, a person usually has angina walking up a flight of stairs. The person should stop half-way and rest before continuing.
- When to get emergency care. Pain that is severe, lasts longer than a few minutes, or is not relieved by rest or drugs may signal a heart attack. Emergency care is needed.

See "Coronary Artery Disease" (p. 739) for the treatment of angina. Increased blood flow to the heart prevents or lowers the risk of heart attack and death.

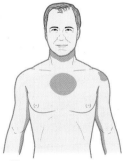

- Chest
- Left shoulder and down both arms
- Neck

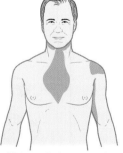

- Chest radiating to neck and jaw
- Left shoulder and down left arm

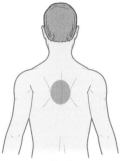

- Back

FIGURE 49-5 *Shaded areas* show common locations and patterns of angina. (Modified from Lewis SL, et al: *Medical-surgical nursing: assessment and management of clinical problems*, ed 10, St Louis, 2017, Elsevier.)

Myocardial Infarction

Myocardial refers to the *heart muscle. Infarction* means *tissue death.* With myocardial infarction (MI) part of the heart muscle dies from sudden blockage of blood flow in a coronary artery. A thrombus (blood clot) in an artery with atherosclerosis blocks blood flow (Fig. 49-6).

MI also is called:

- Heart attack
- Acute myocardial infarction (AMI)
- Acute coronary syndrome (ACS)

CAD, angina, and previous MI are risk factors. See Box 49-2 for signs and symptoms. MI is an emergency. Efforts are made to:

- Relieve pain.
- Reduce the heart's workload.
- Restore blood flow to the heart.
- Stabilize vital signs.
- Give O_2.
- Calm the person.
- Prevent death and life-threatening problems.

The person may need medical or surgical procedures to open or bypass the diseased artery. Cardiac rehabilitation is needed. The goals are to:

- Recover and resume normal activities.
- Prevent another MI.
- Prevent complications such as heart failure or sudden cardiac arrest (sudden cardiac death) (Chapter 58).

See *Focus on Long-Term Care and Home Care: Myocardial Infarction.*

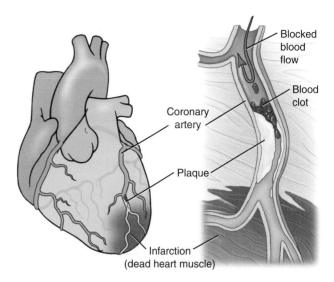

FIGURE 49-6 Myocardial infarction. Blood flow to part of the heart muscle is blocked, causing death of heart tissue.

FOCUS ON LONG-TERM CARE AND HOME CARE

Myocardial Infarction

Home Care

Cardiac rehabilitation continues. The person may go to a gym, health club, or hospital fitness center. Some persons like indoor malls for walking. Normal activities are increased slowly. The person returns to work with the doctor's approval.

BOX 49-2	Myocardial Infarction—Signs and Symptoms

- Chest pain or discomfort
  - Usually in the center or on the left side of the chest
  - Lasts more than a few minutes or goes away and comes back
  - Described as pressure, squeezing, fullness, pain, heartburn, or indigestion
  - Mild or severe
  - Different from usual angina pattern or is not relieved by rest or nitroglycerin
- Upper body discomfort—pain in 1 or both arms, the back, shoulders, neck, jaw, or upper stomach
- *Dyspnea* (difficulty breathing)
  - May be the only symptom or may occur before or with chest pain
  - Can occur with rest or during mild physical activity
- Breaking out in a cold sweat
- Unexplained fatigue (especially in women)
- Nausea and vomiting
- Light-headedness or sudden dizziness

Modified from National Heart, Lung, and Blood Institute; National Institutes of Health; U.S. Department of Health and Human Services: Heart attack, Bethesda, Md, National Institutes of Health.

Heart Failure

Heart failure or congestive heart failure (CHF) occurs when the weakened heart cannot pump normally. Blood backs up. Tissue congestion occurs. Heart failure is caused by conditions that damage or over-work the heart muscle (Box 49-3, p. 742).

When the left side of the heart cannot pump normally, blood backs up into the lungs. Respiratory congestion occurs. When the right side of the heart cannot pump normally, blood backs up into the venous system. Swelling occurs *(edema).* With both left-sided and right-sided failure, the body does not get enough blood. Signs and symptoms occur from the effects on other organs. See Box 49-3, p. 742. *Pulmonary edema* (fluid in the lungs) can result from heart failure. It is an emergency. The person can die.

The goals of treatment are to:

- Treat the cause of heart failure.
- Reduce symptoms.
- Prevent worsening heart failure.
- Improve quality of life.
- Prolong life.

BOX 49-3   Heart Failure

Common Causes
- CAD
- Heart attack
- Hypertension
- Dysrhythmia (abnormal heart rhythm)
- Cardiomyopathy (enlarged, thick, or rigid heart muscle)
- Damaged heart valves
- Congenital heart defects
- Chronic conditions: diabetes, HIV, thyroid problems

Signs and Symptoms
- Dyspnea: worse with exertion or lying down
- Sputum: white, pink, blood-tinged, foamy
- Cough
- Lung sounds: gurgling, wheezing
- Concentration problems, decreased alertness
- Reduced ability to exercise
- Fatigue and weakness
- *Nocturia* (frequent urination at night)
- Nausea
- Appetite: decreased
- Swelling: feet, ankles, legs, abdomen, neck veins
- Weight gain: rapid
- Pulse: rapid, irregular

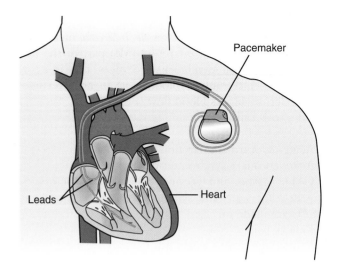

FIGURE 49-7 Pacemaker.

Drugs strengthen the heart, decrease strain on the heart, and reduce fluid buildup. A sodium-controlled diet is ordered. Oxygen is given. Semi-Fowler's position is preferred for breathing. The person must reduce CAD risk factors. If acutely ill, the person needs hospital care.

You assist with these aspects of the person's care.
- Promoting rest and activity as ordered
- Measuring intake and output
- Measuring weight daily
- Assisting with pulse oximetry
- Restricting fluids as ordered
- Promoting a low sodium, fat, and cholesterol diet
- Preventing pressure injuries
- Assisting with range-of-motion and other exercises
- Assisting with transfers and ambulation
- Assisting with self-care activities
- Maintaining good alignment
- Applying elastic stockings

Many older persons have heart failure. Skin breakdown is a risk. Tissue swelling, poor circulation, and fragile skin increase the risk of pressure injuries. Good skin care and regular position changes are needed.

Dysrhythmias

A *dysrhythmia (arrhythmia)* *is an abnormal* (dys) *heart rhythm* (rhythmia). The rhythm may be too fast, too slow, or irregular. Dysrhythmias are caused by changes in the heart's electrical system. Changes may result from hypertension, CAD, MI, or heart failure. Weakening and changes in the heart muscle are other causes. So are drug and alcohol abuse, excess caffeine intake, smoking, stress, and thyroid problems. Some drugs can cause dysrhythmias.

The person may notice the change in the pulse—slow, irregular, skipped beats, pounding, racing. Feeling dizzy or light-headed, chest pain, sweating, and dyspnea are other symptoms. The person may faint (Chapter 58). Some dysrhythmias are minor. Others are life-threatening.

Treatment depends on the type of dysrhythmia. Drugs may be given. A procedure may be needed.
- *Defibrillation* (Chapter 58) or *cardioversion*—an electrical shock is given to stop an abnormal rhythm.
- *Ablation*—areas of tissue in the heart sending abnormal electrical signals are destroyed.

Some abnormal rhythms are treated with a pacemaker (Fig. 49-7). This device monitors and regulates the heart's rhythm. The device is inserted under the skin near the heart. One or more wires (leads) are placed in the heart muscle and connected to the pacemaker. The pacemaker sends signals through the leads to stimulate the heart to beat normally.

For life-threatening dysrhythmias, an implantable cardioverter defibrillator (ICD) may be placed. The ICD delivers a shock when the heart is in a life-threatening rhythm. The shock restores a regular heart rhythm. Some devices are both a pacemaker and an ICD.

See *Focus on Long-Term Care and Home Care: Dysrhythmias.*

FOCUS ON LONG-TERM CARE AND HOME CARE

Dysrhythmias

Home Care

Pacemaker or ICD function is checked regularly. This can be done at home using a phone or Internet connection. A transmitter connects with the pacemaker or ICD. It sends information about heart rhythm and device function to the health team.

RESPIRATORY DISORDERS

The respiratory system brings O_2 into the lungs and removes CO_2 from the body. Respiratory disorders interfere with this function and threaten life.

See *Body Structure and Function Review: The Respiratory System.*

Chronic Obstructive Pulmonary Disease

Chronic obstructive pulmonary disease (COPD) involves 2 disorders—chronic bronchitis and emphysema (Fig. 49-9). These disorders interfere with O_2 and CO_2 exchange in the lungs. They obstruct (block) airflow. Lung function is gradually lost.

Cigarette smoking is the greatest risk factor. Pipe, cigar, and other smoking tobaccos are also risk factors. So is exposure to second-hand smoke. Not smoking is the best way to prevent COPD. COPD has no cure. Air pollution and industrial dusts are other risk factors.

COPD affects the airways and alveoli. Less air gets into the lungs; less air leaves the lungs. These changes occur.
- The airways and alveoli (air sacs) become less elastic. They are like old rubber bands.
- The walls between many alveoli are destroyed.
- Airway walls become thick, inflamed, and swollen.
- The airways secrete more mucus than usual. Excess mucus clogs the airways.

BODY STRUCTURE AND FUNCTION REVIEW
The Respiratory System

Oxygen is needed to live. Every cell needs O_2. The respiratory system (Fig. 49-8) brings O_2 into the lungs and removes CO_2. *Respiration* is the process of supplying the cells with O_2 and removing CO_2 from them. Respiration involves breathing in *(inhalation, inspiration)* and breathing out *(exhalation, expiration)*.

Air enters the body through the *nose.* Then air passes into the *pharynx* (throat), the *larynx* (voice box), and the *trachea* (windpipe). The trachea divides at its lower end into the *right bronchus* and the *left bronchus.* Each bronchus enters a *lung.* The bronchi divide many times into smaller branches *(bronchioles).* They end up in tiny one-celled air sacs called *alveoli.*

O_2 and CO_2 are exchanged between the alveoli and capillaries. Blood in the capillaries picks up O_2 from the alveoli. Then the blood is returned to the left side of the heart and pumped to the rest of the body. Alveoli pick up CO_2 from the capillaries for exhalation.

Each lung is divided into lobes. The right lung has 3 lobes; the left lung has 2. The lungs are separated from the abdominal cavity by a muscle called the *diaphragm.* A bony framework made up of the ribs, sternum, and vertebrae protects the lungs.

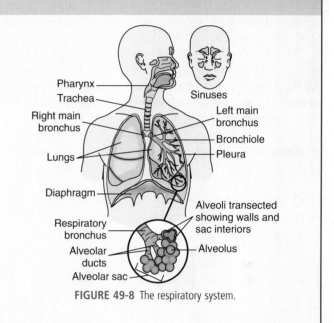

FIGURE 49-8 The respiratory system.

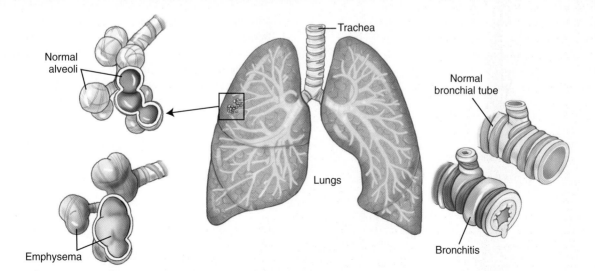

FIGURE 49-9 COPD. Chronic bronchitis causes inflammation and mucus in the airways. Emphysema damages the inner walls of alveoli. (Modified from Brooks ML, Brooks DL: *Exploring medical language: a student-directed approach,* ed 10, St Louis, 2018, Elsevier.)

Chronic Bronchitis. *Bronchitis* means *inflammation* (itis) *of the bronchi* (bronch). With chronic bronchitis, airways are narrowed from inflammation and mucus (see Fig. 49-9).

The main symptom is an on-going cough or a cough that produces a lot of mucus *(smoker's cough)*. The person has difficulty breathing and tires easily. The body cannot get enough O_2. Wheezing and chest tightness can occur.

The person must stop smoking. Oxygen therapy and breathing exercises are common. Drugs are given to open the airways. Respiratory tract infections are prevented. If one occurs, prompt treatment is needed.

Emphysema. In emphysema, the alveoli are damaged (see Fig. 49-9). Alveoli lose their shape and become less elastic. They do not expand and shrink normally. As a result, air is trapped and not exhaled. Over time, more alveoli are involved. O_2 and CO_2 exchange cannot occur in affected alveoli. As more air is trapped in the lungs, the person develops a *barrel chest* (Fig. 49-10).

The person has shortness of breath and a cough. At first, shortness of breath occurs with exertion. Over time, it occurs at rest. Fatigue is common. The body does not get enough O_2. Breathing is easier when sitting upright and slightly forward (Chapter 43).

The person must stop smoking. Respiratory therapy, breathing exercises, oxygen, and drug therapy are ordered.

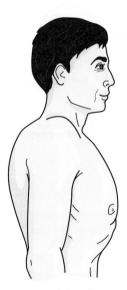

FIGURE 49-10 Barrel chest from emphysema.

Asthma

Asthma comes from the Greek word for *panting*. With asthma, the airway becomes inflamed and narrow. Extra mucus is produced. Coughing, wheezing, chest tightness, and shortness of breath can occur.

Asthma usually is triggered by allergies. Other triggers include air pollutants and irritants, smoking and second-hand smoke, respiratory infections, and exertion.

Asthma is treated with drugs. Sudden attacks *(asthma attacks)* can be mild or severe. Severe attacks may require emergency care.

Sleep Apnea

Apnea is the lack or absence (a) *of breathing* (pnea). In *sleep apnea, pauses in breathing occur during sleep.* Pauses last a few seconds to over a minute and can occur many times during sleep.

The most common cause is blockage of the airway. During sleep, muscles in the throat relax and soft tissues collapse, closing the airway.

Signs and symptoms of sleep apnea include:
* Pauses in breathing during sleep
* Loud snoring
* Waking during sleep with a gasp or shortness of breath
* Difficulty staying asleep
* Day-time sleepiness
* Headache in the morning
* Dry mouth or sore throat after sleeping
* Problems with attention
* Irritability

Life-style changes may help. A healthy diet, exercise, weight loss, no smoking, limiting alcohol before sleep, and having healthy sleep habits are examples. For more severe sleep apnea, surgery or 1 of the following devices may be needed.
* *Continuous positive airway pressure (CPAP).* A mask is attached to a pump. Air pressure is forced through the mask. The air keeps the airway open. The same amount of pressure goes through the mask when the person inhales and exhales.
* *Bilevel positive airway pressure (BiPAP).* This works like a CPAP except more pressure is given when breathing in. Less pressure is given when breathing out. The change in pressure is more comfortable for some persons.

Influenza

Influenza *(flu)* is a respiratory infection caused by viruses. Table 49-1 contrasts *cold* and the *flu*. The flu season is October through March. Children and older persons are at great risk.

Treatment involves fluids and rest. Drugs are ordered for symptom relief and to shorten the flu episode. Pneumonia, ear and sinus infections, and worsening of chronic health problems (heart failure, asthma, diabetes) are complications.

Coughing and sneezing spread flu viruses. The virus is also spread when a person touches a contaminated surface or object and then touches the mouth, eyes, or nose. Follow Standard Precautions.

The flu vaccine is the best prevention. The Centers for Disease Control and Prevention (CDC) recommends the flu vaccine for all persons 6 months old and older unless the person has a severe, life-threatening allergy to the flu vaccine.

See *Focus on Children and Older Persons: Influenza.*

Pneumonia

Pneumonia means inflammation and infection of lung tissue. (Pneumo means lungs.) Affected tissues fill with fluid. O_2 and CO_2 exchange is affected.

Bacteria, viruses, and other microbes are causes. Microbes reach the lungs by being inhaled, aspirated, or carried in the blood to the lungs from an infection in the body.

Risk factors and the signs and symptoms of pneumonia are listed in Box 49-4. Onset may be sudden. The person is very ill.

Drugs are ordered for infection and pain. Fluid intake is increased for fever and to thin secretions. Thin secretions are easier to cough up. Intravenous (IV) therapy and oxygen may be needed. Semi-Fowler's position eases breathing. Rest and mouth care are important. Standard Precautions are followed. Transmission-Based Precautions depend on the cause. Frequent linen changes are needed because of fever.

See *Focus on Children and Older Persons: Pneumonia*, p. 746.

TABLE 49-1	Influenza Versus a Cold	
Signs and Symptoms	Influenza	Cold
Symptom onset	Rapid	Gradual
Fever	Usual; lasts 3 to 4 days	Rare
Aches	Usual; often severe	Slight
Chills	Fairly common	Uncommon
Fatigue, weakness	Usual	Sometimes
Sneezing	Sometimes	Common
Stuffy nose	Sometimes	Common
Sore throat	Sometimes	Common
Chest discomfort; cough	Common; can be severe	Mild to moderate; hacking cough
Headache	Common	Rare

Modified from Centers for Disease Control and Prevention, National Center for Immunization and Respiratory Diseases (NCIRD): Flu symptoms & complications.

BOX 49-4 Pneumonia

Risk Factors
- Age—2 years or younger, 65 years or older
- Smoking
- Excessive alcohol use
- Poor nutrition
- Trouble coughing
- Dysphagia
- Decreased mobility
- Sedative use (drugs for anxiety or sleep)
- Recent cold or the flu
- Some chronic diseases—asthma, COPD, diabetes, cardiovascular disorders
- Weakened immune system from HIV/AIDS, organ transplant, chemotherapy
- Hospital care (especially if on a ventilator)

Signs and Symptoms
- Fever
- Sweating, chills
- Productive cough
- Chest pain with breathing or coughing
- Shortness of breath
- Nausea, vomiting, or diarrhea
- Headache
- Fatigue

FOCUS ON **CHILDREN AND OLDER PERSONS**

Influenza

Older Persons

Older persons may not have the usual flu signs and symptoms. The following may signal flu in older persons.
- Changes in mental status or behavior
- Worsening of other health problems
- A body temperature below the normal range
- Fatigue
- Decreased appetite and fluid intake

Tuberculosis

Tuberculosis (TB) is a bacterial infection in the lungs. It also can occur in the kidneys, spine, and brain. If not treated, the person can die.

TB is spread by airborne droplets with coughing, sneezing, speaking, singing, or laughing (Chapter 17). Nearby persons can inhale the bacteria. Those with close, frequent contact with an infected person are at risk. TB is more likely to occur in close, crowded areas. Age (very young or very old), poor nutrition, and HIV (human immunodeficiency virus) infection are other risk factors.

TB can be present in the body but not cause signs and symptoms (latent TB). *Latent* means *present but not active.* An active infection may not occur for many years. Only persons with an active infection can spread the disease to others.

Chest x-rays and TB testing can detect the disease. Signs and symptoms are tiredness, loss of appetite, weight loss, fever, chills, and night sweats. The person has a bad cough that lasts 3 weeks or longer. Sputum may contain blood. Chest pain occurs.

Drugs for TB are given. Standard Precautions and airborne precautions are needed (Chapter 17). The person must cover the mouth and nose with tissues when sneezing, coughing, or producing sputum. Tissues are discarded in a no-touch waste container. Hand-washing after contact with sputum is essential.

See *Focus on Children and Older Persons: Tuberculosis.*
See *Focus on Long-Term Care and Home Care: Tuberculosis.*

LYMPHATIC DISORDERS

The lymphatic system drains extra fluid from the tissues, helps fight infection, and absorbs and transports fats. Lymphatic disorders affect these functions.

See *Body Structure and Function Review: The Lymphatic System.*

BODY STRUCTURE AND FUNCTION REVIEW

The Lymphatic System

The lymphatic (lymph) system transports lymph throughout the body (Fig. 49-11). *Lymph* is a clear, thin, watery fluid. Lymph contains WBCs, proteins, and fats from the intestines.

The lymphatic system:

- Collects extra lymph from the tissues and returns it to the blood. Water, proteins, and other substances normally leak out of the capillaries into surrounding tissues. The lymphatic system drains the extra fluid from the tissues. Otherwise, the tissues swell.
- Defends the body against infection by producing lymphocytes. *Lymphocytes* are a type of WBC that defends the body against microbes that cause infection.
- Absorbs fats from the intestines and transports them to the blood.

Lymph is formed in the tissues. Lymph is transported by *lymphatic vessels.*

Lymph nodes are shaped like beans. They are found in the neck, underarm, groin area, chest, abdomen, and pelvis. Usually, you cannot see or feel lymph nodes. They swell when producing more lymphocytes to fight infection.

Lymph enters lymph nodes through the lymphatic vessels. The lymph nodes filter bacteria, cancer cells, and damaged cells from the lymph. This prevents such substances from entering the blood and circulating throughout the body.

See Figure 49-11 for the location of the *thymus (thymus gland).* Certain lymphocytes—T lymphocytes (T cells)—develop in the thymus. Such lymphocytes are important for immune system function.

The *tonsils* are in the back of the throat. *Adenoids* are behind the nose. These structures trap microbes in the mouth and nose to help prevent infection.

The *spleen* is the largest structure in the lymphatic system. The spleen:

- Filters and removes bacteria and other substances.
- Destroys old RBCs.
- Saves the iron found in hemoglobin when RBCs are destroyed.
- Stores blood. When needed, the blood is returned to the circulatory system.

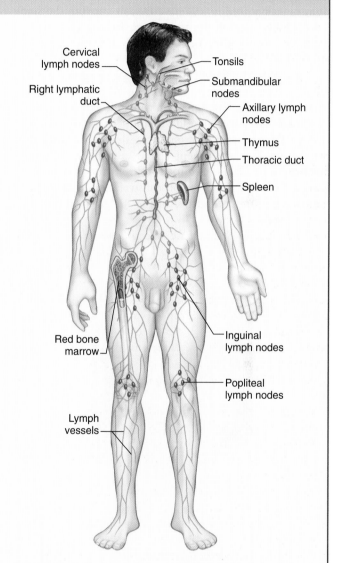

FIGURE 49-11 The lymphatic system. The bean-shaped structures shown in green are lymph nodes. (Modified from Patton KT, Thibodeau GA: *The human body in health and disease,* ed 7, St Louis, 2018, Elsevier.)

Lymphedema

Lymphedema is a buildup of lymph in the tissues causing edema (swelling). It occurs with blockage or damage to the lymph system. Causes include:

- Cancer
- Infection
- Surgical removal of lymph nodes
- Scar tissue from radiation therapy or surgery
- Absent or abnormal lymph nodes present at birth

Lymphedema usually affects an arm or leg (Fig. 49-12). Other body parts can be involved. The person may have a tight or heavy feeling and have trouble moving the body part. Thickening of the skin, pain, itching or burning, and hair loss are also common. Daily activities are often affected.

Damage to the lymph system cannot be reversed. Care measures can prevent lymphedema or keep it from getting worse (Box 49-5). Treatment may include careful exercise, good skin care, and massage therapy. Pressure garments (compression sleeves, lymphedema sleeves or stockings) may be used. The garment applies a certain amount of pressure to the arm or leg to move fluid and prevent fluid buildup. The goals are to control swelling, decrease pain, improve movement and use of the body part, and allow daily activities.

See *Promoting Safety and Comfort: Lymphedema.*

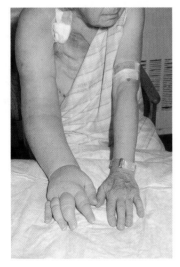

FIGURE 49-12 Lymphedema. (From Swartz MH: *Textbook of physical diagnosis: history and examination,* ed 7, Philadelphia, 2014, Saunders.)

BOX 49-5	Lymphedema—Care Measures

Preventing Infection

- Monitor for signs of skin infection. Report redness, pain, swelling, heat, red streaks below the skin, or fever.
- Apply lotion to keep the skin moist.
- Report small cuts or breaks in the skin. Treatment with an antibacterial ointment is needed.
- Avoid needle-sticks on the affected arm or leg. This includes blood glucose testing (Chapter 38).
- Do not use a hand with lymphedema to test water temperature. Burns are a risk from decreased sensation.
- Report long or jagged toenails. A nurse or doctor (podiatrist) performs toenail care. Nails are cut straight across to prevent ingrown nails and infections.
- Keep the feet clean and dry. Cotton socks are worn.
- The person:
  - Wears gloves for gardening and cooking.
  - Wears sunscreen and shoes when outside.
  - Uses a thimble for sewing.

Promoting Fluid Flow

- Do not use a blood pressure cuff on an arm with or at risk for lymphedema.
- Do not use elastic bandages or stockings with tight bands.
- Position the affected arm or leg higher than heart level if possible.
- Do not apply heat to the affected arm or leg.
- The person:
  - Does not sit with the legs crossed.
  - Changes sitting position at least every 30 minutes.
  - Wears clothes without tight bands or elastic. If jewelry is worn, it is loose.
  - Does not carry bags on an arm with lymphedema.
  - Does not swing the affected arm or leg quickly in circles.
  - Does not let the arm or leg hang down.

Modified from National Cancer Institute: Lymphedema (PDQ®)—patient version, *updated September 19, 2019, National Institutes of Health.*

PROMOTING SAFETY AND COMFORT

Lymphedema

Safety

In persons at risk, actions that block fluid flow or increase fluid buildup can cause lymphedema or make it worse. Never apply a blood pressure cuff to an arm with or at risk for lymphedema. For example, lymph nodes are often removed during breast cancer surgery. Do not use the arm on the surgery side to check blood pressure.

If not sure which arm to use, ask the nurse. Also, ask the person if he or she has an arm that must not be used.

Comfort

Lymphedema can be painful and affect movement. Handle the person gently. Tell the person before you move the body part. Ask the person to tell you if he or she feels pain. Stop movements that cause pain.

Lymphoma

Lymphoma is cancer involving cells in the immune system (lymphocytes). Lymphocytes are a type of WBC that protects the body from infection. They are found in lymph nodes and other lymph tissues.

In cancer, an abnormal cell divides and makes more abnormal cells (Chapter 47). Lymphoma begins with an abnormal lymphocyte. Abnormal lymphocytes cannot protect the body.

There are 2 main types of lymphoma—Hodgkin lymphoma and non-Hodgkin lymphoma. They differ in the types of cells involved, how they spread, and how they respond to treatment.

Signs and symptoms of lymphoma include:
* Painless swelling in the lymph nodes in the neck, underarm, groin, or stomach
* Fever
* Night sweats
* Fatigue
* Weight loss
* Skin rash or itchy skin
* Pain in the chest, abdomen, or bones

Treatment may include chemotherapy, radiation, or both (Chapter 47). Psychological, social, and spiritual support are needed.

FOCUS ON **PRIDE**

The Person, Family, and Yourself

Personal and Professional Responsibility

Apply the information in this chapter to your own life. Are there life-style factors that put you at risk for a cardiovascular or respiratory disorder? A healthy life-style benefits you personally and professionally. You must be healthy and strong to care for others.

Rights and Respect

The right to personal choice promotes independence. Some choices are unhealthy. For example, a person with COPD continues to smoke. Or a person with CAD refuses to exercise or make diet changes. The health team teaches the person the risks and encourages healthy changes. They cannot force changes. However, they must be sure the person understands the risks.

Some persons believe that unhealthy choices improve their quality of life. They are aware of the risks but choose not to change. You may not agree with the person's decision, but you must respect the person. Treat the person with dignity and respect.

Independence and Social Interaction

Infections like the flu, pneumonia, and TB can spread to others. Transmission-Based Precautions may be needed. If family and friends avoid visiting, loneliness can result.

Social and emotional needs are important. As you give care, talk with the person. Be polite. Treat the person with kindness and respect. Tell the nurse about any concerns.

Delegation and Teamwork

A person with angina may have an MI. Hypertension may lead to a stroke. A person may have a severe asthma attack.

Sudden condition changes require the nurse's attention. Assist as directed. You may need to help other patients or residents while the nurse gives care. Help willingly. The entire nursing team must give "extra effort" during an emergency.

Ethics and Laws

Some agencies use color-coded wristbands to promote safety and prevent harm (Chapter 13). They communicate alerts or warnings. "Limb alert" or "forbidden extremity" wristbands communicate that an arm must not be used for blood pressures, intravenous infusions, or blood draws. These are useful for lymphedema.

Know what wristbands are used in your agency. Check for wristbands when providing care. Take pride in using such safety measures to prevent harm.

FOCUS ON **PRIDE**: *Application*

List the risk factors for cardiovascular disorders. Circle those that apply to you. Which factors can you change? Do you plan to make changes to lower your risk? Explain. What would help you make changes?

REVIEW QUESTIONS

Circle the BEST answer.

1 A person with a congenital heart defect
   a Needs heart surgery
   b Has damaged heart valves
   c Has blocked coronary arteries
   d Was born with the defect

2 In hypertension
   a The diastolic pressure is higher than the systolic pressure
   b The systolic pressure is 140 mm Hg or higher
   c The diastolic pressure is 70 mm Hg or higher
   d Chest pain is a common symptom

3 Which is a complication of hypertension?
   a COPD   c Lymphedema
   b Heart attack   d Diabetes

4 A person is being treated for hypertension. Which would you question?
   a No smoking   c Regular exercise
   b A high-sodium diet d A low-fat diet

5 Cardiac rehabilitation involves
   a Exercise
   b Surgery
   c Catheter procedures
   d A vaccine

6 A person has angina. Which is *true?*
   a There is heart muscle damage.
   b Pain is not relieved with rest.
   c It is a risk factor for MI.
   d Pain is always on the left side of the chest.

7 A person complains of sudden squeezing chest pain. You should
   a Report the pain if it is not relieved in 15 minutes
   b Report the pain at once
   c Give the person a nitroglycerin tablet
   d Give the person oxygen

8 A person is having an MI. Which is *true?*
   a Pain is relieved with nitroglycerin.
   b There is no treatment.
   c This is an emergency.
   d The person does not have enough blood.

9 The pain of MI is usually
   a In the center or on the left side of the chest
   b On the right side of the chest
   c In the abdomen
   d In both shoulders

10 A person has heart failure. Which should you question?
   a Encourage fluids
   b Measure intake and output
   c Measure weight daily
   d Perform range-of-motion exercises

11 A person has a dysrhythmia. Tell the nurse at once if
   a You notice a hard, round lump under the skin on the chest
   b The person is dizzy
   c The heart rate is 80
   d The person has a barrel chest

12 The most common cause of COPD is
   a Smoking
   b Allergies
   c Being over-weight
   d A high-sodium diet

13 A person has emphysema. Which is *true?*
   a The person has an infection.
   b Breathing is usually easier lying down.
   c The person has dyspnea and a cough.
   d There is swelling in an arm or leg.

14 Which is least likely to help the person with sleep apnea?
   a Weight loss
   b Quitting smoking
   c Drinking alcohol before sleep
   d CPAP

15 The flu virus is spread by
   a Coughing and sneezing
   b The fecal-oral route
   c Blood
   d Needle sharing

16 Pneumonia is
   a An inflammation of the airway
   b Narrowing of the airway
   c Inflammation and infection of lung tissue
   d A bacterial infection in the lungs

17 Which position eases breathing in the person with pneumonia?
   a Supine
   b Prone
   c Semi-Fowler's
   d Trendelenburg's

18 Tuberculosis is spread by
   a Coughing and sneezing
   b Contaminated drinking water
   c Contact with wound drainage
   d The fecal-oral route

19 A person has TB. You had contact with the person's sputum. What should you do?
   a Wash your hands.
   b Put on gloves.
   c Use an alcohol-based hand sanitizer.
   d Tell the nurse.

20 A person has lymphedema in the left arm. Which should you question?
   a Apply lotion to the skin.
   b Elevate the left arm on pillows.
   c Use the right arm for blood pressure.
   d Apply a hot compress to the left arm.

Answers to Chapter 49 questions are on p. 887.

FOCUS ON **PRACTICE**

Problem Solving

An 82-year-old resident is tired and does not want to eat breakfast. The person is confused. This is not normal behavior. When should you report these changes? Why is it important to monitor for such changes in the elderly?

Digestive and Endocrine Disorders

OBJECTIVES

- Define the key terms and key abbreviations in this chapter.
- Describe the care required for gastro-esophageal reflux disease, vomiting, and inflammatory bowel disease.
- Describe the care required for diverticular disease.
- Describe the care required for gallstones.
- Describe the care required for hepatitis and cirrhosis.
- Describe the care required for diabetes.
- Explain how to promote PRIDE in the person, the family, and yourself.

KEY TERMS

acid reflux See "heartburn"
emesis See "vomitus"
heartburn A burning sensation in the chest or throat; acid reflux
hyperglycemia High *(hyper)* sugar *(glyc)* in the blood *(emia)*

hypoglycemia Low *(hypo)* sugar *(glyc)* in the blood *(emia)*
jaundice Yellowish color of the skin or whites of the eyes
vomitus Food and fluids expelled from the stomach through the mouth; emesis

KEY ABBREVIATIONS

BMs	Bowel movements	**IBD**	Inflammatory bowel disease
GERD	Gastro-esophageal reflux disease	**I&O**	Intake and output
GI	Gastro-intestinal		

Problems can develop in any part of the digestive system. This includes the accessory organs of digestion—liver, gallbladder, and pancreas. The pancreas also is part of the endocrine system.

DIGESTIVE DISORDERS

The digestive system breaks down food into nutrients for the body to absorb. Solid wastes are eliminated. See Chapter 29 for diarrhea, constipation, flatulence, fecal incontinence, and ostomy care.

- *Diarrhea*—the frequent passage of liquid stools
- *Constipation*—the passage of hard, dry stool
- *Flatulence*—the excessive formation of gas or air in the stomach and intestines
- *Fecal incontinence*—the inability to control the passage of feces and gas through the anus
- *Ostomy*—the surgically created opening that connects an internal organ to the body's surface

  See *Body Structure and Function Review: The Digestive System*, p. 752.

BODY STRUCTURE AND FUNCTION REVIEW

The Digestive System

The digestive system *(gastro-intestinal [GI] system)* extends from the mouth to the anus (Fig. 50-1). Digestion begins in the *mouth (oral cavity)*. Using chewing motions, the *teeth* cut, chop, and grind food into small particles for digestion and swallowing. The *tongue* aids in chewing and swallowing. *Salivary glands* in the mouth secrete *saliva*. Saliva moistens food particles to ease swallowing and begin digestion. During swallowing, the tongue pushes food into the *pharynx* (throat).

Contraction of the pharynx pushes food into the *esophagus*. The esophagus extends from the pharynx to the *stomach*. Involuntary muscle contractions *(peristalsis)* move food down the esophagus through the GI tract.

The stomach is a muscular, pouch-like sac. The mucous membrane lining the stomach contains glands that secrete *gastric juices*. Food is mixed and churned with the gastric juices to form a semi-liquid substance called *chyme*. Peristalsis pushes chyme from the stomach into the small intestine.

The first part of the *small intestine* is the *duodenum*. More digestive juices are added to the chyme. One is called *bile*—a greenish liquid made in the *liver*. Bile is stored in the *gallbladder*. Juices from the *pancreas* and small intestine are added to the chyme. Digestive juices chemically break down food into nutrients for absorption.

Peristalsis moves the chyme through the 2 other parts of the small intestine: the *jejunum* and the *ileum*. Most nutrient absorption takes place in the small intestine.

Undigested chyme passes from the small intestine into the *large intestine (large bowel* or *colon)*. The colon absorbs most of the water from the chyme. The remaining semi-solid material is called *feces*. Feces contain a small amount of water, solid wastes, and some mucus and germs. These are the waste products of digestion. Feces pass through the colon into the *rectum* by peristalsis. Feces pass out of the body through the *anus*.

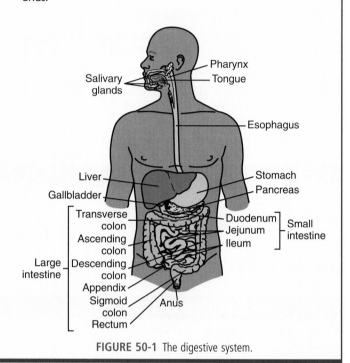

FIGURE 50-1 The digestive system.

Gastro-Esophageal Reflux Disease

Gastro-esophageal reflux disease (GERD) occurs when a muscle at the end of the esophagus does not close properly. Stomach *(gastro)* contents flow back up *(reflux)* into the esophagus *(esophageal)*. Stomach contents contain acid that can irritate and inflame the esophagus lining. This is called *esophagitis*—inflammation *(itis)* of the esophagus.

Heartburn is the most common symptom. *Heartburn (acid reflux) is a burning sensation in the chest or throat.* The person may taste stomach fluid in the back of the mouth. Besides heartburn, other signs and symptoms of GERD include:

- Pain in the chest or upper abdomen
- Hoarseness or sore throat
- *Dysphagia* (difficult or painful swallowing)
- Dry cough
- Bad breath
- Nausea and vomiting

Risk factors include being over-weight, alcohol or coffee use, pregnancy, and smoking. Hiatal hernia is a risk factor. With *hiatal hernia*, the upper part of the stomach is above the diaphragm (Fig. 50-2). Large meals, eating late at night, and lying down after eating can cause gastric reflux. So can chocolate, caffeine drinks, fried and fatty foods, garlic, onions, spicy foods, and tomatoes.

The doctor may order drugs to prevent stomach acid production or to promote stomach emptying. Surgery may be needed. Life-style changes include:

- No smoking or drinking alcohol
- Losing weight
- Eating small meals and eating slowly
- Wearing loose belts and loose-fitting clothes
- Not lying down for at least 3 hours after eating
- Raising the head of the bed 6 to 9 inches so that the head and shoulders are higher than the stomach

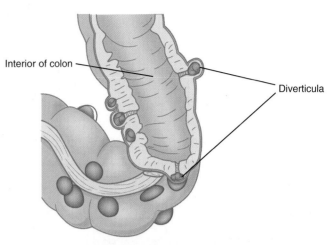

FIGURE 50-3 Diverticulosis. (From Lewis SM, et al: *Medical-surgical nursing: assessment and management of clinical problems,* ed 10, St Louis, 2017, Elsevier.)

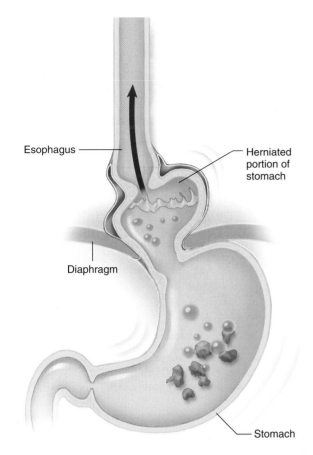

FIGURE 50-2 Hiatal hernia. (Modified from Patton KT, Thibodeau GA: *The human body in health & disease,* ed 7, St Louis, 2018, Elsevier.)

Vomiting

Vomitus (emesis) is the food and fluids expelled from the stomach through the mouth. Vomiting signals illness or injury. Aspirated vomitus can obstruct the airway. Vomiting large amounts of blood can lead to shock (Chapter 58). These measures are needed.

- Follow Standard Precautions and the Bloodborne Pathogen Standard.
- Turn the person's head well to 1 side if the person is supine. This prevents aspiration.
- Place a kidney basin under the chin.
- Move vomitus away from the person.
- Provide oral hygiene. This helps remove the bitter taste of vomitus.
- Eliminate odors.
- Provide for comfort. (See the inside of the back cover.)
- Report your observations.
  - Observe vomitus for blood, color, odor, and undigested food. If it looks like coffee grounds, it contains blood. This signals bleeding.
  - Measure, report, and record the amount of vomitus and your observations.
  - Save a specimen for laboratory study.
  - Dispose of vomitus after the nurse observes it.

Diverticular Disease

Small pouches can develop in the colon. The pouches bulge outward through weak spots in the colon wall (Fig. 50-3). A pouch is called a *diverticulum. (Diverticulare* means *to turn inside out). Diverticulosis* is the condition of having these pouches. *(Osis* means *condition of.)* The pouches can become infected or inflamed—*diverticulitis. (Itis* means *inflammation.)*

Diverticular disease becomes more common with aging. Obesity, smoking, lack of exercise, low-fiber diet, a diet high in animal fat, and some drugs are risk factors.

When feces enter the pouches, they can become inflamed and infected. The person has abdominal pain and tenderness in the lower left abdomen. Fever, nausea and vomiting, chills, cramping, and constipation are likely.

A ruptured pouch is rare. Feces spill into the abdomen. This causes a severe, life-threatening infection. A pouch also can cause a blockage in the intestine (intestinal obstruction). Feces and gas cannot move past the blocked part.

Treatment may include antibiotics, pain-relief drugs, and a liquid diet. Surgery is done for severe disease, obstruction, and ruptured pouches. The diseased part of the bowel is removed. A colostomy may be needed (Chapter 29).

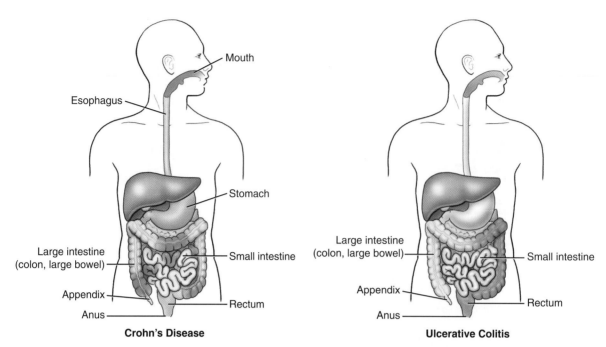

Crohn's Disease

Ulcerative Colitis

FIGURE 50-4 Inflammatory bowel disease. (Affected areas are shown in dark red.) **A,** Crohn's disease. Damaged areas appear in patches. **B,** Ulcerative colitis. The rectum and colon are damaged. (Modified from National Center for Chronic Disease Prevention and Health Promotion: *What is inflammatory bowel disease (IBD)?* Centers for Disease Control and Prevention, March 22, 2018.)

Inflammatory Bowel Disease

Inflammatory bowel disease (IBD) involves chronic inflammation of the GI tract. The 2 types of IBD are shown in Figure 50-4.

- *Crohn's disease.* Any part of the GI tract from the mouth to the anus can be affected. Part of the small intestine is usually involved before the large intestine.
- *Ulcerative colitis.* The large intestine and rectum are affected.

  Signs and symptoms include:
- Persistent diarrhea
- Abdominal pain and cramping
- Fever
- Rectal bleeding and bloody stools
- Appetite: loss of
- Weight loss

IBD often occurs before 30 years of age. Risk factors include a family history of IBD, cigarette smoking, some drugs, and a diet high in fat and refined foods.

Complications include bowel obstruction, ulcers in the GI tract (including the mouth and anus), colon cancer, osteoporosis, and liver disease. Treatment involves diet changes and drug therapy for inflammation, infection, diarrhea, pain, and nutrition. Surgery may be needed to remove damaged parts of the small intestine or colon. A colostomy or ileostomy (Chapter 29) may be necessary.

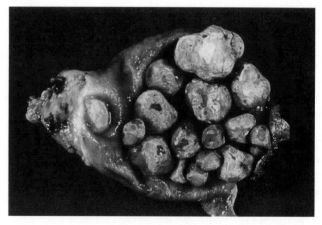

FIGURE 50-5 Inflamed gallbladder with gallstones. (From Damjanov I, Linder J: *Pathology: a color atlas,* St Louis, 2000, Mosby.)

Gallstones

Bile is a liquid made in the liver. It is stored in the gallbladder until needed to digest fat. Gallstones form when the bile hardens into stone-like pieces (Fig. 50-5).

Ducts (tubes) carry bile from the liver through the gallbladder and to the small intestine. Gallstones can lodge in any duct (Fig. 50-6). Bile flow is blocked. The gallbladder and ducts become inflamed. The liver and pancreas may be involved. Severe infections or damage can cause death.

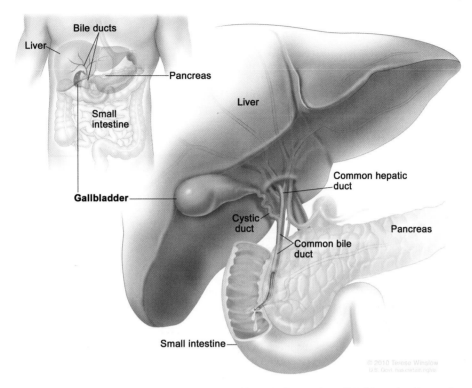

FIGURE 50-6 The gallbladder and ducts that carry bile from the liver to the gallbladder and to the small intestine. (© 2010 Terese Winslow LLC, U. S. Govt. has certain rights.)

Gallstones can be as small as a grain of sand or as big as a golf ball. A person may have 1 large stone or several that vary in size. Persons at risk include those who are:
- Women—especially women who:
  - Are pregnant
  - Use hormone replacement therapy
  - Take birth control pills
- Older persons—the risk increases with aging
- Known to have a family history of gallstones
- American Indians or Mexican Americans
- Over-weight or obese or have had fast weight loss
- Diabetics

A "gallbladder attack" or "gallstone attack" usually occurs suddenly after eating. Signs and symptoms include nausea, vomiting, and pain in the upper right abdomen, back, or right underarm. Removal of the gallbladder is common.

Hepatitis

Hepatitis is inflammation *(itis)* and infection of the liver *(hepat)* caused by a virus. See Table 50-1 (p. 756) for signs and symptoms and persons at risk. Some people have no symptoms. There are 5 major types of hepatitis.

See *Promoting Safety and Comfort: Hepatitis.*

Text continued on p. 758.

PROMOTING SAFETY AND COMFORT

Hepatitis

Safety

Hepatitis is contagious. Protect yourself and others. Practice hand-washing and follow Standard Precautions and the Bloodborne Pathogen Standard. Transmission-Based Precautions are ordered as necessary (Chapter 17). Assist the person with hygiene and hand-washing after BMs, before preparing or eating food, and as needed. Also, people should avoid sharing personal items with an infected person—toothbrush, razor, nail clippers, and so on.

TABLE 50-1	Hepatitis

Signs and Symptoms
- *Jaundice—yellowish color of the skin or whites of the eyes* (Fig. 50-7)
- Fatigue
- Pain: abdominal, joint
- Appetite: loss of
- Nausea and vomiting
- Diarrhea
- Bowel movements (BMs): light, clay-colored
- Urine: dark
- Fever
- Itching: severe
- Weight loss

Type and Cause	Persons at Risk	Treatment, Prevention, and Care Measures
Hepatitis A—spread through contact with the infected person's feces by: - Eating food prepared by the infected person with poor hand-washing after a BM - Drinking untreated water - Eating food washed in untreated water - Placing a finger or object that is contaminated with the infected person's feces into the mouth - Close personal contact with an infected person—sex, providing care	- Travelers to developing countries - Persons who have sex with an infected person - Men who have sex with men - Users of illegal drugs - Homeless persons - Persons who live with or care for someone with hepatitis A - Persons who live with or care for a child recently adopted from a country where hepatitis A is common	- Rest - Drinking plenty of fluids - Healthy diet - No alcohol - Drugs as ordered - Careful handling of bedpans, toilets, commodes, diapers, and rectal thermometers - Checking persons with fecal incontinence, confusion, or dementia for contaminated items and areas - Hepatitis A vaccine to protect against the disease
Hepatitis B—spread through contact with the infected person's blood, semen, or other body fluids by: - Being born to a mother with hepatitis B - Having unprotected sex with an infected person - Sharing drug needles or materials with an infected person - Getting an accidental stick with a needle that was used on an infected person - Being tattooed or pierced with tools not cleaned properly after use on an infected person - Having contact with blood or open sores of an infected person - Using an infected person's razor, toothbrush, or nail clippers	- Are infected with human immunodeficiency virus (HIV) (Chapter 47). - Have lived with a person with hepatitis B. - Had sex with a person with hepatitis B. - Had more than 1 sex partner in the last 6 months. - Had sex with a partner with a history of a sexually transmitted disease (Chapter 51). - Are men who have sex with men. - Are injection drug users. - Have contact with blood, needles, or body fluids at work. - Have lived or traveled to areas where hepatitis B is common—Asia, Pacific Islands, Africa, Eastern Europe. - Have been on kidney dialysis. - Are taking drugs that weaken the immune system. - Have lived or worked in a prison. - Had a blood transfusion or an organ transplant before the mid-1980s. - Are infants born to infected mothers.	- Drugs as ordered - Hepatitis B vaccine to protect against the disease (Chapter 16) - Safe sex - Stop use of illicit drugs - Caution when choosing to have a tattoo or body piercing

TABLE 50-1	Hepatitis—cont'd	
Type and Cause	**Persons at Risk**	**Treatment, Prevention, and Care Measures**
Hepatitis C—spread through contact with an infected person's blood. See hepatitis B.	• Have injected or inhaled illicit drugs. • Had a blood transfusion or an organ transplant before July 1992. • Received a blood clotting factor before 1987. • Have been on kidney dialysis. • Have contact with blood, needles, or body fluids at work. • Have tattoos or body piercings. • Have lived or worked in a prison. • Were born to a mother with hepatitis C. • Are infected with HIV (Chapter 47). • Had more than 1 sex partner in the last 6 months. • Had sex with a partner with a history of a sexually transmitted disease (Chapter 51). • Are men who have or had sex with men. • Are infants born to infected mothers.	• Drugs as ordered • Stop illicit drug use • Safe sex • Caution when choosing to have a tattoo or body piercing
Hepatitis D—spread through an infected person's blood or body fluids by: • Sharing drug needles or materials with an infected person • Having unprotected sex with an infected person • Getting an accidental stick with a needle that was used on an infected person	• Are injection drug users. • Have lived with someone who has hepatitis D. • Had sex with someone who has hepatitis D.	• Drugs as ordered
Hepatitis E—different types are spread by: • Drinking contaminated water. More common in developing countries such as parts of Africa, Asia, Central America, and the Middle East. • Eating under-cooked or wild game such as deer. More common in developed countries such as the United States, Australia, Japan, and parts of Europe and East Asia.	• Adolescents and young adults in developing countries • Older men in developed countries	• Rest • Drinking plenty of fluids • Healthy diet • No alcohol • Drugs as ordered

Modified from National Institute of Diabetes and Digestive and Kidney Diseases: What is viral hepatitis, *May 2017;* Hepatitis A, *September 2019;* Hepatitis B, *May 2017;* Hepatitis C, *May 2017;* Hepatitis D, *May 2017;* Hepatitis E, *June 2017.*

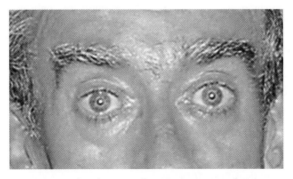

FIGURE 50-7 Jaundice. (From Butcher GP: *Gastroenterology: an illustrated colour text,* London, 2004, Churchill Livingstone.)

Cirrhosis

Cirrhosis is a liver condition caused by chronic liver damage (Fig. 50-8). *(Cirrho* means *yellow-orange. Osis* means *condition.)* Scarred liver tissue blocks blood flow through the liver. Normal liver functions are affected.

- Fighting infection
- Processing, storing, and delivering nutrients to the body
- Cleaning the blood of toxins, fats, cholesterol, and drugs
- Making proteins for blood clotting
- Producing bile for fat digestion

Chronic alcohol abuse, chronic hepatitis B and C, and extra fat in the liver are common causes. Obesity is becoming a common cause. Signs and symptoms may occur as the disease progresses.

- Weakness and fatigue
- Loss of appetite and weight loss
- Nausea and vomiting
- *Ascites*—abdominal bloating from fluid buildup in the abdomen (Fig. 50-9)
- *Edema* (swelling) in the feet and legs
- Itching (severe)
- Spider-like blood vessels on the skin
- Jaundice
- Pain or discomfort in the right upper abdomen

Cirrhosis has many serious complications. Infection, bruising, and bleeding occur. Blood vessels in the esophagus and stomach enlarge and burst. Gallstones may develop. Toxins build up in the brain, causing confusion, personality changes, and memory loss. Liver cancer is a risk.

Treatment is aimed at treating the cause to keep the cirrhosis from getting worse. Complications are treated. A low-sodium diet is needed for edema and ascites. Diuretic drugs (water pills) are ordered to remove fluid. Antibiotics are ordered for infection. The person must avoid alcohol and may need a liver transplant.

The measures listed in Box 50-1 may be part of the person's care plan.

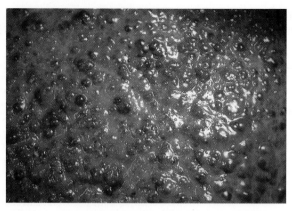

FIGURE 50-8 Liver damage from alcohol. (From Kumar V, Abbas AK, Aster JC: *Robbins and Cotran pathologic basis of disease,* ed 9, Philadelphia, 2015, Saunders.)

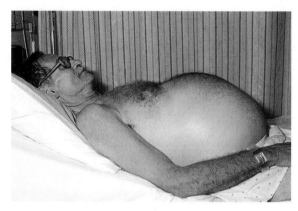

FIGURE 50-9 Fluid in the membrane lining the abdominal cavity *(ascites).* (From Swartz MH: *Textbook of physical diagnosis,* ed 7, Philadelphia, 2014, Saunders.)

BOX 50-1	**Cirrhosis**

General Care

- Follow the care plan to prevent complications from bed rest—pneumonia, blood clots, pressure injuries.
- Provide good skin care and prevent itching.
  - Follow the care plan for what cleanser to use.
  - Apply lotion to the skin.
  - Discourage the scratching of itchy skin.
- Provide mouth care before meals and every 2 hours.
- Follow diet and fluid restriction orders.
- Turn the person at least every 2 hours or as noted on the care plan.
- Promote comfort and the ability to breathe.
  - Semi-Fowler's or Fowler's position
  - Pillows under the arms for support
  - Coughing and deep-breathing exercises
- Assist with ambulation and activities of daily living (ADL) as needed.

Measurements and Observations

- Observe vomitus, urine, and BMs for blood.
- Observe for signs of decreased mental function—confusion, memory loss, behavior changes, and so on.
- Measure vital signs every 2 to 4 hours.
- Measure intake and output (I&O).
- Measure weight daily.

Safety

- Use bed rails according to the care plan.
- Keep the call light and other needed items within reach.
- Complete a safety check before leaving the room. (See the inside of the back cover.)

ENDOCRINE DISORDERS

The endocrine system is made up of glands. The endocrine glands secrete hormones that affect other organs and glands. Diabetes, the most common endocrine disorder, involves the pancreas.

See *Body Structure and Function Review: The Endocrine System (Pancreas).*

BODY STRUCTURE AND FUNCTION REVIEW

The Endocrine System (Pancreas)

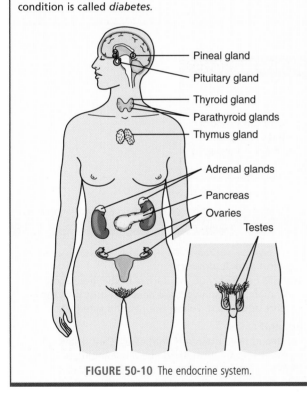

The *endocrine glands* (Fig. 50-10) secrete chemical substances called *hormones* into the bloodstream. Hormones regulate the activities of other organs and glands in the body.

The *pancreas* secretes *insulin.* Insulin regulates the amount of sugar in the blood available for use by the cells. Insulin is needed for sugar to enter the cells. Without insulin, sugar cannot enter the cells. If sugar cannot enter the cells, excess amounts build up in the blood. This condition is called *diabetes.*

- Pineal gland
- Pituitary gland
- Thyroid gland
- Parathyroid glands
- Thymus gland
- Adrenal glands
- Pancreas
- Ovaries
- Testes

FIGURE 50-10 The endocrine system.

Diabetes

In diabetes, the body cannot produce or use insulin properly. Without any or enough insulin, sugar builds up in the blood. Blood glucose (sugar) is high. Cells do not have enough sugar for energy and cannot function.

Types of Diabetes. A family history of the disease is a common risk factor for the 3 types of diabetes.

- *Type 1 diabetes.* Occurs most often in children and young adults but can develop in adults. The pancreas makes no insulin. Too much glucose stays in the blood. Onset is rapid.
- *Type 2 diabetes.* The body does not make enough insulin or use insulin well. The most common type of diabetes, it can occur at any age including childhood. Risk factors include being age 45 or older, having a family history of diabetes, being over-weight or obese, and being physically inactive.
- *Gestational diabetes.* Develops during pregnancy. (*Gestation* comes from *gestare.* It means *to bear.*) This type usually goes away after the baby is born. However, the mother is at risk for type 2 diabetes later in life.

Signs and Symptoms. Signs and symptoms of diabetes are:
- Being very thirsty
- Frequent urination
- Feeling very hungry or tired
- Weight loss without trying
- Sores that heal slowly
- Dry, itchy skin
- Tingling or loss of feeling in the feet
- Blurred vision

Complications. Diabetes must be controlled to prevent complications. High blood glucose levels can cause serious health problems. Heart disease, stroke, kidney disease, eye problems, and nerve damage are examples. So are dental disease and foot problems.

Treatment. Type 1 diabetes is treated with daily insulin therapy, healthy eating (Chapter 30), and exercise. Type 2 diabetes is treated with healthy eating, exercise, and weight loss if needed. The person with type 2 may take oral drugs or need insulin. Types 1 and 2 involve controlling blood pressure, cholesterol, and the risk factors for coronary artery disease.

Good foot care is needed. Corns, blisters, calluses, and other foot problems can lead to an infection and amputation. See Chapters 25 and 40.

The person's blood sugar level can fall too low or go too high.
- *Hypoglycemia means low (hypo) sugar (glyc) in the blood (emia).*
- *Hyperglycemia means high (hyper) sugar (glyc) in the blood (emia).*

Blood glucose is monitored as often as ordered. For example, type 1 testing may be done 4 to 10 times a day. For type 2, testing can range from daily to 4 times a day—before meals and at bedtime.

See Table 50-2 (p. 760) for the causes, signs, and symptoms of hypoglycemia and hyperglycemia. Both can lead to death if not corrected. Call for the nurse at once.

See *Focus on Children and Older Persons: Diabetes,* p. 760.

TABLE 50-2   Hypoglycemia and Hyperglycemia

Hypoglycemia (Low Blood Sugar)		Hyperglycemia (High Blood Sugar)	
Causes	Signs and Symptoms	Causes	Signs and Symptoms
• Too much insulin or diabetic drugs • Increased exercise • Skipping or delaying a meal • Eating too little food • Vomiting • Drinking alcohol	**Mild to Moderate** • Shaky or jittery • Sweaty • Hunger • Headache • Blurred vision • Sleepy or tired • Dizzy or being light-headed • Confused or disoriented • Skin: pale • Uncoordinated movements • Irritable or nervous • Arguing or being combative • Behavior or personality changes • Trouble concentrating • Weakness • Pulse: rapid or irregular **Severe** • Cannot eat or drink • Seizures or convulsions • Unconsciousness	• Not enough insulin or diabetic drugs • Too little exercise • Eating too much food • Emotional stress • Infection or sickness • Undiagnosed diabetes	**Early** • Frequent urination • Increased thirst • Blurred vision • Being tired • Headache • Hunger **Late** • Weakness • Dry mouth • Shortness of breath • Nausea and vomiting • Confusion • Abdominal pain • Coma

---

FOCUS ON CHILDREN AND OLDER PERSONS

Diabetes

Children

Your assignment may include preparing meals for a child with diabetes. Follow the child's diet carefully. Also prepare snacks for the child to take to school. The snack is needed in case the child's blood sugar level drops.

FOCUS ON PRIDE

The Person, Family, and Yourself

Personal and Professional Responsibility

Understanding health problems allows you to safely assist with care. You may want to know more about a person's or your own health problem. Or a person may have a disorder you did not learn about in your training. Ask the nurse for more information. You can also look up the problem in a medical dictionary or on the Internet. Take pride in learning more.

Rights and Respect

Health care workers are at risk for exposure to the hepatitis B virus through blood, needles, and body fluids. The hepatitis B vaccine protects against hepatitis B (Chapter 16). You will be offered the vaccine. You have the right to refuse. You must sign a document saying you refuse. You can have the vaccine at a later time.

Independence and Social Interaction

Many digestive and endocrine disorders require diet changes. Dietary practices are cultural and personal. The person may feel loss of control over an important part of his or her life-style. The person text family need education, support, and encouragement.

Delegation and Teamwork

As a person's needs change, the care plan changes. Good communication and teamwork are needed. Assist with the person's care as directed. Follow the person's care plan.

Ethics and Laws

Some problems need attention right away. Care delays can cause harm. For example, a person who is vomiting uses the call light to signal for help. Minutes pass before anyone responds. The person aspirates. Vomitus obstructs the airway. The person dies.

Prompt responses are needed. Otherwise negligence, neglect, and other legal problems can result (Chapter 5).

FOCUS ON PRIDE: Application

Choose a disorder in this chapter. What life-style changes are needed? Discuss the impact on the person and family. How does the health team help the person and family adjust?

REVIEW QUESTIONS

Circle the BEST answer.

1 A person has gastro-esophageal reflux disease. Which should you question?
  a Loose clothing
  b Supine position after meals
  c Small meals
  d No smoking or alcohol

2 A person with gastro-esophageal reflux disease has these food choices. Which is *best* for the person?
  a Baked chicken
  b Pasta with tomato sauce
  c Fried ravioli
  d Chicken wings with hot sauce

3 A person is vomiting. You should
  a Position the person supine
  b Leave to get the nurse
  c Do nothing
  d Turn the person's head to the side

4 Vomiting is dangerous because of
  a Aspiration
  b Diverticular disease
  c Ascites
  d Jaundice

5 Vomitus looks like coffee grounds. This signals
  a Gastro-esophageal reflux disease
  b Gallstones
  c Bleeding
  d A ruptured pouch

6 A person has diverticular disease. How will you assist with care?
  a Giving antibiotics
  b Promoting normal bowel elimination
  c Dietary teaching and planning
  d Assessing risk factors

7 Gallbladder attacks usually occur
  a On awakening
  b During a fast
  c Suddenly after eating
  d When the person is lying down

8 Which is a sign of gallstones?
  a Extreme thirst
  b Abdominal pain
  c Black, tarry stools
  d Hoarseness and a choking sensation

9 Hepatitis is inflammation of the
  a Liver
  b Gallbladder
  c Pancreas
  d Stomach

10 Which is spread by food or water contaminated with feces from an infected person?
  a Hepatitis A   c Hepatitis C
  b Hepatitis B   d Hepatitis D

11 Hepatitis requires
  a Sterile gloving
  b Double-bagging
  c Standard Precautions
  d Masks, gowns, and goggles

12 Which is a common cause of cirrhosis?
  a Diabetes
  b Alcohol abuse
  c Gallstones
  d GERD

13 A person has cirrhosis. Which should you question?
  a Measure I&O.
  b Weigh the person daily.
  c Apply lotion after bathing.
  d Encourage fluids.

14 A person has cirrhosis. You should observe stools and vomitus for blood.
  a True
  b False

15 Which is a sign of diabetes?
  a Decreased urine output
  b Weight gain
  c Hunger
  d Jaundice

16 A person with diabetes needs
  a A sodium-controlled diet
  b Fluid restriction
  c Surgery
  d Good foot care

17 A person with diabetes is vomiting after a meal. The person is at risk for
  a Hypoglycemia
  b Hyperglycemia
  c Jaundice
  d Bleeding

18 With type 2 diabetes, blood glucose
  a Does not need to be monitored
  b Is low if the disorder is not treated
  c Is often tested before meals and at bedtime
  d Returns to normal after pregnancy

Answers to Chapter 50 questions are on p. 887.

FOCUS ON **PRACTICE**

Problem Solving

A resident with diabetes is confused, weak, and shaky. What do you do? What might these signs and symptoms indicate? How does understanding the person's health problems help you give better care?

OBJECTIVES

- Define the key terms and key abbreviations in this chapter.
- Describe the care required for urinary tract infections.
- Describe the care required for prostate enlargement.
- Describe the care required for urinary diversions.
- Describe the care required for renal calculi.

- Describe the care required for acute and chronic kidney failure.
- Describe sexually transmitted diseases.
- Explain how to promote PRIDE in the person, the family, and yourself.

KEY TERMS

dialysis The process of removing waste products from the blood

dysuria Difficult or painful (dys) urination (uria)

hematuria Blood (hemat) in the urine (uria)

oliguria Scant (olig) urine (uria)

pyuria Pus (py) in the urine (uria)

urinary diversion A surgically created pathway for urine to leave the body

urostomy A surgically created opening (stomy) that connects to the urinary tract (uro)

KEY ABBREVIATIONS

AIDS	Acquired immunodeficiency syndrome	mL	Milliliter
BPH	Benign prostatic hyperplasia	STD	Sexually transmitted disease
CKD	Chronic kidney disease	STI	Sexually transmitted infection
HIV	Human immunodeficiency virus	TURP	Transurethral resection of the prostate
HPV	Human papilloma viruses	UTI	Urinary tract infection

Urinary and reproductive disorders are common. Understanding the disorders gives meaning to the required care.

URINARY SYSTEM DISORDERS

Disorders can occur in urinary system structures—kidneys, ureters, bladder, and urethra. Men can develop prostate problems.

See *Body Structure and Function Review: The Urinary System*.

Urinary Tract Infections

Urinary tract infections (UTIs) are common. Infection in 1 area can spread through the urinary tract. Microbes can enter the system through the urethra. Urological exams, intercourse, poor perineal hygiene, immobility, and poor fluid intake are common causes. Persons with urinary catheters are at high risk (Chapter 28). UTI is a common healthcare-associated infection (Chapter 16).

Women are at high risk. Microbes can easily enter the female urethra and travel a short distance to the bladder. Prostate gland secretions help protect men from UTIs. However, an enlarged prostate increases the risk of UTI.

See Box 51-1 for the types of UTIs and their signs and symptoms. UTIs are treated with antibiotics. Fluids, especially water, are encouraged to flush bacteria from the urinary tract. Normal elimination is promoted. The person should urinate when the urge is felt. For prevention and treatment, proper perineal care and catheter care are needed.

BODY STRUCTURE AND FUNCTION REVIEW

The Urinary System

The urinary system (Fig. 51-1):
- Removes waste products from the blood.
- Maintains water balance.
- Maintains electrolyte balance. *Electrolytes* are substances that dissolve in water—sodium, potassium, calcium, and magnesium.
- Maintains acid-base balance. (See Chapter 10.)

The *kidneys* are 2 bean-shaped organs in the upper abdomen. They lie against the back muscles on each side of the spine.

Each kidney has over a million tiny *nephrons*—the basic working units of the kidney. Each nephron has a cluster of capillaries called a *glomerulus.* Blood passes through the glomeruli and is filtered by the capillaries. Most of the water and other needed substances are re-absorbed by the blood. The rest of the fluid and the waste products form *urine* in the tubule that drains into the *renal pelvis* in the kidney.

A *ureter* is attached to the renal pelvis of each kidney. The ureters carry urine from the kidneys to the *bladder.* Urine is stored in the bladder for urination. Urine passes from the bladder through the *urethra.* Urine passes from the body through the *meatus* at the end of the urethra.

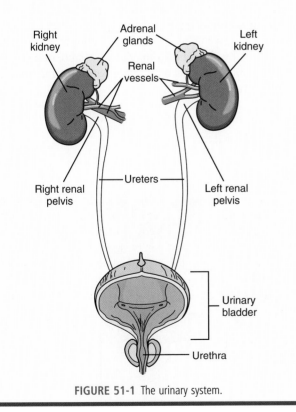

FIGURE 51-1 The urinary system.

BOX 51-1	**Urinary Tract Infections**

Common Signs and Symptoms
- Urinary frequency
- Urgency
- Burning on urination
- *Oliguria*—scant (olig) *urine* (uria)
- *Dysuria*—difficult or painful (dys) *urination* (uria)
- *Hematuria*—blood (hemat) *in the urine* (uria)
- *Pyuria*—pus (py) *in the urine* (uria)
- Cloudy urine
- Urine that appears red, pink, or dark from blood in the urine
- Fever
- Fatigue
- Weakness
- Pressure in the lower abdomen
- Urine odor
- Pelvic pain—women
- Rectal pain—men

Types of Urinary Tract Infections
- Cystitis—a bladder *(cyst)* infection *(itis)* caused by bacteria. Additional symptoms:
  - Pelvic pressure
  - Lower abdominal discomfort
- Pyelonephritis—inflammation *(itis)* of the kidney *(nephr)* (*pyelo* relates to the renal pelvis [see Fig. 51-1]). Additional symptoms:
  - Flank pain—pain in the back between the ribs and the hip (Fig. 51-2)
  - High fever
  - Nausea and vomiting
  - Shaking and chills

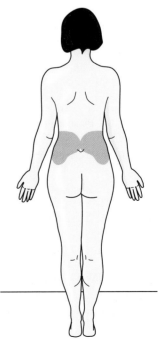

FIGURE 51-2 *Shading* shows the flank area.

Prostate Enlargement

The prostate is a walnut-shaped gland in men. It lies in front of the rectum and just below the bladder (Fig. 51-3). The prostate surrounds the urethra. The prostate grows larger (enlarges) as the man grows older. This is called benign prostatic hyperplasia (BPH). *Benign* means *non-malignant*. *Hyper* means *excessive*. *Plasia* means *formation* or *development*. Benign prostatic hypertrophy is another name for enlarged prostate. (*Trophy* means *growth*.)

Common in older men, BPH symptoms often start after age 50. The enlarged prostate presses against the urethra, obstructing urine flow (see Fig. 51-3). These problems are common.

- Urinary frequency—voiding 8 or more times a day
- Urgency—cannot delay voiding
- Trouble starting a stream
- Weak or "stop and start" urine stream
- Dribbling after voiding
- Frequent voiding during sleep (*nocturia*)
- Urinary retention—the bladder does not empty; urine remains in the bladder
- Urinary incontinence
- Pain during urination (*dysuria*)
- Urine has an unusual color or smell
- Blood in the urine

For mild BPH, drugs can shrink the prostate or stop its growth. Some microwave and laser treatments destroy excess prostate tissue and widen the urethra.

Transurethral resection of the prostate (TURP) is a common surgical procedure for severe BPH. Inserted through the penis, a lighted scope with a wire loop is used to cut prostate tissue and seal blood vessels. The removed tissue is flushed out of the bladder. Flushing fluid enters the bladder through a catheter. Urine and the flushing fluid flow out of the bladder through the same catheter. Some bleeding and blood clots are normal. The person's care plan may include:

- No straining or sudden movements
- Drinking a least 8 cups of water daily
- No straining to have a bowel movement
- A balanced diet to prevent constipation
- No heavy lifting

Urinary Diversion

Cancer and bladder injuries are common reasons for blocked urine flow or surgical removal of the bladder. Urine must be re-routed from the body. A ***urinary diversion*** *is a surgically created pathway for urine to leave the body.*

Often an ostomy is involved. A ***urostomy*** *is a surgically created opening* (stomy) *that connects to the urinary tract* (uro). The 2 main types of urostomies are:

- *Ileal conduit.* A small section of the small intestine (*ileal*) is re-positioned to serve as a channel (*conduit*) for urine. The ureters are connected to the conduit and the conduit is connected to a stoma (Fig. 51-4).
- *Cutaneous ureterostomy.* A *ureter* is brought through the abdominal wall and a stoma (*ostomy*) is created on the skin (*cutaneous*). This type may involve 1 or 2 ureters and stomas (Fig. 51-5).

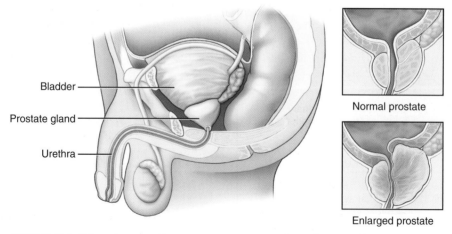

Bladder

Prostate gland

Urethra

Normal prostate

Enlarged prostate

FIGURE 51-3 Enlarged prostate. The prostate presses against the urethra. Urine flow is obstructed.

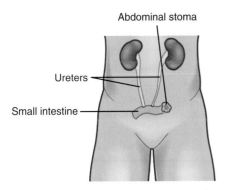

FIGURE 51-4 Ileal conduit. (Modified from Lewis SL, et al: *Medical-surgical nursing: assessment and management of clinical problems,* ed 10, St Louis, 2017, Elsevier.)

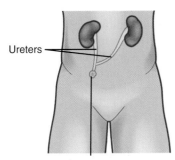

FIGURE 51-5 Cutaneous ureterostomy. The left ureter is connected to the right ureter. One stoma is needed. (Modified from Lewis SL, et al: *Medical-surgical nursing: assessment and management of clinical problems,* ed 10, St Louis, 2017, Elsevier.)

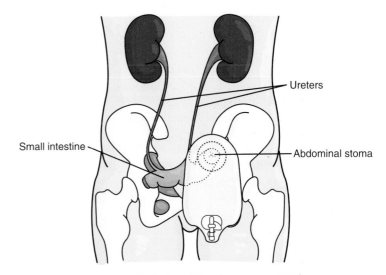

FIGURE 51-6 Ileal conduit with a urostomy pouch.

PROMOTING SAFETY AND COMFORT

Urinary Diversion

Safety
Urine may contain microbes and blood. And you have contact with mucous membranes. Follow Standard Precautions and the Bloodborne Pathogen Standard.

Comfort
The best time to change a pouch is after sleep and before eating or drinking. Urine flow is less when the person has not had anything to eat or drink for 2 to 3 hours.

The stoma does not have sensation. Touching the stoma does not cause pain or discomfort.

Urine drains constantly from the stoma into a pouch applied over the stoma (Fig. 51-6). Pouches are emptied when becoming ⅓ (one-third) to ½ (one-half) full. Pouches become heavy as they fill with urine. For sleep, the person can attach drainage tubing to the pouch for urine to flow to a bigger urine collection device. A heavy pouch can loosen the seal between the pouch and the skin. Urine can leak onto the skin.

Pouches are changed every 5 to 7 days. A pouch is replaced any time it leaks. Urine on the skin can cause irritation, breakdown, and infection.

Good skin care is needed. You must help prevent skin breakdown. Observe and report skin changes around the stoma. See "The Person With an Ostomy" in Chapter 29.

See *Promoting Safety and Comfort: Urinary Diversion.*

Kidney Stones

Kidney stones *(calculi)* are hard, pebble-like materials that develop in 1 or both kidneys (Fig. 51-7, p. 766). They vary in size—from a grain of sand to pea-sized. Larger stones can develop. Stones may be smooth or jagged.

Men are at higher risk than women. A family history of kidney stones increases the risk. So does having kidney stones before. Not drinking enough liquids is another risk factor.

Signs and symptoms include:
- Severe, cramping pain in the back and side just below the ribs (Fig. 51-8, p. 766)
- Pain in the lower abdomen, thigh, and urethra
- Nausea and vomiting
- Fever and chills
- *Dysuria*—difficult or painful *(dys)* urination *(uria)*
- Urinary frequency and urgency
- Pain or burning on urination
- *Hematuria*—blood *(hemat)* in the urine *(uria)*
- Cloudy urine
- Foul-smelling urine

Drugs are given for pain relief. The person needs to drink 2000 to 3000 mL (milliliters) a day. Fluids help flush stones out through the urine. All urine is strained (Chapter 38). Medical or surgical removal of the stone may be necessary. Diet changes may prevent stones.

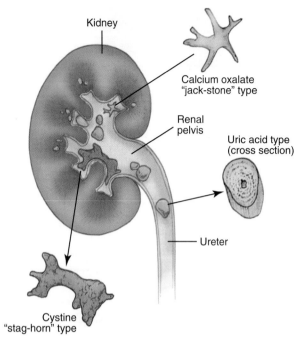

FIGURE 51-7 Kidney stones. Stones vary in shape and size. (Modified from Nix S: *Williams' basic nutrition & diet therapy*, ed 15, St Louis, 2017, Elsevier.)

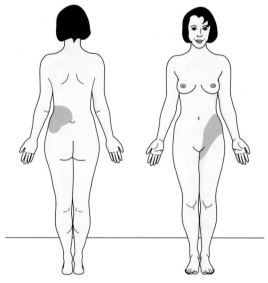

FIGURE 51-8 Shaded areas show where the pain from a left kidney stone is located.

Kidney Failure

In kidney failure (renal failure), the kidneys do not function or are severely impaired. Waste products are not removed from the blood. Fluid is retained. Heart failure and hypertension easily result. The person is very ill.

- *Acute kidney failure.* Onset is rapid in a few days or less. Blood flow to the kidneys is severely decreased, the kidneys are damaged, or the urinary tract is blocked. The causes are many. Usually the person is already critically ill.
- *Chronic kidney disease (CKD).* Kidney function is slowly lost over several months or years. Diabetes and hypertension are the most common causes. Other causes include kidney stones, infection, and a blocked urinary tract. Signs and symptoms may not appear until the disease is advanced (Box 51-2).

Treatment

Treatment for acute kidney failure and CKD involves drugs and fluid and diet restrictions. The person's care plan may include the measures in Box 51-3.

Acute kidney failure may be reversed. CKD has no cure. Kidney failure, also called end-stage renal disease (ESRD), is the last stage of CKD. The person will need a kidney transplant or dialysis. ***Dialysis*** *is the process of removing waste products from the blood.*

- *Hemodialysis* filters blood *(hemo)* through an artificial kidney (Fig. 51-9).
- *Peritoneal dialysis* uses the lining of the abdominal cavity *(peritoneal membrane)* to remove waste and fluid from the blood (Fig. 51-10).

BOX 51-2	Chronic Kidney Disease—Signs and Symptoms

- Appetite—loss of
- Blood in the stools
- Breath odor
- Bruising
- Concentration: problems with
- Drowsiness
- Fatigue
- Feeling ill
- Headaches
- Hiccups
- Muscle cramps or twitching
- Nausea and vomiting
- Numbness in the hands and feet
- Shortness of breath
- Skin—dry, itching; dark or light color
- Sleep problems
- Swelling in the hands and feet
- Thirst: excessive
- Urinary output: decreased
- Weight loss

BOX 51-3	Kidney Failure—Care Measures

- A diet low in protein, potassium, and sodium
- Fluid restriction
- Measuring blood pressure in the supine, sitting, and standing positions
- Measuring daily weight
- Measuring and recording intake and output
- Turning and re-positioning at least every 2 hours
- Measures to prevent pressure injuries
- Range-of-motion exercises
- Measures to prevent itching (bath oils, lotions, creams)
- Measures to prevent injury and bleeding
- Frequent oral hygiene
- Measures to prevent infection
- Deep-breathing and coughing exercises
- Measures to prevent diarrhea or constipation
- Measures to meet emotional needs
- Measures to promote rest

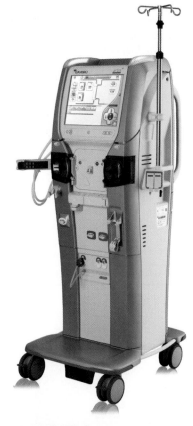

FIGURE 51-9 Dialysis machine. (Image courtesy Baxter International Inc.)

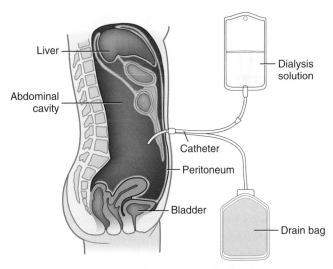

FIGURE 51-10 Peritoneal dialysis system. (Modified from Lewis SL, et al: *Medical-surgical nursing: assessment and management of clinical problems,* ed 10, St Louis, 2017, Elsevier.)

REPRODUCTIVE DISORDERS

Sexual activities involve the structures and functions of the reproductive system (Chapter 10). The male reproductive system:

- Produces and transports sperm.
- Deposits sperm in the female reproductive tract.
- Secretes hormones.
  The female reproductive system:
- Produces eggs (*ova*).
- Secretes hormones.
- Protects and nourishes the fetus during pregnancy.
  Aging affects the reproductive system (Chapters 12 and 55). Injuries, diseases, and surgeries can affect reproductive structures and functions.

Sexually Transmitted Diseases

Sexually transmitted diseases (STDs) are passed from person to person during sexual contact with the penis, vagina, anus, or mouth. Also known as sexually transmitted infections (STIs), the most common STDs/STIs are described in Box 51-4, p. 768.

Signs and symptoms vary depending on the cause. A person may have no symptoms or 1 or more of the following.

- Flu-like symptoms—fever, chills, aches and pains
- Unusual discharge from the penis or vagina
- Sores or bumps on the genital, oral, or anal area
- Itching and redness in the genital area
- Blisters or sores in or around the mouth
- Abnormal vaginal odor or bleeding
- Anal itching, soreness, or bleeding
- Abdominal pain
- Painful or burning urination
- Rash over the trunk, hands, or feet

A person with an STD/STI can spread it to other people through oral, vaginal, or anal sex. Needle sharing (injection drug use) can spread HIV and other blood-borne infections.

STDs/STIs caused by bacteria, yeast, or parasites can be cured with antibiotics or other drugs. Those caused by a virus cannot be cured. The person will always have the virus. However, treatments are available to reduce symptoms and the risk of transmission to others.

Correct use of latex condoms reduces the risk of becoming infected or spreading STDs/STIs. Not having vaginal, anal, or oral sex is the best way to avoid infection. In health care settings, Standard Precautions and the Bloodborne Pathogen Standard are followed.

See *Focus on Children and Older Persons: Sexually Transmitted Diseases,* p. 768.

BOX 51-4	Sexually Transmitted Diseases/Sexually Transmitted Infections

- **Chlamydia**—a bacterial infection, both men and women can become infected. Babies can become infected during childbirth.
  - Women—may occur in the cervix, rectum, or throat.
  - Men—may occur in the urethra, rectum, or throat.

- **Genital herpes**—caused by the herpes simplex virus. Sores can appear on the genital or rectal area, buttocks, and thighs (Fig. 51-11). The virus can spread when sores are not present. Babies can become infected during childbirth.
  - "Outbreaks" occur where the virus entered the body.
  - Sores are blisters that break and become painful before healing.
  - The virus stays in the body for life. Repeated outbreaks are common.

- **Gonorrhea**—a bacterial infection that can infect the genital tract, mouth, or anus. Babies can become infected during childbirth. There may be no symptoms or:
  - Men—pain on urination and discharge from the penis. If untreated, prostate or testicle problems can develop.
  - Women—early symptoms may be mild. Bleeding between menstrual periods, pain on urination, and vaginal discharge are later signs. If untreated, pregnancy and fertility problems can develop.

- **HIV/AIDS**—caused by the human immunodeficiency virus (HIV), the immune system is harmed. White blood cells that fight infection are destroyed. The person is at risk for infections and certain cancers. AIDS (acquired immunodeficiency syndrome) is the final stage of HIV infection. The first signs of HIV may be swollen glands and flu-like symptoms. Severe symptoms may appear months or years later. HIV is often spread:
  - By unprotected sex with an infected person
  - By needle-sharing with injection drug users
  - By contact with an infected person's blood
  - During pregnancy and childbirth

- **Human papilloma viruses (HPV)**—a group of viruses that cause warts on different parts of the body, including the genitals. The most common STD/STI in the United States, sexually active persons are at risk.
  - Low-risk HPV can cause genital warts.
  - High-risk HPV can cause various cancers—cervical, anal, oral and throat, vaginal, vulvar (woman's external genitals), penile.

- **Syphilis**—a bacterial infection that infects the genital areas, lips, mouth, or anus in men and women. Babies can become infected during pregnancy.
  - A single, small, painless sore develops at first. If untreated, a non-itchy skin rash may occur on the hands and feet. Symptoms may come and go for many years.
  - During the late stages, syphilis can cause serious health problems and even death.

- **Trichomoniasis**—caused by a parasite. Men usually do not have symptoms. Women develop vaginitis.
  - Yellow-green or gray vaginal discharge
  - Discomfort during sex
  - Vaginal odor
  - Painful urination
  - Genital itching, burning, and soreness

Modified from MedlinePlus: Sexually transmitted diseases, Bethesda, Md, October 18, 2019, U.S. National Library of Medicine.

FOCUS ON **CHILDREN AND OLDER PERSONS**

Sexually Transmitted Diseases

Older Persons
Many older people are sexually active. They get and can spread STDs/STIs in the same ways as younger persons. However, many do not think they are at risk. Always practice Standard Precautions and follow the Bloodborne Pathogen Standard. Do not assume that older people are too old to have sex.

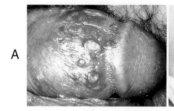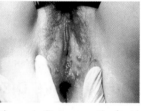

FIGURE 51-11 Herpes. **A,** Sores on the penis. **B,** Sores on the female perineum. (Courtesy United States Public Health Service, Washington, DC.)

FOCUS ON **PRIDE**

The Person, Family, and Yourself

Personal and Professional Responsibility

UTIs are a common healthcare-associated infection. Females are at high risk. Proper perineal care can prevent UTIs (Chapter 24).

You are responsible for providing care that protects the person's health and safety. Take pride in performing safe and careful perineal care.

Rights and Respect

An STD/STI can make the person feel embarrassed, ashamed, or guilty. Do not judge the person. Treat the person with dignity and respect.

Independence and Social Interaction

Persons with late stage CKD cannot live without dialysis. Hemodialysis is often done 3 times a week. Each session can take 4 hours or more. Peritoneal dialysis is often done in the home setting 3 to 5 times a day.

Dialysis takes a lot of time. Work, family time, and other activities are limited by the need for dialysis. These social changes affect quality of life. The person and family need support and encouragement.

Delegation and Teamwork

Kidney stones can cause severe pain. Promote comfort. Be patient, kind, and understanding if the person is behaving rudely. Report pain. Tell the nurse if you need help dealing with the person's behavior.

Ethics and Laws

Urinary and reproductive disorders are personal. Give information only to those directly involved in the person's care. Take pride in protecting the person's right to privacy and confidentiality.

FOCUS ON **PRIDE**: *Application*

Pain, coping with a disorder, and the stress of treatments affect behavior. What other factors affect the person? You cannot control the person's reactions. You can control yours. List helpful responses. What responses are not helpful?

REVIEW QUESTIONS

Circle the BEST answer.

1 A person has cystitis. This is a
   a Kidney infection
   b Kidney stone
   c STD/STI
   d Bladder infection

2 The person with cystitis needs to restrict fluid intake.
   a True
   b False

3 BPH causes urinary problems because
   a The person has a weak urine stream
   b The person voids frequently at night
   c The enlarged prostate presses against the urethra
   d Voidings are in small amounts

4 After a TURP, which measure should you question?
   a No sudden movements
   b No oral fluids
   c No heavy lifting
   d No straining to have a bowel movement

5 A person with a urostomy
   a Has a new pathway for urine to exit the body
   b Needs dialysis
   c Had surgery for an enlarged prostate
   d Has pyuria

6 A person has kidney stones. You need to
   a Strain all urine
   b Empty the pouch
   c Collect a urine specimen
   d Change the urinary drainage bag

7 A person has kidney failure. Which is *true*?
   a Waste products are removed from the blood.
   b The body retains fluid.
   c Urinary diversion is needed.
   d The person has dysuria and hematuria.

8 Chronic kidney disease care includes
   a A diet high in protein, potassium, and sodium
   b Encouraging fluids
   c Measuring weight daily
   d Straining the urine

9 Which statement about STDs/STIs is *true*?
   a Older persons do not get them.
   b They only affect the genital area.
   c Some persons have no signs or symptoms.
   d They can all be cured with antibiotics.

10 STDs/STIs require
   a Masks and protective eyewear
   b Gowns
   c Double-bagging
   d Standard Precautions

Answers to Chapter 51 questions are on p. 887.

FOCUS ON PRACTICE

Problem Solving

A patient has a urinary catheter. Does this affect UTI risk? Describe the care measures for perineal care and catheter care that help lower the risk of UTI.

Mental Health Disorders

OBJECTIVES

- Define the key terms and key abbreviations in this chapter.
- Explain the difference between mental health and mental illness.
- List the causes of mental health disorders.
- Describe anxiety disorders and the defense mechanisms used to relieve anxiety.
- Describe psychotic disorders and schizophrenia.
- Describe mood disorders.

- Describe personality disorders.
- Describe substance use disorder and addiction.
- Describe the common eating disorders.
- Describe suicide and the persons at risk.
- Describe the care required by persons with mental health disorders.
- Explain how to promote PRIDE in the person, the family, and yourself.

KEY TERMS

addiction A chronic disease involving substance-seeking behaviors and use that is compulsive and hard to control despite the harmful effects

alcoholism Alcohol dependence that involves craving, loss of control, physical dependence, and tolerance

anxiety A feeling of worry, nervousness, or fear about an event or situation

compulsion An over-whelming urge to repeat certain rituals, acts, or behaviors

defense mechanism An unconscious reaction that blocks unpleasant or threatening feelings

delusion A false belief

delusion of grandeur An exaggerated belief about one's importance, fame, wealth, power, or talents

delusion of persecution A false belief that one is being mistreated, abused, or harassed

detoxification The process of removing a toxic substance from the body

drug addiction A strong urge or craving to use the substance and cannot stop using; tolerance develops

flashback Reliving the trauma over and over in thoughts during the day and in nightmares during sleep

hallucination Seeing, hearing, smelling, feeling, or tasting something that is not real

mental health Involves a person's emotional, psychological, and social well-being

mental health disorder A serious illness that can affect a person's thinking, mood, behavior, function, and ability to relate to others; mental illness, psychiatric disorder

mental illness See "mental health disorder"

obsession A frequent, upsetting, and unwanted thought, idea, or image

panic An intense and sudden feeling of fear, anxiety, or dread

personality The set of attitudes, values, behaviors, and traits of a person

phobia An intense fear of something that has little or no real danger

psychiatric disorder See "mental health disorder"

psychosis A state of severe mental impairment

stress The response or change in the body caused by any emotional, psychological, physical, social, or economic factor

stressor The event or factor that causes stress

suicide To end one's life on purpose

suicide contagion Exposure to suicide or suicidal behaviors within one's family or one's peer group or through media reports of suicide

withdrawal syndrome The physical and mental response after stopping or severely reducing use of a substance that was used regularly

KEY ABBREVIATIONS

AIDS	Acquired immunodeficiency syndrome	**HIV**	Human immunodeficiency virus
BPD	Borderline personality disorder	**OCD**	Obsessive-compulsive disorder
CDC	Centers for Disease Control and Prevention	**PTSD**	Post-traumatic stress disorder
GAD	Generalized anxiety disorder		

Mental health involves a person's emotional, psychological, and social well-being. Important from childhood through old age, mental health affects how a person:

- Thinks.
- Feels.
- Acts when coping with life.
- Handles stress. *Stress is the response or change in the body caused by any emotional, psychological, physical, social, or economic factor.*
- Relates to others.
- Makes choices.

Mental health disorders are serious illnesses that can affect a person's thinking, mood, behavior, function, and ability to relate to others. Also called *mental illness* and *psychiatric disorder,* early warning signs and risk factors are listed in Box 52-1. A person may experience 1 or more of the signs listed. And a person may have 1 or more risk factors.

Mental health disorders are common. They may be occasional or long-term. Many persons recover completely.

ANXIETY DISORDERS

Anxiety is a feeling of worry, nervousness, or fear about an event or situation. A normal reaction to stress, anxiety helps a person stay alert, remain focused, and cope.

Some anxiety is normal. For example, a person may feel anxious before taking a test at school. Anxiety disorders happen when anxiety cannot be controlled and interferes with every-day activities, work, school, and relationships. The anxiety does not go away and can get worse over time. The person has a sense of danger or doom. Such anxiety is disabling. See Box 52-2 for signs and symptoms.

Anxiety level depends on the stressor. A *stressor is the event or factor that causes stress.* It can be physical, emotional, social, or economic. Past experiences and the number of stressors affect how a person reacts.

Coping and defense mechanisms may help relieve anxiety. Unhealthy coping includes over-eating, drinking, smoking, and fighting. Healthy coping includes discussing the problem, exercising, playing music, and wanting to be alone or with others who are helpful.

Defense mechanisms are unconscious reactions that block unpleasant or threatening feelings (Box 52-3, p. 772). (*Unconscious reactions* are experiences and feelings that cannot be recalled.) Some use of defense mechanisms is normal. In mental health disorders, they are used poorly.

Anxiety disorders often occur with other mental health disorders. Depression, eating disorders, and substance abuse are examples. Anxiety may be linked to health problems. Heart disease, diabetes, thyroid problems, and respiratory disorders are examples.

BOX 52-1	Mental Health Disorders

Early Warning Signs

- Eating or sleeping too much or too little
- Pulling away from people or usual activities
- Having low or no energy
- Feeling numb or like nothing matters
- Having unexplained aches and pains
- Feeling helpless or hopeless
- Smoking, drinking, or using drugs more than usual
- Feeling unusually confused, forgetful, on edge, angry, upset, worried, or scared
- Yelling or fighting with family and friends
- Having severe mood swings that cause relationship problems
- Having persistent thoughts and memories
- Hearing voices or believing things that are not true
- Thinking of harming oneself or others
- Being unable to perform daily tasks

Risk Factors

- Genetics and family history. Mental health disorders tend to run in families.
- Life experiences. Stress or history of abuse are examples.
- Chemical imbalances in the brain.
- Traumatic brain injury.
- Fetal exposure to viruses or toxic chemicals.
- Use of alcohol or recreational drugs.
- Serious health problems.
- Having few friends and feeling lonely or isolated.

Modified from MentalHealth.gov: What is mental health, Washington, D.C., updated April 5, 2019, U.S. Department of Health & Human Services and MedlinePlus: Mental disorders, Washington, D.C., page updated December 3, 2019, U.S. Department of Health & Human Services.

BOX 52-2	Anxiety—Signs and Symptoms

- Weakness
- Breathing problems: shortness of breath, smothering or choking sensations
- Rapid heart rate; pounding heartbeat
- Nausea
- Abdominal pain
- Hot flashes (women)
- Dizziness
- Chest pain
- Nightmares
- Restlessness
- Fatigue
- Difficulty concentrating
- Irritability
- Muscle tension
- Sleep problems
- Sweating
- Trembling or shaking
- Tingling or numb hands

BOX 52-3	Defense Mechanisms

Compensation. *Compensate* means *to make up for, replace,* or *substitute.* A weakness is replaced with a strength.
EXAMPLE: Not good in sports, a child develops another talent.

Conversion. *Convert* means *to change.* An emotion is changed into a physical symptom.
EXAMPLE: Not wanting to read out loud in school, a child complains of a headache.

Denial. *Deny* means *refusing to accept or believe something that is true.* The person refuses to accept unpleasant or threatening things.
EXAMPLE: After a heart attack, a person continues to smoke.

Displacement. *Displace* means *to move* or *take the place of.* Behaviors or emotions are moved from 1 person, place, or thing to a safe person, place, or thing.
EXAMPLE: Angry at your boss, you yell at a friend.

Identification. *Identify* means *to relate* or *recognize.* A person assumes the ideas, behaviors, and traits of another person.
EXAMPLE: A neighbor is a basketball player. A child practices basketball in the backyard.

Projection. *Project* means *to blame another.* Another person or object is blamed for unacceptable behaviors, emotions, ideas, or wishes.
EXAMPLE: After over-sleeping, traffic is blamed for being late for work.

Rationalization. *Rational* means *sensible, reasonable,* or *logical.* An acceptable reason—not the real reason—is given for behaviors or actions.
EXAMPLE: Often late for work, a worker does not get a raise. The worker thinks: "My boss doesn't like me."

Reaction formation. A person acts in a way opposite to how he or she truly feels.
EXAMPLE: A worker does not like the boss. The worker gives the boss a gift.

Regression. *Regress* means *to move back* or *to retreat.* The person retreats or moves back to an earlier time or condition.
EXAMPLE: A 3-year-old wants a baby bottle when a new baby arrives.

Repression. *Repress* means *to hold down* or *keep back.* Unpleasant or painful thoughts or experiences are kept from the conscious mind. They cannot be recalled or remembered.
EXAMPLE: A child was sexually abused. Now 33 years old, there is no memory of the event.

Generalized Anxiety Disorder

The person with generalized anxiety disorder (GAD) has extreme anxiety, fear, or worry. GAD occurs on most days for at least 6 months. The person has worry and concern about many things. Health, work, social situations, and every-day life are examples. Serious problems in such areas can result.

Panic Disorder

Panic is an intense and sudden feeling of fear, anxiety, or dread. The person with panic disorder has sudden, recurring periods of panic when there is no real danger. Such *panic attacks* can last several minutes or longer. Such attacks can be unexpected or brought on by a trigger—fear of an object or situation. The person cannot function. Signs and symptoms of anxiety are severe (see Box 52-2).

The person may feel that he or she is having a heart attack, losing control, or dying. Panic attacks can occur at any time. The person may try to avoid places where panic attacks have occurred. For example, the person had a panic attack in a shopping mall. Malls are avoided.

Obsessive-Compulsive Disorder

The person with obsessive-compulsive disorder (OCD) *has frequent, upsetting, and unwanted thoughts, ideas, or images— obsession.* A person may be obsessed with microbes, dirt, violent thoughts, sexual acts, or things forbidden by religion. To control the obsessions and resulting anxiety, the person has *an over-whelming urge to repeat certain rituals, acts, or behaviors—compulsion.*

Hand-washing, counting, checking on things, cleaning, hoarding, and doing things in a certain order are examples of compulsions. OCD behaviors can take a long time, are very distressing, and can affect daily life.

Phobias

A *phobia is an intense fear of something that has little or no real danger.* Common phobias are fear of:

- Being in an open, crowded, or public place (*agoraphobia—agora* means *marketplace*)
- Being in pain or seeing others in pain (*algophobia—algo* means *pain*)
- Water (*aquaphobia—aqua* means *water*)
- Being in or trapped in an enclosed or narrow space (*claustrophobia—claustro* means *closing*)
- The slightest uncleanliness (*mysophobia—myso* means *anything that is disgusting*)
- Night or darkness (*nyctophobia—nycto* means *night* c *darkness*)
- Fire (*pyrophobia—pyro* means *fire*)
- Strangers (*xenophobia—xeno* means *strange*)

The person avoids what is feared. When faced with the fear, the person has high anxiety and cannot function (see Box 52-2).

BOX 52-4	Post-Traumatic Stress Disorder— Signs and Symptoms

- Flashbacks
- Nightmares or bad dreams
- Frightening thoughts
- Avoiding places, events, or things that remind of the trauma
- Avoiding thoughts or feelings related to the trauma
- Being easily startled or frightened
- Feeling tense or "on edge"
- Sleep problems
- Angry outbursts
- Problems remembering key parts of the trauma
- Negative thoughts about oneself or the world
- Feeling guilt or blame
- Loss of interest in enjoyed activities

Modified from National Institute of Mental Health: Post-traumatic stress disorder, National Institutes of Health, revised May 2019.

FOCUS ON **CHILDREN AND OLDER PERSONS**

Post-Traumatic Stress Disorder

Children

Older children and teenagers may have symptoms similar to adults. They also may show disruptive, disrespectful, or destructive behaviors. There may be feelings of guilt for not preventing injury or deaths. Older children and teens also may have thoughts of revenge.

Children less than 6 years old will have different signs and symptoms than adults.

- Wetting the bed after being toilet-trained
- Forgetting how or not being able to talk
- Acting out the traumatic event during play
- Having frightening dreams
- Being unusually clingy with a parent or other adult

Post-Traumatic Stress Disorder

Post-traumatic stress disorder (PTSD) occurs in some people after a terrifying, traumatic, scary, or dangerous event. There was harm or threat of harm. PTSD can develop at any age after:

- Being harmed or after a loved one was harmed
- Seeing a harmful event happen to a loved one or stranger
- The sudden, unexpected death of a loved one
- Traumatic events
  - War, terrorist attack, bombing
  - Abuse, mugging, rape, torture
  - Kidnapping, being held captive
  - Crashes—vehicle, train, plane
  - Natural disaster—flood, tornado, hurricane, earthquake

Most people recover from their physical and emotional reactions after a traumatic event. Those who do not recover may have PTSD. Persons with PTSD feel stressed or frightened even when not in danger.

Signs and symptoms may begin within 3 months or years after the event (Box 52-4). The signs and symptoms are so severe that they interfere with relationships or work.

Flashbacks are common. A *flashback is reliving the trauma over and over in thoughts during the day and in nightmares during sleep.* During a flashback, the person has symptoms of PTSD. Every-day things can trigger a flashback—words, objects, situations, reminders of the event, or the person's own thoughts. During a flashback, the person may believe that the trauma is happening all over again.

Some people recover within 6 months. For others, PTSD is a chronic condition. Anxiety disorders, depression, and substance abuse may occur with PTSD.

See *Focus on Children and Older Persons: Post-Traumatic Stress Disorder.*

PSYCHOTIC DISORDERS

Psychosis is a state of severe mental impairment. Psychotic disorders cause abnormal thinking and perceptions. (To *perceive* means *to become aware of, know, or understand something through the mind or the senses—sight, hearing, touch, smell, and taste.*) In a psychotic state, the person has lost touch with what is real.

Two main symptoms of a psychosis are:

- *Delusions—false beliefs.* For example, a person believes that a radio station is airing the person's thoughts. Or the person believes he or she is being harmed.
- *Hallucinations—seeing, hearing, smelling, feeling, or tasting something that is not real.* Hearing voices is a common hallucination. "Voices" may comment on the person's behavior or order the person to do things, warn of danger, or talk to other voices.

Schizophrenia is 1 type of psychotic disorder. Other causes of psychosis include alcohol and some drugs, brain tumors, brain infections, and stroke.

Schizophrenia

Schizophrenia is a serious brain illness affecting how a person thinks, feels, and behaves. *Schizophrenia* means split (*schizo*) mind (*phrenia*). Slightly more common in men than women, age of onset is usually between 16 and 30. Schizophrenia in children is rare.

The person with schizophrenia may not make sense when talking. He or she may have hallucinations and delusions that include:

- *Delusions of grandeur—exaggerated beliefs about one's importance, fame, wealth, power, or talents.* For example, a person believes that he or she is a movie star, a famous singer, or a king or queen.
- *Delusions of persecution—false beliefs that one is being mistreated, abused, or harassed.* The person believes that harm is happening or going to happen. For example, a person thinks that others are cheating, poisoning, spying on, or plotting against him or her.

Besides hallucinations and delusions, persons with schizophrenia have experiences not seen in healthy people. Such symptoms can be severe at times but not obvious at other times.

- *Thought disorders.* The person has trouble organizing or logically connecting thoughts. Speech may be garbled and hard to understand. The person may stop speaking in the middle of a thought. Some persons make up words with no meaning.
- *Movement disorders.* These include:
  - Agitated body movements
  - Repeating motions over and over
  - Sitting for hours without moving, speaking, or responding
- *Emotional and behavioral problems.* Normal functions are impaired or absent. The person may:
  - Have a dull voice
  - Have no facial expressions—smile, frown
  - Have trouble being happy
  - Have trouble planning and staying with an activity
  - Withdraw socially—talk little to others, even when important
- *Cognitive problems. Cognitive* relates to *understanding, remembering, and reasoning.* The person may have trouble paying attention or understanding or remembering information. Symptoms make it hard to perform daily tasks.

The person with schizophrenia has severe mental impairment *(psychosis).* Thinking and behavior are disturbed with false beliefs *(delusions)* and hallucinations. That is, the person sees, hears, smells, feels, or tastes things that are not real. The person has problems relating to others. The person may have difficulty organizing thoughts and may make up words. Responses are not appropriate. Communication is disturbed. The person may ramble or repeat what another says. Sometimes speech cannot be understood. The person may withdraw. That is, the person lacks interest in others and is not involved with people or society.

Some persons regress. To *regress* means *to retreat or move back to an earlier time or condition.* For example, a 5-year-old wets the bed when there is a new baby. This is normal. Healthy adults do not act like infants or children.

People with schizophrenia do not tend to be violent. However, if a person becomes violent, it is often directed at oneself. Some persons with schizophrenia attempt suicide (p. 778).

See *Focus on Communication: Schizophrenia.*

FOCUS ON COMMUNICATION

Schizophrenia

Delusions and hallucinations can frighten a person. Good communication is important.

- Speak slowly and calmly.
- Do not pretend to experience what the person does. Help the person focus on reality.
- Do not try to convince the person that the experience is not real. To the person, it is real.

  For example, a person hears voices. You can say: "I don't hear the voices but I believe you do. Try to listen to my voice and not the other voices."

MOOD DISORDERS

Feeling sad, irritable, or in a bad mood from time to time is normal. Mood disorders affect a person's every-day emotional state. They include bipolar disorder and depression. Mood disorders can increase a person's risk of heart disease, diabetes, and other diseases.

Bipolar Disorder

Bipolar means 2 *(bi)* poles or ends *(polar).* The person with bipolar disorder has severe extremes in mood, energy, and function. There are emotional highs or "ups" *(mania)* and emotional lows or "downs" *(depression).* Therefore the disorder is also called manic-depressive disorder.

The disorder runs in families. It usually develops during the late teens or early adulthood. Life-long management is needed. The person may have problems in school or keeping a job.

Signs and symptoms range from mild to severe (Box 52-5). Mood changes are called "episodes." Some people are suicidal.

BOX 52-5   Bipolar Disorder—Signs and Symptoms

Manic Episode

- Feeling very up, high, or happy, or very irritable or touchy
- Feeling jumpy, wired, or more active than usual
- Racing thoughts
- Decreased need for sleep
- Talking fast about many different things ("flight of ideas")
- Excessive appetite for food, drinking, sex, or other pleasurable activities
- Thinking one can do many things at once without getting tired
- Feeling unusually important, talented, or powerful

Depressive Episode

- Feeling very down, sad, or anxious
- Feeling slowed down or restless
- Problems concentrating or making decisions
- Trouble falling asleep, waking up too early, or sleeping too much
- Talking very slowly, feeling that one has nothing to say, or forgetting a lot
- Lack of interest in almost all activities
- Unable to do simple things
- Feeling hopeless or worthless
- Thinking about death or suicide

Modified from National Institute of Mental Health: Bipolar disorder, U.S. Department of Health and Human Services, October 2018.

Depression

Depression is a mood disorder with distressing symptoms that affect feeling, thinking, and daily activities (see Box 52-5). Also called *clinical depression* or *depressive disorder,* 2 common forms are:

* *Major depression.* Symptoms are present most of the day and almost every day for at least 2 weeks. They interfere with work, sleep, studying, eating, and enjoying life. Major depression can occur 1 time in a person's life or more often. Some persons have several episodes.
* *Persistent depressive disorder (dysthymia). Persistent* means *lasting* or *constant. Dys* means *painful* or *disordered. Thymia* means *mind.* Symptoms last for at least 2 years. A person may have episodes of major depression and periods when symptoms are less severe.

Depression can occur with other serious illnesses. Diabetes, cancer, heart disease, stroke, and Parkinson's disease are examples. Depression can make an illness worse. Or an illness can make depression worse. Some drugs used in treatment have the side effect of depression.

See *Focus on Children and Older Persons: Depression.*

FOCUS ON **CHILDREN AND OLDER PERSONS**
Depression
Children
Children with depression may pretend to be sick, refuse to go to school, cling to a parent, or worry about a parent dying. Older children and teenagers may get into trouble at school, sulk, or be irritable. Teenagers may have symptoms of other disorders—anxiety, eating disorders, or substance abuse.
Older Persons
Depression can occur in older persons. They have many losses—death of family and friends, loss of body functions, or loss of independence. Their symptoms of depression may be less obvious (Box 52-6). They may not admit feelings of sadness or grief.
Health problems and drug side effects may cause or involve depression. Depression in older persons is often over-looked or a wrong diagnosis is made. Instead of depression, the person is thought to have a cognitive disorder (Chapter 53). Therefore the depression goes untreated.

BOX 52-6	**Depression in Older Persons— Warning Signs and Symptoms**

* Changes in mood, energy level, or appetite
* Feeling flat or trouble feeling good thoughts
* Problems sleeping or sleeping too much
* Problems concentrating
* Feeling restless or "on edge"
* Angry, irritable, or aggressive behaviors
* On-going headaches, gastro-intestinal problems, or pain
* Need for alcohol or drugs
* Feeling sad or hopeless
* Suicidal thoughts
* High-risk activities
* Obsessive thinking or compulsive behavior
* Thoughts or behaviors that interfere with work, family, or social activities
* Unusual thinking or behaviors about people

Modified from National Institute of Mental Health: Older adults and mental health, revised March 2018.

PERSONALITY DISORDERS

Personality is the set of attitudes, values, behaviors, and traits of a person. Personality development starts at birth. Influencing factors include genes, growth and development (Chapter 11), environment, parenting, and social experiences. People with healthy personalities can cope with normal stresses. They are able to form relationships with family, friends, and co-workers.

Personality disorders involve long-term patterns of thoughts and behaviors that are unhealthy and rigid. Because of their behavior, persons with personality disorders cannot function well in society. They have serious work problems and relationships are often stormy. They have trouble dealing with every-day stresses and issues.

Personality disorders may be seen by the teenage years or earlier. The disorders continue throughout adulthood but become less obvious during middle-age.

There are many types of personality disorders. Two examples are described in this chapter.

Antisocial Personality Disorder

A person has a long-term pattern of manipulating, exploiting, or violating the rights and safety of others. Behavior is often criminal. Setting fires and animal cruelty during childhood are often seen. Symptoms include:

* Being witty and charming
* Flattering and manipulating (conning) others for personal gain or pleasure
* Breaking the law repeatedly—lying, stealing, fighting
* Having no regard for the safety of self and others
* Having problems with substance abuse
* Showing no guilt or remorse (regret, sorrow)
* Being angry
* Feeling superior or more important than others

Borderline Personality Disorder (BPD)

A person has a long-term pattern of unstable moods, behaviors, and emotions. Stormy relationships and impulsive actions often result. (To be *impulsive* means *to be reckless or act in haste without considering the consequences*.) Occurring in both men and women, symptoms may improve after middle-age. Symptoms include:

- Changing interests and values rapidly
- Viewing things in terms of extremes—all good or all bad
- Shifting and changing feelings about other people— liking a person 1 day but not the next
- Having an intense fear of being abandoned
- Being unable to stand being alone
- Feeling empty and bored
- Inappropriate anger
- Impulsive substance use or sexual relationships
- Self-injury such as wrist cutting or over-dosing
- Suicide

SUBSTANCE USE DISORDER

Substance use disorder (substance abuse) is when the use of alcohol or another substance (a drug) leads to health issues or problems at work, school, or home.

The exact cause is unknown. Influencing factors include genetics, how the substance affects the person, peer pressure, anxiety, depression, and stress. The person with substance use disorder may have other mental health problems.

Legal (such as alcohol) and illegal substances (such as heroin) are used. Legal drugs are approved for use in the United States. Illegal drugs are not approved for use. Legal drugs may be bought or obtained illegally. Commonly used substances include:

- *Opiates and other narcotics.* These drugs are strong painkillers that cause drowsiness. Some cause an intense feeling of well-being, happiness, excitement, and joy.
- *Stimulants.* These drugs stimulate the brain and nervous system.
- *Depressants.* Such drugs depress the nervous system, causing drowsiness and reduced anxiety. Alcohol is a depressant.
- *Hallucinogens.* These drugs cause sensations and images (hallucinations) that are not real. LSD is an example.
- *Marijuana.* The drug affects the brain, causing a "high." Seeing brighter colors and mood changes are common. Legal in some states, medical use includes pain management and nausea from cancer therapy.

Signs and symptoms of substance use disorder are listed in Box 52-7.

See *Focus on Children and Older Persons: Substance Use Disorder.*

BOX 52-7	Substance Use Disorder—Signs and Symptoms

Behavior Changes

- Missing school or work; decreased school or work performance
- Getting into trouble: fights, violence, accidents, car crashes, illegal activities
- Using a substance in hazardous situations—driving, using a machine
- Secretive or suspicious behaviors; hiding substance use
- Appetite: changes in
- Sleep pattern: changes in
- Personality and attitude: changes in
- Mood swings
- Irritability
- Angry outbursts
- Hyperactivity
- Agitation
- Giddiness
- Motivation: lacking
- Fearful, anxious, or paranoid behaviors for no reason

Physical Changes

- Eyes: bloodshot, abnormal pupil size
- Weight: loss or gain
- Appearance: decline in
- Smells: body, breath, clothing
- Tremors
- Speech: slurred
- Coordination: impaired

Social Changes

- Sudden change in friends, hangouts, or hobbies
- Legal problems related to substance use
- Unexplained need for money
- Financial problems
- Continued substance use despite harmful effects on health, work, or family

Modified from U.S. Department of Health & Human Services: Mental health and substance use disorders, MentalHealth.gov, updated March 22, 2019.

FOCUS ON CHILDREN AND OLDER PERSONS

Substance Use Disorder

Children

According to the Centers for Disease Control and Prevention (CDC), alcohol is the most commonly used and abused substance among teenagers. As a consequence, under-age drinking is more likely to result in:

- School problems—absences, failing grades
- Social problems—fighting, not taking part in activities
- Legal problems—driving arrests, hurting someone while drunk
- Physical problems—hang-overs, illness
- Unwanted, unplanned, unprotected sexual activity
- Disrupted normal growth and sexual development
- Physical and sexual assault
- Risk for suicide and homicide
- Alcohol-related car crashes
- Alcohol-related injuries—burns, falls, drowning
- Memory problems
- Drug abuse
- Changes in brain development with life-long effects
- Death from alcohol poisoning

Older Persons

Older persons are at risk for substance use disorder. Reasons include:

- Long-term and many prescription drugs
- Not taking drugs properly
- Multiple health problems
- Physical changes from aging
- Using over-the-counter drugs and dietary supplements
- Drug interactions

Alcohol use is another risk factor. Even small amounts of alcohol can make older persons feel "high." Older persons are at risk for falls, fractures, vehicle crashes, and other injuries from drinking. They have:

- Slower reaction times
- Hearing and vision problems
- A lower tolerance for alcohol

Mixing alcohol with some prescribed drugs can be harmful, even fatal. Alcohol also makes some health problems worse. High blood pressure is an example.

Addiction

Addiction is a chronic disease involving substance-seeking behaviors and use that is compulsive and hard to control despite the harmful effects. The person must have the substance. Persons addicted to drugs or alcohol cannot stop taking the substance without treatment.

- *Drug addiction—a strong urge or craving to use the substance. The person cannot stop using the drug. Tolerance develops—needing more of the drug for the same effect.*
- *Alcoholism—alcohol dependence that involves:*
  - *Craving—*a strong need to drink
  - *Loss of control—*not being able to stop drinking once started
  - *Physical dependence—*withdrawal symptoms
  - *Tolerance—*the need for more alcohol for the same effect

The following signal addiction.

- The substance is taken in larger amounts. Or it is taken longer than intended.
- The person tries to cut down or stop using the substance.
- The person craves or has a strong urge for the substance.
- Dangerous activities occur during or after substance use. See Box 52-7.
- Much time is spent using the substance or recovering from its effects. Or the person spends much time trying to obtain the substance. This interferes with family, work, school, or interests. Substance use continues despite problems.
- The person continues to use the substance even when it causes depression or anxiety or worsens other health problems.
- Substance use causes impaired memory *(blackouts)*.
- The person has tolerance to the substance.
  - The substance has less and less effect on the person.
  - More of the substance is needed for the same effect.
- The person has withdrawal symptoms. *Withdraw means to stop, remove, or take away. Withdrawal syndrome is the physical and mental response after stopping or severely reducing use of a substance that was used regularly.* The body responds with anxiety, restlessness, insomnia, irritability, poor attention, and physical illness.

Treatment

Substance use disorder is not easy to treat. The process is long-term. The person may *relapse*—use the substance again after stopping. Treatment may involve:

- Emergency treatment. An over-dose is life-threatening. Treatment depends on the substance used.
- Detoxification (detox). A *toxin* is a harmful substance that can cause death or serious illness. *Detoxification is the process of removing a toxic substance from the body.*
- Drug therapy. A drug with a similar action on the body is slowly given to reduce withdrawal effects.
- Counseling. See "Care and Treatment" on p. 779.

Complications

Besides death from an over-dose, other complications can occur from substance abuse. They include:

- Sudden death. This can occur from 1 use of the substance.
- Stroke.
- Lung disease.
- Cancer. Cancers of the mouth and stomach are linked to alcohol abuse.
- Infection. HIV/AIDS (human immunodeficiency virus/acquired immunodeficiency syndrome) and hepatitis B and C are risks from shared needles (Chapter 50).
- Job loss.
- Depression.
- Memory and concentration problems.
- Problems with police and legal issues.
- Relationship problems.
- Unsafe sexual practices. Unwanted pregnancy, sexually transmitted disease, HIV/AIDS, or hepatitis can result.
- Suicide.

EATING DISORDERS

An eating disorder involves a severe disturbance in eating behavior with thoughts and emotions related to eating. Eating disorders often develop during the teen years. However, they can develop during childhood or later in life. The person may have other mental health disorders—depression, anxiety disorders, substance use disorder.

Eating disorders include:

- *Anorexia nervosa.* *Anorexia* means no (a) appetite (orexis). *Nervosa* relates to *nerves* or *emotions*. The person has an intense fear of gaining weight. A fat body image is felt despite being quite thin (Fig. 52-1). The person eats in small amounts and only certain foods are eaten. The person may force vomit or use laxatives to lose weight. Serious health problems can result. Death is a risk from cardiac arrest or suicide.

- *Bulimia nervosa.* Binge eating occurs—eating large amounts of food. The over-eating is followed by forced vomiting and intense exercise. Enemas and laxatives are used to promote defecation to rid the body of food. Diuretic abuse may occur. Diuretics cause the kidneys to produce large amounts of urine. Extra fluid is lost, resulting in weight loss.

- *Binge-eating disorder.* The person often eats large amounts of food. Eating is out of control. Binge eating is not followed by purging, fasting, or exercise. Often the person is over-weight or obese. High blood pressure, heart disease, diabetes, and joint pain can occur.

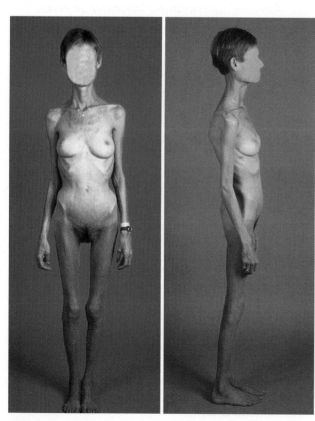

FIGURE 52-1 A person with anorexia nervosa. (Courtesy George D. Comerci, MD, Tucson.)

SUICIDE

Suicide means to end one's life on purpose. People direct violence at themselves with the intent to end their lives. Their actions result in death. According to the CDC, suicide is the 10th leading cause of death in the United States. Some people attempt suicide. A *suicide attempt* is when people harm themselves with the intent to end their lives. However, they do not die because of their actions.

People of all genders, ages, and ethnic groups can be at risk. See Box 52-8 for risk factors and warning signs. *If a person mentions or talks about suicide, take the person seriously. Call for the nurse at once. Do not leave the person alone.*

BOX 52-8	Suicide

Risk Factors
- Prior suicide attempt
- Depression, anxiety, and other mental health disorders
- Substance use disorder
- Family history of a mental health disorder or substance abuse
- Family history of suicide
- Family violence (including physical or sexual abuse)
- Guns or other firearms in the home
- Being in prison or jail
- Exposure to the suicidal behavior of others (family, friends, media figures)
- Medical illness
- Being between the ages of 15 and 24 or over age 60

Warning Signs
- Talking about wanting to die or to kill oneself
- Talking about feeling empty, hopeless, or having no reason to live
- Planning or looking for a way to kill oneself—searching on-line, saving pills, obtaining lethal items (guns, ropes, knives)
- Talking about guilt or shame
- Talking about feeling trapped or feeling without solutions
- Feeling unbearable pain—physical, emotional
- Talking about being a burden to others
- Using alcohol or drugs often
- Acting anxious or agitated
- Withdrawing from family and friends
- Changing eating or sleeping habits
- Showing rage or talking about revenge
- Taking risks that could lead to death, such as reckless driving
- Talking or thinking about death
- Posting suicidal messages on social media sites
- Having extreme mood swings—a sudden change from very sad to very calm or happy
- Giving away important belongings
- Saying good-bye to family or friends
- Putting legal affairs in order—will, advance directive

Modified from National Institute of Mental Health: Suicide in America: frequently asked questions, *NIH publication No. TR 18-6389, Bethesda, Md, National Institutes of Health, February 2018.*

Agencies treating persons with mental health disorders must identify persons at risk for suicide. They must:

- Identify specific factors or features that increase or decrease the risk for suicide.
- Meet the person's immediate safety needs.
- Provide the most appropriate setting to treat the person.
- Provide crisis information to the person and family. A crisis "hotline" phone number is an example.
  See *Focus on Communication: Suicide.*
  See *Focus on Children and Older Persons: Suicide.*

FOCUS ON COMMUNICATION

Suicide

A person thinking about suicide may say:
- "I just don't want to live anymore."
- "I wish I was dead."
- "I wish I had never been born."
- "Everyone would be better off without me."

A person may ask you not to tell anyone about the suicidal thoughts. Protecting personal information is important. But the person's safety is the priority. Never promise that you will not tell anyone. *Call for the nurse at once if a person talks about suicide.*

FOCUS ON CHILDREN AND OLDER PERSONS

Suicide

Children

Suicide is a leading cause of death among children and young adults. Besides the risk factors and warning signs listed in Box 52-8, others include:
- Having problems at school—lower grades, lacking interest in school, refusing to go to school, bullying
- Writings or drawings about death or suicide

Older Persons

According to the National Institute of Mental Health, older adults are at risk for suicide. Many older persons suffer from depression (p. 775). Depression often occurs with other serious illnesses. Heart disease, stroke, diabetes, cancer, and Parkinson's disease are examples. The person also may have social and financial problems.

Most older victims did not report depression to their doctors. Or depression was not diagnosed.

Suicide Contagion

Suicide contagion is exposure to suicide or suicidal behaviors within one's family or one's peer group or through media reports of suicide. The exposure has led to suicides and suicidal behaviors in persons at risk. Adolescents and young adults are at risk for suicide contagion.

Following suicide exposure, those close to the victim need evaluation by a mental health professional. They include family, friends, peers, and co-workers. Persons at risk for suicide need mental health services.

CARE AND TREATMENT

Treatment of mental health disorders involves having the person explore thoughts and feelings. Psychotherapy and behavior, group, occupational, art, and family therapies are used. Often drugs are ordered.

The care plan reflects the needs of the total person. This includes physical, safety and security, and emotional needs.

Communication is important. Be alert to nonverbal communication—the person's and your own. The person may respond to stress with anxiety, panic, anger, or violence. Protect yourself. Once you are safe, the health team can protect the person and others. To protect yourself:

- Call for help. Do not try to handle the situation on your own.
- Keep a safe distance between you and the person.
- Be aware of your setting. Do not let the person block your exit.
  See *Focus on Communication: Care and Treatment.*

FOCUS ON COMMUNICATION

Care and Treatment

Nonverbal communication involves eye contact, tone of voice, facial expressions, body movements, and posture. Persons with depression often have little eye contact, poor posture, and speak softly. Some do not talk much at all. Facial expressions may not change. Some persons cry.

Persons with anxiety may be restless, unable to sit still, and talk fast. Eye contact may be prolonged and intense. Others have poor eye contact. The eyes may dart about. Be alert to nonverbal cues. Report what you observe.

Your nonverbal communication is important. When interacting with persons with mental health disorders:
- Face the person.
- Maintain eye contact.
- Position yourself near the person but not too close. Do not invade the person's space.
- Crouch, sit, or stand at the person's level if safe to do so.
- Show interest and concern through your posture and facial expressions.
- Speak calmly.

FOCUS ON **PRIDE**

The Person, Family, and Yourself

Personal and Professional Responsibility

Just as a person does not choose to have a physical illness, a person does not choose a mental health disorder. How you view the disorder affects how you treat the person. Treat the person with kindness, respect, and compassion. Provide quality care.

Rights and Respect

Agencies have strict rules to protect the person's rights to privacy and confidentiality (Chapters 2, 5, and 6). Do not talk about the person with your family or friends. Never give information to someone not involved in the person's care. This includes the person's family. Direct questions to the nurse. Follow agency policies. Take pride in protecting the person's rights.

Independence and Social Interaction

Social support is important in treating mental health disorders. Interacting with others is a healthy way to manage stress. Family and friends provide a sense of worth and belonging. The care plan includes how they are involved in the person's care.

Supporting a person with a mental health disorder can be demanding. The family needs support. Many communities offer support groups for families. You can offer encouragement. Tell the family that you value the support they give.

Delegation and Teamwork

Teamwork is important. A person may become hostile, violent, or threaten or attempt suicide. The health team must react quickly to protect the person and others. If someone calls for help, respond at once. Assist as the nurse directs. Take pride in working as a team to ensure safety.

Ethics and Laws

Mental health disorders can affect the person's judgment. Unsafe actions can cause harm. The person must be protected. In the following case, failure to protect the person resulted in patient harm and charges of negligence.

A patient sued a hospital after setting her bed and herself on fire. The patient was in the hospital for alcohol abuse and mental illness. She had a history of mental illness, suicide threats, and alcohol abuse.

While in the hospital:
- *Many packs of cigarettes were taken from her.*
- *Arm, leg, and waist restraints were applied when she became agitated. She was also given a sedative.*
- *After she calmed down, some restraints were removed at her request. They were removed from her right wrist, left ankle, and waist.*
- *She asked to go outside to smoke. A nurse left after asking her to wait a few minutes.*
- *While the nurse was out of the room, the patient set her bed on fire with a cigarette and lighter.*
- *The patient suffered severe burns to her left arm and chest. (The burns required skin grafting. Scars were left at the burn and skin graft sites.)*
- *The patient's lawsuit claimed negligence because:*
  - *The nurse left her.*
  - *Restraints were removed.*
  - *The cigarettes and lighter were not found.*

The jury found in favor of the patient. She was awarded $350,000 for past and future pain, suffering, and disfigurement.

(Wilson v Boscobel Area Health Care Center.)

FOCUS ON **PRIDE**: *Application*

Why are persons with mental health disorders at risk for violations of their rights? How must the health team protect the person's rights?

REVIEW QUESTIONS

*Circle **T** if the statement is **TRUE** and **F** if it is **FALSE**.*

1 T F   Unexplained aches and pains can warn of a mental health disorder.
2 T F   Anxiety is an intense and sudden feeling of fear or dread.
3 T F   Panic occurs suddenly for no obvious reason.
4 T F   Children and older persons can experience depression.
5 T F   Sudden death can occur from 1 use of a substance.
6 T F   Persons with binge-eating disorder are often obese.
7 T F   A person is talking about suicide. You can leave the person alone to get the nurse.

Circle the BEST answer.

8 Stress is
   a A way to cope with or adjust to every-day living
   b A response or change in the body caused by some factor
   c A mental health disorder
   d An unwanted thought or idea

9 Defense mechanisms are used to
   a Blame others
   b Make excuses for behavior
   c Return to an earlier time
   d Block unpleasant feelings

10 These statements are about defense mechanisms. Which is *true*?
   a Using them signals a mental health disorder.
   b They relieve anxiety.
   c They prevent mental health disorders.
   d Persons with mental health disorders use them well.

REVIEW QUESTIONS—cont'd

11 A phobia is
   a The event that causes stress
   b A false belief
   c An intense fear of something
   d A ritual

12 A person cleans and cleans. This behavior is
   a A delusion
   b A hallucination
   c A compulsion
   d An obsession

13 A person has nightmares about a trauma. The person is having
   a Flashbacks
   b Phobias
   c Panic attacks
   d Anxiety

14 A woman believes she is married to a rock singer. This is called a
   a Fantasy
   b Delusion of grandeur
   c Delusion of persecution
   d Hallucination

15 A man believes someone is trying to kill him. This is called a
   a Fantasy
   b Delusion of grandeur
   c Delusion of persecution
   d Hallucination

16 Schizophrenia
   a Involves obsessions and compulsions
   b Can be cured with drugs and therapy
   c Usually begins in late adulthood
   d Is a serious psychotic disorder

17 Bipolar disorder means that the person
   a Is very suspicious
   b Has anxiety
   c Is very unhappy and feels unwanted
   d Has severe extremes in mood

18 In bipolar disorder, an "emotional high" is called
   a Depression
   b A hallucination
   c Mania
   d An obsession

19 Which is a sign of depression in older persons?
   a Hallucinations
   b Appetite changes
   c Increased energy and activity
   d Garbled speech

20 In antisocial personality disorder, the person
   a Lacks regard for the rights and safety of others
   b Has a sad, anxious, or empty mood
   c Withdraws from people and interests
   d Is paranoid and avoids social situations

21 Which statement about substance use disorder is *true?*
   a Legal substances cannot cause addiction.
   b Substance abuse causes problems at work, home, or school.
   c Complications of substance abuse are minor.
   d There is no treatment for substance abuse.

22 A person has withdrawal syndrome. This means that
   a The person has a physical and mental response when the drug is not taken
   b The person needs higher doses of the drug
   c The effect is reduced with the same amount of drug
   d The person has a relapse after treatment

23 Binge eating followed by forced vomiting occurs in
   a Anorexia nervosa
   b Binge-eating disorder
   c Bulimia nervosa
   d Borderline personality disorder

24 Suicide risk
   a Decreases with aging
   b Increases with mental health disorders
   c Decreases with suicide contagion
   d Is low for young adults

25 A person talks about suicide. What should you do?
   a Call for the nurse.
   b Identify factors that increase the risk of suicide.
   c Ask what method the person plans to use.
   d Restrain the person.

26 A patient's family member asks what to say when the person talks about suicide. You should
   a Give advice
   b Direct the question to the nurse
   c Suggest a local support group
   d Call a crisis hotline

Answers to Chapter 52 questions are on p. 888.

FOCUS ON **PRACTICE**

Problem Solving

A patient is being treated for bipolar disorder. The patient is pacing, appears restless, and is talking very fast about work that needs to be done at home. The patient says: "I don't need to be here. I'm leaving and you can't stop me!" What will you do? How will you protect yourself if the patient becomes violent?

OBJECTIVES

- Define the key terms and key abbreviations in this chapter.
- Describe confusion and its causes.
- List the measures that help confused persons.
- Explain the difference between delirium and dementia.
- Describe the signs, symptoms, and behaviors of Alzheimer's disease (AD).

- Explain the care required by persons with AD and other dementias.
- Describe the effects of AD on the family.
- Explain validation therapy.
- Explain how to promote PRIDE in the person, the family, and yourself.

KEY TERMS

cognitive function Involves memory, thinking, reasoning, ability to understand, judgment, and behavior

confusion A state of being disoriented to person, time, place, situation, or identity

delirium A state of sudden, severe confusion and rapid changes in brain function

delusion A false belief

dementia The loss of cognitive function that interferes with daily life and activities

elopement When a patient or resident leaves the agency without staff knowledge

hallucination Seeing, hearing, smelling, feeling, or tasting something that is not real

paranoia A disorder (*para*) of the mind (*noia*); false beliefs (delusions) and suspicion about a person or situation

sundowning Signs, symptoms, and behaviors of AD increase during hours of darkness

KEY ABBREVIATIONS

AD Alzheimer's disease
ADL Activities of daily living

CMS Centers for Medicare & Medicaid Services
NIA National Institute on Aging

Changes in the brain and nervous system occur with certain diseases and with age. See Box 53-1. Cognitive function may be affected. (*Cognitive* relates to *knowledge*.) *Cognitive function involves memory, thinking, reasoning, ability to understand, judgment, and behavior.* Changes in function affect quality of life.

CONFUSION

Confusion is a state of being disoriented to person, time, place, situation, or identity. Disoriented means to be apart from (dis) *one's awareness* (oriented). Memory and the ability to make good judgments are often lost. A person may not know people, the time, or the place. Daily activities may be affected. Behavior changes are common—anger, restlessness, depression, irritability.

Disease, brain injury, infections, fever, alcohol or drug use, and drug side effects are some causes of confusion. Hypoxia (Chapter 43), hypoglycemia (Chapter 50), sleep problems (Chapter 35), and seizures (Chapter 58) are other causes. Poor nutrition and fluid and electrolyte imbalances (Chapters 30 and 31) can cause confusion.

Depending on the cause, onset may be fast or slow. Report sudden onset of confusion at once. Confusion may be temporary or permanent. Treatment is aimed at the cause. Some measures help improve function (Box 53-2). You must meet the person's basic needs.

BOX 53-1 Nervous System Changes From Aging

- Nerve cells are lost.
- Nerve conduction slows.
- Reflexes, responses, and reaction times are slower.
- Vision, hearing, taste, smell, and touch decrease.
- Sensitivity to pain decreases.
- Blood flow to the brain is reduced.
- Sleep patterns change.
- Memory is shorter; forgetfulness occurs.
- Dizziness can occur.

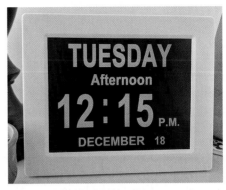

FIGURE 53-1 A large clock can help persons who are confused.

BOX 53-2 Confusion—Care Measures

- Follow the care plan.
- Provide for safety.
- Face the person. Speak clearly.
- Call the person by name each time you have contact.
- State your name. Show your name tag.
- Give the date and time each morning. Repeat as needed during the day or evening.
- Explain what you are going to do and why.
- Give clear, simple directions and answers to questions.
- Break tasks into small steps.
- Ask clear and simple questions. Allow time to respond.
- Make sure the person can see a calendar and clock (Fig. 53-1). Remind the person of holidays, birthdays, and other events.
- Have the person wear needed eyeglasses and hearing aids.
- Use touch to communicate (Chapter 7).
- Place familiar objects and photos within view.
- Provide newspapers, magazines, TV, radio, phone, and other electronic devices. Read to the person if appropriate.
- Discuss current events.
- Maintain the day-night cycle.
  - Open window coverings during the day. Close them at night.
  - Use night-lights in rooms, bathrooms, hallways, and other areas at night.
  - Have the person wear day-time clothes during the day.
- Provide a calm, relaxed, and peaceful setting. Prevent loud noises, rushing, and crowded hallways and dining rooms.
- Follow the person's routine. Meals, bathing, exercise, TV, bedtime, and other activities have a schedule. This promotes a sense of order and what to expect.
- Do not re-arrange furniture or the person's belongings.
- Encourage the person to take part in self-care.

Delirium

Delirium is a state of sudden, severe confusion and rapid changes in brain function. Usually temporary and reversible, it occurs with physical or mental illness. Other causes include surgery, drug or alcohol abuse, drug side effects, severe lack of sleep, and electrolyte imbalances. Infections such as urinary tract infections (Chapter 27) and pneumonia (Chapter 49) can cause delirium.

Onset is usually fast—within hours or a few days. Signs and symptoms (Box 53-3) may come and go during the day and worsen at night. Delirium often lasts for about 1 week. However, it may take several weeks for normal mental function to return.

Delirium signals illness. It is an emergency. The cause must be found and treated.

See *Focus on Children and Older Persons: Delirium.*

BOX 53-3 Delirium—Signs and Symptoms

- Alertness: changes in (usually more alert in the morning and less alert at night)
- Sensation: changes in
- Awareness: changes in
- Movement: very active or slow moving
- Drowsiness
- Confusion about time or place
- Memory: decreased short-term memory and recall (cannot remember events since the delirium began)
- Thinking: changes in
- Concentration: problems with
- Speech: does not make sense
- Incontinence
- Emotional changes: agitation, anger, depression, euphoria, irritability

Modified from MedlinePlus: Delirium, Bethesda, Md, U.S. National Library of Medicine, National Institutes of Health. Page updated November 22, 2019.

FOCUS ON CHILDREN AND OLDER PERSONS

Delirium

Older Persons
Older persons in a hospital or long-term care setting are at risk for delirium. Do not assume the nurse knows about a problem. Report the signs and symptoms in Box 53-3 or a change in the person's normal behavior at once.

DEMENTIA

Dementia is the loss of cognitive function that interferes with daily life and activities. (*De* means *from. Mentia* means *mind.*) Changes in personality, mood, behavior, and communication are common. Dementia is a group of symptoms, not a specific disease.

Dementia is caused by damage to brain cells. Some conditions cause thinking and memory problems that can be reversed when the cause is treated. Depression, drug side effects, excess alcohol use, thyroid problems, and vitamin deficiencies are examples. Head injury and blood clots, tumors, or infections in the brain are other treatable causes.

Permanent dementias result from changes in the brain (Box 53-4). There is no cure. Function declines over time.

Dementia is not a normal part of aging. The risk increases with age. Persons over 65 and those with a family history of dementia are at higher risk.

Early warning signs include:
- Memory loss (losing things, forgetting names)
- Problems with common tasks (for example, dressing, cooking, driving)
- Problems with language and communication; forgetting simple words
- Getting lost in familiar places
- Misplacing things and putting things in odd places (for example, putting a watch in the oven)
- Personality, mood, and behavior changes
- Poor or decreased judgment (for example, going out in the snow without shoes)
See *Focus on Children and Older Persons: Dementia.*

Mild Cognitive Impairment

Mild cognitive impairment (MCI) causes slight changes in memory or thinking. For example, the person loses things often, forgets important events or appointments, or forgets which words to use. Changes are greater than those with normal aging. The person can do normal activities and care for himself or herself. The person is at risk for dementia.

ALZHEIMER'S DISEASE

Alzheimer's disease (AD) is the most common type of permanent dementia. Many brain cells are destroyed and die. Connections between nerve cells are lost. Over time, the brain shrinks from nerve cell death and tissue loss (Fig. 53-2). Two abnormal structures are thought to cause damage.
- Plaques—protein pieces that build up in the spaces between nerve cells.
- Tangles—twisted protein fibers that build up inside cells.

With aging, most people develop some plaques and tangles. In AD, plaque and tangle development is severe. Memory areas of the brain are often affected before other areas.

AD onset is gradual. Usually symptoms appear after age 60. Persons with AD can live for 4 to 8 years or longer.

BOX 53-4	Types of Permanent Dementia

- Alzheimer's disease—most common type. See "Alzheimer's Disease."
- Vascular dementia—stroke or other blood vessel problems damage vessels that supply blood to the brain.
- Lewy body dementia—abnormal protein deposits in the brain (Lewy bodies) affect chemicals in the brain.
- Fronto-temporal disorders—nerve cells in certain areas of the brain (front and sides) break down.
- Mixed dementia—2 or more types of dementia occur together.

FOCUS ON CHILDREN AND OLDER PERSONS

Dementia

Older Persons

Depression is a common mental health disorder in older persons. Confusion and attention problems from depression may be mistaken for dementia. Dementia, depression, aging, and some drug side effects have similar signs and symptoms. See "Depression" in Chapter 52.

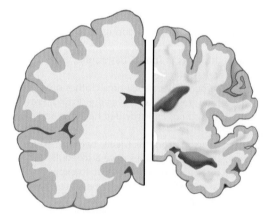

Healthy brain   Severe AD

FIGURE 53-2 Nerve cell death and tissue loss shrink the brain in the person with AD. (Redrawn from National Institute on Aging: *Alzheimer's disease fact sheet,* National Institutes of Health, U.S. Department of Health and Human Services, content reviewed May 22, 2019.)

Risk Factors

The greatest risk factor is increasing age. The risk increases after age 65. About one-third ($\frac{1}{3}$) of people age 85 and older have AD. A family history of AD increases the person's risk. More persons with AD are women because women live longer than men.

The National Institute on Aging (NIA) recommends the following to maintain cognitive health.

- Get regular exercise.
- Eat a healthy diet.
- Spend time with family and friends.
- Keep the mind active.
- Control type 2 diabetes (Chapter 50).
- Maintain healthy blood pressure (Chapter 49) and cholesterol levels (Chapter 30).
- Maintain a healthy weight.
- Do not smoke.
- Get help for depression (Chapter 52).
- Avoid excess alcohol intake.
- Get enough sleep.

Signs of AD

According to the Alzheimer's Association, one of the most common early symptoms of AD is forgetting newly learned information. There is a slow decline in memory, thinking, and reasoning.

Box 53-5 lists early signs and symptoms of AD. AD is not a normal part of aging. See Box 53-6 for the differences between AD and normal age-related changes.

BOX 53-5	Alzheimer's Disease—Early Signs and Symptoms

Memory loss that disrupts daily life
- Forgets newly learned information
- Forgets important dates or events
- Asks for the same information over and over
- Relies more on memory aids—reminder notes, electronic devices
- Relies on family members for things usually handled alone

Problems with planning or problem solving
- Has trouble making a plan or working with numbers
- Has problems following a recipe
- Has trouble keeping track of monthly bills
- Difficulty concentrating
- Takes longer to do things than before

Problems completing familiar tasks
- Has a hard time with tasks in the home, at work, or with recreation
- Has problems driving to familiar places
- Has trouble managing a budget
- Forgets the rules to a favorite game

Confusion with time or place
- Loses track of dates, seasons, and passing of time
- Has trouble understanding something that is not happening right away
- Forgets where he or she is
- Forgets how he or she got to a certain place

Problems with vision and spatial relationships
- Difficulty reading
- Difficulty judging distance
- Has problems with color or contrast
- Has trouble driving

Problems with speaking or writing
- Has trouble following or joining a conversation
- Stops in the middle of a conversation and does not know how to continue
- Repeats himself or herself
- Has trouble finding the right word
- Calls things by the wrong name—calling a "watch" a "hand-clock" is an example

Misplacing items and being unable to find them
- Puts things in strange places
- Loses things and is unable to retrace steps to find them
- Accuses others of stealing

Decreased or poor judgment
- Changes in judgment or decision-making
- Poor judgment with money—giving away large amounts is an example
- Pays less attention to hygiene and grooming

Withdrawal from work or social activities
- No longer does hobbies, social activities, work projects, or sports
- Has trouble keeping up with a favorite sports team
- Has trouble remembering how to do a hobby
- Avoids being social

Mood and personality changes
- Is confused
- Is depressed
- Is suspicious, afraid, or anxious
- Is easily upset at home, at work, with friends, or in places where he or she is less comfortable

Modified from Alzheimer's Association: 10 early signs and symptoms of Alzheimer's, 2019.

BOX 53-6	Alzheimer's Disease and Normal Aging

Signs of AD
- Poor judgment and decision making.
- Cannot manage a budget.
- Loses track of the date or season.
- Problems having a conversation.
- Misplaces things. Cannot retrace steps to find them.

Normal Age-Related Changes
- Makes a bad decision once in a while.
- Misses a monthly payment.
- Forgets which day it is but remembers later.
- Sometimes forgets which word to use.
- Loses things from time to time.

Modified from Alzheimer's Association: 10 early signs and symptoms of Alzheimer's, 2019.

Stages of AD

Signs and symptoms become more severe as AD progresses. The disease ends in death. AD is described in 3 stages. See Box 53-7 and Figure 53-3.

Behavior and Function Changes

AD changes how a person behaves and acts. Besides the signs and symptoms in Boxes 53-5 and 53-7, these common behaviors and changes of AD are described in the following pages.

- Wandering and getting lost
- Sundowning
- Hallucinations
- Delusions
- Paranoia
- Catastrophic reactions
- Agitation and aggression
- Communication changes
- Screaming
- Repetitive behaviors
- Rummaging and hiding things
- Changes in intimacy and sexuality
Besides brain changes, the following can affect behavior.
- Health problems—illness, pain, infection, drugs, lack of sleep, constipation, hunger, thirst, poor vision or hearing, alcohol abuse, too much caffeine
- Emotions—sadness, fear, feeling overwhelmed, stress, anxiety
- Changes in routine
- Problems in the person's setting:
  - A strange setting. The person does not know the setting well.
  - Too much noise (TV, music, people talking at once) can cause confusion and frustration.
  - Not understanding signs. The person may think that a WET FLOOR sign means to urinate on the floor.
  - Mirrors. The person may think that a mirror image is another person in the room.

See *Promoting Safety and Comfort: Behavior and Function Changes.*

BOX 53-7	Alzheimer's Disease—Stages

Mild AD
- Memory loss
- Poor judgment, bad decisions
- Loss of spontaneity and initiative
- Taking longer to do daily tasks
- Repeating questions
- Problems handling money and paying bills
- Wandering and getting lost
- Losing things or misplacing them in odd places
- Mood and personality changes
- Anxiety or aggression

Moderate AD
- Increased memory loss and confusion
- Cannot learn new things
- Problems with language, reading, writing, and working with numbers
- Trouble with thoughts and thinking logically
- Shortened attention span
- Problems coping with new situations
- Problems with tasks having multiple steps—getting dressed is an example
- Problems recognizing family and friends
- Hallucinations, delusions, and paranoia
- Impulsive behavior—undressing at inappropriate times or places and using vulgar language are examples
- Outbursts of anger
- Restlessness, agitation, anxiety, tearfulness
- Wandering—especially in the late afternoon or evening
- Repetitive statement or movements, occasional muscle twitches

Severe AD
- Depends on others for care
- In bed most or all of the time
- Cannot communicate
- Weight loss
- Seizures
- Skin infections
- Difficulty swallowing
- Groaning, moaning, or grunting
- Increased sleeping
- Loss of bowel and bladder control

Modified from National Institute on Aging: What are the signs of Alzheimer's disease? National Institutes of Health, content reviewed May 16, 2017.

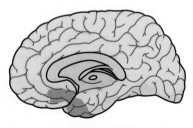

Very Early AD

A

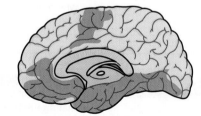

Mild to Moderate AD

B

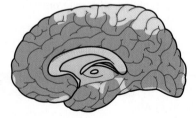

Severe AD

C

FIGURE 53-3 A, Very early AD. **B,** Mild to moderate AD. **C,** Severe AD. (NOTE: Blue shading shows the areas of the brain affected.) (Redrawn from National Institute on Aging: *Alzheimer's disease: Unraveling the mystery,* Bethesda, Md, September 2008, National Institutes of Health.)

PROMOTING SAFETY AND COMFORT

Behavior and Function Changes

Safety

Some behaviors are caused by illness, injury, or drugs—not AD. Without treatment, life may be threatened. Always report changes in behavior.

Wandering and Getting Lost. Persons with AD are not oriented to person, time, and place. They may wander off and not find their way back. Wandering is by foot, car, bike, or other means. They may be with you one moment and gone the next.

Judgment is poor. They cannot tell what is safe or dangerous. Life-threatening accidents are great risks. They can walk into traffic or a nearby river, lake, ocean, or forest. If not properly dressed, heat or cold exposure is a risk.

TEAMWORK AND TIME MANAGEMENT

Wandering and Getting Lost

Patients and residents may try to wander to another nursing unit or out of the agency. *Leaving the agency without staff knowledge is called elopement.* Serious injury and death have resulted. State and federal guidelines to prevent elopement are followed.

All staff must be alert to persons who wander. Wandering is allowed in safe areas (Fig. 53-4). Unsafe areas include kitchens, shower rooms, and utility rooms.

Tell other staff that a person wanders. You cannot be with the person all the time. All staff can help monitor the person. Help other staff in the same way. If you see a person wandering into an unsafe area, gently guide the person to a safe place (Fig. 53-5). Tell the nurse.

FOCUS ON LONG-TERM CARE AND HOME CARE

Wandering and Getting Lost

Home Care

A person who wanders should not be left alone. The following may prevent wandering from home.

* Keep doors locked. A keyed deadbolt or locks at the top and bottom of doors (Fig. 53-6) may be used. Or door knob covers are used. The device turns instead of the door knob. In case of emergency, a caregiver must be present to help the person exit.
* Place STOP, DO NOT ENTER, or CLOSED signs on doors.
* Place a poster, curtain, or brightly colored streamers across the door. Or wallpaper the door to match the walls. The person does not focus on the exit.
* Install safety devices on windows to limit how much windows open.
* Use a door chime that sounds when a door is opened.
* Secure the yard with a fence and a locked gate.
* Keep shoes, keys, suitcases, coats, hats, and other items used when leaving the home out of sight.

Wandering may have no cause. Or the person is looking for something or someone—the bathroom, the bedroom, a child, or a partner. Pain, drug side effects, stress, restlessness, too much stimulation, and anxiety are other causes. A wandering pattern may reflect a life-long routine—leaving work, getting children from school, and so on. Sometimes finding the cause prevents wandering.

See *Teamwork and Time Management: Wandering and Getting Lost.*

See *Focus on Long-Term Care and Home Care: Wandering and Getting Lost.*

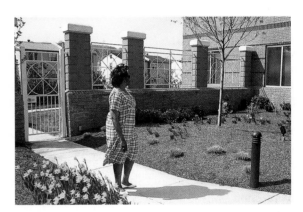

FIGURE 53-4 An enclosed garden allows persons with AD to wander in a safe setting.

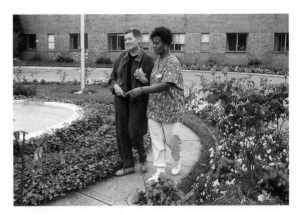

FIGURE 53-5 Guide the person who wanders to a safe area.

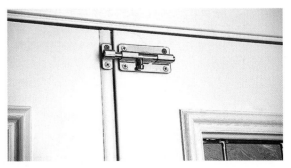

FIGURE 53-6 A slide lock is at the top of the door. The person is not likely to look for a lock here.

MedicAlert® + Alzheimer's Association Safe Return®. *MedicAlert® + Alzheimer's Association Safe Return®* is a nationwide 24-hour emergency service for persons who wander or have a medical emergency. The purpose is to find and safely return persons who wander and become lost. A small fee is charged.

A family member provides required information and a photo. The person receives an ID (wallet card and bracelet or necklace). If reported missing, the person's information is sent to the police. When the person is found, someone calls the toll-free number on the ID. *MedicAlert® + Alzheimer's Association Safe Return®* then calls the family member or caregiver. The person is returned home.

Sundowning. With *sundowning, signs, symptoms, and behaviors of AD increase during hours of darkness.* As daylight ends and darkness starts, confusion and restlessness increase. So do anxiety, agitation, and other symptoms. Behavior is worse after sundown. It may continue during the night.

Brain changes affecting the sleep-wake cycle may cause sundowning. Other possible causes include:
- Fatigue
- Hunger or thirst
- Depression
- Pain
- Boredom
- Confusion and fear (poor light and shadows cause the person to see things that are not there)

Hallucinations and Delusions. A *hallucination is seeing, hearing, smelling, feeling, or tasting something that is not real.* Senses are dulled. Affected persons see animals, insects, or people that are not present. Some hear voices. They may feel bugs crawling or feel that they are being touched.

Poor vision or hearing may be a cause. The person should wear needed eyeglasses and hearing aids. Other causes include infection, pain, and drugs.

Delusions are false beliefs. To the person, the beliefs are real. People with AD think they are another person. Some believe they are in jail, are being killed, or are being attacked. A person may believe the caregiver is someone else. Many other false beliefs can occur.

Paranoia. *Paranoia is a disorder* (para) *of the mind* (noia). *The person has false beliefs (delusions) and suspicion about a person or situation.* Paranoia is a type of delusion. The person believes others are mean, lying, not fair, or "out to get" him or her. The person may be suspicious, fearful, or jealous.

Paranoia may worsen as memory loss gets worse. The NIA uses these examples.
- The person forgets where he or she put something. The person thinks the item was stolen.
- The person forgets you are a caregiver. The person thinks you are a stranger and does not trust you.
- The person forgets people whom he or she has met. The person believes strangers are harmful.
- The person forgets the directions you give. The person thinks you are trying to trick him or her.

The person may express loss through paranoia. Reasons for the loss do not make sense. Therefore the person blames or accuses others.

See *Promoting Safety and Comfort: Paranoia.*

PROMOTING SAFETY AND COMFORT
Paranoia

Safety

Behaviors may not mean paranoia. Fears of harm, strangers, stealing, mistreatment, and so on may be real. Some people abuse vulnerable adults (Chapter 5). This includes sexual and financial abuse.

Abuse may be by phone, mail, e-mail, or in person. The abuser may be a friend or family member. Financial abuse occurs when money or belongings are stolen. Financial abuse can include:
- Forging checks or cashing checks without permission
- Taking retirement and Social Security benefits
- Using the person's credit cards or bank accounts
- Changing names on wills, bank accounts, insurance policies, or titles to homes or cars
- "Scams" such as identity theft, phone prizes, and threats
- Borrowing money and not paying it back
- Giving away or selling the person's property without permission
- Forcing the person to sign over property

Protect the person from harm, abuse, and mistreatment. Report the following at once.
- What the person is saying
- The person seems afraid or worried about money
- Missing items
- The person's behaviors
- Signs and symptoms of problems
- Visitors or family members acting strangely

Catastrophic Reactions. These are extreme responses to normal events or things. The person reacts as if there is a disaster or tragedy. The person may scream, cry, or be agitated or combative (ready to fight). These reactions are common from too many stimuli. Eating, music or TV playing, and being asked questions all at once can overwhelm the person.

Agitation and Aggression. When agitated, the person is restless or worried and cannot settle down. The person may pace, move about, or not sleep. Agitation may lead to aggression. The person may yell, scream, swear, hit, pinch, grab, or try to hurt someone. Common causes are:

- Pain or discomfort.
- Anxiety, depression, or stress.
- Loneliness.
- Drug interactions.
- Fatigue.
- Too many stimuli. Too much noise or too many people in the room are examples.
- Hunger or thirst.
- Elimination needs, constipation, and incontinence.
- Feeling lost or abandoned.
- A feeling of loss. Missing driving or caring for children are examples.
- Care measures (bathing, dressing) that upset or frighten the person.
- Feeling pressured to do something that is now hard or impossible. Remembering an event or person are examples.
- Change in routine, caregiver, or setting.
- Caregivers. A caregiver may rush the person or be impatient. Or mixed verbal and nonverbal messages are sent. For example, a caregiver talks too fast or too loud. Consider how your behaviors affect the person.

Communication Changes. Communication skills gradually decline. The person has trouble expressing thoughts and emotions. Communication changes include:

- Struggling to find the right word
- Problems understanding the meaning of words
- Attention problems during conversations
- Losing one's train of thought when talking
- Problems blocking background noises—radio, TV, music, phones, others talking, and so on
- Frustration with communication problems
- Being sensitive to touch, tone, and voice volume

As the person loses the ability to talk clearly, other communication methods may be used. Facial expressions and gestures are examples. In time, the person cannot understand others and communicate verbally.

See *Caring About Culture: Communication Changes.*
See *Focus on Communication: Communication Changes.*

CARING ABOUT CULTURE
Communication Changes

For some, English is a second language. For example, the first language learned is Spanish, Italian, French, Russian, Chinese, or Japanese. With AD, the person may forget or no longer understand English. He or she uses and understands only the first language learned.

FOCUS ON COMMUNICATION
Communication Changes

To promote communication with the person with AD, see Box 53-8 (p. 790). Avoid:

- *Giving orders.* For example: "Sit down and eat" is bossy. It does not show respect. Instead say: "Let me help you sit down."
- *Wanting the truth.* For example, do not say: "Don't you remember?" or "What day is it?" Instead say: "Today is Friday."
- *Correcting errors.* For example, do not say: "I just told you it's time to get dressed. You already had breakfast." Instead say: "Let me help you get dressed."
- *Pointing out errors.* Instead of saying: "You missed a button," say: "Let's try it this way."
- *Giving many choices.* For example: "What would you like for dinner?" involves many choices. Instead, limit choices. Say: "Do you want potatoes or rice?"
- *Asking open-ended questions.* For example, do not say: "How do you feel?" Instead, ask "yes" or "no" questions. You can say: "Are you tired?"

Screaming. At first, persons with AD have problems finding the right words. As AD progresses, they speak in short sentences or just words. Often speech is not understandable.

Screaming to communicate is common in persons who are very confused and have poor communication skills. They may scream a word or a name. Or they just make screaming sounds.

Possible causes include hearing and vision problems, pain or discomfort, fear, and fatigue. Too much or not enough stimulation is another cause. A person may react to a caregiver or family member by screaming. The following measures and those in Box 53-8 may be helpful.

- Provide a calm, quiet setting.
- Play soft music.
- Have the person wear hearing aids and eyeglasses.
- Have a family member or favorite caregiver comfort and calm the person.
- Use touch to calm the person.

BOX 53-8	Communication—Persons With AD or Other Dementias

- Treat the person with dignity and respect.
- Approach the person in a calm, quiet manner.
- Approach the person from the front—not from the side or the back. This avoids startling the person.
- Make eye contact to get the person's attention. Maintain eye contact.
- Have the person's attention before you start speaking.
- Identify yourself and other people by name.
- Call the person by name.
- Avoid pronouns (he, she, them, it, and so on). For example, instead of saying: "She is here," say: "Mary is here."
- Follow the rules and measures to promote communication (Chapter 7).
- Do not talk about the person as if he or she is not there.
- Control distractions and noise. TV, radio, and music are examples.
- Speak in a calm, gentle voice.
- Be aware of your body language. Smile and avoid frowning, grimacing, or other negative actions. Standing with the arms folded tightly signals tension or anger.
- Use gestures or cues. Point to objects.
- Watch the person's facial expressions and gestures. Expressions may show sadness, anger, or frustration. Pulling at under-garments may signal incontinence or elimination needs.
- Comfort the person with touch. Hold the person's hand while you talk.
- Speak slowly. Use simple words and short sentences.
- Do not "baby talk" or use a "baby voice."
- Ask or say 1 thing at a time. Present 1 idea, statement, or question at a time.
- Give simple, step-by-step instructions.
- Explain all procedures and activities.
- Repeat instructions as needed. Allow time to respond or react.
- Ask simple questions with simple answers. Do not ask complex questions.
- Let the person speak. Do not interrupt or rush the person.
- Give the person time to respond.
- Try other words if the person does not seem to understand.
- Provide the word the person is looking for if he or she is struggling to communicate a thought.
- Do not criticize, correct, interrupt, argue, or try to reason with the person.
- Give consistent responses.
- Practice the measures in Chapter 46.
  - To promote hearing
  - To communicate with speech-impaired persons
  - For blind and visually impaired persons

Repetitive Behaviors. *Repetitive* means *to do over and over.* The person repeats the same motions, words, or questions over and over. For example, the same napkin is folded over and over. Or the person says the same words or asks the same question over and over. Such behaviors are not harmful. However, they can annoy caregivers and the family.

Rummaging and Hiding Things. To *rummage* means *to search for things by moving things around, turning things over, or looking through something such as a drawer or closet.* The behavior may have no meaning. Or the person is looking for a certain item but cannot tell you what or why. Or boredom or hunger is the cause.

The person may hide things, throw things away, or lose things. Eyeglasses, hearing aids, and dentures must stay with the person. Always make sure these items are safe. Money, jewelry, and other important items usually are sent home with the family.

Changes in Intimacy and Sexuality. *Intimacy* is a special bond between people who love and respect each other. It includes the way people talk and act toward each other. *Sexuality* involves the way partners physically express feelings for each other (Chapter 55). The person with AD may:

- Depend on and cling to a partner.
- Not remember life with a partner.
- Not remember feelings for a partner.
- Fall in love with another person.
- Have side effects from drugs that affect sexual interest.
- Have memory loss, brain changes, or depression that affects sexual interest.
- Have abnormal sexual behaviors.

Sexual behaviors are labeled abnormal because of how and when they occur—wrong person, wrong place, or wrong time. Persons with AD cannot control behavior.

Healthy persons do not undress or expose themselves in front of others. They do not masturbate or engage in sexual acts in public. They know their sexual partners. Persons with AD often mistake someone else for a sexual partner. The person kisses and hugs the other person.

Being overly *(hyper)* interested in sex is called *hypersexuality.* The person may try to seduce others or masturbate often. These behaviors may not mean that the person wants to have sex. If masturbating in public, lead the person to his or her room. Provide for privacy and safety.

The nurse encourages the partner to show affection. Their normal practices are encouraged. Examples include hand holding, hugging, kissing, touching, and dancing.

Some behaviors are not sexual. Touching, scratching, and rubbing the genitals can signal infection, pain, or discomfort in the urinary or reproductive systems. Poor hygiene and incontinence are other causes. Good hygiene prevents itching. Clean the person promptly and thoroughly after elimination. Do not let the person stay wet or soiled.

CARE OF PERSONS WITH AD AND OTHER DEMENTIAS

The person may be cared for at home until symptoms become severe. Adult day care may help. Often assisted living or nursing center care is required. Other illnesses may require hospital care. The person may need hospice care as death nears (Chapter 59). You may care for persons with AD or other dementias in such settings. The person and family need your support and understanding.

People with AD do not choose the behaviors, signs, and symptoms of the disease. They cannot control what is happening to them. *The disease is responsible, not the person.*

Currently AD has no cure. Symptoms worsen over many years. Over time, the person depends on others for care. Safety, hygiene, food and fluids, elimination, and activity needs must be met. So must comfort and sleep needs. Good skin care and alignment prevent skin breakdown and contractures. The person's care plan and the agency's safety plan will include many of the measures listed in Box 53-9.

The person can have other health problems and injuries. However, the person may not be aware of pain, fever, constipation, incontinence, or other signs and symptoms. Carefully observe the person. Report any change in usual behavior.

Infection is a risk. Infection can occur from poor hygiene. This includes poor skin care, oral hygiene, and perineal care after elimination. Inactivity and immobility can cause pneumonia and pressure injuries.

You must treat persons with AD with dignity and respect. They have the same rights as everyone else.

See *Focus on Long-Term Care and Home Care: Care of Persons With AD and Other Dementias,* p. 794.

See *Teamwork and Time Management: Care of Persons With AD and Other Dementias,* p. 794.

See *Focus on Surveys: Care of Persons With AD and Other Dementias,* p. 794.

Text continued on p. 795.

BOX 53-9	Care of Persons With AD and Other Dementias

Environment
- Follow set routines.
- Place picture signs by room doors, bathrooms, dining rooms, and other areas (Fig. 53-7, p. 794).
- Keep personal items where the person can see and reach them.
- Stay within the person's sight to the extent possible.
- Place memory aids (large clocks and calendars) where the person can see them.
- Keep noise levels low.
- Play music and show movies from the person's past.

Safety
- Reassure the person that you are there to help.
- Remove harmful, sharp, and breakable items from the area. This includes knives, scissors, glasses, dishes, razors, and tools.
- Provide plastic eating and drinking utensils. They help prevent breakage and cuts.
- Practice electrical safety measures (Chapter 13). Also remove electric appliances from the bathroom. Hair dryers, curling irons, make-up mirrors, and electric shavers are examples.
- Provide safe storage for:
  - Personal care items (shampoo, deodorant, lotion, and so on)
  - Cleaners and drugs
  - Dangerous equipment and tools
  - Cigarettes, cigars, pipes, matches, and other smoking materials
  - Car keys
- Keep childproof caps on drug containers and cleaners.
- Remove knobs from stoves or place safety covers on the knobs (Fig. 53-8, p. 794).

Safety—cont'd
- Remove dangerous appliances, power tools, and firearms and weapons from the home.
- Supervise the person who smokes.
- Practice safety measures to prevent:
  - Falls (Chapter 14)
  - Fires (Chapter 13)
  - Burns (Chapter 13)
  - Poisoning (Chapter 13)
- Lock doors to kitchens, utility rooms, and housekeeping closets. Keep them locked.

Wandering
- Follow agency policy for locking doors and windows.
- Keep door alarms and electronic doors turned on. Respond to alarms at once.
- Follow agency policy for fire exits.
- Have the person wear an ID bracelet or *MedicAlert® + Alzheimer's Association Safe Return®* ID at all times.
- Know when the person is more likely to wander.
- Follow the care plan for daily routine, activities, and exercise. Meet food, fluid, and elimination needs.
- Involve the person in activities—folding napkins, dusting a table, sorting socks, rolling yarn, sweeping, sanding blocks of wood, or watering plants.
- Do not use restraints. They tend to increase confusion and disorientation. See Chapter 15.
- Do not argue with the person who wants to leave. The person will not understand.
- Go with the person who insists on going outside. Provide proper clothing. Guide the person inside after a few minutes.
- Allow wandering in enclosed and safe areas.

Continued

BOX 53-9   Care of Persons With AD and Other Dementias—cont'd

Sundowning

- Complete treatments and activities early in the day.
- Encourage exercise and activity early in the day.
- Avoid too many activities in a day.
- Allow for rest during the day if needed. If a nap is needed, it should be short and not late in the day.
- Keep the person on a schedule. Waking up, meal times, and bedtime should involve a set routine.
- Avoid caffeine (coffee, tea, colas, chocolate), sweets, and alcohol late in the day.
- Provide a calm, quiet setting late in the day.
- Do not restrain the person.
- Meet nutrition and elimination needs. Unmet needs can increase restlessness.
- Use night-lights at night.
- Do not try to reason with the person. He or she will not understand.
- Do not ask the person to explain the problem. Communication changes impair understanding and speech.
- Promote sleep at night. See "Sleep."

Hallucinations and Delusions

- Have the person wear eyeglasses and hearing aids as needed.
- Do not argue with the person. He or she will not understand.
- Reassure the person. Say that you will keep the person safe.
- Distract the person with an item or activity. Or take the person to another room or for a walk.
- Turn off TV or movies when violent and disturbing programs are on. The person may believe the story is real.
- Comfort the person if he or she seems afraid. Use touch to calm and reassure the person (Fig. 53-9, p. 794).
- Eliminate noises that can be misinterpreted. TV, radio, music, furnaces, and air conditioners are examples.
- Check lighting. Eliminate glares, shadows, or reflections.
- Cover or remove mirrors. The person could misinterpret his or her reflection.
- Remove anything that could be used to hurt the self or others.
- Report behavior changes. They may signal a physical illness.

Paranoia

- Do not react if the person blames you for something.
- Do not argue with the person.
- Tell the person that he or she is safe.
- Use touch or gently hug the person to show you care.
- Search for missing things to distract the person. Talk about what you found. For example, talk about a photo you found.

Catastrophic Reactions

- Approach the person from the front. Do not startle from behind or the side.
- Be calm. Do not appear rushed. Give the person time to calm down.
- Use touch correctly. Know how the person responds to touch. Touch can comfort some people. Others do not like being touched.
- Explain in simple terms what you want the person to do. For example: "It's time for bed. I'll help you into bed."
- Do not argue with the person.
- Follow the person's daily routine, including naps and bedtime.
- Distract the person with an item or activity.

Agitation and Aggression

- Look at how your behaviors affect the person.
- Provide a calm, quiet setting.
- Follow the care plan and a set routine for ADL (activities of daily living). Meet basic needs.
- Observe for early signs of agitation and aggression. Try to remove the cause before behaviors worsen.
- Do not ignore the problem. Try to find the cause.
- Allow personal choice to the extent possible.
- Try to distract the person. A snack or activity may help.
- Reassure the person.
  - Speak calmly.
  - Listen to concerns.
  - Try to show that you understand the person's anger or fears.
- Keep personal items within the person's sight. Photos and treasures are examples.
- Reduce glares, noise, and clutter.
- Limit the number of people in the room.
- Use gentle touch.
- Provide soothing music.
- Read to the person with a gentle voice.
- Try taking the person for a walk.
- Provide quiet times.
- Limit the amount of caffeine (coffee, tea, colas, chocolate) and sweets.
- See Chapter 7 for dealing with the angry person.
- See Chapter 13 for workplace violence.

Repetitive Behaviors

- Allow harmless acts. Holding a purse, folding napkins, and petting a stuffed animal are examples.
- Distract the person. See Chapter 35.
- Take the person for a walk.
- Know when repetitive behaviors are likely. For example, a person constantly calls for a nurse at bedtime.
- Use a calm voice and gentle touch.
- Do not argue with the person.
- Answer questions. You may have to answer the same question many times.
- Follow the care plan for memory aids. Clocks, calendars, and photos are examples.

Rummaging and Hiding Things

- Keep harmful items and products out of sight and reach.
- Remove spoiled items from refrigerators and cabinets. The person may look for food and snacks. He or she may not know or be able to taste spoiled food.
- Guide the person away from other patient or resident rooms.
- Keep wastebaskets covered or out of sight. The person may rummage through a wastebasket or throw things away.
- Check wastebaskets, linens, and food trays. Look for items thrown away or hidden.
- Keep bathroom doors closed and toilet seats down. The person cannot flush things down the toilet.
- Allow rummaging in a safe place. The agency may have a drawer, closet, bag, box, basket, or chest with safe items.

BOX 53-9   Care of Persons With AD and Other Dementias—cont'd

Sleep

- Develop a regular bedtime. Bedtime should be the same each evening.
- Perform activities that use more energy early in the day.
- Provide a quiet, peaceful mood in the evening—dimmed lights, low noise level, and soft music.
- Follow bedtime rituals.
- Use night-lights in rooms, hallways, bathrooms, and other areas. They help the person see and prevent accidents and disorientation.
- Limit caffeine.
- Limit naps during the day.
- Follow the person's exercise plan. Play music to the exercise.
- Reduce noises.

Oral Care

- Allow the person to do as much as possible.
- Explain what to do 1 step at a time. For example: "Pick up the toothpaste. Take off the cap. Squeeze the toothpaste on the toothbrush. Put the toothbrush in your mouth. Brush."
- Show the person how to brush the teeth step-by-step.
- Help the person clean dentures.
- Try a long-handled, angled, or electric toothbrush.

Bathing

- Follow the care plan for how often to give a bath or shower. Bathing 2 to 3 times a week is enough. A partial bath is done on other days.
- Follow the person's habits and routines.
  - Use the person's preferred bathing method—tub bath, shower. Follow the care plan. Some persons may need complete bed baths.
  - Perform the bath at the same time—in the morning, before bed.
- Practice safety measures. See Chapter 24.
  - Do not leave the person alone in the bath or shower.
  - Check for a comfortable water temperature.
  - Use a hand-held shower head.
  - Use a bath mat and grab (safety) bars.
  - Use a sturdy shower chair.
  - Do not use bath oils. They make the tub slippery and may increase risk of urinary tract infection.
- Expect that bathing will be a difficult task. Plan ahead to calm the person. Before the bath:
  - Gather supplies—soap, washcloths, towels, shampoo, and so on.
  - Make sure the bathroom is warm and well lit.
  - Play soft music if this relaxes the person.
  - Be matter-of-fact. Say: "It is time for a bath now." Try the bath when the person is calm. Never use force.
  - Provide privacy.
- Promote comfort and independence. During the bath or shower:
  - Be gentle and respectful.
  - Tell the person what you will do step-by-step.
  - Do not rush the person.
  - Allow the person to do as much as possible. This shows dignity and helps the person feel in control.
  - Give the person a washcloth to hold.
  - Put a towel over the shoulders or lap. The person feels less exposed. Clean under the towel with a washcloth.
  - Talk to the person about something else. This may distract the person if he or she is upset.
- Dry the skin well after bathing to prevent a rash or infection. Dry well between skin folds.

Hygiene and Grooming

- Provide good skin care.
- Provide incontinence care as needed. Apply a barrier cream or moisturizer (cream, lotion, paste) as directed by the nurse and care plan.
- Help the person apply make-up if this is a routine. Do not apply eye make-up.
- Use an electric razor for shaving. Help the person as needed.
- Keep the nails clean and trimmed without rough edges.

Dressing and Undressing

- Choose clothing that is comfortable and simple to put on. Front-opening garments are easy to put on. Pullover tops are harder. And the person may become frightened when the head is inside a garment.
- Select clothing that closes with Velcro. Such items are easy to put on and take off. Buttons, zippers, snaps, and other closures can frustrate the person.
- Apply slip-on shoes that will not slide off or shoes with Velcro straps.
- Offer simple clothing choices (Fig. 53-10, p. 794). Let the person choose between 2 shirts or 2 blouses, 2 pants or 2 slacks, and so on.
- Lay clothing out in the order it will be put on. Hand the person 1 item at a time. Tell or show the person what to do. Do not rush.

Meals

- Maintain a routine. Have meals at usual times. Serve food in a familiar place and in a consistent way.
- Serve favorite foods.
- Respect personal, cultural, and religious food preferences.
- Use the meal as a time for social interaction. Keep a warm and happy tone of voice.
- Play music during the meal.
- Be patient. Give the person time to eat.
- Provide finger foods.
- Avoid coffee, tea, and cola. The caffeine can increase restlessness, confusion, and agitation.
- Cut food and pour liquids as needed.
- Tell the nurse about changes in eating habits and appetite.
- Watch for signs of dysphagia (Chapter 30) and dehydration (Chapter 31).

Other Basic Needs

- Follow a daily routine. This helps the person know when certain things will happen.
- Promote urinary and bowel elimination and prevent incontinence.
- Promote exercise and activity during the day. This helps reduce wandering and sundowning behaviors. The person may also sleep better.
- Provide a quiet, restful setting. Soft music is better than loud TV programs.
- Have equipment ready for any procedure. This lessens the time for care measures.
- Observe for signs and symptoms of health problems (Chapter 8). Common health problems include:
  - Dental problems (Chapter 23)
  - Incontinence (Chapters 27 and 29)
  - Constipation and diarrhea (Chapter 29)
  - Dehydration (Chapter 31)
  - Flu and pneumonia (Chapter 49)
  - Fever—may signal infection, dehydration, heat-related illness (Chapter 58), or constipation
- Prevent infection.

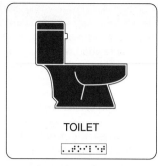

DINING ROOM

TOILET

FIGURE 53-7 Signs give cues to persons with dementia.

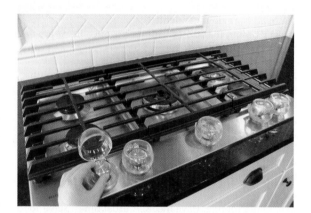

FIGURE 53-8 Safety covers are on stove knobs.

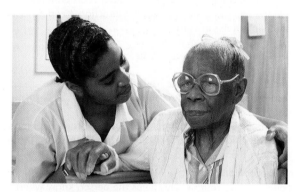

FIGURE 53-9 Use touch to calm the person.

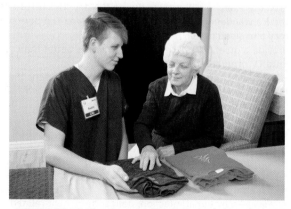

FIGURE 53-10 The person is offered simple clothing choices.

FOCUS ON LONG-TERM CARE AND HOME CARE

Care of Persons With AD and Other Dementias

Long-Term Care

Many nursing centers have secure memory care units (Chapter 1). Entrances and exits are locked. Residents cannot wander away. They have a safe setting to move about. Some persons have aggressive behaviors that disrupt or threaten others. They need a secured unit.

According to the Centers for Medicare & Medicaid Services (CMS), persons on a secured unit must be protected from involuntary seclusion (Chapter 5). The agency must identify the reason for placement on the unit. The reason must *not* be:

- For staff convenience or discipline.
- Based on a diagnosis alone. Placement is made on an individual basis.
- By request of the family or the person's representative without a medical reason.

The person's medical record must include:

- The reason for placement on the unit.
- How the resident or resident's representative was involved in the decision.
- If the secured unit is the least restrictive approach to protect the person.
- The person's reaction to placement on the unit.
- On-going review and revision of the care plan as needed. For example, are interventions meeting the resident's needs? Is a secured unit still needed?

At some point, the secured unit is no longer needed. For example, a person's condition progresses to severe AD (see Box 53-7). The person cannot sit or walk. Wandering is not a concern. The person is transferred to another unit.

TEAMWORK AND TIME MANAGEMENT

Care of Persons With AD and Other Dementias

The entire staff must protect the person from harm. Look for dangers in the person's room and in hallways, lounges, and dining and other areas. Remove the danger if you can and tell the nurse at once. If you cannot remove the danger, also tell the nurse at once.

FOCUS ON SURVEYS

Care of Persons With AD and Other Dementias

To ensure quality of life, surveyors look at all aspects of dementia care. For example:

- Are bathing, dressing, and grooming needs met?
- Is independence promoted? For example, does the staff give cues so the person can dress himself or herself?
- Is the person reminded to use the toilet at regular times?
- Is the person in a calm, quiet setting for meals?
- Are enough fluids offered to prevent dehydration?
- Does the staff respond to the person in a dignified manner?
- Is a safe setting provided?
- Does the staff provide supervision for safe behaviors?

Federal laws require that nursing assistant education and training include dementia management and preventing abuse. Annual in-service training also is required. Surveyors will review employee records to make sure requirements are met.

Activities

Persons with dementia need to feel useful, worthwhile, and active. This promotes self-esteem. Therapies and activities focus on strengths and past successes. For example:

- A person who used to cook helps clean fruit.
- Once a good dancer, activities are planned so the person can dance.
- A person who likes to clean helps with dusting.

Supervised activities meet the person's needs and cognitive abilities. Activities are based on what the person enjoys and can do. Some people like crafts, exercise, gardening, and listening and moving to music. Others like sing-alongs, board games, and reminiscing. (*Reminiscence* or *to reminisce* is *to talk about or recall past events.*) Some like to string beads, fold towels, or roll dough.

Massage, soothing touch, music, and aromatherapy are comforting and relaxing.

The Family

The person may live at home or with a partner, children, or other family members. Or someone stays with the person. Home care may help for a while. Adult day care and assisted living are options (Chapters 1 and 57). Nursing center care is needed when:

- The family cannot meet the person's needs.
- The person no longer knows the caregiver.
- Family members have health problems.
- Money problems occur.
- The person's behavior presents dangers to self and others.

Doctor's visits, drugs, home care, and assisted living are costly. So is nursing center care. The person's medical care can drain finances.

Home care and nursing center care are stressful. The family has physical, emotional, social, and financial stresses. Adult children are in the *sandwich generation.* Their own children need attention while an ill parent needs care. Caring for 2 families is stressful. Often adult children have jobs too.

Caregivers can suffer from anger, anxiety, guilt, depression, and sleep problems. Some cannot concentrate or are irritable. Health problems can develop. They need to focus on their own health. They need a healthy diet, exercise, and plenty of rest. Asking family and friends for help is hard for some people.

Caregivers need support and encouragement. The NIA suggests how family members can take care of themselves. See Box 53-10. AD support groups are sponsored by hospitals, nursing centers, and the Alzheimer's Association. The Alzheimer's Association has chapters across the country. Support groups offer encouragement and advice. Members share feelings, anger, frustration, guilt, and other emotions. They also share coping and caregiving ideas.

The family often feels hopeless. No matter what is done, the person gets worse. Much time, money, energy, and emotion are needed to care for the person. Anger and resentment may result. Guilt feelings are common. The

---

BOX 53-10	**Family Caregivers—Taking Care of Yourself**

- Ask for help when you need it. Asking for something specific may be useful. For example:
  - "Can you make Mom's dinner Sunday night?"
  - "Can you stay with Dad from 2 to 4 Monday afternoon?"
  - "Can Mom stay at your house Saturday afternoon?"
- Join a support group.
- Take breaks every day.
- Spend time with friends.
- Maintain hobbies and interests.
- Eat healthy foods and exercise often.
- See a doctor regularly.
- Keep health, legal, and financial information current.
- Remember that these feelings are normal—being sad, lonely, frustrated, confused, angry. Say to yourself:
  - "I'm doing the best I can."
  - "What I'm doing would be hard for anyone."
  - "I'm not perfect and that's okay."
  - "I can't control some things."
  - "I need to do what works for right now."
  - "Even when I do everything I can, there will still be problem behaviors. They are caused by the illness, not what I do."
  - "I will enjoy our peaceful times together."
  - "I will get counseling if caregiving becomes too much."
- Meet spiritual needs—attending religious services, believing that larger forces or a higher power is at work.
- Understand that you may feel powerless and hopeless about what is happening.
- Understand that you may feel a sense of loss and sadness.
- Understand why you are caring for a person with AD. Was the choice made out of love, loyalty, duty, religious obligation, money concerns, fear, habit, or self-punishment?
- Let yourself feel "uplifts." Examples include good feelings about the person, support from caring people, and time for your interests.

Modified from National Institute on Aging: Alzheimer's caregiving: caring for yourself, Bethesda, Md, content reviewed May 17, 2017, National Institutes of Health.

---

family knows that the person did not choose the disease and its signs, symptoms, and behaviors. Sometimes behaviors are embarrassing. The family may be upset and angry that the loved one cannot show love or affection.

The family is an important part of the health team. They help plan care when possible. The nurse and support group help the family learn how to provide a safe home setting and give needed care. They learn how to bathe, feed, dress, and give oral care.

In nursing centers, some family members take part in unit activities. For many persons, family members provide comfort. They also need support and understanding from the health team.

See *Focus on Long-Term Care and Home Care: The Family,* p. 796.

Validation Therapy

Validation therapy is a way to communicate with persons with dementia. *Validate* means *to show that a person's feelings and needs are fair and have meaning.* Behaviors signal the need to express feelings and needs—safety, security, comfort, love and belonging, feeling useful, and so on. Caregivers help the person express feelings and needs verbally or nonverbally. With validation, the person's reality (what the person thinks is real and true) is accepted. The person is treated with dignity and self-worth.

Validation therapy is based on these principles.
- All behavior has meaning.
- A person may have unresolved issues and emotions from the past.
- A person's mind may return to the past to resolve issues and emotions.
- Caregivers need to listen and provide empathy.
- Attempts are not made to correct thoughts or bring the person back to reality (reality orientation). For example:
  - A person talks about waiting for the bus to go to work. The caregiver does not say: "You don't work anymore." Instead, the caregiver says: "Tell me about your work."
  - A resident says she is at the train station waiting for her husband. Killed in a war, her husband never came home. The caregiver does not remind the resident of what happened. Instead, the caregiver asks the resident about her husband.
  - A patient was 3 years old when his father died. He holds a ball constantly. He calls for his father and repeats "play ball, play ball." The caregiver does not remind the patient that his father is not alive. Instead, the caregiver says: "Tell me about playing ball."

Validation therapy is useful for some persons. If used in your agency, you will be trained to use validation therapy correctly.

FOCUS ON **PRIDE**—cont'd

The Person, Family, and Yourself

E thics and Laws

Persons with AD may become agitated or angry. The person cannot control words and actions. Some behaviors are hard to deal with. The following is a real example of a poor response to the person's behavior.

While a licensed nursing assistant (LNA) was feeding a resident with AD, the resident threw the tray on the floor. The LNA called the resident a degrading name and swore at her.

The Board of Nursing concluded that the LNA abused and improperly cared for the resident. The unprofessional conduct violated the Administrative Rules of the Board of Nursing because of:

- *Abusing or neglecting a patient*
- *Performing unsafe or unacceptable patient care*
- *Failing to conform to acceptable standards of practice*
- *Engaging in conduct likely to harm the public*
  The nursing assistant's license was reprimanded.

(Author note: A *reprimand* means that the Board considered her conduct to be improper. However, the Board did not limit her right to work as an LNA.)

(State of Vermont Board of Nursing, 2000.)

You must control your reactions to stress. Be professional. Tell the nurse if you feel frustrated, angry, or impatient. You may need an assignment change. Never take out your anger on the person. The person must be protected from physical and verbal abuse and mistreatment.

FOCUS ON **PRIDE**: *Application*

Caregivers affect the person's quality of life. Describe care that values the person. What qualities must the caregiver have? How must the caregiver treat the person?

REVIEW QUESTIONS

*Circle **T** if the statement is TRUE and **F** if it is FALSE.*

1   T   F   Cognitive function involves memory, thinking, reasoning, understanding, judgment, and behavior.

2   T   F   The onset of delirium is gradual.

3   T   F   Depression can cause cognitive changes.

4   T   F   A person with AD is agitated and restless. A caregiver may have caused the behaviors.

5   T   F   A person with AD keeps moving an empty cup back and forth across the table. You should take the cup away.

6   T   F   A person with AD hides things. You should check wastebaskets before emptying them.

7   T   F   The person with AD can control behavior.

8   T   F   The person with AD can tell you about pain, constipation, and other discomforts.

9   T   F   The person with AD is at risk for infection from poor hygiene after elimination.

10   T   F   A set routine is important for the person with AD.

11   T   F   You can use gestures or point to things to communicate with persons who have AD.

12   T   F   Restraints help improve the behaviors of AD.

13   T   F   Family members continue their hobbies and holiday events. They are abusing the person with AD.

Circle the BEST answer.

14 A person is confused after surgery. The confusion is likely to be
  a   Permanent
  b   Temporary
  c   Caused by dementia
  d   Caused by a brain injury

15 A person is confused. Which should you question?
  a   Restrain in bed at night.
  b   Give clear, simple directions.
  c   Use touch to communicate.
  d   Open drapes during the day.

16 A person has AD. Which is *true?*
  a   AD is a normal part of aging.
  b   Diet and drugs can cure the disease.
  c   AD and delirium are the same.
  d   AD ends in death.

17 During the final stage of AD, the person is likely to
  a   Wander and become lost
  b   Follow simple commands
  c   Need total assistance with ADL
  d   Repeat questions over and over

18 Which is common in persons with AD?
  a   Paralysis
  b   Dyspnea
  c   Headache
  d   Sleep disturbances

Continued

REVIEW QUESTIONS—cont'd

19 A person has AD. To communicate, you should
   a Give orders
   b Limit choices
   c Correct mistakes
   d Ask open-ended questions

20 A person with AD is screaming. You know that this is
   a A way to communicate
   b An agitated reaction
   c Caused by a delusion
   d A repetitive behavior

21 Which statement about sundowning is *true?*
   a AD behaviors improve at night.
   b Encouraging activity late in the day can help.
   c Being tired or hungry can increase restlessness.
   d Dim lighting or darkness is calming.

22 A person with AD has delusions. Which should you question?
   a Distract the person with an activity.
   b Tell the person you will provide protection.
   c Tell the person the beliefs are not real.
   d Use touch to calm the person.

23 Which can cause delusions in persons with AD?
   a Mirrors
   b Eyeglasses
   c Hearing aids
   d Night-lights

24 A person with AD keeps telling you that someone is stealing things. What should you do?
   a Nothing. The person has paranoia.
   b Tell the nurse. Someone could be abusing the person.
   c Replace missing items.
   d Send other items home with the family.

25 A person with AD is at risk for elopement. Which should you question?
   a Make sure door alarms are turned on.
   b Make sure an ID bracelet is worn.
   c Assist with exercise as ordered.
   d Remind the person not to wander.

26 Which can help with rummaging?
   a Keep the person's room locked.
   b Provide safe places to rummage.
   c Ask the person to explain the behavior.
   d Hide items the person looks for.

27 Which is *unsafe* for persons with AD?
   a Safety plugs are placed in electrical outlets.
   b Cleaners and drugs are locked up.
   c The person keeps smoking materials.
   d Sharp objects are removed from the setting.

28 A person with AD is upset. Which is a correct response?
   a Try to reason with the person.
   b Ask what is bothering the person.
   c Ignore the problem.
   d Provide reassurance and try to find the cause.

29 You are caring for a person with AD. You should avoid
   a Trying to bring the person back to reality
   b Offering support to the family
   c Following a set routine
   d Providing a quiet setting

30 Validation therapy involves
   a Support groups and counseling for persons with severe AD
   b Drugs to treat AD
   c Helping the person with AD express needs and feelings
   d Orienting the person with AD to reality

Answers to Chapter 53 questions are on p. 888.

FOCUS ON **PRACTICE**

Problem Solving

A person has moderate AD. While preparing for a bath, the person becomes upset and repeats: "Go away" over and over. How will you respond? How might you meet hygiene needs?

Intellectual and Developmental Disabilities

A *disability is any lost, absent, or impaired physical or mental function.* Intellectual and developmental disabilities (IDDs) affect physical, intellectual, and emotional development. An IDD can be a physical or mental impairment or both.

- *Intellectual disability—involves severe limits in intellectual function and adaptive behavior occurring before age 18.*

- *Developmental disability—a severe and chronic disability that involves a mental or physical impairment or both.* According to the *Developmental Disabilities Assistance and Bill of Rights Act of 2000,* a developmental disability occurs before the age of 22. The person has limited functioning in at least 3 of these areas.
  - Self-care
  - Communication—receiving and expressing language
  - Learning
  - Mobility
  - Self-direction
  - Ability to live independently
  - Ability to financially support oneself

BOX 54-1	Intellectual and Developmental Disabilities—Causes and Warning Signs

Causes
- Genetics
  - Abnormal genes inherited from 1 or both parents. (*Inherited* means to be passed down from parents to children.)
  - Problems when genes combine during fertilization.
- Fetal exposure to certain substances. Alcohol, drugs, and lead are examples.
- Infections during pregnancy. German measles is an example.
- Problems during childbirth.
  - Lack of oxygen to the brain
  - Head injury during birth
- Premature birth.

Causes—cont'd
- Problems after birth.
  - Infections
  - Head injuries
  - Near drowning
  - Poisoning

Warning Signs
- Delays in sitting up, crawling, or walking
- Delays in talking or having difficulty speaking
- Trouble remembering things
- Trouble understanding the rules of social behavior
- Trouble "seeing" or "understanding" the outcomes of actions
- Trouble solving problems

"Causes" modified from The Arc of the United States: Causes and prevention of intellectual disabilities, Silver Springs, Md, revised March 1, 2011. "Warning Signs" modified from National Institute of Child Health and Human Development: What are the signs of IDDs? Bethesda, Md, last reviewed December 1, 2016.

Occurring during the developmental period (Chapter 11), IDDs begin before, during, or after birth or during childhood. They may affect day-to-day function and usually last throughout life. IDDs can be mild to severe. Some causes and warning signs are listed in Box 54-1.

Some IDDs involve birth defects. A *birth defect is a problem that develops during pregnancy, often during the first 3 months. It may involve a body structure or function.* Spina bifida (p. 804) is an example of a structural defect. Down syndrome is a functional (developmental) defect. Birth defects may affect how a body looks, functions, or both.

Children with IDDs become adults. *Independence to the extent possible* is the goal for these persons. This includes having a job and living in the community. Many need life-long help, support, and special services.

- Personal services:
  - Self-care
  - Adaptive (assistive) devices for eating, dressing, bathing, mobility, and other needs
  - Health care including drug therapy or surgery
  - Home and vehicle needs
  - Therapies: physical, occupational, speech and language, respiratory, recreation, and other
  - Hearing and vision aids
- Housing—family, independent living, group homes, or long-term care centers
- Finances and employment
- Education:
  - Understanding and expressing language
  - Job training
- Protection of their rights:
  - The *Americans With Disabilities Act of 1990 (ADA)*
  - The *Developmental Disabilities Assistance and Bill of Rights Act of 2000*

An IDD affects the family throughout life. The infant or child may become a teenager, young adult, middle-age adult, and older. Both the child and parents grow older. Often it is hard to provide care, handle, move, or financially support the disabled person. A parent may become ill, injured, or disabled or may die. Still the disabled person needs care.

See *Focus on Long-Term Care and Home Care: Intellectual and Developmental Disabilities.*

FOCUS ON LONG-TERM CARE AND HOME CARE

Intellectual and Developmental Disabilities

Long-Term Care

Changes from aging (Chapter 12) may occur earlier when IDDs are severe. Some adults with IDDs need nursing center care. They are further protected by the *Omnibus Budget Reconciliation Act of 1987 (OBRA)*. OBRA requires that centers provide age-appropriate activities. Staff must have special training to meet care needs.

Some severely disabled children live in agencies for the developmentally disabled.

INTELLECTUAL DISABILITIES

Intellectual function relates to *learning, thinking, reasoning, and solving problems. Adapt* means *to change* or *adjust.* The person has low intellectual function. Adaptive behavior is impaired (Box 54-2). Adaptive behaviors are skills needed to function in every-day life—to live, work, and play.

The Arc is a national organization focusing on people with intellectual and related disabilities. The Arc describes an intellectual disability as:

- An IQ score of about 70 or below. (*IQ* means *intelligence quotient.*) The person learns at a slower rate than normal. Learning ability is less than normal.
- A significant limit in at least 1 adaptive behavior. See Box 54-2.
- Onset before age 18.

Brain development is impaired. According to the Arc, alcohol is the leading preventable cause of intellectual disabilities. See Box 54-1 for other causes.

Intellectual disabilities can be mild to severe. Persons mildly affected are slow to learn in school. As adults, they can function in society with some support. For example, they need help finding a job. Support is not needed every day. Others need much support every day at home and at work. Still others need constant support in all areas.

See *Focus on Communication: Intellectual Disabilities.*

BOX 54-2 | **Adaptive Behaviors**

- Communication—receiving and expressing language
- Reading
- Writing
- Money concepts and managing money
- Social skills—interpersonal skills, responsibility, not being tricked by others, following rules, obeying laws
- Activities of daily living—eating, dressing, mobility, elimination, preparing meals, taking drugs, using the phone, using transportation, housekeeping, job skills, and maintaining a safe setting

Modified from The Arc: Introduction to intellectual disabilities, *Washington, D.C., March 1, 2011.*

FOCUS ON COMMUNICATION

Intellectual Disabilities

Mental retardation was a common term for intellectual disabilities. However, the term is offensive and out-dated. *Intellectual disabilities* is the preferred term.

In June 2003, the President's Committee on Mental Retardation was changed to the "President's Committee for People with Intellectual Disabilities." The name was changed to:

- Update and improve the image of people with intellectual disabilities.
- Help reduce discrimination against such persons.
- Reduce confusion between "mental illness" and "mental retardation."

Signed in 2010, *Rosa's Law* replaces *mental retardation* with *intellectual disability* in federal health, education, and labor laws. The law is named after Rosa Marcellino, who has Down syndrome. At age 9 when the law was signed, she did not like the word "retarded."

Do not use "mental retardation" and "mentally retarded." Use "intellectual disabilities" and "intellectually disabled."

Sexuality

Persons with IDDs may have physical, emotional, and social needs and desires. Reproductive organs develop. Some have life partners. Others marry and have children. Some persons can control sexual urges. Others cannot—the type and site of sexual responses may be inappropriate.

The Arc's beliefs about sexuality include the right to:

- Develop friendships and emotional and sexual relationships. This involves the right to:
  - Love and be loved.
  - Choose to end a relationship.
- Dignity and respect.
- Privacy and confidentiality.
- Freely choose associations.
- Sexual expression.
- Learn about sex, marriage and family, abstinence, safe sex, sexual orientation, sexual abuse, sexually transmitted diseases, and emotional abuse.
- Be protected from sexual harassment and abuses—physical, sexual, emotional.
- Decide about having and raising children.
- Make birth control decisions.
- Have control over one's own body.
- Protection from sterilization because of the disability. *Sterilization* means to remove or block sex organs so the person cannot have children.

DOWN SYNDROME

Down syndrome (DS) is named for the doctor who identified the syndrome. DS is a genetic cause of mild to moderate intellectual disabilities. At fertilization, a male sex cell (sperm) unites with a female sex cell (ovum). Each cell has 23 chromosomes. The fertilized cell has 46 chromosomes. In DS, an extra chromosome is present. The fertilized cell has 47 chromosomes.

The DS child has certain features caused by the extra chromosome (Fig. 54-1, p. 802).

- Small head, ears, and mouth
- Eyes that slant upward
- Flat face and wide, flat nose
- Short, wide neck
- Large tongue
- Short height
- Short, wide hands with short fingers
- Poor muscle tone

Children with DS may have heart defects and thyroid gland problems. They tend to have hearing and vision problems and to be over-weight. They are at risk for ear and respiratory infections. Dementia may appear in adults with DS.

Persons with DS need the support and services listed on p. 800. Most learn self-care skills. They also need health and sex education. Weight gain and constipation are problems. They need a healthy diet and regular exercise.

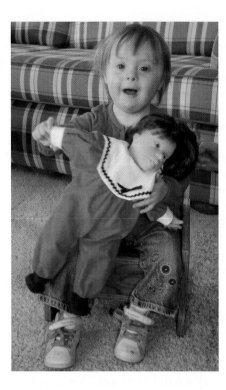

FIGURE 54-1 A child with Down syndrome. (From Hockenberry MJ, Wilson D, Rodgers CC: *Wong's nursing care of infants and children*, ed 11, St Louis, 2019, Elsevier.)

FRAGILE X SYNDROME

Fragile X syndrome (Fragile X) is the most common form of inherited IDD. There is a change in the gene that makes a protein needed for brain development. The body makes little or none of the protein.

Girls usually have milder symptoms than boys do. Fragile X has no cure. The following signs and symptoms are treated with educational, speech, behavior, physical, and drug therapies.

- *Learning.* Learning disabilities range from mild to severe.
- *Physical.* Physical features develop during puberty. The person may have a long or large face, ears, and jaw. Joints may be loose and flexible. This allows extending the elbow, thumb, and knee further than normal. Poor muscle tone, flat feet, and large body size are other signs.
- *Social and emotional.* Behavior problems are common.
  - Boys: attention problems, aggression
  - Girls: shyness
- *Speech and language.* Boys may have more severe delays than girls.

AUTISM SPECTRUM DISORDER

Autism spectrum disorder (ASD) is a developmental disorder that begins in early childhood and lasts throughout life. *Autos* means *self. Spectrum* means *a wide range.* Persons with ASD may have a wide range of symptoms (Box 54-3). They often seem to be in their "own world." Symptoms usually appear before the age of 3.

BOX 54-3	Autism Spectrum Disorder—Signs and Symptoms

Social Skills
- Does not respond to his or her name by 12 months of age.
- Avoids eye contact.
- Prefers to play alone.
- Does not share interests with others.
- Only interacts for a desired goal.
- Has flat or inappropriate facial expressions.
- Does not understand personal space boundaries.
- Avoids or resists physical contact.
- Is not comforted by others when distressed.
- Has trouble understanding the feelings of others.
- Has trouble talking about his or her feelings.

Communication
- Has delayed speech and language skills.
- Repeats words or phrases over and over (echolalia—echo means to repeat; lalia means disorder of speech).
- Reverses pronouns. For example, the child says "you" instead of "I."
- Gives unrelated answers to questions.
- Does not point or respond to pointing.
- Uses few or no gestures. For example, does not wave good-bye.
- Talks in a flat, robot-like, or sing-song voice.
- Does not engage in imaginary play. For example, does not pretend to feed a doll.
- Does not understand jokes, sarcasm, or teasing.

Unusual Interests and Behaviors
- Lines up toys or other objects.
- Plays with toys the same way every time.
- Likes parts of objects.
- Is very organized.
- Gets upset by small changes.
- Has narrow interests.
- Follows certain routines.
- Rocks, spins in circles, or flaps hands.
- Repeats motions over and over again.

Other
- Is hyperactive (very active).
- Acts without thinking (impulsive).
- Has a short attention span.
- Can be aggressive.
- Causes self-injury.
- Has temper tantrums.
- Has unusual eating and sleeping habits.
- Has unusual mood or emotional reactions.
- Lacks fear or has more fear than expected.
- Has unusual reactions to how things sound, smell, taste, look, or feel.

Modified from Centers for Disease Control and Prevention: Autism spectrum disorder (ASD), *Atlanta, Ga, page reviewed August 27, 2019.*

The cause of ASD is unknown. Genetics and environment play important roles.

Early diagnosis and treatment are important. ASD treatment involves a variety of life-long therapies depending on the person's changing needs. Examples include behavior, speech, language, and communication therapies; physical, occupational, and recreational therapies; diet therapy; and drug therapy.

A daily routine is helpful for persons with ASD. A change in routine can be very upsetting. As adults, some persons with ASD work and live independently. Others need family support and community services. Some live in group homes or residential facilities.

Other disorders may occur with ASD. Fragile X syndrome and seizure disorders are examples.

CEREBRAL PALSY

Cerebral palsy (CP) is a group of disorders affecting the ability to move and maintain balance and posture. Areas of the brain (*cerebral*) that control movement and posture do not develop correctly or are damaged. *Palsy* means *weakness* or *problems using the muscles.*

Brain damage can occur before, during, or after birth. Brain damage more than 28 days after birth may be caused by a brain infection or serious head injury.

A movement disorder, CP causes the person problems controlling muscles. Signs and symptoms range from mild to severe (Box 54-4). One or both sides of the body may be affected.

Spastic CP is the most common type. *Spastic means uncontrolled contractions of skeletal muscles.* The person has increased muscle tone, causing stiff muscles and awkward movements. Different body parts may be involved—legs; arms and legs; 1 side of the body; both arms and legs, the trunk, and face. Posture, balance, and movement are

affected. The person may be able to walk with adaptive (assistive) devices or not be able to walk at all (Fig. 54-2). When the arms are affected, there are problems with eating, writing, dressing, and other activities of daily living.

The person may have other health problems.

- Seizure disorders
- Intellectual disabilities
- Delayed growth and development
- Spinal deformities and arthritis
- Impaired vision
- Hearing loss
- Speech and language disorders
- Drooling
- Incontinence
- Pain or difficulty feeling sensations
- Learning problems
- Infections and long-term illnesses—heart and lung diseases, pneumonia
- Contractures
- Malnutrition
- Dental problems
- Inactivity

CP has no cure. The health team develops a plan to help the person reach his or her full potential. Treatment may involve drugs, surgery, braces, crutches, and various therapies—physical, occupational, speech and language, and so on.

BOX 54-4 **Cerebral Palsy—Signs and Symptoms**

3 to 6 Months of Age
- Head falls back when picked up while lying on the back.
- Feels stiff.
- Feels floppy.
- Seems to over-extend the back and neck when held.
- Legs get stiff and cross or scissor when picked up.

6 Months of Age and Older
- Does not roll over in either direction.
- Cannot bring the hands together.
- Has difficulty bringing the hand to the mouth.
- Reaches out with 1 hand while keeping the other fisted.

10 Months of Age and Older
- Crawls in a lop-sided manner. Pushes off with 1 hand and leg; drags the other hand and leg.
- Scoots on buttocks or hops on knees.
- Does not crawl on all fours.

Modified from Centers for Disease Control and Prevention: 11 things to know about cerebral palsy, *Atlanta, Ga, page reviewed September 23, 2019.*

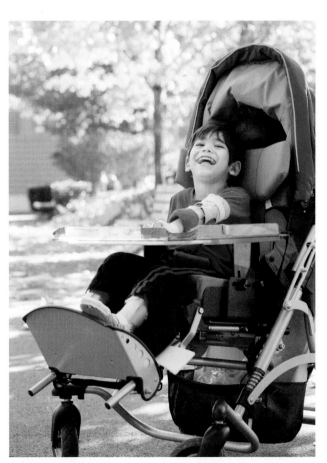

FIGURE 54-2 A child with cerebral palsy. (Copyright © jarenwicklund/ iStock/Thinkstock.com.)

SPINA BIFIDA

Spina bifida (SB) is a defect in which the brain, bones in the spine (vertebrae), or spinal cord do not form properly. *(Spina* means *backbone. Bifid* means *split in 2 parts.)* The defect occurs during the first month of pregnancy. Hydrocephalus often occurs with SB.

The lower back is a common site for SB. Types of SB include:

- *Spina bifida occulta. Occult* means *hidden.* A defect occurs in the vertebrae. A layer of skin covers and hides the defect. The spinal cord and nerves are not damaged. The person has a dimple or tuft of hair on the back (Fig. 54-3). The most common and mildest form of SB, often there are no symptoms. Foot weakness and bowel and bladder problems can occur.
- *Closed neural tube defect.* During the first month of pregnancy, the brain and spinal cord develop from the neural tube. In this defect, the spinal cord is malformed. Depending on the defect, symptoms vary from none to paralysis and urinary and bowel problems.
- *Meningocele. Meningo* means *membrane. Cele* means *hernia* or *swelling.* Meninges are the connective tissue that cover and protect the brain and spinal cord. A sac of fluid without the spinal cord comes through an opening in the back (Fig. 54-4, *A* and Fig. 54-5). The sac does not contain nerve tissue. The spinal cord and nerves may be normal with no damage. Or there is paralysis and bowel and bladder problems. Surgery corrects the defect.
- *Myelomeningocele (or meningomyelocele). Myelo* means *spinal cord.* A sac of fluid containing nerves and part of the spinal cord comes through an opening in the back (see Fig. 54-4, *B*). Nerve damage occurs. Loss of function occurs below the level of damage. Leg paralysis and lack of sensation are common. So is the lack of bowel and bladder control. The defect is closed with surgery.

Children with SB are at high risk for bladder, bowel, and mobility problems. Skin breakdown, depression, and social and sexual issues are other risks. Some children have learning problems.

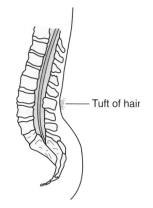

FIGURE 54-3 Spina bifida occulta.

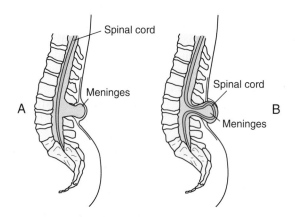

FIGURE 54-4 A, Meningocele. **B,** Meningomyelocele.

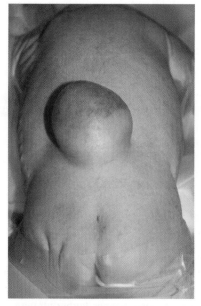

FIGURE 54-5 Meningocele. (From Swaiman KF et al: *Swaiman's pediatric neurology, principles and practice,* ed 6, Philadelphia, 2017, Elsevier.)

HYDROCEPHALUS

With hydrocephalus, cerebrospinal fluid collects in and around the brain. *(Hydro* means *water. Cephalo* means *head.)* The head enlarges (Fig. 54-6). Pressure inside the head increases. Intellectual disabilities and neurological damage occur without treatment. Vision problems, seizures, and learning disabilities can occur.

If untreated, hydrocephalus usually causes death. Treatment involves a shunt placed in the brain. It allows cerebrospinal fluid to drain from the brain. The shunt is a long, flexible tube. It goes from the brain into a body cavity to drain (Fig. 54-7). The shunt must remain open *(patent)*. If blocked, the cerebrospinal fluid cannot drain from the brain.

Hydrocephalus can be present at birth. Genetic problems and problems with fetal development are causes. Hydrocephalus also can occur at any age after birth. Injury, stroke, infections, tumors, and bleeding in the brain are causes.

FETAL ALCOHOL SPECTRUM DISORDERS

Drinking alcohol during pregnancy can cause a group of conditions called fetal alcohol spectrum disorders (FASDs). Children born with FASD have a mix of problems—medical, behavioral, educational (learning), and social. Signs and symptoms are listed in Box 54-5.

Types of FASD depend on the signs and symptoms present. For example, a person might have an intellectual disability and problems with learning and behavior. Or a person may have problems with the heart, kidneys, or bones. Fetal alcohol syndrome (FAS) is the most serious type. Fetal death is possible. Persons with FAS may have a mix of the signs and symptoms listed in Box 54-5.

FASDs are life-long with no cure. Treatment depends on the person's needs. Drugs for some symptoms, behavior and education therapy, and parent training are common.

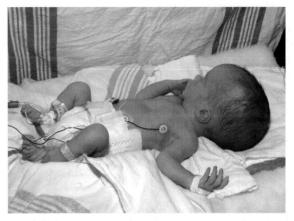

FIGURE 54-6 Hydrocephalus. (From Kliegman RM, Stanton BF, St Geme JW III, Schor NF: *Nelson textbook of pediatrics,* ed 20, Elsevier, 2016.)

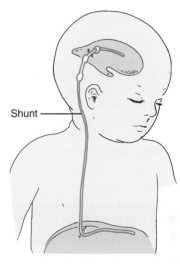

FIGURE 54-7 A shunt drains fluid from the brain. (Modified from Hockenberry MJ, Wilson D, Rodgers CC: *Wong's nursing care of infants and children,* ed 11, St Louis, 2019, Elsevier.)

BOX 54-5	**Fetal Alcohol Spectrum Disorders—Signs and Symptoms**
• Abnormal facial features such as a smooth ridge between the nose and upper lip • Small head size • Shorter-than-average height • Low body weight • Poor coordination • Hyperactive behavior • Attention problems • Poor memory	• Learning disabilities and difficulty in school (especially with math) • Speech and language delays • Intellectual disabilities • Poor reasoning and judgment skills • Sleep and sucking problems as a baby • Vision or hearing problems • Problems with the heart, kidneys, or bones

FOCUS ON PRIDE

The Person, Family, and Yourself

Personal and Professional Responsibility

Caring for persons with IDDs is a joy and a challenge. The person may struggle with speech, learning, mobility, or self-care. Care needs can be great. Despite these challenges, the person often has a positive outlook on life and brings joy to others.

Do not allow challenges to affect your attitude. Instead, let your attitude overcome the challenges. Take pride in your decision to have a positive attitude.

Rights and Respect

Persons with IDDs have the right to enjoy and maintain a good quality of life. That involves friendships, health and safety, and the right to make choices and take risks. Treat the person with dignity and respect. Allow personal choice. Always provide quality care.

Independence and Social Interaction

The Arc believes that children with IDDs should be included in community life. They should have the opportunity to live in a family home. They should learn and play with children without disabilities.

As adults, they should control their lives as much as possible. They should speak, make choices, and act for themselves. They should live in a home, have friends, do meaningful work, and enjoy adult activities. Independence to the greatest extent possible is the goal.

Delegation and Teamwork

Some persons respond better to care from certain people. For example, you are patient and kind but a person refuses to eat. A visiting family member is able to get the person to eat.

Do not be offended if the person responds to someone else. It does not mean you have done something wrong. And it does not mean the person does not like you. The person may prefer another person at that time.

Do not let your pride get in the way of meeting the person's needs. Another caregiver may need to assist the person. Learn from the person. He or she may take a different approach or know the person's preferences. Thank him or her for helping.

Ethics and Laws

Persons with IDDs must be protected from abuse, mistreatment, and neglect (Chapters 2 and 5). They may have limited communication skills. Or they may fear what will happen if they tell. Changes in mood or behavior, frequent injuries, poor hygiene, weight loss, and anxiety around a caregiver are signs of abuse. See Chapter 5 for others. Tell the nurse right away if you suspect abuse. Take pride in protecting the person's safety and well-being.

FOCUS ON PRIDE: Application

What factors affect quality of life? Are these the same for persons with IDDs? How do family members, caregivers, friends, and others affect the person's quality of life and self-worth?

REVIEW QUESTIONS

Circle the BEST answer.

1 All IDDs
   a Are preventable
   b Occur from trauma
   c Are caused by birth defects
   d Begin before, during, or after birth or in childhood

2 These statements are about IDDs. Which is *true*?
   a Self-care, learning, and mobility are always affected.
   b The disability is life-long.
   c Physical and intellectual impairments are mild.
   d The person cannot hold a job.

3 The person with an intellectual disability
   a Has delayed development of sexual organs
   b Does not have the skills to live, work, and play
   c Learns at a slower rate than normal
   d Needs care in a special setting

4 Intellectual disabilities
   a Are always severe
   b Begin before 18 years of age
   c Are caused by an extra chromosome
   d Affect the motor region of the brain

5 Down syndrome occurs
   a At fertilization
   b During the first month of pregnancy
   c Any time before, during, or after birth
   d From trauma

6 Down syndrome always involves some degree of
   a Cerebral palsy
   b Autism
   c Impaired mobility
   d Intellectual disability

7 Fragile X syndrome is
   a The result of brain injury
   b Caused by drug and alcohol use
   c Inherited from parents
   d Caused by an infection

8 Autism spectrum disorder begins
   a At fertilization
   b During pregnancy
   c At birth
   d In early childhood

9 The person with autism spectrum disorder has
   a Impaired movement
   b Paralysis and brain damage
   c Social and communication problems
   d Poor muscle tone

REVIEW QUESTIONS—cont'd

10 Which statement about cerebral palsy is *true*?
   a CP is caused by brain damage or abnormal brain development.
   b Children with CP have distinct facial features.
   c Drugs and therapies can cure CP.
   d CP is a genetic disorder.

11 The spastic type of cerebral palsy involves problems with
   a Learning
   b Drooling
   c Posture, balance, and movement
   d Communication

12 Spina bifida involves
   a Brain damage
   b A defect in the spinal column
   c Seizures
   d Intellectual disabilities

13 The person with spina bifida may have
   a Bowel and bladder problems
   b A short attention span
   c Hearing and vision problems
   d Speech and language problems

14 Hydrocephalus often occurs with
   a Down syndrome
   b Cerebral palsy
   c Spina bifida
   d Autism

15 Hydrocephalus is treated with
   a Braces and crutches
   b A shunt
   c Drugs
   d Social services

16 The child with fetal alcohol syndrome
   a Has a seizure disorder
   b Always has a physical disability
   c Has a mix of symptoms
   d Must stop drinking alcohol

Answers to Chapter 54 questions are on p. 888.

FOCUS ON **PRACTICE**

Problem Solving

A child with autism spectrum disorder becomes agitated when taken to an activity area with other children. Is this behavior expected? What will you do?

OBJECTIVES

- Define the key terms and key abbreviations in this chapter.
- Describe sex, sexuality, and sexual relationships.
- Explain why sexuality is important throughout life.
- Explain how aging, injury, and illness can affect sexuality.
- Explain how the nursing team can promote sexuality.

- Explain why some persons become sexually aggressive.
- Describe how to deal with sexually aggressive persons.
- Explain how to promote PRIDE in the person, the family, and yourself.

KEY TERMS

bisexual A person who is attracted to males and females

erectile dysfunction (ED) The inability of the male to have or maintain an erection

gay A person who is attracted to members of the same sex

gender identity A person's sense or feelings of being male, female, a combination of male and female, or neither male nor female

heterosexual A person who is attracted to members of the other sex

sex Physical interactions between people involving the body and reproductive organs

sexual orientation Emotional, romantic, and physical attraction to men, women, or both sexes

sexuality The physical, emotional, social, cultural, and spiritual factors that affect a person's feelings, attitudes, and behaviors about one's gender identity and sexual behavior

transgender Describes people who express their sexuality or gender identity in ways that do not fit with their biological sex (male, female)

KEY ABBREVIATIONS

ED	Erectile dysfunction	OBRA	Omnibus Budget Reconciliation Act of 1987

Patients and residents are viewed as whole persons with basic needs. Their physical, emotional, social, and spiritual needs are considered. So are their needs for love, affection, sexual intimacy, and sense of well-being. Sexuality involves the whole person. Illness, injury, and aging can affect sexuality.

NOTE: Definitions and descriptions related to sexuality vary. Some are very complex. Terms used in society continue to change over time as more information becomes known. Those used in this chapter are broad and dictionary-based.

See *Body Structure and Function Review: The Reproductive System.*

SEX AND SEXUALITY

Sex is the physical interactions between people involving the body and reproductive organs. **Sexuality** *is the physical, emotional, social, cultural, and spiritual factors that affect a person's feelings, attitudes, and behaviors about one's gender identity and sexual behavior.* Sexuality involves the personality and the body—how a person behaves, thinks, dresses, and responds to others.

Sexuality development begins when a baby's biological sex—male or female—is known. One's sex—being male or female—is based on reproductive organs and structures. Names, colors, and toys are chosen accordingly. For example, blue is commonly used for boys. Pink is commonly

BODY STRUCTURE AND FUNCTION REVIEW

The Reproductive System

The Male Reproductive System

The male reproductive system is shown in Figure 55-1. The 2 *testes (testicles)* are the male sex glands. Male sex cells *(sperm)* are produced in the testes. So is *testosterone,* the male hormone. This hormone is needed for reproductive organ function and for the development of male secondary sex characteristics (Chapter 11).

The *prostate gland* lies just below the bladder. The *urethra* runs through the prostate gland. The urethra is contained within the penis.

The *penis* is outside of the body. The penis has *erectile* tissue. When a man is sexually excited, blood fills the erectile tissue. The penis enlarges and becomes hard and erect for sexual activity.

The Female Reproductive System

Figures 55-2 and 55-3 show the female reproductive system. The female sex glands are called *ovaries.* The 2 ovaries contain *ova* or eggs—the female sex cells. The ovaries secrete the female hormones *estrogen* and *progesterone.* These hormones are needed for reproductive system function and the development of female secondary sex characteristics (Chapter 11).

The *uterus* is a hollow, muscular organ. The uterus serves as a place for the *fetus* (unborn baby) to grow and receive nourishment. The *cervix* of the uterus projects into a muscular canal called the *vagina.* The vagina opens to the outside of the body. The vagina receives the penis during intercourse. It also is part of the birth canal. Glands in the vaginal wall keep it moistened with secretions.

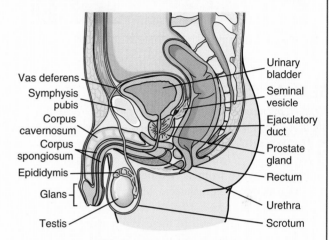

FIGURE 55-1 Male reproductive system.

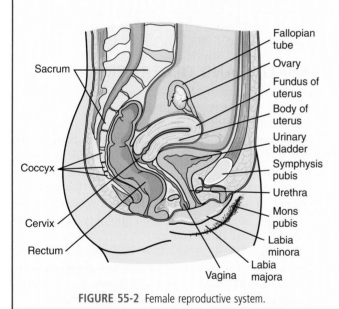

FIGURE 55-2 Female reproductive system.

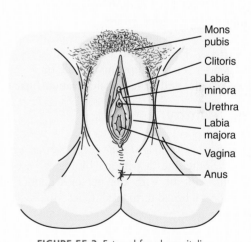

FIGURE 55-3 External female genitalia.

used for girls. Dolls are for girls. Trains are for boys. By the age of 3, children can identify males and females. They learn male and female roles from adults (Fig. 55-4, p. 810). Children learn that boys and girls behave in certain ways.

As children develop and grow older, interest increases about the body and how it works. Teens are more aware of their bodies. Their bodies respond to stimulation. They engage in sexual behaviors. They kiss, embrace, pet, or have intercourse. Pregnancy and sexually transmitted diseases (Chapter 51) are great risks.

Sex and sexuality have more meaning as young adults mature. Attitudes and feelings are important. Partners are selected. Decisions are made about sex before marriage and birth control.

Sexuality is important throughout life. Attitudes and needs change with aging. They are affected by life events. These include divorce, death of a partner, injury, illness, and surgery.

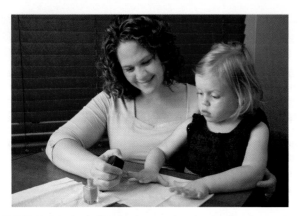

FIGURE 55-4 This little girl is learning female roles from her mother.

SEXUAL ORIENTATION

Sexual orientation refers to the emotional, romantic, and physical attraction to men, women, or both sexes.

- *Heterosexual—a person who is attracted to members of the other sex. (Hetero means another or different.)* Men are attracted to women. Women are attracted to men. Sexual behavior is male-female.
- *Gay—a person who is attracted to members of the same sex.* Men are attracted to men. Women are attracted to women. *Lesbian* refers to a gay woman. Gay people were previously called "homosexuals." That term is considered out-dated and offensive by many gay persons and gay rights groups.
- *Bisexual—a person who is attracted to males and females. (Bi means 2.)* Persons who are bisexual have same-gender relationships (male-male or female-female) and male-female relationships.

Gender Identity

Gender identity refers to a person's sense or feelings of being male, female, a combination of male and female, or neither male nor female. Sometimes a person's biological sex (male or female) does not fit with the person's gender identity. Transgender is a broad term used to describe such persons. *Transgender describes people who express their sexuality or gender identity in ways that do not fit with their biological sex (male, female).*

Some people express gender identity by their behaviors, clothing, hair-style, grooming, voice, and so on. There may be name and pronoun changes. For example, Jamie and "she" and "her" are used instead of James and "he" and "him." Or Allison is changed to Allen with pronoun changes.

Physical transitions involve body changes from male to female or female to male. Hormone and surgical measures are involved.

INJURY, ILLNESS, AND SURGERY

Injury, illness, and surgery can affect sexual function. Sometimes the nervous, circulatory, and reproductive systems are involved. Sexual ability may change. Most chronic illnesses affect sexual function. Heart disease, stroke, diabetes, and chronic obstructive pulmonary disease are examples. Some drugs affect sexual desire or performance.

Reproductive system surgeries have physical and mental effects. Removal of the uterus, ovaries, or a breast affects women. Prostate or testes removal affects erections.

Erectile dysfunction (ED) is the inability of the male to have or maintain an erection. The many causes include diabetes, spinal cord injuries, prostate problems, alcoholism, cardiovascular disorders, drug abuse, and psychological factors. Some drugs for high blood pressure cause ED. So do other drugs. Some drugs treat ED.

Emotional changes are common in men and women. A person may feel unclean, unwhole, unattractive, or mutilated. The person may feel unfit for closeness and love. Therefore some problems are emotional. Time and understanding are helpful. So is a caring partner. Some persons need counseling.

Changes in sexual function greatly affect the person. Fear, anger, worry, and depression are seen in behaviors and comments. The person's feelings are normal and expected. The care plan has measures to help the person deal with his or her feelings.

SEXUALITY AND OLDER PERSONS

Love, affection, and intimacy are needed throughout life (Fig. 55-5). Older persons love, fall in love, and have intimate relationships and activities.

Older persons have many losses. Children leave home. Family and friends die. People retire. Health problems occur. Strength decreases. Appearance changes.

Reproductive organs change with aging (Chapter 12). Frequency of sex may decrease. Reasons relate to weakness, fatigue, and pain. Reduced mobility, aging, and chronic illness are other factors.

Some older people do not have intercourse. This does not mean loss of sexual needs or desires. Often needs are expressed in other ways. They hold hands, touch, caress, and embrace. These bring closeness and intimacy.

Sexual partners are lost through death, divorce, and relationship break-ups. Or a partner needs hospital or nursing center care. These situations occur in adults of all ages.

MEETING SEXUAL NEEDS

The nursing team promotes the meeting of sexual needs. The measures in Box 55-1 may be part of the person's care plan.

See *Focus on Long-Term Care and Home Care: Meeting Sexual Needs.*

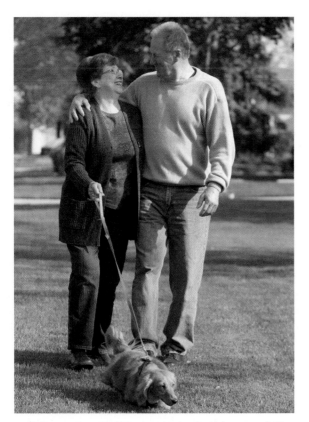

FIGURE 55-5 Love and affection are important to persons of all ages.

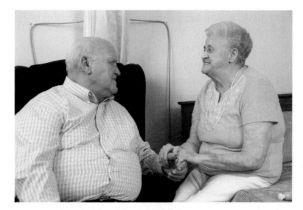

FIGURE 55-6 Relationships continue even when nursing center care is needed.

BOX 55-1 Promoting Sexuality

- Let the person practice grooming routines. Assist as needed. See Chapter 25.
- Let the person choose clothing. Patient gowns can embarrass the person. Street clothes are worn if the person's condition permits.
- Protect the right to privacy. Do not expose the person. Drape and screen the person.
- Treat the person with dignity and respect. The person may not share your sexual attitudes, values, or practices. The person may have a premarital or extramarital relationship. Do not judge or gossip about the person.
- Allow privacy. If the person has a private room, close the door for privacy. Some agencies have DO NOT DISTURB signs for doors. Let the person and partner know how much time they have alone. For example, remind them about meal times and care measures. Tell other staff that the person wants time alone.
- Knock before you enter any room. This simple courtesy shows respect for privacy.
- Consider the person's roommate. Privacy curtains do not block sound. Arrange for privacy when the roommate is out of the room. A roommate may offer to leave for a while. Or the nurse finds a private area.
- Allow privacy for masturbation. It is a normal form of sexual expression. Close the privacy curtain and the door. Knock before you enter the room. This saves you and the person embarrassment. Sometimes confused persons masturbate in public areas. Lead the person to a private area. Or distract him or her with an activity.

INAPPROPRIATE SEXUAL BEHAVIOR

Patients and residents may have inappropriate sexual behaviors. Such behaviors may be innocent and non-aggressive. Others are aggressive.

Some persons flirt, make sexual advances or comments, or ask for sexual favors. Some expose themselves, masturbate, or touch or grab a staff member's breast, buttocks, or genitals. This can anger and embarrass the staff member. These reactions are normal. Often there are reasons for the person's behavior. Understanding this helps you deal with the matter.

Inappropriate sexual behaviors have many causes. They include:

- Nervous system disorders
- Confusion, disorientation, and dementia
- Drug side effects
- Fever
- Poor vision

Some sexually inappropriate behaviors are innocent. The person may confuse someone with his or her partner. Or the person cannot control the behavior. The healthy person controls sexual urges. Changes in the brain and mental function make control difficult.

Sometimes touch is used to gain attention. For example, a resident cannot speak or move his or her right side. Your buttocks are within reach. To get your attention, the person touches your buttocks. The behavior is not sexual.

Some persons engage in masturbation. That is, they touch and fondle their own genitals for sexual pleasure. Sometimes masturbation is an aggressive behavior. However, touching the genitals may signal a health problem. Urinary or reproductive system disorders can cause genital soreness and itching. So can poor hygiene and being wet or soiled from urine or feces.

Sexually aggressive behaviors—touching, grabbing, offensive comments—may be about power, control, or fears about sexual function. For example, a person wants to prove attractiveness and the ability to perform sexually. You must be professional about the matter.

- Ask the person not to touch you. State the places where you were touched.
- Stand back from the person or move the person's hand away if you are being touched or grabbed. Tell the person: "Don't do that."
- Tell the person that you will not do what the person wants.
- Tell the person what behaviors make you uncomfortable. Politely ask the person not to act that way.
- Tell the person how to address you. For example, tell the person your name. Ask the person not to call you honey, sweetheart, and so on.
- Allow privacy if the person is becoming aroused. Provide for safety. Complete a safety check of the room (see the inside of the back cover). Tell the person when you will return.
- Discuss the matter with the nurse. The nurse can help you understand the behavior.
- Follow the care plan. It has measures to deal with sexually aggressive behaviors. They are based on the cause of the behavior.

See *Focus on Communication: Inappropriate Sexual Behavior.*

FOCUS ON COMMUNICATION

Inappropriate Sexual Behavior

Dealing with sexually inappropriate behavior is hard. This is true for young and older staff and for new and experienced staff. Ask yourself these questions.

- Does the person have a health problem that affects impulse control? If yes, the behavior may not have a sexual purpose.
- Is the person's behavior on purpose? Is the intent sexual? If yes, you must confront the behavior. Be direct and matter-of-fact. For example, you can say:
  - "You brushed your hand across my breast (or other body part) twice this morning. Please don't do that again."
  - "No, I cannot kiss you. It would be unprofessional."
  - "You exposed yourself to me again today. Please do not do that again."

The sexually aggressive person needs the nurse's attention. Report what happened and when. Also report what you said and did. The nurse must deal with the problem. If other staff report such behaviors, the nurse views the problem in a broader way.

Protecting the Person

The person must be protected from unwanted sexual comments and advances. This is sexual abuse (Chapter 5). Tell the nurse right away. No one is allowed to sexually abuse another person. This includes staff members, patients, residents, family members or other visitors, and volunteers.

SEXUALLY TRANSMITTED DISEASES

Some diseases are spread by sexual contact. They are discussed in Chapter 51.

FOCUS ON PRIDE

The Person, Family, and Yourself

Personal and Professional Responsibility
Touching a person's body without the person's consent is abuse and a crime (Chapter 5). You must be extra cautious when care involves the genitals, buttocks, or breasts. Without consent, you may be accused of sexual abuse.

To obtain consent, explain what you will do before starting procedures and step-by-step. If the person asks you to stop, you must stop. Obtaining consent and explaining procedures are professional responsibilities. The person has control over care, knows what to expect, and is more at ease. The person's rights are protected. And you protect yourself from being accused of sexual abuse.

Rights and Respect
Each member of the health team must maintain an appropriate relationship with the person. Professional sexual misconduct is a serious violation of the person's rights (Chapters 2 and 5). Report any suspected inappropriate sexual behavior. This includes staff comments or behaviors that may seem sexual. Take pride in protecting the person from mistreatment and abuse.

Independence and Social Interaction
Sexuality includes emotional, social, cultural, spiritual, and physical factors. To promote sexuality:

- Assist the person with hygiene and grooming before visitors arrive.
- Compliment the person's appearance. Comment on hair, clothing, jewelry, nails, and other grooming measures.
- Talk with the person about family. Years of marriage and number of children are common topics. Respect privacy if the person does not want to talk.
- Use touch to show you care. A touch on the arm, shoulder, or upper back can communicate care without crossing boundaries (Chapter 5).

FOCUS ON **P R I D E—cont'd**

The Person, Family, and Yourself

Delegation and Teamwork

The health team must try to determine the cause of inappropriate sexual behaviors. If the cause can be corrected, the behavior may stop. If not, the care plan includes measures to manage the behavior. A professional response is always needed.

Tell the nurse about aggressive sexual behaviors. The problem cannot be ignored. Rely on the nursing team for advice, guidance, and support.

Ethics and Laws

The following is a real case of a nursing assistant who violated the person's right to freedom from abuse and mistreatment.

A certified nursing assistant (CNA) had his certificate revoked by the Arizona State Board of Nursing. The Board found that he violated the state's Nurse Practice Act because of the following actions.

- *He was convicted of "Driving Under the Influence."*
- *He agreed to a $150 penalty on his CNA certificate for several incidents of resident abuse. He also admitted to removing an impaction from a female resident, which he knew was not within the scope of CNA duties.*

Ethics and Laws—cont'd

- *While employed at a nursing home in 2005:*
  - *A female resident reported that he was "rough with her and 'hurt her groin.'" The resident demanded a transfer to another facility.*
  - *An alert and oriented resident reported that the CNA "'raped' her by placing his hand inside her private parts." The resident also stated that she "could smell alcohol on his breath."*
  - *His employment was terminated for policy violation and "causing a resident undue stress and fear when he assisted her to expel an impaction."*
- *While employed in a group home in 2005, it was reported that he violated agency policy regarding alcohol use.* (Arizona State Board of Nursing, 2006.)

No one is allowed to sexually abuse another person. Report concerns of abuse to the nurse.

FOCUS ON **PRIDE**: *Application*

Self-image affects sexuality. Identify ways you can promote the person's self-image.

REVIEW QUESTIONS

Circle the BEST answer.

1 Sex involves
   a The organs of reproduction
   b Attitudes and feelings
   c Cultural and spiritual factors
   d Masturbation

2 Sexuality is important to
   a Small children
   b Teenagers and young adults
   c Middle-age adults
   d Persons of all ages

3 Erectile dysfunction
   a Occurs in men and women
   b Involves transgender behaviors
   c Affects sexual performance
   d Is an inappropriate sexual behavior

4 Reproductive organs change with aging.
   a True   b False

5 To help promote a resident's sexuality you can
   a Stay in the room while the resident talks to a romantic friend
   b Provide a patient gown
   c Help with hair-styling
   d Enter the room without knocking

6 Two residents are holding hands. Nursing staff should keep them apart.
   a True   b False

7 Married residents want some time alone. Which measure would you question?
   a Close the room door.
   b Put a DO NOT DISTURB sign on the door.
   c Tell other staff that they want some time alone.
   d Close the privacy curtain so no one can hear them.

8 Married residents should each have a room. This is an OBRA requirement.
   a True   b False

9 A person is masturbating in the dining room. You should
   a Do nothing
   b Scold the person
   c Quietly take the person to his or her room
   d Restrain the person

10 A person touches you sexually. You should
   a Ignore the behavior
   b Do what the person asks
   c Tell your co-workers
   d Ask the person not to touch you

Answers to Chapter 55 questions are on p. 888.

FOCUS ON **PRACTICE**

Problem Solving

You are a student in the clinical setting needing to practice the bathing skill. A nursing assistant and an older resident are preparing for a bath. You introduce yourself and ask if you can assist. The resident says: "Morgan always gives me my bath." The nursing assistant says: "You don't have any modesty left at your age. The student can give your bath today." The resident is quiet. What will you do?

OBJECTIVES

- Define the key terms and key abbreviations in this chapter.
- Describe how to meet the safety and security needs of infants and children.
- Identify the signs and symptoms of illness in infants.
- Explain how to help mothers with breast-feeding.
- Describe 3 forms of baby formulas.
- Explain how to bottle-feed babies.
- Explain how to burp a baby.
- Describe how to give cord care.

- Describe the purposes of circumcision, needed observations, and the required care.
- Explain how to bathe infants.
- Explain why infants are weighed.
- Describe the care needed by mothers after childbirth.
- Perform the procedures described in this chapter.
- Explain how to promote PRIDE in the person, the family, and yourself.

KEY TERMS

breast-feeding Feeding a baby milk from the mother's breasts; nursing
circumcision The surgical removal of foreskin from the penis
episiotomy Incision *(otomy)* into the perineum
lochia The vaginal discharge that occurs after childbirth
meconium A dark green to black, tarry bowel movement
nursing See "breast-feeding"

postpartum After *(post)* childbirth *(partum)*
prenatal care The health care a woman receives while pregnant
umbilical cord The structure that connects the mother and fetus (unborn baby); it carries blood, oxygen, and nutrients from the mother to the fetus

KEY ABBREVIATIONS

BM	Bowel movement	F	Fahrenheit
C	Centigrade	ID	Identification
CPSC	Consumer Product Safety Commission	SIDS	Sudden infant death syndrome
C-section	Cesarean section	SUID	Sudden unexpected infant death

Mothers and newborns usually have short hospital stays. Some need home care after discharge because of:

- Complications before or after childbirth
- Health problems
- Needing help with other young children
- A multiple birth (twins, triplets, and so on)
- Needing help with meals and housekeeping

Babies depend on others for basic needs—physical, safety and security, and love and belonging. A review of growth and development will help you care for babies (Chapter 11).

See *Promoting Safety and Comfort: Caring for Mothers and Babies.*

PROMOTING SAFETY AND COMFORT

Caring for Mothers and Babies

Safety
Some care measures in this chapter involve exposing and touching a baby's private areas—the perineum and rectum. Sexual abuse has occurred in health care settings. Perform such care measures with a parent present. Always act in a professional manner.

Contact with urine or feces (stools) is likely when assisting with diaper changing and bathing. Urine and feces (stools) may contain microbes or blood. Follow Standard Precautions and the Bloodborne Pathogen Standard (Chapter 16).

NOTE: A task may require more than 1 pair of gloves. Change gloves as needed. Use careful judgment. Remember to practice hand hygiene after removing gloves.

SAFETY AND SECURITY

Babies cannot protect themselves. They need to feel safe and secure. They feel secure when warm and when wrapped and held snugly. Babies cry to communicate. They cry when soiled, hungry, hot or cold, tired, uncomfortable, or in pain. To promote safety and security, respond to their cries—feed them, change diapers as needed, comfort them, talk to them, and so on.

Follow the infant safety measures in Box 56-1. Follow the measures in Chapters 13 and 14 to protect children from burns, poisoning, choking and suffocation, and falls. Also see Appendix D, p. 893.

See *Focus on Long-Term Care and Home Care: Safety and Security*, p. 816.

Text continued on p. 818.

BOX 56-1	**Infant Safety**

General Safety

- Keep the baby warm. Check windows for drafts. Close windows securely.
- Keep your fingernails short. Do not wear non-natural nails. Long nails can scratch the baby.
- Do not wear rings or bracelets. Jewelry can scratch the baby.
- Respond to the baby's crying. Babies communicate by crying. Responding to their cries helps them feel safe and secure.
- Keep 1 hand on a child lying in a crib or on a scale, bed, table, or other surface or furniture (Fig. 56-1).
- Keep pins and small objects out of the baby's reach.
- Do not shake powder directly over the baby. The powder can get into the baby's eyes and lungs. Shake some on your hand away from the baby.
- Do not tie a pacifier around the baby's neck.

Holding a Baby

- Use both hands to lift a newborn. Use 1 hand to support the head and upper back. Use your other hand to support the legs. Do not lift a newborn by the arms.
- Hold the baby securely. Use the cradle hold, football hold, or shoulder hold (Fig. 56-2, p. 816).
- Support the baby's head and neck when lifting or holding the baby. Neck support is necessary for the first 3 months after birth.
- Handle the baby with gentle, smooth movements. Avoid sudden or jerking movements. Do not startle the baby.
- Hold and cuddle infants. It is comforting and helps them learn to feel love and security.

Crib and Furniture Safety

- Make sure the crib is within hearing distance of the caregivers.
- Do not put a pillow, quilts, bumper pads, or soft toys in the crib. They can cause suffocation.
- Place infants on a firm surface to sleep. Do not lay an infant on soft bedding products. This includes fluffy, plush products such as sheepskin, quilts, comforters, pillows, and toys. Soft products can cause suffocation.
- Report crib or furniture problems at once. Loose nuts, bolts, screws or bent, broken, or open mattress hooks are examples.
- See "Crib Safety" on p. 818.
- See Appendix D (p. 893) for nursery equipment safety. Nursery equipment must be safe and in good repair.

Sleep

- Remove bibs and necklaces before sleep.
- Lay babies on their backs for sleep. *Do not lay babies on their stomachs for sleep. This can interfere with chest expansion and breathing. The baby can suffocate.* Infants can lie on their sides and stomachs when awake and supervised.
- Make sure there is no soft bedding under the baby.
- Maintain a comfortable temperature. Babies must not get too hot during sleep. Do not use clothing that may cover the infant's head or cause over-heating.

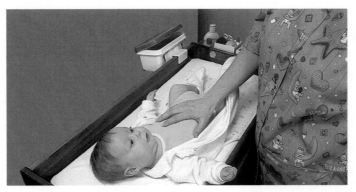

FIGURE 56-1 Keep 1 hand on a child lying on a raised surface.

FOCUS ON LONG-TERM CARE AND HOME CARE

Safety and Security

Home Care

Injuries in the home are preventable. Safety measures can protect infants and children from harm.

- Supervise infants and children at all times.
- Use childproof locks or door knob covers leading to non-childproof areas (Fig. 56-3).
- Use safety gates at the top and bottom of stairs.
- Do not let children climb on furniture. Also prevent furniture from tipping.
- Remove or pad furniture with sharp or rough edges.
- Check that the crib meets federal safety standards.
- Store harmful items where children cannot reach them. Keep items in locked storage areas.
- Keep child-resistant caps on drugs and other harmful substances.
- Keep cords and strings out of reach and away from cribs and playpens.
- Use outlet safety covers or outlet plugs on electrical outlets (Chapter 13). A choking hazard, use outlet plugs with caution. The plug must not be easily removed by children.
- Keep the hot water heater temperature below 120°F (Fahrenheit) (48°C [centigrade]) to prevent burns.

- Supervise children in or near water. Prevent children from entering areas that contain water.
- Follow safety measures for car seats.
  - Use a federally approved car seat. Choose a seat based on the child's age and size (Fig. 56-4).
  - Follow the car seat manufacturer's weight and height limits. The child should use the car seat for as long as possible—until weight or height limits are outgrown.
  - Use the seat correctly. Follow the manufacturer's instructions for how to install.
  - Keep the seat rear-facing for as long as possible. See Figure 56-4.
- Check that the child's clothing is safe and fits well. Drawstrings, ribbons, and cords are hazards (Fig. 56-5). Loose clothing, long clothing, and items around the neck are dangerous.
- Check that all toys are age-appropriate and are not damaged.
- Keep small items away from children. Make sure the child cannot fit items in the mouth.
- Follow the safety measures in Appendix D, p. 893.

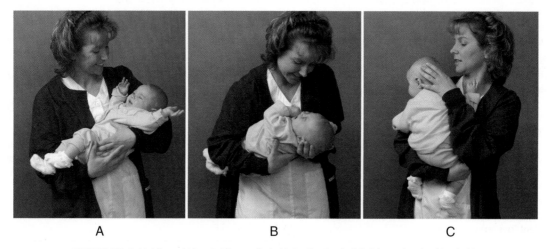

FIGURE 56-2 Holding a baby. **A,** The cradle hold. **B,** The football hold. **C,** The shoulder hold.

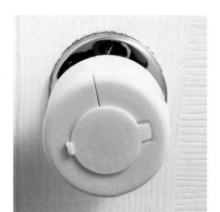

FIGURE 56-3 Door knob cover. The device turns instead of the door knob.

Using the correct car seat or booster seat can be a lifesaver: make sure your child is always buckled in an age- and size-appropriate car seat or booster seat.

Birth | 1 | 2 | 3 | 4 | 5 | 6 | 7 | 8 | 9 | 10 | 11 | 12+

Age by Years*

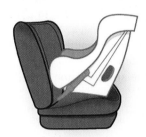 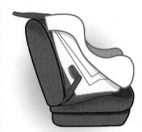 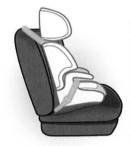 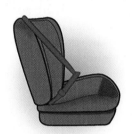

REAR-FACING CAR SEAT	FORWARD-FACING CAR SEAT	BOOSTER SEAT	SEAT BELT
Birth until age 2-4	**After outgrowing rear-facing seat until at least age 5**	**After outgrowing forward-facing seat and until seat belts fit properly**	**Once seat belts fit properly without a booster seat**
Buckle children in a rear-facing car seat until they reach the maximum weight or height limit of their car seat. Keep children rear-facing as long as possible.	When children outgrow their rear-facing car seat, they should be buckled in a forward-facing car seat until they reach the maximum weight or height limit of their car seat.	Once children outgrow their forward-facing seat, they should be buckled in a booster seat until seat belts fit properly. Proper seat belt fit usually occurs when children are 4 feet 9 inches tall and age 9-12.	Children no longer need to use a booster seat once seat belts fit them properly. Seat belts fit properly when the lap belt lays across the upper thighs (not the stomach) and the shoulder belt lays across the chest (not the neck).

Keep children ages 12 and under properly buckled in the back seat. Never place a rear-facing car seat in front of an active air bag.

Recommended age ranges for each seat type vary to account for differences in child growth and height/weight limits of car seats and booster seats. Use the car seat or booster seat owner's manual to check installation and the seat height and weight limits, and proper seat use.

Child safety seat recommendations: American Academy of Pediatrics.
Graphic design: adapted from National Highway Traffic Safety Administration.

FIGURE 56-4 Car seat guidelines. (From Centers for Disease Control and Prevention, Department of Health and Human Services.)

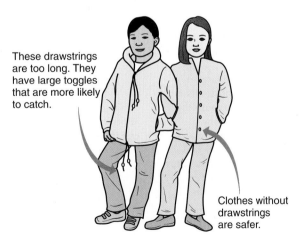

These drawstrings are too long. They have large toggles that are more likely to catch.

Clothes without drawstrings are safer.

FIGURE 56-5 Drawstrings, ribbons, and cords can get caught in many things and strangle the child.

Crib Safety

Cribs and crib linens present safety hazards. They can strangle and suffocate the baby. Mattresses, linens, and bumper pads pose many dangers. For safety:

- The mattress is firm and fits tightly.
- The mattress is covered with a fitted crib sheet that fits snugly.
- Sheets for larger beds are not used.
- Sheets are not used if they are frayed, worn, or have loose threads or stitching.
- Bumper pads are not used.
- Blankets or pillows are not placed between the mattress and fitted crib sheet.
- Pillows, blankets, comforters, quilts, sheepskin, sleep positioners, and pillow-like stuffed toys and other soft products are not placed in the crib.
- Plastic trash bags, dry-cleaning bags, or plastic packaging materials are not used to protect the mattress. The plastic can cling to the baby's face, nose, and mouth. This prevents breathing and causes suffocation.

Report any hazard to the nurse.

See *Focus on Long-Term Care and Home Care: Crib Safety.*

Sudden Unexpected Infant Death

Sudden unexpected infant death (SUID) is any sudden and unexpected death in an infant younger than 1 year old. The death may be explained or unexplained. The most common causes of SUID are:

- *Sudden infant death syndrome (SIDS)*—the sudden, unexplained death of an infant younger than 1 year old. SIDS is the leading cause of death in children between 1 month and 1 year of age. Most SIDS deaths occur between 1 and 4 months of age. It usually occurs during sleep.
- Accidental suffocation or strangulation in bed.
- Unknown causes.

Crib and sleep safety help prevent sudden infant death. See Figure 56-6 and Box 56-2, p. 820.

Regular wellness visits are important for infant and child health. Vaccines and breast-feeding (p. 821) protect against sudden infant death.

The mother's health during pregnancy affects the baby's risk. Women should receive regular prenatal care. *Prenatal care is the health care a woman receives while pregnant.* Mothers must avoid smoking, alcohol, and illegal drug use during pregnancy and after childbirth.

FOCUS ON LONG-TERM CARE AND HOME CARE

Crib Safety

Home Care

Cribs must meet federal safety standards. The American Academy of Pediatrics lists these safety standards and guidelines.

- Cribs with drop-side rails are not used. Cribs manufactured since June 2011 meet safety standards that ban a drop-side rail. Older cribs may not meet current safety standards.
- Crib slats (bars) are no more than 2⅜ inches apart. The baby's head can get caught in larger spaces, causing suffocation and death.
- Head-boards and foot-boards must not have cut-outs. The baby's head, arms, or legs can get trapped in cut-outs.
- Corner posts are flush with the end panels. Or they are very tall (as on a canopy bed). Clothing and ribbons can catch on corner posts and strangle a baby.
- Screws, bolts, nuts, plastic parts, and other hardware are original from the manufacturer and in place. Loose, missing, or replacement parts from a hardware store can cause the crib to collapse. This can trap and suffocate the baby.
- There are no rough edges or sharp points on metal parts. There are no cracks or splinters in wood.
- The mattress is the same size as the crib. There are no gaps to trap arms, legs, or the body. No more than 2 fingers should fit between the mattress and the sides or ends of the crib.

- Plastic wrapping from a new mattress is removed and destroyed. Plastic wrapping can suffocate a child.
- The crib is away from windows. Strangulation can occur from cords on window coverings. The Consumer Product Safety Commission (CPSC) recommends cordless window coverings.
- The following guide is used for when to lower the mattress and change beds.
  - *Before the baby can sit:* lower the mattress so the baby cannot fall out by leaning against a side or pulling over a side.
  - *Before the child can stand:* lower the mattress to the lowest position.
  - *When the child is 35 inches tall or when the height of the side rail is about nipple-level:* use a different bed. Falls occur most often when a child tries to climb out of the crib.

Check the crib after assembly and then weekly for loose joints, missing or broken parts, or sharp edges. Do not use the crib if parts are missing or broken.

What Does A **Safe Sleep Environment** Look Like?

The image below shows a safe infant sleep environment.

Baby's sleep area is in the same room, next to where parents sleep.

Use a firm and flat sleep surface, such as a mattress in a safety-approved crib*, covered by a fitted sheet

Baby should not sleep in an adult bed, on a couch, or on a chair alone, with you, or with anyone else.

Do not smoke or let anyone else smoke around your baby.

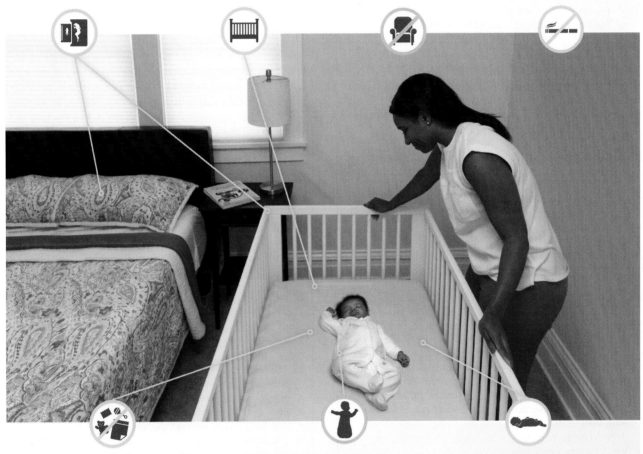

Do not put pillows, blankets, sheepskins, or crib bumpers anywhere in your baby's sleep area.

Keep soft objects, toys, and loose bedding out of your baby's sleep area. Make sure nothing covers the baby's head.

Dress your baby in sleep clothing, such as a wearable blanket. Do not use a loose blanket, and do not overbundle.

Always place your baby on his or her back to sleep, for naps and at night.

 NIH *Eunice Kennedy Shriver* National Institute of Child Health and Human Development

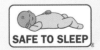 **SAFE TO SLEEP**

---

* A crib, bassinet, portable crib, or play yard that follows the safety standards of the Consumer Product Safety Commission (CPSC) is recommended. For information on crib safety, contact the CPSC at **1-800-638-2772** or http://www.cpsc.gov.

FIGURE 56-6 A safe sleep setting can reduce SIDS risk. (From Eunice Kennedy Shriver National Institute of Child Health and Human Development: *What does a safe sleep environment look like?*, U.S. Department of Health and Human Services.)

BOX 56-2	Sudden Infant Death Syndrome

Risk Factors
- Sleeping on the stomach.
- Sleeping on soft surfaces—adult mattress, couch, chair.
- Sleeping on or under soft or loose bedding or coverings.
- Getting too hot during sleep.
- Being exposed to cigarette smoke before or after birth.
- Sleeping in an adult bed with parents, other children, or pets. The danger increases if:
  - The adult smokes, has recently had alcohol, or is tired.
  - The baby is covered by a blanket or quilt.
  - The baby sleeps with more than 1 person.
  - The baby is younger than 11 to 14 weeks old.

Safety Measures
- Lay babies on their backs to sleep—for naps and at night.
- Use a firm, flat sleep surface.
  - Use a crib that meets CPSC safety standards.
  - Use a tight-fitting mattress covered by a fitted sheet.
- Do not use any other bedding or soft items in the sleep area—soft objects, toys, crib bumpers, loose bedding. See "Crib Safety."
- Place babies to sleep in the same room as the parents but not in the same bed. Do so for at least the first 6 months. It is best to do so for the first year.
- Do not smoke or allow smoking around babies or in their setting—home, car, and so on.
- Offer a pacifier for sleep.
  - Do not attach the pacifier to anything that could cause suffocation, choking, or strangulation. Strings, clothing, stuffed toys, and blankets are examples.
  - Wait until babies breast-feed well before using a pacifier. For formula-fed babies, a pacifier can be offered at any time. Do not force the baby to use one.
- Do not let babies get too hot during sleep. Dress babies in a wearable blanket. Do not use a loose blanket or over-bundle the baby. Watch for signs of over-heating—sweating, the chest feels hot to the touch. Do not cover the face or head.
- Do not use products that claim to reduce SIDS risk—wedges, positioning devices, heart and breathing monitors.
- Provide supervised time on the stomach (tummy time) when babies are awake.

Modified from National Institutes of Health: Known risk factors for SIDS and other sleep-related causes of infant death; Ways to reduce the risk of SIDS and other sleep-related causes of infant death, U.S. Department of Health and Human Services.

SIGNS AND SYMPTOMS OF ILLNESS

Babies can become ill quickly. Signs and symptoms may be sudden. You must be very alert. Report any of the signs and symptoms in Box 56-3 at once. Be alert to any change in the baby's behavior—sleep pattern, cry, appetite, or activity.

Tell the nurse when a sign or symptom began. You may need to measure the baby's temperature, pulse, and respirations (Chapter 33). The nurse tells you what temperature site to use—tympanic, rectal, temporal artery, or axillary. Apical pulses are taken on infants and young children.

BOX 56-3	Illness in Babies—Signs and Symptoms

- The baby has *jaundice*—a yellowish color to the skin and whites of the eyes.
- The baby looks sick.
- The baby has redness or drainage around the cord stump (p. 829) or circumcision (p. 829).
- The baby has a fever (Chapter 33).
- The baby is limp and slow to respond.
- The baby is hard to wake up.
- The baby is less active than usual.
- The baby cries all the time or does not stop crying.
- The baby is flushed, pale, or perspiring.
- The baby has noisy, rapid, difficult, or slow respirations.
- The baby is coughing or sneezing.
- The baby has reddened or irritated eyes.
- The baby turns the head to 1 side or puts a hand to 1 ear (signs of an earache).
- The baby screams for a long time.
- The baby is feeding poorly or has skipped feedings.
- The baby has vomited most of the feeding or vomits between feedings.
- The baby has watery stools or hard, formed stools.
- Stools are light-colored, green, or foul-smelling.
- The baby has fewer wet diapers.
- The baby has a rash.

HELPING MOTHERS BREAST-FEED

Breast-feeding (nursing) is feeding a baby milk from the mother's breasts.

- The baby can feed at the mother's breast.
- The mother can pump milk from her breasts. The baby is fed breast-milk from a bottle.

Babies usually breast-feed every 2 to 3 hours during the first month (8 to 12 times a day). They are fed on demand. That is, they are fed when hungry, not on a schedule. Breast-milk is digested faster than formula. Therefore nursing is needed more often.

The following signal hunger.

- Being more alert and active
- Putting the hands or fists to the mouth
- Making sucking motions with the mouth
- Turning the head to look for the breast (rooting reflex)
- Crying (may be a late sign)

Babies nurse for a short time the first few days. These early feedings are important. The mother makes a rich, thick, yellowish milk called *colostrum*. Colostrum protects the baby from infection and helps the gastro-intestinal system grow and function. By day 3 to 5, mature milk is formed. Nursing time takes longer—about 15 to 20 minutes at each breast. The rate varies for each baby. With time, feedings often are shorter and less frequent.

A feeding ends when:

- The baby's sucking slows.
- The baby pulls off the breast.
- The baby is no longer interested in feeding.

Weight, elimination, and behavior are monitored. Babies are getting enough milk if they:

- Gain weight steadily after the first week of age.
- Pass enough clear or pale urine (p. 826). Urine is not deep yellow or orange.
- Have enough bowel movements (p. 826).
- Have short sleeping periods and wakeful, alert periods.
- Are satisfied and content after feedings.

Nurses help new mothers learn to breast-feed and about breast care. Tell the nurse if the mother or baby is having problems nursing.

Mothers may need help getting ready to nurse. They may need help with hand-washing and positioning. Provide for privacy and make sure the call light is within reach before leaving the room. Follow the care plan and the measures in Box 56-4.

See *Focus on Long-Term Care and Home Care: Helping Mothers Breast-Feed*, p. 822.

BOX 56-4	Assisting With Breast-Feeding

- Practice hand hygiene and Standard Precautions. Remember, the human immunodeficiency virus (HIV) can be transmitted through breast-milk (Chapter 47).
- Place milk, juice, or water near the mother. Most mothers become thirsty while breast-feeding.
- Help the mother wash her hands. She needs clean hands before handling her breasts.
- Help the mother to a comfortable position. The cradle position, side-lying position, and football hold are the basic positions for breast-feeding (Fig. 56-7, p. 822).
- Change the baby's diaper if necessary. Bring the baby to the mother.
- Make sure the mother holds the baby close to her breast.
- Have the mother use her nipple to stroke the baby's cheek or lower lip. This stimulates the *rooting reflex* (Chapter 11). The baby turns his or her head toward the breast and starts to suck.
- Make sure the baby's nose is not blocked by the mother's breast. One nostril must be clear for breathing. If the nose seems blocked, have the mother do 1 of the following.
  - Re-position the baby. She can raise the baby's hips. Or she can move the baby's head back slightly.
  - Use her thumb to keep breast tissue away from the baby's nose with her thumb (Fig. 56-8, p. 822).
- Give her a baby blanket to cover the baby and her breast. This promotes privacy.
- Encourage nursing from both breasts at each feeding. If the last feeding ended at the right breast, the next feeding is started at the right breast. The mother can use a ribbon or diaper pin on her bra strap to remind her which breast to start with.

- Remind her how to remove the baby from the breast. To break the suction between the baby and the breast, she can insert a finger into a corner of the baby's mouth (Fig. 56-9, p. 822).
- Help the mother burp the baby (p. 825). The baby is burped after nursing at 1 breast. Then the baby is burped after nursing at the other breast.
- Remind the mother to air-dry her nipples after a feeding.
- Change the baby's diaper after the feeding.
- Lay the baby in the crib if he or she has fallen asleep. *Lay the baby on his or her back. Do not lay the baby on the stomach.*
- Help the mother prevent dry and cracked nipples. Follow the nurse's directions and the care plan.
  - Milk is left on the nipple after a feeding. The milk is allowed to air-dry.
  - The mother applies prescribed ointment or cream after each feeding if the nipples are cracked. If directed, remind her to wash her breasts with water before a feeding to remove the ointment or cream.
  - Soap is not used to clean the breasts and nipples.
  - Breasts and nipples are washed and dried gently.
- Help the mother straighten clothing after the feeding if necessary.
- Remind the mother to wash her breasts with a clean washcloth and warm water. Soap is not used. It can cause the nipples to dry and crack. Nipples are air-dried after washing to prevent cracking and soreness.
- Encourage the mother to wear a nursing bra day and night. The bra supports the breasts and promotes comfort.
- Encourage the mother to place nursing pads in the bra. The pads absorb leaking milk.

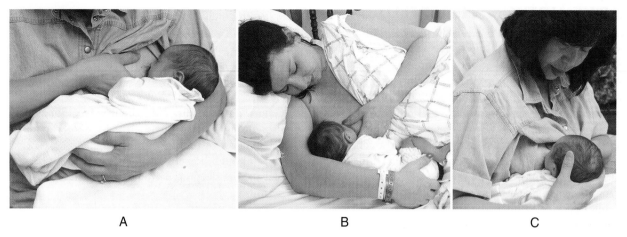

A   B   C

FIGURE 56-7 Basic breast-feeding positions. **A,** Cradle position. **B,** Side-lying position. **C,** Football hold. (From James SR, Nelson KA, Ashwill JW: *Nursing care of children: principles and practice*, ed 4, St Louis, 2013, Saunders.)

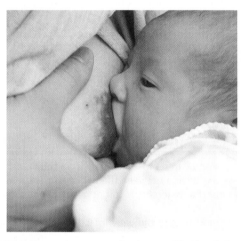

FIGURE 56-8 The mother supports her breast with 1 hand. The thumb is on top of the breast to keep breast tissue away from the baby's nose. (From James SR, Nelson KA, Ashwill JW: *Nursing care of children: principles and practice*, ed 4, St Louis, 2013, Saunders.)

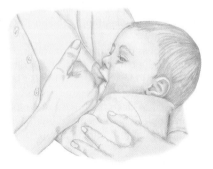

FIGURE 56-9 The mother inserts a finger into the corner of the baby's mouth to remove the baby from the breast. (From James SR, Ashwill JW, Droske SC: *Nursing care of children: principles and practice*, ed 2, Philadelphia, 2002, Saunders.)

FOCUS ON LONG-TERM CARE AND HOME CARE

Helping Mothers Breast-Feed

Home Care

Nursing mothers need good nutrition (Chapter 30). Calorie needs are the same as before pregnancy. This promotes weight loss after pregnancy. Some seafoods contain mercury. Tilefish, shark, swordfish, and king mackerel are examples. These are avoided when breast-feeding. White (albacore) tuna is limited to no more than 6 ounces per week.

Fluid needs increase when breast-feeding. The mother should:

- Drink plenty of fluids. Drink when thirsty. Drinking a glass of water or other fluid after each breast-feeding promotes hydration. More fluids are needed if urine is dark yellow and for other signs of dehydration (Chapter 31).
- Limit drinks with added sugars. Soda and fruit drinks are examples.
- Limit caffeine. A moderate amount (1 to 2 cups daily) does not affect most breast-fed babies. Sleep problems and fussiness can occur from too much caffeine.
- Avoid alcohol. Alcohol passes into breast-milk.

BOTTLE-FEEDING BABIES

Babies who are not breast-fed use formula. The doctor prescribes the formula. It provides the nutrients the infant needs.

Formula comes in 3 forms.

- *Ready-to-feed.* Ready to use, it is poured from the container into a baby bottle (Fig. 56-10). The container may have more than 1 feeding. Refrigerate after opening. Use the contents within 48 hours.
- *Powdered.* Container directions tell how much powder and water to use.
- *Liquid concentrate.* Container directions tell you how much liquid and water to use.

Bottles are prepared 1 at a time or in batches for the whole day. To prepare a bottle:

- Practice hand hygiene.
- Use water from a safe water source as directed by the nurse.
  - Bottled water.
  - Tap water. State and local health departments determine tap water safety.
  - Boiled tap water. Bring cold tap water to a boil for 1 minute. Cool to room temperature for no more than 30 minutes.
- Follow the container directions carefully. Measure exact amounts.
- Pour the correct amount of water and formula into the bottle.
- Gently shake or swirl the bottle to mix.
- Check the temperature by placing drops on the inside of your wrist. The formula should feel warm, not hot.
- Cap extra bottles (Fig. 56-11). Store them in the refrigerator. Use stored bottles within 24 hours.

Cleaning Baby Bottles

Protect the baby from infection. Baby bottles, caps, nipples, and other items must be as clean as possible. Disposable equipment is used in hospitals. Reusable equipment is common in homes. It is carefully washed in hot, soapy water or in a dishwasher. Complete rinsing is needed to remove all soap. Some bottles have plastic liners that are discarded after 1 use.

See *Delegation Guidelines: Cleaning Baby Bottles.*
See *Promoting Safety and Comfort: Cleaning Baby Bottles.*
See procedure: *Cleaning Baby Bottles,* p. 824.

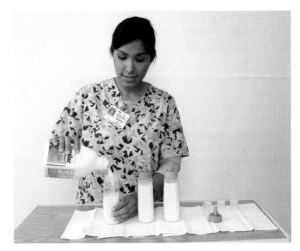

FIGURE 56-10 Ready-to-feed formula is poured from the container into the bottle.

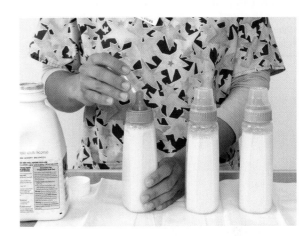

FIGURE 56-11 Bottles are capped for storage in the refrigerator.

DELEGATION GUIDELINES
Cleaning Baby Bottles

Cleaning baby bottles is a routine nursing task. Before cleaning bottles, you need this information from the nurse.
- What basin and bottle brush to use
- What dishwashing soap to use
- What other items to clean—funnel, can opener, and so on
- Where to place items to air-dry

PROMOTING SAFETY AND COMFORT
Cleaning Baby Bottles

Safety
Baby bottles, caps, nipples, and other items must be thoroughly rinsed to remove all soap. Otherwise, the baby takes in soap with the feeding. This can cause serious stomach and intestinal irritation.

Cleaning Baby Bottles

PRE-PROCEDURE

1   Follow *Delegation Guidelines: Cleaning Baby Bottles*, p. 823. See *Promoting Safety and Comfort: Cleaning Baby Bottles*, p. 823.
2   Practice hand hygiene.
3   Collect the following.
    • Bottles, nipples, caps, and any other bottle parts (rings, valves, and so on)
    • Wash basin—clean, used only for washing baby-feeding items

    • Bottle brush—clean, used only for washing baby-feeding items
    • Dishwashing soap
    • Other items used to prepare formula
    • Towel

PROCEDURE

4   Practice hand hygiene.
5   Take apart the bottles. Separate the parts of each bottle—bottle, nipple, cap, and any other parts.
6   Rinse the bottles, nipples, caps, and other bottle parts in warm or cold running water.
7   Place the items in the basin.
8   Fill the basin with hot water. Add dishwashing soap.
9   Wash the bottles, nipples, caps, and other bottle parts. Wash any other items used to prepare formula.
10 Clean inside baby bottles with the bottle brush (Fig. 56-12).

11 Squeeze hot, soapy water through the nipples (Fig. 56-13). This removes formula.
12 Rinse all items thoroughly. Squeeze water through the nipples to remove soap.
13 Lay a clean towel on the counter.
14 Stand bottles upside down to drain. Place nipples, caps, and other items on the towel. Let the items air-dry.
15 Rinse the basin and bottle brush well. Let them air-dry after use.

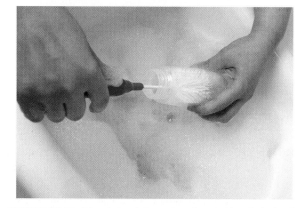

FIGURE 56-12 A bottle brush is used to clean inside a baby bottle.

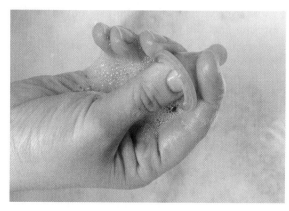

FIGURE 56-13 Water is squeezed through the nipple during washing and rinsing.

Feeding the Baby

Formula-fed babies usually want to be fed every 2 to 4 hours. They are fed on demand. The amount of formula taken increases as they grow older. The nurse or the mother tells you how much formula a baby needs at each feeding. Babies usually take as much formula as they need. The baby stops sucking and turns away from the bottle when satisfied.

Most babies do not like cold formula out of the refrigerator. To warm a bottle, hold the bottle under warm running tap water or in a container of warm water. Turn the bottle to warm the formula evenly.

The formula should feel warm. To test the temperature, sprinkle a few drops on the inside of your wrist. Allow the formula to cool if it is hot. The guidelines in Box 56-5 will help you bottle-feed babies.

Solid foods are given around 6 months. Usually baby rice or oatmeal cereal is the first solid food given. The cereal is mixed with breast-milk or formula to a thin consistency. Other solid foods are added as the baby grows. The nurse tells you what foods the baby can have.

See *Promoting Safety and Comfort: Feeding the Baby.*

PROMOTING SAFETY AND COMFORT

Feeding the Baby

Safety

Do not set the bottle out to warm at room temperature. This takes too long and allows the growth of microbes. Do not heat formula in microwave ovens. The formula can heat unevenly and burn the baby's mouth.

BOX 56-5	Bottle-Feeding Babies

- Warm a refrigerated bottle. The formula should feel warm to the inside of your wrist (Fig. 56-14).
- Assume a comfortable position for the feeding.
- Hold the baby close to you. Relax and snuggle the baby.
- Stroke the baby's cheek or lip with the nipple. The baby's head will turn to the nipple.
- Tilt the bottle so that the neck of the bottle and the nipple are always full (Fig. 56-15). Otherwise some air is in the neck or nipple. The baby sucks air into the stomach, causing cramping and discomfort.
- Do not prop the bottle and lay the baby down for the feeding (Fig. 56-16).

- Burp the newborn after every ½ to 1 ounce of formula. (Measurements are marked on the bottle.) Older babies are burped less often—after every 2 to 3 ounces. Also burp the baby at the end of the feeding.
- Do not leave the baby alone with a bottle.
- Do not force the baby to finish the bottle.
- Discard remaining formula. Do not save or reheat it for another feeding.
- Wash the bottle, cap, nipple, and any other bottle parts after the feeding (see procedure: *Cleaning Baby Bottles*).

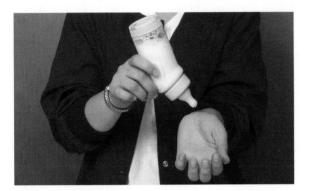

FIGURE 56-14 Testing formula temperature. Formula should feel warm on the inside of your wrist.

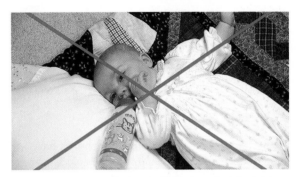

FIGURE 56-16 Do NOT prop the bottle to feed the baby.

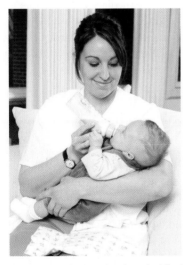

FIGURE 56-15 The bottle is tilted so that formula fills the bottle neck and nipple.

BURPING THE BABY

Babies take in air during feedings. Air in the stomach and intestines causes cramping and discomfort. This can lead to vomiting. Burping helps to get rid of the air. Most babies burp mid-way and after a feeding.

To burp a baby, gently pat or rub the baby's back with circular motions. Figure 56-17 (p. 826) shows how to position the baby for burping.

- *Over the shoulder.* First place a clean diaper or towel over your shoulder. This protects your clothing if the baby "spits up." Then hold the infant over your shoulder.
- *On your lap.* Support the baby in a sitting position on your lap. Hold the towel or diaper in front of the baby. *Remember to support the infant's head and neck for the first 3 months after birth.*
- *On the baby's stomach.* First place a clean diaper or towel on your lap where the baby's head will be. Position the baby on your lap with his or her stomach down.

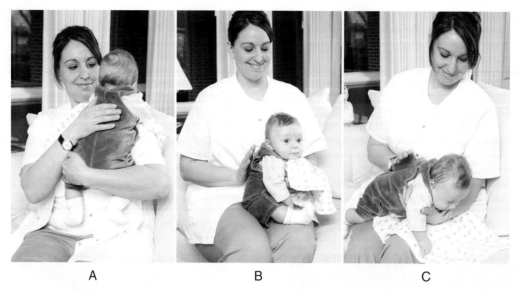

FIGURE 56-17 Burping a baby. **A,** The baby is held over the shoulder. **B,** The baby is supported in the sitting position. **C,** The baby is laid on the stomach.

DIAPERING A BABY

In the first 1 or 2 days after birth, newborns have meconium stools. *Meconium is a dark green to black, tarry bowel movement.* By day 3 or 4, stools are greenish brown to yellowish brown in color and less sticky. By day 4 or 5:

- *Breast-fed babies*—have yellow and seedy-looking stools. They are soft or runny. Breast-fed babies usually have a bowel movement (BM) with every feeding.
- *Formula-fed babies*—have yellow to brown stools. Formula-fed babies have fewer stools than breast-fed babies and their stools are firmer. They may have 1 or 2 stools a day.

Over time, an elimination pattern develops. Some babies have 1, 2, or 3 stools a day. Stools are usually soft and unformed. Hard, formed stools signal constipation. Watery stools mean diarrhea. Diarrhea is very serious in infants. Their fluid balance is upset quickly (Chapter 31). Tell the nurse at once if you suspect constipation or diarrhea.

Babies wet at least 6 to 8 times a day. Diapers are changed when wet or when stools are present.

Cloth diapers are re-used. With Velcro fasteners, no diaper pins are needed. The danger of sticking the baby or yourself with a diaper pin is avoided. To care for cloth diapers:

- Rinse a soiled cloth diaper. Rinse stools into the toilet.
- Store soiled diapers in a diaper pail.
- Wash them daily or every 2 days.
- Do not wash them with other laundry items.
- Wash them in hot water. Use a baby laundry detergent.
- Put them through the wash cycle a second time without detergent. This helps remove all soap.
- Hang them outside to dry if possible for a fresh, clean smell. Otherwise, dry them in the dryer.

Disposable diapers are secured with Velcro or tape strips. Fold soiled diapers so the soiled area is on the inside. Then discard the diaper in the trash container. Do not flush it down the toilet. Using disposable diapers costs more than using cloth ones.

Changing diapers often helps prevent diaper rash. Moisture, stools, and urine irritate the baby's skin. When changing diapers, make sure the baby is clean and dry before applying a clean diaper. If a diaper rash develops, tell the nurse at once.

See *Delegation Guidelines: Diapering a Baby.*
See *Promoting Safety and Comfort: Diapering a Baby.*
See procedure: *Diapering a Baby.*

DELEGATION GUIDELINES
Diapering a Baby

Diapering a baby is a routine nursing task. Before changing a baby's diaper, you need this information from the nurse and the care plan.

- The size and type of diaper to use (cloth or disposable)
- If you need to give cord care (p. 829) or circumcision care (p. 829)
- What lotion or cream to use
- What observations to report and record:
  - Color and amount of urine—small, medium, large
  - Color, amount, consistency, and odor of stools
  - Condition of the baby's skin and genital area
  - Redness or irritation of the skin or genital area
  - Blood or discharge on the diaper
- When to report observations
- What concerns about the baby to report at once

PROMOTING SAFETY AND COMFORT

Diapering a Baby

Safety

Older babies can tear and pull disposable diapers apart. They can choke or suffocate on diaper material if placed in the nose or mouth. Observe babies closely. Change any torn or damaged diaper at once.

Diaper pins for cloth diapers must point away from the abdomen. If a pin opens toward the abdomen, it can pierce the skin and damage organs. Keep your hand between the pin and the baby's skin when removing or applying a pin.

Keep the baby safe during diapering. The baby may squirm, wiggle, or kick and cry. To prevent falls:

- Gather all needed supplies before you begin.
- Place the baby on a firm surface. If the baby is on a table, make sure it is sturdy.
- Always keep 1 hand on a baby who is on a table or other raised surface.
- Never look away from the baby.

Diapering a Baby

QUALITY OF LIFE

- Knock before entering the baby's room.
- Address the baby and parents by name.
- Introduce yourself by name and title.

- Explain the procedure to the parents before starting and during the procedure.
- Protect the baby's rights during the procedure.
- Handle the baby gently during the procedure.

PRE-PROCEDURE

1 Follow *Delegation Guidelines: Diapering a Baby.* See *Promoting Safety and Comfort: Diapering a Baby.*
2 Practice hand hygiene.
3 Collect the following.
   - Gloves
   - Clean diaper
   - Waterproof changing pad
   - Washcloth
   - Disposable wipes or cotton balls
   - Basin of warm water
   - Baby soap
   - Baby lotion or cream

PROCEDURE

4 Put on the gloves.
5 Place the changing pad under the baby.
6 Unfasten the dirty diaper. Place diaper pins out of the baby's reach.
7 Wipe the genital area with the front of the diaper (Fig. 56-18, *A*, p. 828). Wipe from the front to the back (top to bottom).
8 Note the color and amount of urine and stools. Fold the diaper so urine and stools are inside. Set the diaper aside.
9 Clean the genital area from front to back (top to bottom). Use a wet washcloth, disposable wipes, or cotton balls (Fig. 56-18, *B*, p. 828). Wash with mild soap and water for a large amount of stools or if the baby has a rash. Rinse thoroughly and pat the area dry. Remove and discard the gloves. Practice hand hygiene. Put on clean gloves.
10 Clean the circumcision (p. 829). Follow the nurse's instructions for cord care (p. 829).
11 Apply cream or lotion to the genital area and buttocks. Do not use too much. Caking can occur.
12 Raise the baby's legs. Slide a clean diaper under the buttocks.

13 Fold a cloth diaper as shown in Figure 56-19 (p. 828).
   a *For a boy:* the extra thickness is in the front (see Fig. 56-19, *A*).
   b *For a girl:* the extra thickness is at the back (see Fig. 56-19, *B*).
   c Bring the diaper between the baby's legs.
14 Make sure the diaper is snug around the hips and abdomen.
   a It is loose near the penis if the circumcision has not healed.
   b It is below the umbilicus if the cord stump has not healed.
15 Secure the diaper in place (Fig. 56-20, p. 828). Use the tape strips or Velcro on disposable diapers (see Fig. 56-20, *A*). Make sure the tabs stick in place. Use baby pins or Velcro for cloth diapers. Pins point away from the abdomen (see Fig. 56-20, *B*).
16 Apply a diaper cover or waterproof pants if cloth diapers are worn.
17 Put the baby in the crib, infant seat, or other safe place.

POST-PROCEDURE

18 Rinse stools from the cloth diaper into the toilet and flush.
19 Store used cloth diapers in a covered pail. Put a disposable diaper in the trash.
20 Remove and discard the gloves. Practice hand hygiene.
21 Put on clean gloves.
22 Clean, rinse, dry, and return other items to their proper place.

23 Remove and discard the gloves. Practice hand hygiene.
24 Complete a safety check of the room. See the inside of the back cover.
25 Report and record your observations.

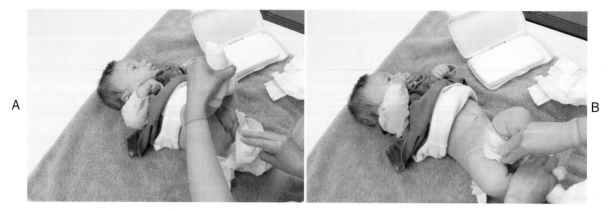

FIGURE 56-18 A, The front of the diaper is used to wipe the genital area from front (top) to back (bottom). **B,** A disposable wipe is used to clean the genital area from front (top) to back (bottom).

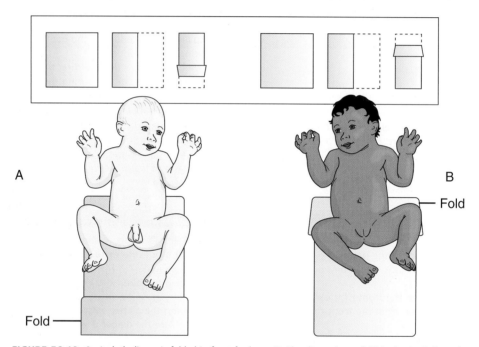

FIGURE 56-19 A, A cloth diaper is folded in front for boys. **B,** The diaper has a fold in the back for girls.

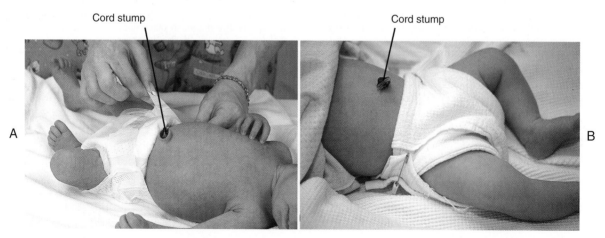

FIGURE 56-20 Securing a diaper. **A,** A disposable diaper is secured in place with tape strips. **B,** Diaper pins secure a cloth diaper. Pins point away from the abdomen. NOTE: The diapers in A and B are below the cord stump.

UMBILICAL CORD CARE

The *umbilical cord connects the mother and fetus (unborn baby). It carries blood, oxygen, and nutrients from the mother to the fetus* (Fig. 56-21). The cord is not needed after birth. Shortly after delivery, the cord is clamped and cut. A cord stump is left on the baby (see Fig. 56-20). The stump dries up and falls off usually within 2 weeks after birth. Slight bleeding can occur when the cord comes off.

The cord provides a place for microbes to grow. Keep the cord clean and dry. Cord care is done at each diaper change. Cord care is continued for 1 or 2 days after the cord comes off. It involves the following.

- Do not get the stump wet.
- Keep the diaper below the cord as in Figure 56-20. This prevents the diaper from irritating the stump. It also keeps the cord from becoming wet from urine.
- Give sponge baths until the cord falls off. Then the baby can have a tub bath.
- Do not pull the cord off—even if it looks ready to fall off.
- Report the following.
  - Swelling, redness, odor, or drainage from the stump
  - Bleeding from the cord or navel area
  - Fever
  - Crying when the cord or skin near the cord is touched

See *Promoting Safety and Comfort: Umbilical Cord Care.*

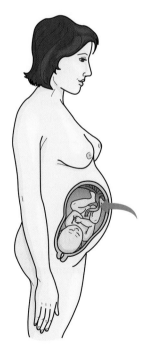

FIGURE 56-21 The umbilical cord connects the mother and fetus.

PROMOTING SAFETY AND COMFORT
Umbilical Cord Care

Safety

For cord care, a common practice involved wiping the base of the stump with alcohol at every diaper change. The alcohol promoted drying. It is now thought that the stump heals faster if left to air-dry. When giving cord care, follow the nurse's directions. The nurse may have you wash the stump with water if it is dirty or sticky. If so, dry it thoroughly after washing.

CIRCUMCISION CARE

Boys are born with foreskin on the penis. *The surgical removal of foreskin from the penis is called a* **circumcision** (Chapter 24). The procedure is optional. The parents decide whether or not to circumcise.

Circumcision is thought to:
- Allow for easier hygiene.
- Prevent urinary tract infections in infants.
- Lower the risk of cancer of the penis.
- Prevent problems with foreskin retraction. Some foreskin is too tight to be pulled back (retracted) over the penis.
- Decrease the risk of sexually transmitted diseases.

The procedure is usually done within 10 days after birth. Circumcision is a religious ceremony in the Jewish and Islamic faiths.

The tip of the penis is often sore and may look red, swollen, or bruised. However, the entire penis should not be swollen. And the circumcision should not interfere with voiding. Carefully observe for signs of bleeding and infection. There should be no odor, drainage, or fever. A slight yellowish discharge or crust at the tip of the penis is normal. It does not signal infection. Report any concerns at once. The area should heal in 7 to 10 days.

Circumcision care involves the following.
- Clean the penis at each diaper change. This is very important after a BM.
- Use mild soap and water, plain water, or commercial wipes as the nurse directs.
- Apply a petrolatum gauze dressing or petrolatum jelly to the penis as the nurse directs. This protects the penis from urine and stools. It also prevents the penis from sticking to the diaper. Use a cotton swab to apply the petrolatum jelly (Fig. 56-22, p. 830).
- Apply the diaper loosely. This prevents the diaper from irritating the penis.

See *Promoting Safety and Comfort: Circumcision Care,* p. 830.

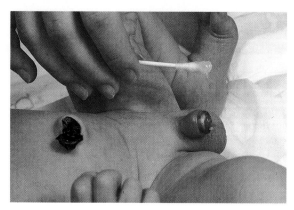

FIGURE 56-22 Petrolatum jelly is applied to the circumcised penis.

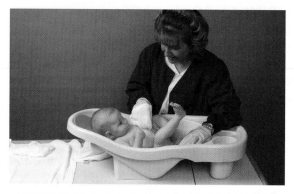

FIGURE 56-23 The baby is given a bath in a baby bathtub.

PROMOTING SAFETY AND COMFORT

Circumcision Care

Safety

In the uncircumcised baby, foreskin covers the penis (Chapter 24). Foreskin does not retract (pull back) until later in childhood. *Do not retract a baby's foreskin.* Forcing the foreskin to retract can cause pain, tearing, and bleeding. When bathing, gently clean the penis with soap and water.

BATHING AN INFANT

Infants do not need a bath every day. Bathing too often can cause dry skin. Bathing 3 times a week is common. Areas with creases need special attention—under the arms, behind the ears, around the neck, and the genital area. Also wash and dry well between the fingers and toes.

Baths comfort and relax babies. They provide a wonderful time to hold, touch, and talk to babies. Stimulation is important for development. Being touched and held helps babies learn safety, security, and love and belonging.

Planning for the bath is important. You cannot leave the baby alone if you forget something. Gather needed equipment, supplies, and the baby's clothes before you start the bath. Everything you need must be within your reach.

There are 2 bath procedures for babies. Sponge baths are given until the cord stump falls off and the umbilicus and circumcision heal. *The cord must not get wet.* A bath in a baby bathtub is given after the cord site and circumcision heal (Fig. 56-23).

See *Focus on Long-Term Care and Home Care: Bathing an Infant.*

See *Delegation Guidelines: Bathing an Infant.*

See *Promoting Safety and Comfort: Bathing an Infant.*

See procedure: *Giving a Baby a Sponge Bath.*

See procedure: *Giving a Baby a Bath in a Baby Bathtub,* p. 833.

FOCUS ON LONG-TERM CARE AND HOME CARE

Bathing an Infant

Home Care

Families have routines. Some babies are bathed in the morning. The baby is more alert and ready to interact at this time. Others bathe in the evening. Evening baths:

- Comfort and relax the baby. This helps some babies sleep longer at night.
- Allow a parent who works during the day to be involved in the bath.

Sometimes 1 parent bathes the baby so the other parent can rest or tend to other children. Follow the family's routine when working in the home.

DELEGATION GUIDELINES

Bathing an Infant

Bathing an infant is a routine nursing task. Before bathing an infant, you need this information from the nurse and the care plan.

- How often to bathe the baby.
- What type of bath to give—sponge bath or a bath in a baby bathtub.
- What water temperature to use—usually 100°F to 105°F (37.7°C to 40.5°C).
- When to bathe the infant.
- If you should use baby soap or plain water. Usually soap is not used unless the baby is dirty or smells.
- If you should apply lotion after the bath.
- What observations to report and record:
  - Bruising
  - Rashes
  - Skin irritation
  - Redness
  - Swelling
  - Open skin areas
  - See "Umbilical Cord Care," p. 829
  - See "Circumcision Care," p. 829
- When to report observations.
- What concerns about the baby to report at once.

PROMOTING SAFETY AND COMFORT

Bathing an Infant

Safety

To protect an infant during a bath, follow these safety measures.

- Turn up the thermostat and close windows and doors about 20 minutes before the bath. Room temperature should be 75°F to 80°F for the bath. The room may be too warm for you. Remove a sweater or lab coat or roll up your sleeves before starting the bath.
- Measure bath water temperature with a water thermometer. The nurse tells you what temperature to use (usually 100°F to 105°F [37.7°C to 40.5°C]). Or test water temperature with the inside of your wrist (Fig. 56-24). The water should feel warm and comfortable. Babies have delicate skin and are easily burned.
- Never leave the baby alone on a table or in the baby bathtub.
- Always keep 1 hand on the baby if you must look away for a moment.
- Hold the baby securely during the bath. Babies are slippery when they are wet. A wet, squirming baby is hard to hold.
- Keep the baby's face out of the water.

Comfort

Keep the baby warm and comfortable during the bath. For a sponge bath, cover the table or other bathing surface with a towel. You can also wrap the baby in a towel and expose only the body parts being washed. When in a baby bathtub, pour warm water over the baby's body during the bath.

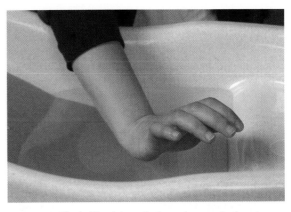

FIGURE 56-24 The inside of the wrist is used to test bath water temperature.

Giving a Baby a Sponge Bath

QUALITY OF LIFE

- Knock before entering the baby's room.
- Address the baby and parents by name.
- Introduce yourself by name and title.

- Explain the procedure to the parents before starting and during the procedure.
- Protect the baby's rights during the procedure.
- Handle the baby gently during the procedure.

PRE-PROCEDURE

1. Follow *Delegation Guidelines: Bathing an Infant*. See *Promoting Safety and Comfort: Bathing an Infant*.
2. Practice hand hygiene.
3. Place the following items in your work area.
   - Baby bathtub
   - Water thermometer
   - Bath towel
   - 2 hand towels
   - Receiving blanket
   - Washcloth
   - Items for diaper changing (see procedure: *Diapering a Baby*, p. 827)

   - Clean clothing for the baby
   - Cotton balls
   - Baby soap (if needed)
   - Baby shampoo
   - Baby lotion
   - Petrolatum gauze or petrolatum jelly (if needed)
   - Gloves
4. Identify the baby. Check the ID (identification) bracelet against the assignment sheet. Use 2 identifiers (Chapter 13). Follow agency policy.
5. Provide for privacy.

PROCEDURE

6. Fill the baby bathtub with 2 to 3 inches of warm water. Water temperature should be 100°F to 105°F (37.7°C to 40.5°C). Measure water temperature with the water thermometer or use the inside of your wrist. The water should feel warm and comfortable.
7. Put on gloves.

8. Undress the baby. Leave the diaper on.
9. Wash the baby's eye lids (Fig. 56-25, p. 832).
   a. Dip a cotton ball into the water.
   b. Squeeze out excess water.
   c. Wash 1 eye lid from the inner part to the outer part.
   d. Repeat this step for the other eye with a new cotton ball.

Continued

Giving a Baby a Sponge Bath—cont'd

PROCEDURE—cont'd

10 Moisten the washcloth and make a mitt (Chapter 24). Clean the outside of the ear and then behind the ear. Repeat this step for the other ear. Be gentle. *Do not use cotton swabs to clean inside the ears.*

11 Rinse and squeeze out the washcloth. Make a mitt with the washcloth.

12 Wash the baby's face (Fig. 56-26). Clean inside the nostrils with the washcloth. *Do not use cotton swabs to clean inside the nose.* Pat the face dry.

13 Pick up the baby. Hold the baby over the baby bathtub using the football hold. Support the baby's head and neck with your wrist and hand.

14 Wash the baby's head (Fig. 56-27).

  a Squeeze a small amount of water from the washcloth onto the baby's head. Or bring water to the baby's head using a cupped hand.

  b Apply a small amount of baby shampoo to the head.

  c Wash the head with circular motions.

  d Rinse the head by squeezing water from a washcloth over the baby's head. Or bring water to the baby's head using a cupped hand. Rinse thoroughly. Do not get soap in the baby's eyes.

  e Use a small hand towel to dry the head.

15 Lay the baby on the table.

16 Remove the diaper.

17 Wash the front of the body with a washcloth or your hands. Do not get the cord wet. Also wash the arms, hands, fingers, legs, feet, and toes. Wash the genital area and all creases and folds. Rinse thoroughly. Pat dry.

18 Follow the nurse's instructions for cord care. Clean the circumcision.

19 Turn the baby to the prone position. Wash the back and buttocks. Use a washcloth or your hands. Rinse thoroughly. Pat dry.

20 Apply baby lotion as directed by the nurse.

21 Apply petrolatum gauze or petrolatum jelly to the penis as the nurse directs.

22 Remove and discard the gloves. Practice hand hygiene.

23 Put a clean diaper and clean clothes on the baby.

24 Wrap the baby in the receiving blanket. Put the baby in the crib or other safe area.

POST-PROCEDURE

25 Practice hand hygiene. Put on gloves.

26 Clean, rinse, dry, and return equipment and supplies to the proper place. Do this step when the baby is settled.

27 Remove and discard the gloves. Practice hand hygiene.

28 Complete a safety check of the room. (See the inside of the back cover.)

29 Report and record your observations.

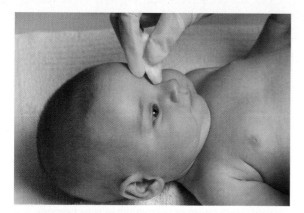

FIGURE 56-25 Wash the baby's eyes with cotton balls. The eye lids are cleaned from the inner to the outer part.

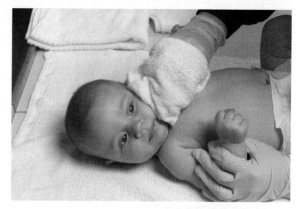

FIGURE 56-26 The baby's face is washed with a mitted washcloth.

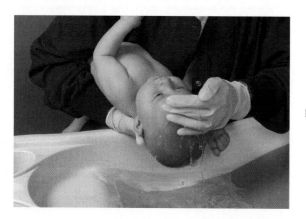

FIGURE 56-27 The baby's head is washed over the baby bathtub.

Giving a Baby a Bath in a Baby Bathtub

QUALITY OF LIFE

- Knock before entering the baby's room.
- Address the baby and parents by name.
- Introduce yourself by name and title.

- Explain the procedure to the parents before beginning and during the procedure.
- Protect the baby's rights during the procedure.
- Handle the baby gently during the procedure.

PROCEDURE

1 Follow steps 1 through 16 in procedure: *Giving a Baby a Sponge Bath* (p. 831).
2 Hold the baby as in Figure 56-28.
  a Place 1 hand under the baby's shoulders. Your thumb should be over the baby's shoulder. Your fingers should be under the arm.
  b Support the buttocks with your other hand. Slide your hand under the thighs. Hold the far thigh with your other hand.
3 Lower the baby into the water feet first.
4 Wash the front of the baby's body. Also wash the arms, hands, fingers, legs, feet, and toes. Wash the genital area and all creases and folds.

5 Reverse your hold. Use your other hand to hold the baby. Keep the baby's face out of the water.
6 Wash the baby's back and buttocks. Rinse thoroughly.
7 Reverse your hold again. Hold the baby with your other hand.
8 Lift the baby out of the water and onto a towel.
9 Wrap the baby in the towel. Also cover the baby's head.
10 Pat the baby dry. Dry all creases and folds.
11 Follow steps 20 through 29 in procedure: *Giving a Baby a Sponge Bath.* (Omit step 21—applying petrolatum gauze or petrolatum jelly.)

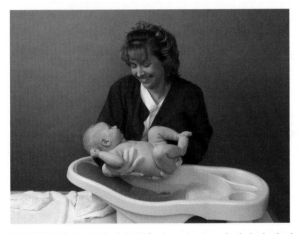

FIGURE 56-28 The baby is held for lowering into the baby bathtub.

NAIL CARE

The baby's fingernails and toenails are kept short. Otherwise, the baby can scratch himself or herself and others. Nails are best cut after a bath or when the baby is sleeping. The sleeping baby is quiet and will not squirm or fuss. Use infant nail clippers and a soft emery board.

- Hold the finger or toe with 1 hand.
- Press the skin under the nail. This moves the skin out of the way to avoid pinching or cutting the skin.
- Trim the nails with an infant nail clipper.
  - *Fingernails:* clip following the natural shape of the nail.
  - *Toenails:* clip straight across as for an adult (Chapter 25).
- Smooth rough or sharp edges with a soft emery board.

WEIGHING INFANTS

The infant's birth weight is a baseline for measuring growth. The nurse uses weight measurements in the assessment step of the nursing process. They also are used to measure the amount of breast-milk taken in during breast-feeding. The baby is weighed before and after breast-feeding. The difference in the weights is the amount of milk taken in during breast-feeding. It tells the nurse if the baby is getting enough milk.

See *Focus on Math: Weighing Infants.*
See *Delegation Guidelines: Weighing Infants,* p. 834.
See *Promoting Safety and Comfort: Weighing Infants,* p. 834.
See procedure: *Weighing an Infant,* p. 834.

FOCUS ON MATH

Weighing Infants

Weight can be measured in pounds or kilograms (Chapter 36). For weighing infants, the following may be used.

- Pounds (lb) and ounces (oz). There are 16 ounces in 1 pound. (NOTE: Ounces used for weight are different than ounces used for liquid measurements [Chapter 31].)
- Kilograms (kg). See Chapter 36 for converting kilograms and pounds.
- Grams (g). There are 1000 grams in 1 kilogram. Grams are often used for "before" and "after" feeding weights.

Know what is used in your agency. Follow agency policy for reporting and recording.

For a "before" and "after" feeding weight, subtract the infant's "before" weight from the "after" weight. The nurse uses the weight difference to calculate the amount of breast-milk taken in.

For example, a baby's "before" feeding weight is 2720 grams. After feeding, the baby weighs 2750 grams. You report a weight change of 30 grams.

2750 grams (after feeding) – 2720 grams (before feeding)
= 30 grams (weight change)

DELEGATION GUIDELINES
Weighing Infants

Measuring weight is a routine nursing task. Before weighing an infant, you need this information from the nurse and the care plan.
- When to weigh the baby.
- What measurement to use—pounds and ounces, kilograms, grams.
- If the baby is breast-fed or bottle-fed. Breast-fed babies wear the same diaper for "before" and "after" feeding weight measurements. The clothes and blanket are removed.
- When to report the weight measurement.
- What concerns about the baby to report at once.

PROMOTING SAFETY AND COMFORT
Weighing Infants
Safety

You must meet the baby's safety needs. Protect the baby from chills. Keep the room warm and free of drafts. Also protect the baby from falling. Always keep a hand over the baby when measuring weight. Remember to keep 1 hand on the baby if you need to look away.

Weighing an Infant

QUALITY OF LIFE

- Knock before entering the baby's room.
- Address the baby and parents by name.
- Introduce yourself by name and title.
- Explain the procedure to the parents before beginning and during the procedure.
- Protect the baby's rights during the procedure.
- Handle the baby gently during the procedure.

PRE-PROCEDURE

1. Follow *Delegation Guidelines: Weighing Infants*. See *Promoting Safety and Comfort: Weighing Infants*.
2. Practice hand hygiene.
3. Collect the following.
   - Baby scale (Fig. 56-29)
   - Paper for the scale
   - Items for diaper changing (see procedure: *Diapering a Baby*, p. 827)
   - Gloves
4. Identify the baby. Check the ID bracelet against the assignment sheet. Use 2 identifiers (Chapter 13). Follow agency policy.

PROCEDURE

5. Place the paper on the scale. Adjust the scale to zero (0).
6. Put on the gloves.
7. Undress the baby and remove the diaper. Clean the genital area.
8. Remove and discard the gloves and practice hand hygiene. Put on clean gloves.
9. Lay the baby on the scale. Keep 1 hand over the baby to prevent falling.
10. Read the digital display or move the weights until the scale is balanced (Chapter 36).
11. Note the measurement.
12. Take the baby off of the scale.
13. Diaper and dress the baby. Lay the baby in the crib.
14. Discard the paper and soiled diaper.
15. Disinfect the scale following agency policy.
16. Remove and discard the gloves. Practice hand hygiene.

POST-PROCEDURE

17. Return the scale to its proper place.
18. Practice hand hygiene.
19. Complete a safety check of the room. See the inside of the back cover.
20. Report and record your observations.

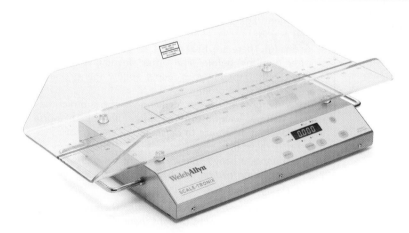

FIGURE 56-29 Digital infant scale. (Courtesy Welch Allyn, Skaneateles Falls, N.Y.)

CARE OF THE MOTHER

Postpartum means after (post) *childbirth* (partum). The postpartum period starts with the birth of the baby. It ends 6 weeks later. The mother's body returns to its normal state during this time. The mother adjusts physically and emotionally to childbirth.

The uterus returns almost to its pre-pregnant size. This is called *involution of the uterus.* If the mother does not breast-feed, she can expect a menstrual period within 4 to 6 weeks. Breast-feeding is not an effective method of birth control. Without birth control measures, the mother can get pregnant again.

Lochia

After childbirth, a vaginal discharge called **lochia** *occurs. (Lochia* comes from the Greek word *lochos.* It means *childbirth.)* Lochia consists of blood and other matter left in the uterus from childbirth. The lochia changes color and decreases in amount during the postpartum period.

- *Lochia rubra*—is dark or bright red *(rubra)* discharge. Mainly blood, it is seen during the first 3 to 4 days.
- *Lochia serosa*—is pinkish-brown *(serosa)* drainage. It lasts until about 10 days after birth.
- *Lochia alba*—is whitish *(alba)* drainage. It continues for 10 to 14 days or more after birth.

Lochia increases with breast-feeding and activity. When she stands after lying or sitting, the mother may feel a gush of lochia. She wears a sanitary napkin (sanitary pad) to absorb the lochia. Normally lochia smells like menstrual flow. Foul-smelling lochia signals infection.

Good perineal care is important. Sanitary pads are changed often. When wiping after elimination, the mother wipes from front (top) to back (bottom). Sanitary napkins are applied and removed from front to back (top to bottom). Good hand-washing is essential after perineal care, changing sanitary napkins, and elimination. Standard Precautions and the Bloodborne Pathogen Standard are followed.

Episiotomies

Some mothers have episiotomies. An *episiotomy is an incision* (otomy) *into the perineum. (Episeion means pubic region.)* The doctor performs this procedure during childbirth. It increases the size of the vaginal opening for the baby. The incision is sutured after delivery. The doctor may order sitz baths for comfort and hygiene (Chapter 42). Like other incisions, complications can develop. These include infection and wound separation *(dehiscence).* Tell the nurse at once if the mother complains of pain, discomfort, or a discharge.

Cesarean Section Delivery

Some mothers deliver by *cesarean section (C-section).* The baby is delivered through an incision made into the abdominal wall. The doctor performs a C-section when:

- The baby must be delivered to save the baby's or mother's life.
- The baby is too large to pass through the birth canal or is in an abnormal position.
- The mother has a vaginal infection that could be transmitted to the baby.
- A normal vaginal delivery will be difficult for the baby or mother.

The C-section incision needs to heal. See Chapter 40 for wound healing and wound care.

Postpartum Complications

Complications can occur during pregnancy, labor, and delivery. They also can occur in the postpartum period. Report any sign or symptom listed in Box 56-6 at once.

BOX 56-6 | **Postpartum Complications—Signs and Symptoms**

- Temperature of 100.4°F or greater
- Pain: abdominal or perineal
- Discharge:
  - Foul smelling from the vagina
  - From an episiotomy
  - From a C-section incision
- Bleeding from an episiotomy or C-section incision
- Redness, swelling: episiotomy or C-section incision
- Saturating a sanitary napkin within 1 hour of application
- Lochia:
  - Red lochia after lochia has changed color to pinkish-brown or white
  - Lochia with large clots
- Urination: burning
- Leg pain, tenderness, or swelling
- Sadness or feelings of depression
- Breast pain, tenderness, or swelling

Postpartum Depression. Many women have emotional reactions called "baby blues" after childbirth. Hormone changes, life-style changes, and lack of sleep are causes. Symptoms last for a few days to up to 2 weeks. The mother may:

- Have mood swings.
- Feel sad, anxious, irritable, or over-whelmed.
- Have crying spells.
- Have trouble concentrating.
- Lose her appetite.
- Have problems sleeping.

Postpartum depression is a form of depression (Chapter 52) that occurs after childbirth. Signs and symptoms are more severe and last longer than "baby blues." See Box 56-7. Postpartum depression can interfere with the mother's ability to care for the baby or herself. Treatment is needed. Report signs and symptoms of depression at once.

See *Focus on Long-Term Care and Home Care: Postpartum Depression.*

BOX 56-7	Postpartum Depression—Signs and Symptoms

- Feeling sad, hopeless, empty, or over-whelmed
- Crying more than usual or for no reason
- Feeling worried or anxious
- Feeling moody, irritable, or restless
- Sleep problems—sleeping too much or being unable to sleep
- Trouble concentrating, remembering details, or making decisions
- Having anger or rage
- Loss of interest in activities usually enjoyed
- Headaches, stomach problems, muscle aches
- Eating too much or too little
- Withdrawing from or avoiding family and friends
- Having trouble bonding with the baby
- Doubting the ability to care for the baby
- Thinking about harming oneself or the baby

Modified from National Institute of Mental Health: Postpartum depression facts, Bethesda, Md, U.S. Department of Health and Human Services.

FOCUS ON LONG-TERM CARE AND HOME CARE

Postpartum Depression

Home Care
Rest and self-care are important after childbirth. These measures can help the mother at home.
- Resting as much as possible. Sleeping when the baby sleeps.
- Performing personal hygiene and grooming measures. Taking a shower and hair care are examples.
- Spending time alone with her partner. Or planning time to go out or visit friends.
- Avoiding doing too much. The mother may need help from a supportive partner, family member, or friend. When feeling depressed, someone else may need to help care for the baby.

FOCUS ON **PRIDE**

The Person, Family, and Yourself

Personal and Professional Responsibility
A newborn may go to the nursery while the mother rests or leave the room for a test or procedure. You must return the baby to the correct parent. Follow agency policy to identify the mother and newborn. You must not rely on the parent to identify the baby. Safe identification is a professional responsibility.

Rights and Respect
A parent's preferences for newborn care may differ from yours. Your opinion must not affect the care you give. Respect parent preferences.

Independence and Social Interaction
Parents must learn to care for their baby. The nurse teaches parents about newborn care. They watch the nurse. Then they try it on their own. Parents gain confidence by giving care independently.

Parents who rely on the staff may not know how to provide care at home. Avoid doing everything for the parents. Tell the nurse if the parents rely on the staff too much.

Delegation and Teamwork
Alarm systems protect the security of newborns. The baby wears an electronic security bracelet. An alarm sounds when the baby is carried toward an exit. Alarms and exits are checked at once. All staff members respond. If a baby is missing, security staff send out a message to the entire agency. Procedures are followed to find the baby. The entire agency works as a team to protect the newborn.

Ethics and Laws
Having a baby is usually a happy time. However, this is not always the case. The health team must monitor closely for signs of mistreatment. A parent may not be interested in the baby. Or the parent may be unwilling to learn how to care for the baby. The baby must be protected from abuse and neglect. Tell the nurse about any concerns at once.

FOCUS ON **PRIDE**: Application
New parents have to adjust to many new things. Explain the health team's role in helping parents adjust. How can you provide support and encouragement?

REVIEW QUESTIONS

Circle **T** *if the statement is* TRUE *and* **F** *if it is* FALSE.

1 **T F** A baby's crib should be within hearing distance of caregivers.

2 **T F** A baby needs a pillow for sleep.

3 **T F** A baby is placed on his or her back for sleep.

4 **T F** Exposure to smoke increases the risk of SIDS.

5 **T F** A yellowish crust at the tip of a circumcised penis is a sign of infection.

6 **T F** A baby's diapers are changed whenever they are wet.

7 **T F** A baby's cord and circumcision have not healed. The baby should have a sponge bath.

8 **T F** Cotton swabs are used to clean inside a baby's ears.

9 **T F** A breast-fed baby needs a "before" and "after" feeding weight. The baby is weighed with the diaper on.

10 **T F** Postpartum depression is normal after childbirth.

Circle the BEST *answer.*

11 A baby's head and neck are supported for the first
   a 7 to 10 days
   b Month
   c 3 months
   d 6 months

12 Which is unsafe when holding a newborn?
   a Holding the infant securely
   b Cuddling the infant
   c Using 2 hands
   d Lifting the infant by the arms

13 You see the following in an infant's home. Which is *unsafe?*
   a Electrical outlets have safety covers.
   b A cord hangs near the crib.
   c Drugs have child-resistant caps.
   d Cleaning supplies are in locked cabinets.

14 Which is *safe?*
   a A crib without bumper pads
   b A crib with a loose crib sheet
   c A crib with a soft blanket and stuffed toys
   d A crib with a drop-side rail

15 You observe the following. Which is normal?
   a The baby looks flushed and is perspiring.
   b The baby has watery stools.
   c The baby's eyes are red and irritated.
   d The baby spits up a small amount when burped.

16 A breast-feeding mother should
   a Nurse the infant every 4 to 6 hours
   b Avoid wearing a bra
   c Clean her breasts with soap and water
   d Stimulate the rooting reflex

17 A breast-fed baby is burped
   a Every 5 minutes
   b After nursing from a breast
   c After 1 ounce of breast-milk
   d After half the formula is taken

18 You are shopping for baby formula. Which should you buy?
   a The one that is on sale
   b The ready-to-feed type
   c The one ordered by the doctor
   d The powdered form

19 When warming a baby bottle
   a Warm the bottle in the microwave
   b Leave the formula out to warm at room temperature
   c Check that the formula is warm on the inside of your wrist
   d Boil the formula in a pan for 5 minutes

20 When bottle-feeding a baby
   a Tilt the bottle so the formula fills the neck of the bottle and the nipple
   b Save remaining formula for the next feeding
   c Burp the baby every 5 minutes
   d Leave the baby alone with the bottle

21 A newborn's cord has not yet healed. The diaper should be
   a Loose over the cord
   b Snug over the cord
   c Below the cord
   d Disposable

22 A circumcision is cleaned
   a Once a day
   b With an alcohol wipe
   c 3 times a day
   d At every diaper change

23 Bath water for a newborn should be
   a 85°F to 90°F
   b 90°F to 95°F
   c 95°F to 100°F
   d 100°F to 105°F

24 When bathing an infant
   a Have needed supplies within reach
   b Retract the foreskin to rinse the penis
   c Leave the baby alone in the tub
   d Lower the room temperature to 70°F

25 A mother has a red vaginal discharge the first few days after childbirth. This
   a Is a menstrual period
   b Signals a postpartum complication
   c Is lochia rubra
   d Is from her episiotomy

26 A cesarean delivery involves
   a A vaginal incision
   b A perineal incision
   c An abdominal incision
   d A normal delivery through the birth canal

Answers to Chapter 56 questions are on p. 888.

FOCUS ON **PRACTICE**

Problem Solving

A mother had a vaginal delivery yesterday. She just finished breast-feeding and stands to the lay the baby down. As she stands, she says: "I just felt a gush of blood. Is that normal?" How will you respond? Describe normal and abnormal vaginal discharge after birth.

OBJECTIVES

- Define the key terms and key abbreviations in this chapter.
- Describe the purpose of assisted living.
- Describe assisted living residents and their rights.
- Identify the types of assisted living residences and the living areas offered.
- Describe requirements and features of assisted living units.
- Describe the requirements for assisted living staff.
- Describe the usual needs and abilities of assisted living residents.

- Describe an assisted living service plan.
- Explain how to safely assist with meals, housekeeping, and laundry.
- Explain how to assist with drugs.
- Identify the reasons for transferring, discharging, or evicting a person.
- Explain how to promote PRIDE in the person, the family, and yourself.

KEY TERMS

assisted living A housing option for older persons who need help with activities of daily living but do not need 24-hour nursing care and supervision

medication reminder Reminding the person to take drugs, observing them being taken as prescribed, and recording that they were taken

service plan A written plan listing the services needed, the help needed, and who provides services

KEY ABBREVIATIONS

ADL Activities of daily living

ALR Assisted living residence

Many older people cannot or do not want to live alone. Some need help with self-care or taking drugs. Some have physical or cognitive problems and disabilities. *Assisted living is a housing option for older persons who need help with activities of daily living (ADL) but do not need 24-hour nursing care and supervision.*

Assisted living residences (ALRs) offer quality of life with independence, companionship, and social involvement. A home-like setting is provided.

ALRs may be part of a retirement community, nursing center, senior citizen housing, or a stand-alone facility. Licensing requirements and residents' rights vary from state to state.

See *Promoting Safety and Comfort: Assisted Living.*

PROMOTING SAFETY AND COMFORT
Assisted Living

Safety
Residents have the same diseases and illnesses as persons at home, in hospitals, and in nursing centers. Infections are risks. This includes sexually transmitted and other communicable diseases. Follow Standard Precautions and the Bloodborne Pathogen Standard when in contact with blood, body fluids, secretions, and excretions, or when contact with potentially contaminated items and surfaces is likely.

ASSISTED LIVING RESIDENTS

Assisted living residents usually have stable health and do not need 24-hour nursing care. They usually need some help with 1 or more ADL.

- Personal care—bathing, dressing, grooming, elimination
- Meals—cooking, eating
- Taking drugs
- Housekeeping
- Personal safety
- Transportation

ALR resident requirements vary. For example, an ALR may require that residents be able to walk. Others allow wheelchair use. An ALR may serve residents with mild memory loss but not those with severe memory impairments.

Resident Rights

ALR residents have rights and liberties as United States citizens. They also gain special rights under state laws and rules (Box 57-1) for ALRs. Such rights are similar to those in Chapter 2. If unable to exercise his or her rights, family members, legal representatives, or ombudsmen act on the person's behalf.

ALR SERVICES AND LIVING AREAS

Assisted living residences usually offer:

- 3 meals a day
- Help with ADL—bathing, dressing, grooming, toileting, eating, walking
- Housekeeping, laundry, and maintenance
- A 24-hour communications system for an emergency or to call for help
- 24-hour security
- Transportation
- Social, educational, recreational, and spiritual services
- Help with shopping, banking, and money management
- Some health services
- Exercise and wellness programs
- Medication (drug) management or help taking drugs
- Supervision for persons with memory problems or other disabilities

Living areas vary. A small cottage or apartment has a bedroom, bathroom, living area, kitchen, and laundry areas (Figs. 57-1 and 57-2). Some people just want a bedroom and bathroom. Box 57-2 (p. 840) lists some common features of ALRs.

See *Focus on Long-Term Care and Home Care: ALR Services and Living Areas*, p. 840.

BOX 57-1	Assisted Living Resident Rights

A resident has the right to:

- Not be discriminated against based on race, national origin, religion, gender, sexual orientation, age, disability, marital status, or diagnosis.
- Receive ALR services that support and respect the person's individuality, choices, strengths, and abilities.
- Receive privacy in:
  - Personal care
  - Correspondence, communication, and visits
  - Financial and personal matters
- Maintain, use, and display personal items. Such items must not pose a safety hazard.
- Take part in or refuse to take part in activities—social, recreational, rehabilitative, religious, political, community.
- Review his or her medical record.
- Take part in developing a service plan (p. 840). The resident may have his or her family or representative involved.
- Have help from others (family, representative) in understanding, protecting, or exercising resident rights.

Modified from Resident Rights, Arizona Administrative Code (R9-10-810).

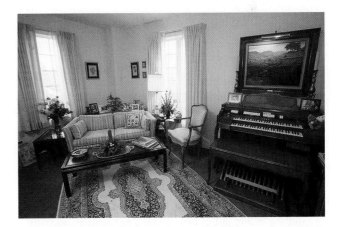

FIGURE 57-1 A living area in an assisted living apartment.

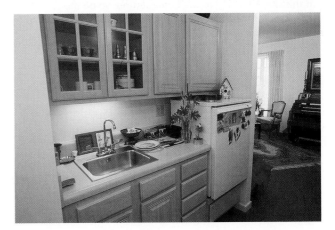

FIGURE 57-2 A kitchen in an assisted living apartment.

BOX 57-2	Assisted Living Residences—Common Features

Physical
- Attractive and home-like decor
- An easy to understand and follow floor plan
- Wide doors, hallways, and bathrooms for walker and wheelchair use
- Elevators in 2-story or higher buildings
- Hand rails in hallways and stairways
- Easy to reach cupboards and shelves
- Flooring material for easy walking and easy walker and wheelchair use
- Good general and task lighting
- Clean and odor-free
- Clearly marked exits
- Smoke alarms and a fire sprinkling system

Personal Areas
- Resident doors lock
- 24-hour emergency communication system
- Private bathroom large enough for a walker or wheelchair

Personal Areas—cont'd
- Grab bars/safety bars in bathrooms
- Furnishings—personal and provided
- Access to phone, cable, TV, and Internet
- Kitchen with a refrigerator, sink, and cooking means

Activities
- Daily schedule of activities—within the ALR and the community
- Volunteers or families help residents with activities
- Transportation to appointments, shopping, and activities
- Barber and beauty services

Food
- Menus vary daily
- 3 meals a day and snacks
- Common dining areas
- Meal times vary to meet resident needs
- Special diets and requests available

Modified from Assisted Living Federation of America: Guide to choosing an assisted living community.

FOCUS ON LONG-TERM CARE AND HOME CARE

ALR Services and Living Areas

Home Care
Unlike assisted living residents, home care patients may still need medical care. They may need help with:
- Prescribed exercises
- Changing wound dressings
- Taking drugs, fluids, or feedings intravenously
- Measuring vital signs
- Managing urinary catheters or ostomies
- Taking drugs correctly
- Personal care, dressing, and grooming
- Getting in and out of bed, showers or bathtubs, and cars

The home care patient may need help with meals, food safety, housekeeping, and laundry. The measures described in this chapter apply to the home setting. So do the measures for medication assistance if that role is allowed by your state and agency.

STAFF REQUIREMENTS

Staff requirements vary among states. Some require a nursing assistant training and competency evaluation program (NATCEP). Staff also may need additional training in these areas.
- The needs, goals, and rights of ALR residents
- Elder abuse and neglect
- Memory and dementia problems
- Using service plans
- Menu planning and food preparation, service, and storage
- Housekeeping and sanitation
- Assisting with drugs

Criminal background and fingerprint checks are common requirements. The ALR cannot employ a person with a criminal record.

SERVICE PLANS

Similar to a care plan, a *service plan* is a written plan listing:
- *The services needed*
- *The help needed*
- *Who provides the services*

The plan relates to ADL, activities and social services, dietary needs, taking drugs, and special needs.

For example, the service plan states that you will help the person get dressed. For physical therapy, a physical therapist will visit in the resident's room. And a family member will assist with the person's drugs.

The plan is reviewed when the person's condition, wants, or service needs change. Services are added or reduced as needed.

Meals

Three meals a day and snacks are provided. Special dietary needs are met. Menus are posted for residents to see.

Dining options range from cafeteria style to fine dining. Residents eat in the dining room with others. Or they can eat in their rooms if they wish.

Food Safety

Certain measures are needed to handle, prepare, and store food. They protect against infection. See Chapter 30. Also practice these safety measures.

- Follow the safe handling instructions on food labels (Fig. 57-3).
- Scrape and rinse eating and cooking items before washing or placing them in the dishwasher.
- Use liquid detergent and hot water to wash eating and cooking items. Wash the least soiled items first. These are usually glasses, cups, and flatware. Follow with plates, bowls, and serving pieces. Wash cookware last. Rinse well with hot water.
- Place washed items in a drainer to dry. Air-drying is more aseptic than towel drying.
- Use dishwasher soap for a dishwasher.
- Do not wash pots and pans and cast iron, wood, and some plastic items in a dishwasher.
- Clean appliances, counters, tables, and other surfaces after each meal. Use hot, soapy water and paper towels or clean cloths.
- Remove grease spills and splashes. Use a liquid surface cleaner.
- Clean sinks with a sink cleaner.
- Save or discard left-overs.
- Dispose of garbage and other soiled supplies after each meal. Use a garbage disposal for food and liquid garbage but not bones.
- Recycle paper, boxes, cans, and plastic containers according to ALR policy.
- Empty garbage at least once a day.

Housekeeping

Housekeeping measures help prevent infection. And they keep living units neat and clean.

- Make beds and straighten bedrooms.
- Wipe up spills right away.
- Use a dust mop or broom to sweep. Use a dustpan to collect dust and crumbs.
- Sweep daily or more often as needed.

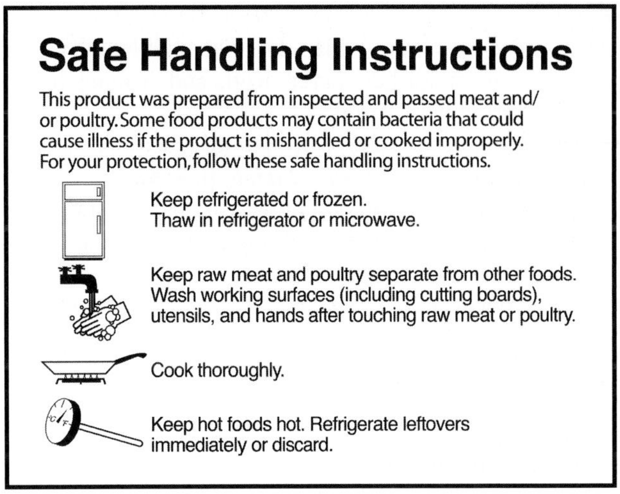

Safe Handling Instructions

This product was prepared from inspected and passed meat and/or poultry. Some food products may contain bacteria that could cause illness if the product is mishandled or cooked improperly. For your protection, follow these safe handling instructions.

Keep refrigerated or frozen. Thaw in refrigerator or microwave.

Keep raw meat and poultry separate from other foods. Wash working surfaces (including cutting boards), utensils, and hands after touching raw meat or poultry.

Cook thoroughly.

Keep hot foods hot. Refrigerate leftovers immediately or discard.

FIGURE 57-3 Safe handling instructions for meat and poultry. They are required by the U.S. Department of Agriculture. (Redrawn from [USDA] United States Department of Agriculture, Food Safety and Inspection Service.)

- Make sure toilets flush after each use.
- Rinse the sink after washing, shaving, or oral hygiene.
- Clean the tub or shower after each use.
- Remove and dispose of hair from the sink, tub, or shower.
- Hang towels to dry. Or place them in a hamper.
- Clean bathroom surfaces with a disinfectant or water and detergent.
  - The toilet bowl, seat, and outside areas of the toilet
  - The floor
  - The sides, walls, and curtain or door of the tub or shower
  - Towel racks and toilet paper, toothbrush, and soap holders
  - The sink and mirror
  - Window sills
- Mop or vacuum the bathroom floor every day.
- Empty bathroom wastebaskets every day.
- Put out clean towels and washcloths every day.
- Wash bath mats, the wastebasket, and laundry hamper at least weekly.
- Replace toilet paper and facial tissues as needed.
- Open bathroom windows for a short time. Also use air fresheners.
- Dust furniture at least weekly.
- Vacuum floors at least weekly and as needed.

Laundry

Clean linens may be provided. For personal laundry, residents can use a washer, dryer, iron, and ironing board. When assisting with laundry:

- Wear gloves to handle soiled laundry (see *Promoting Safety and Comfort: Assisted Living*, p. 838).
- Separate white, colored, and dark items. Separate sturdy and delicate fabrics. Also separate by the amount of dirt, soiling, or stain.
- Empty pockets.
- Fasten buttons, zippers, snaps, hooks, and other closures.
- Wash very dirty or heavily soiled or stained items separately.
- Follow detergent directions.
- Follow care label directions and the person's preferences for the correct:
  - Wash cycle and water temperature
  - Drying temperature and cycle
- Fold, hang, or iron clothes as the person prefers. See *Teamwork and Time Management: Laundry.*

TEAMWORK AND TIME MANAGEMENT

Laundry

Residents may share washers and dryers. If assisting with laundry, remove clothes from washers and dryers promptly. Others may need the machines.

Sometimes laundry is left in a washer or dryer. First, try to find the person who left the laundry. Politely tell the person that the machine is done and that you have laundry to do. Offer to remove the laundry if the other person is busy. If you cannot find that person, do the following.

- *If left in a washer*—place wet items on a clean surface, not in the dryer. Some items may need to dry flat, hang to dry, or need certain dryer settings. Or the resident may have drying preferences.
- *If left in a dryer*—fold and place items on a clean surface. While laundry is in the washer or dryer, tend to other tasks. Assist with ADL, do housekeeping, prepare meals, and so on.

Nursing Services

Some ALRs provide limited nursing services. The nurse assesses each person and monitors health. The nurse guides and assists you with delegated tasks as needed. If a person cannot manage his or her own drugs, the nurse gives them.

Medication Assistance

Drugs must be taken as prescribed. The 6 rights of drug administration are:

- The right drug
- The right dose (amount)
- The right route (by mouth, injection, applied to the skin, inhalation, vaginally, or rectally)
- The right time
- The right person
- The right documentation (recording)

Your role depends on your state's laws, ALR policy, and your training and education. *Remember, you do not give drugs (Chapter 3). Also remember that the person has the right to refuse to take prescribed drugs.* Your role may involve:

- Reminding the person to take a drug
- Reading the drug label to the person
- Opening containers if the person cannot do so
- Checking the dosage against the drug label
- Providing water, juice, milk, crackers, applesauce, or other food and fluids
- Making sure the person takes the right drug, the right amount, at the right time, and in the right way (route)
- Recording that the person took or refused to take the drug (right documentation)
- Storing drugs

Self-directed medication management is when residents manage and take their own drugs. The person knows drugs by name, color, or shape. The person knows what drugs to take, the correct doses, and when and how to take them. The person questions changes in the usual drug routine. For example, a pill is not broken in half. Or a pill looks different. Report comments or questions to the nurse.

Pill organizers (Fig. 57-4) have sections for days and times. They are for a week or month. The person, a family member or representative, or a nurse prepares the pill organizer. Drugs are taken on the right day and at the right time.

Some pharmacies offer pre-sorted dose packets. The person's drugs are sorted into packets according to the day and time of day to take the drugs. The person does not need to use pill bottles or pill organizers. Usually a month's supply is provided.

You may need to remind some people. A *medication reminder means reminding the person to take drugs, observing them being taken as prescribed, and recording that they were taken.* Setting clock or phone alarms for when to take drugs is useful for some people.

See *Focus on Communication: Medication Assistance.*
See *Delegation Guidelines: Medication Assistance.*

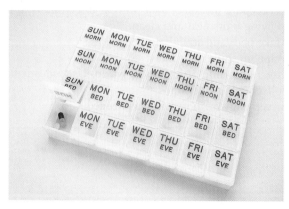

FIGURE 57-4 Pill organizer.

Medication Assistance

To remind a person to take his or her drugs, you can say:
- "Ms. Parks, it's time to take your 8 o'clock pills."
- "Mr. Ladd, you need to take your pills in about 10 minutes."
- "Mrs. Young, are you ready to take your medicine?"
  To read a drug label to a person, read the following.
- The name of the person on the drug label
- The name of the drug
- How to take the drug (by mouth, with food, with a full glass of water, apply to the skin, rectally, and so on)
- The dosage
- When to take the drug (before meals, with meals, after meals, at bedtime, and so on)
- How often to take the drug
- Warnings and other information on the drug label

DELEGATION GUIDELINES

Medication Assistance

Some agencies use "10 rights of medication assistance." The added 4 are:
- *Right education.* The nurse provides information about the drug.
- *Right to refuse.* The person has the right to refuse any drug. The nurse advises the person about problems that can result if the drug is not taken.
- *Right assessment.* Vital signs may be measured before a drug is given.
- *Right evaluation.* The nurse assesses if the drug had the desired effect or any side effects.
  These added rights are nursing responsibilities. The nurse may delegate taking vital signs to you. If so, the nurse may:
- Ask you to report the vital signs before assisting the person.
- Give you guidance about how to proceed. For example, a person takes a drug that affects heart rate. The nurse may tell you that the drug should not be taken if the pulse is less than 60 beats per minute.
  A person may refuse to take a drug. If so, report the refusal to the nurse. The nurse will follow the "right to refuse" described above.

Medication Record. A medication record is kept. The record includes:
- The person's name
- Drug name, dose, directions, and route of administration
- Date and time to take the drug
- Date and time help was given
- Signature or initials of the person assisting

Drug Errors. Report any drug error to the nurse. Also complete an incident report. An error means 1 or more of the following.
- Taking another person's drugs
- Taking the wrong drug
- Taking the wrong dose
- Taking an extra dose
- Missing or skipping a dose
- Taking a drug at the wrong time
- Taking a drug by the wrong route
- Not taking a drug when ordered
- Not recording that a drug was taken

Storing Drugs. Drugs are kept in a secure place. This prevents others from taking them. The ALR may keep drugs in a locked area. Some persons store their own drugs. If sharing a room, each person's ability to safely have drugs is assessed. Drugs are in a locked container if safety is a factor.

Drugs must have the original pharmacy label. They are stored as directed on the label. For example, some drugs are refrigerated. Others are kept away from light. The label also has an expiration date. The ALR has procedures for disposing of expired or discontinued drugs.

Activities and Recreation

Residents are urged to take part in activity and recreational programs. Social, physical, and community activities promote well-being and independence. An activities director plans, organizes, and conducts the ALR's activity program. ALR and community events and activities are noted on a calendar.

Special Services and Safety Needs

Sometimes emergencies occur. Some people need help getting out of bed or transferring to a wheelchair. Then they can leave the building with little or no help. The ALR and the person agree on how and who will meet the person's needs.

TRANSFER, DISCHARGE, AND EVICTION

Residents can be transferred, discharged, or evicted. The ALR must tell the person about the action. Reasons are:
- The ALR can no longer meet the person's needs. The person is a threat to the health and safety of self or others. Or the ALR cannot provide needed care.
- The person fails to pay for services.
- The person fails to comply with ALR policies or rules.
- The person wants to transfer.
- The ALR closes.

FOCUS ON **PRIDE**

The Person, Family, and Yourself

P ersonal and Professional Responsibility

Moving to an ALR can bring mixed emotions. The person may be happy and excited. Fear, anxiety, and uncertainty are also common. The move may bring the family peace of mind. The person is in a clean, safe setting. Needs are met.

Be professional and caring. Your interactions should assure the resident and family that you will provide safe, dignified care.

R ights and Respect

Federal and state laws protect the person's rights. The person has the right to quality of life, privacy, protection against restraint and abuse, and access to information. The person also has rights regarding the transfer, discharge, or eviction from the ALR. See Box 57-1. Take pride in protecting the person's rights.

I ndependence and Social Interaction

People choose assisted living for many reasons. Many need some help. Many like the social interaction with other residents. The ALR's activities and services offer other benefits.

To promote independence, assist as needed while allowing as much privacy and personal choice as possible. Follow the resident's service plan.

D elegation and Teamwork

Good teamwork is needed when new residents arrive. The person and family should see that the staff is helpful and works together to meet the person's needs.

E thics and Laws

How you assist with drugs depends on your state's laws, ALR policy, and your training. There are legal limits to your role. If you act beyond those limits, you could be practicing nursing without a license. You can lose your job and your ability to work as a nursing assistant. Follow the limits for your state and agency.

FOCUS ON **PRIDE**: *Application*

Identify the changes a new ALR resident faces. How might the person respond? Describe positive and negative feelings. How do the following affect the transition?

- The person's attitude
- The family's involvement and support level
- The ALR's appearance
- The ALR staff's conduct

REVIEW QUESTIONS

*Circle **T** if the statement is TRUE and **F** if it is FALSE.*

1   T   F   ALRs provide 24-hour nursing care.

2   T   F   Some ALR residents have memory problems.

3   T   F   ALR residents must speak English.

4   T   F   ALRs provide 24-hour security.

5   T   F   ALR residents can refuse care.

6   T   F   ALR residents must organize their own activities.

7   T   F   Resident doors must remain unlocked.

8   T   F   ALRs provide an emergency communication system.

9   T   F   Food safety involves following safe handling instructions on food labels.

Circle the BEST answer.

10   A person wants to attend a concert. Which is *true?*
   a   The ALR must approve the concert.
   b   The person must return by 10 PM.
   c   An attendant must go with the person.
   d   The ALR must respect the person's choice.

11   Assisted living staff must
   a   Complete a nursing assistant training and competency evaluation program
   b   Meet state requirements
   c   Assist with drugs
   d   Provide transportation for residents

12   A service plan
   a   Describes nursing care needs
   b   Lists the drugs the person needs to take
   c   Describes needed services and who provides them
   d   Lists service fees and charges

13   Which statement about ALR dining is *true?*
   a   Residents are allowed to eat in their rooms.
   b   Residents must cook their own meals.
   c   The family provides meals if a special diet is needed.
   d   Eating in the dining room is discouraged.

14   When assisting with housekeeping
   a   Dust and vacuum daily
   b   Wipe up spills right away
   c   Clean the bathroom only as needed
   d   Put out clean washcloths and towels weekly

REVIEW QUESTIONS—cont'd

15 You assist with laundry. Which is *true*?
   a Care label directions are followed.
   b Clothes are washed in hot water.
   c Clothes are ironed.
   d Gloves are not needed for soiled laundry.

16 Usually ALR nursing assistants are allowed to
   a Give drugs
   b Give medication reminders
   c Refill drugs
   d Prepare pill organizers

17 Drugs are kept
   a In the person's closet
   b In the person's drawer
   c In a secure place
   d With the family

18 The ALR cannot provide a person with all needed services. Which is *true*?
   a The ALR must hire more staff.
   b The family must provide the needed care.
   c The ALR can ask the person to transfer.
   d The person's service plan needs to change.

Answers to Chapter 57 questions are on p. 888.

FOCUS ON PRACTICE

Problem Solving

Your state and ALR allow you to assist with drugs. The roles on p. 842 are allowed. A resident asks you to apply eye drops and apply a "heart patch." What do you do? Explain what you can and cannot do.

OBJECTIVES

- Define the key terms and key abbreviations in this chapter.
- Describe the rules of emergency care.
- Identify the signs of cardiac arrest and the emergency care required.
- Describe the emergency care for respiratory arrest.
- Describe the emergency care for heart attack.
- Describe the emergency care for hemorrhage, fainting, and shock.

- Describe the emergency care for stroke.
- Explain how to care for a person during a seizure.
- Describe the emergency care for concussions.
- Describe the emergency care for cold- and heat-related illnesses.
- Describe the emergency care for burns.
- Explain how to promote PRIDE in the person, the family, and yourself.

KEY TERMS

anaphylaxis A life-threatening sensitivity to an antigen

cardiac arrest See "sudden cardiac arrest"

cardiopulmonary resuscitation (CPR) An emergency procedure performed when the heart and breathing stop

convulsion See "seizure"

fainting The sudden loss of consciousness from an inadequate blood supply to the brain; syncope

first aid The emergency care given to an ill or injured person before medical help arrives

frostbite An injury to the body caused by freezing of the skin and underlying tissues

hemorrhage The excessive loss *(rrhage)* of blood *(hemo)* in a short time

hypothermia Abnormally low *(hypo)* body temperature *(thermia)*

respiratory arrest Breathing stops but heart action continues for several minutes

resuscitate To revive from apparent death or unconsciousness using emergency measures

seizure Violent and sudden contractions or tremors of muscle groups caused by abnormal electrical activity in the brain; convulsion

shock Results when tissues and organs do not get enough blood

sudden cardiac arrest (SCA) The heart stops suddenly and without warning; cardiac arrest

KEY ABBREVIATIONS

AED	Automated external defibrillator	RRS	Rapid Response System
CPR	Cardiopulmonary resuscitation	SCA	Sudden cardiac arrest
EMS	Emergency Medical Services	VF; V-fib	Ventricular fibrillation

Emergencies can occur anywhere. Sometimes you can save a life if you know what to do.

The information in this chapter is basic. First aid and cardiopulmonary resuscitation (CPR) courses provide more training and practice. Most agencies require nursing assistants to be CPR certified. *You need a CPR course for health care providers.* Ask your instructor about courses in your area or on-line.

CPR guidelines are updated as new information becomes available. You are responsible for following current guidelines. Updates can be found on-line at the American Heart Association's website.

EMERGENCY CARE

First aid is the emergency care given to an ill or injured person before medical help arrives. The goals of first aid are to:
- Prevent death.
- Prevent injuries from becoming worse.

In an emergency, the Emergency Medical Services (EMS) system is activated. Emergency personnel (paramedics, emergency medical technicians) give advanced emergency care. They treat, stabilize, and transport persons with life-threatening problems. They have guidelines for care and communicate with doctors in hospital emergency rooms. EMS ambulances have emergency drugs, equipment, and supplies.

To activate the EMS system, do 1 of the following.
- Dial 911.
- Call the local fire or police department.
- Call the phone operator.

Each emergency is different. The rules in Box 58-1 apply to any emergency. Hospitals and other agencies have procedures for advanced emergency care. In hospitals, a Rapid Response System (RRS) is activated when a person shows signs of a life-threatening condition. An RRS team may include a doctor, a nurse, and a respiratory therapist. The RRS team brings emergency drugs, supplies, and equipment to the bedside. The goal is to prevent death.

See *Focus on Communication: Emergency Care.*

See *Promoting Safety and Comfort: Emergency Care.*

BOX 58-1   Emergency Care Rules

- Call for help. Or have someone activate the EMS system. *Do not hang up until the operator has hung up.* Give the following information.
  - Your location—street address and city, cross streets or roads, and landmarks
  - Phone number you are calling from
  - What seems to have happened (for example: heart attack, crash, fire)—police, fire equipment, and ambulances may be needed
  - How many people need help
  - Conditions of victims, obvious injuries, and life-threatening situations
  - What aid is being given
- Wait for help if the scene is not safe enough to approach.
- Know your limits. Do not do more than you are able. Do not perform an unfamiliar procedure. Do what you can under the circumstances.
- Stay calm. This helps the person feel more secure.
- Know where to find emergency supplies.
- Follow Standard Precautions and the Bloodborne Pathogen Standard to the extent possible.
- Check for life-threatening problems. Check for breathing, a pulse, and bleeding.
- Keep the person lying down or as you found him or her. Moving the person could make an injury worse.
- Move the person only if the setting is unsafe. Examples include:
  - A burning car or building
  - A building that might collapse
  - Stormy conditions with lightning
  - In water
  - Near electrical wires
- Perform necessary emergency measures.
- Do not remove clothes unless you have to. To remove clothing, tear or cut garments along the seams. (For CPR, remove clothing or move it out of the way. See p. 848.)
- Keep the person warm. Cover the person with a blanket, coats, or sweaters.
- Reassure the person. Explain what is happening and that help was called.
- Do not give the person fluids.
- Keep on-lookers away. They invade privacy and tend to stare, give advice, and comment about the person's condition. The person may think the situation is worse than it is.

FOCUS ON COMMUNICATION

Emergency Care

Some illnesses and injuries are life-threatening. To find out what happened and the person's condition, you can say:
- "Are you okay?"
- "Tell me what's wrong."
- "Where does it hurt?"
- "If you can, please point to where it hurts."
- "Can you move your arms and legs?"

PROMOTING SAFETY AND COMFORT

Emergency Care

Safety

Contact with blood, body fluids, secretions, and excretions is likely. Follow Standard Precautions and the Bloodborne Pathogen Standard to the extent possible.

For an emergency in an agency, call for the nurse at once. You may need to activate the EMS system or the RRS. Or you take the person's vital signs (Chapter 33). Assist as the nurse instructs.

Comfort

Mental comfort is important. Help the person feel safe and secure. Give reassurance. Explain the care you provide. Use a calm approach.

SUDDEN CARDIAC ARREST

Sudden cardiac arrest (SCA) or *cardiac arrest is when the heart stops suddenly and without warning.* Within seconds, breathing stops too. Blood and oxygen are not supplied to the body. Brain and other organ damage occurs within minutes.

SCA is a sudden, unexpected, and dramatic event. It can occur anywhere and at any time—while driving, shoveling snow, playing golf or tennis, watching TV, eating, or sleeping. Common causes include cardiovascular disorders, dysrhythmias (arrhythmias), and congenital heart defects (Chapter 49). Electrical shock, chest trauma, and substance use (Chapter 52) are other causes. The person is at risk for an abnormal heart rhythm called ventricular fibrillation (p. 852). The heart cannot pump blood. A normal rhythm must be restored or the person will die.

Signs of Sudden Cardiac Arrest

There are 3 major signs of SCA.

- *No response.*
- *No breathing or no normal breathing.* The person may have *agonal gasps (agonal respirations)* early during SCA. (*Agonal* means *to struggle.* Agonal relates to death and dying.) Agonal gasps do not bring enough oxygen into the lungs. Agonal gasps are not normal breathing.
- *No pulse.*

The skin is cool, pale, and gray. The person is not coughing or moving.

To check for SCA:

1   *Check for a response.* In an adult, tap or gently shake the person. Call the person by name, if known. Shout: "Are you okay?" Get help and emergency equipment if there is no response.
2   *Check for breathing and a pulse at the same time.* Do so for 5 to 10 seconds.
    - Look for no breathing or only gasping.
    - In an adult, check the carotid pulse (Fig. 58-1).

CPR

Cardiopulmonary resuscitation (CPR) is an emergency procedure performed when the heart and breathing stop. *Cardio* relates to the *heart.* *Pulmonary* relates to the *lungs.* To *resuscitate means to revive from apparent death or unconsciousness using emergency measures.* CPR must be started at once when a person has SCA. CPR provides blood and oxygen to the heart, brain, and other organs until advanced emergency care is given.

CPR involves:

- Giving chest compressions
- Opening the airway and giving breaths
- Defibrillation

    See *Focus on Communication: CPR.*
    See *Focus on Long-Term Care and Home Care: CPR.*
    See *Promoting Safety and Comfort: CPR.*

FOCUS ON COMMUNICATION

CPR

Getting help is a critical part of CPR. Advanced emergency care is needed at once. Follow the agency's procedure for activating the RRS or EMS. Outside the work setting, use a phone to call 911. For an adult:

- *If you are alone and have a phone*—call while giving care.
- *If you are alone without a phone*—leave the person to call 911 before starting CPR.
- *If you are not alone*—have someone call 911.

FOCUS ON LONG-TERM CARE AND HOME CARE

CPR

Long-Term Care

In nursing centers, a nurse decides when to activate the EMS system. The nurse tells you how to help. For SCA, the nurse may start CPR. Some agencies allow nursing assistants to start CPR. Others do not. Know your agency's policy.

Death is expected in persons with terminal illnesses. Usually these persons are not resuscitated (Chapter 59). This information is found in the care plan.

PROMOTING SAFETY AND COMFORT

CPR

Safety

The area must be safe for you to approach. If unsafe, wait for help to arrive. Do not approach the person. Only move the person if needed for safety and if safe enough to do so.

If the person has injuries, special measures are used to position the person for CPR and open the airway for breathing (p. 850). Such measures are learned during a CPR certification course.

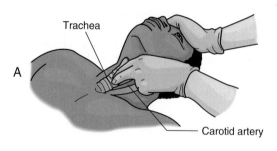
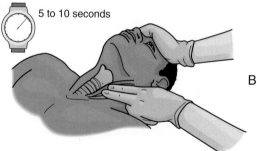

FIGURE 58-1 Checking the carotid pulse. **A,** Place 2 fingers on the trachea. **B,** Move the fingertips down into the groove of the neck to the carotid artery. Feel for a pulse for at least 5 seconds but no more than 10 seconds.

Chest Compressions

Chest compressions force blood through the circulatory system. When pressure is applied to the chest, the sternum compresses the heart (Fig. 58-2). For effective compressions, the person must be supine on a hard, flat surface.

To position the hands for compressions on an adult:

- Expose the chest. Remove clothing or move it out of the way.
- Place the heel of 1 hand (usually the dominant hand) in the center of the bare chest (Fig. 58-3, *A*). The hand is between the nipples on the lower half of the sternum.
- Place the heel of the other hand on top of the heel of the first hand (Fig. 58-3, *B*).

When giving compressions, the arms are straight. The shoulders are directly over the hands. Fingers are interlocked. See Figure 58-4. Press down and release pressure without removing the hands. Releasing pressure allows the chest to recoil—to return to its normal position. Recoil lets the heart fill with blood. Do not lean on the chest.

Compressions are given fast—at a rate of 100 to 120 per minute. The chest is pressed down at least 2 inches for an adult. Compressions are stopped only when necessary and for a short time—less than 10 seconds. Without compressions, blood does not flow to the heart, brain, and other organs.

See *Promoting Safety and Comfort: Chest Compressions.*

PROMOTING SAFETY AND COMFORT

Chest Compressions

Safety

The person must be on a hard, flat surface—floor or back-board. For the person in bed, place a board under the person. Logroll the person so there is no twisting of the spine. Place the arms alongside the body.

In a hospital, the RRS team brings a back-board. The head-board can be removed in some hospital beds for use as a back-board. Other hospital beds have a CPR button that lowers and deflates the mattress for a hard surface.

In a home setting, you may have to move the person to the floor.

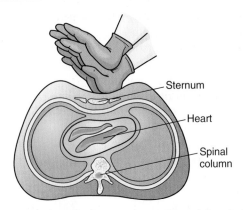

FIGURE 58-2 The heart lies between the sternum and the spinal column. The heart is compressed when pressure is applied to the sternum.

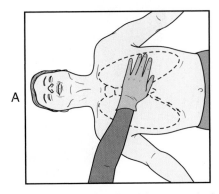 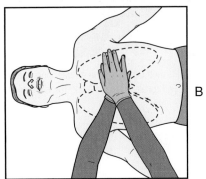

FIGURE 58-3 Hand position for adult CPR. **A,** The heel of the dominant hand is in the center of the chest. It is between the nipples and on the lower half of the sternum. **B,** The heel of the non-dominant hand is on top of the dominant hand.

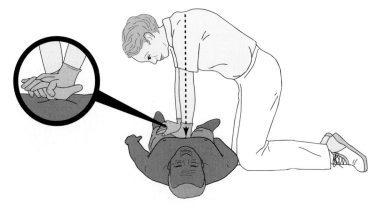

FIGURE 58-4 Giving chest compressions. The arms are straight. The shoulders are over the hands. The fingers are interlocked.

Airway and Breathing

The airway is often obstructed (blocked) during SCA. The tongue falls to the back of the throat and blocks the airway. The airway must be open to give breaths. The head tilt–chin lift method is used to open the airway. See Figure 58-5.

The rescuer breathes air into the person's mouth. To give mouth-to-mouth breaths to an adult (Fig. 58-6):

1 Keep the airway open with the head tilt–chin lift method.
2 Pinch the nostrils shut to keep air from coming out of the nose. Use the fingers on the hand on the person's forehead.
3 Take a normal breath.
4 Place your mouth tightly over the person's mouth. Seal the mouth with your lips.
5 Blow air into the person's mouth. The breath is given over 1 second. *The chest should rise as the lungs fill with air.*
6 Repeat the head tilt–chin lift if the chest did not rise.
7 Remove your mouth from the person's mouth. Take in another breath.
8 Give another breath. Watch for the chest to rise.

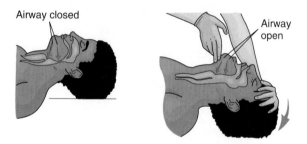

FIGURE 58-5 The head tilt–chin lift method opens the airway. One hand is on the forehead. Pressure is applied to tilt the head back. The chin is lifted with the fingers of the other hand.

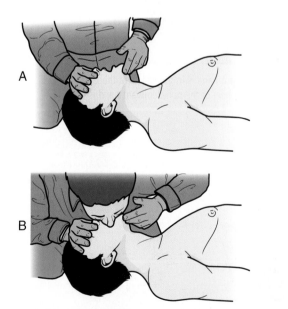

FIGURE 58-6 Mouth-to-mouth breathing. **A,** The airway is opened. The nostrils are pinched shut. **B,** The person's mouth is sealed by the rescuer's mouth.

Masks. A mask or other barrier device is used to give breaths when possible (Fig. 58-7, *A*). The device prevents contact with the person's mouth and blood, body fluids, secretions, or excretions. Place the mask over the person's mouth and nose (Fig. 58-7, *B*). Make a tight seal. Open the airway and blow through the mouth-piece to give breaths.

EMS and hospital staff often use a bag valve mask (Fig. 58-8) to give breaths. The device consists of a hand-held bag attached to a mask. The mask is held securely to the face. The bag is squeezed to give breaths. The bag can be connected to an oxygen source.

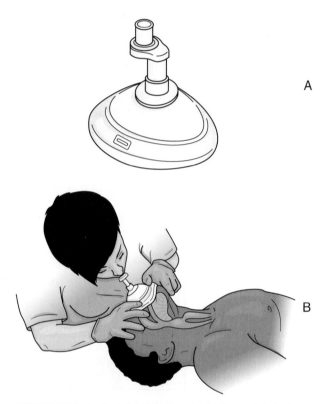

FIGURE 58-7 A, Mask for giving breaths. **B,** The mask is in place.

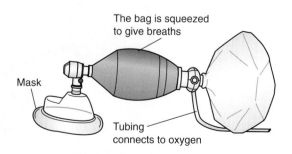

FIGURE 58-8 A bag valve mask.

Adult CPR Cycle

In an adult, a cycle of CPR involves 30 chest compressions and 2 breaths. Continue cycles of 30 compressions followed by 2 breaths until the person responds or help takes over. CPR is paused briefly to use a defibrillator (p. 852). Then CPR continues with compressions first. See Figure 58-9 for the sequence of CPR for an adult.

CPR is done by 1, 2, or more rescuers (Fig. 58-10). With more rescuers, a team approach promotes effective CPR. For example, with 2 rescuers:

- Rescuer 1 checks for a response. If no response, rescuer 1 tells rescuer 2 to call 911 and get an automated external defibrillator (AED) (p. 852).
- Rescuer 2 leaves to call for help and get an AED.
- Rescuer 1 gives CPR alone until rescuer 2 returns.
- Rescuer 2 returns and uses the AED.
- Rescuer 2 resumes compressions after AED use. (Rescuer 1 needs a break from compressions.)
- Rescuer 1 gives 2 breaths after every 30 compressions.
- Both rescuers continue CPR. They switch roles about every 2 minutes to avoid fatigue and inadequate compressions. They follow the AED's prompts to repeat AED use.

See *Focus on Communication: Adult CPR Cycle.*

FOCUS ON COMMUNICATION

Adult CPR Cycle

Good communication is needed when 2 rescuers give CPR. The rescuer giving compressions counts out loud so the other rescuer is ready to give breaths. Clear communication prevents delays and lessens interruptions in chest compressions.

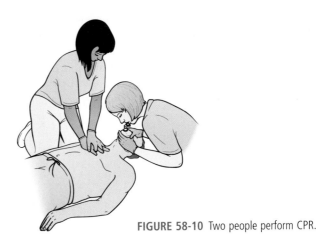

FIGURE 58-10 Two people perform CPR.

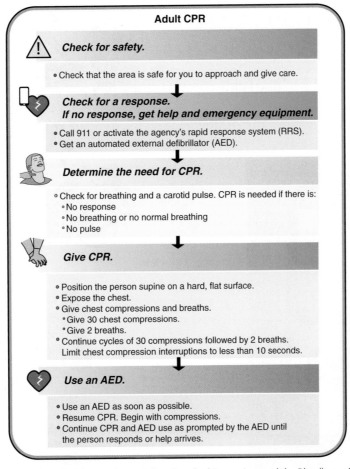

Adult CPR

⚠️ ***Check for safety.***

- Check that the area is safe for you to approach and give care.

Check for a response.
If no response, get help and emergency equipment.

- Call 911 or activate the agency's rapid response system (RRS).
- Get an automated external defibrillator (AED).

Determine the need for CPR.

- Check for breathing and a carotid pulse. CPR is needed if there is:
  - No response
  - No breathing or no normal breathing
  - No pulse

Give CPR.

- Position the person supine on a hard, flat surface.
- Expose the chest.
- Give chest compressions and breaths.
  - Give 30 chest compressions.
  - Give 2 breaths.
- Continue cycles of 30 compressions followed by 2 breaths. Limit chest compression interruptions to less than 10 seconds.

⚡ ***Use an AED.***

- Use an AED as soon as possible.
- Resume CPR. Begin with compressions.
- Continue CPR and AED use as prompted by the AED until the person responds or help arrives.

FIGURE 58-9 Sequence of adult CPR. (NOTE: Follow Standard Precautions and the Bloodborne Pathogen Standard to the extent possible. This includes the use of gloves and a mask or other barrier device.)

Defibrillation

Ventricular fibrillation (VF, V-fib) is an abnormal heart rhythm (Fig. 58-11). It causes SCA. Rather than beating in a regular rhythm, the heart quivers and does not pump blood.

A defibrillator delivers a shock to the heart. The shock stops the VF (V-fib). This may allow a regular rhythm to return. Defibrillation as soon as possible after the onset of VF (V-fib) increases the chance of survival.

Automated external defibrillators (AEDs) are found in health care agencies and in many public places (Fig. 58-12). Some persons have them at home.

See Box 58-2 for how to use an AED on an adult. Use an AED as soon as possible. You will learn more about AEDs in a CPR certification course.

See *Focus on Children and Older Persons: Defibrillation.*

BOX 58-2	Using an AED

Follow these steps to use an AED on an adult.
1. Open the AED case.
2. Turn on the AED (Fig. 58-13, *A*).
3. Apply adult electrode pads to the chest (Fig. 58-13, *B*). Follow the AED's instructions and diagram.
4. Attach the connecting cables to the AED (Fig. 58-13, *C*).
5. Clear away from the person. Make sure no one is touching the person (Fig. 58-13, *D*).
6. Let the AED check the heart rhythm.
7. Make sure everyone is clear of the person if the AED advises a "shock" (see Fig. 58-13, *D*). Loudly tell others not to touch the person. Say: "Everyone, clear!" Look to make sure no one is touching the person.
8. Press the SHOCK button if the AED advises a "shock" (Fig. 58-13, *E*).
9. Resume CPR beginning with compressions. Continue cycles of CPR.
10. Repeat steps 5 through 8 when prompted by the AED—after about 2 minutes of CPR. (NOTE: With 2 rescuers, rescuers switch roles at this step to avoid fatigue and inadequate compressions.)
11. Continue CPR and use of the AED until help takes over or the person responds.

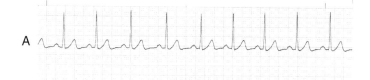

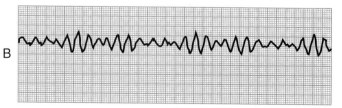

FIGURE 58-11 A, Normal rhythm. **B,** Ventricular fibrillation. (From Ignatavicius DD, Workman ML, Rebar CR: *Medical-surgical nursing: concepts for interprofessional collaborative care*, ed 9, St Louis, 2018, Elsevier.)

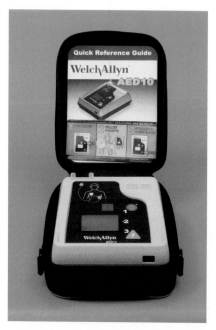

FIGURE 58-12 An automated external defibrillator (AED).

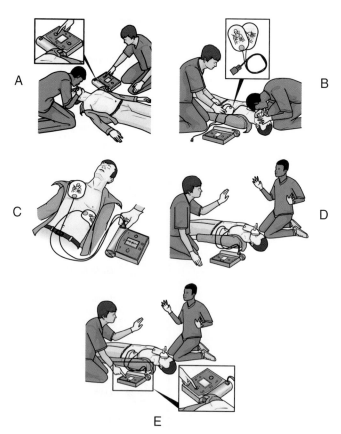

FIGURE 58-13 Using an AED. **A,** The rescuer turns on the AED. **B,** Electrode pads are placed on the chest. **C,** The cables are connected to the AED. **D,** The rescuers "clear" the person. The rescuers make sure no one is touching the person. **E,** The SHOCK button is pressed to deliver a shock.

FOCUS ON CHILDREN AND OLDER PERSONS

Defibrillation

Children

Some AEDs are designed for adults and children. A key or switch is used to lower the shock dosage for a child (Fig. 58-14). Or child pads are applied. Follow the manufacturer's instructions.

For children 8 years old and older, adult pads (adult dose) may be used. A lower shock dosage is used for children younger than 8 years. Use child pads (child dose) if possible. If not, adult pads (adult dose) may be used. Place the pads so they do not over-lap.

For infants, a manual defibrillator is best. Trained staff and EMS use the defibrillator. If one is not available, an AED with child pads (child dose) may be used. If neither is available, adult pads (adult dose) may be used. If needed, place pads on the chest and back so they do not touch.

Recovery Position

The recovery position is used after CPR when the person is breathing and has a pulse (Fig. 58-15). The person may not be responding. The position helps keep the airway open and prevents aspiration.

Logroll the person into the recovery position. Keep the head, neck, and spine straight. A hand supports the head. *Do not use this position if the person might have neck injuries or other trauma.*

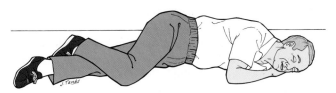

FIGURE 58-15 Recovery position.

Hands-Only CPR

With SCA, survival depends on others nearby. In public, bystanders may worry that they will not do CPR correctly or may cause injury. The "hands-only" method of CPR involves only chest compressions. Breaths are not given. There are only 2 steps.

1 Call 911.
2 Push hard and fast in the center of the chest.

The hands-only method is for persons in public who are not trained in CPR. With training and practice, you will learn all of the steps of CPR. As a health care provider, you will use the CPR method learned in your CPR certification course.

See *Focus on Children and Older Persons: Hands-Only CPR.*

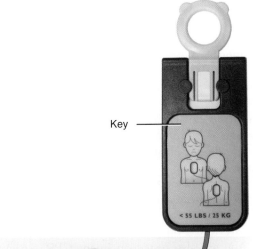
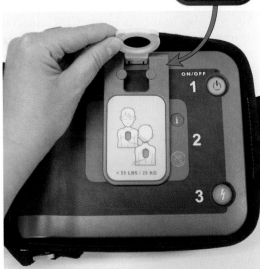

Key

FIGURE 58-14 On this AED, a key is inserted to lower the shock dosage for a child. Pads are placed on the chest and back so they do not over-lap.

FOCUS ON CHILDREN AND OLDER PERSONS

Hands-Only CPR

Children

The hands-only CPR method is intended for adults and adolescents with SCA. In infants and children, SCA caused by heart disease is rare. Usually a respiratory disease or injury causes the heart and breathing to stop. Motor vehicle crashes, drowning, suffocation, burns, smoke inhalation, falls, and poisoning are causes. Sudden infant death syndrome (SIDS) is the leading cause of death in children between 1 month and 1 year of age (Chapter 56).

For infants and children, breaths should be given with CPR. However, if the rescuer is unable or unwilling to deliver breaths, the hands-only method may be used.

Child and Infant CPR

CPR for children and infants differs from adult CPR. For CPR, these age ranges are used.

- *Child*—from 1 year of age to puberty. Puberty is marked by secondary sex characteristics (Chapter 11).
- *Infant*—from birth (outside the delivery room) until 1 year (12 months) of age. Special guidelines are used for newborns.

To check for a response in an infant, tap the infant's foot and shout. Infants cannot answer you. However, shouting should startle the responsive infant.

It may be hard to find a pulse in a child or infant. If you do not feel a pulse within 10 seconds, start CPR. If you feel a pulse, count it. Start CPR if the pulse is 60 beats per minute or less and the child or infant has signs of poor circulation. Such signs include:

- Cold arms and legs
- Unresponsive or decreased level of consciousness
- Weak pulse
- Pale, mottled (blotchy), or bluish skin
  See *Focus on Math: Child and Infant CPR.*

FOCUS ON **MATH**

Child and Infant CPR

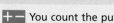 You count the pulse for no more than 10 seconds. To calculate the number of beats per minute:

- Multiply the number counted by 12 when you count for 5 seconds.
- Multiply the number counted by 6 when you count for 10 seconds.
  For example, when checking for a child's pulse you count 4 beats in 5 seconds. Multiply 4 beats (the number of beats in 5 seconds) by 12 to calculate the number of beats per minute.

  4 (number of beats in 5 seconds) × 12 = 48 beats per minute

  You calculate 48 beats per minute. This is less than 60 beats per minute. You give compressions.

  As a quick guide, give compressions if the number of beats counted is less than or equal to the number of seconds counted. *For example:*

- *Give compressions if you count 10 beats or less in 10 seconds.*
- *Give compressions if you count 9 beats or less in 9 seconds, and so on.*

All Age-Groups

Some CPR steps are the same for all persons. For *all* age-groups:

- Check that the area is safe for you to approach and give care.
- Check for a response. Get help and emergency equipment if there is no response.
- Check for breathing and a pulse. This takes less than 10 seconds.
- Give CPR for signs of SCA (p. 848).
- Give chest compressions at a rate of 100 to 120 per minute.
- Allow the chest to recoil after each compression. Do not lean on the chest.
- Limit interruptions in chest compressions to less than 10 seconds.
- Give breaths that make the chest rise over 1 second.
- Use an AED as soon as 1 is available.
  See Table 58-1 for the differences between CPR in adults and adolescents, children, and infants.

CPR Skills Testing

CPR certification courses involve:

- Training
- Skills practice
- A multiple-choice test
- A skills test

The American Heart Association's CPR training may be done in a classroom or on-line. For on-line training, a skills test with an evaluator is completed after the on-line portion.

A current training manual (print or electronic) is required. The manual includes the steps you must perform to pass the skills test.

You are tested on providing adult CPR and using an AED. You are also tested on infant CPR. An evaluator watches you perform the skills on a mannequin. To receive certification, you must pass the multiple-choice test and the skills test.

TABLE 58-1	CPR—Differences by Age-Group		
CPR Basics	**Adults and Adolescents**	**Children** (1 Year to Puberty)	**Infants** (Birth to 1 Year)
Getting help and an AED	• *If alone with a phone*—call 911 while giving care. Get an AED if possible. • *If alone without a phone*—leave the person to call 911 and get an AED before starting CPR. • *If not alone*—have someone call 911 and get an AED. • *In an agency*—follow agency procedures to activate the RRS or EMS and get emergency equipment.	• *If alone and the arrest was sudden and witnessed*—use the guidelines for adults and adolescents. • *If alone and the arrest was not witnessed*—give 2 minutes of CPR before leaving to call 911 and get an AED. • *If not alone*—have someone call 911 and get an AED. • *In an agency*—follow agency procedures to activate the RRS or EMS and get emergency equipment.	
Pulse check	• Carotid artery (neck)	• Carotid artery (neck) or femoral artery (groin) (Chapter 33) • CPR for pulse of 60 or less and poor circulation	• Brachial artery (upper arm) (Fig. 58-16) • CPR for pulse of 60 or less and poor circulation
Hand placement for compressions	• 2 hands on the lower half of the sternum	• 2 hands on the lower half of the sternum • 1 hand may be used if the child is small and the chest is compressed enough (Fig. 58-17)	• *1 rescuer*—2 fingers in the center of the chest just below the nipple line (Fig. 58-18) • *2 or more rescuers*—2-thumb-encircling hands method in the center of the chest just below the nipple line (Fig. 58-19)
Depth of compressions	• At least 2 inches	• About 2 inches (at least ⅓ of the depth of the chest)	• About 1½ inches (at least ⅓ of the depth of the chest)
Compressions and breaths	• 30 compressions followed by 2 breaths • 100 to 120 compressions per minute	• *1 rescuer*—30 compressions followed by 2 breaths • *2 or more rescuers*—15 compressions followed by 2 breaths • 100 to 120 compressions per minute	
Airway and breathing	• Mouth-to-mouth method or mask	• Mouth-to-mouth method or mask	• Mouth-to-mouth-and-nose method or mask (Fig. 58-20, p. 856 and see Fig. 58-19)

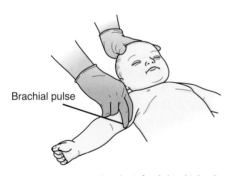

FIGURE 58-16 Locating the infant's brachial pulse.

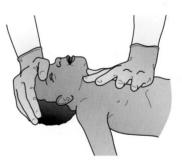

FIGURE 58-17 For a small child (1 year of age or older), the heel of 1 hand can be used for CPR. The fingers are off the chest.

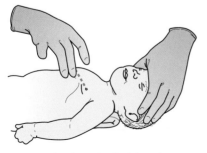

FIGURE 58-18 Locating hand position for infant chest compressions. Imagine a line between the nipples. Find the sternum. For 1-rescuer CPR, place 2 fingers on the sternum just below the imaginary line.

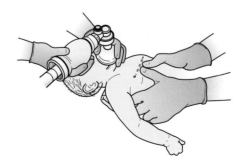

FIGURE 58-19 The 2-thumb-encircling hands method for chest compressions. This method is used when 2 rescuers perform infant CPR.

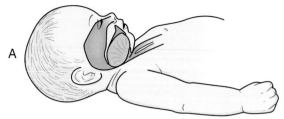

A

The tongue is at the back of the throat blocking the airway.

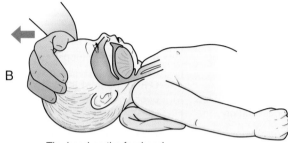

B

The hand on the forehead is used to tilt the head back.

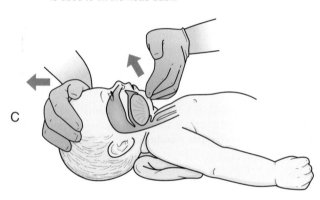

C

The fingers on the other hand are under the bony part of the jaw (near the chin). The fingers lift the jaw to bring the chin forward.

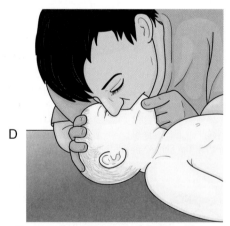

D

The mouth and nose are covered to give breaths.

FIGURE 58-20 Opening the airway and giving breaths to an infant.

CHOKING

Foreign bodies can obstruct (block) the airway. This is called *choking* or *foreign-body airway obstruction (FBAO).* Air cannot pass into the lungs. The body does not get enough oxygen. It can lead to cardiac arrest.

Airway obstruction can be mild or severe. With severe airway obstruction, air does not move in and out of the lungs. If the obstruction is not removed, the person will die. Abdominal thrusts are used to relieve severe airway obstruction. See Chapter 13 for emergency care of the choking person.

RESPIRATORY ARREST

Respiratory arrest is when breathing stops but heart action continues for several minutes. If breathing is not restored, cardiac arrest occurs. Respiratory arrest can occur from:

- Blocked airflow—choking (Chapter 13), drowning, suffocation
- Problems affecting nerves, muscles, or areas of the brain that control breathing—amyotrophic lateral sclerosis (ALS), spinal cord injuries, stroke (Chapter 48); drug or alcohol over-dose; drug side effects
- Lung disorders and problems—pneumonia, chronic obstructive pulmonary disease (Chapter 49), pulmonary embolism (Chapter 39), chest injuries
- Inhaling harmful substances—smoke, chemicals, fumes

Rescue Breathing

Rescue breaths are given when there is a pulse but no breathing or only agonal gasping. To give rescue breaths:

- Open the airway (p. 850).
- Give 1 breath every 5 to 6 seconds for adults.
- Give 1 breath every 3 to 5 seconds for infants and children.
- Give each breath over 1 second. The chest should rise when breaths are given.

Follow the rules in Box 58-1. This includes activating the EMS system. Check the pulse every 2 minutes. If no pulse, begin CPR. If the pulse is 60 or less in an infant or child, begin CPR.

HEART ATTACK

Heart attack (myocardial infarction) occurs when part of the heart muscle dies from the sudden blockage of blood flow in a coronary artery (Chapter 49). Signs and symptoms include:

* Chest pain (not relieved by rest)
* Pain or discomfort in 1 or both arms, the back, neck, jaw, or stomach
* Shortness of breath
* Perspiration (sweating) and cold, clammy skin
* Feeling light-headed
* Nausea and vomiting

If you suspect a heart attack, have the person sit and rest. Loosen tight clothing. Activate the EMS system at once. Prompt treatment can reduce the amount of heart muscle damage. Follow the rules in Box 58-1. Start CPR for cardiac arrest.

HEMORRHAGE

Life and body functions need an adequate blood supply. If a blood vessel is cut or torn, bleeding occurs. The larger the blood vessel, the greater the bleeding and blood loss. *Hemorrhage is the excessive loss* (rrhage) *of blood* (hemo) *in a short time.* If bleeding is not stopped, the person will die.

Hemorrhage is internal or external. You cannot see internal hemorrhage. The bleeding is inside body tissues and body cavities. Pain, shock, vomiting blood, coughing up blood, cold and moist skin, and loss of consciousness signal internal hemorrhage. There is little you can do for internal bleeding.

* Follow the rules in Box 58-1. This includes activating the EMS system.
* Keep the person warm, flat, and quiet until help arrives.
* Do not give fluids.

If not hidden by clothing, external bleeding is usually seen. Bleeding from an artery occurs in spurts. There is a steady flow of blood from a vein. To control bleeding:

* Follow the rules in Box 58-1. This includes activating the EMS system.
* Do not remove any objects that have pierced or stabbed the person.
* Place a sterile dressing directly over the wound. Or use any clean material (handkerchief, towel, cloth, or sanitary napkin).
* Apply firm pressure directly over the bleeding site (Fig. 58-21). Do not release pressure until the bleeding stops. If needed, wrap an elastic bandage firmly over the dressing or material.
* Do not remove the dressing or material. If bleeding continues, apply more dressings on top and apply more pressure.
* Bind the wound when bleeding stops. Tape or tie the dressing in place. You can tie the dressing with such things as clothing, a scarf, or a necktie.

See *Promoting Safety and Comfort: Hemorrhage.*

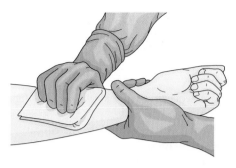

FIGURE 58-21 Direct pressure is applied to the wound to stop bleeding.

> ### PROMOTING SAFETY AND COMFORT
> #### *Hemorrhage*
>
> **Safety**
> Contact with blood is likely with hemorrhage. Follow Standard Precautions and the Bloodborne Pathogen Standard to the extent possible. Wear gloves if possible. Practice hand hygiene as soon as you can.

SHOCK

Shock results when tissues and organs do not get enough blood. Blood loss, allergic reaction, poisoning, heart attack (myocardial infarction), burns, and severe infection are causes. Signs and symptoms include:

* Low or falling blood pressure
* Rapid and weak pulse
* Rapid respirations
* Cold, moist, and pale skin
* Thirst
* Nausea and vomiting
* Restlessness
* Confusion and loss of consciousness as shock worsens

Shock is possible in any acutely ill or severely injured person. Follow the rules in Box 58-1. Keep the person lying down. If no injuries from trauma, raise the feet about 6 to 12 inches. Lower the feet if the position causes pain. Maintain an open airway and control bleeding. Start CPR for cardiac arrest.

Anaphylactic Shock

Some people are allergic or sensitive to foods, insects, chemicals, and drugs. For example, allergies to *penicillin* are common. An *antigen* is a substance that the body reacts to. The body releases chemicals to fight or attack the antigen. The person may react with an area of redness, swelling, or itching. Or the reaction may involve the entire body.

Anaphylaxis is a life-threatening sensitivity to an antigen. (*Ana* means *without. Phylaxis* means *protection.*) The reaction can occur within seconds.

Signs and symptoms of anaphylaxis include:
- An itchy rash
- Swelling of the face, eyes, or lips
- Flushed or pale skin
- Feeling warm
- Dyspnea or wheezing from airway narrowing or a swollen tongue or throat
- Feeling that there is a "lump" in the throat
- A fast and weak pulse
- Nausea, vomiting, or diarrhea
- A feeling of dread or doom
- Dizziness or fainting
- Signs and symptoms of shock

Anaphylactic shock is an emergency. The EMS system must be activated. Drugs are needed to reverse the allergic reaction. Keep the person lying down and the airway open. Start CPR for cardiac arrest. Give rescue breathing for respiratory arrest.

Some persons carry *epinephrine*—a drug used to treat life-threatening allergic reactions. The person injects the drug into the outer thigh. One dose is given for anaphylaxis. The person may give a second dose if:
- There is no response to the first dose.
- EMS arrival will take longer than 5 to 10 minutes.

FAINTING

Fainting (syncope) is the sudden loss of consciousness from an inadequate blood supply to the brain. Hunger, fatigue, fear, and pain are common causes. Some people faint at the sight of blood or injury. Standing in 1 position too long and being in a warm, crowded room are other causes. Hemorrhage and other serious problems can cause fainting.

Dizziness, perspiration (sweating), weakness, and vision changes are warning signs. The person looks pale. The pulse is weak. Respirations are shallow if consciousness is lost.

If a person has warning signs of fainting:
- Have the person sit or lie down to prevent fainting.
  - If sitting, the person bends forward and places the head between the knees (Fig. 58-22).
  - If lying down, raise the person's legs.
- Loosen tight clothing (belts, ties, scarves, collars, and so on).

If fainting occurs:
- Activate the EMS system.
- Keep the person lying down. Raise the feet about 12 inches.
- Start CPR for cardiac arrest. Give rescue breathing for respiratory arrest.
- Help the person to a sitting position after recovery from fainting. Do not let the person get up quickly. Observe for fainting again.

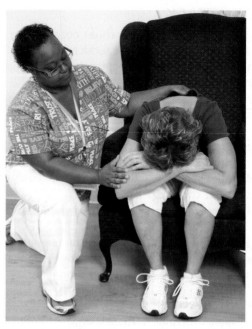

FIGURE 58-22 The person bends forward and lowers her head to prevent fainting.

STROKE

Stroke (cerebrovascular accident) occurs when the brain is suddenly deprived of its blood supply (Chapter 48). Usually only part of the brain is affected. A stroke may be caused by a thrombus, an embolus, or hemorrhage if a blood vessel in the brain ruptures.

Signs of stroke vary (Chapter 48). They depend on the size and location of brain injury. The National Institute of Neurological Disorders and Stroke lists these major signs.
- Sudden numbness or weakness of the face, arm, or leg, especially on 1 side of the body
- Sudden confusion or trouble speaking or understanding speech
- Sudden trouble seeing in 1 or both eyes
- Sudden trouble walking, dizziness, or loss of balance or coordination
- Sudden, severe headache with no known cause

If you suspect a stroke, activate the EMS system at once. The most effective stroke treatments must be given within 3 hours of symptom onset. Find out when the symptoms began. Tell the EMS staff the time. Follow the rules in Box 58-1. Keep the person comfortable, warm, and quiet. Give emergency care for seizures if necessary. Start CPR for cardiac arrest. Give rescue breathing for respiratory arrest.

SEIZURES

Seizures (convulsions) are violent and sudden contractions or tremors of muscle groups caused by abnormal electrical activity in the brain. Movements are uncontrolled. The person may lose consciousness. Causes include head injury during birth or from trauma, high fever, brain tumors, poisoning, and nervous system disorders or infections. Lack of blood flow to the brain can also cause seizures.

Epilepsy

Epilepsy is a brain disorder in which clusters of nerve cells sometimes signal abnormally. There are brief changes in the brain's electrical function. The person can have strange sensations, emotions, and behavior. Sometimes there are seizures, muscle spasms, and loss of consciousness.

A single seizure does not mean epilepsy. In epilepsy, seizures recur from a permanent brain injury or defect.

Epilepsy develops more often in children and older adults. However, epilepsy can begin at any age. It can occur with any problem affecting the brain. Such causes include:

- Brain injury during or after birth (Chapter 54)
- Problems with brain development before birth
- The mother having an injury or infection during pregnancy
- Traumatic brain injury (accidents, gunshot wounds, sports injuries, falls, blows to the head)
- Brain tumor
- Poison—such as lead and alcohol
- Infection—such as meningitis and encephalitis
- Stroke
- Dementia

There is no cure at this time. Drugs control seizures in many people. Surgery may be done when drug therapy does not work.

When controlled, epilepsy usually does not affect learning and activities of daily living. Activity and job limits occur in severe cases. For example, a person has seizures at any time. The person may not be allowed to drive. This may limit job choices. Also, the person is at risk for accidents and injuries. Safety measures are needed. They are needed for the home, workplace, transportation, and recreation.

Types of Seizures

Seizures are generalized or focal.

- *Generalized seizures*—affect both sides of the brain. There are 2 types.
  - *Absence (petit mal) seizures*—cause staring and rapid blinking. The seizure lasts a few seconds.
  - *Tonic-clonic (grand mal) seizures*—have 2 phases. In the *tonic* phase, muscles become stiff. The person loses consciousness and falls to the floor. The *clonic* phase follows. Muscles contract and relax. Jerking and shaking movements occur. The person may be incontinent. After the seizure, the person is often tired.
- *Focal (partial) seizures*—affect 1 area of the brain. A body part may twitch or have sensation changes. A strange taste or smell is an example. The person may be confused or unable to respond for a few minutes.

Emergency Care for Seizures

You cannot stop a seizure. However, you can protect the person from injury.

- Follow the rules in Box 58-1. See Box 58-3 for when to activate the EMS system.
- Do not leave the person alone.
- Lower the person to the floor. This protects the person from falling.

BOX 58-3	Seizures—Activating EMS

Activate the EMS system for any of the following.
- This is the person's first seizure.
- The person has trouble breathing after the seizure.
- The person has difficulty awaking after the seizure.
- The seizure lasts longer than 5 minutes.
- The person has another seizure soon after the first seizure.
- The person is or may be injured.
- The seizure happened in water.
- The person has diabetes or heart disease.
- The person is pregnant.

Modified from National Center for Chronic Disease Prevention and Health Promotion, Centers for Disease Control and Prevention: Seizure first aid, page reviewed January 10, 2019.

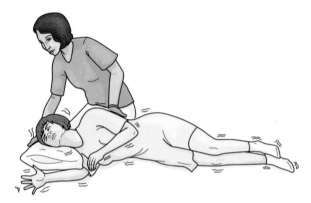

FIGURE 58-23 A pillow protects the person's head during a seizure.

- Note the time the seizure started.
- Place something soft under the head (Fig. 58-23). It prevents the head from striking the floor. You can use a pillow, a cushion, or a folded blanket, towel, or jacket. Or cradle the person's head in your lap.
- Remove eyeglasses and loosen tight jewelry and clothing around the neck. Ties, scarves, collars, and necklaces are examples.
- Turn the person onto the side. Make sure the head is turned to the side. See Figure 58-23.
- Do not put any object or your fingers between the teeth. The person can bite down on your fingers or injure his or her teeth or jaw.
- Do not try to stop the seizure or control movements.
- Move furniture, equipment, and sharp objects out of the way. The person may strike these objects during the seizure.
- Note the time the seizure ends.
- Make sure the mouth is clear of food, fluids, and saliva after the seizure.
- Do not give food or fluids until the person is fully alert.
- Do not let the person drive after a seizure.
- Monitor the person's breathing. Gasping or pauses may occur when chest muscles tighten during a seizure. Rescue breathing and CPR usually are not needed. Breathing should return to normal after the seizure.

CONCUSSIONS

Head injuries can be minor or serious and life-threatening. Concussion is the most common brain injury. Concussion comes from the Latin word *concutere* that means *to shake violently*. A concussion results from a bump or blow to the head or jolt to the head or body. The head and brain move quickly back and forth.

Symptoms can last for days, weeks, or longer. Symptoms affect:
* Thinking—difficulty thinking clearly, concentrating, remembering new information
* Physical function—headache, fuzzy or blurred vision, nausea and vomiting, dizziness, sensitivity to noise or light, balance problems, tired feeling, no energy
* Mood—irritability, sadness, nervousness, anxiety
* Sleep—more or less sleep than usual, trouble falling asleep

Some people have repeated concussions. Football players are examples. Long-term effects from repeated concussions include chronic problems with concentration, memory, headaches, and balance.

Emergency Care for Concussions

The following danger signs in adults signal the need for emergency care.
* Headache—gets worse or does not go away
* Weakness, numbness, or decreased coordination
* Nausea or vomiting more than once
* Slurred speech
* Very sleepy; drowsy; cannot be awakened
* One eye pupil is larger than the other
* Convulsions or seizures
* Cannot recognize people, places, or things
* Increased confusion, restlessness, or agitation
* Unusual behavior
* Loss of consciousness

Emergency care for a concussion includes the following.
* Follow the rules in Box 58-1. This includes activating the EMS system.
* Start CPR for cardiac arrest. Give rescue breathing for respiratory arrest.
* Place your hands on both sides of the head to keep the head aligned with the spine. Prevent movement.
* Apply firm pressure with a clean cloth to a bleeding area. See "Hemorrhage" on p. 857. Be careful not to move the person's head.
* Do not apply direct pressure to the skull if the skull may be fractured. Cover the wound with sterile gauze dressing.
* Do not remove any object from a wound.
* Logroll the person as a unit onto the side if vomiting occurs.
* Apply ice packs to swollen areas.

See *Focus on Children and Older Persons: Emergency Care for Concussions.*

FOCUS ON CHILDREN AND OLDER PERSONS

Emergency Care for Concussions

Children
Children can receive a bump, blow, or jolt to the head or body. Emergency care is needed if the child:
* Has the danger signs listed for adults.
* Will not stop crying.
* Cannot be consoled (comforted).
* Will not nurse or eat.

COLD- AND HEAT-RELATED ILLNESSES

When over-exposed to cold or heat, a person can become seriously ill. The person can die.

Cold-Related Illnesses

Hypothermia and frostbite are 2 cold-related illnesses.

Hypothermia. *Hypothermia is abnormally low* (hypo) *body temperature* (thermia). Prolonged exposure to cold temperatures is the most common cause. Other causes include being cold and wet or being under cold water for too long. A body temperature below 95°F (Fahrenheit) is an emergency.

Persons who spend a lot of time outdoors in cold weather are at risk. So are babies and older persons, especially if in a very cold house or sleeping in a cold room.

Signs and symptoms of hypothermia include:
* Cold hands and feet
* Pale skin
* Shivering
* Speech problems: slurring or slowed speech
* Sleepiness
* Confusion
* Movement problems: moving slowly, trouble walking, being clumsy
* Heart rate: slow
* Respirations: slow
* Losing consciousness

Emergency care for hypothermia includes the following:
* Activate the EMS system.
* While waiting for medical help to arrive:
  * Move the person to a warmer place, if possible.
  * Wrap the person in warm blankets, towels, or coats.
  * Give the person something warm to drink. Do not give the person drinks containing alcohol or caffeine (coffee, tea).
  * Do not rub the person's arms or legs.
  * Do not try to warm the person in a bath or shower.
  * Do not use a heating pad.

Frostbite. *Frostbite is an injury to the body caused by freezing of the skin and underlying tissues.* The nose, ears, cheeks, chin, fingers, and toes are the most common sites for frostbite. Damage can be permanent. Severe cases may require amputation (Chapter 48).

Signs and symptoms of frostbite include:

- White or grayish-yellow skin
- Skin that feels unusually firm or waxy
- Numbness

Emergency care of frostbite includes:

- Seeking medical care.
- Getting into a warm room as soon as possible.
- Not walking on toes or feet with frostbite.
- Putting the affected part in warm water (not hot water).
- Using body heat to warm the part. For example, warming fingers in the underarm.
- Not rubbing or massaging the part.
- Not using a heating pad, heat lamp, stove, fireplace, or other heat source to warm the part. Affected areas are numb and unable to sense heat. The area is easily burned.

Heat-Related Illnesses

Sweating is the body's way of cooling itself. When sweating is not enough for cooling, body temperature can rise to dangerous levels. Brain and other organ damage can occur.

Staying out in the heat too long is a common cause. Exercising and working outside during hot, humid weather are other causes. Persons at risk include infants, young children, and older persons. Other risk factors include obesity, fever, dehydration, heart disease, mental health disorders, poor circulation, prescription drug use, and alcohol use.

See Table 58-2 for the heat-related illnesses, signs and symptoms, and emergency care.

BURNS

Burns can severely disable a person. They can also cause death. Most burns occur in the home. Infants, children, and older persons are at risk. Common causes of burns and fires are:

- Scalds from steam or hot liquids
- Playing with matches and lighters
- Electrical injuries
- Cooking accidents (barbecues, microwave ovens, stoves, ovens)
- Falling asleep while smoking
- Fireplaces
- Space heaters
- No smoke alarms or non-functioning smoke alarms
- Sunburns
- Fireworks
- Chemicals

TABLE 58-2	Heat-Related Illnesses	
Heat-Related Illness	Signs and Symptoms	Emergency Care

Heat stroke	• Body temperature of 103°F or higher
	• Hot, red, dry, or damp skin
	• Pulse: strong and fast
	• Headache
	• Dizziness
	• Nausea
	• Confusion
	• Loss of consciousness
		• Activate the EMS system.
		• Move the person to a cooler place.
		• Remove excess clothing.
		• Cool the person.
		  • Bathe or shower in cool water.
		  • Spray with a garden hose.
		  • Sponge or mist with cool water.
		  • Apply cool, wet cloths to the head, neck, underarms, and groin.
		• Do not give the person anything to drink.

Heat exhaustion	• Heavy sweating • Cold, pale, and clammy skin • Pulse: fast and weak • Nausea or vomiting • Muscle cramps • Tiredness • Weakness • Dizziness • Headache • Fainting	• Move the person to a cooler place. • Loosen clothing. • Apply cool, wet cloths to the head, neck, underarms, and groin. Or bathe or shower in cool water. • Give sips of water. • Seek medical care.

Heat cramps	• Heavy sweating during exercise
	• Muscle pain
	• Muscle spasms
		• Stop physical activity.
		• Move to a cool place.
		• Drink water or a sports drink.
		• Seek medical help if:
		  • Cramps last longer than 1 hour.
		  • The person is on a low-sodium diet.
		  • The person has heart problems.

Sunburn	• Painful, red, and warm skin • Blisters	• Move out of the sun. • Apply cool cloths to sunburned areas. • Apply moisturizing lotion to sunburned areas. • Do not break the blisters.

Modified from Centers for Disease Control and Prevention: Warning signs and symptoms of heat-related illness, page reviewed September 1, 2017, Atlanta, Ga.

Types of Burns

The skin has 2 layers: the epidermis and dermis. Burns are described as:

- *Superficial (first degree) burns*—involve the epidermis only. They are painful, but the burn is not severe. There is redness and swelling.
- *Partial thickness (second degree) burns*—involve the epidermis and part of the dermis. They are very painful. Nerve endings are exposed. There is redness, swelling, and blistering.
- *Full thickness (third degree) burns*—involve the entire epidermis and dermis. Fat, muscle, and bone may be injured or destroyed. These burns are not painful. Nerve endings are destroyed. The burned skin is white or black.

Some burns are severe (Fig. 58-24). Severity depends on burn size and depth, the body part involved, and age. Burns to the face, hands, feet, groin, buttocks, or over a joint are more serious than burns to an arm or leg. Infants, young children, and older persons are at high risk for complications and death.

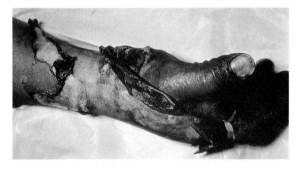

FIGURE 58-24 A severe burn. (From Ignatavicius DD, Workman ML, Rebar, CR: *Medical-surgical nursing: patient-centered collaborative care,* ed 9, St Louis, 2018, Elsevier.)

Emergency Care for Burns

Emergency care for severe burns includes the following.

- Follow the rules in Box 58-1. This includes activating the EMS system.
- Do not touch the person if he or she is in contact with an electrical source. Have the power source turned off. Do not approach the person or try to remove the electrical source with any object until the power source is turned off.
- Remove the person from the fire or burn source.
- Stop the burning process. Put out flames with water or roll the person in a blanket. Or smother flames with a coat, sheet, or towel.
- Apply cold or cool water for 10 to 15 minutes. Water temperature is between 59°F and 77°F (15°C and 25°C [centigrade]). Do not put ice directly on the burn.
- Remove hot clothing that is not sticking to the skin. If you cannot remove hot clothing, cool the clothing with water.
- Remove jewelry and any tight clothing that is not sticking to the skin.
- Provide rescue breathing and CPR as needed.
- Cover burns with sterile, dry dressings. Or use a sheet or any other clean cloth.
- Do not put oil, butter, salve, or ointments on the burns.
- Keep blisters intact. Do not break blisters.
- Elevate the burned area above heart level if possible.
- Cover the person with a blanket or coat to prevent heat loss.

POISONING

A *poison* is any substance harmful to the body when swallowed, inhaled, injected, or absorbed through the skin. For contact with a poison, call the Poison Control Center (1-800-222-1222). Follow the rules in Box 58-1. Also follow the directions from the Poison Control Center. See Chapter 13.

FOCUS ON **PRIDE**

The Person, Family, and Yourself

Personal and Professional Responsibility

Practicing CPR skills improves confidence. Never practice CPR on another person. Serious damage can be done. Practice on a mannequin. Take pride in learning CPR. Your training can save a life.

Rights and Respect

Protect the right to privacy. Do not expose the person unnecessarily. The person may be in a lounge, dining area, or public place. Do what you can to provide privacy. As always, treat the person with dignity and respect.

Independence and Social Interaction

Quality of life and independence are important. In an emergency, choices may be few. However, they are given when possible. For example, the person has the right to choose a hospital.

The EMS staff has guidelines if a person refuses care. For example, the person must be competent and able to legally make medical decisions. The person must also be informed of the risks, benefits, and alternatives to recommended care.

Delegation and Teamwork

On-lookers can threaten privacy and confidentiality. Your main concern is the person's illness or injuries. You cannot give care and manage on-lookers. Ask someone else to deal with on-lookers. If someone else is giving care, keep on-lookers away from the person. Work together to protect the person's privacy.

Ethics and Laws

People are curious. They want to know what happened, the extent of injuries or illness, and if the person will be okay. Do not discuss the situation. Do not offer ideas of what is wrong. Information about care, treatment, and condition is confidential. Keep the person's information private. It is the right thing to do.

FOCUS ON **PRIDE**: *Application*

Emergencies are stressful. A calm, professional approach helps the person and family feel more secure. Describe professional conduct in an emergency. Explain how you will prepare yourself to respond.

REVIEW QUESTIONS

Circle the BEST answer.

1 The goals of first aid are to
   a Call for help and keep the person warm
   b Prevent death and prevent injuries from becoming worse
   c Stay calm and give emergency care
   d Calm the person and keep bystanders away

2 When giving first aid, you should
   a Know your own limits
   b Move the person
   c Give the person fluids
   d Keep the person cool

3 Sudden cardiac arrest is
   a The same as stroke
   b The sudden stopping of heart action
   c The sudden loss of consciousness
   d When organs and tissues do not get enough blood

4 The signs of sudden cardiac arrest are
   a Restlessness, rapid breathing, and a weak pulse
   b Confusion, hemiplegia, and slurred speech
   c No response, no normal breathing, and no pulse
   d Dizziness, pale skin, and slow breathing

5 A person is not responsive. To check for breathing
   a Use the head tilt–chin lift method to open the airway
   b Look for no breathing or agonal gasping
   c Look, listen, and feel for air moving in and out of the lungs
   d Take 10 to 15 seconds to listen for breathing

6 Which pulse is checked for an unresponsive adult?
   a The carotid pulse
   b The apical pulse
   c The brachial pulse
   d The femoral pulse

7 Which hand placement is correct for adult chest compressions?
   a 1 hand in the center of the chest
   b 2 hands below the sternum
   c 2 hands on the lower half of the sternum
   d 2 fingers on the lower half of the sternum

8 Which compression rate is used for adult, child, and infant CPR?
   a 30 compressions per minute
   b 100 to 120 compressions per minute
   c 15 compressions per minute
   d 60 to 100 compressions per minute

9 For adult CPR
   a Give 2 breaths after every 15 compressions
   b Give 2 breaths after every 30 compressions
   c Give 1 breath after every 5 compressions
   d Give 2 breaths when you are tired from giving compressions

10 Two rescuers are giving adult CPR. When should the AED be used?
   a After 5 cycles of CPR
   b After 2 minutes of CPR
   c As soon as the AED arrives
   d When EMS staff arrives

Continued

REVIEW QUESTIONS—cont'd

11 Two rescuers are giving a child CPR. Breaths are given
   a After every compression
   b After every 5 compressions
   c After every 15 compressions
   d After every 30 compressions

12 When 2 rescuers give an infant CPR
   a Use the 2-thumb-encircling hands method for compressions
   b Give 30 compressions followed by 2 breaths
   c Check for a carotid pulse
   d Give CPR if the heart rate is less than 100 beats per minute

13 Rescue breathing for an adult involves
   a Giving each breath over 2 seconds
   b Watching the abdomen rise with each breath
   c Giving a breath every 3 to 5 seconds
   d Giving a breath every 5 to 6 seconds

14 Which statement about heart attack is *true*?
   a It is the same as cardiac arrest.
   b It can cause cardiac arrest.
   c Symptoms resolve with rest.
   d It is a severe response to an antigen.

15 Arterial bleeding
   a Cannot be seen
   b Oozes from the wound
   c Is dark red
   d Occurs in spurts

16 A person is hemorrhaging from the forearm. Your *first* action is to
   a Lower the arm
   b Apply pressure to the brachial artery
   c Tape a dressing in place
   d Apply direct pressure to the wound

17 Which is a sign of shock?
   a High blood pressure
   b Slow pulse
   c Slow and deep respirations
   d Cold, moist, and pale skin

18 A person in shock needs
   a Rescue breathing
   b Clothes removed
   c To be kept lying down
   d The recovery position

19 A person is about to faint. What should you do?
   a Have the person sit or lie down.
   b Take the person outside for fresh air.
   c Have the person stand very still.
   d Raise the head if the person is lying down.

20 Emergency care for stroke involves
   a Asking when the person's symptoms began
   b Giving the person sips of water
   c Controlling bleeding
   d Positioning the person bent forward with the head lowered

21 A person is having a tonic-clonic (grand mal) seizure. You should
   a Place an object between the person's teeth
   b Loosen tight jewelry and clothing around the neck
   c Try to stop the person's movements
   d Place the person's head on a firm surface

22 After falling down stairs, a person is confused and has a headache. You should
   a Place the person in the recovery position
   b Give the person a pain-relief drug
   c Prevent movement of the head and neck
   d Help the person to bed to lie down

23 Which emergency measure is *correct*?
   a Apply a heating pad for hypothermia.
   b Massage fingers with frostbite.
   c Give cold water to drink for a heat stroke.
   d Apply cool, wet cloths for heat exhaustion.

24 While waiting for help to arrive, cover a severe burn with
   a A sterile, dry dressing or clean cloth
   b Butter or oil
   c Salve or an ointment
   d Nothing

25 A person swallowed a chemical. You should
   a Have the person drink a glass of water
   b Have the person try to vomit
   c Call the Poison Control Center
   d Contact the chemical's manufacturer

Answers to Chapter 58 questions are on p. 888.

FOCUS ON **PRACTICE**
Problem Solving

A resident has a tonic-clonic (grand mal) seizure during an activity. What emergency care will you provide? How will you and the nursing team provide for the person's privacy?

End-of-Life Care

OBJECTIVES

- Define the key terms and key abbreviations in this chapter.
- Describe palliative care and hospice care.
- Describe the factors affecting attitudes about death.
- Describe how different age-groups view death.
- Describe the 5 stages of dying.
- Explain how to meet the needs of the dying person and family.
- Explain the purposes of the *Patient Self-Determination Act*.

- Describe 3 advance directives.
- Identify the signs of approaching death and the signs of death.
- Explain how to assist with post-mortem care.
- Perform the procedure in this chapter.
- Explain how to promote PRIDE in the person, the family, and yourself.

KEY TERMS

advance directive A document stating a person's wishes about health care when that person cannot make his or her own decisions
autopsy The examination of the body after death
end-of-life care The support and care given during the time surrounding death
palliative care Care to relieve or reduce the intensity of uncomfortable symptoms without producing a cure
post-mortem care Care of the body after *(post)* death *(mortem)*

reincarnation The belief that the spirit or soul is reborn in another human body or in another form of life
rigor mortis The stiffness or rigidity *(rigor)* of skeletal muscles that occurs after death *(mortis)*
terminal illness An illness or injury from which the person will not likely recover

KEY ABBREVIATIONS

DNR	Do Not Resuscitate	OBRA	Omnibus Budget Reconciliation Act of 1987
ID	Identification		

End-of-life care describes the support and care given during the time surrounding death. Sometimes death is sudden. Often it is expected. Some people gradually fail. End-of-life care may involve days, weeks, or months. The person may need hospital, nursing center, or home care. Hospice care is common.

Death and dying may cause staff discomfort because of feeling helpless and failing to cure. They remind us that our loved ones and we will die.

Your feelings about death affect the care you give. You will help meet the dying person's physical, psychological, social, and spiritual needs. Therefore you must understand

the dying process. Then you can approach the dying person with caring, kindness, and respect.

See *Teamwork and Time Management: End-of-Life Care.*

> ### TEAMWORK AND TIME MANAGEMENT
> *End-of-Life Care*
>
> Dying persons need a lot of time from nurses. Often it is a busy time before and after someone dies. Offer to take equipment and supplies to and from the room. Also help with other patients or residents.

TERMINAL ILLNESS

Many illnesses and diseases have no cure. The body cannot function after some injuries. Recovery is not expected. The disease or injury ends in death. *An illness or injury from which the person will not likely recover is a* **terminal illness.**

Doctors cannot predict the time of death. A person may have days, months, weeks, or years to live. People expected to live for a short time have lived for years. Others have died earlier than expected.

Modern medicine has prolonged life in many cases. Research will bring new cures. However, hope and the will to live strongly influence living and dying. Many people have died for no apparent reason after losing hope or the will to live.

Types of Care

Terminally ill persons may need palliative care or hospice care. The person may opt for palliative care and then change to hospice care.

- *Palliative care. Palliate* means *to soothe or relieve.* *Palliative care relieves or reduces the intensity of uncomfortable symptoms without producing a cure.* The focus is on comfort. The intent is to improve quality of life and provide family support. Palliative care can be given along with disease treatment.
- *Hospice care.* The focus is on the physical, emotional, social, and spiritual needs of dying persons and their families (Chapter 1). Often the person has less than 6 months to live. Cure or life-saving measures are not concerns. Pain relief and comfort are stressed. The goal is to improve quality of life. Follow-up care and support groups for survivors are hospice services. Hospice also supports the health team in dealing with a person's death.

ATTITUDES ABOUT DEATH

Experiences, culture, religion, and age influence attitudes about death. Many people fear death. Others do not believe they will die. Some look forward to and accept death. Attitudes about death often change as a person grows older and with changing needs.

Many adults and children have not been present when someone dies. Some have not attended a visitation (wake) or funeral. They have not seen the process of dying and death. Therefore it may be frightening, morbid, and a mystery.

Cultural and Spiritual Needs

Practices and attitudes about death differ among cultures. See *Caring About Culture: Death Rites.* In some cultures, dying people are cared for at home by the family. Some families prepare the body for burial.

Spiritual needs relate to the human spirit and to religion and religious beliefs. They involve finding meaning in one's life. Some people resolve issues with family and friends. Many people strengthen religious beliefs when dying. Religion can comfort the dying person and the family.

Attitudes about death are often closely related to religion. Some believe life after death is free of suffering and hardship. They also believe in reunion with loved ones. Many believe sins and misdeeds are punished in the afterlife. Others do not believe in the afterlife. To them, death is the end of life.

There are also religious beliefs about the body's form after death. Some believe the body keeps its physical form. Others believe that only the spirit or soul is present in the afterlife. *Reincarnation is the belief that the spirit or soul is reborn in another human body or in another form of life.*

Many religions have rites and rituals during the dying process and at the time of death and after. Prayers, blessings, scripture readings, and religious music are common sources of comfort. So are visits from a cleric.

See *Focus on Communication: Cultural and Spiritual Needs.*

🌸 CARING ABOUT CULTURE

Death Rites

In *Vietnam,* dying persons may be helped to recall past good deeds and to achieve a fitting mental state. Death at home may be preferred. In some areas, a coin or jewels (a wealthy family) or rice (a poor family) is put in the dead person's mouth. The belief is that they will help the soul go through encounters with gods and devils and the soul will be born rich in the next life.

White is the color for mourning in *China.* Funeral rights depend on age and status.

In *India,* Hindu persons are often accepting of God's will. The person's desire to be clear-headed as death nears must be assessed in planning treatment. The family and person need a time and place for prayer. The Hindu priest reads from Holy Sanskrit books. Some priests tie strings (meaning a blessing) around the waist. Cremation is usually preferred.

(NOTE: Each person is unique. A person may not follow all of the beliefs and practices of his or her culture. Follow the care plan.)

Modified from D'Avanzo CE: Pocket guide to cultural health assessment, ed 4, St Louis, 2008, Mosby.

FOCUS ON COMMUNICATION

Cultural and Spiritual Needs

Your cultural or religious practices and beliefs may differ from those of patients and residents. Do not judge the person by your standards. Do not make negative comments or insult the person's beliefs. Respect the person as a whole. This includes his or her beliefs and customs.

Age

Adults may fear pain and suffering, dying alone, and the invasion of privacy. They also may fear loneliness and separation from loved ones. Worries about the care and support of those left behind are common. Adults often resent death because it affects plans, hopes, dreams, and ambitions.

See *Focus on Children and Older Persons: Age.*

Age

Children

Infants and toddlers do not understand death. They know or sense that something has changed. They sense a caregiver's absence or a different caregiver. They also sense changes in when and how their needs are met. They may feel a sense of loss.

Between about 3 and 6 years old, children think death is temporary. It can be reversed. The dead person continues to live and function and can come back to life. Such ideas come from fairy tales, cartoons, movies, video games, and TV. Children this age often blame themselves when someone or something dies. To them, death is punishment for being bad. They know when family members or pets die. They notice dead birds or bugs. Answers to questions about death often cause fear and confusion. Children who are told "He is sleeping" may be afraid to go to sleep.

School-age children learn that death is final. They do not think they will die. Death happens to others, especially adults. It can be avoided. Children relate death to punishment and body mutilation. It also involves witches, ghosts, goblins, and monsters. Understanding increases as children grow older and have more experiences with death.

Older Persons

Older persons know death will occur. Many have lost family and friends. Some welcome death as freedom from pain, suffering, and disability. Depending on religious beliefs, death means reunion with those who have died. Like younger adults, many fear dying alone.

THE STAGES OF DYING

Dr. Elisabeth Kübler-Ross described 5 stages of dying. They also are called the "stages of grief." *Grief* is the person's response to loss.

- *Stage 1: Denial.* The person refuses to believe that he or she is dying. "No, not me" is a common response. The person believes a mistake was made. Information about the illness or injury is not heard. The person cannot deal with any problem or decision about the matter. This stage can last for a few hours, days, or much longer. Some people remain in denial.
- *Stage 2: Anger.* The person thinks "Why me?" There is anger and rage. Dying persons envy and resent those with life and health. Family, friends, and the health team are often targets of anger. The person blames others and finds fault with those who are loved and needed the most. It can be hard to deal with the person during this stage. Anger is normal and healthy. Do not take anger personally. Control any urge to attack back or avoid the person.
- *Stage 3: Bargaining.* Anger has passed. The person now says: "Yes, me but…" The person may bargain with God or a higher power for more time. Promises are made in exchange for more time. The person may want to see a child marry, see a grandchild, have another Christmas, or live for a special event. Usually more promises are made as the person makes "just one more" request. Bargaining is usually private and spiritual.
- *Stage 4: Depression.* The person thinks "Yes, me" and is very sad. The person mourns lost things and the future loss of life. The person may cry or say little. Sometimes the person talks about people and things that will be left behind.
- *Stage 5: Acceptance.* The person is calm, at peace, and accepts death. The person has said what needs to be said. Unfinished business is complete. This stage may last for many months or years. Reaching the acceptance stage does not mean death is near.

Dying persons do not always pass through each stage. A person may stay in one stage. Some move back and forth between stages. For example, a person moves from acceptance back to bargaining and then moves forward to acceptance.

COMFORT NEEDS

End-of-life care involves physical, mental and emotional, and spiritual comfort. See "Cultural and Spiritual Needs." Comfort goals are to:

- Prevent or relieve suffering to the extent possible.
- Respect and follow end-of-life wishes.

Dying persons may want family and friends present. They may want to talk about fears, worries, and anxieties. Some want to be alone. Often they need to talk during the night. Things are quiet, distractions are few, and there is more time to think. You need to listen and use touch.

- *Listening.* The person may need to talk and share worries and concerns. Let the person express feelings and emotions. Do not worry about saying the wrong thing or finding comforting words. You do not need to say anything. Being there is what counts.
- *Touch.* Touch shows care and concern when words cannot. Sometimes the person does not want to talk but needs you nearby. Do not feel that you must talk. Silence, along with touch, is a powerful and meaningful way to communicate.

Some people want to see a spiritual leader. Or they want to take part in religious practices. Provide privacy during prayer and spiritual times. Be courteous to the spiritual leader. The person has the right to have religious items nearby—medals, pictures, statues, writings, and so on. Handle them with care and respect.

See *Focus on Communication: Comfort Needs.*

See *Focus on Children and Older Persons: Comfort Needs*, p. 868.

Comfort Needs

Knowing what to say to the dying person is hard for many health team members. Unless you have been near death yourself, do not say: "I understand what you are going through." The statement is a communication barrier. Instead, you can say:

- "Would you like to talk? I have time to listen."
- "You seem sad. Can I help?"
- "Can I quietly sit with you for a while?"

FOCUS ON CHILDREN AND OLDER PERSONS

Comfort Needs

Older Persons

Persons with Alzheimer's disease (AD) become more and more disabled. Those with advanced AD cannot share their concerns, discomforts, or problems. It is hard to provide emotional and spiritual comfort.

Focus on the person's senses—hearing, touch, sight—to promote comfort. Comforting touch or massage can be soothing. So can soft music or sounds from nature—birds chirping, gentle breezes, ocean waves, and so on.

Physical Needs

Dying may take a few minutes, hours, days, or weeks. Body processes slow. The person is weak. Levels of consciousness change. The person is independent to the extent possible. As the person weakens, basic needs are met by others. Every effort is made to promote physical and psychological comfort. The person is allowed to die in peace and with dignity.

Pain. Pain can range from none to severe. Report signs and symptoms of pain at once (Chapter 35). Some persons cannot tell you about pain. Watch for signs of pain or discomfort. Report:

- Restlessness, agitation
- Frowning, grimacing
- Sighing
- Moaning
- Whimpering, crying
- Tense muscles
- Rapid pulse

Skin care, personal and oral hygiene, back massages, and good alignment promote comfort. So do frequent position changes and supportive devices. Turn the person slowly and gently. Follow the care plan to prevent and control pain. The nurse can give pain-relief drugs.

Breathing Problems. Shortness of breath and difficulty breathing *(dyspnea)* are common end-of-life problems. Semi-Fowler's position and oxygen (Chapter 43) are helpful. An open window for fresh air may be helpful. So might a fan circulating air.

Noisy breathing—the *death rattle*—is common as death nears. This is from mucus collecting in the airway. These measures may help.

- The side-lying position
- Suctioning by the nurse
- Drugs to reduce the amount of mucus

Vision, Hearing, and Speech. Vision blurs and gradually fails. The person turns toward light. A darkened room may frighten the person. The eyes may be half-open. Secretions may collect in the eye corners.

Because of failing vision, explain who you are and what you are doing to the person or in the room. The room should be lit to meet the person's needs. Avoid bright lights and glares.

Good eye care is needed (Chapter 24). If the eyes stay open, a nurse may apply a protective ointment. Then the eyes are covered with moist pads to prevent injury.

Hearing is one of the last functions lost. Many people hear until the moment of death. Even unconscious persons may hear. Always assume that the person can hear. Speak in a normal voice. Give reassurance and explain care. Offer words of comfort. Avoid upsetting topics. Do not talk about the person.

Speech becomes harder. It may be hard to understand the person. Sometimes the person cannot speak. Anticipate needs. Do not ask questions with long answers. Ask a few "yes" or "no" questions. Despite speech problems, you must talk to the person.

Mouth, Nose, and Skin. Oral hygiene promotes comfort. Give routine mouth care if the person can eat and drink. Give frequent oral hygiene as death nears and when taking oral fluids is difficult. Oral hygiene is needed if mucus collects in the mouth and the person cannot swallow. A lip balm may be used for dry lips.

Crusting and irritation of the nostrils can occur. Nasal secretions, an oxygen cannula, and a naso-gastric tube are common causes. Carefully clean the nose. Apply lubricant as directed by the nurse and the care plan.

Circulation fails. Body temperature changes as death nears. The skin is cool, pale, and mottled (blotchy). Sweating increases. Skin care, bathing, and preventing pressure injuries are necessary. Linens and gowns are changed as needed. Although the skin feels cool, only light bed coverings are needed. Blankets may cause warmth and restlessness. However, observe for signs of cold—shivering, hunching shoulders, and pulling covers. Prevent drafts and provide more blankets.

Nutrition. Nausea, vomiting, and loss of appetite are common at the end of life. Drugs for nausea and vomiting are ordered.

You may need to feed the person. Favorite foods may help loss of appetite. So may small, frequent meals.

As death nears, loss of appetite is common. The person may choose not to eat or drink. Do not force the person to eat or drink. Tell the nurse.

Elimination. Urinary and fecal incontinence may occur. Use incontinence products or waterproof underpads as directed. Give perineal care as needed. Constipation and urinary retention are common. A catheter may be needed. Follow the care plan for catheter care and bowel elimination.

The Person's Room. Provide a comfortable and pleasant room. It should be well ventilated. Remove unnecessary equipment. Some equipment is upsetting to see (suction machines, drainage containers). If possible, keep such items out of the person's sight.

Mementos, pictures, cards, flowers, and religious items provide comfort. The person and family arrange the room as they wish. This helps meet love, belonging, and esteem needs. The room should reflect the person's choices.

Mental and Emotional Needs

Mental and emotional needs are very personal. Some persons are calm and at peace. Others are anxious or depressed or have specific fears and concerns. Examples include:

* Severe pain
* When and how death will occur
* What will happen to loved ones
* Dying alone

Simple measures may be soothing—touch, holding hands, back massage, soft lighting, music at a low volume.

THE FAMILY

The family usually gathers at the bedside to comfort the person and each other. This is a hard time for the family. It may be hard to find comforting words. To show you care, use touch and be available, courteous, and considerate.

Sometimes the family keeps a *vigil*. That is, someone is always with the person even at night. They watch over or pray for the person. Provide for the family's comfort.

Respect the right to privacy. The person and family need time together. However, do not neglect care because the family is present. Most agencies let family members help give care. Or you can suggest that they take a beverage or meal break.

The family may be very tired, sad, and tearful. Watching a loved one die is very painful. So is dealing with the eventual loss of that person. The family goes through stages like the dying person. They need support, understanding, courtesy, and respect. A spiritual leader may provide comfort. Communicate this request to the nurse at once.

LEGAL ISSUES

Much attention is given to the right to die. Many people do not want machines or other measures keeping them alive. Consent is needed for any treatment. When able, the person makes care decisions. Some people make end-of-life wishes known.

Advance Directives

The *Patient Self-Determination Act* and the *Omnibus Budget Reconciliation Act of 1987 (OBRA)* give persons the right to accept or refuse treatment. They also give the right to make advance directives. An *advance directive is a document stating a person's wishes about health care when that person cannot make his or her own decisions.* Advance directives usually forbid certain care if there is no hope of recovery. Quality of care cannot be less because of the person's advance directives.

Agencies must inform all persons of the right to advance directives on admission. The medical record documents whether or not the person has made them.

Living wills and durable power of attorney for health care are common advance directives.

See *Focus on Surveys: Advance Directives.*

FOCUS ON SURVEYS

Advance Directives

Federal and state laws require that agencies educate staff about policies and procedures for advance directives. A surveyor may ask you about advance directives. For example:

* Did you receive information from the agency about advance directives?
* When did you receive such information?
* What do advance directives mean to you?
* What care do you give when a person has an advance directive?

Living Wills. A living will is about measures that support or maintain life when death is likely. Tube feedings, ventilators, and resuscitation are examples. A living will may instruct doctors:

* Not to start measures that prolong dying
* To remove measures that prolong dying

Durable Power of Attorney for Health Care. This advance directive gives the power to make health care decisions to another person. That person is often called a *health care proxy*. Usually this is a family member, friend, or lawyer. When a person cannot make health care decisions, the health care proxy can do so. This advance directive does not cover property or financial matters.

"Do Not Resuscitate" Orders. "Do Not Resuscitate" (DNR) or "No Code" orders mean that the person will not be resuscitated (Chapter 58). The person is allowed to die with peace and dignity. The orders are written after consulting with the person and family. The family and doctor make the decision if the person is not mentally able to do so.

You may not agree with care and resuscitation decisions. However, you must follow the person's or family's wishes and the doctor's orders. These may be against your personal, religious, and cultural values. If so, talk to the nurse. You may need an assignment change.

SIGNS OF DEATH

In the weeks or days before death, the dying process may involve:

- Restlessness and agitation
- Shortness of breath; pauses in breathing
- Depression
- Anxiety
- Drowsiness
- Confusion
- Constipation or incontinence
- Nausea and loss of appetite
- Healing problems
- Swelling in the hands, feet, or other body areas

As death nears, the following signs may occur fast or slowly.

- Movement, muscle tone, and sensation are lost. This usually starts in the feet and legs. Mouth muscles relax, the jaw drops. The mouth may stay open. The facial expression is often peaceful.
- Gastro-intestinal functions slow down. Abdominal distention, fecal incontinence, nausea, and vomiting are common.
- Body temperature changes. The person feels cool or cold, looks pale, and perspires heavily.
- Circulation fails. The pulse is fast or slow, weak, and irregular. Blood pressure starts to fall.
- The respiratory system fails. Slow or rapid and shallow respirations are observed. Mucus collects in the airway. Breathing sounds are noisy and gurgling (*death rattle*).
- Pain decreases as the person loses consciousness. However, some people are conscious until the moment of death.

The signs of death include *no pulse*, *no respirations*, and *no blood pressure*. A doctor determines that death has occurred. He or she pronounces the person dead. If a doctor is not present in a nursing center, a nurse calls the doctor to report the signs of death. The time and place are noted for the death certificate.

CARE OF THE BODY AFTER DEATH

Care of the body after (post) *death* (mortem) *is called post-mortem care.* You may be asked to assist the nurse. Post-mortem care begins when the person is pronounced dead.

Post-mortem care is done to maintain a good appearance of the body. Discoloration and skin damage are prevented. Valuables and personal items are gathered for the family.

Within 2 to 4 hours after death, rigor mortis develops. *Rigor mortis is the stiffness or rigidity* (rigor) *of skeletal muscles that occurs after death* (mortis). The body is positioned in normal alignment before rigor mortis sets in. The body should appear in a comfortable and natural position when the family sees the body.

Sometimes an autopsy is done. An *autopsy is the examination of the body after death.* (*Autos* means *self. Opsis* means *view.*) It is done to determine the cause of death. Post-mortem care is not done. Doing so could remove or destroy evidence.

Post-mortem care involves bathing soiled areas and positioning the body in good alignment. When moving the body, air in the lungs, stomach, and intestines can be expelled. When air is expelled, sounds are produced. Do not let those sounds alarm or frighten you. They are normal and expected.

See *Delegation Guidelines: Care of the Body After Death.*

See *Promoting Safety and Comfort: Care of the Body After Death.*

See procedure: *Assisting With Post-Mortem Care.*

DELEGATION GUIDELINES

Care of the Body After Death

In some agencies the funeral director performs post-mortem care. In others it is a nursing responsibility. To assist with post-mortem care, you need this information from the nurse.

- If dentures are inserted or placed in a denture cup
- If tubes and dressings are removed or left in place
- If rings are removed or left in place
- If the family wants to view the body
- Special agency policies and procedures

PROMOTING SAFETY AND COMFORT

Care of the Body After Death

Safety
Standard Precautions and the Bloodborne Pathogen Standard are followed. You may have contact with blood, body fluids, secretions, and excretions.

Assisting With Post-Mortem Care

PRE-PROCEDURE

1 Follow *Delegation Guidelines: Care of the Body After Death.* See *Promoting Safety and Comfort: Care of the Body After Death.*
2 Practice hand hygiene.
3 Collect the following.
   - Post-mortem kit (shroud or body bag, gown, ID [identification] tags, gauze squares, safety pins)
   - Disposable bed protectors
   - Wash basin
   - Bath towel and washcloths

   - Denture cup
   - Items for shaving facial hair (Chapter 25)
   - Tape
   - Dressings
   - Gloves
   - Cotton balls
   - Valuables envelope
4 Provide for privacy.
5 Raise the bed for body mechanics.
6 Make sure the bed is flat.

PROCEDURE

7 Put on the gloves.
8 Position the body supine. Arms and legs are straight. A pillow is under the head and shoulders. Or raise the head of the bed 15 to 20 degrees if this is agency policy.
9 Close the eyes. Gently pull the eyelids over the eyes. Apply moist cotton balls gently over the eyelids if the eyes do not stay closed.
10 Insert dentures or put them in a labeled denture cup. Follow agency policy.
11 Close the mouth. If necessary, place a rolled towel under the chin to keep the mouth closed.
12 Remove all jewelry, except for wedding rings if this is agency policy. List the jewelry that you removed. Place the jewelry and the list in a valuables envelope.
13 Place a cotton ball over the rings. Tape them in place as the nurse directs.
14 Remove drainage containers.
15 Remove tubes and catheters with gauze squares as the nurse directs.
16 Shave facial hair if agency policy or if desired by the family. Some men normally grow facial hair (beard, mustache). If so, do not shave facial hair.
17 Bathe soiled areas with plain water. Dry thoroughly.
18 Place a disposable bed protector under the buttocks.
19 Remove soiled dressings. Replace them with clean ones.
20 Put a clean gown on the body. Position the body as in step 8.

21 Brush and comb the hair if necessary.
22 Cover the body to the shoulders with a sheet if the family will view the body.
23 Gather belongings. Put them in a bag labeled with the person's name. Include eyeglasses, hearing aids, and other valuables.
24 Remove supplies, equipment, and linens. Straighten the room. Provide soft lighting.
25 Remove and discard the gloves. Practice hand hygiene.
26 Let the family view the body. Provide for privacy. Return to the room after they leave.
27 Practice hand hygiene. Put on gloves.
28 Fill out the ID tags. Tie 1 to the ankle or to the right big toe.
29 Place the body in the body bag or cover it with a sheet. Or apply a shroud (Fig. 59-1, p. 872).
   a Position the shroud under the body.
   b Bring the top down over the head.
   c Fold the bottom up over the feet.
   d Fold the sides over the body.
   e Pin or tape the shroud in place.
30 Attach the second ID tag to the shroud, sheet, or body bag.
31 Leave the denture cup with the body.
32 Pull the privacy curtain around the bed. Or close the door.

POST-PROCEDURE

33 Remove and discard the gloves. Practice hand hygiene.
34 Clean the unit after the body has been removed. Wear gloves for this step.
35 Remove and discard the gloves. Practice hand hygiene.

36 Report the following.
   - The time the body was taken by the funeral director
   - What was done with jewelry, other valuables, and personal items
   - What was done with dentures

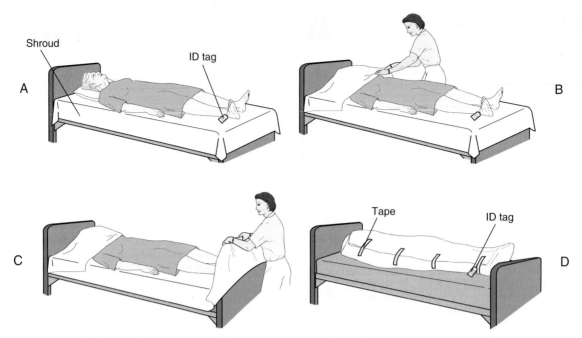

FIGURE 59-1 Applying a shroud. **A,** Position the shroud under the body. **B,** Bring the top down over the head. **C,** Fold the bottom up over the feet. **D,** Fold the sides over the body. Tape or pin the sides together. Attach the ID tag.

FOCUS ON **PRIDE**

The Person, Family, and Yourself

Personal and Professional Responsibility

To give quality care to the dying person:

- Promote comfort. Report complaints or signs of pain at once. Follow the comfort measures in the care plan.
- Protect the person's privacy.
- Provide support to the person and family. Be kind. Show compassion and respect.
- Offer the family time alone with the person.

Take pride in supporting the person and family during a difficult time. The family has many emotions during the dying process and after a loved one's death (Fig. 59-2).

Rights and Respect

Understanding the person's needs and desires allows you to give better care. Respect the person's right to die in peace and with dignity. The right to privacy and the right to be treated with dignity and respect apply after death.

Independence and Social Interaction

The person is encouraged to take part in care to the extent possible. Some days the person can do more than other days. Follow the nurse's directions and the care plan. Do not force the person to do more than he or she can physically or mentally do.

Delegation and Teamwork

Over time, the health team often bonds with the person. This is common in hospice and long-term care. The person's death is difficult for the staff. Sadness and grief may occur.

Tell the nurse if you have trouble coping with a person's death. Support others who need help. A kind word, a hug, or taking time to listen show concern. Take pride in being a part of a caring and supportive team.

Ethics and Laws

The dying person has rights under OBRA.

- *The right to privacy before and after death.* The person has the right not to have his or her body seen by others. Proper draping and screening are important.
- *The right to visit others in private.* If the person is too weak to leave the room, the roommate may have to do so. Moving the dying person to a private room provides privacy. The family can also stay as long as they like.
- *The right to confidentiality before and after death.* The final moments and cause of death are confidential. So are statements, conversations, and family reactions.
- *The right to be free from abuse, mistreatment, and neglect.* The person has the right to kind and respectful care before and after death. Report signs of abuse, mistreatment, or neglect at once.
- *Freedom from restraint.* Restraints are used only if ordered by the doctor. Dying persons are often too weak to be dangerous to themselves or others.
- *The right to personal possessions.* The person may want photos and religious items nearby. Protect the person's property from loss or damage before and after death. The person may have family treasures or mementos.
- *The right to a safe and home-like setting.* Everyone must keep the setting safe and home-like. Try to keep equipment and supplies out of view. The room should be free from unpleasant odors and noises. Do your best to keep the room neat and clean.
- *The right to personal choice.* The dying person may refuse treatment. Advance directives are common. The health team must respect choices to refuse treatment or not prolong life.

FOCUS ON **PRIDE**: *Application*

Genuine concern for the dying person is shown in the care you give. How can you show respect at the end of life and with post-mortem care? How can you show care and concern for the grieving family?

ROGER'S BELL

Mom neared the end of her travail,
she suffered much...so thin, so frail.
I worried a lot: "What if she fell?"
Then I remembered "Roger's bell!"
I put the bell beside her bed.
"Just ring it anytime," I said,
"and I'll be there to help you stand,
or rub your back, or hold your hand."
I'd tell Mom most every night
to ring that bell if things weren't right.
And once or twice she rang the bell,
she did it for me, I could tell.
The final weeks were Carol's hell...
yet she ignored the nightstand bell.

The bell was quiet the day she died,
when friends she barely knew had cried.
I went to the nightstand...said a prayer,
picked up the bell...Do I dare?
"Why have it there beside your bed,
when now I need your help instead?"
She answered, "If you're sad and lonely too,
ring the bell and I'll be there with you!"
– Now Mom doesn't need my steady hand,
– she marches on...leading the band.
Her ordeal is over, her task complete,
and she watches over me, till again we meet.

–Bob Pinkerton

FIGURE 59-2 When he was dying of cancer, Linda Pinkerton Davis gave her husband, Roger, a nightstand bell. Several years later, Linda gave "Roger's bell" to her mom, Carol. Carol's husband wrote the poem after her death. (Printed with permission from Robert Pinkerton, July 2017.)

REVIEW QUESTIONS

Circle the BEST answer.

1 Which is *true?*
   a Death from terminal illness is sudden.
   b Doctors know when death will occur.
   c An illness is terminal when recovery is not likely.
   d All severe injuries end in death.

2 Which statement is *true?*
   a Attitudes about death change as a person ages.
   b Culture does not influence attitudes about death.
   c Young children understand death well.
   d A family member's death does not affect a toddler.

3 Reincarnation is the belief that
   a There is no afterlife
   b The spirit or soul is reborn into another human body or form of life
   c The body keeps its physical form in the afterlife
   d Only the spirit or soul is present in the afterlife

4 A 5-year-old usually views death as
   a Temporary
   b Final
   c Adults do
   d Going to sleep

5 Adults and older persons usually fear
   a Reincarnation
   b The 5 stages of dying
   c Advance directives
   d Dying alone

6 Persons in the stage of denial
   a Are angry
   b Are calm and at peace
   c Refuse to believe they are dying
   d Are sad and quiet

7 A person tries to gain more time during the stage of
   a Anger
   b Bargaining
   c Depression
   d Acceptance

8 When caring for the dying person, you should
   a Use touch and listen
   b Do most of the talking
   c Ask questions with long answers
   d Speak in a loud voice

9 As death nears, the last sense lost is usually
   a Sight
   b Taste
   c Smell
   d Hearing

10 The dying person's care includes the following. Which should you question?
   a Eye care
   b Mouth care
   c Active range-of-motion exercises
   d Position changes

Continued

REVIEW QUESTIONS—cont'd

11 The dying person is positioned in
   a The supine position
   b The Fowler's position
   c Good body alignment
   d The dorsal recumbent position

12 A "DNR" order means that
   a CPR will not be done
   b The person has a living will
   c Life-prolonging measures will be carried out
   d The person is kept alive as long as possible

13 Which signals approaching death?
   a Increased pain
   b Slow and shallow respirations
   c Increased blood pressure
   d Warm and dry skin

14 The signs of death are
   a Convulsions and incontinence
   b No pulse, respirations, or blood pressure
   c Loss of consciousness and convulsions
   d The eyes stay open, no muscle movements, and the body is rigid

15 Post-mortem care is done
   a After rigor mortis sets in
   b When the funeral director arrives for the body
   c After the family has viewed the body
   d After the doctor pronounces the person dead

Answers to Chapter 59 questions are on p. 888.

FOCUS ON PRACTICE

Problem Solving

A person is nearing the end of life. You want to provide mouth care. The family arrives. Is this a good time to give care? What will you say to the family?

Getting a Job

- Define the key terms and key abbreviations in this chapter.
- Identify the sources for jobs and places to work.
- Describe what employers look for when hiring staff.
- Describe the qualities and traits needed to work in home care settings.
- Describe how to prove completion of a nursing assistant training and competency evaluation program (NATCEP).
- Explain how to complete a job application.
- Describe in-person, phone, and video interviews.

- Explain how to prepare and dress for an interview.
- Identify common interview questions.
- Explain how to conduct yourself during an interview.
- Describe the questions you cannot be asked during an interview or on a job application.
- Explain what to do after an interview.
- Explain how to accept or decline a job offer.
- Explain how to promote PRIDE in the person, the family, and yourself.

KEY TERMS

discrimination Unjust treatment based on age, race, gender, and other personal qualities
job application An agency's official form listing questions that require factual answers from the person seeking employment; employment form

job interview When an employer asks a job applicant questions about his or her education and career
reasonable accommodation To assist or change a position or workplace to allow an employee to do his or her job despite having a disability

KEY ABBREVIATIONS

EEOC	Equal Employment Opportunity Commission
NATCEP	Nursing assistant training and competency evaluation program

OBRA	Omnibus Budget Reconciliation Act of 1987

Successfully completing a nursing assistant training and competency evaluation program (NATCEP) is a step toward employment. This chapter will help you find a job in a professional and efficient manner.

SOURCES OF JOBS

There are easy ways to learn about jobs and places to work.
- The Internet—job sites and social media sites
- Newspaper ads
- Local and state employment services
- Agencies you would like to work at
- Phone book yellow pages
- People you know—instructor, family, and friends
- Your school's or college's job placement counselors
- Job fairs
- Your clinical experience site

Your clinical experience site is an important source. The staff observe students as future employees. They look for good work ethics. They watch how students treat patients, residents, and co-workers. They look for the qualities and traits of a nursing assistant described in Chapter 6. If your clinical agency is not hiring, the staff may suggest other places to apply.

WHAT EMPLOYERS LOOK FOR

If you owned a business, who would you hire? Your answer helps you better understand the agency's point of view. Agencies want staff who:
- Are dependable
- Are well-groomed
- Have needed job skills and training
- Have values and attitudes that fit with the agency

To function well, you need good work ethics. Review Chapter 6 and the "Ethics and Laws" sections in the *Focus on PRIDE* boxes at the end of each chapter. They will help you develop positive attitudes and work practices.

You must be at work on time and when scheduled. Undependable people cause everyone problems. Other staff have extra work. Fewer staff give care. Quality of care suffers. You want co-workers to work when scheduled. Otherwise, you have extra work. You have less time to spend with patients and residents. Likewise, co-workers expect you to work when scheduled.

You have 1 chance to make a good first impression. A well-groomed applicant communicates many things to the employer. So does a sloppy person with wrinkled or dirty clothes. See p. 880 for how to dress for an interview.

See *Focus on Long-Term Care and Home Care: What Employers Look For.*

FOCUS ON LONG-TERM CARE AND HOME CARE

What Employers Look For

Home Care

Besides the qualities and traits already described and those in Chapter 6, home care requires:

- *The ability to work alone.* Usually a nurse is not with you. If problems occur, you can reach the nurse by phone. You must provide skillful and safe care.
- *Self-discipline.* You must arrive at homes on time. Plan how to complete personal care and housekeeping tasks. Avoid temptations. This includes watching TV, talking on the phone, visiting, and having a cup of coffee.
- *Honesty.* You might need to shop for the person. Be honest and thrifty with the person's money. Accurately report what you bought, the cost with receipts, amount spent, and amount returned.
- *Respect for the person's property.* You will handle valuables and personal property in home care settings. You will use furnishings, appliances, linens, and household items for care and housekeeping. Treat personal and family property with respect. Prevent damage. Read the manufacturer's instructions before using any appliance. Clean the appliance after use.

Job Skills and Training

The agency checks the nursing assistant registry for your NATCEP test results and requests proof of successful completion of a nursing assistant training program. To prove training program completion, an agency will accept 1 or more of the following.

- A certificate of program completion
- A high school, college, or technical school transcript
- An official grade report (report card)

Give the agency a *copy* of your certificate, transcript, or grade report. Never give the original to anyone. Keep originals in a safe place for future use. Some agencies want a transcript sent directly from the school or college.

JOB APPLICATIONS

A *job application (employment form) is an agency's official form listing questions that require factual answers from the person seeking employment* (Fig. 60-1). Personal information (legal name, address, phone number), work history, education, qualifications, and references are examples. The same information is required of all applicants.

You get a job application from the *personnel office (human resources office)* or on-line through an agency's website. For a paper application, use a pen with black ink to complete the form. You can complete the application at the agency or take it home to return by mail or in person. You must be well-groomed and behave pleasantly when seeking or returning a job application. It may be your first chance to make a good impression.

On-line job applications require an electronic device—computer, tablet, phone. Follow the agency's website instructions for completing an on-line application.

Completing a Job Application

To complete a job application, see Box 60-1, p. 879. The application may be your first chance to impress the agency. A neat, readable, and complete application gives a good image. A sloppy or incomplete one does not. A job application is easier to complete with a file of your education and work history. The file should contain:

- A copy of your high school diploma or general equivalency diploma (GED).
- A copy of any grade reports, college degrees, certificates, or military training.
- A copy of your nursing assistant training program certificate of completion.
- NATCEP test results.
- Nursing assistant registry information for each state in which you are certified (licensed, registered).
- Copies of communications with your state's nursing assistant registry agency.
- Copies of court records for criminal convictions.
- A copy of your Social Security card.
- Names, addresses, and phone numbers of references.
- Names, addresses, and phone numbers of current and past employers. Include:
  - Your job title
  - Dates employment started and ended
  - Your supervisor's name
  - Hourly salary
- Proof of in-services attended and continuing education units (CEUs).

When requesting a job application, also ask for the agency's nursing assistant job description (Chapter 3).

EMPLOYMENT APPLICATION

All information listed on this application will be considered and handled as personal and confidential. Please print or write legibly.

AN EQUAL OPPORTUNITY EMPLOYER

This employer provides equal opportunity to all persons without regard to disability, race, color, religion, gender, age, or national origin.

Name

Date of Application

Address

City

State

Zip

Home Phone

Cell Phone

Social Security Number

GENERAL INFORMATION

Position applied for:

Available to work: ☐ Full-time ☐ Part-time ☐ Temporary   Date available to start work:

Will transportation be a problem for you? _____ ☐ No ☐ Yes

Do you have the legal right to work in the United States? _____ ☐ No ☐ Yes

Were you given a job description? _____ ☐ No ☐ Yes

Do you understand the functions of the job? _____ ☐ No ☐ Yes

Can you perform the functions of the job with or without reasonable accommodation? _____ ☐ No ☐ Yes

Have you ever been convicted of a felony? _____ ☐ No ☐ Yes

If yes, explain:

EDUCATION

	Name and Address of School	Major/Degree(s)	Number of Years Completed	Did you Graduate?
High School				
Community College				
4 Year Institution				
Vocational				
Other (specify)				

Describe specialized training, skills, seminars, courses, in-services, continuing education, or extra-curricular actvities:

FIGURE 60-1 A sample job application.

EMPLOYMENT RECORD

Beginning with your current employer, please list your work experience over the last ten years. You may include pertinent volunteer activities.

Name and Address of Employer

Start Date _____ End Date _____

Phone _____

Job Title _____ Supervisor _____ Phone _____

Start Salary _____ End Salary _____

Duties

Reason for Leaving

Name and Address of Employer

Start Date _____ End Date _____

Phone _____

Job Title _____ Supervisor _____ Phone _____

Start Salary _____ End Salary _____

Duties

Reason for Leaving

Name and Address of Employer

Start Date _____ End Date _____

Phone _____

Job Title _____ Supervisor _____ Phone _____

Start Salary _____ End Salary _____

Duties

Reason for Leaving

REFERENCES

Only include persons familiar with your work ability. Do not include family.

Name and Title _____ Address _____ Phone _____

Name and Title _____ Address _____ Phone _____

Name and Title _____ Address _____ Phone _____

Name and Title _____ Address _____ Phone _____

SIGNATURE

I certify that the information provided on this application is true and complete. I understand that any false information or omissions may result in rejection of my application or job loss at any time during employment. I authorize verification of my education and past employment. I release all persons, schools, and past employers from liability for supplying such information.

I understand that the employer will conduct a criminal background check.

I understand that the use of illegal drugs is prohibited during employment. I am willing to submit to drug testing before and during employment.

_____ _____

Signature   Date

FIGURE 60-1, cont'd

| BOX 60-1 | Guidelines for Completing a Job Application |

- Read and follow the directions. They may ask you to print using black ink. Following directions on the job application gives insight about your ability to follow directions on the job.
- Write neatly. Writing must be readable. A messy application gives a bad image. Readable writing gives the correct information. The agency cannot contact you if unable to read your phone number. You may miss getting the job.
- Complete the entire form. If an item does not apply to you, write "N/A" for non-applicable. Or draw a line through the space. This shows that you read the section. It also shows that you did not skip the item on purpose.
- Report any felony convictions as directed. Write "no" or "none" as appropriate. Criminal background and fingerprint checks are common requirements (Chapter 3).
- Give information about employment gaps. If you did not work for a time, the agency wonders why. Providing this information shows you are honest. Some reasons are an illness, school, raising children, or caring for a family member.
- Tell why you left a job, if asked. Be brief but honest. People leave jobs for one that pays better. Some leave for career advancement. Others leave for reasons given for employment gaps. If fired from a job, give an honest but positive answer. Do not talk badly about the former agency.

- Give references. List the names, titles, addresses, and phone numbers of at least 4 non-family references. Have this information with you before completing an application. (Always ask references if an agency can contact them.) You may get the job faster if the agency can check references quickly. The agency should not have to wait for missing or incomplete information. This wastes your time and the agency's time. Also, the agency wonders if you are hiding something with incomplete reference information.
- Be prepared to provide the following.
  - Social Security number
  - Proof of the legal right to work in the United States
  - Proof of successful NATCEP completion; training program completion and test results
  - Identification—driver's license or government-issued ID card
- Give honest answers. Lying on an application is fraud. It is grounds for being fired.
- Complete a final review of your application. Make sure you have provided all required information.

THE JOB INTERVIEW

A *job interview is when an employer asks a job applicant questions about his or her education and career.* The agency gets to know and evaluate you. You learn about the agency.

The interview may be when you complete the job application. Some agencies review applications before scheduling interviews. An interview may be conducted by 1 person or 2 or more people.

When an interview is scheduled, write down the interviewer's name and the interview date and time. If you need directions to the agency, ask for them when the interview is scheduled.

When expecting a call from the agency, answer your phone. Do not let your phone go to voice mail. If the caller has to leave a message, you need an appropriate and professional greeting. Besides a voice message, the agency may contact you through a text, e-mail, or other message. Return messages within 24 hours.

Types of Interviews

Interviews may be in-person, by phone, or by video. You need good communication skills. (See Chapters 7 and 8.)
- *In-person interview.* You and the interviewer meet in the same room face-to-face. Appropriate dress and body language are needed.
- *Phone interview.* A phone interview may be used to decide if an in-person interview will follow. If distance is a factor, a phone interview may work for the agency and you.
- *Video interview.* You use a computer or other electronic device at home or another site. Appropriate dress and body language are needed.

For phone and video interviews:
- Use a quiet room. Turn off phones, music, TV, and other devices. Do not use a room where phones ring, people are talking, or pets are present.
- Be ready to answer the phone or turn on the electronic device at the scheduled time.
- Have your electronic device charged. Consider plugging into a power source to prevent the device from turning off.
- Speak clearly and slowly. Do not shout.
- Listen carefully. Let the interviewer finish speaking before you answer.
- Smile. Smile even for a phone interview. Attitude and facial expression affect your voice tone.

Preparing for the Interview

Box 60-2 (p. 880) lists common interview questions. Prepare your answers ahead of time. Also prepare a list of your skills for the interviewer.

You must present a good image. You need to be neat, clean, and well-groomed. How you dress is important. Follow the guidelines in Box 60-3, p. 880.

Show that you are dependable. No matter the type of interview, be on time. For an in-person interview, do a practice run (dry run). Go to the agency some day before the interview. Note how long it takes to get there and where to park. Also find the personnel office. A practice run gives an idea of the time needed from your home to the personnel office.

BOX 60-2   Common Interview Questions

What the Interviewer May Ask

- Tell me about yourself.
- Tell me about your career goals.
- What are you doing to reach these goals?
- Describe what *professional* behavior means to you.
- Tell me about your last job. Why did you leave?
- What did you like the most about your last job? The least?
- What would your supervisor and co-workers tell me about you? Your dependability? Your skills? Your flexibility?
- Which functions are hard for you? How do you handle this difficulty?
- How do you set priorities?
- How have your experiences prepared you for this job?
- What would you like to change about your last job?
- How do you handle problems with patients, residents, families, and co-workers?
- Why do you want to work here?
- Why should this agency hire you?

What to Ask the Interviewer

- Which job functions are the most important?
- What employee qualities and traits are important to you?
- What nursing care pattern is used here (Chapter 1)?
- Who will I work with?
- When are performance evaluations done? Who does them? How are they done?

What to Ask the Interviewer—cont'd

- What performance factors are evaluated?
- How does the supervisor handle problems?
- What are the most common reasons that nursing assistants lose their jobs here? What are common reasons for resigning? (To *resign* means *to leave a job*.)
- How do you see this job in the next year? In the next 5 years?
- What is the greatest reward from this job? The greatest challenge?
- What do you like the most about nursing assistants who work here? The least?
- Why should I work here rather than in another agency?
- How much will I make an hour?
- What hours will I work?
- What uniforms are required?
- What benefits do you offer?
  - Health and dental insurance?
  - Continuing education?
  - Vacation time?
- Do you have a new employee orientation program? How long is it?
- May I have a tour of the agency and the unit I will work on? Can I meet the nurse manager and unit staff?
- Can I have a few minutes to talk to the nurse manager?

BOX 60-3   Grooming and Dressing for an Interview

- Bathe and brush your teeth. Wash your hair. Men should shave facial hair or groom beards and mustaches.
- Use deodorant or antiperspirant.
- Make sure your hands and fingernails are clean.
- Apply make-up in a simple, attractive manner.
- Style your hair in a neat and attractive way.
- Do not wear jeans, shorts, leggings, yoga pants, tank tops, halter tops, or other casual clothing. Also do not wear bright colors; animal or other distracting prints; or lacy, sheer, tight, or low-cut garments.
- Iron clothing. Sew on loose buttons and mend garments.
- Wear clothing that covers tattoos (body art).
- Wear a simple dress or a skirt or slacks and blouse (women). Wear slacks and a shirt (men). A jacket or tie is optional. A long-sleeved white or light blue shirt is best. See Figure 60-2.
- Wear socks (men and women) or hose or tights (women). Hose should be free of runs and snags.
- Make sure shoes are clean and in good repair.
- Avoid heavy perfumes, colognes, and after-shave lotions. A light fragrance is okay.
- Wear only simple jewelry that complements your clothes. Avoid adornments in body piercings. For multiple ear piercings, wear only 1 set of earrings.
- Brush your teeth again before leaving for the interview. Do not smoke or chew gum before the interview. You must have fresh breath.
- Stop in the restroom when you arrive at the agency. Check your hair, make-up, clothes, and hands.

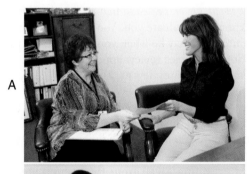

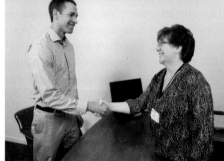

FIGURE 60-2 Dress for an interview. **A,** This woman wears a simple blouse and slacks. **B,** This young man wears a simple shirt and slacks.

Arriving at the Agency. When you arrive at the agency, turn off your phone and other devices. Tell the receptionist your name, why you are there, and the interviewer's name. Then sit quietly in the waiting area. Do not smoke, chew gum, or use your phone or other devices for calls, e-mails, text messages, or other reasons. While waiting, review your answers to the common interview questions. Waiting may be part of the interview. The interviewer may ask staff about how you acted while waiting. Smile and be polite and friendly.

During the Interview

Politely greet and address the interviewer as Miss, Mrs., Ms., Mr., or Doctor. For an in-person interview, a firm hand-shake is correct for men and women. Stand until asked to sit. Sit with good posture and in a professional way. If offered a beverage, you may accept. Be sure to thank the person.

Good eye contact is needed for in-person and video interviews. Look directly at the interviewer to answer or ask questions. Poor eye contact sends negative information—shy, insecure, dishonest, or lacking interest.

Watch your body language (Chapter 7)—facial expressions, gestures, posture, and body movements. What you say is important. However, your body tells a great deal. Avoid distracting habits—slumping; biting nails; playing with jewelry, clothing, or your hair; crossing your arms; and crossing and swinging legs back and forth. Focus on the interview. Do not touch or read things on the person's desk.

Give complete and honest answers. Speak clearly and with confidence. Avoid short and long answers. "Yes" and "no" answers give little information. Briefly explain "yes" and "no" responses.

The interviewer will ask about your skills. Share your skills list. An agency-required skill may not be on your list. Explain that you are willing to learn if your state allows nursing assistants to perform the skill.

Review the job description with the interviewer. Ask questions. Advise the interviewer of functions you cannot perform because of training, legal, ethical, or religious reasons. Honesty now prevents problems later.

Find the right job for you. An employer wants to hire staff who will be happy in the job and the agency. Box 60-2 lists some questions for you to ask at the end of the interview. The interviewer's answers will help you decide if the job is right for you.

The interview usually lasts 15 to 20 minutes. You may be offered a job at this time. Or you are told when to expect a call or letter. Follow-up is acceptable. Ask when you can check on your application. Always thank the interviewer. Say that you look forward to hearing from him or her. Shake the person's hand after an in-person interview.

See *Focus on Long-Term Care and Home Care: During the Interview.*

FOCUS ON LONG-TERM CARE AND HOME CARE

During the Interview

Home Care
You need to ask more questions when interviewing with a home care agency.
- What part of the community does the agency serve?
- What neighborhoods will you go to?
- How far will you have to travel between homes?
- Do you use your own car or an agency car?
- How are you paid for mileage and tolls?
- Will you use public transportation? If yes, who pays for bus or train fares? If the agency pays, are you given fare money beforehand or repaid later?

Questions You Cannot Be Asked. The U.S. Equal Employment Opportunity Commission (EEOC) is a government agency. To guard against discrimination in hiring, the EEOC has guidelines for questions that cannot be asked during an interview or on a job application. *Discrimination involves unjust treatment based on age, race, gender, and other personal qualities.* See Box 60-4, p. 882.

See *Focus on Communication: Questions You Cannot Be Asked.*

FOCUS ON COMMUNICATION

Questions You Cannot Be Asked

If asked a question listed in Box 60-4, you have the right to decline to answer. Decline politely. You can say: "I'm sorry, but the EEOC does not allow you to ask that question. What else can I answer for you?"

BOX 60-4	Interview Questions Not Allowed by the EEOC

- *Age.* Generally, you cannot be asked your age, your birth date, or any question that refers to your age. However, under OBRA, you must be at least 16 years old. Some states have limits on the tasks allowed for persons under 18 years of age.
- *Color, race, or national origin.* This includes questions related to your place of birth or that of your parents; language spoken; or how you learned to read, write, or speak a language.
- *Religion or spiritual beliefs.* You cannot be asked about your religion, religious practices, church, priest or pastor, or religious holidays observed.
- *Gender.* No questions are allowed about gender or your sexuality.
- *Disabilities.* You cannot be asked if you have disabilities or what they are. This includes treatment for alcoholism. However, you can be asked if you can perform the job with reasonable accommodation. *Reasonable accommodation means to assist or change a position or workplace to allow an employee to do his or her job despite having a disability.*

- *Pregnancy or plans for pregnancy.* You cannot be asked if you are pregnant, planning to get pregnant, or about your pregnancy history.
- *Marital status.* You cannot be asked if you are married, single, divorced, separated, engaged, or widowed.
- *Children.* You cannot be asked if you have children, how many children or their ages, or who will care for children while you are at work.
- *Arrest record.* You cannot be asked about arrests. However, you can be asked about criminal convictions.
- *Finances.* You cannot be asked about credit cards or bank accounts or if you own your home or car.
- *Number of sick days used in the last year.* You cannot be asked about your medical history. However, you may have to take a medical exam or have some tests done after a job offer is made.
- *Citizenship.* You cannot be asked if you are a United States citizen. You cannot be asked to provide proof of citizenship. However, if hired, you can be asked to provide proof of the legal right to work in the United States.

December 12

Dear [Interviewer's name],

Thank you for the interview yesterday. I enjoyed meeting you and learning more about the nursing center. I was impressed by the friendliness of the staff and would enjoy working in that environment.

Again, thank you. I look forward to hearing from you soon.

Sincerely,
[Your full name]

FIGURE 60-3 Sample thank-you note written after a job interview.

After the Interview

A thank-you letter or note is advised within 24 hours after the interview (Fig. 60-3). Write neatly and clearly. Use a computer or other electronic device or a typewriter if your writing is hard to read. The thank-you note should include:
- The date
- The interviewer's formal name with Miss, Ms., Mrs., Mr., or Dr.
- A statement thanking the person for the interview
- Comments about the interview, the agency, and your eagerness to hear about the job
- Your signature, using your first and last names

ACCEPTING OR DECLINING A JOB OFFER

You can apply to many places and have many interviews. Think about all offers before accepting one. You might have more questions about an agency. Ask them before accepting a job. To help you decide, discuss the offer with a family member, friend, co-worker, or your instructor.

When you accept a job, agree on a starting date, pay rate, and work hours. Ask where to report on your first day. Ask for all information in writing. That way you and the agency have the same understanding of the job offer. Use the written offer later if questions arise. Also ask for the employee handbook and other agency information. Read everything before you start working.

Accept the best job for you. To decline a job offer, thank the person for offering you a job. If asked why you are refusing, give a positive response. For example: "Thank you for offering me a job. I'm going to accept a job closer to my home."

Sometimes a job is not offered. You may not hear from the agency. Or the agency calls, writes, or e-mails saying that you will not be offered the job. If this happens, thank the person for letting you know. Ask that the agency keep your application active. For example: "Thank you for letting me know. I'm disappointed but please keep me in mind for other openings."

DRUG TESTING

State laws vary about drug testing. Drug testing may be part of the application process. If so, review the job application before signing it. The application usually states 1 of the following (see Fig. 60-1).
- Drug testing is part of the application screening process for new staff.
- A job offer depends on passing a drug test.

FOCUS ON **PRIDE**

The Person, Family, and Yourself

P ersonal and Professional Responsibility

Agencies invest much time and money in new staff. Changing jobs often can reflect poorly on you. Before applying, find out about the agency. This helps you decide if the agency is a good fit for you. Also, your interest in the agency can make a good impression during an interview.

R ights and Respect

You have the right to protection from discrimination. Application and interview questions must relate to your ability to do the job. See Box 60-4 for questions that are not allowed.

Job-related questions are allowed if asked to all applicants, regardless of age or gender. These questions are allowed.

- What languages do you read, write, and speak fluently?
- Can you perform the duties of this job? Do you need any special accommodations to perform the job?
- Have you ever been convicted of a crime?

Know your rights. Plan how to respond if you suspect a question violates your rights.

I ndependence and Social Interaction

Some agencies perform social media background checks. State laws vary about what information can be accessed—public or private. Age, gender, disability, color, race, national origin, or religion must not be considered in hiring decisions. Employers must focus only on information related to the job.

Show good judgment when using social media (Chapter 5). Be professional. Agencies may view postings on social media sites.

D elegation and Teamwork

Non–health care work experiences, education, and training are important. They give employers information about your dependability, teamwork, and work quality. Draw from your experiences. Give examples of your positive work ethics.

E thics and Laws

Agencies watch for safe and ethical conduct. They must act when conduct is unsafe or unethical. Background checks, drug testing, and interview questions help agencies decide if an applicant will meet safety and ethical standards. This is a real example of a nursing assistant who did not meet standards for safe and ethical behavior.

A certified nursing assistant (CNA) began working at an Arizona hospital. While employed, she received Employee Corrective Action reports for:

- *Poor communication with co-workers*
- *Arguing with an RN who gave her instructions*
- *Not being able to work in a team environment*
- *Excess time off the nursing unit for breaks*
- *Not taking the initiative in answering call lights, collecting equipment, or transferring patients' belongings*
- *Excess socializing with staff in other departments*
- *Not meeting standards relating to customer service relations*

E thics and Laws—cont'd

Four years after being terminated from the hospital, she applied for a job at another Arizona hospital. A pre-employment urine drug screen was positive for benzodiazepine. The CNA reported the drug test to the Arizona State Board of Nursing. The CNA reported that she had a headache the night before her interview at the hospital. She admitted taking Valium (benzodiazepine) that was prescribed for her mother. The CNA explained that "she knew this was wrong, that this was a one-time occurrence and that it would not happen again."

The Board requested that the CNA submit to a urine drug screen. It was positive for benzodiazepine. The CNA did not have a prescription for that drug.

The Board revoked the CNA's certificate for unprofessional conduct. The Arizona State Board of Nursing found that the CNA's actions violated these aspects of the state's Nurse Practice Act.

- *Conduct or a practice that is or might be harmful or dangerous to the health of a patient or the public*
- *Committing an act that deceives, defrauds, or harms the public*
- *Obtaining, possessing, using, or selling any narcotic, controlled substance, or illegal drug in violation of any federal or state criminal law, or in violation of the policy of any employer*
- *Using violent or abusive behavior in any work setting*
- *Failing to cooperate with the Board during an investigation*
- *Practicing in any other manner that gives the Board reasonable cause to believe that the health of a patient or the public may be harmed*

(Arizona State Board of Nursing, 2005.)

Poor conduct outside of work can affect your job. Take pride in making good choices inside and outside the workplace.

FOCUS ON **PRIDE**: *Application*

Being prepared for an interview is helpful. You may be nervous about what questions will be asked, how you will answer, and if you will make a good impression. Describe how you will prepare yourself for a job interview. How will you respond to a question not allowed by the EEOC?

REVIEW QUESTIONS

Circle the BEST answer.

1 When should you ask questions about your job description?
   a After completing the job application
   b Before completing the job application
   c When your interview is scheduled
   d During the interview

2 Lying on a job application is
   a Negligence
   b Fraud
   c Libel
   d Defamation

3 When completing a job application
   a Use pencil
   b Leave spaces blank that do not apply to you
   c Give information about employment gaps
   d List family members as references

4 Being dependable means to
   a Work when scheduled
   b Be courteous and polite
   c Have needed job skills
   d Have a good attitude

5 What should you wear to a job interview?
   a A uniform
   b Party clothes
   c Slacks and a shirt or blouse
   d What is most comfortable

6 For a phone interview you should
   a Shout answers so they are heard
   b Take another call during the interview
   c Have the interviewer leave a message
   d Use a quiet room

7 Which is poor behavior during a job interview?
   a Crossing your arms and legs
   b Good eye contact with the interviewer
   c Shaking hands with the interviewer
   d Asking the interviewer questions

8 Which is the *best* response to an interview question?
   a Brief explanations
   b "Yes" or "no"
   c Long answers
   d A written response

9 An interviewer asks the following. Which should you decline to answer?
   a Tell me about yourself.
   b Are you married?
   c Have you ever been convicted of a crime?
   d What are your career goals?

10 After an interview
   a Ask if the agency plans to hire you
   b Ask to be paid for your time at the interview
   c Write a thank-you note
   d Do not apply to any other agencies

11 When accepting a job offer, avoid discussing
   a Starting date
   b Personal finances
   c Pay rate
   d Work hours

12 Drug testing may be required before an agency hires you.
   a True
   b False

Answers to Chapter 60 questions are on p. 888.

FOCUS ON **PRACTICE**

Problem Solving

You are asked the following questions at a job interview. How will you respond to each?
- Why did you decide to become a nursing assistant?
- What are your strengths and weaknesses?
- Describe a problem in your clinical training. How did you resolve it?
- Give an example of when you had to prioritize. How did you decide what to do first, second, and so on?

Review Question Answers

CHAPTER 1:
HEALTH CARE
AGENCIES
1 d
2 b
3 a
4 c
5 b
6 b
7 a
8 d
9 a
10 b
11 a
12 a
13 c
14 c
15 b
16 d

CHAPTER 2:
THE PERSON'S
RIGHTS
1 F
2 T
3 T
4 F
5 T
6 F
7 T
8 F
9 T
10 F
11 F
12 F
13 d
14 b
15 c
16 d
17 b
18 a
19 a
20 d
21 b
22 c
23 d
24 a
25 d
26 c
27 b
28 b

CHAPTER 3:
THE NURSING
ASSISTANT
1 T
2 F
3 T
4 F
5 F
6 F
7 a
8 d

9 c
10 c
11 b
12 a
13 c
14 b
15 d

CHAPTER 4:
DELEGATION
1 F
2 T
3 T
4 T
5 F
6 T
7 c
8 a
9 d
10 b
11 d
12 c
13 d
14 a

CHAPTER 5:
ETHICS AND
LAWS
1 b
2 c
3 d
4 a
5 b
6 a
7 c
8 a
9 d
10 c
11 b
12 a
13 b
14 d
15 d
16 c
17 b
18 a
19 c
20 b
21 c
22 a

CHAPTER 6:
STUDENT AND
WORK ETHICS
1 T
2 T
3 F
4 T
5 T
6 T
7 F
8 T
9 F

10 T
11 F
12 d
13 c
14 a
15 b
16 a
17 d
18 a
19 c
20 a
21 b
22 d
23 a
24 c
25 d
26 b

CHAPTER 7:
COMMUNICATING
WITH THE
PERSON
1 c
2 d
3 b
4 a
5 c
6 c
7 c
8 d
9 d
10 b
11 a
12 b
13 a
14 d
15 c
16 d
17 b
18 a
19 b
20 c
21 a
22 d

CHAPTER 8:
HEALTH TEAM
COMMUNICATIONS
1 F
2 T
3 F
4 T
5 F
6 T
7 F
8 F
9 T
10 F
11 d
12 c
13 c
14 a
15 d

16 a
17 c
18 a
19 b
20 c
21 b
22 d
23 a
24 a
25 c

CHAPTER 9:
MEDICAL
TERMINOLOGY
1 c
2 b
3 c
4 d
5 d
6 b
7 b
8 a
9 a
10 a
11 d
12 b

CHAPTER 10:
BODY
STRUCTURE
AND FUNCTION
1 a
2 b
3 a
4 c
5 c
6 a
7 b
8 c
9 d
10 d
11 c
12 b
13 a
14 b
15 b
16 b
17 c
18 d
19 a
20 d
21 b
22 a

CHAPTER 11:
GROWTH AND
DEVELOPMENT
1 b
2 d
3 b
4 a
5 c
6 b

7 b
8 a
9 c
10 c
11 c
12 b
13 d
14 d
15 a
16 c
17 b
18 d
19 c
20 a

CHAPTER 12: THE
OLDER PERSON
1 a
2 a
3 b
4 c
5 d
6 c
7 a
8 c
9 a
10 d
11 b
12 d
13 b
14 a
15 d
16 b
17 a
18 a
19 c
20 a

CHAPTER 13:
SAFETY
1 a
2 d
3 c
4 a
5 b
6 c
7 d
8 b
9 a
10 c
11 c
12 d
13 b
14 a
15 c
16 b
17 c
18 b
19 a
20 d
21 d
22 b
23 c

24 a
25 c
26 d
27 b
28 d

CHAPTER 14:
PREVENTING
FALLS
1 a
2 c
3 c
4 a
5 b
6 c
7 d
8 b
9 c
10 b
11 a
12 c
13 c
14 b
15 d

CHAPTER 15:
RESTRAINT
ALTERNATIVES
AND RESTRAINTS
1 F
2 T
3 T
4 F
5 F
6 T
7 T
8 T
9 F
10 F
11 T
12 F
13 F
14 T
15 F
16 d
17 c
18 b
19 c
20 a
21 b
22 a
23 c
24 d

CHAPTER 16: PREVENTING INFECTION

1 F
2 T
3 T
4 F
5 F
6 T
7 F
8 F
9 F
10 F
11 T
12 T
13 b
14 b
15 a
16 c
17 a
18 b
19 d
20 c
21 a
22 a
23 c
24 d
25 b

CHAPTER 17: ISOLATION PRECAUTIONS

1 c
2 a
3 a
4 c
5 c
6 c
7 d
8 c
9 b
10 c

CHAPTER 18: BODY MECHANICS

1 a
2 b
3 c
4 a
5 a
6 c
7 b
8 a
9 d
10 c
11 b
12 b
13 c
14 a

CHAPTER 19: MOVING THE PERSON

1 c
2 b
3 a
4 b

5 a
6 a
7 b
8 c
9 d
10 b
11 a
12 d
13 d
14 c

CHAPTER 20: TRANSFERRING THE PERSON

1 b
2 d
3 c
4 b
5 b
6 c
7 a
8 d
9 d
10 b
11 c
12 b
13 c
14 a

CHAPTER 21: THE PERSON'S UNIT

1 T
2 T
3 F
4 T
5 F
6 T
7 T
8 T
9 F
10 T
11 d
12 c
13 b
14 d
15 c
16 a
17 b
18 a
19 b
20 c
21 b
22 c

CHAPTER 22: BEDMAKING

1 F
2 F
3 T
4 F
5 T
6 T
7 F
8 T
9 d
10 b
11 a

12 b
13 d
14 a
15 c

CHAPTER 23: ORAL HYGIENE

1 F
2 T
3 F
4 F
5 F
6 T
7 c
8 d
9 c
10 c

CHAPTER 24: DAILY HYGIENE AND BATHING

1 T
2 F
3 T
4 F
5 T
6 T
7 T
8 F
9 F
10 T
11 T
12 T
13 c
14 a
15 b
16 a
17 d
18 c
19 a
20 d
21 d
22 b
23 b
24 a

CHAPTER 25: GROOMING

1 T
2 T
3 T
4 F
5 F
6 F
7 F
8 T
9 T
10 F
11 d
12 b
13 b
14 c
15 a
16 d
17 d
18 c
19 b

20 d
21 b
22 a

CHAPTER 26: DRESSING AND UNDRESSING

1 d
2 d
3 b
4 a
5 a
6 d
7 a
8 c

CHAPTER 27: URINARY NEEDS

1 c
2 d
3 a
4 a
5 b
6 b
7 d
8 a
9 d
10 c
11 b
12 c
13 d
14 a

CHAPTER 28: URINARY CATHETERS

1 c
2 d
3 a
4 a
5 c
6 b
7 d
8 c
9 a
10 b
11 a
12 d

CHAPTER 29: BOWEL NEEDS

1 b
2 a
3 b
4 c
5 c
6 a
7 c
8 d
9 b
10 b
11 a
12 d
13 c
14 d

CHAPTER 30: NUTRITION NEEDS

1 b
2 b
3 d
4 c
5 d
6 a
7 a
8 c
9 b
10 a
11 d
12 b
13 c
14 c
15 d
16 c
17 a
18 d
19 d
20 d

CHAPTER 31: FLUID NEEDS

1 d
2 b
3 b
4 a
5 d
6 b
7 c
8 d
9 b
10 a

CHAPTER 32: NUTRITIONAL SUPPORT AND IV THERAPY

1 c
2 a
3 a
4 b
5 d
6 a
7 a
8 c
9 c
10 d
11 b
12 b
13 a
14 d
15 b
16 c
17 b
18 a

CHAPTER 33: VITAL SIGNS

1 b
2 a
3 b
4 c
5 a
6 d
7 c

8 b
9 d
10 c
11 c
12 a
13 c
14 d
15 b

CHAPTER 34: EXERCISE AND ACTIVITY

1 T
2 F
3 T
4 F
5 F
6 T
7 T
8 T
9 b
10 b
11 c
12 d
13 c
14 a
15 c
16 a
17 d
18 a
19 b
20 a

CHAPTER 35: COMFORT, REST, AND SLEEP

1 T
2 T
3 F
4 T
5 T
6 T
7 F
8 F
9 T
10 F
11 T
12 F
13 T
14 T
15 b
16 d
17 c
18 d
19 a
20 b
21 d
22 c
23 b
24 a

CHAPTER 36: ADMISSIONS, TRANSFERS, AND DISCHARGES
1 T
2 F
3 T
4 F
5 F
6 T
7 T
8 T
9 F
10 T
11 b
12 a
13 c
14 c
15 a
16 d

CHAPTER 37: ASSISTING WITH THE PHYSICAL EXAMINATION
1 b
2 c
3 c
4 d
5 a

CHAPTER 38: COLLECTING AND TESTING SPECIMENS
1 c
2 d
3 b
4 a
5 a
6 c
7 b
8 a
9 d
10 a
11 b
12 c
13 a
14 d
15 b

CHAPTER 39: THE PERSON HAVING SURGERY
1 F
2 T
3 F
4 F
5 F
6 T
7 T
8 F
9 T
10 T
11 c
12 b
13 b

14 a
15 d
16 c
17 a
18 b
19 c
20 a
21 a
22 d
23 b
24 d
25 a

CHAPTER 40: WOUND CARE
1 a
2 c
3 a
4 c
5 b
6 d
7 a
8 c
9 c
10 b
11 a
12 c
13 b
14 d
15 b
16 c

CHAPTER 41: PRESSURE INJURIES
1 T
2 T
3 T
4 T
5 T
6 F
7 T
8 F
9 F
10 T
11 F
12 F
13 T
14 b
15 d
16 d
17 a
18 a
19 c
20 c
21 b
22 b
23 d
24 a
25 b
26 a
27 d
28 c
29 c
30 d
31 c
32 b

CHAPTER 42: HEAT AND COLD APPLICATIONS
1 d
2 b
3 b
4 a
5 c
6 a
7 b
8 c
9 a
10 b
11 d
12 c
13 a
14 b

CHAPTER 43: OXYGEN NEEDS
1 a
2 c
3 c
4 b
5 b
6 d
7 c
8 d
9 a
10 b
11 a
12 b
13 d
14 c
15 d
16 b
17 a
18 c

CHAPTER 44: RESPIRATORY SUPPORT AND THERAPIES
1 c
2 d
3 d
4 b
5 b
6 a
7 d
8 c
9 a
10 b
11 c
12 b

CHAPTER 45: REHABILITATION NEEDS
1 T
2 F
3 T
4 T
5 F
6 T
7 F
8 T
9 T
10 c
11 b
12 a
13 d
14 c
15 c

CHAPTER 46: HEARING, SPEECH, AND VISION PROBLEMS
1 b
2 c
3 d
4 b
5 a
6 c
7 c
8 d
9 a
10 b
11 a
12 c
13 a
14 b
15 c
16 a
17 d
18 d
19 c
20 b

CHAPTER 47: CANCER, IMMUNE SYSTEM, AND SKIN DISORDERS
1 F
2 T
3 T
4 T
5 T
6 F
7 T
8 T
9 T
10 F
11 b
12 a
13 b
14 a
15 c
16 d
17 a
18 c
19 d
20 b

CHAPTER 48: NERVOUS SYSTEM AND MUSCULO-SKELETAL DISORDERS
1 a
2 b
3 d
4 c
5 d
6 b
7 a
8 a
9 c
10 b
11 a
12 c
13 a
14 d
15 b
16 b
17 d
18 d
19 a
20 a
21 c

CHAPTER 49: CARDIOVASCULAR, RESPIRATORY, AND LYMPHATIC DISORDERS
1 d
2 b
3 b
4 b
5 a
6 c
7 b
8 c
9 a
10 a
11 b
12 a
13 c
14 c
15 a
16 c
17 c
18 a
19 a
20 d

CHAPTER 50: DIGESTIVE AND ENDOCRINE DISORDERS
1 b
2 a
3 d
4 a
5 c
6 b
7 c
8 b
9 a
10 a
11 c
12 b
13 d
14 a
15 c
16 d
17 a
18 c

CHAPTER 51: URINARY AND REPRODUCTIVE DISORDERS
1 d
2 b
3 c
4 b
5 a
6 a
7 b
8 c
9 c
10 d

CHAPTER 52: MENTAL HEALTH DISORDERS

1 T
2 F
3 T
4 T
5 T
6 T
7 F
8 b
9 d
10 b
11 c
12 c
13 a
14 b
15 c
16 d
17 d
18 c
19 b
20 a
21 b
22 a
23 c
24 b
25 a
26 b

CHAPTER 53: CONFUSION AND DEMENTIA

1 T
2 F
3 T
4 T
5 F
6 T
7 F
8 F
9 T
10 T
11 T
12 F
13 F
14 b
15 a
16 d
17 c
18 d
19 b
20 a
21 c
22 c
23 a
24 b
25 d
26 b
27 c
28 d
29 a
30 c

CHAPTER 54: INTELLECTUAL AND DEVELOPMENTAL DISABILITIES

1 d
2 b
3 c
4 b
5 a
6 d
7 c
8 d
9 c
10 a
11 c
12 b
13 a
14 c
15 b
16 c

CHAPTER 55: SEXUALITY

1 a
2 d
3 c
4 a
5 c
6 b
7 d
8 b
9 c
10 d

CHAPTER 56: CARING FOR MOTHERS AND BABIES

1 T
2 F
3 T
4 T
5 F
6 T
7 T
8 F
9 T
10 F
11 c
12 d
13 b
14 a
15 d
16 d
17 b
18 c
19 c
20 a
21 c
22 d
23 d
24 a
25 c
26 c

CHAPTER 57: ASSISTED LIVING

1 F
2 T
3 F
4 T
5 T
6 F
7 F
8 T
9 T
10 d
11 b
12 c
13 a
14 b
15 a
16 b
17 c
18 c

CHAPTER 58: EMERGENCY CARE

1 b
2 a
3 b
4 c
5 b
6 a
7 c
8 b
9 b
10 c
11 c
12 a
13 d
14 b
15 d
16 d
17 d
18 c
19 a
20 a
21 b
22 c
23 d
24 a
25 c

CHAPTER 59: END-OF-LIFE CARE

1 c
2 a
3 b
4 a
5 d
6 c
7 b
8 a
9 d
10 c
11 c
12 a
13 b
14 b
15 d

CHAPTER 60: GETTING A JOB

1 d
2 b
3 c
4 a
5 c
6 d
7 a
8 a
9 b
10 c
11 b
12 a

National Nurse Aide Assessment Program (NNAAP®)
Written Examination Content Outline

The NNAAP® Written Examination is comprised of seventy (70) multiple choice questions. Ten (10) of these questions are pre-test (non-scored) questions on which statistical information will be collected.

I. Physical Care Skills
   A. Activities of Daily Living   9 questions
     1. Hygiene
     2. Dressing and Grooming
     3. Nutrition and Hydration
     4. Elimination
     5. Rest/Sleep/Comfort
   B. Basic Nursing Skills   23 questions
     1. Infection Control
     2. Safety/Emergency
     3. Therapeutic/Technical Procedures
     4. Data Collection and Reporting
   C. Restorative Skills   5 questions
     1. Prevention
     2. Self Care/Independence

II. Psychosocial Care Skills
   A. Emotional and Mental Health Needs   6 questions
   B. Spiritual and Cultural Needs   2 questions
III. Role of the Nurse Aide
   A. Communication   4 questions
   B. Client Rights   4 questions
   C. Legal and Ethical Behavior   2 questions
   D. Member of the Health Care Team   5 questions

National Nurse Aide Assessment Program (NNAAP®)
Skills Evaluation

List of Skills
1. Hand hygiene (hand washing)
2. Applies one knee-high elastic stocking
3. Assists to ambulate using transfer belt
4. Assists with use of bedpan
5. Cleans upper or lower denture
6. Counts and records radial pulse
7. Counts and records respirations
8. Donning and removing PPE (gown and gloves)
9. Dresses client with affected (weak) right arm
10. Feeds client who cannot feed self
11. Gives modified bed bath (face and one arm, hand and underarm)
12. Measures and records electronic blood pressure (state specific)
13. Measures and records urinary output
14. Measures and records weight of ambulatory client
15. Performs modified passive range of motion (PROM) for one knee and one ankle
16. Performs modified passive range of motion (PROM) for one shoulder
17. Positions on side
18. Provides catheter care for female
19. Provides foot care on one foot
20. Provides mouth care
21. Provides perineal care (peri-care) for female
22. Transfers from bed to wheelchair using transfer belt
23. Measures and records manual blood pressure (state specific)

Appendix B

MINIMUM DATA SET—SELECTED PAGES

Resident _____ Identifier _____ Date _____

Section G	Functional Status

G0110. Activities of Daily Living (ADL) Assistance
Refer to the ADL flow chart in the RAI manual to facilitate accurate coding

Instructions for Rule of 3
- When an activity occurs three times at any one given level, code that level.
- When an activity occurs three times at multiple levels, code the most dependent, exceptions are total dependence (4), activity must require full assist every time, and activity did not occur (8), activity must not have occurred at all. Example, three times extensive assistance (3) and three times limited assistance (2), code extensive assistance (3).
- When an activity occurs at various levels, but not three times at any given level, apply the following:
  - When there is a combination of full staff performance, and extensive assistance, code extensive assistance.
  - When there is a combination of full staff performance, weight bearing assistance and/or non-weight bearing assistance code limited assistance (2).

If none of the above are met, code supervision.

1. ADL Self-Performance
Code for **resident's performance** over all shifts - not including setup. If the ADL activity occurred 3 or more times at various levels of assistance, code the most dependent - except for total dependence, which requires full staff performance every time

Coding:

Activity Occurred 3 or More Times
0. **Independent** - no help or staff oversight at any time
1. **Supervision** - oversight, encouragement or cueing
2. **Limited assistance** - resident highly involved in activity; staff provide guided maneuvering of limbs or other non-weight-bearing assistance
3. **Extensive assistance** - resident involved in activity, staff provide weight-bearing support
4. **Total dependence** - full staff performance every time during entire 7-day period

Activity Occurred 2 or Fewer Times
7. **Activity occurred only once or twice** - activity did occur but only once or twice
8. **Activity did not occur** - activity did not occur or family and/or non-facility staff provided care 100% of the time for that activity over the entire 7-day period

2. ADL Support Provided
Code for **most support provided** over all shifts; code regardless of resident's self-performance classification

Coding:
0. **No** setup or physical help from staff
1. **Setup** help only
2. **One** person physical assist
3. **Two+** persons physical assist
8. ADL activity itself **did not occur** or family and/or non-facility staff provided care 100% of the time for that activity over the entire 7-day period

	1. Self-Performance	2. Support
	↓ Enter Codes in Boxes ↓	
A. Bed mobility - how resident moves to and from lying position, turns side to side, and positions body while in bed or alternate sleep furniture	☐	☐
B. Transfer - how resident moves between surfaces including to or from: bed, chair, wheelchair, standing position (**excludes** to/from bath/toilet)	☐	☐
C. Walk in room - how resident walks between locations in his/her room	☐	☐
D. Walk in corridor - how resident walks in corridor on unit	☐	☐
E. Locomotion on unit - how resident moves between locations in his/her room and adjacent corridor on same floor. If in wheelchair, self-sufficiency once in chair	☐	☐
F. Locomotion off unit - how resident moves to and returns from off-unit locations (e.g., areas set aside for dining, activities or treatments). **If facility has only one floor,** how resident moves to and from distant areas on the floor. If in wheelchair, self-sufficiency once in chair	☐	☐
G. Dressing - how resident puts on, fastens and takes off all items of clothing, including donning/removing a prosthesis or TED hose. Dressing includes putting on and changing pajamas and housedresses	☐	☐
H. Eating - how resident eats and drinks, regardless of skill. Do not include eating/drinking during medication pass. Includes intake of nourishment by other means (e.g., tube feeding, total parenteral nutrition, IV fluids administered for nutrition or hydration)	☐	☐
I. Toilet use - how resident uses the toilet room, commode, bedpan, or urinal; transfers on/off toilet; cleanses self after elimination; changes pad; manages ostomy or catheter; and adjusts clothes. Do not include emptying of bedpan, urinal, bedside commode, catheter bag or ostomy bag	☐	☐
J. Personal hygiene - how resident maintains personal hygiene, including combing hair, brushing teeth, shaving, applying makeup, washing/drying face and hands (**excludes** baths and showers)	☐	☐

Resident _____   Identifier _____   Date _____

Section G	Functional Status

G0120. Bathing

How resident takes full-body bath/shower, sponge bath, and transfers in/out of tub/shower (**excludes** washing of back and hair). Code for **most dependent** in self-performance and support

Enter Code	A. Self-performance
☐	0. **Independent** - no help provided 1. **Supervision** - oversight help only 2. **Physical help limited to transfer only** 3. **Physical help in part of bathing activity** 4. **Total dependence** 8. **Activity itself did not occur** or family and/or non-facility staff provided care 100% of the time for that activity over the entire 7-day period

Enter Code	B. Support provided
☐	(Bathing support codes are as defined in item **G0110 column 2, ADL Support Provided**, above)

G0300. Balance During Transitions and Walking

After observing the resident, **code the following walking and transition items for most dependent**

Coding:
- 0. **Steady at all times**
- 1. **Not steady, but <u>able</u> to stabilize without staff assistance**
- 2. **Not steady, <u>only able</u> to stabilize with staff assistance**
- 8. **Activity did not occur**

↓ **Enter Codes in Boxes**

Box	
☐	A. **Moving from seated to standing position**
☐	B. **Walking** (with assistive device if used)
☐	C. **Turning around** and facing the opposite direction while walking
☐	D. **Moving on and off toilet**
☐	E. **Surface-to-surface transfer** (transfer between bed and chair or wheelchair)

G0400. Functional Limitation in Range of Motion

Code for limitation that interfered with daily functions or placed resident at risk of injury

Coding:
- 0. **No impairment**
- 1. **Impairment on one side**
- 2. **Impairment on both sides**

↓ **Enter Codes in Boxes**

Box	
☐	A. **Upper extremity** (shoulder, elbow, wrist, hand)
☐	B. **Lower extremity** (hip, knee, ankle, foot)

G0600. Mobility Devices

↓ **Check all that were normally used**

Box	
☐	A. **Cane/crutch**
☐	B. **Walker**
☐	C. **Wheelchair** (manual or electric)
☐	D. **Limb prosthesis**
☐	Z. **None of the above** were used

G0900. Functional Rehabilitation Potential
Complete only if A0310A = 01

Enter Code	A. **Resident believes he or she is capable of increased independence** in at least some ADLs
☐	0. **No** 1. **Yes** 9. **Unable to determine**

Enter Code	B. **Direct care staff believe resident is capable of increased independence** in at least some ADLs
☐	0. **No** 1. **Yes**

From Centers for Medicare & Medicaid Services: MDS 3.0, http://www.cms.gov/Medicare/Quality-Initiatives-Patient-Assessment-Instruments/NursingHomeQualityInits/MDS30RAIManual.html.

Appendix C

CARE AREA ASSESSMENT (CAA)—SAMPLE PAGE

Resident _____ Identifier _____ Date _____

Section V	Care Area Assessment (CAA) Summary

V0200. CAAs and Care Planning

1. Check column A if Care Area is triggered.

2. For each triggered Care Area, indicate whether a new care plan, care plan revision, or continuation of current care plan is necessary to address the problem(s) identified in your assessment of the care area. The Care Planning Decision column must be completed within 7 days of completing the RAI (MDS and CAA(s)). Check column B if the triggered care area is addressed in the care plan.

3. Indicate in the Location and Date of CAA Documentation column where information related to the CAA can be found. CAA documentation should include information on the complicating factors, risks, and any referrals for this resident for this care area.

A. CAA Results

Care Area	A. Care Area Triggered	B. Care Planning Decision	Location and Date of CAA documentation
	↓ Check all that apply ↓		
01. Delirium	☐	☐	
02. Cognitive Loss/Dementia	☐	☐	
03. Visual Function	☐	☐	
04. Communication	☐	☐	
05. ADL Functional/Rehabilitation Potential	☐	☐	
06. Urinary Incontinence and Indwelling Catheter	☐	☐	
07. Psychosocial Well-Being	☐	☐	
08. Mood State	☐	☐	
09. Behavioral Symptoms	☐	☐	
10. Activities	☐	☐	
11. Falls	☐	☐	
12. Nutritional Status	☐	☐	
13. Feeding Tube	☐	☐	
14. Dehydration/Fluid Maintenance	☐	☐	
15. Dental Care	☐	☐	
16. Pressure Ulcer	☐	☐	
17. Psychotropic Drug Use	☐	☐	
18. Physical Restraints	☐	☐	
19. Pain	☐	☐	
20. Return to Community Referral	☐	☐	

B. Signature of RN Coordinator for CAA Process and Date Signed

1. Signature

2. Date ☐☐ – ☐☐ – ☐☐☐☐
Month   Day   Year

C. Signature of Person Completing Care Plan Decision and Date Signed

1. Signature

2. Date ☐☐ – ☐☐ – ☐☐☐☐
Month   Day   Year

From Centers for Medicare & Medicaid Services: MDS 3.0, http://www.cms.gov/Medicare/Quality-Initiatives -Patient-Assessment-Instruments/NursingHomeQualityInits/MDS30RAIManual.html.

INFANT AND CHILD SAFETY

Home Safety*

The following home safety measures can protect infants and children from harm.

Kitchen

- Knives, forks, scissors, and other sharp tools are kept in a drawer with a childproof latch.
- The stove has a lock and knob protectors.
- A dishwasher lock is installed.
- Childproof latches are installed on all cabinet doors.
- Chairs and step stools are away from the stove.
- When cooking, pot handles on the stove are turned inward or placed on back burners where children cannot reach them.
- Tablecloths and placemats are not used. Infants and children can pull things off the table and onto themselves.
- Glass objects and appliances with sharp blades are stored out of reach.
- The garbage can is behind a cabinet door with a childproof latch.
- Appliances are unplugged when not in use, with cords out of reach.
- Matches and lighters are stored in a locked cabinet.
- Cleaning supplies, bug sprays, dishwasher detergent, and dishwashing liquids are in the original containers and in a locked cabinet. A cabinet under the sink is not a safe storage area.
- Bottles containing alcohol are in the original containers and in a locked cabinet.
- Plastic garbage bags and sandwich bags are out of reach.
- Refrigerator magnets and other small objects are out of reach.
- There is a working fire extinguisher. Family members know how to use it.

Bathroom

- The thermostat on the hot water heater is set below 120°F (49°C).
- Razors, nail clippers, and other sharp items are stored in a locked cabinet.
- Drug bottles are closed tightly with child-resistant caps and stored in the original containers and in a locked cabinet.
- Childproof latches are installed on all drawers and cabinets.
- Toilets are closed and have toilet-lid locks.
- Sinks, tubs, and basins are empty when not in use.
- Outlets have ground fault circuit interrupters. These protect against electrical injuries if an electrical appliance gets wet.
- Hair dryers, curling irons, and electric razors are unplugged when not in use.
- There are slip-resistant strips on the floors of showers and bathtubs.
- There are anti-slip pads under rugs to hold them securely to the floor.
- Cosmetics and cleaners are stored in the original containers and in a locked cabinet.
- Bottles of mouthwash, perfumes, hair dyes, hair sprays, nail polishes, and nail polish removers are stored in the original containers and in a locked cabinet.

Stairways

- Hardware-mounted safety gates are at the top and bottom of every stairway. Gates meet current safety standards.
- Stairways are clear of tripping hazards such as loose carpeting or toys.
- Banisters and railings have guards if a child can fit through the rails.
- The railings and banisters are secure.
- The door to the basement steps is kept locked.
- There is enough light in the stairway.
- Children are supervised around stairs.

---

*Home Safety modified and adapted from kidshealth.org: *First Aid & Safety.*

Doors, Windows, Walls, and Floors

- Doors have finger-pinch guards.
- Rubber tips are removed from door stops or 1-piece door stops are installed.
- Doorknob covers or childproof locks are used on doors leading outside and to non-childproof areas.
- Glass doors have decorative markers so they are not mistaken for open doors.
- Sliding doors have childproof locks.
- Safety bars or window guards are installed on upper-story windows.
- Window stops are present to keep windows from closing all the way.
- Window blind and curtain cords are kept out of reach. The U.S. Consumer Product Safety Commission (CPSC) recommends cordless window coverings.
- Cribs, playpens, beds, or other furniture are not placed near a window.
- Window guards are placed on windows that are not emergency exits.
- Windows are opened from the top down.
- Walls are in good condition with no peeling or cracking paint.
- Mirrors and frames are hung securely.
- Rugs are secured to floors, fitted with anti-slip pads underneath, or removed.
- Floors are free of clutter.

Furniture

- Bookshelves and other furniture are secured to the wall or floor to prevent tipping.
- Children are not allowed to climb on furniture. This includes using shelves as steps.
- Toys or things that attract children are not placed on the top of furniture.
- Protective padding is placed on corners of coffee tables, furniture, and countertops with sharp edges.
- Baby equipment has not been recalled.
- Flatscreen TVs are mounted securely on the wall. Older, heavy TVs are on low, stable furniture.
- Stops are on all removable drawers to prevent them from falling out.

Child's Bedroom and Clothing

- The changing table has a safety belt.
- Painted cribs, bassinets, and high chairs made before 1978 are not used. (Paint was lead based before 1978.)
- The crib meets federal safety standards. See "Cribs," p. 899 and Chapter 56.
- There are no soft pillows, large stuffed animals, bumper pads, or soft bedding in the crib.
- Infants are not put to sleep on an adult or child's bed, water bed, couch, pillow, or other soft surface. Death from entrapment and suffocation are risks.
- Strings or ribbons have been removed from hanging mobiles and crib toys.
- Electric cords (including baby monitor cords) are at least 3 feet away from the crib or bed.
- Dressers are secured to walls or floors with drawers closed.
- Lids on toy chests and toy storage containers have a lid support to prevent slamming shut. Toy chests do not lock.
- Night-lights do not touch any fabric such as bedspreads or curtains.
- Sleepwear is flame-retardant.
- Drawstrings are removed from clothing.
- Children are not allowed to wear necklaces, strings, cords, ribbons, or other such items around the neck.
- Bibs are removed before naptime and bedtime.
- Clothing fits well. Clothing is not loose and does not touch or drag the floor.

Garage and Laundry Area

- Gardening, automotive, and lawn care tools and supplies are stored safely away from children.
- Hazardous automotive, pool, and gardening products are in a locked area.
- Recycling containers storing glass and metal are out of reach.
- Garbage cans are securely covered.
- Cleaning products are in the original containers and stored in a locked cabinet.
- Buckets used for cleaning are out of reach.
- Laundry detergent pods are in the original container and in a locked cabinet away from children.
- Washer and dryer doors are kept closed.
- Laundry chutes are locked with childproof locks.

Outdoors, Backyard, and Pool
- Walkways and outdoor stairways are well lit. They are clear of toys, objects, or things blocking a clear path.
- Sidewalks and outdoor stairways are without cracks and missing pieces.
- Playground equipment is safe with no loose parts, splinters, sharp edges, or rust.
- The surface beneath playground equipment is cushioned with material such as sand, mulch, wood chips, or approved rubber surfacing mats to absorb the shock of a fall.
- Outdoor toys are in a secure, dry place when not used.
- Toys are kept away from pools, spas, hot tubs, or whirlpools. Children playing with such toys could fall into the water.
- Toys are removed from pools after swimming.
- Climb-proof fencing is at least 5 feet high on all sides of the pool. The fence has a self-closing gate with a childproof lock.
- The ladder is removed from an above-ground pool when not in use.
- Door, window, and pool alarms are on. They alert you if a child wanders into an unsafe area.
- Inflatable flotation devices are not relied on to keep a child afloat. Children near water must be constantly supervised.
- Buckets, pails, containers, and wading pools are empty and upside down when not in use.

Vehicle Safety
- Children are not left alone in any vehicle even if the windows are down. They can develop heat-related illness, suffocate, and die from high temperatures within minutes.
- Seat-belt laws are followed.
- Car seat safety measures are followed. (See p. 899.)
- Vehicle doors and the trunk are locked. Keys are kept out of children's sight and reach.
- Trunk access is kept closed.
- Children are not allowed to play in vehicles.
- Children do not ride as passengers on tractors, mowers, mini-bikes, or all-terrain vehicles.
- Children under age 17 do not ride all-terrain vehicles. A helmet and eye protection are worn. Three-wheeled all-terrain vehicles are never used.

Electrical
- Un-used outlets are covered.
- Electrical items are unplugged when not in use.
- Major electrical appliances are grounded.
- Cord holders keep cords fastened against walls.
- There are no potential electrical fire hazards such as over-loaded electrical sockets and electrical wires running under carpets.
- Equipment with old or frayed cords and damaged extension cords are removed.
- Computers, TVs, and stereo equipment are against walls. This prevents children from touching cords.
- Electronic toys are checked for signs of danger. Toys that spark, feel hot, or smell unusual are repaired or discarded.

Heating and Cooling Elements
- Radiators and baseboard heaters are covered with childproof screens.
- Gas fireplaces are secured with a valve cover or key.
- Working fireplaces have a screen and other barriers in place when in use.
- Chimneys have been cleaned recently.
- Electric space heaters are at least 3 feet from beds, curtains, or anything flammable.

Emergency Equipment and Numbers
- A list of emergency phone numbers is stored in or kept near each phone in the home.
- Fire extinguishers are on every floor and in the kitchen, the basement, the garage, and any workshop area.
- Upper floors of the home have an emergency ladder.
- Smoke alarms are on each floor of the home, outside each sleeping area, and inside each bedroom.
- Smoke alarms are tested monthly and batteries changed every 6 months.
- The home has a carbon monoxide alarm. (See Chapter 13.)

Firearm Safety
- Guns are stored in a securely locked case out of children's reach. All firearms are stored unloaded and in the uncocked position.
- Ammunition is stored in a separate place and in a securely locked container out of reach.
- Keys for gun storage, ammunition, and gun-cleaning supplies are kept where children cannot find them.
- Trigger locks or other childproof devices are used.
- Gun safety is practiced. Adults have taken a firearm safety course to use the firearm safely and correctly.
- Children are taught that guns are not toys, they are not to touch or play with guns, and they should tell an adult if they find one.
- Gun-cleaning supplies are locked up. Cleaning supplies are often poisonous.

Other Safety Measures

- Infants and children are supervised at all times.
- Infants and children are supervised by an adult when in the bathtub or near water. Siblings do not supervise.
- Medication (drug) bottles, loose pills, coins, scissors, magnets, and any other small or sharp objects are out of reach.
- Smoking is not allowed in the home.
- Testing has been done for lead, radon, asbestos, mercury, mold, and carbon monoxide when such substances may be present.
- There are no potentially poisonous houseplants.
- Children are supervised around dogs and other pets.

Nursery Equipment Safety*

Nursery equipment must be safe, in good repair, and used properly. Use the following guidelines to check nursery equipment in an agency or home setting.

Carriers

- The carrier has:
  - Straps that prevent the baby from falling or crawling out
  - A firm, padded head support
  - Durable fabric with strong stitching or large, heavy fasteners to prevent slipping
- There is enough depth to support the baby's back.
- Leg openings are small enough to prevent the baby from slipping out but large enough to prevent chafing.
- A framed carrier has a kickstand that locks in the open position. The folding mechanism is free of areas that could pinch the baby's fingers. There is padding on the metal frame around the baby's face.
- Follow these safety measures when using carriers.
  - Never use a framed carrier before an infant is 4 to 5 months old. Do not use it as an infant seat. It can tip over without warning.
  - Use restraining straps at all times if the carrier has them.
  - If you need to lean over, bend from the knees rather than the waist to prevent the baby from falling out of the carrier.
  - Check the carrier often for loose fasteners or ripped seams.

Infant Seats

- The seat has a wide, sturdy base for stability.
- The base has a slip-resistant surface.
- Locking mechanisms are secure. Push down on the unit to make sure it is sturdy.
- Supporting devices lock securely.
- The safety belt is secure and the fabric is washable.
- Follow these safety measures when using infant seats.
  - Never place the baby in an infant seat on a table or other raised surface.
  - Use the safety belt every time you place the baby in the seat.
  - Do not place the seat on soft surfaces such as beds or sofas. The seat may tip over and the baby can suffocate.
  - The seat is never used to transport a baby in a vehicle.

Baby Bathtubs

- The bathtub has slip-resistant backing to keep it from moving.
- There are no rough edges that can scratch the baby.
- The tub stays firm in the center when filled with water.
- Bath rings, baby flotation devices, and bath seats are avoided. The baby can drown if the device tips.
- Foam cushions are avoided. Pieces can be torn off and swallowed.
- Follow these bathing safety measures.
  - Always check the water temperature before putting the baby in the bathtub. Water that is too hot can burn babies.
  - Only adults should give babies baths. Baths can be dangerous. Babies can drown in less than 1 inch of water.
  - Always keep 1 hand on the baby while he or she is in water.
  - Always take the baby with you if you step away from the bathtub.
  - Gather bathing supplies ahead of time, including shampoo, soap, washcloth, towel, clean clothes, a clean diaper, and wipes.
  - Always empty the bathtub and turn it upside down when it is not being used. A plug at the bottom of the tub makes draining easier.

---

*Nursery Equipment Safety modified and adapted from kidshealth.org: *Choosing Safe Baby Products.*

Changing Tables

- The table is sturdy. The base is wide enough to prevent tipping.
- The table has safety straps to prevent falls.
- The table has drawers or shelves that are easy to reach without leaving the baby unattended. Supplies are within your reach but out of the baby's reach.
- A flat changing surface is surrounded on all 4 sides by a guard-rail that is at least 2 inches high. The surface is lower in the middle than on the sides to keep the baby from rolling.
- Follow these safety measures.
  - Use the safety belt when you change the baby.
  - Never leave the infant unattended, even if you think he or she is secure.
  - Stop using the changing table when the baby reaches the manufacturer's age or weight limit. Age 2 or 30 pounds is common.

Gates

- The gate has a pressure bar or other fastener that will resist forces exerted by a child.
- A hardware-mounted gate is used at the top of stairs. Pressure-mounted or free-standing gates can fall if the child pushes hard enough.
- The gate has a straight top edge with rigid bars or a tight mesh screen.
- There is less than 2 inches between the floor and the gate bottom to prevent a child from going underneath.
- Rigid vertical slats or rods are no more than $2\frac{3}{8}$ inches apart to prevent head entrapment between the slats.
- There are no sharp edges or pieces that could cut a child's hand. Wooden gates are smooth to prevent splinters.
- There are no openings to use for climbing.
- The gate should be at least three quarters ($\frac{3}{4}$) of the child's height.
- Accordion-style gates are not used. They can trap a child's head.
- Follow these safety measures when using gates.
  - Keep large toys away from the gate. A child can use the toy to climb over.
  - Pressure-mounted and free-standing gates may be used for doors between rooms unless there are stairs between the rooms. Place the pressure bar away from the child.
  - Gates that swing out are never to be used at the top of stairways.
  - Stop using the gate if the child can open or climb over it.

Playpens

- Playpens have top rails that automatically lock when lifted into the normal-use position.
- The locks for lowering a side are out of the baby's reach.
- The sides are at least 20 inches high, measured from the floor of the playpen.
- Playpen mesh has small weave (less than $\frac{1}{4}$-inch openings).
- The mesh has no tears, holes, or loose threads.
- The mesh is securely attached and checked regularly for breaks and tears.
- A wooden playpen has slats spaced no more than $2\frac{3}{8}$ inches apart.
- The playpen has well-protected hinges and supports.
- There is padding on the tops of the rails.
- The bottom of the playpen has a 1-inch firm mattress or pad.
- Follow these safety measures when using playpens.
  - Never leave a baby in a mesh playpen with the side lowered. Entrapment between the mesh side and floor board is a risk.
  - Never use soft bedding or pillows.
  - Do not replace the mattress or pad. The new mattress may not fit the playpen well.
  - Check all padded parts regularly for tears. Cover or repair tears.
  - Do not place the playpen near windows. Cords on window coverings can strangle the baby.
  - Do not use a playpen with large diamond-shaped openings. Entrapment is a risk.
  - Never tie or string toys from the sides of the playpen.
  - Stop using the playpen when the child can easily climb out—when the child is 34 inches tall or weighs 30 pounds.

Strollers and Carriages

- There is a wide base to prevent tipping.
- The device has a reliable restraining belt. A 5-point harness is safest.
- Brakes securely lock the wheels.
- The shopping basket is low on the back. It is located in front of the rear wheels.
- When used in the reclined position, the leg openings can be closed.
- No stroller parts can pinch a child's fingers or are a choking hazard.
- The leg openings are small enough to prevent an infant from slipping through.
- The stroller steers in a straight line when pushed with 1 hand.
- Handlebars are at waist level or slightly lower.
- Follow these safety measures.
  - Never exceed age, weight, and height limits.
  - Position newborns almost flat. Newborns cannot support the head and neck.
  - Never leave a child unattended.
  - Always use the safety harness.
  - Avoid using a pillow or blanket as a mattress.
  - Apply the brakes when not moving.
  - Never hang purses or diaper bags on the handles.
  - Fold and unfold the stroller or carriage away from children to avoid pinching fingers.

Walkers

- Walkers are not used. Walkers are a leading cause of injury in babies. Injury risks include:
  - Falling over objects or down stairs.
  - Rolling into dangerous objects or areas. Hot stoves, heaters, and pools are examples.
  - Reaching higher than normal and touching dangerous items. Stovetops, kitchen knives, and hot coffee cups are examples.

Toys

- Small toys are kept away from children. Make sure toys are too large to fit into the child's mouth. Objects should have a diameter of $1\frac{3}{4}$ inches or more. This includes marbles, balls, and games with balls.
- Battery cases on battery-operated toys are secured with screws.
- Toys are strong and durable. They do not have:
  - Sharp ends, small parts, and small ends that can extend into the back of a baby's mouth
  - Strings longer than 7 inches
  - Parts that can pinch fingers
- Riding toys are stable and secure to prevent tipping.
- Safety gear is worn for bicycles, skateboards, scooters, in-line skates, and other devices with wheels. A helmet and knee pads, elbow pads, and wrist guards are examples.
- Follow these safety measures for toys.
  - Follow manufacturers' age recommendations.
  - Read all warning labels.
  - Make sure toys have not been recalled for safety reasons.
  - Do not give an infant or toddler painted toys made before 1978. The paint may contain lead.
  - Never give balloons or latex gloves to children younger than 8 years.
  - Never give a baby vending machine toys. They often contain small parts.
  - Check toys and play equipment for cracks, chips, breaks, sharp edges, loose parts, and other damage.
  - Check carnival toys carefully. They are not required to meet safety standards.
  - Keep older children's toys away from infants and younger children.

Cribs

- Side rails are fixed and not adjustable. The U.S. Consumer Product Safety Commission (CPSC) banned the sale of drop-side cribs.
- Slats are spaced no more than $2\frac{3}{8}$ inches apart.
- No slats are missing, loose, or cracked.
- The mattress is firm and fits snugly.
- The mattress pad fits tightly and the plastic mattress packaging is removed.
- Crib corner posts are either flush with the top of the head-board and foot-board or are over 16 inches.
- The crib meets federal safety standards for strength, durability, and testing. The crib has not been recalled by the manufacturer.
- Follow these safety measures when using cribs.
  - Always place a baby on his or her back to sleep.
  - Remove a baby's bib when in the crib.
  - Check that all screws and hardware are present and tight.
  - Never place soft bedding or soft toys in the crib.
  - Bumper pads are not used.
  - Remove a mobile from the crib when 1 of the following occur.
    - The child can push on the hands and knees.
    - The child reaches 5 months of age.
  - Do not hang toys by strings.
  - Use flame-retardant sheets and sleepwear.
  - Never place a crib near a window or drapes. A baby can become entangled in window covering cords.

Child Safety Seats (Car Seats)

- The car seat is federally approved and fits the child's height and weight.
- Parts and manufacturer labels—including the manufacturer's name, model number, and date made—are intact.
- The seat has not been in a motor vehicle accident.
- The seat is less than 6 years old. Check the manufacturer's recommended expiration date.
- Follow these safety measures for using car seats.
  - Do not use a car seat that does not have the manufacturer's instructions.
  - Infants and toddlers ride rear-facing until they have reached the weight and height limits recommended by the manufacturer.
  - Children in forward-facing seats are harnessed in until they reach the weight or height for that seat.
  - A booster seat is used for children who have outgrown the forward-facing harness seat.
  - Children use a booster seat until the vehicle's lap-and-shoulder belt fits properly. This usually occurs when the child has reached 4 feet, 9 inches in height—between 8 and 12 years of age.
  - Follow the car seat guidelines in Chapter 56.

Glossary

A

abbreviation A shortened form of a word or phrase

abduction Moving a body part away from the mid-line of the body

abrasion A partial-thickness wound caused by the scraping away or rubbing of the skin

abuse
- The willful infliction of injury, unreasonable confinement, intimidation, or punishment that results in physical harm, pain, or mental anguish
- Depriving the person (or the person's caregiver) of the goods or services needed to attain or maintain well-being

accountable To answer to one's self and others about his or her choices, decisions, and actions

acetone See "ketone"

acid reflux See "heartburn"

activities of daily living (ADL) The activities usually done during a normal day in a person's life

acute illness An illness of rapid onset and short duration; the person is expected to recover

acute pain Pain that is sharp or severe; may be felt suddenly from injury, disease, trauma, or surgery

addiction A chronic disease involving substance-seeking behaviors and use that is compulsive and hard to control despite the harmful effects

adduction Moving a body part toward the mid-line of the body

admission Official entry of a person into a health care setting

adolescence The time between puberty and adulthood; a time of rapid growth and physical, sexual, emotional, and social changes

advance directive A document stating a person's wishes about health care when that person cannot make his or her own decisions

afebrile Without (a) a fever (febrile)

affected side The side of the body with weakness from illness or injury; weak side

alcoholism Alcohol dependence that involves craving, loss of control, physical dependence, and tolerance

allergy A sensitivity to a substance that causes the body to react with signs and symptoms

alopecia Hair loss

AM care See "early morning care"

ambulation The act of walking

amputation The removal of all or part of an extremity

anaphylaxis A life-threatening sensitivity to an antigen

anesthesia The loss (an) of all sensation (esthesia), especially pain, produced by a drug

anorexia The loss of appetite

anterior At or toward the front of the body or body part; ventral

antibiotic A drug that kills certain microbes that cause infection

anticoagulant A drug that prevents or slows down (anti) blood clotting (coagulate)

antisepsis The processes, procedures, and chemical treatments that kill microbes or prevent them from causing an infection; anti means against and sepsis means infection

antiseptic A chemical applied to the skin to prevent the growth and reproduction of microbes

anxiety A feeling of worry, nervousness, or fear about an event or situation

aphasia The total or partial loss (a) of the ability to use or understand language (phasia)

apical-radial pulse Taking the apical and radial pulses at the same time

apnea The lack or absence (a) of breathing (pnea)

arrhythmia See "dysrhythmia"

arterial ulcer An open wound on the foot, ankle, or lower leg caused by poor arterial blood flow

artery A blood vessel that carries blood away from the heart

arthritis Joint (arthr) inflammation (itis)

arthroplasty The surgical replacement (plasty) of a joint (arthro)

asepsis The absence (a) of disease-producing microbes; sepsis means infection

aspiration Breathing fluid, food, vomitus, or an object into the lungs

assault Intentionally attempting or threatening to touch a person's body without the person's consent

assessment Collecting information about the person; see "nursing process"

assisted living A housing option for older persons who need help with activities of daily living but do not need 24-hour nursing care and supervision

assisted living residence (ALR) Provides housing, personal care, support services, health care, and social activities in a home-like setting to persons needing some help with daily activities

atelectasis The collapse of a portion of a lung

atrophy The decrease in size or wasting away of tissue

autopsy The examination of the body after death

avoidable pressure injury A pressure injury that develops from the improper use of the nursing process

B

bariatrics The field of medicine focused on the treatment and control of obesity

base of support The area on which an object rests

battery Touching a person's body without his or her consent

bedfast Confined to bed

bed mobility How a person moves to and from a lying position, turns from side to side, and re-positions in a bed or other sleeping furniture

bed rail A device that serves as a guard or barrier along the side of the bed; side rail

bed rest Restricting a person to bed and limiting activity for health reasons

benign tumor A tumor that does not spread to other body parts

biohazardous waste Items contaminated with blood, body fluids, secretions, or excretions; bio means life and hazardous means dangerous or harmful

biopsy A procedure in which a piece of tissue is removed for testing

Biot's respirations Rapid and deep respirations followed by 10 to 30 seconds of apnea

birth defect A problem that develops during pregnancy, often during the first 3 months; it may involve a body structure or function

bisexual A person who is attracted to males and females

blindness The absence of sight

blood pressure (BP) The amount of force exerted against the walls of an artery by the blood

body alignment The way the head, trunk, arms, and legs align with one another; posture

body language Messages sent through facial expressions, gestures, posture, hand and body movements, gait, eye contact, and appearance

body mechanics Using the body in an efficient and careful way

body temperature The amount of heat in the body that is a balance between the amount of heat produced and the amount lost by the body

bony prominence An area where the bone sticks out or projects from the flat surface of the body; pressure point

boundary crossing
- A brief act or behavior of being over-involved with the person
- The intent of the act or behavior is to meet the person's needs

boundary sign An act, behavior, or thought that warns of a boundary crossing or boundary violation

boundary violation An act or behavior that meets your needs, not the person's

bradycardia A slow (*brady*) heart rate (*cardia*); less than 60 beats per minute

bradypnea Slow (*brady*) breathing (*pnea*); respirations are fewer than 12 per minute

braille A touch reading and writing system that uses raised dots for each letter of the alphabet; the first 10 letters also represent the numbers 0 through 9

breast-feeding Feeding a baby milk from the mother's breasts; nursing

Broca's aphasia See "expressive aphasia"

bullying Repeated attacks or threats of fear, distress, or harm by a bully toward a target

burnout A job stress resulting in being physically or mentally exhausted, having doubts about your abilities, and having doubts about the value of your work

C

calorie The fuel or energy value of food

cancer See "malignant tumor"

capillary A very tiny blood vessel; nutrients, oxygen, and other substances pass from the capillaries into the cells

cardiac arrest See "sudden cardiac arrest"

cardiopulmonary resuscitation (CPR) An emergency procedure performed when the heart and breathing stop

carrier A human or animal that is a reservoir for microbes but does not develop the infection

case management A nursing care pattern; services for the person's care needs are obtained and monitored from admission through discharge and into the home or long-term care setting

catheter A tube used to drain or inject fluid through a body opening

catheterization The process of inserting a catheter

cell The basic unit of body structure

certification Official recognition by a state that standards or requirements have been met

cerumen Earwax

chairfast Confined to a chair

chart See "medical record"

chemical restraint Any drug used for discipline or convenience and not required to treat medical symptoms

Cheyne-Stokes respirations Respirations gradually increase in rate and depth and then become shallow and slow; breathing may stop (*apnea*) for 10 to 20 seconds

child abuse and neglect The intentional harm or mistreatment of a child under 18 years old:
- Involves any recent act or failure to act on the part of a parent or caregiver
- Results in death, serious physical or emotional harm, sexual abuse, or exploitation
- Presents a likely or immediate risk for harm

cholesterol A soft, waxy substance found in the bloodstream and all body cells

chronic illness A long-term health condition that may not have a cure; it can be controlled and complications prevented with proper treatment

chronic pain Pain that continues for a long time (longer than 12 weeks, occurs off and on, or is persistent [constant])

chronic wound A wound that does not heal easily and within about 3 months

circadian rhythm Daily rhythm based on a 24-hour cycle that involves behavior, sleep, eating, and waking patterns; the day-night cycle or body rhythm

circulatory ulcer An open sore on the lower legs or feet caused by decreased blood flow through the arteries or veins; vascular ulcer

circumcised The fold of skin (foreskin) covering the glans of the penis was surgically removed

circumcision The surgical removal of foreskin from the penis

civil law Laws concerned with relationships between people

clean technique See "medical asepsis"

clinical record See "medical record"

closed fracture The bone is broken but the skin is intact; simple fracture

code of ethics Rules, or standards of conduct, for group members to follow

cognitive function Involves memory, thinking, reasoning, ability to understand, judgment, and behavior

colonized The presence of bacteria on the wound surface or in wound tissue; the person does not have signs and symptoms of an infection

colostomy A surgically created opening (*stomy*) between the colon (*colo*) and the body's surface

coma A state of being unaware of one's setting and being unable to react or respond to people, places, or things

comatose Being unable to respond to stimuli

comfort A state of well-being; the person has no physical or emotional pain and is calm and at ease

comminuted fracture The bone is shattered or broken into 3 or more pieces

communicable disease A disease caused by a pathogen that spreads easily; contagious disease

communication The exchange of information—a message sent is received and correctly interpreted by the intended person

compound fracture See "open fracture"

compress A soft pad applied over a body area

compulsion An over-whelming urge to repeat certain rituals, acts, or behaviors

condom catheter A soft sheath that slides over the penis and is used to drain urine

confidentiality Trusting others with personal and private information

conflict A clash between opposing interests or ideas

confusion A state of being disoriented to person, time, place, situation, or identity

congenital To be born with

constipation The passage of a hard, dry stool

constrict To narrow

contagious disease See "communicable disease"

contamination The process of becoming unclean

contracture Decreased motion and stiffness of a joint caused by shortening (contracting) of a muscle

convenience Any action taken to control or manage a person's behavior that requires less effort by the staff; the action is not in the person's best interest

convulsion See "seizure"

cotton drawsheet A drawsheet made of cotton; it helps keep the mattress and bottom linens clean

courtesy A polite, considerate, or helpful comment or act

crime An act that violates a criminal law

criminal law Laws concerned with offenses against the public and society in general

cross-contamination Passing microbes from 1 person to another by contaminated hands, equipment, or supplies

culture The characteristics of a group of people—language, values, beliefs, habits, likes, dislikes, customs—passed from 1 generation to the next

cyanosis Bluish (*cyano*) color; bluish color (*cyano*) to the skin, lips, mucous membranes, and nail beds

D

dandruff Excessive amounts of dry, white flakes from the scalp

deafness Hearing loss in which it is impossible for the person to understand speech through hearing alone

deconditioning The loss of muscle strength from inactivity

defamation Injuring a person's name and reputation by making false statements to a third person

defecation The process of excreting feces from the rectum through the anus; a bowel movement

defense mechanism An unconscious reaction that blocks unpleasant or threatening feelings

dehydration The excessive loss of water from tissues; a decrease in the amount of water in body tissues

delegate To authorize or direct a nursing assistant to perform a nursing task

delegated nursing responsibility A nursing task that a nurse transfers to a nursing assistant when it does not require a nurse's professional knowledge or judgment

delegation The process a nurse uses to direct a nursing assistant to perform a nursing task; allowing a nursing assistant to perform a nursing responsibility that is beyond the nursing assistant's usual role and not routinely done by the nursing assistant

delirium A state of sudden, severe confusion and rapid changes in brain function

delusion A false belief

delusion of grandeur An exaggerated belief about one's importance, fame, wealth, power, or talents

delusion of persecution A false belief that one is being mistreated, abused, or harassed

dementia The loss of cognitive and social function caused by changes in the brain; the loss of cognitive function that interferes with daily life and activities

denture A removable replacement for missing teeth

detoxification The process of removing a toxic substance from the body

development Changes in mental, emotional, and social function

developmental disability A severe and chronic disability that involves a mental or physical impairment or both

developmental task A skill that must be completed during a stage of development for development to continue

diabetic foot ulcer An open wound on the foot caused by complications from diabetes

dialysis The process of removing waste products from the blood

diaphoresis Profuse (excessive) sweating

diarrhea The frequent passage of liquid stools

diastole The period of heart muscle relaxation; the heart is at rest

diastolic pressure The pressure in the arteries when the heart is at rest

digestion The process that breaks down food physically and chemically so it can be absorbed for use by the cells

dilate To expand or open wider

disability Any lost, absent, or impaired physical or mental function

disaster A sudden, catastrophic event in which people are injured and killed and property is destroyed

discharge Official departure of a person from a health care setting

discipline Any action taken by the agency to punish or penalize a patient or resident

discomfort See "pain"

discrimination Unjust treatment based on age, race, gender, and other personal qualities

disinfectant A liquid chemical that can kill many or all pathogens except spores

disinfection The process of killing pathogens

distal The part farthest from the center or from the point of attachment

distraction To focus the person's attention on something unrelated to pain

dorsal See "posterior"

dorsal recumbent position The back-lying or supine position; the supine position with the legs together (*dorsal* means *the back of something*; *recumbent* means *to lie down*); horizontal recumbent position

dorsiflexion Bending the toes and foot up at the ankle

drawsheet A small sheet placed over the middle of the bottom sheet

drug abuse Using a drug for non-medical or non-therapy effects

drug addiction A strong urge or craving to use the substance and cannot stop using; tolerance develops

dysphagia Difficulty (*dys*) swallowing (*phagia*)

dyspnea Difficult, labored, or painful (*dys*) breathing (*pnea*)

dysrhythmia An abnormal (*dys*) heart rhythm (*rhythmia*); arrhythmia

dysuria Painful or difficult (*dys*) urination (*uria*); burning on urination

E

early morning care Routine care given before breakfast; AM care

edema The swelling of body tissues with water

ejaculation The release of semen

elder abuse Any knowing, intentional, or negligent act by a caregiver or any other person to an older adult that causes harm or serious risk of harm

elective surgery Surgery done by choice to improve life or well-being

electrical shock When electrical current passes through the body

electrolytes Minerals dissolved in water

electronic health record (EHR) An electronic version of a person's medical record; electronic medical record

electronic medical record (EMR) See "electronic health record"

elopement When a patient or resident leaves the agency without staff knowledge

embolus A blood clot (*thrombus*) that travels through the vascular system until it lodges in a blood vessel

emergency surgery Surgery done at once to save life or function

emesis See "vomitus"

enabler A device that limits freedom of movement but is used to promote independence, comfort, or safety

end-of-life care The support and care given during the time surrounding death

end-of-shift report A report that the nurse gives at the end of the shift to the on-coming shift; change-of-shift report

endorsement A state recognizes the certificate, license, or registration issued by another state; reciprocity or equivalency

enema The introduction of fluid into the rectum and lower colon

enteral nutrition Giving nutrients into the gastro-intestinal (GI) tract (*enteral*) through a feeding tube

entrapment Getting caught, trapped, or entangled in spaces created by the bed rails, the mattress, the bed frame, the head-board, or the foot-board

enuresis Involuntary loss or leakage of urine during sleep; bed-wetting

epidermal stripping Removing the epidermis (outer skin layer) as tape is removed from the skin

episiotomy Incision (*otomy*) into the perineum

equivalency See "endorsement"

erectile dysfunction (ED) The inability of the male to have or maintain an erection

ergonomics The science of designing a job to fit the worker; *ergo* means *work*, *nomos* means *law*

eschar Thick, leathery dead tissue that may be loose or adhered to the skin; it is often black or brown

esteem The worth, value, or opinion one has of a person

ethics Knowledge of what is right conduct and wrong conduct

evaluation To measure if goals in the planning step were met; see "nursing process"

evening care Care given in the evening at bedtime; PM care

excoriation Loss of the epidermis (top skin layer) caused by scratching or when skin rubs against skin, clothing, or other material

expressive aphasia Difficulty expressing or sending out thoughts through speech or writing; Broca's aphasia

extension Straightening a body part

external rotation Turning the joint outward

F

fainting The sudden loss of consciousness from an inadequate blood supply to the brain; syncope

false imprisonment Unlawful restraint or restriction of a person's freedom of movement

febrile With a fever

fecal impaction The prolonged retention and buildup of feces in the rectum

fecal incontinence The inability to control the passage of feces and flatus through the anus

feces The semi-solid mass of waste products in the colon that is expelled through the anus; stool or stools

fever Elevated body temperature

first aid The emergency care given to an ill or injured person before medical help arrives

flashback Reliving the trauma over and over in thoughts during the day and in nightmares during sleep

flatulence The excessive formation of gas or air in the stomach and intestines

flatus Gas or air passed through the anus

flexion Bending a body part

flow rate The number of drops per minute (*gtt/min*) or milliliters per hour (*mL/hr*)

Foley catheter See "indwelling catheter"

footdrop The foot falls down at the ankle; permanent plantar flexion

Fowler's position A semi-sitting position; the head of the bed is raised between 45 and 60 degrees

fracture A broken bone

fraud Saying or doing something to trick, fool, or deceive a person

freedom of movement Any change in place or position of the body or any part of the body that the person can control

friction The rubbing of 1 surface against another

frostbite An injury to the body caused by freezing of the skin and underlying tissues

full visual privacy Having the means to be completely free from public view while in bed

functional incontinence The person has bladder control but cannot use the toilet in time

functional nursing A nursing care pattern focusing on tasks and jobs; each nursing team member is assigned certain tasks and jobs

G

gait belt See "transfer belt"

gangrene A condition in which there is death of tissue

garment An item of clothing

gastrostomy tube A feeding tube inserted through a surgically created opening (*stomy*) in the stomach (*gastro*); stomach tube

gavage The process of giving a tube feeding

gay A person who is attracted to members of the same sex

gender identity A person's sense or feelings of being male, female, a combination of male and female, or neither male nor female

general anesthesia A treatment with certain drugs that produces a deep sleep and the absence of all sensation, especially pain

genupectoral position See "knee-chest position" (*genu* means *knee; pectoral* refers to the *chest*)

geriatrics The field of medicine concerned with the problems and diseases of old age and older persons; the care of aging people

gerontology The study of the aging process

global aphasia Difficulty expressing or sending out thoughts and difficulty understanding language; mixed aphasia

glucometer A device for measuring (*meter*) blood glucose (*gluco*); glucose meter

glucosuria Sugar (*glucose*) in the urine (*uria*)

gossip To spread rumors or talk about the private matters of others

graduate A measuring container for fluid

gravity A natural force that pulls things downward

groin Where a thigh and the abdomen meet

ground That which carries leaking electricity to the earth and away from an electrical item

growth The physical changes that are measured and that occur in a steady, orderly manner

guided imagery Creating and focusing on a relaxing image

H

hallucination Seeing, hearing, smelling, feeling, or tasting something that is not real

harassment To trouble, torment, offend, or worry a person by one's behavior or comments

hazard Any thing in the person's setting that could cause injury or illness

hazardous chemical Any chemical that is a physical hazard or a health hazard

healthcare-associated infection (HAI) An infection that develops in a person cared for in any setting where health care is given; the infection is related to receiving health care

health team The many health care workers whose skills and knowledge focus on the person's total care; interdisciplinary health care team

hearing loss Not being able to hear the range of sounds associated with normal hearing

heartburn A burning sensation in the chest or throat; acid reflux

hematoma A swelling (*oma*) that contains blood (*hemat*)

hematuria Blood (*hemat*) in the urine (*uria*)

hemiplegia Paralysis (*plegia*) on 1 side (*hemi*) of the body

hemoglobin The substance in red blood cells that carries oxygen and gives blood its red color

hemoptysis Bloody (*hemo*) sputum (*ptysis* means *to spit*)

hemorrhage The excessive loss (*rrhage*) of blood (*hemo*) in a short time

hemothorax Blood (*hemo*) in the pleural space (*thorax*)

heterosexual A person who is attracted to members of the other sex

high-Fowler's position A semi-sitting position; the head of the bed is raised 60 to 90 degrees

hirsutism Excessive body hair

holism A concept that considers the whole person; the whole person has physical, social, psychological, and spiritual parts that are woven together and cannot be separated

horizontal recumbent position See "dorsal recumbent position"

hormone A chemical substance secreted by the endocrine glands into the bloodstream

hospice A health care agency or program that promotes comfort and quality of life for the dying person and his or her family

hospital bed system The bed frame and its parts—mattress, bed rails, head- and foot-boards, and bed attachments

hydration Having an adequate amount of water in body tissues

hygiene The cleanliness practices that promote health and prevent disease

hyperextension Excessive straightening of a body part

hyperglycemia High (*hyper*) sugar (*glyc*) in the blood (*emia*)

hypertension High blood pressure

hyperventilation Breathing (*ventilation*) is rapid (*hyper*) and deeper than normal

hypoglycemia Low (*hypo*) sugar (*glyc*) in the blood (*emia*)

hypotension Low blood pressure

hypothermia Abnormally low (*hypo*) body temperature (*thermia*)

hypoventilation Breathing (*ventilation*) is slow (*hypo*), shallow, and sometimes irregular

hypoxemia A reduced amount (*hypo*) of oxygen (*ox*) in the blood (*emia*)

hypoxia Cells do not have enough (*hypo*) oxygen (*oxia*)

I

ileostomy A surgically created opening (*stomy*) between the ileum (small intestine [*ileo*]) and the body's surface

immunity Protection against a disease or condition; the person will not get or be affected by the disease

implementation To perform or carry out nursing interventions (nursing measures, nursing actions, nursing tasks) in the care plan; see "nursing process"

incident Any event that has harmed or could harm a patient, resident, visitor, or staff member

incision A cut produced surgically by a sharp instrument; it creates an opening into an organ or body space

indwelling catheter A catheter left in the bladder so urine drains constantly into a drainage bag; retention or Foley catheter

infancy The first year of life

infection A disease state resulting from the invasion and growth of microbes in the body

infection control Practices and procedures that prevent the spread of infection

infestation Being in or on a host

informed consent The process by which a person receives and understands information about a treatment or procedure and is able to decide if he or she will receive it

inherited That which is passed down from parents to children

insomnia A chronic condition in which the person cannot sleep or stay asleep all night

intact skin Normal skin and skin layers without damage or breaks

intake The amount of fluid taken in; input

intellectual disability Involves severe limits in intellectual function and adaptive behavior occurring before age 18

internal rotation Turning the joint inward

intimate partner violence (IPV) Physical violence, sexual violence, stalking, or psychological aggression by a current or former partner

intravenous (IV) therapy Giving fluids through a needle or catheter inserted into a vein; IV and IV infusion

intubation Inserting an artificial airway

invasion of privacy Violating a person's right not to have his or her name, photo, or private affairs exposed or made public without giving consent

involuntary seclusion Separating a person from others against his or her will, keeping the person to a certain area, or keeping the person away from his or her room without consent

J

jaundice Yellowish color of the skin or whites of the eyes

jejunostomy tube A feeding tube inserted into a surgically created opening (*stomy*) in the *jejunum* of the small intestine

job application An agency's official form listing questions that require factual answers from the person seeking employment; employment form

job description A document that describes what the agency expects you to do

job interview When an employer asks a job applicant questions about his or her education and career

joint The point at which 2 or more bones meet to allow movement

K

ketone A substance appearing in urine from the rapid breakdown of fat for energy; acetone, ketone body

ketone body See "ketone"

knee-chest position The person kneels and rests the body on the knees and chest; the head is turned to 1 side, the arms are above the head or flexed at the elbows, the back is straight, and the body is flexed about 90 degrees at the hips; genupectoral position

Kussmaul respirations Very deep and rapid respirations

L

laceration An open wound with torn tissues and jagged edges

laryngeal mirror An instrument used to examine the mouth, teeth, and throat

lateral Away from the mid-line; at the side of the body or body part

lateral position The person lies on 1 side or the other; side-lying position

lateral transfer When a person moves between 2 horizontal surfaces

law A rule of conduct made by a government body

libel Making false statements in print, in writing (including e-mail and text messages), through pictures or drawings, through broadcast (radio, TV, or video), posted on-line on websites, or through video sites and social media sites

lice See "pediculosis"

licensed practical nurse (LPN) A nurse who has completed a practical nursing program and has passed a licensing test; called *licensed vocational nurse (LVN)* in California and Texas

licensed vocational nurse (LVN) See "licensed practical nurse (LPN)"

lithotomy position The woman lies on her back with the hips at the edge of the exam table, her knees are flexed, her hips are externally rotated, and her feet are in stirrups

local anesthesia The loss of sensation, produced by a drug, in a small area

lochia The vaginal discharge that occurs after childbirth

logrolling Turning the person as a unit, in alignment, with 1 motion

low vision Vision loss that cannot be corrected with eyeglasses, contact lenses, drugs, or surgery; vision loss interferes with every-day activities

lymphedema A buildup of lymph in the tissues causing edema (swelling)

M

malignant tumor A tumor that invades and destroys nearby tissues and can spread to other body parts; cancer

malpractice Negligence by a professional person

mechanical ventilation Using a machine to move air into and out of the lungs

meconium A dark green to black, tarry bowel movement

medial At or near the middle or mid-line of the body or body part

medical asepsis Practices used to reduce the number of microbes and prevent their spread from 1 person or place to another person or place; clean technique

medical record The legal account of a person's condition and response to treatment and care; chart or clinical record

medical symptom An indication or characteristic of a physical or psychological condition

medication reminder Reminding the person to take drugs, observing them being taken as prescribed, and recording that they were taken

melena A black, tarry stool

menarche The first menstruation and the start of menstrual cycles

menopause The time when menstruation stops and menstrual cycles end; there has been at least 1 year without a menstrual period

menstruation The process in which the lining of the uterus (*endometrium*) breaks up and is discharged from the body through the vagina

mental health Involves a person's emotional, psychological, and social well-being

mental health disorder A serious illness that can affect a person's thinking, mood, behavior, function, and ability to relate to others; mental illness, psychiatric disorder

mental illness See "mental health disorder"

metabolism How the body uses nutrients to provide energy and maintain body functions

metastasis The spread of cancer to other body parts

microbe See "microorganism"

microorganism A small (*micro*) living thing (*organism*) seen only with a microscope; microbe

milestone A behavior or skill that occurs in a stage of development

misappropriation The dishonest use of property

mite A very small spider-like organism

mixed aphasia See "global aphasia"

mixed incontinence The combination of stress incontinence and urge incontinence

mole A brown, tan, or black spot on the skin that is flat or raised and round or oval

morbid obesity Weighing 100 pounds or more over one's normal weight

morning care Care given after breakfast; hygiene measures are more thorough at this time

mouth care See "oral hygiene"

musculo-skeletal disorders (MSDs) Injuries and disorders of the muscles, tendons, ligaments, joints, and cartilage

N

nasal speculum An instrument (*speculum* means *mirror*) used to examine the inside of the nose (*nasal*)

naso-enteral tube A feeding tube inserted through the nose (*naso*) into the small bowel (*enteral*)

naso-gastric (NG) tube A feeding tube inserted through the nose (*naso*) into the stomach (*gastro*)

need Something necessary or desired for maintaining life and mental well-being

neglect When a caregiver or responsible person fails to:
- Protect a vulnerable person from harm
- Provide food, water, clothing, shelter, health care, and other activities of daily living to a vulnerable person

negligence An unintentional wrong in which a person did not act in a reasonable and careful manner and a person or the person's property was harmed

nocturia Frequent urination (*uria*) at night (*noc*)

non-pathogen A microbe that does not usually cause an infection

nonverbal communication Communication that does not use words

normal flora Microbes that live and grow in a certain area

nursing See "breast-feeding"

nursing assistant A person who has passed a nursing assistant training and competency evaluation program (NATCEP); performs delegated nursing tasks under the supervision of a licensed nurse

nursing care plan A written guide about the person's nursing care; care plan

nursing diagnosis A health problem that can be treated by nursing measures; see "nursing process"

nursing intervention An action or measure taken by the nursing team to help the person reach a goal; nursing action, nursing measure, nursing task

nursing process The method nurses use to plan and deliver nursing care; its 5 steps are assessment, nursing diagnosis, planning, implementation, and evaluation

nursing task Nursing care or a nursing function, procedure, skill, or activity

nursing team Those who provide nursing care—RNs, LPNs/LVNs, and nursing assistants

nutrient A substance that is ingested, digested, absorbed, and used by the body

nutrition The processes involved in the ingestion, digestion, absorption, and use of food and fluids by the body

O

obesity Having an excess amount of total body fat; body weight is 20% or more above what is normal for the person's height and age

objective data Information that is seen, heard, felt, or smelled by an observer; signs

observation Using the sense of sight, hearing, touch, and smell to collect information

obsession A frequent, upsetting, and unwanted thought, idea, or image

obstetrics The field of medicine concerned with the care of women during pregnancy, labor, and childbirth and for 6 to 8 weeks after birth

oliguria Scant amount (*olig*) of urine (*uria*); less than 500 mL in 24 hours

ombudsman Someone who supports or promotes the needs and interests of another person

open fracture The broken bone has pierced the skin; compound fracture

ophthalmoscope A lighted instrument (*scope*) used to examine the internal eye (*ophthalmo*) structures

opposition Touching an opposite finger with the thumb

optimal level of function A person's highest potential for mental and physical performance

oral hygiene The practices that promote healthy tissues and structures of the mouth; mouth care

organ Groups of tissue with the same function

orthopnea Breathing (*pnea*) deeply and comfortably only when sitting (*ortho*)

orthopneic position Sitting up (*ortho*) and leaning over a table to breathe (*pneic*)

orthostatic hypotension See "postural hypotension"

orthotic A device used to support a muscle, promote a certain motion, or correct a deformity; *ortho* means *to straighten*

ostomy A surgically created opening that connects an internal organ to the body's surface; see "colostomy" and "ileostomy"

otoscope A lighted instrument (*scope*) used to examine the external ear (*oto*) and the eardrum (tympanic membrane)

output The amount of fluid lost

over-flow incontinence Small amounts of urine leak from a full bladder

oxygen concentration The amount (percent [%]) of hemoglobin containing oxygen

P

pack Wrapping a body part with a wet or dry application

padded waterproof drawsheet A drawsheet made of an absorbent top and waterproof bottom used to protect the mattress and bottom linens from dampness and soiling

pain To ache, hurt, or be sore; discomfort

palliative care Care to relieve or reduce the intensity of uncomfortable symptoms without producing a cure

panic An intense and sudden feeling of fear, anxiety, or dread

paralysis Loss of muscle function, sensation, or both

paranoia A disorder (*para*) of the mind (*noia*); false beliefs (delusions) and suspicion about a person or situation

paraphrasing Re-stating the person's message in your own words

paraplegia Paralysis in the legs and lower trunk (*para* means *beyond; plegia* means *paralysis*)

parenteral nutrition Giving nutrients through a catheter inserted into a vein; *para* means *beyond; enteral* relates to the *bowel*

patent Open and unblocked

pathogen A microbe that is harmful and can cause an infection

patient-focused care A nursing care pattern; services are moved from departments to the bedside

pediatrics The field of medicine concerned with the growth, development, and care of children—newborns to teenagers

pediculosis Infestation with wingless insects that feed on blood; lice

pediculosis capitis Infestation of the scalp (*capitis*) with lice

pediculosis corporis Infestation of the body (*corporis*) with lice

pediculosis pubis Infestation of the pubic (*pubis*) hair with lice

peer A person of the same age-group and background

penetrating wound An open wound that breaks the skin and enters a body area, organ, or cavity

percussion hammer An instrument used to tap body parts to test reflexes (*percussion* means *to strike hard*); reflex hammer

percutaneous endoscopic gastrostomy (PEG) tube A feeding tube inserted into the stomach (*gastro*) through a small incision (*stomy*) made through (*per*) the skin (*cutaneous*); a lighted instrument (*scope*) is used to see inside a body cavity or organ (*endo*)

pericare See "perineal care"

perineal care Cleaning the genital and anal areas; pericare

peristalsis Involuntary muscle contractions in the digestive system that move food down the esophagus through the alimentary canal; the alternating contraction and relaxation of intestinal muscles

personal protective equipment (PPE) The clothing or equipment worn by the staff for protection against a hazard

personality The set of attitudes, values, behaviors, and traits of a person

person's unit The space, furniture, and equipment used by the person in the agency

phantom pain Pain that seems to come from a body part that is no longer there

phobia An intense fear of something that has little or no real danger

physical restraint Any manual method or physical or mechanical device, material, or equipment attached to or near the person's body that he or she cannot remove easily and that restricts freedom of movement or normal access to one's body

pivot To turn one's body from a set standing position

planning Setting priorities and goals; see "nursing process"

plantar flexion The foot (*plantar*) is bent (*flexion*); bending the foot down at the ankle

plaque A thin film that sticks to the teeth; it contains saliva, microbes, and other substances

pleural effusion The escape and collection of fluid (*effusion*) in the pleural space

PM care See "evening care"

pneumonia Inflammation and infection of lung tissue

pneumothorax Air (*pneumo*) in the pleural space (*thorax*)

poison Any substance harmful to the body when ingested, inhaled, injected, or absorbed through the skin

pollutant A harmful chemical or substance in the air or water

polyuria Abnormally large amounts (*poly*) of urine (*uria*)

position change alarm Any physical or electronic device that monitors a person's movement and alerts staff of movement

posterior At or toward the back of the body or body part; dorsal

post-mortem care Care of the body after (*post*) death (*mortem*)

post-operative After (*post*) surgery; post-op

postpartum After (*post*) childbirth (*partum*)

postural hypotension Abnormally low (*hypo*) blood pressure when the person suddenly stands up (*postural*); orthostatic hypotension

posture See "body alignment"

prefix A word element at the beginning of a word; it changes the meaning of the word

prenatal care The health care a woman receives while pregnant

pre-operative Before (*pre*) surgery; pre-op

pressure injury Localized damage to the skin and underlying soft tissue; the injury is usually over a bony prominence or related to a medical or other device and results from pressure or pressure in combination with shear

pressure point See "bony prominence"

primary caregiver The person mainly responsible for providing or assisting with the child's basic needs

primary nursing A nursing care pattern; an RN is responsible for the person's total care

priority The most important thing at the time

professional boundary That which separates helpful actions and behaviors from those that are not helpful

professionalism Following laws, being ethical, having good work ethics, and having the skills to do your work

professional sexual misconduct An act, behavior, or comment that is sexual in nature

progress note Describes the care given and the person's response and progress

pronation Turning the joint downward

prone position The person lies on the abdomen with the head turned to 1 side

prosthesis An artificial replacement for a missing body part

protected health information Identifying information and information about the person's health care that is maintained or sent in any form (paper, electronic, oral)

proximal The part nearest to the center or to the point of attachment

psychiatric disorder See "mental health disorder"

psychiatry The field of medicine concerned with mental health disorders

psychosis A state of severe mental impairment

puberty The period when reproductive organs begin to function and secondary sex characteristics appear

pulse The beat of the heart felt at an artery as a wave of blood passes through the artery

pulse deficit The difference between the apical and radial pulse rates

pulse oximetry Measures (*metry*) the oxygen (*oxi*) concentration in arterial blood

pulse rate The number of heartbeats or pulses in 1 minute

puncture wound An open wound made by a sharp object

purulent drainage Thick green, yellow, or brown drainage

pyuria Pus (*py*) in the urine (*uria*)

Q

quadriplegia Paralysis in the arms, legs, and trunk (*quad* means *4*; *plegia* means *paralysis*); tetraplegia

R

radiating pain Pain felt at the site of tissue damage and that spreads to other areas

range of motion (ROM) The movement of a joint to the extent possible without causing pain

reasonable accommodation To assist or change a position or workplace to allow an employee to do his or her job despite having a disability

receptive aphasia Difficulty understanding language; Wernicke's aphasia

reciprocity See "endorsement"

recording The written account of care and observations; charting, documentation

referred pain Pain from a body part that is felt in another body part

reflex The body's response (function or movement) to a stimulus; an involuntary movement

reflex incontinence Urine is lost at predictable intervals when a specific amount of urine is in the bladder

regional anesthesia The loss of sensation, produced by a drug, in a large area

registered nurse (RN) A nurse who has completed a 2-, 3-, or 4-year nursing program and has passed a licensing test

regurgitation The backward flow of stomach contents into the mouth

rehabilitation The process of restoring the person to his or her highest possible level of physical, psychological, social, and economic function

reincarnation The belief that the spirit or soul is reborn in another human body or in another form of life

relaxation To be free from mental and physical stress

religion Spiritual beliefs, needs, and practices

remove easily The manual method, device, material, or equipment used to restrain the person that can be removed intentionally by the person in the same manner it was applied by the staff

reporting The oral account of care and observations

representative A person with the legal right to act on the patient's or resident's behalf when he or she cannot do so for himself or herself

respiration The process of supplying cells with oxygen and removing carbon dioxide from them; breathing air into (*inhalation*) and out of (*exhalation*) the lungs

respiratory arrest When breathing stops; breathing stops but heart action continues for several minutes

respiratory depression Slow, weak respirations at a rate of fewer than 12 per minute

rest To be calm, at ease, and relaxed with no anxiety or stress

restorative aide A nursing assistant with special training in restorative nursing and rehabilitation skills

restorative nursing care Care that helps persons regain health and strength for safe and independent living

resuscitate To revive from apparent death or unconsciousness using emergency measures

retention catheter See "indwelling catheter"

reverse Trendelenburg's position The head of the bed is raised and the foot of the bed is lowered

rigor mortis The stiffness or rigidity (*rigor*) of skeletal muscles that occurs after death (*mortis*)

root A word element containing the basic meaning of the word

rotation Turning the joint

routine nursing task A nursing task that is part of a nursing assistant's routine job description and commonly assigned to the nursing assistant; a nursing task that was learned in a nursing assistant training and competency evaluation program (NATCEP)

S

sanguineous drainage Bloody (*sanguis*) drainage

scabies A skin disorder caused by a female mite

sedation A state of quiet, calmness, or sleep produced by a drug

seizure Violent and sudden contractions or tremors of muscle groups caused by abnormal electrical activity in the brain; convulsion

self-actualization Experiencing one's potential

self-esteem Thinking well of oneself and seeing oneself as useful and having value

self-neglect A person's behaviors and way of living that threaten his or her health, safety, and well-being

semi-Fowler's position The head of the bed is raised 30 degrees; or the head of the bed is raised 30 degrees and the knee portion is raised 15 degrees

semi-prone side position See "Sims' position"

serosanguineous drainage Thin, watery drainage (*sero*) that is blood-tinged (*sanguineous*)

serous drainage Clear, watery fluid (*serum*)

service plan A written plan listing the services needed, the help needed, and who provides services

sex Physical interactions between people involving the body and reproductive organs

sexual orientation Emotional, romantic, and physical attraction to men, women, or both sexes

sexuality The physical, emotional, social, cultural, and spiritual factors that affect a person's feelings, attitudes, and behaviors about one's gender identity and sexual behavior

shear When layers of the skin rub against each other; when the skin remains in place and underlying tissues move and stretch, tearing underlying capillaries and blood vessels and causing tissue damage

shearing When the skin sticks to a surface while muscles slide in the direction the body is moving

shock Results when tissues and organs do not get enough blood

side-lying position See "lateral position"

signs See "objective data"

simple fracture See "closed fracture"

Sims' position A left side-lying position in which the upper leg (right leg) is sharply flexed so it is not on the lower leg (left leg) and the lower arm (left arm) is behind the person; semi-prone side position

skin breakdown Changes or damage to intact skin—normal skin and skin layers

skin tear A break or rip in the outer layers of the skin; the epidermis (top skin layer) separates from the underlying tissues

slander Making false statements through the spoken word, sounds, sign language, or gestures

sleep A state of reduced consciousness, reduced voluntary muscle activity, and lowered metabolism

sleep apnea Pauses (a) in breathing (pnea) that occur during sleep

sleep deprivation The amount and quality of sleep are not adequate, causing reduced function and alertness

sleepwalking When the person leaves the bed and walks about while sleeping

slough Dead tissue that is shed from the skin; it is usually light colored, soft, and moist; may be stringy at times

spastic Uncontrolled contractions of skeletal muscles

sphygmomanometer A cuff and measuring device used to measure blood pressure (*sphygmo* means *pulse*; *manometer* is *a device for measuring pressure*)

spore A bacterium protected by a hard shell

sputum Mucus from the respiratory system when expectorated (expelled) through the mouth

stage A period of time (age range) in which a person learns certain skills

standard of care The skills, care, and judgments required by a health team member under similar conditions

stasis ulcer See "venous ulcer"

sterile The absence of *all* microbes

sterile field A work area free of *all* pathogens and non-pathogens (including spores)

sterile technique See "surgical asepsis"

sterilization The process of destroying *all* microbes

stethoscope An instrument used to listen to the sounds produced by the heart, lungs, and other body organs

stimulus Anything that excites or causes a body part to function, become active, or respond

stoma A surgically created opening seen on the body's surface; see "colostomy" and "ileostomy"

stomatitis Inflammation (*itis*) of the mouth (*stomat*)

stool Excreted feces

straight catheter A catheter that drains the bladder and then is removed

stress The response or change in the body caused by any emotional, psychological, physical, social, or economic factor

stress incontinence When urine leaks during exercise and certain movements that cause pressure on the bladder

stressor The event or factor that causes stress

subjective data Things a person tells you about that you cannot observe through your senses; symptoms

suction The process of withdrawing or sucking up fluid (secretions)

sudden cardiac arrest (SCA) The heart stops suddenly and without warning; cardiac arrest

suffix A word element at the end of a word; it changes the meaning of the word

suffocation When breathing stops from the lack of oxygen

suicide To end one's life on purpose

suicide contagion Exposure to suicide or suicidal behaviors within one's family or one's peer group or through media reports of suicide

sundowning Signs, symptoms, and behaviors of Alzheimer's disease (AD) increase during hours of darkness

supination Turning the joint upward

supine position The back-lying or dorsal recumbent position

suppository A cone-shaped, solid drug that is inserted into a body opening; it melts at body temperature

supra-pubic catheter A catheter surgically inserted into the bladder through an incision above (*supra*) the pubis bone (*pubic*)

surgical asepsis The practices used to remove *all* microbes; sterile technique

surgical site infection (SSI) An infection that occurs after surgery in the body part where the surgery took place

survey The formal review of an agency through the collection of facts and observations

surveyor A person who collects information by observing and asking questions

symptoms See "subjective data"

syncope A brief loss of consciousness; fainting

system Organs that work together to perform special functions

systole The period of heart muscle contraction; the heart is pumping blood

systolic pressure The pressure in the arteries when the heart contracts

T

tachycardia A rapid (*tachy*) heart rate (*cardia*); more than 100 beats per minute

tachypnea Rapid (*tachy*) breathing (*pnea*); respirations are more than 20 per minute

tartar Hardened plaque

team nursing A nursing care pattern; an RN leads a team of nursing staff; the RN decides the amount and kind of care each person needs

teamwork Staff members work together as a group; each person does his or her part to give safe and effective care

teen dating violence (TDV) The physical, sexual, psychological, or emotional violence within a dating relationship as well as stalking

terminal illness An illness or injury from which the person will not likely recover

tetraplegia See "quadriplegia" (*tetra* means *4*; *plegia* means *paralysis*)

thermometer A device used to measure (*meter*) temperature (*thermo*)

thrombus A blood clot

tinnitus A ringing, roaring, hissing, or buzzing sound in the ears or head

tissue A group of cells with similar functions

tort A wrong committed against a person or the person's property

tracheostomy A surgically created opening (*stomy*) in the neck into the trachea (*tracheo*)

transfer How a person moves to and from a surface; moving the person to another health care setting; moving the person to a new room within the agency

transfer belt A device applied around the waist and used to support a person who is unsteady or disabled; gait belt

transgender Describes people who express their sexuality or gender identity in ways that do not fit with their biological sex (male, female)

transient incontinence Temporary or occasional incontinence that is reversed when the cause is treated

treatment The care provided to maintain or restore health, improve function, or relieve symptoms

Trendelenburg's position The head of the bed is lowered and the foot of the bed is raised

tumor A new growth of abnormal cells that is benign or malignant

tuning fork An instrument vibrated to test hearing

U

ulcer A shallow or deep crater-like sore of the skin or mucous membrane

umbilical cord The structure that connects the mother and fetus (unborn baby); it carries blood, oxygen, and nutrients from the mother to the fetus

unaffected side The side of the body opposite the affected side; strong side

unavoidable pressure injury A pressure injury that occurs despite efforts to prevent one through proper use of the nursing process

uncircumcised Foreskin covers the head of the penis

under-garment An item of clothing worn next to the skin under clothing

urge incontinence The loss of urine in response to a sudden, urgent need to void; the person cannot get to a toilet in time

urgent surgery Surgery needed for health; it can be delayed for a few days

urinary diversion A surgically created pathway for urine to leave the body

urinary frequency Voiding at frequent intervals

urinary incontinence (UI) The involuntary loss or leakage of urine

urinary retention Not being able to completely empty the bladder

urinary urgency The need to void at once

urination The process of emptying urine from the bladder; voiding

urostomy A surgically created opening (*stomy*) that connects to the urinary tract (*uro*)

V

vaccination Giving a vaccine to produce immunity against an infectious disease

vaccine A preparation containing dead or weakened microbes

vaginal speculum An instrument (*speculum*) used to open the vagina (*vaginal*) to examine it and the cervix

vascular ulcer See "circulatory ulcer"

vector A carrier (animal, insect) that transmits disease

vehicle Any substance that transmits microbes

vein A blood vessel that returns blood to the heart

venous ulcer An open sore on the lower legs or feet caused by poor venous blood flow; stasis ulcer

ventral See "anterior"

verbal communication Communication that uses written or spoken words

vertigo Dizziness

vital signs Temperature, pulse, respirations, and blood pressure; pulse oximetry and pain are included in some agencies

voiding See "urination"

vomitus Food and fluids expelled from the stomach through the mouth; emesis

vulnerable adult A person 18 years old or older who has a disability or condition that makes him or her at risk to be wounded, attacked, or damaged

W

Wernicke's aphasia See "receptive aphasia"

will A legal document of how a person wants property distributed after death

withdrawal syndrome The physical and mental response after stopping or severely reducing use of a substance that was used regularly

word element A part of a word

work ethics Behavior in the workplace

workplace violence Violent acts (including assault and threat of assault) directed toward persons at work or while on duty

wound A break in the skin or mucous membrane

Key Abbreviations

AD Alzheimer's disease; autonomic dysreflexia

ADA American Dental Association; Americans With Disabilities Act of 1990

ADL Activities of daily living

ADU Accessory dwelling unit

AE Anti-embolism; anti-embolic

AED Automated external defibrillator

AIDS Acquired immunodeficiency syndrome

ALR Assisted living residence

ALS Amyotrophic lateral sclerosis

AMD Age-related macular degeneration

APRN Advanced practice registered nurse

ASC Ambulatory surgery center

ASD Autism spectrum disorder

ASL American Sign Language

BM; BMs Bowel movement; bowel movements

BON Board of nursing

BP Blood pressure

BPD Borderline personality disorder

BPH Benign prostatic hyperplasia

C Centigrade

CAA Care Area Assessment

CAD Coronary artery disease

CAUTI Catheter-associated urinary tract infection

CBC Complete blood count

CCRC Continuing care retirement community

CDC Centers for Disease Control and Prevention

C. diff *Clostridioides difficile; Clostridium difficile*

CHF Congestive heart failure

CKD Chronic kidney disease

cm Centimeter

CMS Centers for Medicare & Medicaid Services

CNA Certified nursing assistant; certified nurse aide

CNS Central nervous system

CO Carbon monoxide

CO₂ Carbon dioxide

COPD Chronic obstructive pulmonary disease

CP Cerebral palsy

CPR Cardiopulmonary resuscitation

CPSC Consumer Product Safety Commission

C-section Cesarean section

CVA Cerebrovascular accident

DNR Do Not Resuscitate

DOB Date of birth

DON Director of nursing

DS Down syndrome

ECG Electrocardiogram

ECHO Elder Cottage Housing Opportunity

ED Erectile dysfunction

EEOC Equal Employment Opportunity Commission

EHR Electronic health record

EKG Electrocardiogram

EMR Electronic medical record

EMS Emergency Medical Services

EPA Environmental Protection Agency

EPHI; ePHI Electronic protected health information

ET Endotracheal

F Fahrenheit

FAS Fetal alcohol syndrome

FASDs Fetal alcohol spectrum disorders

FBAO Foreign-body airway obstruction

FDA Food and Drug Administration

Fragile X Fragile X syndrome

ft Foot; feet

GAD Generalized anxiety disorder

GERD Gastro-esophageal reflux disease

GI Gastro-intestinal

gtt Drops

gtt/min Drops per minute

HAI Healthcare-associated infection

HBV Hepatitis B virus

HCS Hazard Communication Standard

Hg Mercury

HIPAA Health Insurance Portability and Accountability Act of 1996

HIV Human immunodeficiency virus

HPV Human papilloma viruses

IBD Inflammatory bowel disease

ICD Implanted cardioverter defibrillator

ID Identification

IDCP Interdisciplinary care planning

IDD Intellectual and developmental disability

in Inch; inches

I&O Intake and output

IPV Intimate partner violence

IQ Intelligence quotient

ISTAP International Skin Tear Advisory Panel

IV Intravenous

JA Juvenile arthritis

lb Pound; pounds
L/min Liters per minute
LNA Licensed nursing assistant
LPN Licensed practical nurse
LVN Licensed vocational nurse

MDRO Multidrug-resistant organism
MDS Minimum Data Set
mg Milligram
MI Myocardial infarction
mL Milliliter
mL/hr Milliliters per hour
mm Millimeter
mm Hg Millimeters of mercury
MRN Medical record number
MRSA Methicillin-resistant *Staphylococcus aureus*
MS Multiple sclerosis
MSD Musculo-skeletal disorder
MSDS Material safety data sheet

NATCEP Nursing assistant training and competency
evaluation program
NFPA National Fire Protection Association
NG Naso-gastric
NIA National Institute on Aging
NPO *Nil per os*; nothing by mouth
NPIAP National Pressure Injury Advisory Panel

O_2 Oxygen
OAB Over-active bladder
OASIS Outcome and Assessment Information Set
OBRA Omnibus Budget Reconciliation Act of 1987
OCD Obsessive-compulsive disorder
OPIM Other potentially infectious materials
OR Operating room
OSHA Occupational Safety and Health Administration
oz Ounce

PACU Post-anesthesia care unit
PASS *Pull* the safety pin, *aim* low, *squeeze* the lever, *sweep*
back and forth
PEG Percutaneous endoscopic gastrostomy
PHI Protected health information
post-op Post-operative
PPE Personal protective equipment
PPS Prospective Payment Systems
pre-op Pre-operative
PROM Passive range of motion
PTSD Post-traumatic stress disorder

RA Rheumatoid arthritis
RACE Rescue, alarm, confine, extinguish
RBC Red blood cell
RN Registered nurse
RNA Registered nurse aide
ROM Range-of-motion; range of motion
RRS Rapid Response System
RT Respiratory therapist

SB Spina bifida
SCA Sudden cardiac arrest
SCD Sequential compression device
SDS Safety data sheet
SIDS Sudden infant death syndrome
SNF Skilled nursing facility
SpO_2 Saturation of peripheral oxygen (oxygen
concentration)
SRNA State registered nurse aide
SSE Soapsuds enema
SSI Surgical site infection
STD Sexually transmitted disease
STI Sexually transmitted infection
STNA State tested nurse aide
SUID Sudden unexpected infant death

TB Tuberculosis
TBI Traumatic brain injury
TDV Teen dating violence
TED Thrombo-embolic disease
TIA Transient ischemic attack
TJC The Joint Commission
TPN Total parenteral nutrition
TPR Temperature, pulse, and respirations
TURP Transurethral resection of the prostate

U/A Urinalysis
UI Urinary incontinence
USDA United States Department of Agriculture
UTI Urinary tract infection

VF; V-fib Ventricular fibrillation
VRE Vancomycin-resistant *Enterococci*

WBC White blood cell

Index

Page numbers followed by *b*, *t*, and *f* indicate boxes, tables, and figures, respectively.